Y0-EMG-592

# CONNECT CORE CONCEPTS IN HEALTH BRIEF

**EIGHTEENTH EDITION**

**Claire E. Insel**
*California Institute of Human Nutrition*

**Walton T. Roth**
*Stanford University*

**Paul M. Insel**
*Stanford University*

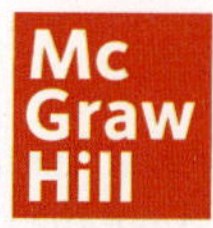

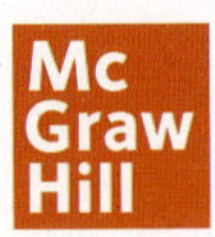

CONNECT CORE CONCEPTS IN HEALTH: BRIEF, EIGHTEENTH EDITION

Published by McGraw Hill LLC, 1325 Avenue of the Americas, New York, NY 10019. 

This book is printed on acid-free paper.

1 2 3 4 5 6 7 8 9 LWI 28 27 26 25 24 23

ISBN 978-1-264-42792-5 (bound edition)
MHID 1-264-42792-1 (bound edition)
ISBN 978-1-265-49368-4 (loose-leaf edition)
MHID 1-265-49368-5 (loose-leaf edition)

Portfolio Manager: *Erika Lo*
Senior Product Development Manager: *Dawn Groundwater*
Senior Product Developer: *Kirstan Price*
Marketing Manager: *Robin Stalheim*
Content Project Managers: *Mary E. Powers (Core), Vanessa McClune (Assessment)*
Manufacturing Project Manager: *Laura Fuller*
Senior Designer: *Beth Blech*
Content Licensing Specialist: *Sarah Flynn*
Cover Image: *BAZA Production/Shutterstock*
Compositor: *Aptara®, Inc.*

All credits appearing on page or at the end of the book are considered to be an extension of the copyright page.

**Library of Congress Cataloging-in-Publication Data**

Names: Insel, Claire E., author. | Roth, Walton T., author. | Insel, Paul M., author.
Title: Connect core concepts in health : brief / Claire E. Insel, California Institute of Human Nutrition; Walton T. Roth, Stanford University; Paul M. Insel, Stanford University.
Description: Eighteenth edition. | New York, NY : McGraw Hill LLC, [2024] | Includes index.
Identifiers: LCCN 2022037245 (print) | LCCN 2022037246 (ebook) | ISBN 9781264427925 (hardcover) | ISBN 9781265493684 (spiral bound) | ISBN 9781265497118 (ebook) | ISBN 9781265488468 (ebook other)
Subjects: LCSH: Health.
Classification: LCC RA776 .C83 2024 (print) | LCC RA776 (ebook) | DDC 613–dc23/eng/20220808
LC record available at https://lccn.loc.gov/2022037245
LC ebook record available at https://lccn.loc.gov/2022037246



mheducation.com/highered

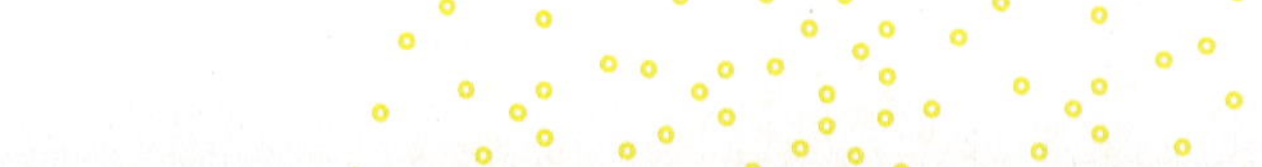

# BRIEF CONTENTS


## PART ONE

### ESTABLISHING A BASIS FOR WELLNESS

CHAPTER 1 Taking Charge of Your Health *1*
CHAPTER 2 Stress: The Constant Challenge *23*
CHAPTER 3 Psychological Health *42*
CHAPTER 4 Sleep *66*

## PART TWO

### UNDERSTANDING SEXUALITY

CHAPTER 5 Intimate Relationships and Communication *86*
CHAPTER 6 Sexuality, Pregnancy, and Childbirth *108*
CHAPTER 7 Contraception and Abortion *145*

## PART THREE

### SUBSTANCE USE DISORDERS: MAKING RESPONSIBLE DECISIONS

CHAPTER 8 Drug Use and Addiction *169*
CHAPTER 9 Alcohol and Nicotine *192*

## PART FOUR

### GETTING FIT

CHAPTER 10 Nutrition Basics *224*
CHAPTER 11 Exercise for Health and Fitness *259*
CHAPTER 12 Weight Management *283*

## PART FIVE

### PROTECTING YOURSELF FROM DISEASE

CHAPTER 13 Cardiovascular Health and Cancer *306*
CHAPTER 14 Immunity and Infection *344*

## PART SIX

### LIVING WELL IN THE WORLD

CHAPTER 15 Environmental Health *380*
CHAPTER 16 Conventional and Complementary Medicine *399*
CHAPTER 17 Personal Safety *424*

## PART SEVEN

### ACCEPTING PHYSICAL LIMITS

CHAPTER 18 The Challenge of Aging *448*

Index *473*

# CONTENTS

Preface xiv

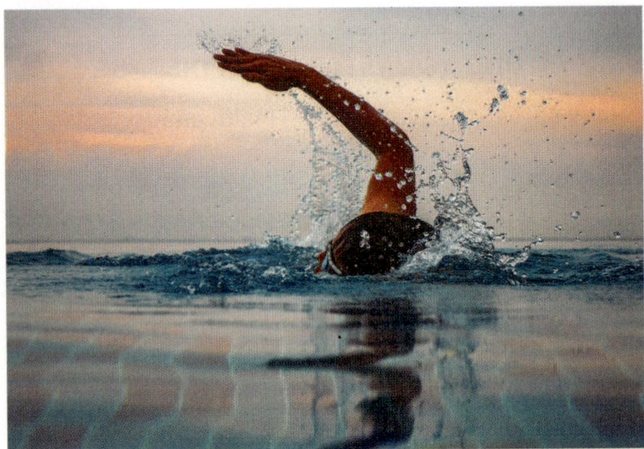
Narong Pimsook/EyeEm/Getty Images

PART ONE

ESTABLISHING A BASIS FOR WELLNESS

1 TAKING CHARGE OF YOUR HEALTH 1

WELLNESS AS A HEALTH GOAL 1
Dimensions of Wellness 2
The Long and the Short of Life Expectancy 3

PROMOTING NATIONAL HEALTH 7
Health Insurance Options 7
The Healthy People Initiative 8
Health Issues for Diverse Populations 8

FACTORS THAT INFLUENCE WELLNESS 11
Health Habits 12
Genetics/Family History 12
Environment 12
Access to Health Care 12
Personal Health Behaviors 12

REACHING WELLNESS THROUGH LIFESTYLE MANAGEMENT 13
Getting Serious about Your Health 13
Building Motivation to Change 13
Enhancing Your Readiness to Change 14
Dealing with Relapse 16
Developing Skills for Change: Creating a Personalized Plan 17
Putting Your Plan into Action 19
Staying with It 19

BEING HEALTHY FOR LIFE 19
*Tips for Today and the Future* 19
*Summary* 20
*For More Information* 20
*Selected Bibliography* 21

2 STRESS: THE CONSTANT CHALLENGE 23

WHAT IS STRESS? 23
Physical Responses to Stressors 24
Cognitive and Psychological Responses to Stressors 26

STRESS AND HEALTH 27
The General Adaptation Syndrome 28
More Recent Ideas about Stress 28
Psychoneuroimmunology 29
Stress and Specific Conditions 29

COMMON SOURCES OF STRESS 30
Major Life Changes 31
Daily Hassles 31
College Stressors 31
Job-Related Stressors 31
Social Stressors 31
Other Stressors 32

MANAGING STRESS 34
Social Support 34
Volunteering 34
Communication 34
Exercise 34
Nutrition 35
Time Management 35
Cultivating Spiritual Wellness 35
Confiding in Yourself through Writing 36
Thinking and Acting Constructively 36
Relaxation and Body Awareness Techniques 38
Counterproductive Coping Strategies 38
Getting Help 39
*Tips for Today and the Future* 39
*Summary* 40
*For More Information* 40
*Selected Bibliography* 40

## 3 PSYCHOLOGICAL HEALTH 42

**DEFINING PSYCHOLOGICAL HEALTH** 42
Positive Psychology 42
What Psychological Health Is Not 44

**MEETING LIFE'S CHALLENGES WITH A POSITIVE SELF-CONCEPT** 44
Growing Up Psychologically 44
Achieving Healthy Self-Esteem 45
Psychological Defense Mechanisms–Healthy and Unhealthy 47
Being Optimistic 48
Maintaining Honest Communication 48
Finding a Social Media Balance 49
Dealing with Loneliness 49
Dealing with Anger 49

**PSYCHOLOGICAL DISORDERS** 50
Anxiety Disorders 52
Attention-Deficit/Hyperactivity Disorder 53
Mood Disorders 54
Schizophrenia 55

**SUICIDE** 56

**MODELS OF HUMAN NATURE AND THERAPEUTIC CHANGE** 58
The Biological Model 58
The Behavioral Model 58
The Cognitive Model 59
The Psychodynamic Model 59
Evaluating the Models 59
Other Psychotherapies 60

**GETTING HELP** 60
Self-Help 60
Peer Counseling and Support Groups 60
Online Help and Apps 60
Professional Help 61
*Tips for Today and the Future* 62
*Summary* 62
*For More Information* 64
*Selected Bibliography* 64

## 4 SLEEP 66

**SLEEP BIOLOGY** 66
Sleep Stages 66
Natural Sleep Drives 68

**CHANGES IN SLEEP BIOLOGY ACROSS THE LIFE SPAN** 71
Changes in Circadian Rhythm 72
Sleep Cycles, Age, and Gender 72

**SLEEP AND ITS RELATION TO HEALTH** 72
Mood and Depression 72
Dementia 73
Athletic Performance 73
Musculoskeletal Pain 73
Obesity and Weight Management 74
Cardiovascular Disease 74
Diabetes 74
Public Health Impact 74

**GETTING STARTED ON A HEALTHY SLEEP PROGRAM** 75
Step I: Take an Inventory 75
Step II: Identify Sleep Disrupters 76
Step III: Improve Sleep Fitness 78

**SLEEP DISORDERS** 79
Chronic Insomnia 79
Restless Leg Syndrome 81
Sleep Apnea 81
Narcolepsy 82
*Tips for Today and the Future* 82
*Summary* 83
*For More Information* 84
*Selected Bibliography* 84


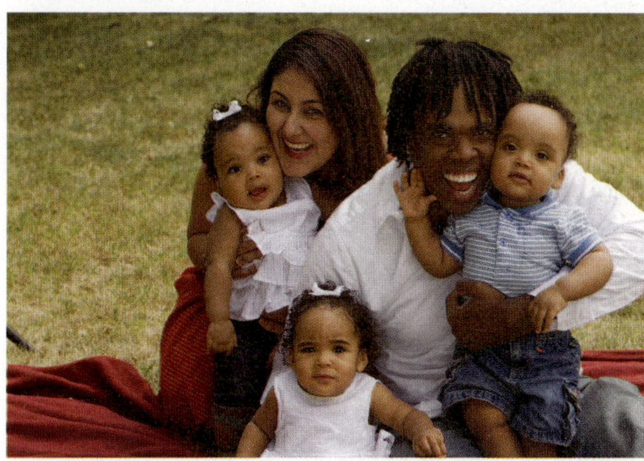

digitalskillet/Shutterstock


**PART TWO**

# UNDERSTANDING SEXUALITY

## 5 INTIMATE RELATIONSHIPS AND COMMUNICATION 86

**DEVELOPING INTERPERSONAL RELATIONSHIPS** 86
Self-Concept, Developing from Childhood 86
Nonsexual Intimate Relationships: Family, Friends, Peers 87
Love, Sex, and Intimacy 88
Challenges in Relationships 89
Unhealthy Intimate Relationships 91
Ending a Relationship 91

**COMMUNICATION** 92
Nonverbal Communication 92
Digital Communication and Our Social Networks 92
Communication Skills 93
Conflict and Conflict Resolution 93

**PAIRING AND SINGLEHOOD** 95
Choosing a Partner 95
Dating 95

Online Dating and Relationships 95
Sexual Orientation and Gender Identity in Society 97
Singlehood 98
Living Together 99

MARRIAGE 100
The Benefits of Marriage 100
Issues and Trends in Marriage 100
Separation and Divorce 101

FAMILY LIFE 101
Becoming a Parent 101
Parenting 101
Single Parents 102
Stepfamilies/Blended Families 103
Successful Families 103
*Tips for Today and the Future* 104
*Summary* 104
*For More Information* 105
*Selected Bibliography* 105

6 SEXUALITY, PREGNANCY, AND CHILDBIRTH 108

SEXUALITY, HUMAN STYLE 108
Opposites? Hardly 108
When Sex Became Gender 109
Cultural Norms and Biological Variations 109

SEXUAL ANATOMY: VARIATIONS ON A COMMON THEME 109
Human Sexual Anatomy: The Basic Plan 110
Female Sex Organs 110
Male Sex Organs 112

HUMAN SEXUAL DEVELOPMENT: PUBERTY AND ADULTHOOD 114
Aging and Human Sexuality 116
Atypical Sexual Development 117

SEXUAL AROUSAL AND RESPONSE 118
Sexual Arousal 118
The Sexual Response Cycle 118
Sexual Behavior 120
Sexual Disorders 121

GENDER AND SEXUALITY: BIOLOGIC SEX, GENDER ROLES, GENDER IDENTITY, SEXUAL ORIENTATION 123
Gender Nonconforming 123
Transgender 123
Sexual Orientation 124
The Origins of Sexual Orientation 124

SEXUALITY AND THE LIFE CYCLE 124
Childhood Sexual Behavior 125
Adolescent Sexuality 125
Adult Sexuality 125
Sexuality in Illness and Disability 125
Force and Sexual Coercion 125
Responsible Sexual Behavior 127

CONCEPTION 128
Fertilization 128
Twins 129

INFERTILITY 129
Female Infertility 129
Male Infertility 129
Treating Infertility 129

PREGNANCY 130
Physical Changes with Pregnancy 130
Emotional Responses to Pregnancy 132

FETAL DEVELOPMENT 132
The First Trimester 132
The Second Trimester 133
The Third Trimester 134
Diagnosing Fetal Abnormalities 134

THE IMPORTANCE OF PRENATAL CARE 135
Regular Checkups 135
Blood Tests 135
Prenatal Nutrition 135
Avoiding Drugs and Other Environmental Hazards 135
Prenatal Activity and Exercise 136
Preparing for Birth 137

COMPLICATIONS OF PREGNANCY AND PREGNANCY LOSS 137
Ectopic Pregnancy 137
Spontaneous Abortion 138
Stillbirth 138
Preeclampsia 138
Placenta Previa 138
Placental Abruption 138
Gestational Diabetes 138
Preterm Labor and Birth 138
Labor Induction 139
Low Birth Weight and Premature Birth 139
Infant Mortality and SIDS 139

CHILDBIRTH 139
Choices in Childbirth 139
Labor and Delivery 139
The Postpartum Period 141
*Tips for Today and the Future* 142
*Summary* 143
*For More Information* 143
*Selected Bibliography* 144

7 CONTRACEPTION AND ABORTION 145

TYPES OF CONTRACEPTION 146

WHICH CONTRACEPTIVE METHOD IS RIGHT FOR YOU? 147

PERMANENT CONTRACEPTION 149
Male Sterilization: Vasectomy 149
Female Sterilization 149

**LONG-ACTING REVERSIBLE CONTRACEPTION** *150*
Intrauterine Devices (IUDs) *150*
Contraceptive Implants *151*

**SHORT-ACTING REVERSIBLE CONTRACEPTION** *151*
Oral Contraceptives: The Pill *152*
Contraceptive Skin Patch *152*
Vaginal Contraceptive Ring *153*
Injectable Contraceptives *153*
Male (External) Condoms *154*
Female (Internal) Condoms *155*
Diaphragm with Spermicide *156*
Cervical Cap *157*
Contraceptive Sponge *157*
Vaginal Spermicides and Gels *157*

**BEHAVIORAL METHODS OF CONTRACEPTION** *158*
Abstinence *158*
Withdrawal *158*
Fertility Awareness-Based Methods *158*

**CONTRACEPTION AFTER PREGNANCY** *159*

**EMERGENCY CONTRACEPTION** *159*

**ABORTION** *160*

**UNDERSTANDING ABORTION** *162*
Personal and Social Indicators *162*
Fetal and Maternal Indicators *162*
Personal Considerations for the Pregnant Woman *162*
Personal Considerations for the Partner *162*
Considering Adoption *163*

**METHODS OF ABORTION** *163*
First-Trimester Abortion *163*
Second-Trimester Abortion *164*

**POSTABORTION CONSIDERATIONS** *164*

**THE POLITIZATION OF ABORTION** *165*
*Tips for Today and the Future* *166*
*Summary* *166*
*For More Information* *167*
*Selected Bibliography* *167*

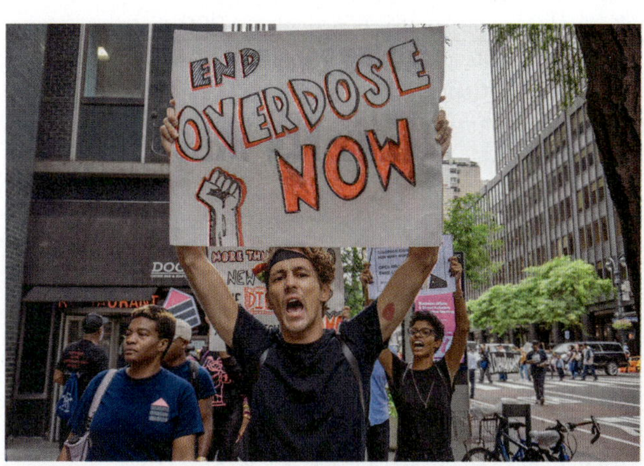

Erik McGregor/Pacific Press Media Production Corp./Alamy Stock Photo

## PART THREE

## SUBSTANCE USE DISORDERS: MAKING RESPONSIBLE DECISIONS

### 8 DRUG USE AND ADDICTION *169*

**ADDICTION** *169*
What Is Addiction? *170*
Diagnosing Substance Misuse and Substance Use Disorder *171*
The Development of Substance Use Disorder *172*
Behavioral Addictions *172*

**WHY PEOPLE USE AND MISUSE DRUGS** *173*
The Allure of Drugs *173*
Risk Factors for Drug Misuse and Addiction *173*

**RISKS ASSOCIATED WITH DRUG MISUSE** *175*

**HOW DRUGS AFFECT THE BODY** *175*
Changes in Brain Chemistry *175*
Physical Factors *176*
Psychological Factors *176*
Social Factors *176*

**GROUPS OF PSYCHOACTIVE DRUGS** *176*
Opioids *176*
Central Nervous System Depressants *178*
Central Nervous System Stimulants *179*
Marijuana and Other Cannabis Products *181*
Hallucinogens *182*
Inhalants *183*
Prescription Drug Misuse *183*
New Psychoactive Substances *183*

**PREVENTING DRUG-RELATED PROBLEMS** *184*
Drugs, Society, and Families *184*
Legalizing Drugs *184*
Treating Drug Addiction *184*
Preventing Drug Misuse *187*
*Tips for Today and the Future* *188*
*Summary* *188*
*For More Information* *188*
*Selected Bibliography* *190*

### 9 ALCOHOL AND NICOTINE *192*

**ALCOHOL AND THE BODY** *192*
Common Alcoholic Beverages *192*
Absorption *193*
Metabolism and Excretion *193*
Alcohol Intake and Blood Alcohol Concentration *194*

**ALCOHOL'S IMMEDIATE AND LONG-TERM EFFECTS** *195*
Immediate Effects *195*
Drinking and Driving *197*
Long-Term Effects of Chronic Misuse *199*
Alcohol Use during Pregnancy *200*
Possible Health Benefits of Alcohol? *201*

**EXCESSIVE USE OF ALCOHOL** 201
Alcohol Use Disorder: From Mild to Severe 201
Binge Drinking 202
Severe Alcohol Use Disorder 202
Sex and Race Differences 205
Supporting Someone with an Alcohol Problem 206

**WHO USES TOBACCO?** 206

**WHY PEOPLE USE TOBACCO** 206
Nicotine Addiction 206
Social and Psychological Factors 208
Genetic Factors 208
Why Start in the First Place? 209

**HEALTH HAZARDS** 209
Tobacco Smoke: A Toxic Mix 209
The Immediate Effects of Smoking 210
The Long-Term Effects of Smoking 210
Additional Health, Cosmetic, and Economic Concerns 212
Risks Associated with Other Forms of Tobacco Use 213

**THE EFFECTS OF SMOKING ON THE NONSMOKER** 214
Environmental Tobacco Smoke 214
Smoking and Pregnancy 215

**WHAT CAN BE DONE TO COMBAT SMOKING?** 216
Action at Many Levels 216
FDA Regulation of Tobacco 216
Individual Action 216

**HOW A TOBACCO USER CAN QUIT** 216
Benefits of Quitting 216
Options for Quitting 217
*Tips for Today and the Future* 218
*Summary* 220
*For More Information* 220
*Selected Bibliography* 221


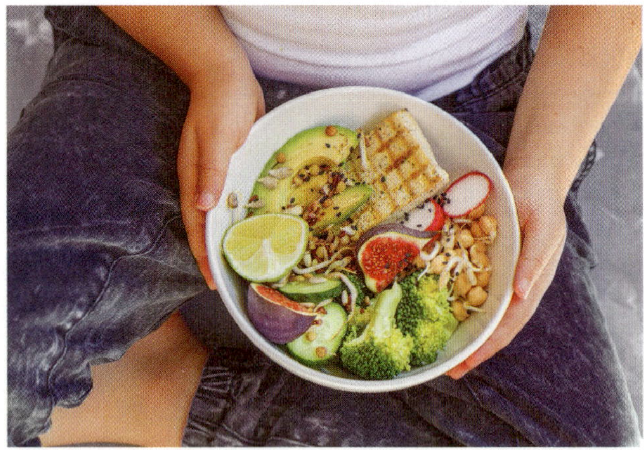
Nina Firsova/Alamy Stock Photo


## PART FOUR

## GETTING FIT

### 10 NUTRITION BASICS 224

**COMPONENTS OF A HEALTHY DIET** 224
Proteins—The Basis of Body Structure 225
Fat—Another Essential Nutrient 226
Carbohydrates—An Important Source of Energy 228
Fiber—A Closer Look 229
Vitamins—Organic Micronutrients 230
Minerals—Inorganic Micronutrients 232
Water—Vital but Underappreciated 233
Other Substances in Food 234

**NUTRITIONAL GUIDELINES: PLANNING YOUR DIET** 234
Dietary Reference Intakes (DRIs) 235
Dietary Guidelines for Americans 235
USDA's MyPlate 239
DASH Eating Plan 242
Choosing a Plant-Based Diet 242
Dietary Challenges for Various Population Groups 243

**A PERSONAL PLAN: MAKING INFORMED CHOICES ABOUT FOOD** 244
Reading Food Labels 245
Calorie Labeling: Restaurants and Vending Machines 246
Dietary Supplements 246
Protecting Yourself against Foodborne Illness 247
Organic Foods 247
Guidelines for Fish Consumption 250
Additives in Food 250
Food Biotechnology 250
Food Allergies and Food Intolerances 250
*Tips for Today and the Future* 251
*Summary* 251
*For More Information* 253
*Selected Bibliography* 253

### 11 EXERCISE FOR HEALTH AND FITNESS 259

**THE BENEFITS OF EXERCISE** 259
Improved Cardiorespiratory Functioning 259
More Efficient Metabolism and Improved Cell Health 259
Improved Body Composition 260
Disease Prevention and Management 260
Improved Psychological and Emotional Wellness 262
Improved Immune Function 262
Prevention of Injuries and Low-Back Pain 262
Improved Wellness for Life 262

**WHAT IS PHYSICAL FITNESS?** 262
Cardiorespiratory Endurance 262
Muscular Strength and Endurance 263
Flexibility 263
Body Composition 263
Skill-Related Components of Fitness 263

**COMPONENTS OF AN ACTIVE LIFESTYLE** 264
Increasing Physical Activity and Exercise 264
Reducing Sedentary Time 265

**DESIGNING YOUR EXERCISE PROGRAM** 266
First Steps 267
Cardiorespiratory Endurance Exercise 269
Exercises for Muscular Strength and Endurance 271
Flexibility Exercises 273
Training in Specific Skills 274
Putting It All Together 274

**GETTING STARTED AND STAYING ON TRACK** 274
Selecting Instructors, Equipment, and Facilities 274
Eating and Drinking for Exercise 276
Managing Your Fitness Program 276
*Tips for Today and the Future* 280
*Summary* 280
*For More Information* 281
*Selected Bibliography* 281

**12 WEIGHT MANAGEMENT** 283

**FACTORS THAT INFLUENCE WEIGHT** 283
Genetic Factors 283
Fat Cells 284
Metabolism 284
Hormones 285
Gut Microbiota 285
Sleep 285
Food Marketing and Public Policy 286
Food Perceptions and Behaviors 286

**EVALUATING BODY WEIGHT AND BODY COMPOSITION** 286
Body Composition 286
Defining Healthy Weight, Overweight, and Obesity 287
Body Mass Index 288
Estimating Body Composition 289
Body Fat Distribution 290
What Is the Right Weight for You? 290

**BODY FAT AND WELLNESS** 290
Diabetes 291
Heart Disease and Other Chronic Conditions 291
Problems Associated with Very Low Levels of Body Fat 292

**BODY IMAGE AND EATING DISORDERS** 293
Severe Body Image Problems 293
Eating Disorders 293

**ADOPTING A HEALTHY LIFESTYLE FOR SUCCESSFUL WEIGHT MANAGEMENT AND DISEASE PREVENTION** 296
Dietary Patterns and Eating Habits 296
Physical Activity and Exercise 298
Emotions and Coping Strategies 298

**APPROACHES TO OVERCOMING A WEIGHT PROBLEM** 299
Weight-Loss Plans and Products 299
Weight-Loss Programs 300
Prescription Drugs and Surgery 301
Gaining Weight 301
*Tips for Today and the Future* 301
*Summary* 302
*For More Information* 302
*Selected Bibliography* 303

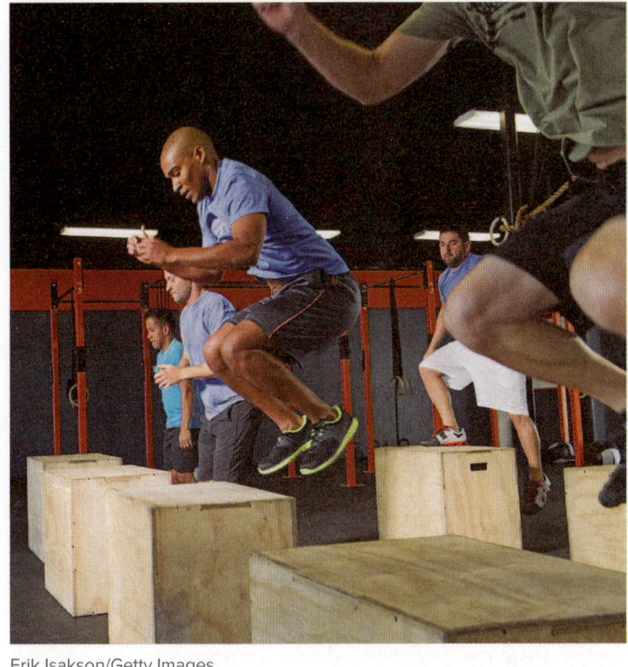

Erik Isakson/Getty Images

**PART FIVE**

**PROTECTING YOURSELF FROM DISEASE**

**13 CARDIOVASCULAR HEALTH AND CANCER** 306

**THE CARDIOVASCULAR SYSTEM** 306

**MAJOR FORMS OF CARDIOVASCULAR DISEASE** 309
Atherosclerosis 309
Coronary Artery Disease and Heart Attack 310
Stroke 313
Peripheral Arterial Disease 315
Congestive Heart Failure 316
Other Forms of Heart Disease 316

**RISK FACTORS FOR CARDIOVASCULAR DISEASE** 317
Major Risk Factors That Can Be Changed 317
Contributing Risk Factors That Can Be Changed 321
Major Risk Factors That Can't Be Changed 322
Possible Risk Factors Currently Being Studied 322

**PROTECTING YOURSELF AGAINST CARDIOVASCULAR DISEASE** 324
Eat Heart-Healthy 324
Exercise Regularly 324
Avoid Tobacco Products 325
Manage Your Blood Pressure, Cholesterol Levels, and Stress/Anger 325

**BASIC FACTS ABOUT CANCER** *326*
Tumors *326*
Metastasis *326*
The Stages of Cancer *326*
Remission *326*
The Incidence of Cancer *326*

**THE CAUSES OF CANCER** *327*
The Role of DNA *327*
Tobacco and Alcohol Use *328*
Dietary Factors *328*
Inactivity and Obesity *329*
Carcinogens in the Environment *329*

**DETECTING, DIAGNOSING, AND TREATING CANCER** *330*
Detecting Cancer *330*
Diagnosing Cancer *330*
Treating Cancer *330*

**COMMON TYPES OF CANCER** *332*
Lung Cancer *332*
Colon and Rectal Cancer *333*
Breast Cancer *333*
Prostate Cancer *334*
Cancers of the Female Reproductive Tract *335*
Skin Cancer *336*
Testicular Cancer *338*
*Tips for Today and the Future* *339*
*Summary* *339*
*For More Information* *341*
*Selected Bibliography* *341*

## 14 IMMUNITY AND INFECTION *344*

**THE BODY'S DEFENSE SYSTEM** *344*
Physical and Chemical Barriers *344*
The Immune System: Cells, Tissues, and Organs *345*
Immunization *347*
Allergy: A Case of Mistaken Identity *349*

**THE SPREAD OF DISEASE** *350*
Symptoms and Contagion *350*
The Chain of Infection *350*
Epidemics and Pandemics *351*

**PATHOGENS, DISEASES, AND TREATMENTS** *352*
Bacteria *352*
Viruses *357*
Fungi *359*
Protozoa *359*
Parasitic Worms *359*
Emerging Infectious Diseases *359*
Immune Disorders *360*

**SUPPORTING YOUR IMMUNE SYSTEM** *360*

**THE MAJOR STIs** *361*
HIV and AIDS *361*
Chlamydia *367*
Gonorrhea *368*
Pelvic Inflammatory Disease *369*
Human Papillomavirus *369*
Genital Herpes *371*
Hepatitis A, B, and C *372*
Syphilis *372*
Other Sexually Transmitted Infections *373*

**WHAT YOU CAN DO ABOUT SEXUALLY TRANSMITTED INFECTIONS** *374*
Education *374*
Diagnosis and Treatment *374*
Prevention *374*
*Tips for Today and the Future* *374*
*Summary* *374*
*For More Information* *376*
*Selected Bibliography* *377*

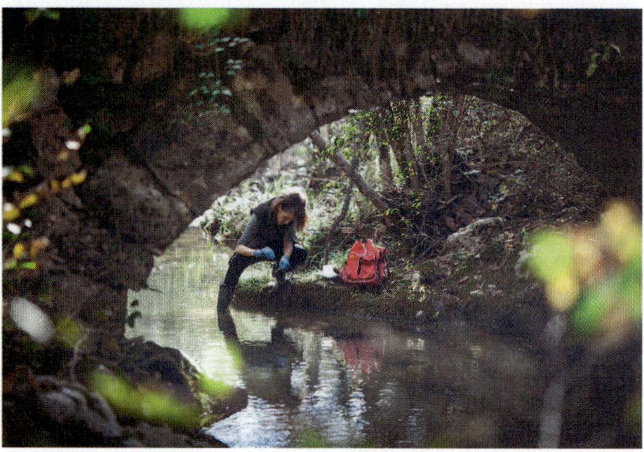
CasarsaGuru/Getty Images

**PART SIX**

## LIVING WELL IN THE WORLD

## 15 ENVIRONMENTAL HEALTH *380*

**ENVIRONMENTAL HEALTH DEFINED** *380*

**POPULATION GROWTH AND CONTROL** *381*

**ENVIRONMENTAL IMPACTS OF ENERGY USE AND PRODUCTION** *382*
Environmental Threats of Extreme Energy Sources *382*
Renewable Energy *383*
Alternative Fuels *383*
Hybrid and Electric Vehicles *384*

**AIR QUALITY AND POLLUTION** *384*
Air Quality and Smog *384*
The Greenhouse Effect and Global Warming *384*
Thinning of the Ozone Layer *386*
Indoor Air Quality (IAQ) *387*
Preventing Air Pollution *387*

**WATER QUALITY AND POLLUTION** *387*
Water Contamination and Treatment *387*
Water Shortages *388*

Sewage *389*
Protecting the Water Supply *389*

**SOLID WASTE POLLUTION** *389*
Disposing of Solid Waste *389*
Reducing Solid Waste *390*

**CHEMICAL POLLUTION AND HAZARDOUS WASTE** *391*
Asbestos *391*
Lead *391*
Pesticides *391*
Mercury *392*
Other Chemical Pollutants *393*
Preventing Chemical Pollution *394*

**RADIATION POLLUTION** *394*
Nuclear Weapons and Nuclear Energy *394*
Medical Uses of Radiation *395*
Radiation in the Home and Workplace *395*
Avoiding Radiation *395*

**NOISE POLLUTION** *395*
*Tips for Today and the Future* *396*
*Summary* *397*
*For More Information* *397*
*Selected Bibliography* *398*

**16 CONVENTIONAL AND COMPLEMENTARY MEDICINE** *399*

**SELF-CARE** *399*
Self-Assessment *399*
Knowing When to See a Physician *400*
Self-Treatment *400*

**PROFESSIONAL CARE** *402*

**CONVENTIONAL MEDICINE** *403*
Premises and Assumptions of Conventional Medicine *403*
Pharmaceuticals and the Placebo Effect *404*
The Providers of Conventional Medicine *406*
Primary Care Physicians *407*
Choosing a Specialist *407*
Getting the Most Out of Your Medical Care *407*

**INTEGRATIVE HEALTH** *411*
Alternative Medical Systems *411*
Mind–Body Medicine *413*
Biologically Based Products *414*
Manipulative and Body-Based Practices *414*
Other CAM Practices *416*
When Does CAM Become Conventional Medicine? *416*
Evaluating Complementary and Alternative Therapies *417*

**PAYING FOR HEALTH CARE** *417*
The Affordable Care Act *418*
How Health Insurance Works *419*
*Tips for Today and the Future* *421*
*Summary* *421*
*For More Information* *421*
*Selected Bibliography* *422*

**17 PERSONAL SAFETY** *424*

**UNINTENTIONAL INJURIES** *425*
What Causes an Injury? *425*
Home Injuries *425*
Motor Vehicle Injuries *428*
Leisure Injuries *431*
Weather-Related Injuries *431*
Work Injuries *433*

**VIOLENCE AND INTENTIONAL INJURIES** *433*
Factors Contributing to Violence *434*
Assault *435*
Homicide *435*
Gang-Related Violence *435*
Hate Crimes *436*
School Violence *436*
Workplace Violence *436*
Terrorism *437*
Family and Intimate-Partner Violence *437*
Sexual Violence *439*
What You Can Do about Violence *442*

**PROVIDING EMERGENCY CARE** *444*
*Tips for Today and the Future* *444*
*Summary* *445*
*For More Information* *445*
*Selected Bibliography* *446*

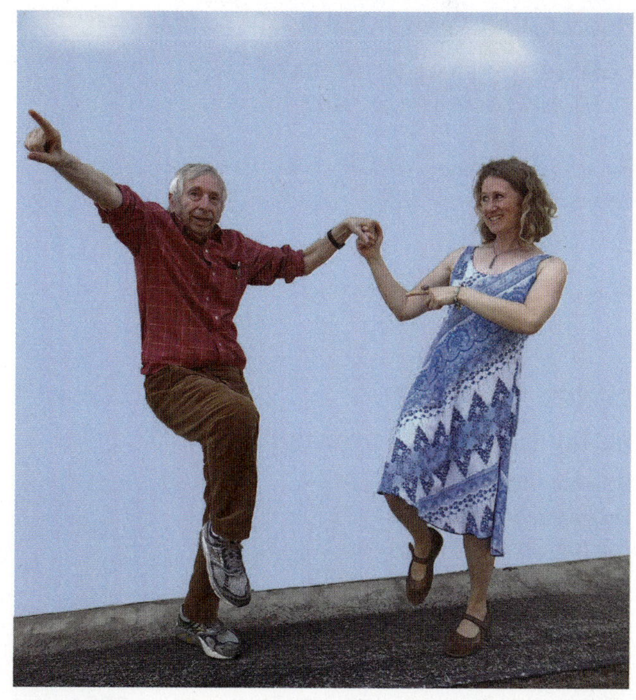
Marcia Seyler

PART SEVEN

## ACCEPTING PHYSICAL LIMITS

18 THE CHALLENGE OF AGING 448

PERSPECTIVES ON AGING 448
Life-Enhancing Measures 449

DEALING WITH THE CHANGES OF AGING 452
Changing Roles and Relationships 452
Adapting to Physical Changes 452
Psychological and Cognitive Changes 454

LIFE IN AN AGING SOCIETY 455
The Aging Minority 456
Family and Community Resources for Older Adults 457
Government Aid and Policies 457

WHAT IS DEATH? 458
Defining Death 458
Learning about Death 459
Denying versus Acknowledging Death 459

PLANNING FOR DEATH 460
Making a Will 460
Giving the Gift of Life 460
Considering Options for End-of-Life Care 461
Difficult Decisions at the End of Life 462
Planning a Funeral or Memorial Service 463

COPING WITH IMMINENT DEATH 465
The Tasks of Coping 465
Supporting a Person in the Last Phase of Life 465

COPING WITH LOSS 465
Experiencing Grief 465
Supporting a Grieving Person 467
When a Young Adult Loses a Friend 467
Helping Children Cope with Loss 467

COMING TO TERMS WITH DEATH 467
*Tips for Today and the Future* 469
*Summary* 469
*For More Information* 470
*Selected Bibliography* 471

Index 473

## BOXES

### BEHAVIOR CHANGE STRATEGY

Behavior Change Contract 21
Dealing with Social Anxiety 63
Lab Exercise: Sleep Case Scenarios 83
Changing Your Drug Habits 189
Kicking the Tobacco Habit 219
Improving Your Diet by Choosing Healthy Beverages 252
Planning a Personal Exercise Program 278
Reducing the Saturated and Trans Fats in Your Diet 325
Incorporating More Fruits and Vegetables into Your Diet 340
Talking about Condoms and Safer Sex 375
Adhering to Your Physician's Instructions 422

### CRITICAL CONSUMER

Evaluating Sources of Health Information 15
Choosing and Evaluating Mental Health Professionals 61
Home Pregnancy Tests 131
Alcohol Advertising 204
Using Food Labels 245
Using Dietary Supplement Labels 248
What to Wear 275
Apps and Wearables for Weight Management 300
Sunscreens and Sun-Protective Clothing 337
Know Your Status: Getting an HIV Test 366
Endocrine Disruption: A "New" Toxic Threat 393
Avoiding Health Fraud and Quackery 412
Choosing a Health Insurance Plan 420
A Consumer Guide to Funerals 464

### DIVERSITY MATTERS

Can Racial Categories Be Used in Medicine? 10
Diverse Populations, Discrimination, and Stress 32
Ethnicity, Race, Culture, and Psychological Health 51
Marriage Equality 98
Barriers to Contraceptive Use 148
The Trouble with Substance Use Surveys 185
Metabolizing Alcohol: Our Bodies Work Differently 194
Is BMI Biased? 288
Gender, Race/Ethnicity, and Cardiovascular Disease 323
Race/Ethnicity, Poverty, and Cancer 328
HIV/AIDS around the World 362
Poverty, Gender, and Environmental Health 392
Health Care Visits and Gender 408
Injuries among Young Men 426
Why Do Women Live Longer? 456

### TAKE CHARGE

Financial Wellness 4
Life Expectancy and the Obesity Epidemic 5
Mindfulness Meditation 37
Realistic Self-Talk 47
Digital Devices: Help or Harm for a Good Night's Sleep? 70
Delayed Sleep Phase 79
Guidelines for Effective Communication 94
Strategies of Strong Families 104
Communicating about Sexuality 127
Physical Activity during Pregnancy 137
A Deeper Look 161
If Someone You Know Has a Drug Problem . . . 186
Dealing with an Alcohol Emergency 196
Strategies to Quit Smoking 218
Choosing More Whole-Grain Foods 229

**CHAPTER 6**

- New presentation of the development of sex organs, focusing on how homologous tissues and structures develop
- Revised discussion of human sexuality, including the relationship between sex and gender, and the shift away from biological determinism
- New section of gender and sexuality, including the role of culture, the shift away from a binary view, and the distinction between biologic sex and gender
- Revised discussion of how racism and bias affect pregnancy and related outcomes

**CHAPTER 7**

- Updated Diversity Matters box to include how underrepresented racial and ethnic groups have faced harmful reproductive policies and historical practices that lead to mistrust of the medical establishment
- New discussion of personal considerations that are factors in an individual's decision to continue a pregnancy
- New discussion of how the Hyde Amendment and the Supreme Court's ruling on *Dobbs v. Jackson Women's Health Organization* disproportionately impact underrepresented populations and people experiencing poverty

**CHAPTER 8**

- New coverage of the effects of pandemic-related stress on U.S. rates of drug misuse, including the trends in overdose deaths among different demographic groups.
- New Diversity Matters box covering problems related to substance-use surveys that identify specific demographic populations.

**CHAPTER 9**

- New section on alcohol-related health disparities along racial and ethnic lines, including how to address the effects of trauma in treatment plans for American Indians
- Updated discussion refuting stereotypes about people facing severe alcohol use disorder
- Updated data and discussion of the prevalence, risk factors, and treatment considerations across racial and ethnic groups
- Updated discussion of the relationship between genetics and the prevalence of cigarette smoking
- Updated information on the impact of cigarette marketing, promotions, and sponsorship targeting the LGBTQIA+ community

**CHAPTER 12**

- New Diversity Matters box covering the potential biases in the body mass index (BMI) and the implications for the health of diverse populations
- New section on the Health at Every Size (HAES) movement and the fight against stigmatizing people with overweight

**CHAPTER 13**

- Revised discussion of the rates of hypertension among racially and ethnically diverse populations, according to the U.S. National Health and Nutrition Examination Survey
- Updated data on the prevalence and risk factors for individuals from diverse racial, ethnic, and genetic backgrounds
- Updated Diversity Matters box highlighting key considerations for identifying and treating cardiovascular disease in women and across racial/ethnic groups
- Updated to reflect the American Cancer Society's most recent data, including new reporting on American Indian or Alaska Native people
- Updated to include data about cancer risk, incidence rates, and testing disparities among different racial and ethnic populations

**CHAPTER 14**

- Updated data on key populations disproportionately affected by HIV
- New feature on vaccine hesitancy explains how the history of institutional racism has made some underrepresented racial and ethnic groups skeptical about vaccination

**CHAPTER 15**

- Updated data on how and those experiencing poverty and residents of urban areas are disproportionately impacted by pollution

**CHAPTER 16**

- New section explores the drivers of healthcare inequity and the unequal treatment of Black, Latino, and Indigenous communities
- Updated data on the effects of the Affordable Care Act on various racial and ethnic groups

**CHAPTER 17**

- New section on the prevalence and risks of gun violence and homicide across various racial and ethnic populations
- New section on hate crimes and police violence due to racism and discrimination against members of the transgender community
- New discussion of racism and prejudice as a learned behavior
- Updated data on the incidence of interpersonal violence experienced by people across races, ethnicities, and genders

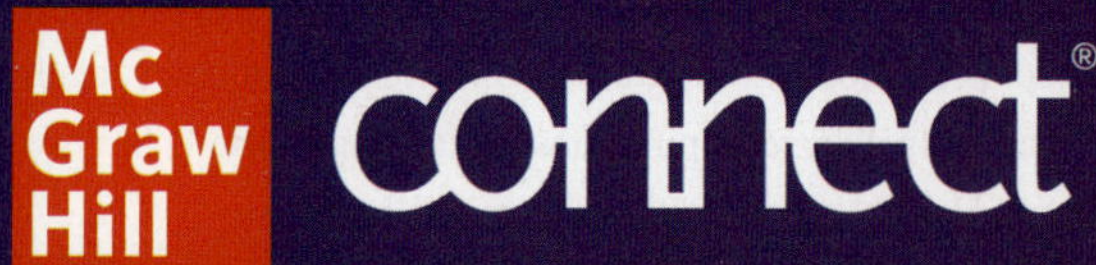

# Instructors
## The Power of Connections

### A complete course platform

Connect enables you to build deeper connections with your students through cohesive digital content and tools, creating engaging learning experiences. We are committed to providing you with the right resources and tools to support all your students along their personal learning journeys.

**65%** Less Time Grading

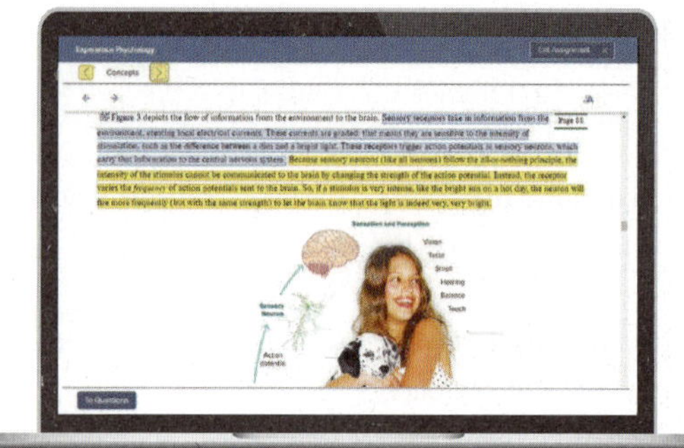

Laptop: Getty Images; Woman/dog: George Doyle/Getty Images

### Every learner is unique

In Connect, instructors can assign an adaptive reading experience with SmartBook® 2.0. Rooted in advanced learning science principles, SmartBook 2.0 delivers each student a personalized experience, focusing students on their learning gaps, ensuring that the time they spend studying is time well-spent. **mheducation.com/highered/connect/smartbook**

### Affordable solutions, added value

Make technology work for you with LMS integration for single sign-on access, mobile access to the digital textbook, and reports to quickly show you how each of your students is doing. And with our Inclusive Access program, you can provide all these tools at the lowest available market price to your students. Ask your McGraw Hill representative for more information.

### Solutions for your challenges

A product isn't a solution. Real solutions are affordable, reliable, and come with training and ongoing support when you need it and how you want it. Visit **supportateverystep.com** for videos and resources both you and your students can use throughout the term.

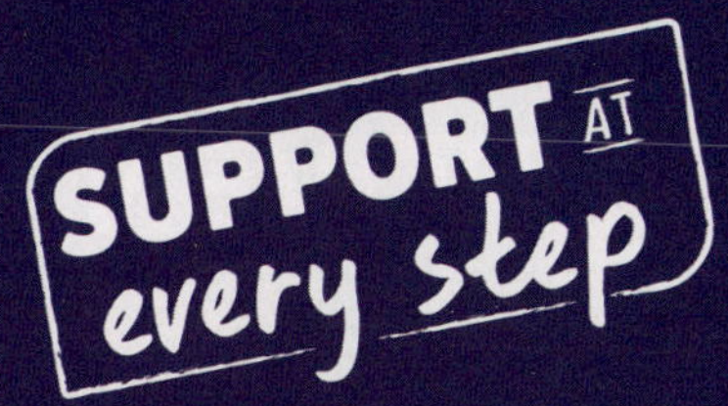


# Students
## Get Learning that Fits You

### Effective tools for efficient studying

Connect is designed to help you be more productive with simple, flexible, intuitive tools that maximize your study time and meet your individual learning needs. Get learning that works for you with Connect.

### Study anytime, anywhere

Download the free ReadAnywhere® app and access your online eBook, SmartBook® 2.0, or Adaptive Learning Assignments when it's convenient, even if you're offline. And since the app automatically syncs with your Connect account, all of your work is available every time you open it. Find out more at **mheducation.com/readanywhere**

***"I really liked this app—it made it easy to study when you don't have your text-book in front of you."***

- Jordan Cunningham,
Eastern Washington University

iPhone: Getty Images

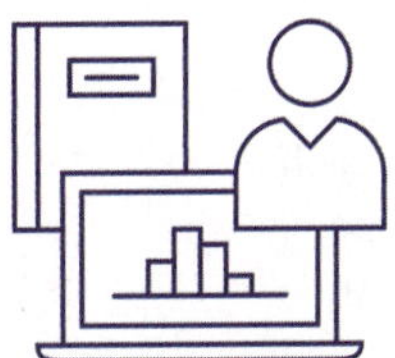

### Everything you need in one place

Your Connect course has everything you need—whether reading your digital eBook or completing assignments for class—Connect makes it easy to get your work done.

### Learning for everyone

McGraw Hill works directly with Accessibility Services Departments and faculty to meet the learning needs of all students. Please contact your Accessibility Services Office and ask them to email accessibility@mheducation.com, or visit **mheducation.com/about/accessibility** for more information.

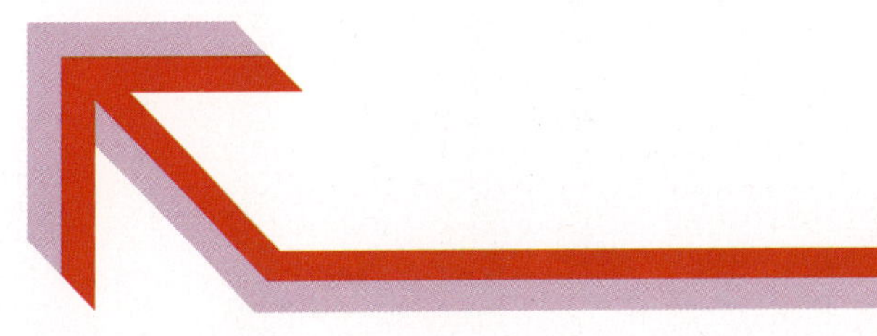

# PROVEN, SCIENCE-BASED CONTENT

Now in its eighteenth edition, *Connect Core Concepts in Health* remains the leading health textbook in U.S. higher education. In 2020, *Connect Core Concepts in Health* won the Textbook and Academic Authors McGuffey Award for Excellence and Longevity. The book's unique psychological approach to mind-body health encourages students to take proactive self-assessments. Students can stay current on the latest studies while learning how to negotiate cross-cultural ideas of what it means to be healthy and how to live in our diverse, consumer-oriented society. McGraw Hill digital and teaching learning tools also integrate *Connect Core Concepts in Health's* authoritative, science-based content.

**Assess Yourself** helps students analyze their own health and health-related behavior.

**Take Charge** challenges students to take meaningful action toward personal improvement.

**Critical Consumer** helps students navigate the numerous and diverse health-related products available on the market.

**Diversity Matters** introduces the many ways that cultural and gendered ideas of health come to influence our health strengths, risks, and behaviors.

**Wellness on Campus** focuses on health issues, challenges, and opportunities that students are likely to encounter on a regular basis.

**Behavior Change Strategy** offers specific behavior management/modification plans related to the chapter topic.

**Ask Yourself: Questions for Critical Thinking and Reflection** encourages critical reflection on students' own health-related behaviors.

**Quick Stats** updated for the seventeenth edition, focuses attention on particularly striking statistics related to the chapter content.

**Tips for Today and the Future** ends each chapter with a quick, bulleted list of concrete actions readers can take now and in the near future.

# CONNECT IS PROVEN EFFECTIVE

McGraw Hill connect

***McGraw Hill Connect®*** is a digital teaching and learning environment that improves performance over a variety of critical outcomes; it is easy to use and proven effective. Connect® empowers students by continually adapting to deliver precisely what they need, when they need it, and how they need it, so your class time is more engaging and effective. Connect for *Core Concepts in Health* offers a wealth of interactive online content, including health labs and self-assessments, video activities on timely health topics, and practice quizzes with immediate feedback.

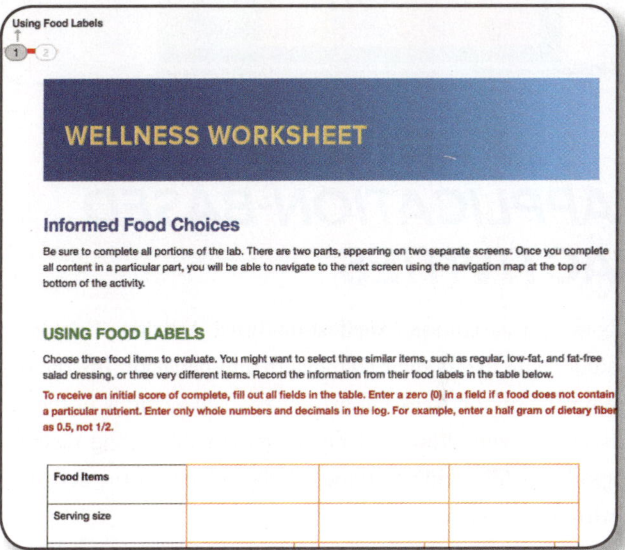


## PERSONALIZED LEARNING

McGraw Hill SMARTBOOK®

Available within Connect, ***SmartBook®*** makes study time as productive and efficient as possible by identifying and closing knowledge gaps. SmartBook identifies what an individual student knows and doesn't know based on the student's confidence level, responses to questions, and other factors. SmartBook builds an optimal, personalized learning path for each student, so students spend less time on concepts they already understand and more time on those they don't. As a student engages with SmartBook, the reading experience continuously adapts by highlighting the most impactful content that person needs to learn at that moment. This ensures that every minute spent with SmartBook is returned to the student as the most value-added minute possible. The result? More confidence, better grades, and greater success.

SmartBook is optimized for phones and tablets. Its interactive features are also accessible for students with disabilities. Just like our ebook and ReadAnywhere app, SmartBook is available both online and offline.

Read or study when it's convenient for you with McGraw Hill's free **ReadAnywhere** app. Available for iOS or Android smartphones or tablets, ReadAnywhere gives users access to McGraw Hill tools, including the eBook and SmartBook or Adaptive Learning Assignments in Connect. Take notes, highlight, and complete assignments offline–all of your work will sync when you open the app with WiFi access. Log in with your McGraw Hill Connect username and password to start learning–anytime, anywhere!

McGraw Hill NutritionCalc Plus

**NutritionCalc Plus** is a powerful dietary analysis tool featuring more than 30,000 foods from the reliable and accurate ESHA Research nutrient database, which is comprised of data from the latest USDA Standard Reference database, manufacturers' data, restaurant data, and data from literature sources. NutritionCalc Plus allows users to track food and activities and then analyze their choices with a robust selection of intuitive reports. The interface was updated to accommodate ADA requirements and a modern mobile experience native to today's students.

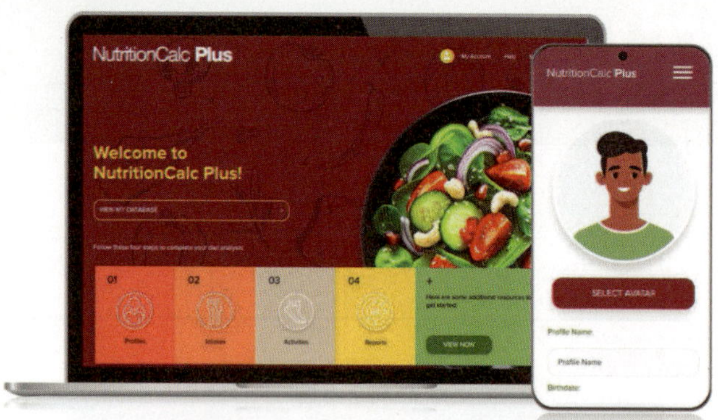


## APPLICATION-BASED ACTIVITIES

New to this edition, **Application-Based Activities** help your students to assess their own health and behavior. Instructors have the option to assign privacy-enabled versions of the activities, which allow students to opt out of sharing their responses while being credited for completion of the activities within Connect.

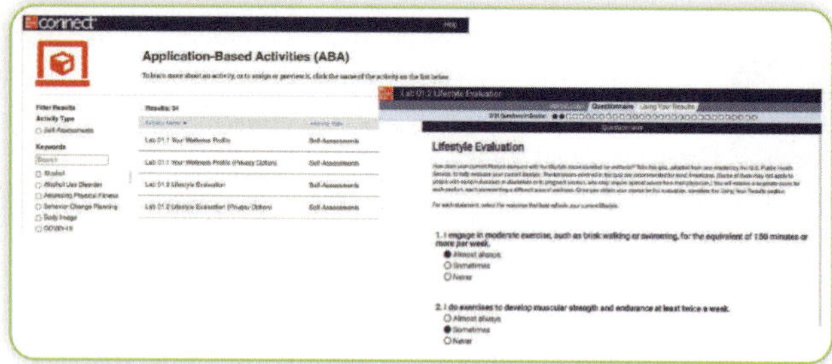


## WRITING ASSIGNMENT

McGraw Hill's **Writing Assignment** tool delivers a learning experience that improves students' written communication skills and conceptual understanding with every assignment. Assign, monitor, and provide feedback on writing more efficiently and grade assignments within McGraw Hill Connect®. Writing Assignment gives students an all-in-one place interface, so you can provide feedback more efficiently.

Features include:

- Saved and reusable comments (text and audio)
- Ability to link to resources in comments
- Rubric building and scoring
- Ability to assign draft and final deadline milestones
- Tablet ready and tools for all learners

## VIDEO CAPTURE POWERED BY GOREACT™

With just a smartphone, tablet, or webcam, students and instructors can capture video with ease. **Video Capture** Powered by GoReact does not require any extra equipment or complicated training. All it takes is five minutes to set up and start recording! Use Video Capture to create your own custom video capture assignment, including lab activities, exercise technique demonstrations, presentations, self-review, and peer review. With customizable rubrics, time-coded comments, and visual markers, students will see feedback at exactly the right moment, and in context, to help improve their skills.

## CONCEPT CLIPS

Short videos on topics like the stress response and sleep stages are also new to this edition. Assignable and assessable through Connect, **Concept Clips** provide step-by-step presentations to promote student comprehension.

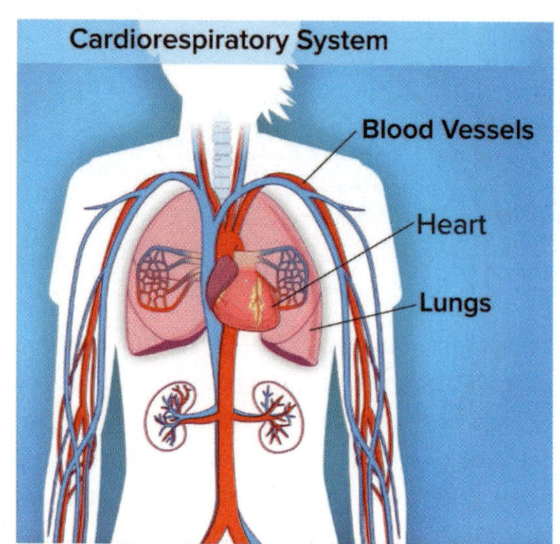


## CURRENT ISSUES

Also in Connect, **NewsFlash** activities tie current news stories to key personal health concepts. After interacting with a contemporary news story, students are assessed on their understanding and their ability to make the connections between real-life events and course content. Examples of NewsFlash topics include the Covid-19 pandemic's effect on mental health, racial health disparities, dangers of sedentary time, colon cancer screening, and low-fat versus low-carb diets.

# CHAPTER-BY-CHAPTER CHANGES

The eighteenth edition focuses current events, health trends, and content changes informed by the Covid-19 pandemic. All data and statistics have been updated to reflect the most current data available.

**Chapter 1: Taking Charge of Your Health**

- Updated life expectancy data, including the impact of Covid-19, one of the leading causes of death in 2020 and 2021.
- Updated data on obesity and drug overdose deaths, and their impact on life expectancy.
- Revised figure showing the percentage of Americans who engage in unhealthy behaviors (e.g., obesity, tobacco use, excessive alcohol use) using updated data.
- Updated "Vital Statistics" table presenting the current leading causes of death among Americans ages 15–24.
- New Diversity Matters box, reviewed by social and medical scientists, that addresses the challenges in using social categories in health data.
- Revised Wellness on Campus box detailing the top sources of stress among college students, newly categorized by gender (cis men, cis women, transgender and gender nonconforming).

**Chapter 2: Stress: The Constant Challenge**

- New discussion of allostatic load and how frequent stress can be harmful.
- New discussion of the adaptive calibration model.
- Updated data from the Center for Collegiate Mental Health on trends in depression and self-harm among college students.

**Chapter 3: Psychological Health**

- Expanded discussion of the relationship between psychological health and discrimination among LGBTQIA+ persons.
- Expanded discussion of the challenges faced by immigrants and underrepresented racial and ethnic groups.
- Updated data on depression, self-injury, and suicidal thoughts among U.S. adults.
- Updated discussion of mental health treatment options, including those available through telehealth and video visits.

**Chapter 4: Sleep**

- New figure showing the stages of the sleep cycle.
- Updated discussion of the effects of the Covid-19 pandemic on sleep, including the link between anxiety and insomnia.
- Updated discussion of the effects of sleep on weight.

**Chapter 5: Intimate Relationships and Communication**

- Updated data on support for marriage equality.
- Revised discussion of emotional intelligence and the connection between empathy and prejudice.
- Updated data on rates of child abuse and neglect, including the long-term effects and correlation to socioeconomic status.
- New Wellness on Campus box about the effects of the Covid-19 pandemic on sex and dating.

**Chapter 6: Sex and Pregnancy**

- New discussion of human sexuality, including the relationship between sex and gender, and the shift away from biological determinism.
- Reorganized discussion of how society and culture have shaped gender roles, gender identity, and even puberty and our biology.
- New discussion of the development of sex organs, reducing the focus on difference and beginning with humans as made of homologous tissues and structures.
- Inclusion of the importance of self-awareness and body exploration.
- Updated discussion of the physical and psychological aspects of the menstrual cycle.
- New discussion of sexual cycles in men.
- Updated and revised section about gender and the sexual response.
- Updated discussion of sexual coercion and consent.

**Chapter 7: Contraception and Abortion**

- New chapter presentation combines contraception and abortion.
- Most current data reflecting public opinion about abortion.
- Revised and updated section on emergency contraception.
- Newly updated section about abortion laws, including the effects of the Supreme Court's ruling on *Dobbs v. Jackson Women's Health Organization*.

**Chapter 8: Drug Use and Addiction**

- Revised and updated terminology reflects language used in the American Psychiatric Association's *Diagnostic and Statistical Manual of Mental Disorders* (*DSM-5-TR*).
- Updated discussion of gambling and gaming disorders.

- New coverage of the effects of pandemic-related stress on U.S. rates of drug misuse, including the trends in overdose deaths among different demographic groups.
- Updated data from the most current National Survey of Substance Abuse Treatment Services.
- New Diversity Matters box covering problems related to substance-use surveys that identify specific demographic populations.

**Chapter 9: Alcohol and Nicotine**

- Revised and updated terminology to reflect the language used in the American Psychiatric Association's *Diagnostic and Statistical Manual of Mental Disorders* (*DSM-5-TR*).
- Updated data about the correlation between alcohol and aggressive behavior.
- Revised passage on moderate alcohol consumption and coronary health, including new research rejecting the theory that light to moderate drinking fosters heart health.
- New data from the current National Institute on Alcohol Abuse and Alcoholism incorporated.
- New section on alcohol-related health disparities along racial and ethnic lines.
- New chapter presentation and organization emphasizes e-cigarettes and vaping in addition to tobacco cigarettes.
- New data from a 2021 investigation by the Centers for Disease Control and Prevention about vaping among middle and high school students.
- Updated data on smoking prevalence, including new research that links genetics to cigarette smoking prevalence.
- Updated data about tobacco and vaping imagery in entertainment media.
- New figure showing the brain and the reward pathways affected by nicotine.
- Updated data about smoking as a risk factor for severe illness from Covid-19.

**Chapter 10: Nutrition Basics**

- Updated discussion of the health risks and sources of trans fats.
- Revised and expanded to reflect recommendations from the *2020–2025 Dietary Guidelines* and the American Heart Association.

**Chapter 11: Exercise for Health and Fitness**

- Updated data about the effects of physical activity on premature death risk.
- Updated to include the Health and Retirement Study.

**Chapter 12: Weight Management**

- New chapter presentation and organization that improves clarity and linkage between topics.
- Updated inclusion of the role of social pressure in unhealthy thought patterns and weight.
- New section on how behavior is influenced by biocultural perspectives and perceptions of food.
- New figures illustrating body composition and how it can vary across people of the same height and weight.
- New Diversity Matters box exploring the appropriate uses, drawbacks, and potential biases of body mass index.

**Chapter 13: Cardiovascular Health and Cancer**

- Updated guidance on cholesterol screening and goals based on the American College of Cardiology and the American Heart Association.
- Updated findings on the effects of Covid-19 on the cardiovascular system.
- Updated to include data about cancer risk, incidence rates, and testing disparities among different racial and ethnic populations.

**Chapter 14: Immunity and Infection**

- New special feature about vaccine effectiveness and vaccine hesitancy.
- Updated explanation about mRNA vaccine technology.
- New discussion of Covid-19, including the development of new variants and the role of vaccination in ending the pandemic.
- Updated explanation about masking to reduce the spread of illness.
- Updated data about HIV in the United States and throughout the world.
- Updated sections on the treatment, incidence, and risk factors for gonorrhea, human papillomavirus, herpes, and syphilis.

**Chapter 15: Environmental Health**

- Revised explanation about the scientific analysis of climate change.
- Updated discussion of recycling and electronics waste.

**Chapter 16: Conventional and Complementary Medicine**

- Updated discussion of health equity in the United States and worldwide.
- Updated discussion of the impact of the Affordable Care Act, including the most recent enrollment data and demographic trends.

**Chapter 17: Personal Safety**

- Updated numbers for leading causes of death, including a deeper look at drug overdose and motor vehicle fatalities.
- Updated data about homicides and firearm injuries and deaths.
- New section drawing on Department of Justice statistics about hate crimes and terrorism, including an updated discussion of right-wing terrorist networks.
- Revised coverage of intimate partner violence and rape, including updated trends and data.

**Chapter 18: The Challenge of Aging**

- Revised discussion of depression and suicide among the elderly.

# YOUR COURSE, YOUR WAY

McGraw Hill create

**McGraw Hill Create®** is a self-service website that allows you to create customized course materials using McGraw Hill's comprehensive, cross-disciplinary content and digital products. You can even access third-party content such as readings, articles, cases, videos, and more.

- Select and arrange content to fit your course scope and sequence.
- Upload your own course materials.
- Select the best format for your students–print or eBook.
- Select and personalize your cover.
- Edit and update your materials as often as you'd like.

Experience how McGraw Hill's Create empowers you to teach your students your way: http://create.mheducation.com.

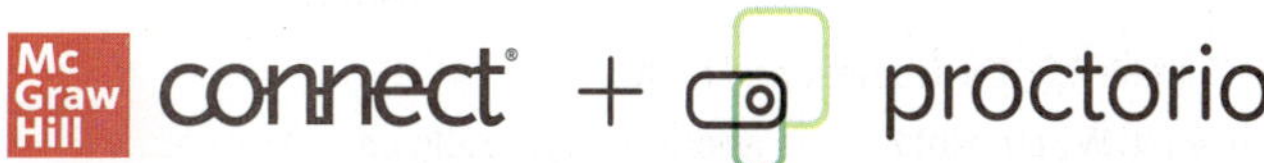


**Remote proctoring and browser-locking capabilities,** hosted by Proctorio within Connect, provide control of the assessment environment by enabling security options and verifying the identity of the student.

Seamlessly integrated within Connect, these services allow instructors to control students' assessment experience by restricting browser activity, recording students' activity, and verifying students are doing their own work.

Instant and detailed reporting gives instructors an at-a-glance view of potential academic integrity concerns, thereby avoiding personal bias and supporting evidence-based claims.

## INSTRUCTOR RESOURCES

*Core Concepts in Health* offers an array of instructor resources for the personal health course:

**Instructor's manual.** The instructor's manual provides a wide variety of tools and resources for presenting the course, including learning objectives and ideas for lectures and discussions.

**Test bank.** By increasing the rigor of the test bank development process, McGraw Hill has raised the bar for student assessment. Each question has been tagged for level of difficulty, Bloom's taxonomy, and topic coverage. Organized by chapter, the questions are designed to test factual, conceptual, and higher-order thinking.

**Test Builder.** Available within Connect, Test Builder is a cloud-based tool that enables instructors to format tests that can be printed and administered within a Learning Management System. Test Builder offers a modern, streamlined interface for easy content configuration that matches course needs, without requiring a download.

Test Builder enables instructors to:

- Access all test bank content from a particular title
- Easily pinpoint the most relevant content through robust filtering options
- Manipulate the order of questions or scramble questions and/or answers
- Pin questions to a specific location within a test
- Determine your preferred treatment of algorithmic questions
- Choose the layout and spacing
- Add instructions and configure default settings

**PowerPoint.** The PowerPoint presentations highlight the key points of the chapter and include supporting visuals. All slides are WCAG compliant.

# ACKNOWLEDGMENTS

We are grateful for the contributors and reviewers who provided feedback and suggestions for enhancing this eighteenth edition:

## ACADEMIC CONTRIBUTORS

Laura Acosta, DCN, RDN, LD/N
University of Florida
*Weight Management*

Anna Altshuler, MD, MPH
California Pacific Medical Center
*Contraception and Abortion*

Sarah Brunnig, MS, MPH, RDN
University of Florida
*Nutrition Basics*

Boyce Burge, PhD
California Institute of Human Nutrition
*Cancer*

Thomas D. Fahey, EdD
California State University–Chico
*Exercise for Health and Fitness*

Nancy Kemp, MD, MA
Board Certified in Hospice and Palliative Medicine
*Aging: An Ongoing Process*
*Dying and Death*

Candice McNeil, MD, MPH
Wake Forest University School of Medicine
*Sexually Transmitted Infections*

Carol Chapnick Mukhopadhyay, PhD
San Jose State University
*Sex and Your Body*

Michael Joshua Ostacher, MD, MPH, MMSc
Stanford University School of Medicine
*Psychological Health*

Samantha M. Portis, PhD
Brown University
*Alcohol: The Most Popular Drug*

Johanna Rochester, PhD
ICF
*Environmental Health*
*Immunity and Infection*

Maria I. Rodriguez, MD MPH
Oregon Health and Science University
*Contraception and Abortion*

Pir Rothenberg, PhD
California Institute of Human Nutrition
*Stress*
*Personal Safety*

Lily K. Stern, MD
Cedars-Sinai Medical Center
*Cardiovascular Health*

Jeroen Vanderhoeven, MD
Swedish Medical Center
*Pregnancy and Childbirth*

Joseph Winer, PhD
Stanford University
*Sleep*

## ACADEMIC ADVISORS AND REVIEWERS

Elizabeth Ash, Morehead State University
Michael Ash, Morehead State University
Candy Carr-Smith, Community College of Baltimore County, Essex
Freelun Chen, Borough of Manhattan Community College
Karl DeBate, Hillsborough Community College - Dale Mabry Campus
Robert Flores, Moreno Valley College
Michael Grez, Harold Washington College
Robert M. Hess, Community College of Baltimore County, Catonsville
Matt Hutchins, Indiana State University
Andre Ifill, The Community College of Baltimore County Catonsville
John Janowiak, Appalachian State University
Eve A. Laidacker, Montgomery County Community College
Mechelle Medhurst, Cuesta Community College SLO
Craig Newton, CCBC Catonsville
Ayanna Walker, California University of PA
Matthew Warner, Indiana State University

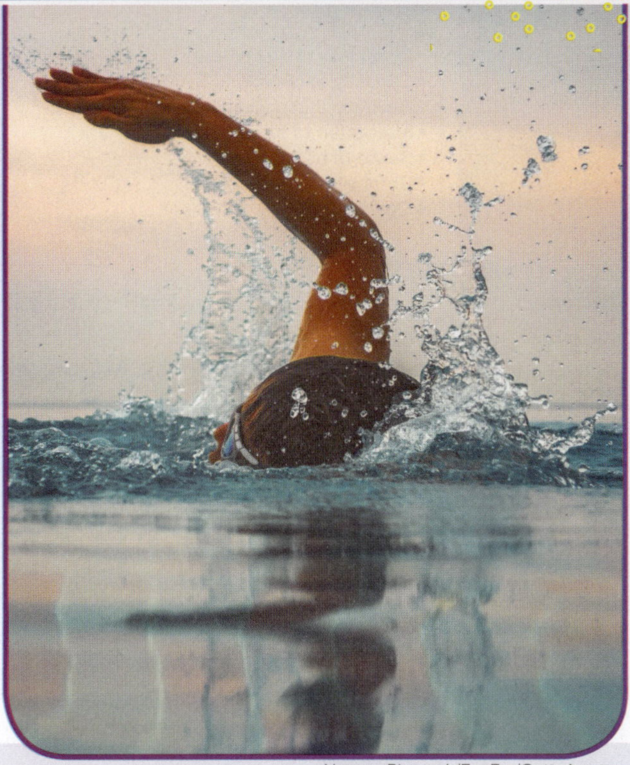

Narong Pimsook/EyeEm/Getty Images

## CHAPTER OBJECTIVES

- Define wellness as a health goal
- Explain two major efforts to promote national health
- Describe factors that influence wellness
- Explain methods for achieving wellness through lifestyle management
- List ways to promote lifelong wellness for yourself and your environment

CHAPTER 1

# Taking Charge of Your Health

When was the last time you felt truly healthy? Not just free from illness, but energized, hungry, and flexible, like all your muscles just got a good stretching or workout? Many of us do not feel this way. We're overweight; we smoke; we eat a lot of sugar; we don't sleep well.

The good news? There is always something we could be improving. This book can help you learn about the many aspects of life that work together to get you feeling on top of your game.

## WELLNESS AS A HEALTH GOAL

Generations of people have viewed good health simply as the absence of disease, and that view largely prevails today. The word **health** typically refers to the overall condition of a person's body or mind and to the presence or absence of illness or injury. **Wellness** expands this idea of good health to include living a rich, meaningful, and energetic life. Beyond the simple presence or absence of disease, wellness can refer to optimal health and vitality—to living life to its fullest. Although we use the words *health* and *wellness* interchangeably, they differ in two important ways. *Health* can be determined or influenced by factors beyond your control, such as your genes, age, and family history. *Wellness* is determined largely by the decisions you make about how you live. These decisions affect **risk factors** that contribute to disease or injury. We cannot control risk factors such as age and family history, but behaviors such as eating a healthy diet and choosing not to smoke are well within our control.

**TERMS**

**health** The overall condition of body or mind and the presence or absence of illness or injury.

**wellness** Optimal health and vitality, encompassing all the dimensions of well-being.

**risk factor** A condition that increases your chances of disease or injury.

PHYSICAL WELLNESS
- Eating well
- Exercising
- Getting enough sleep
- Avoiding harmful habits
- Practicing safer sex
- Recognizing symptoms of disease
- Getting regular checkups
- Avoiding injuries

EMOTIONAL WELLNESS
- Optimism
- Trust
- Self-esteem
- Self-acceptance
- Self-confidence
- Ability to understand and accept one's feelings
- Ability to share feelings with others

INTELLECTUAL WELLNESS
- Openness to new ideas
- Capacity to question
- Ability to think critically
- Motivation to master new skills
- Sense of humor
- Creativity
- Curiosity
- Lifelong learning

INTERPERSONAL WELLNESS
- Communication skills
- Capacity for intimacy
- Ability to establish and maintain satisfying relationships
- Ability to cultivate a support system of friends and family

CULTURAL WELLNESS
- Creating relationships with those who are different from you
- Maintaining and valuing your own cultural identity
- Avoiding stereotyping based on race, ethnicity, gender, religion, or sexual orientation

SPIRITUAL WELLNESS
- Capacity for love
- Compassion
- Forgiveness
- Altruism
- Joy and fulfillment
- Caring for others
- Sense of meaning and purpose
- Sense of belonging to something greater than oneself

ENVIRONMENTAL WELLNESS
- Having abundant, clean natural resources
- Having safe and healthy neighborhoods to live and work in
- Maintaining sustainable development
- Recycling whenever possible
- Reducing pollution and waste

FINANCIAL WELLNESS
- Having a basic understanding of how money works
- Living within one's means
- Avoiding debt, especially for unnecessary items
- Saving for the future and for emergencies

OCCUPATIONAL WELLNESS
- Enjoying what you do
- Feeling valued by your manager
- Building satisfying relationships with coworkers
- Taking advantage of opportunities to learn and be challenged

FIGURE 1.1 **Qualities and behaviors associated with the dimensions of wellness.** Carefully review each dimension and consider your personal wellness strengths and weaknesses.

## Dimensions of Wellness

The process of achieving wellness is continual and dynamic, involving change and growth. Figure 1.1 lists specific qualities and behaviors associated with nine dimensions of wellness.

**Physical Wellness** Your physical wellness includes not just your body's overall condition and the absence of disease but also your fitness level and your ability to care for yourself. The higher your fitness level, the higher your level of physical wellness. Similarly, as you develop the ability to take care of your own physical needs, you ensure greater physical wellness. The decisions you make now, and the habits you develop over your lifetime, will determine the length and quality of your life.

**Emotional Wellness** Trust, self-confidence, optimism, satisfying relationships, and self-esteem are some of the qualities of emotional wellness. Emotional wellness is dynamic and involves the ups and downs of living. It fluctuates with your intellectual, physical, spiritual, cultural, and interpersonal health. Maintaining emotional wellness requires exploring thoughts and feelings. *Self-acceptance* is your personal satisfaction with yourself—it might exclude society's expectations—whereas *self-esteem* relates to the way you think others perceive you; *self-confidence* can be a part of both acceptance and esteem. Achieving emotional wellness means finding solutions to emotional problems, with professional help if necessary.

**Intellectual Wellness** Those who enjoy intellectual wellness constantly challenge their minds. An active mind is essential to wellness because it detects problems and seeks solutions to questions about the self and the larger world. People with active minds often discover new things about themselves.

**Interpersonal Wellness** Satisfying and supportive relationships are important to physical and emotional wellness. Learning good communication skills, developing the capacity for intimacy, and cultivating a supportive network are all important to interpersonal (or social) wellness. Social wellness requires participating in and contributing to your community and to society.

**Cultural Wellness** Cultural wellness refers to the way you interact with others who are different from you in terms of ethnicity, religion, gender, sexual orientation, age, and customs. It involves creating relationships with others and suspending judgment of other's behavior until you have "walked in their shoes." It also includes accepting and valuing the different cultural ways people interact in the world. The extent to which you value your own and others' cultural identities is one measure of cultural wellness.

**Spiritual Wellness** To enjoy spiritual wellness is to possess a set of guiding beliefs, principles, or values that give meaning and purpose to your life, especially in difficult times. The spiritually well person focuses on the positive aspects of life and finds spirituality to be an antidote for negative feelings such as cynicism, anger, and pessimism. Organized religions help many people develop spiritual health. Religion, however, is not the only source or form of spiritual wellness. Many people find meaning and purpose in their lives through their loved ones or on their own—through nature, art, meditation, or good works.

**Environmental Wellness** Your environmental wellness is defined by the livability of your surroundings. Personal health depends on the health of the planet—from the safety of the food supply to the degree of violence in society. To improve your environmental wellness, you can learn about and protect yourself against hazards in your surroundings and work to make your world a cleaner, safer, and more beautiful place.

**Financial Wellness** Financial wellness refers to your ability to live within your means and manage your money in a way that gives you peace of mind. It includes balancing your income and expenses, staying out of debt, saving for the future, and understanding your emotions about money. See the "Financial Wellness" box.

**Occupational Wellness** Occupational wellness refers to the level of happiness and fulfillment you gain through your work. Although high salaries and prestigious titles are gratifying, they alone may not bring about occupational wellness. An occupationally well person enjoys their work, feels a connection with others in the workplace, and takes advantage of opportunities to learn and be challenged. Another important aspect of occupational wellness is recognition from managers and colleagues. An ideal job draws on your interests and passions, as well as your vocational skills, and allows you to feel that you are making a contribution in your everyday work.

## The Long and the Short of Life Expectancy

Studies suggest that our genes can determine up to 25% of the variability in life span. A genomic study found correlations among genes, behavior, and how long we might expect to live. The strongest correlations between genes and mortality are susceptibility to coronary artery disease and modifiable behaviors such as cigarette smoking.

Education helps us live longer. Consider smoking to understand the effect of education on life span. People with more education smoke less, so they have a lowered risk for lung cancer. Smoking a pack of cigarettes per day over 20 years reduces **life expectancy** by seven years. Each year spent in higher education correlates to an additional year of life.

Other factors, such as obesity and drug use, also strongly correlate to life span (Figure 1.2). Except for smoking, no other

> **TERMS**
>
> **life expectancy** The period of time a member of a given population is expected to live.

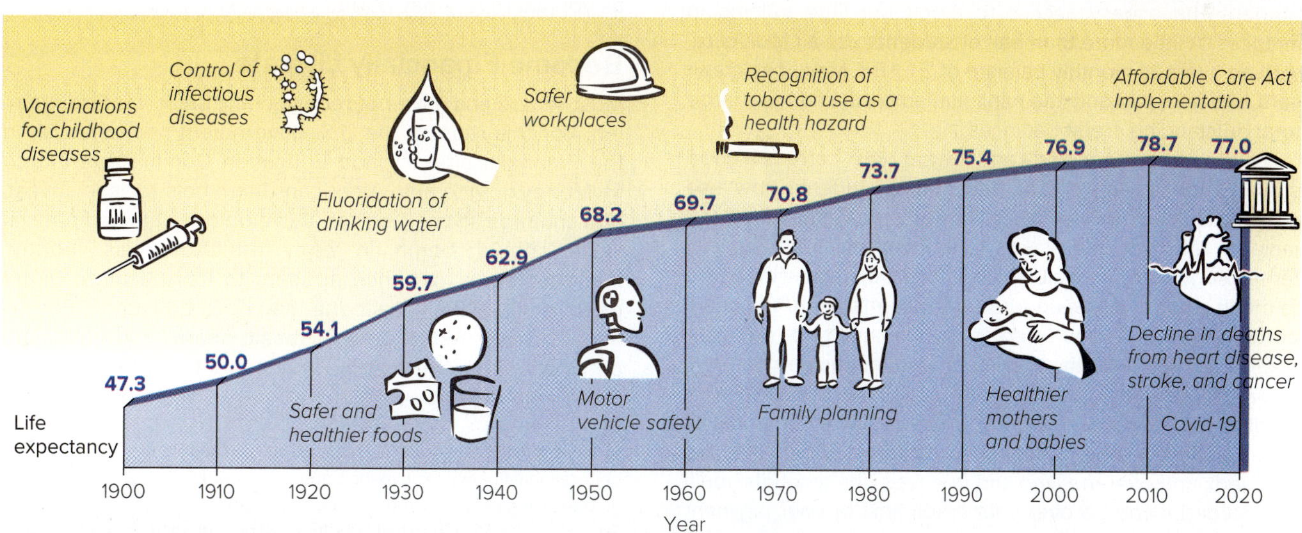


FIGURE 1.2 **Public health, life expectancy, and quality of life.** Public health achievements during the 20th century are credited with adding more than 25 years to life expectancy for Americans, greatly improving quality of life, and dramatically reducing deaths from infectious diseases. Public health improvements continue into the 21st century, including greater roadway safety and a steep decline in childhood lead poisoning. Between 2014 and 2017, U.S. life expectancy declined, likely due to the opioid and obesity epidemics. In 2020 and 2021, Covid-19 played a large role in another decline in life expectancy, the largest drop since World War II. In both those years, the disease ranked as the third leading underlying cause of death.

SOURCES: Centers for Disease Control and Prevention. 2011. "Ten great public health achievements—United States, 2001–2010." *MMWR* 60, no.19: 619–623; Centers for Disease Control and Prevention. 1999. Ten great public health achievements—United States, 1900–1999. *MMWR* 48, no.12: 241–243; Murphy S. L., et al. 2021. "Mortality in the United States, 2020." *NCHS Data Brief, no 427*. Hyattsville, MD: National Center for Health Statistics.

## TAKE CHARGE
## Financial Wellness

Many students feel less prepared to manage their money than to handle almost any other aspect of college life. Compared to a 2016 study on students' financial behaviors, an identical 2019 study reveals that fewer students reported paying bills on time, saving money, and avoiding spending money they don't have. Compared to college graduates and those who did not complete college, students were least likely to know their credit score; they also scored lower on tests about financial literacy and money management skills. *Financial wellness* means having a healthy relationship with money. Here are strategies for establishing that relationship:

### Follow a Budget

A budget is a way of tracking where your money goes and making sure you're spending it on the things that are most important to you. To start one, list your monthly income and expenditures. If you aren't sure where you spend your money, track your expenses for a few weeks or a month. Then organize them into categories, such as housing, food, transportation, entertainment, services, personal care, clothes, books and school supplies, health care, credit card and loan payments, and miscellaneous. Knowing where your money goes is the first step in gaining control of it.

Now total your income and expenditures and examine your spending patterns. Use this information to set guidelines and goals for yourself. If your expenses exceed your income, identify ways to make some cuts.

### Be Wary of Credit Cards

Students have easy access to credit but little training in finances. A little more than half of students use a credit card, with an average monthly balance of $1,183. Many pay credit card bills late, pay only the minimum amount, and have large total outstanding credit balances.

Shifting away from credit and toward debit cards is a good strategy for staying out of debt. More students now use mobile payment services like PayPal and Venmo, and the majority link their debit cards to it. Familiarity with financial terminology helps as well. Basic financial literacy with regard to credit cards involves understanding terms like *APR* (annual percentage rate—the interest you're charged on your balance), *credit limit* (the maximum amount you can borrow), *minimum monthly payment* (the smallest payment your creditor will accept each month), *grace period* (the number of days you have to pay your bill before interest or penalties are charged), and *over-the-limit* and *late fees* (the amounts you'll be charged if you go over your credit limit or your payment is late).

### Manage Your Debt

One-fifth of students with a debt are behind on their payments. When it comes to student loans, having a direct, personal plan for repayment can save time and money, reduce stress, and help you prepare for the future. However, only about 10% of students surveyed feel they have all the information needed to pay off their loans. Work with your lender and make sure you know how to access your balance, when to start repayment, how to make payments, what your repayment plan options are, and what to do if you have trouble making payments. Information on managing federal student loans is available from https://studentaid.ed.gov/sa/.

If you have credit card debt, stop using your cards and start paying them off. If you can't pay the whole balance, try to pay more than the minimum payment each month. It can take a very long time to pay off a loan by making only the minimum payments. For example, paying off a credit card balance of $2000 at 10% interest with monthly payments of $20 would take 203 months—nearly 17 years. Check out an online credit card calculator like http://money.cnn.com/calculator/pf/debt-free/. If you carry a balance and incur finance charges, you are paying back much more than your initial loan.

### Start Saving

If you start saving early, the same miracle of compound interest that locks you into years of credit card debt can work to your benefit (for an online compound interest calculator, visit http://www.interestcalc.org). Experts recommend "paying yourself first" every month—that is, putting some money into savings before you pay your bills. If you work for a company with a 401(k) retirement plan, contribute as much as you can every pay period.

### Become Financially Literate

Most Americans have not received any basic financial training. For this reason, the U.S. government has established the Financial Literacy and Education Commission (http://MyMoney.gov) to help Americans learn how to save, invest, and manage money better. Developing lifelong financial skills should begin in early adulthood, as money-management experience appears to have a more direct effect on financial knowledge than does education. For example, when tested on their basic financial literacy, students who had checking accounts had higher scores than those who did not.

SOURCES: Smith, C., and G. A. Barboza. 2013. The role of transgenerational financial knowledge and self-reported financial literacy on borrowing practices and debt accumulation of college students. Social Science Research Network (http://ssrn.com/abstract=2342168); EverFi. 2016. *Money Matters on Campus: Examining Financial Attitudes and Behaviors of Two-Year and Four-Year College Students* (www.moneymattersoncampus.org); Sallie Mae and Ipsos Public Affairs. 2019. *Majoring in Money 2019*. (https://www.salliemae.com/assets/about/who_we_are/Majoring-In-Money-Report-2019.pdf).

## TAKE CHARGE
## Life Expectancy and the Obesity Epidemic

Life expectancy consistently increased each decade in the United States since 1900 (see Figure 1.3). But the upward trend has reversed, and some researchers point to the significant increase in obesity among Americans as a potential cause. According to estimates released in 2020, about 42% of adults and 19% of children are obese. The problem isn't confined to the United States: The World Health Organization reports that at least 2.8 million people worldwide die each year due to overweight or obesity.

Along with increases in obesity come increased rates of diabetes, chronic liver disease, heart disease, stroke, and other chronic diseases that are leading causes of death. For people with obesity, an infection with Covid-19 means a greater risk of hospitalization, more severe illness, the need for intensive care and a ventilator, and death. Of course, medical interventions for these conditions have improved over time, lessening the impact of obesity to date. Still, medical treatments may be reaching their limits in preventing early deaths related to obesity. Moreover, people are becoming obese at earlier ages, exposing them to the adverse effects of excess body fat over a longer period of time.

What can be done? For an individual, body composition is influenced by a complex interplay of personal factors, including heredity, metabolic rate, hormones, age, and dietary and activity habits. But many outside forces—social, cultural, and economic—shape our behavior, and some experts recommend viewing obesity as a public health problem that requires an urgent and coordinated public health response. A response in health care technology such as gastric bypass surgery, medications, and early screening for obesity-related diseases has helped in the past, but if obesity trends persist, especially among children, average life spans may begin to decrease.

What actions might be taken? Suggestions from health promotion advocates include the following:

- Change food pricing to promote healthful options; for example, tax sugary beverages and offer incentives to farmers and food manufacturers to produce and market affordable healthy choices and smaller portion sizes.
- Limit advertising of unhealthy foods targeting children.
- Require daily physical education classes in schools.
- Fund strategies to promote physical activity by creating more walkable communities, parks, and recreational facilities.
- Train health professionals to provide nutrition and exercise counseling, and mandate health insurance coverage for treatment of obesity as a chronic condition.
- Promote the expansion of work site programs for improving diet and physical activity habits.
- Encourage increased public investment in obesity-related research.

In addition to indirectly supporting these actions, you can directly do the following:

- Analyze your own food choices, and make appropriate changes. Nutrition is discussed in detail in Chapter 10, but you can start by shifting away from consuming foods high in sugar and refined grains.
- Be more physically active. Take the stairs rather than the elevator, ride a bike instead of driving a car, and reduce your overall sedentary time.
- Educate yourself about current recommendations and areas of debate in nutrition.
- Speak out, vote, and become an advocate for healthy changes in your community.

See Chapters 10–12 for more on nutrition, exercise, and weight management.

SOURCES: Hales, C. M., et al. 2020. Prevalence of obesity and severe obesity among adults: United States, 2017–2018. NCHS Data Brief, No 360. Hyattsville, MD: National Center for Health Statistics (https://www.cdc.gov/nchs/data/databriefs/db360-h.pdf); Ludwig, D. S. 2016. Lifespan weighed down by diet. *JAMA* (published online April 4, 2016, DOI:10.1001/jama.2016.3829); Olshansky, S. J., et al. 2005. A potential decline in life expectancy in the United States in the 21st century. *New England Journal of Medicine* 352(11): 1138–1145; National Center for Health Statistics. 2016. *Health, United States, 2015: With Special Feature on Racial and Ethnic Health Disparities*. Hyattsville, MD: National Center for Health Statistics; World Health Organization. 2021. *Obesity* (https://www.who.int/news-room/facts-in-pictures/detail/6-facts-on-obesity); U.S. Department of Agriculture. 2020. *Dietary Guidelines for Americans, 2020–2025* (DietaryGuidelines.gov).

modifiable risk factor contributes more to shortening the life span than obesity. (See box "Life Expectancy and the Obesity Epidemic.")

In the United States, opioid use disorders stand out as a contributor to years of life lost, and this has been exacerbated by the pandemic. In 2020, there were about 107,600 drug-related deaths, three-quarters of which involved opioids. Alcohol-related deaths also surged during the pandemic, by 25%.

In the early 20th century, **morbidity** and **mortality rates** (rates of illness and death, respectively) from common

**TERMS**

**morbidity rate** The relative incidence of disease among a population.

**mortality rate** The number of deaths in a population in a given period; usually expressed as a ratio, such as 75 deaths per 1000 members of the population.

VITAL STATISTICS

**Table 1.1** Leading Causes of Death in the United States, 2020–2021

| RANK | CAUSE OF DEATH | NUMBER OF DEATHS | PERCENTAGE OF TOTAL DEATHS | LIFESTYLE FACTORS |
|---|---|---|---|---|
| 1 | Heart disease | 693,021* | 20.0 | D I S A O |
| 2 | Malignant neoplasms (cancer) | 604,553* | 17.5 | D I S A O |
| 3 | Covid-19 | 415,399* | 13.3 | D I S A O |
| 4 | Unintentional injuries (accidents) | 219,487* | 6.4 | I S A |
| 5 | Cerebrovascular diseases (stroke) | 160,264 | 4.7 | D I S A O |
| 6 | Chronic lower respiratory diseases | 152,657 | 4.5 | S O |
| 7 | Alzheimer's disease | 134,242 | 4.0 | |
| 8 | Diabetes mellitus | 102,188 | 3.0 | D I S O |
| 9 | Chronic liver disease and cirrhosis | 56,408* | 1.6 | A O |
| 10 | Kidney disease | 52,547 | 1.6 | S O |
| 11 | Influenza and pneumonia | 41,835* | 1.2 | D I S A |
| 12 | Intentional self-harm (suicide) | 45,979 | 1.4 | A |
| 13 | Hypertension (high blood pressure) | 41,907 | 1.2 | D I S A O |
| 14 | Parkinson's disease | 40,284 | 1.2 | |
| 15 | Septicemia (systemic blood infection) | 40,050 | 1.2 | A |
| | All other causes | 573,841 | 17.0 | |
| | All causes | 3,383,729 | 100.0 | |

**Key**
D Diet plays a part.
I Inactive lifestyle plays a part.
S Smoking plays a part.
A Excessive alcohol use plays a part.
O Obesity is a contributing factor.

NOTE: *Asterisked numbers represent 2021 data; corresponding percentages represent number of deaths from particular cause out of total 2021 deaths (3,458,697).

SOURCES: Murphy, S. L., et al. 2021. Mortality in the United States, 2020. *NCHS Data Brief* 427. Hyattsville, MD: National Center for Health Statistics. (https://dx.doi.org/10.15620/cdc:112079); Ahmad, F. B., J. A. Cisewski, and R. N. Anderson. 2022. Provisional Mortality Data–United States, 2021. *Morbidity and Mortality Weekly Report* 71: 597–600.

**infectious diseases** (e.g., pneumonia, tuberculosis, and diarrhea) were much higher than Americans experience today. By 1980, life expectancy had nearly doubled, due largely to the development of vaccines and antibiotics to fight infections and to public health measures such as water purification and sewage treatment to improve living conditions. In 2020, Covid-19 contributed to an almost 17% increase in the national death rate; in other words, there were half a million more deaths in 2020 than in 2019. The major difference between life span (how long we live) and **health span** (how long we stay healthy) is freedom from chronic or disabling disease.

The good news is that people also have some control over whether they develop **chronic diseases.** Table 1.1 and Figure 1.3 both show **lifestyle choices** that most affect the length and the quality of our lives. The need to make good choices is especially

**TERMS**

**infectious disease** A disease that can spread from person to person, caused by microorganisms such as bacteria and viruses.

**health span** How long we stay healthy and free from chronic or disabling disease.

**chronic disease** A disease that develops and continues over a long period, such as heart disease, cancer, or diabetes.

**lifestyle choice** A conscious behavior that can increase or decrease a person's risk of disease or injury; such behaviors include smoking, exercising, and eating a healthful diet.

**Ask Yourself**

**QUESTIONS FOR CRITICAL THINKING AND REFLECTION**

How often do you feel exuberant? Vital? Joyful? What makes you feel that way? Conversely, how often do you feel downhearted, de-energized, or depressed? What makes you feel that way? Have you ever thought about how you might increase experiences of vitality and decrease experiences of discouragement?

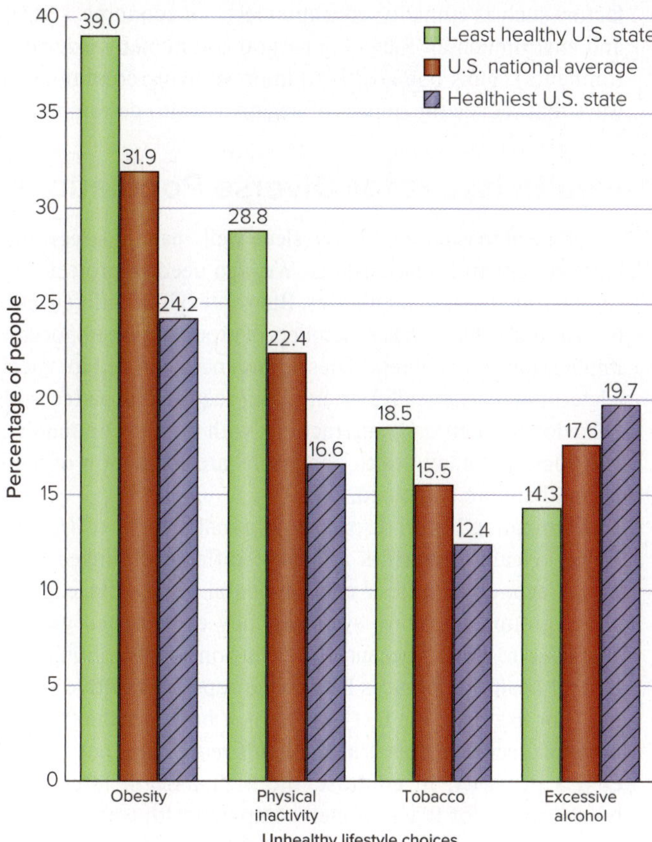


**FIGURE 1.3 Key behaviors to avoid for a longer, healthier life.** America's Health Ranking reports assess the nation's health state by state, based on factors including behaviors, public policies, access to health care, poverty, education, and environmental conditions. The poorer, less educated areas of the country also fare the worst.

**SOURCE:** United Health Foundation. 2022. *America's Health Rankings Annual Report, 2021*. (https://assets.americashealthrankings.org/app/uploads/americashealthrankings-2021annualreport.pdf)

true for teens and young adults. For Americans aged 15–24, for example, the leading cause of death is unintentional injuries (accidents), with the greatest number of deaths linked to car crashes, followed by drug overdose deaths (Table 1.2).

# PROMOTING NATIONAL HEALTH

Wellness is a personal concern, but the U.S. government has financial and humanitarian interests in it, too. A healthy population is the nation's source of vitality, creativity, and wealth. Poor health drains the nation's resources and raises health care costs for all. The primary **health promotion** strategies at the government and community levels are public health policies and agencies that identify and discourage unhealthy and high-risk behaviors and that encourage and provide incentives for positive health behaviors. At the federal level in the United States, the National Institutes of Health (NIH) and the Centers for Disease Control and Prevention (CDC) are charged with promoting the public's health. These and other agencies translate research results into interventions and communicate research findings to health care providers and the public. There are also health promotion agencies and programs at the state, community, workplace, and college levels. Take advantage of health promotion resources at all levels that are available to you.

## Health Insurance Options

The Affordable Care Act (ACA), also called "Obamacare," was signed into law on March 23, 2010. The ACA has survived over 2000 challenges in state and federal courts as well as at least 70 Republican-led votes to dismantle it in Congress.

**Finding a Plan** Under the ACA, health insurance marketplaces, also called health exchanges, facilitate the purchase of health insurance at the state level. The health exchanges provide a selection of government-regulated health care plans that students and others may choose from. Those who are below income requirements are eligible for federal help with the

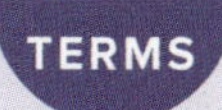


**health promotion** The process of enabling people to increase control over their health and its determinants, and thereby improve their health.

VITAL STATISTICS

**Table 1.2** Leading Causes of Death among Americans Aged 15–24, 2020

| RANK | CAUSE OF DEATH | NUMBER OF DEATHS | PERCENTAGE OF TOTAL DEATHS |
|---|---|---|---|
| 1 | Unintentional injuries (accidents): | 15,117 | 42.2 |
| | Motor vehicle | 6,741 | 44.6 (of accidents) |
| | Unintentional poisoning (drug overdose) | 6,664 | 44.1 (of accidents) |
| | All other unintentional injuries | 1,712 | 11.3 (of accidents) |
| 2 | Homicide | 6,466 | 18.1 |
| 3 | Suicide | 6,062 | 16.9 |
| 4 | Cancer | 1,306 | 3.6 |
| 5 | Heart disease | 870 | 2.4 |
| | All causes | 35,816 | 100.0 |

**SOURCE:** Centers for Disease Control and Prevention. 2021. Fatal Injury Data: Leading Causes of Death 1999–2020 (https://www.cdc.gov/injury/wisqars/index.html).

premiums. Many employers and universities also offer health insurance to their employees and students. Small businesses and members of certain associations may also be able to purchase insurance through membership in a professional group.

**Benefits to College Students** The ACA continues to permit students to stay on their parents' health insurance plans until age 26—even if they are married or have access to coverage through an employer. Students not on their parents' plans who do not want to purchase insurance through their schools can do so through a health insurance marketplace.

Young, healthy people may be tempted to buy a "catastrophic" health plan. Such plans tend to have low premiums but require you to pay all medical costs up to a certain amount, usually several thousand dollars. This can be risky if you select a plan that does not cover the ACA's 10 essential benefits. They are: preventive care, outpatient care, emergency services, hospitalization, maternity care, lab tests, mental health and substance use treatment, prescription drugs, rehabilitative services and devices, lab services, and pediatric care. It's recommended that everyone select a plan that covers all of these important types of care.

Students whose income is below a certain level may qualify for Medicaid. Check with your state. Lawfully present immigrants, which includes those with worker visas and student visas, qualify for insurance coverage through the exchanges. You can browse plans and apply for coverage at HealthCare.gov.

## The Healthy People Initiative

The national Healthy People initiative aims to prevent disease and improve Americans' quality of life. *Healthy People* reports, published each decade since 1980, set national health goals based on 10-year agendas. *Healthy People 2030* proposes the eventual achievement of the following broad national health objectives:

- Eliminate preventable disease, disability, injury, and premature death.
- Achieve health equity, eliminate disparities, and improve health literacy.
- Create social, economic, and physical environments that promote good health for all.
- Promote healthy development and healthy behaviors across every stage of life.
- Engage leadership and the public to design effective health policies.

This continues a trend set by *Healthy People 2020*. Both emphasize the importance of health determinants—factors that affect the health of individuals, demographic groups, or entire populations. Health determinants are social (including factors such as ethnicity, education level, or economic status) and environmental (including natural and human-made environments). Thus one goal is to improve living conditions in ways that reduce the impact of negative health determinants.

**TERMS**

**health disparity** A health difference linked to social, economic, or environmental disadvantage that adversely affects a group of people.

## Health Issues for Diverse Populations

We all need to exercise, eat and sleep well, manage stress, and cultivate positive relationships. We also need to protect ourselves from disease and injuries. But some of our differences—both as individuals and as members of groups—have important implications for wellness. These differences can be biological (determined genetically) or cultural (acquired as patterns of behavior through daily interactions with family, community, and society); many health conditions are a function of biology and culture combined.

Eliminating health disparities is a major focus of *Healthy People*. **Health disparities** are those differences linked with social, economic, and/or environmental disadvantage. They affect groups who have systematically experienced greater obstacles to health because of exclusion or discrimination. Not all health differences between groups are health disparities. For example, the fact that women have a higher rate of breast cancer than men is a health *difference* but is not considered a disparity. In contrast, the higher death rates from breast cancer for Black women compared with white women is considered a health disparity. Health disparities especially came to light during the Covid-19 pandemic.

**Sex and Gender** *Sex* refers to the biological and physiological characteristics that define male, female, and intersex people. In contrast, *gender* encompasses how people identify themselves and also the roles, behaviors, activities, and attributes that a given society considers appropriate for them. Examples of gender-related characteristics that affect wellness include the higher rates of smoking and drinking found among men and the lower earnings found among women (compared with men doing similar work). Transgender people have higher rates of drinking and smoking, are more likely to experience violent crime, and are less likely to use health care services.

Although men are more biologically likely than women to suffer from certain diseases (a sex issue), men are less likely to visit their physicians for regular exams (a gender issue). Men have higher rates of death from injuries, suicide, and homicide, whereas women are at greater risk for Alzheimer's disease and depression. On average, men and women also differ in body composition and certain aspects of physical performance.

**Race and Ethnicity** Among America's racial and ethnic groups, striking disparities exist in health status, access to and quality of health care, and life expectancy. However, measuring the relationships between ethnic or racial backgrounds and health issues is complicated for several reasons. First, separating the effects of race and ethnicity from socioeconomic status is difficult. In some studies, controlling for social conditions reduces health disparities. For example, a study from the Exploring Health Disparities in Integrated Communities project found that in a racially integrated community where Blacks and whites had the same earnings, disparities were eliminated or reduced in the areas of hypertension, female obesity, and diabetes.

In other studies, even when patients shared equal status in terms of education and income, insurance coverage, and clinical need, disparities in care persisted. For example, compared with whites, Blacks and Hispanics are less likely to get appropriate medication for heart conditions or to have coronary artery bypass surgery; they are also less likely to receive kidney transplants or dialysis.

Second, the classification of race (a social construct) itself is complex (see the box "Can Racial Categories Be Used in Medicine?"). Despite these limitations, it is still useful to identify and track health risks among population groups. Some diseases are concentrated in certain gene pools, the result of each ethnic group's relatively distinct history. In addition to such genetic differences, many sociocultural differences occur along ethnic lines. Traditional diets; the fabric of family and interpersonal relationships; attitudes toward tobacco, alcohol, and other drugs; and health beliefs and practices are factors that may have ethnic components, and all have implications for wellness.

In tracking health status, the federal government collects data on what it defines as five race groups (African American/Black, American Indian or Alaska Native, Asian American, Native Hawaiian or Other Pacific Islander, and European American/white) as well as two categories of ethnicity (Hispanic or Latino; not Hispanic or Latino); Hispanics may identify as being of any race group.

- ***African Americans*** have the same leading causes of death as the general population, but they have a higher infant mortality rate and lower rates of suicide and osteoporosis. Health issues of special concern for African Americans include high blood pressure, stroke, diabetes, asthma, and obesity. African American men are at significantly higher risk of prostate cancer than men in other groups.

- ***American Indians and Alaska Natives*** typically embrace a tribal identity, such as Sioux, Navaho, or Hopi. American Indians and Alaska Natives have lower death rates from heart disease, stroke, and cancer than the general population, but they have higher rates of early death from causes linked to smoking and alcohol use, including injuries and cirrhosis. Diabetes is a special concern for many groups.

- ***Asian Americans*** include people who trace their ancestry to countries in the Far East, Southeast Asia, or the Indian subcontinent. Asian Americans have lower rates of coronary heart disease and obesity. However, health differences exist among these groups. For example, Southeast Asian American men have higher rates of smoking and lung cancer, and Vietnamese American women have higher rates of cervical cancer.

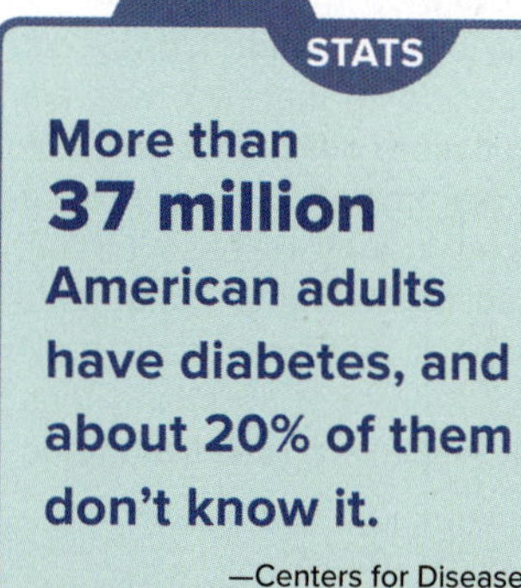
QUICK STATS

**More than 37 million American adults have diabetes, and about 20% of them don't know it.**

—Centers for Disease Control and Prevention, 2021

- ***Native Hawaiian and Other Pacific Islander Americans*** trace their ancestry to the original peoples of Hawaii, Guam, Samoa, and other Pacific Islands. Pacific Islander Americans have a higher overall death rate than the general population and higher rates of diabetes and asthma. Smoking and obesity are special concerns for this group.

- ***Latinos*** are a diverse group, with roots in Mexico, Puerto Rico, Cuba, and South and Central America. Many Latinos are of mixed Spanish and American Indian descent or of mixed Spanish, Indian, and African American descent. Latinos on average have lower rates of heart disease, cancer, and suicide than the general population; areas of concern include gallbladder disease, obesity, diabetes, and lack of health insurance.

Poverty and low educational attainment are key factors underlying ethnic health disparities, but they do not fully account for the differences. Access to appropriate health care can be a challenge. Nonwhite racial and ethnic groups, regardless of income, are more likely to live in areas that are medically underserved, with fewer sources of high-quality or specialist care. Language and cultural barriers, environmental health, and racism and discrimination can also prevent people from receiving appropriate health services.

**Income and Education** Income and education are closely related. Groups with the highest poverty rates and the least education have the worst health status. They have higher rates of infant mortality, traumatic injury, violent death, and many diseases, including heart disease, diabetes, tuberculosis, HIV infection, and some cancers. They are also more likely to lack proper nutrition, experience overweight, smoke, drink, and misuse drugs. And to complicate and magnify all these factors, they are also exposed to more day-to-day stressors and have less access to health care services. Researchers estimate that about 250,000 deaths per year can be attributed to low educational attainment, 175,000 to individual and community poverty, and 120,000 to income inequality.

**Disability** People with disabilities have activity limitations or need assistance due to a physical or mental impairment. About one in four people in the United States has some level of disability, and the rate is rising, especially among younger segments of the population. People with disabilities are more likely to have obesity, heart disease, diabetes, and to smoke. Many also lack access to health care services.

**Geographic Location** About one in four Americans currently lives in a rural area—a place with fewer than 10,000 residents. People living in rural areas are less likely to be physically active, use seat belts, or obtain screening tests for preventive health care. They have less access to timely emergency services and much higher rates of some diseases and injury-related deaths than people living in urban areas. They are also more likely to lack health insurance.

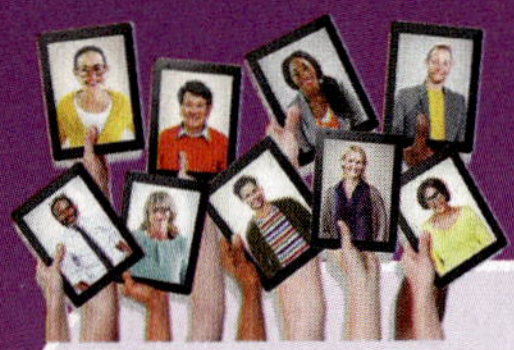

## DIVERSITY MATTERS
# Can Racial Categories Be Used in Medicine?

As you read, pay attention to the terms and statistics. Terms often take shortcuts to refer to complicated situations or groups of people who can't all fit neatly under one name. For example, in the United States, "Black" can refer to two people from opposite ends of the earth with very different genetic profiles; they can have fewer genes in common than with a person designated "white." In Brazil, what people call themselves can change in a day: if the person next to you is darker, you might call yourself "white;" if lighter, you might identify as "Brown" or "Black."

We have entered an age where terms keep evolving and consensus around them is waning. For example, *Latinx* is a term that allows for not having to specify gender. But critics note that the word seems to be used mostly in academic settings, and that, linguistically and culturally, *Latinx* feels unnatural for many Spanish and Portuguese speakers. Similarly, many Native peoples take offense at the label *Indians*, but others say they prefer it.

Remember that American ideas of race stem from 18th-century European scientific and religious classifications that presupposed fixed and unblended races. But race is not fixed. It does not represent a set of genes that matches those of every other member of that race. We are a species that moves around and mingles our genes. There is no neat line to draw around people of one color. Humans come in a wide variety of hues, which a single color term cannot capture.

Nor can we classify people based on a single feature. When we consider one feature of *phenotype* (for example, of skin color, a visible trait), we see that not everyone who shares that feature also shares others, such as hair or nose type.

## What Categories Can Reveal

If our racial categories are not based much in biology, they still point to social divisions that have very real effects. For example, the people most vulnerable to disease are typically the ones with fewer resources—less wealth, less access to health care, and less control over where they live. By April 2020, a racial breakdown of Covid-19 cases and deaths showed that in addition to older people, non-Euro ethnic groups were disproportionately affected. When race was reported, 34% of cases involved Black and African Americans, although they make up only 13% of the total population. They also were far more likely to be hospitalized, and they died at higher rates.

We can also classify people by genetic traits that cause hereditary conditions and disorders. For example, the gene mutation that causes Tay-Sachs disease is commonly found in Eastern European Jews, Southern Louisiana Cajuns, and French Canadians. Genetic counselors can provide culturally relevant care by asking clients about racial and ethnic identity to identify Tay-Sachs risk.

In other situations, it might make sense to group people by blood type—A, B, AB, or O. In the case of a blood transfusion, only a person with type AB positive can receive all blood types. For everyone else, receiving a noncompatible blood type has a much greater biological impact than getting blood from someone with a different skin color.

## How Far We Have Come and Still Need to Go

Early Western medical research was performed mostly by Euro-American, heterosexual males on Euro-American, heterosexual males. Now the medical community has recognized that some of this information may not help people outside those categories. For example, the National Kidney Foundation recently dropped race from its algorithm for diagnosing chronic kidney disease after concluding that race was actually making it more difficult for Black people to be diagnosed. Because a certain marker in kidney disease (creatinine) was statistically higher in adults identified as Black, a different scale had been used for them. But assuming that they did not need referrals, treatment, and transplants as early as other people meant that many cases went egregiously undiagnosed and untreated.

Many statistical breakdowns by race and gender continue to use simplified categories. Some studies allow for self-reported race but don't offer a full range of categories; in some studies, race is determined only by the researchers conducting them. Ancestry is continuous, not a fixed category. Consequently, someone identifying as "Black" may have only 30% African ancestry.

Keep in mind that health information about groups of people is based on generalizations. Not everyone fits into these crude categories. However, using general groupings can allow further and more detailed investigations. As social categories, statistical breakdowns by race point to inequalities and inconsistencies within our health care system (and society). Reporting on this information is therefore useful for bringing about change: We could change how doctors treat patients and how patients understand resources available to them. We could provide easier access and more resources to people not getting them; we could help all people, no matter their community, get the education and support needed to make healthy lifestyle choices.

SOURCES: Torregrosa, L. L. 2021. Many Latinos say 'Latinx' offends or bothers them. *NBC News Think*, December 21; Mukhopadhyay, C., R. Henze, and Y. T. Moses. 2014. *How Real Is Race? A Sourcebook on Race, Culture, and Biology*, 2nd ed. Lanham, MD: AltaMira Press; Delgado, C., et al. 2021. Reassessing the inclusion of race in diagnosing kidney diseases: An interim report from the NKF-ASN Task Force. *American Journal of Kidney Disease* 78(1): 103–115; Artiga, S., et al. 2020. Growing data underscore that communities of color are being harder hit by COVID-19. *Kaiser Family Foundation,* 21 April; Kottak, C. P. 2022. *Anthropology: Appreciating Human Diversity*, 19th ed. New York: McGraw Hill; Centers for Disease Control and Prevention. 2022. Distribution of COVID-19 deaths and populations, by jurisdiction, age, and race and Hispanic origin.

## WELLNESS ON CAMPUS
### Wellness Matters for College Students

Most college students, in their late teens and early twenties, appear to be healthy. But appearances can be deceiving. Each year, thousands of students lose productive academic time to physical and emotional health problems—some of which can continue to plague them for life.

The following table shows the top health issues affecting students' academic performance, according to the Fall 2021 American College Health Association–National College Health Assessment III.

**Percentage of Students by Gender**

| CHALLENGES IN THE PAST 12 MONTHS | CIS MEN | CIS WOMEN | TRANS/GENDER NONCONFORMING |
|---|---|---|---|
| Procrastination | 46.0 | 48.3 | 61.6 |
| Finances | 13.5 | 14.8 | 21.1 |
| Family | 7.6 | 11.7 | 19.8 |
| Career | 13.3 | 13.5 | 18.9 |
| Health of someone close to me | 7.9 | 11.5 | 15.0 |
| Intimate relationships | 10.3 | 11.3 | 14.4 |
| Physical appearance | 4.5 | 6.7 | 13.3 |
| Death of a family member, friend, or someone close to me | 7.7 | 11.0 | 12.3 |
| Faculty | 6.4 | 6.6 | 11.0 |
| Roommate/housemate | 4.2 | 6.3 | 10.1 |

Although the reporting agency has gathered information about survey respondents' gender identity for 12 years, only now is the survey including it in the findings. This decision reflects a growing number of students identifying as transgender or gender nonconforming, and the realization that some significant health disparities exist between them and their cisgender peers.

Although some troubles—such as the death of a friend or family member—cannot be controlled, students can moderate their physical and emotional impact by choosing healthy behaviors. For example, there are many ways to manage procrastination, the top health challenge affecting students (see Chapter 2). By reducing unhealthy choices (such as using alcohol to relax) and by increasing healthy choices (such as using time management and relaxation techniques), students can reduce the impact of procrastination stress on their lives.

The survey also estimated that, based on students' reporting of their height and weight, over 22% of college students are overweight and 14.3% are obese.

Although students may not see (or feel) the effects of their dietary habits today, the long-term health risks are significant. Overweight and obese persons run a higher-than-normal risk of developing diabetes, heart disease, and cancer later in life. Overeating, choosing unhealthy, processed foods, and staying sedentary are behaviors we can do something about. Still, the first step toward weight loss and overall health improvement is to value and appreciate our bodies, no matter the size and shape. Seeking a counselor or partner in wellness can help us find the right customized path.

#### Other Choices, Other Problems

Other health issues reported in the 2021 National College Health Assessment III include the following:

- Only 41% of students reported that they used a condom during vaginal intercourse in the past 30 days.
- About 11% of students had seven or more drinks the last time they partied.
- Almost 8% of students had smoked cigarettes at least once during the past 3 months; 14% used an e-cigarette; and 23% used marijuana.

What choices do you make in these situations? Remember: It's never too late to change. The sooner you trade an unhealthy behavior for a healthy one, the longer you'll be around to enjoy the benefits.

SOURCE: American College Health Association. 2022. *American College Health Association–National College Health Assessment III: Reference Group Executive Summary Fall 2021*. Hanover, MD: American College Health Association (https://www.acha.org/documents/ncha/NCHA-III_FALL_2021_REFERENCE_GROUP_EXECUTIVE_SUMMARY.pdf).

Children living in dangerous neighborhoods—rural or urban—are less likely to play outside and are four times more likely to be overweight than children living in safer areas.

**Sexual Orientation and Gender Identity** Lesbian, gay, bisexual, and transgender (LGBT) health was added as a new topic area in *Healthy People 2020*. Questions about sexual orientation and gender identity have not been included in many health surveys, making it difficult to estimate the number of LGBT people and to identify their special health needs. However, research suggests that LGBT individuals may face health disparities due to discrimination and denial of their civil and human rights. LGBT youth have high rates of tobacco, alcohol, and other drug misuse as well as an elevated risk of suicide; they are more likely to be homeless and are less likely to have health insurance and access to appropriate health care providers and services.

## FACTORS THAT INFLUENCE WELLNESS

Optimal health and wellness come mostly from a healthy lifestyle—patterns of behavior that promote and support your health and promote wellness now and as you get older. In the pages that follow, you'll find current information and suggestions you can use to build a healthier lifestyle; also, see the "Wellness Matters for College Students" box.

Our behavior, family health history, environment, and access to health care are all important influences on wellness. These factors, which vary for both individuals and groups, can interact in ways that produce either health or disease.

## Health Habits

Research continually reveals new connections between our habits and health. For example, heart disease is associated with smoking, stress, a hostile attitude, a poor diet, and being sedentary. Poor health habits take hold before many Americans reach adulthood.

Other habits, however, are beneficial. Regular exercise can help prevent heart disease, high blood pressure, diabetes, osteoporosis, and depression. Exercise can also reduce the risk of colon cancer, stroke, and back injury. A balanced and varied diet helps prevent many chronic diseases. As we learn more about how our actions affect our bodies and minds, we can make informed choices for a healthier life.

## Genetics/Family History

Your **genome** consists of the complete set of genetic material in your cells—about 25,000 genes, half from each of your parents. **Genes** control the production of proteins that serve both as the structural material for your body and as the regulators of all your body's chemical reactions and metabolic processes. The human genome varies only slightly from person to person, and many of these differences do not affect health. However, some differences have important implications for health, and knowing your family's health history can help you determine which conditions may be of special concern for you.

Errors in our genes are responsible for about 3500 clearly hereditary conditions, including sickle-cell disease and cystic fibrosis. Altered genes also play a part in heart disease, cancer, stroke, diabetes, and many other common conditions. However, in these more common and complex disorders, genetic alterations serve only to increase an individual's risk, and the disease itself results from the interaction of many genes with other factors. An example of the power of behavior and environment can be seen in the more than 60% increase in the incidence of diabetes that has occurred among Americans since 1990. This huge increase is not due to any sudden change in our genes; it is the result of increasing rates of obesity caused by poor dietary choices and lack of physical activity.

QUICK STATS

**Death rates increased for 6 of the 10 leading causes of death in 2020, including a nearly 17% increase in deaths from accidents.**

—National Center for Health Statistics, 2022

TERMS

**genome** The complete set of genetic material in an individual's cells.

**gene** The basic unit of heredity, containing chemical instructions for producing a specific protein.

## Environment

Your environment includes substances and conditions in your home, workplace, and community. Are you frequently exposed to environmental tobacco smoke or the radiation in sunlight? Do you live in an area with high rates of crime and violence? Do you have access to nature?

Today environmental influences on wellness also include conditions in other countries and around the globe, particularly climate changes occurring as a result of global warming. The burning of fossil fuels causes not only climate change but also outdoor air pollution, which damages our hearts and lungs; a growing collection of studies is discovering how air pollution also damages our brains. The devastation and smoke caused by wildfires are also growing problems. Indoor air pollution caused by toxic gases (e.g., carbon monoxide and radon), household cleaning products, formaldehyde, and mold can also lead to serious health problems for people who are exposed. Industrial waste, including lead and cancer-causing chemicals, can leach into our water and compromise our health (see Chapter 15).

## Access to Health Care

Adequate health care helps improve both quality and quantity of life through preventive care and the treatment of disease. For example, vaccinations prevent many dangerous infections, and screening tests help identify key risk factors and diseases in their early treatable stages. As described earlier, inadequate access to health care is tied to factors such as low income, lack of health insurance, and geographic location. Cost is one of many issues surrounding the development of advanced health-related technologies.

## Personal Health Behaviors

In many cases, behavior can tip the balance toward good health, even when heredity or environment is a negative factor. For example, breast cancer can run in families, but it also may be associated with being overweight and inactive. A woman with a family history of breast cancer is less likely to develop the disease if she controls her weight, exercises regularly, and has regular mammograms to help detect the disease in its early, most treatable stage.

Similarly, a young man with a family history of obesity can maintain a normal weight by balancing calorie intake against activities that burn calories. If your life is highly stressful, you can lessen the chances of heart disease and stroke by managing and coping with stress (see Chapter 2). If you live in an area with severe air pollution, you can reduce the risk of lung disease by not smoking. You can also take an active role in improving your environment. Behaviors like these can make a difference in how great an impact heredity and environment will have on your health.

## REACHING WELLNESS THROUGH LIFESTYLE MANAGEMENT

As you consider the behaviors that contribute to wellness, you may be doing a mental comparison with your own behaviors. If you are like most young adults, you probably have some healthy habits and some habits that place your health at risk. For example, you may be physically active and have a healthful diet but spend excessive hours on your cell phone or on social media. You may be careful to wear your seat belt in your car but you haven't yet gotten a vaccine for Covid-19. Moving in the direction of wellness means cultivating healthy behaviors and working to overcome unhealthy ones. This approach to lifestyle management is called **behavior change.**

As you may already know, changing an unhealthy habit can be harder than it sounds. When you embark on a behavior change plan, it may seem like too much work at first. But as you make progress, you will gain confidence in your ability to take charge of your life. You will also experience the benefits of wellness—more energy, greater vitality, deeper feelings of appreciation and curiosity, and a higher quality of life.

**QUICK STATS**

**About 107,600 Americans died of drug overdoses in 2021, a 15% increase from the year before**

—CDC, 2022

### Getting Serious about Your Health

Before you can start changing a wellness-related behavior, you have to know that the behavior is problematic and that you *can* change it. To make good decisions, you need information about relevant topics and issues, including what resources are available to help you change.

**Examine Your Current Health Habits** How is your current lifestyle affecting your health today and in the future? Think about which of your current habits enhance your health and which detract from it. Begin your journey toward wellness with self-assessment: Talk with friends and family members about what they have noticed about your lifestyle and your health, and take the quiz in the box titled "Wellness: Evaluate Your Lifestyle." Challenge any unrealistically optimistic attitudes or ideas you may hold—for example, "To protect my health, I don't need to worry about quitting smoking until I'm 40 years old" or "Being overweight won't put *me* at risk for diabetes." Health risks are very real and can become significant while you're young; health habits are important throughout life.

Many people consider changing a behavior when friends or family members express concern, when a landmark event occurs (such as turning 30), or when new information—like receiving high cholesterol results—raises their awareness of risk. If you find yourself reevaluating some of your behaviors as you read this text, take advantage of the opportunity to make a change in a structured way.

**Choose a Target Behavior** Changing any behavior can be demanding. Start small by choosing one behavior you want to change—called a **target behavior**—and working on it until you succeed. Your chances of success will be greater if your first goal is simple, such as replacing less healthy snacks (potato chips) for healthy ones (nuts and raisins). As you change one behavior, make your next goal a little more significant, and build on your success.

**Learn about Your Target Behavior** Once you've chosen a target behavior, you need to learn its risks and benefits—both now and in the future. Ask these questions:

- How is your target behavior affecting your level of wellness today?
- Which diseases or conditions does this behavior place you at risk for?
- What effect would changing your behavior have on your health?

As a starting point, use this text and the resources listed in the "For More Information" section at the end of each chapter. See the "Evaluating Sources of Health Information" box for additional guidelines.

**Find Help** Have you identified a particularly challenging target behavior or condition—something like overuse of alcohol, binge eating, or depression—that interferes with your ability to function or places you at a serious health risk? If so, you may need help to change a behavior or address a disorder that is deeply rooted or too serious for self-management. Don't let the problem's seriousness stop you; many resources are available to help you solve it. On campus, the student health center or campus counseling center can provide assistance. To locate community resources, consult the yellow pages, your physician, or the internet.

### Building Motivation to Change

Knowledge is necessary for behavior change, but it isn't usually enough to make people act. Millions of people have sedentary lifestyles, for example, even though they know it's bad for their health. This is particularly true of young adults, who feel healthy despite their unhealthy behaviors. To succeed at behavior change, you need strong motivation. The sections that follow address some considerations.

**Examine the Pros and Cons of Change** Health behaviors have short-term and long-term benefits and costs. Consider the benefits and costs of an inactive lifestyle. In the short

**TERMS**

**behavior change** A lifestyle management process that involves cultivating healthy behaviors and working to overcome unhealthy ones.

**target behavior** An isolated behavior selected as the object for a behavior change program.

term, such a lifestyle allows you more time to watch TV, use social media, do your homework, and hang out with friends, but it leaves you less physically fit and less able to participate in recreational activities. Over the long term, it increases the risk of heart disease, cancer, stroke, and premature death.

To successfully change your behavior, you must believe that the benefits of change outweigh the costs.

Carefully examine the pros and cons of continuing your current behavior and of changing to a healthier one. Focus on the effects that are most meaningful to you, including those that are tied to your personal identity and values. For example, engaging in regular physical activity and getting adequate sleep can support an image of yourself as an active person who is a good role model for others. To complete your analysis, ask friends and family members about the effects of your behavior on them.

The short-term benefits of behavior change can be an important motivating force. Although some people are motivated by long-term goals, such as avoiding a disease that may hit them in 30 years, most are more likely to be moved to action by shorter-term, more personal goals. Feeling better, doing better in school, improving at a sport, reducing stress, and increasing self-esteem are common short-term benefits of health behavior change.

### Boost Self-Efficacy

A big factor in your eventual success is whether you feel confident in your ability to change. **Self-efficacy** refers to your belief in your ability to successfully take action and perform a specific task. Strategies for boosting self-efficacy include developing an internal locus of control, using visualization and self-talk, and getting encouragement from supportive people.

**LOCUS OF CONTROL** Who do you believe is controlling your life? Is it your parents, friends, or school? Is it "fate"? Or is it you? **Locus of control** refers to the extent to which we believe we have control over the events in our lives. People who believe they are in control of their lives are said to have an *internal locus of control.* Those who believe that factors beyond their control determine the course of their lives are said to have an *external locus of control.*

For lifestyle management, an internal locus of control is an advantage because it reinforces motivation and commitment. An external locus of control can sabotage efforts to change behavior. For example, if you believe that you are destined to die of breast cancer because your mother died from the disease, you may view regular screening mammograms as a waste of time. In contrast, if you believe that you can take action to reduce your risk of breast cancer despite hereditary factors, you will be motivated to follow guidelines for early detection of the disease.

If you find yourself attributing too much influence to outside forces, gather more information about your wellness-related behaviors. List all the ways that making lifestyle changes will improve your health. If you believe you'll succeed, and if you recognize that you are in charge of your life, you're on your way to wellness.

**VISUALIZATION AND SELF-TALK** One of the best ways to boost your confidence and self-efficacy is to visualize yourself successfully engaging in a new, healthier behavior. Imagine yourself going for an afternoon run three days a week or no longer smoking cigarettes. Also visualize yourself enjoying all the short-term and long-term benefits that your lifestyle change will bring.

You can also use *self-talk,* the internal dialogue you carry on with yourself, to increase your confidence in your ability to change. Counter any self-defeating patterns of thought with more positive or realistic thoughts: "I am a strong, capable person, and I can maintain my commitment to change."

**ROLE MODELS AND SUPPORTIVE PEOPLE** Social support can make a big difference in your level of motivation and your chances of success. Perhaps you know people who have reached the goal you are striving for. They could be role models or mentors for you, providing information and support for your efforts. Gain strength from their experiences, and tell yourself, "If they can do it, so can I." Find a partner who wants to make the same changes you do and who can take an active role in your behavior change program. For example, an exercise partner can provide companionship and encouragement when you might be tempted to skip your workout.

### Identify and Overcome Barriers to Change

Don't let past failures at behavior change discourage you. They can be a great source of information you can use to boost your chances of future success. Make a list of the problems and challenges you faced in any previous behavior change attempts. To this, add the short-term costs of behavior change that you identified in your analysis of the pros and cons of change. Once you've listed these key barriers to change, develop a practical plan for overcoming each one. For example, if you are not getting enough sleep when you're with certain friends, decide in advance how you will turn down their next late-night invitation.

**TERMS**

**self-efficacy** The belief in your ability to take action and perform a specific task.

**locus of control** The extent to which a person believes they have control over the events in their life.

## Enhancing Your Readiness to Change

The transtheoretical, or "stages of change," model has been shown to be an effective approach to lifestyle self-management. According to this model, you move through distinct stages of action as you achieve your target behavior. First, determine your target behavior, the final stage where your goals are accomplished; then determine what stage you are in now so that you can choose appropriate strategies to progress through the cycle of change. This will help you enhance your readiness and intention to change. Read the following sections to determine what stage you are in. Let's use exercise as an example of changing sedentary behavior to active, engaging behavior.

## CRITICAL CONSUMER
### Evaluating Sources of Health Information

Surveys indicate that college students are smart about evaluating health information. They trust the health information they receive from health professionals and educators and are skeptical about popular information sources, such as magazine articles and websites.

How good are you at evaluating health information? Here are some tips.

#### General Strategies

Whenever you encounter health-related information, take the following steps to make sure it is credible:

- ***Go to the original source.*** Media reports often simplify the results of medical research. Find out for yourself what a study really reported, and determine whether it was based on good science. What type of study was it? Was it published in a recognized medical journal? Was it an animal study, or did it involve people? Did the study include a large number of people? What did the authors of the study actually report?
- ***Watch for misleading language.*** Reports that tout "breakthroughs" or "dramatic proof" are probably hype. A study may state that a behavior "contributes to" or is "associated with" an outcome; this does not prove a cause-and-effect relationship.
- ***Distinguish between research reports and public health advice.*** Do not change your behavior based on the results of a single report or study. If an agency such as the National Cancer Institute urges a behavior change, however, follow its advice. Large, publicly funded organizations issue such advice based on many studies, not a single report.
- ***Remember that anecdotes are not facts.*** A friend may tell you he lost weight on some new diet, but individual success stories do not mean the plan is truly safe or effective. Check with your physician before making any serious lifestyle changes.
- ***Be skeptical.*** If a report seems too good to be true, it probably is. Be wary of information contained in advertisements. An ad's goal is to sell a product, even if there is no need for it.
- ***Make choices that are right for you.*** Friends and family members can be a great source of ideas and inspiration, but you need to make health-related choices that work best for you.

#### Internet Resources

Online sources pose special challenges; when reviewing a health-related website, ask these questions:

- ***What is the source of the information?*** Websites maintained by government agencies, professional associations, or established academic or medical institutions are likely to present trustworthy information. Many other groups and individuals post accurate information, but it is important to look at the qualifications of the people who are behind the site. (Check the home page or click the "About Us" link.)
- ***How often is the site updated?*** Look for sites that are updated frequently. Check the "last modified" date of any web page.
- ***Is the site promotional?*** Be wary of information from sites that sell specific products, use testimonials as evidence, appear to have a social or political agenda, or ask for money.
- ***What do other sources say about a topic?*** Be cautious of claims or information that appear at only one site or come from a chat room, bulletin board, newsgroup, or blog.
- ***Does the site conform to any set of guidelines or criteria for quality and accuracy?*** Look for sites that identify themselves as conforming to some code or set of principles, such as those established by the Health on the Net Foundation or the American Medical Association. These codes include criteria such as use of information from respected sources and disclosure of the site's sponsors.

**Precontemplation** At this stage, you think you have no problem and don't intend to change your behavior. Your friends have commented that you should exercise more, but you are resistant. You have tried to exercise in the past and now think your situation is hopeless. You are unaware of risks associated with being sedentary, and you also blame external factors like other people for your condition. You believe that there are more important reasons *not* to change than there are reasons to change.

To move forward in this stage, try raising your awareness. *Research* the importance of exercise, for example. Look up articles, websites, and other resources that address the issue. How does exercise affect the body and mind? *Look also at the mechanisms you use to resist change,* such as denial or rationalization. Find ways to counteract these mechanisms of resistance.

*Seek social support.* Friends and family members can help you identify target behaviors (e.g., fitting exercise into your time schedule or encouraging you while you work out). *Other resources* might include exercise classes or stress management workshops offered by your school.

**Contemplation** You now know you have a problem and within six months intend to do something about it, such as join a gym or take an exercise class. You realize that getting more exercise will help decrease your stress level. You acknowledge the benefits of behavior change but are also aware that the barriers to change may be difficult to overcome. You consider possible courses of action but don't know how to proceed.

To take charge, start by *keeping a journal.* Record what you have done so far and include your plan of action. *Do a cost-benefit analysis:* Identify the costs (e.g., it will cost money to take an exercise class) and benefits (e.g., I will probably stick to my goal if someone else is guiding me through the exercise). *Identify barriers to change* (e.g., I hate getting sweaty when I have no opportunity to shower). Knowing these obstacles can help you overcome them. Next, *engage your emotions.* Imagine what your life will be like if you don't change.

Other ways to move forward in the contemplation stage include *creating a new self-image* and thinking before you act. *Imagine what you'll be like* after changing your unhealthy behavior. Try to think of yourself in those new terms right now. *Learn why you engage in the unhealthy behavior.* Determine what "sets you off" and train yourself not to act reflexively.

**Preparation** You plan to take action within a month, or you may already have begun to make small changes in your behavior, like taking the stairs instead of the elevator. You may have discovered a place to go jogging but have not yet gone regularly or consistently.

*Work on creating a plan.* Include a start date, goals, rewards, and specific steps you will take to change your behavior. *Make change a priority.* Create and sign a contract with yourself. *Practice visualization and self-talk.* Say, "I see myself jogging three times a week and going to yoga on Fridays." "I know I can do it because I've met challenging goals before." *Take small steps.* Successfully practicing your new behavior for a short time—even a single day—can boost your confidence and motivation.

**Action** You outwardly modify your behavior and your environment. Maybe you start riding your bike to school or work. You put your stationary bicycle in front of the TV, and you leave your yoga mat out on your bedroom floor. The action stage requires the greatest commitment of time and energy, and people in this stage are at risk of relapsing into old, unhealthy patterns of behavior. *Monitor your progress.* Keep up with your journal entries. *Make changes* that will discourage the unwanted behavior—for example, park your car farther from your house or closer to the stairs. *Find alternatives* to your old behavior. Make a list of things you can do to replace the behavior.

*Reward yourself.* Rewards should be identified in your change plan. *Praise yourself* and focus on your success. *Involve your friends.* Tell them you want to change, and ask for their help. Don't get discouraged. Real change is difficult.

**Maintenance** You have maintained your new, healthier lifestyle for at least six months by working out and riding your bike. Lapses have occurred, but you have been successful in quickly reestablishing the desired behavior. The maintenance stage can last months or years.

*Keep going.* Continue using the positive strategies that worked in earlier stages. And *be prepared for lapses.* If you find yourself skipping exercise class, don't give up on the whole project. Try inviting a friend to join you and then keep the date. *Be a role model.* Once you successfully change your behavior, you may be able to help someone do the same thing.

**Termination** For some behaviors, you may reach the sixth and final stage of termination. At this stage, you have exited the cycle of change and are no longer tempted to lapse back into your old behavior. You have a new self-image and total control with regard to your target behavior.

## Dealing with Relapse

People seldom progress through the stages of change in a straightforward, linear way. Rather, they tend to move to a certain stage and then slip back to a previous stage before resuming their forward progress. Research suggests that most people make several attempts before they successfully change a behavior, and four out of five people experience some degree of backsliding. For this reason, the stages of change are best conceptualized as a spiral in which people cycle back through previous stages but are farther along in the process each time they renew their commitment (Figure 1.4).

If you experience a lapse (a single slip) or a relapse (a return to old habits), don't give up. Relapse can be demoralizing, but it is not the same as failure; failure means stopping before you reach your goal and never changing your target behavior. During the early stages of the change process, it's a good idea to plan for relapse so that you can avoid guilt and self-blame and get back on track quickly. Forgive yourself for

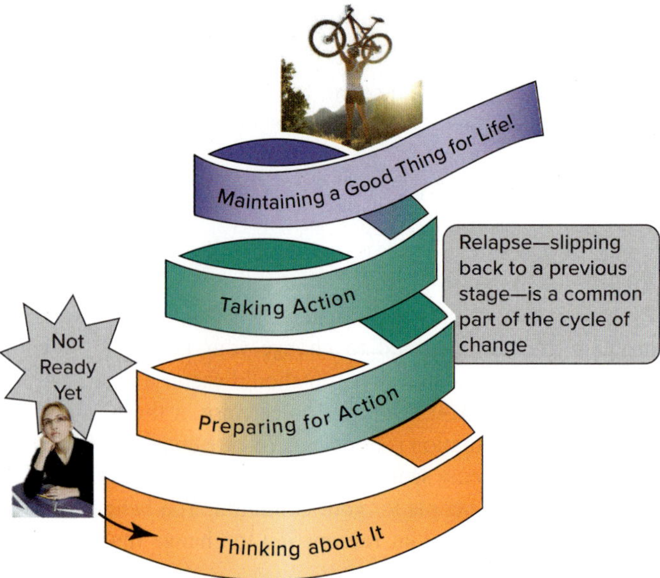


**FIGURE 1.4 The stages of change: A spiral model.**

SOURCE: Adapted from Centers for Disease Control and Prevention. n.d. *PEP Guide: Personal Empowerment Plan for Improving Eating and Increasing Physical Activity.* Dallas, TX: The Cooper Institute. Bottom left: Glow Images; Top right: UpperCut Images/Alamy Stock Photo

the slip, give yourself credit for the progress you have already made, and move on.

If relapses keep occurring or you can't seem to control them, you may need to return to a previous stage of the behavior change process. If this is necessary, reevaluate your goals and strategy. A different or less stressful approach may help you avoid setbacks when you try again.

## Developing Skills for Change: Creating a Personalized Plan

Once you are committed to making a change, put together a plan of action. Your key to success is a well-thought-out plan that sets goals, anticipates problems, and includes rewards.

**1. Monitor Your Behavior and Gather Data** Keep a record of your target behavior and the circumstances surrounding it. Record this information for at least a week or two. Keep your notes in a health journal or notebook or on your computer (see the sample journal entries in Figure 1.5). Record each occurrence of your behavior, noting what the activity was, when and where it happened, what you were doing, and how you felt at that time.

Tracking your activities will help, for example, if your goal is to start an exercise program, and you want to determine how to make time for workouts.

**2. Analyze the Data and Identify Patterns** After you have collected data on the behavior, analyze the data to identify patterns. When are you most likely to overeat? To skip a meal? What events trigger your appetite? Perhaps you are especially hungry at midmorning or when you put off eating dinner until 9:00. Perhaps you overindulge in food and drink when you go to a particular restaurant or when you're with certain friends. Note the connections between your feelings and such external cues as time of day, location, situation, and the actions of others around you.

**3. Be "SMART" about Setting Goals** If your goals are too challenging, you will have trouble making steady progress and will be more likely to give up altogether. If, for example, you are in poor physical condition, it will not make sense to set a goal of being ready to run a marathon within two months. If you set goals you can live with, it will be easier to stick with your behavior change plan and be successful.

Experts suggest that your goals meet the "SMART" criteria; that is, your behavior change goals should be

- ***Specific.*** Avoid vague goals like "eat more fruits and vegetables." Instead use specific terms, such as "eat two cups of fruit and three cups of vegetables every day."

- ***Measurable.*** Your progress will be easier to track if your goals are quantifiable, so give your goal a number. You might measure your goal in terms of time ("walk briskly for 20 minutes a day"), distance ("run two miles, three days per week"), or some other amount ("drink eight glasses of water every day").

- ***Attainable.*** Set goals that are within your physical limits. For example, if you are a poor swimmer, you might not be able to meet a short-term fitness goal by swimming laps. Walking or biking might be better options.

- ***Realistic.*** Manage your expectations when you set goals. For example, a long-time smoker may not be able to quit cold turkey. A more realistic approach might be to use nicotine replacement patches or gum for several weeks while getting help from a support group.

Date November 5 Day M [TU] W TH F SA SU

| Time of day | M/S | Food eaten | Cals. | H | Where did you eat? | What else were you doing? | How did someone else influence you? | What made you want to eat what you did? | Emotions and feelings? | Thoughts and concerns? |
|---|---|---|---|---|---|---|---|---|---|---|
| 7:30 | M | 1 C Crispix cereal<br>1/2 C skim milk<br>coffee, black<br>1 C orange juice | 110<br>40<br>—<br>120 | 3 | home | looking at news headlines on my phone | alone | I always eat cereal in the morning | a little keyed up & worried | thinking about quiz in class today |
| 10:30 | S | 1 apple | 90 | 1 | hall outside classroom | studying | alone | felt tired & wanted to wake up | tired | worried about next class |
| 12:30 | M | 1 C chili<br>1 roll<br>1 pat butter<br>1 orange<br>2 oatmeal cookies<br>1 soda | 290<br>120<br>35<br>60<br>120<br>150 | 2 | campus food court | talking | eating w/ friends; we decided to eat at the food court | wanted to be part of group | excited and happy | interested in hearing everyone's plans for the weekend |

M/S = Meal or snack H = Hunger rating (0–3)

**FIGURE 1.5** **Sample health journal entries.**

• ***Time frame-specific.*** Give yourself a reasonable amount of time to reach your goal, state the time frame in your behavior change plan, and set your agenda to meet the goal within the given time frame.

Using these criteria, sedentary people who want to improve their health and build fitness might set a goal of being able to run three miles in 30 minutes, to be achieved within a time frame of six months. To work toward that goal, they might set a number of smaller, intermediate goals that are easier to achieve. For example, their list of goals might look like this:

| WEEK | FREQUENCY (DAYS/WEEK) | ACTIVITY | DURATION (MINUTES) |
|---|---|---|---|
| 1 | 3 | Walk < 1 mile | 10–15 |
| 2 | 3 | Walk 1 mile | 15–20 |
| 3 | 4 | Walk 1–2 miles | 20–25 |
| 4 | 4 | Walk 2–3 miles | 25–30 |
| 5–7 | 3–4 | Walk/run 1 mile | 15–20 |
| ⋮ | | | |
| 21–24 | 4–5 | Run 2–3 miles | 25–30 |

For some goals and situations, it may make more sense to focus on something other than your outcome goal. If you are in an early stage of change, for example, your goal may be to learn more about the risks associated with your target behavior or to complete a cost-benefit analysis. If your goal involves a long-term lifestyle change, such as reaching a healthy weight, focus on developing healthy habits rather than targeting a specific weight loss. Your goal in this case might be exercising for 30 minutes every day, reducing portion sizes, or eliminating late-night snacks.

**4. Devise a Plan of Action** Develop a strategy that will support your efforts to change. Your plan of action should include the following steps:

• ***Get what you need.*** Identify resources that can help you. For example, you can join a community walking club or sign up for a smoking cessation program. You may need to buy running shoes or nicotine replacement patches. Get the items you need right away; waiting can delay your progress.

• ***Modify your environment.*** If you have cues in your environment that trigger your target behavior, control them. For example, if you typically have alcohol at home, getting rid of it can help prevent you from indulging. If you usually study with a group of friends in an environment that allows smoking, move to a nonsmoking area. If you always buy a snack at a certain vending machine, change your route so that you don't pass by it.

• ***Control related habits.*** You may have habits that contribute to your target behavior. Modifying these habits can help change the behavior. For example, if you usually plop down on the sofa while watching TV, try putting an exercise bike in front of the set so that you can burn calories while watching your favorite programs.

• ***Reward yourself.*** Giving yourself instant, real rewards for good behavior will reinforce your efforts. Plan your rewards; decide in advance what each one will be and how you will earn it. Tie rewards to achieving specific goals or subgoals. For example, you might treat yourself to a movie after a week of avoiding snacks. Make a list of items or events to use as rewards. They should be special to you and preferably unrelated to food or alcohol.

• ***Involve the people around you.*** Tell family and friends about your plan and ask them to help. To help them respond appropriately to your needs, create a specific list of dos and don'ts. For example, ask them to support you when you make time to exercise or avoid second helpings at meals.

• ***Plan for challenges.*** Think about situations and people that might derail your program and develop ways to cope with them. For example, if you think it will be hard to stick to your usual exercise program during exams, schedule short bouts of physical activity (such as a brisk walk) as stress-reducing study breaks.

## Ask Yourself

**QUESTIONS FOR CRITICAL THINKING AND REFLECTION**

Think about the last time you made an unhealthy choice instead of a healthy one. How could you have changed the situation, the people in the situation, or your own thoughts, feelings, or intentions to avoid making that choice? What can you do in similar situations in the future to produce a different outcome?

**5. Make a Personal Contract** A serious personal contract—one that commits you to your word—can result in a better chance of follow-through than a casual, offhand promise. Your contract can help prevent procrastination by specifying important dates and can also serve as a reminder of your personal commitment to change.

Your contract should include a statement of your goal and your commitment to reaching it. The contract should also include details such as the following:

- The date you will start
- The steps you will take to measure your progress
- The strategies you will use to promote change
- The date you expect to reach your final goal

Have someone—preferably someone who will be actively helping you with your program—sign your contract as a witness.

You can apply the general behavior change planning framework presented in this chapter to any target behavior. Additional examples of behavior change plans appear in the

## Ask Yourself

**QUESTIONS FOR CRITICAL THINKING AND REFLECTION**

Have you tried to change a behavior in the past, such as exercising more or quitting smoking? How successful were you? Do you feel the need to try again? If so, what would you do differently to improve your chances of success?

Behavior Change Strategy sections at the end of many chapters in this text. In these sections, you will find specific plans for quitting smoking, starting an exercise program, and making other positive lifestyle changes.

### Putting Your Plan into Action

When you're ready to put your plan into action, you need commitment—the resolve to stick with the plan no matter what temptations you encounter. Remember all the reasons you have to make the change—and remember that *you* are the boss. Use all your strategies to make your plan work. Make sure your environment is change-friendly, and get as much support and encouragement from others as possible. Keep track of your progress in your health journal and give yourself regular rewards. And don't forget to give yourself a pat on the back—congratulate yourself, notice how much better you look or feel, and feel good about how far you've come and how you've gained control of your behavior.

### Staying with It

As you continue with your program, don't be surprised when you run up against obstacles; they're inevitable. In fact, it's a good idea to expect problems and give yourself time to step back, see how you're doing, regroup, and make some changes before going on.

## BEING HEALTHY FOR LIFE

Your first few behavior change projects may never go beyond the planning stage. Those that do may not all succeed. But as you begin to see progress and changes, you'll start to experience new and surprising positive feelings about yourself. You'll probably find that you're less likely to buckle under stress. You may accomplish things you never thought possible—running a marathon, traveling abroad, or finding a rewarding relationship. Being healthy takes extra effort, but the paybacks in energy and vitality are priceless.

Once you've started, don't stop. Remember that maintaining good health is an ongoing process. Tackle one area at a time, but make a careful inventory of your health strengths and weaknesses and lay out a long-range plan. Take on the easier problems first, and then use what you have learned to attack more difficult areas. Keep informed about the latest health news and trends; research is continually providing new information that directly affects daily choices and habits.

You can't completely control every aspect of your health. At least three other factors—heredity, health care, and environment—play important roles in your well-being. After you quit smoking, for example, you may still be inhaling smoke from other people's cigarettes. Your resolve to eat better foods may suffer a setback when you have trouble finding healthy choices on campus.

But you can make a difference—you can help create an environment around you that supports wellness for everyone. You can support nonsmoking areas in public places. You can speak up in favor of more nutritious foods and better physical fitness facilities. You can provide nonalcoholic drinks at your parties.

You can also work on larger environmental challenges: air and water pollution, traffic congestion, overcrowding and overpopulation, global warming and climate change, toxic and nuclear waste, and many others. These difficult issues need the attention and energy of people who are informed and who care about good health. On every level, from personal to planetary, we can all take an active role in shaping our environment.

### TIPS FOR TODAY AND THE FUTURE

You are in charge of your health. Many of the decisions you make every day have an impact on the quality of your life, both now and in the future. By making positive choices, large and small, you help ensure a lifetime of wellness.

**RIGHT NOW YOU CAN:**

- Go for a 15-minute walk.
- Have a piece of fruit for a snack.
- Call a friend and arrange a time to catch up with each other.
- Think about whether you have a health behavior you'd like to change. If you do, consider the elements of a behavior change strategy. For example, begin a mental list of the pros and cons of the behavior, or talk to someone who can support you in your attempts to change.

**IN THE FUTURE YOU CAN:**

- Stay current on health- and wellness-related news and issues.
- Participate in health awareness and promotion campaigns in your community—for example, support smoking restrictions at local venues.
- Be a role model for (or at least be supportive of) someone else who is working on a health behavior you have successfully changed.

## SUMMARY


- Wellness is the ability to live life fully, with vitality and meaning. Wellness is dynamic and multidimensional. It incorporates physical, emotional, intellectual, interpersonal, cultural, spiritual, environmental, financial, and occupational dimensions.
- As chronic diseases have emerged as major health threats in the United States, people must recognize that they have greater control over, and greater responsibility for, their health than ever before.
- With new health insurance options and the Healthy People initiative, the U.S. government is seeking to achieve a better quality of life for all Americans.
- Health-related disparities that have implications for wellness can be described in the context of sex and gender, race and ethnicity, income and education, disability, geographic location, and sexual orientation and gender identity.
- Although heredity, environment, and health care all play roles in wellness and disease, behavior can mitigate their effects.
- To make lifestyle changes, you need information about yourself, your health habits, and resources available to help you change.
- You can increase your motivation for behavior change by examining the benefits and costs of change, boosting self-efficacy, and identifying and overcoming key barriers to change.
- The "stages of change" model describes six stages that people move through as they try to change their behavior: precontemplation, contemplation, preparation, action, maintenance, and termination.
- You can develop a specific plan for change by (1) monitoring your behavior by keeping a journal; (2) analyzing those data; (3) setting specific goals; (4) devising strategies for modifying the environment, rewarding yourself, and involving others; and (5) making a personal contract.
- To start and maintain a behavior change program, you need commitment, a well-developed plan, social support, and a system of rewards.
- Although you cannot control every aspect of your health, you can make a difference in helping create an environment that supports wellness for everyone.


## FOR MORE INFORMATION

The internet addresses listed here were accurate at the time of publication.

*Centers for Disease Control and Prevention (CDC).* The CDC provides a wide variety of health information for researchers and the general public.

http://www.cdc.gov

*Federal Deposit Insurance Corporation.* "Money Smart" is a free source of information, unaffiliated with commercial interests, that includes eight modules on topics such as "borrowing basics" and "paying for college and cars."

https://www.fdic.gov/resources/consumers/money-smart/index.html

*Federal Trade Commission: Health Claims.* Takes you through a variety of consumer health topics, including fitness equipment, generic drugs, and fraudulent health claims.

https://www.ftc.gov/business-guidance/advertising-marketing/health-claims

*Healthfinder.* A gateway to online publications, websites, support and self-help groups, and agencies and organizations that produce reliable health information.

http://healthfinder.gov

*Healthy People.* Provides information on Healthy People objectives and priority areas.

http://www.healthypeople.gov

*MedlinePlus.* Provides links to news and reliable information about health from government agencies and professional associations; also includes a health encyclopedia and information about prescription and over-the-counter drugs.

http://medlineplus.gov

*National Health Information Center (NHIC).* Puts consumers in touch with the organizations that are best able to provide answers to health-related questions.

http://www.health.gov/nhic/

*National Institutes of Health (NIH).* Provides information about all NIH activities as well as consumer publications, hotline information, and an A-to-Z listing of health issues with links to the appropriate NIH institute.

http://www.nih.gov

*National Wellness Institute.* Serves professionals and organizations that promote health and wellness.

http://www.nationalwellness.org

*Office of Minority Health.* Promotes improved health among racial and ethnic minority populations.

http://minorityhealth.hhs.gov

*Office on Women's Health.* Provides information and answers to frequently asked questions.

http://www.womenshealth.gov

*Surgeon General.* Includes information on activities of the Surgeon General and the text of many key reports on topics such as tobacco use, physical activity, and mental health.

http://www.surgeongeneral.gov

*World Health Organization (WHO).* Provides information about health topics and issues affecting people around the world.

http://www.who.int/en

## BEHAVIOR CHANGE STRATEGY
### Behavior Change Contract

**1.** I, ____________________, agree to ________________________________________

________________________________________________________________

**2.** I will begin on ____________________ and plan to reach my goal of ____________________

____________________ by ____________________

**3.** To reach my final goal, I have devised the following schedule of mini-goals. For each step in my program, I will give myself the reward listed.

| Mini-goal | Target date | Reward |
|---|---|---|
| ____________ | ____________ | ____________ |
| ____________ | ____________ | ____________ |
| ____________ | ____________ | ____________ |

My overall reward for reaching my goal will be ____________________

**4.** I have gathered and analyzed data on my target behavior and have identified the following strategies for changing my behavior:

________________________________________________________________

________________________________________________________________

**5.** I will use the following tools to monitor my progress toward my final goal: ____________________

________________________________________________________________

________________________________________________________________

I sign this contract as an indication of my personal commitment to reach my goal: ____________________

________________________________________________________________

I have recruited a helper who will witness my contract and ____________________

________________________________________________________________

________________________________________________________________

## SELECTED BIBLIOGRAPHY


American Cancer Society. 2022. *Cancer Facts and Figures–2022.* Atlanta, GA: American Cancer Society. (https://www.cancer.org/content/dam/cancer-org/research/cancer-facts-and-statistics/annual-cancer-facts-and-figures/2022/2022-cancer-facts-and-figures.pdf).

American College Health Association. 2022. *American College Health Association–National College Health Assessment III: Reference Group Executive Summary Fall 2021.* Hanover, MD: American College Health Association. (https://www.acha.org/documents/ncha/NCHA-III_FALL_2021_REFERENCE_GROUP_EXECUTIVE_SUMMARY.pdf).

American Heart Association. 2022. *Heart Disease and Stroke Statistics.* Dallas, TX: American Heart Association. (https://www.empoweredtoserve.org/en/about-us/heart-and-stroke-association-statistics).

Bakalar, N. 2019. Air pollution may damage the brain. *The New York Times,* 25 November (https://www.nytimes.com/2019/11/25/well/mind/air-pollution-brain-dementia-alzheimer-memory.html).

Bardo, A. R., and S. M. Lynch. 2019. Cognitively intact and happy life expectancy in the United States. *The Journals of Gerontology: Series B:* gbz080 (https://doi-org.laneproxy.stanford.edu/10.1093/geronb/gbz080).

Benjamin, E. J., et al. 2019. Heart disease and stroke statistics—2019 update: a report from the American Heart Association. *Circulation* 139(10): e56–528.

Bennett, I. M., et al. 2009. The contribution of health literacy to disparities in self-rated health status and preventive health behaviors in older adults. *Annals of Family Medicine* 7(3): 204–211.

Bleich, S. N., et al. 2012. Health inequalities: Trends, progress, and policy. *Annual Review of Public Health* 33: 7–40.

Centers for Disease Control and Prevention. 2020. *2020 Final Death Statistics: Covid-19 as an Underlying Cause of Death vs. Contributing Cause* (https://www.cdc.gov/nchs/pressroom/podcasts/2022/20220107/20220107.htm).

Centers for Disease Control and Prevention. 2020. Disability Impacts All of Us. (https://www.cdc.gov/ncbddd/disabilityandhealth/infographic-disability-impacts-all.html).

Centers for Disease Control and Prevention. 2020. *Division of Diabetes Translation at a Glance.* (http://www.cdc.gov/chronicdisease/resources/publications/aag/diabetes.htm).

Centers for Disease Control and Prevention. 2022. National Diabetes Statistics Report. Atlanta, GA: Centers for Disease Control and Prevention, U.S. Dept of Health and Human Services. (https://www.cdc.gov/diabetes/data/statistics-report/index.html).

Centers for Disease Control and Prevention. 2022. *Obesity, Race/Ethnicity, and COVID-19* (https://www.cdc.gov/obesity/data/obesity-and-covid-19.html).

Centers for Disease Control and Prevention. 2022. U.S. *Overdose Deaths in 2021 Increased Half as Much as in 2020 - But Are Still Up 15%.* (https://www.cdc.gov/nchs/pressroom/nchs_press_releases/2022/202205.htm).

Cleveland Clinic. 2017. Cleveland Clinic study finds obesity as top cause of preventable life-years lost. (https://newsroom.clevelandclinic.org/2017/04/22/cleveland-clinic-study-finds-obesity-top-cause-preventable-life-years-lost/).

Curtin, S. C., et al. 2018. Recent increases in injury mortality among children and adolescents aged 10–19 year in the United States: 1999–2016. *National Vital Statistics Reports* 67(4): 1–16.

Everett, B. G, et al. 2013. The nonlinear relationship between education and mortality: An examination of cohort, race/ethnic, and gender differences. *Population Research and Policy Review* 32(6).

Flegal, K. M., et al. 2016. Trends in obesity among adults in the United States, 2005–2014. *JAMA* 315(21): 2284–2291.

Frieden, T. R. 2016. Foreword. *MMWR* 65(Suppl.) Doi: http://dx.doi.org/10.15585/mmwr.su6501a1.

Goldman, D. 2020. Obesity, Second to Smoking as the Most Preventable Cause of US Deaths, Needs New Approaches (https://healthpolicy.usc.edu/article/obesity-second-to-smoking-as-the-most-preventable-cause-of-us-deaths-needs-new-approaches/).

Horneffer-Ginter, K. 2008. Stages of change and possible selves: Two tools for promoting college health. *Journal of American College Health* 56(4): 351–358.

Joshi, P. K., et al. 2017. Genome-wide meta-analysis associates HLA-DQA1/DRB1 and LPA and lifestyle factors with human longevity. *Nature Communications* 8(1): 910. Doi: 10.1038/s41467-017-00934-5.

Lange, K. W., and Y. Nakamura. 2020. Lifestyle factors in the prevention of COVID-19. *Global Health Journal* 4(4): 146–152.

Luczak, S. E., et al. 2017. A review of the prevalence and co-occurrence of addictions in US ethnic/racial groups: Implications for genetic research. *The American Journal on Addictions* 26(5): 424–436.

National Center for Health Statistics. 2019. Health, United States Spotlight: Racial and Ethnic Disparities in Heart Disease. Hyattsville, MD: National Center for Health Statistics. (https://www.cdc.gov/nchs/hus/spotlight/HeartDiseaseSpotlight_2019_0404.pdf).

National Conference of State Legislatures. 2021. Legal cases and state legislative actions related to the ACA (https://www.ncsl.org/research/health/state-laws-and-actions-challenging-ppaca.aspx).

O'Loughlin, J., et al. 2007. Lifestyle risk factors for chronic disease across family origin among adults in multiethnic, low-income, urban neighborhoods. *Ethnicity and Disease* 17(4): 657–663.

Office of Disease Prevention and Health Promotion. 2022. *Healthy People 2030 Framework.* (https://www.healthypeople.gov/2020/About-Healthy-People/Development-Healthy-People-2030/Proposed-Framework).

Pinkhasov, R. M., et al. 2010. Are men shortchanged on health? Perspective on health care utilization and health risk behavior in men and women in the United States. *International Journal of Clinical Practice* 64(4): 475–487.

Printz, C. 2012. Disparities in cancer care: Are we making progress? A look at how researchers and organizations are working to reduce cancer health disparities. *Cancer* 118(4): 867–868.

Prochaska, J. O., J. C. Norcross, and C. C. DiClemente. 1995. *Changing for Good: The Revolutionary Program That Explains the Six Stages of Change and Teaches You How to Free Yourself from Bad Habits.* New York: Morrow.

Thorpe, R. J., et al. 2008. Social context as an explanation for race disparities in hypertension: Findings from the Exploring Health Disparities in Integrated Communities (EHDIC) Study. *Social Science and Medicine* 67(10): 1604-1611.

The U.S. Burden of Disease Collaborators. 2018. The state of US health, 1990–2016: Burden of diseases, injuries, and risk factors among US States. *JAMA* 319(14): 1444–1472.

U.S. Department of Health and Human Services. 2022. *Healthy People 2030: Lesbian, Gay, Bisexual, and Transgender Health* (https://health.gov/healthypeople/objectives-and-data/browse-objectives/lgbt).

U.S. National Library of Medicine. 2022. Is longevity determined by genetics? (https://ghr.nlm.nih.gov/primer/traits/longevity).

White, A. M., I. P. Castle, and P. A. Powell. 2022. Alcohol-related deaths during the COVID-19 pandemic. *JAMA* (Doi:10.1001/jama.2022.4308).

Williams, D. R. 2012. Miles to go before we sleep: Racial inequities in health. *Journal of Health and Social Behavior* 53(3): 279–295.

Yudell, M., et al. 2016. Taking race out of human genetics. *Science* 351(6273): 564.

**Design Elements:** Assess Yourself icon: Aleksey Boldin/Alamy Stock Photo; Diversity Matters icon: Rawpixel Ltd/Getty Images; Wellness on Campus icon: Radius Images/Alamy Stock Photo; Take Charge icon: VisualCommunications/Getty Images; Critical Consumer icon: pagadesign/Getty Images.

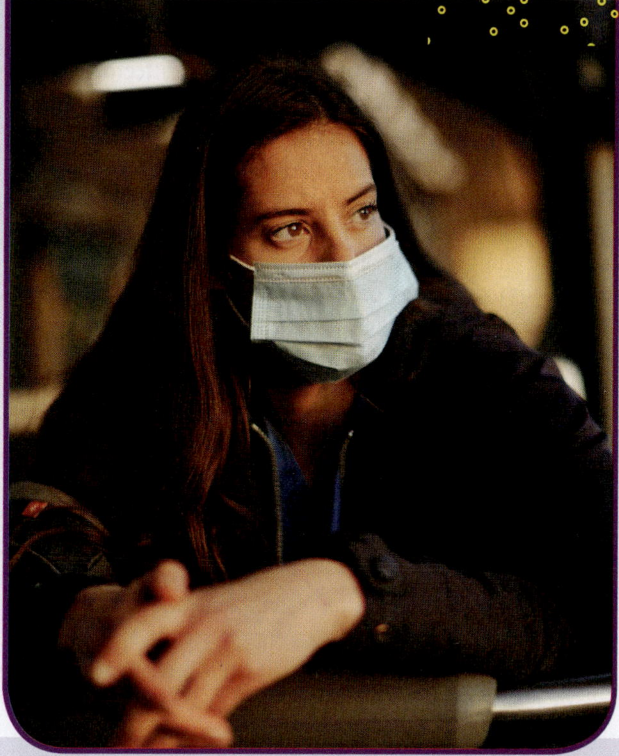
Tempura/Getty Images

## CHAPTER OBJECTIVES

- Explain what stress is
- Describe the relationship between stress and health
- List common sources of stress
- Describe and apply techniques for managing stress

CHAPTER 2

# Stress: The Constant Challenge

Like the term *wellness, stress* is a word many people use without understanding its precise meaning. Stress is popularly viewed as an uncomfortable response to a negative event, which probably describes *nervous tension* more than the cluster of physical and psychological responses that actually constitutes stress. In fact, stress is not limited to negative situations; it is also a response to pleasurable physical challenges and the achievement of personal goals.

Whether stress is experienced as pleasant or unpleasant depends largely on the situation and the individual. Learning effective responses to stress can enhance psychological health and help prevent a number of serious diseases, and stress management can be an important part of daily life.

As a college student, you may be in one of the most stressful times of your life. This chapter explains the physiological and psychological reactions that make up the stress response and describes how these reactions can put your health at risk. The chapter also discusses the most common sources of stress and offers methods of managing stress in your life.

## WHAT IS STRESS?

In common usage, the term *stress* refers to two things: the mental states or events that trigger physical and psychological reactions (e.g., "That relationship is way too much stress"), *and* the reactions themselves (e.g., "I feel a lot of stress every time I walk into that classroom"). We use the more precise term **stressor** for a physical or psychological event that triggers physical and emotional reactions and the term **stress response** for the reactions themselves. Thoughts or feelings about an approaching event can be just as stressful as the event itself. A first date or a final exam can be a stressor that leads to sweaty palms and a pounding heart,

TERMS

**stressor** Any physical or psychological event or condition that produces usually negative reactions.

**stress response** The physical and emotional reactions to a stressor.

symptoms of the stress response. We use the term **stress** to describe the general physical and emotional state that accompanies the stress response (e.g., "I take a day at the beach when I feel stressed").

Each individual's experience of stress depends on many factors, including the nature of the stressor and how it is perceived. Stressors take many different forms. Like a fire in your home, some occur suddenly and neither last long nor repeat. Others, like air pollution or quarreling parents, can continue for a long time. The memory of a stressful occurrence, such as the memory of the loss of a loved one, can itself be a stressor years after the event. Responses to stressors can include a wide variety of physical, cognitive, behavioral, and emotional changes. A short-term response might be an upset stomach or insomnia; a long-term response might be a change in your personality or social relationships.

## Physical Responses to Stressors

Imagine a close call: As you step off the curb, a car careens toward you. With just a fraction of a second to spare, you leap safely out of harm's way. In that split second of danger and in the moments that follow, you experience a predictable series of physical reactions. Your body goes from a relaxed state to one prepared for physical action to cope with a threat to your life.

**TERMS**

**stress** The general physical and emotional state that the stressor produces.

**nervous system** The brain, spinal cord, and nerves.

**autonomic nervous system** The part of the nervous system that controls certain basic body processes; consists of the sympathetic and parasympathetic divisions.

**parasympathetic division** The part of the autonomic nervous system that moderates the excitatory effect of the sympathetic division, slowing metabolism and restoring energy supplies.

**sympathetic division** Division of the autonomic nervous system that reacts to danger or other challenges by accelerating body processes.

**endocrine system** The system of glands, tissues, and cells that secrete hormones into the bloodstream to influence metabolism and other body processes.

**hormone** A chemical messenger produced in the body and transported in the bloodstream to target cells or organs for specific regulation of their activities.

**cortisol** A steroid hormone secreted by the cortex (outer layer) of the adrenal gland that triggers an energy source for your large muscles; also called *hydrocortisone*.

**epinephrine** A hormone secreted by the medulla (inner core) of the adrenal gland that affects the functioning of organs involved in responding to a stressor; also called *adrenaline*.

**fight, flight, or freeze reaction** A defense reaction that prepares a person for conflict or escape by triggering hormonal, cardiovascular, metabolic, and behavioral changes.

Two systems in your body are responsible for your physical response to stressors: the nervous system and the endocrine system. Through rapid chemical reactions affecting almost every part of your body, you are primed to act quickly and appropriately in times of danger.

### The Nervous System

The **nervous system** consists of the brain, spinal cord, and nerves. Part of the nervous system is under voluntary control, as when you tell your arm to reach for an orange. The part that is *not* under conscious supervision—for example, the part that controls the digestion of the orange—is the **autonomic nervous system.** In addition to digestion, it controls your heart rate, breathing, blood pressure, and hundreds of other involuntary functions. The autonomic nervous system consists of two divisions:

- The **parasympathetic division** is in control when you are relaxed. It aids in digesting food, storing energy, and promoting growth.
- The **sympathetic division** is activated when your body is stimulated, for example, by exercise, and when you face an emergency and experience severe pain, anger, or fear.

Sympathetic nerves use the neurotransmitter norepinephrine (or *noradrenaline*) to affect nearly every organ, sweat gland, blood vessel, and muscle to enable your body to handle an emergency. In general, the sympathetic division commands your body to stop storing energy and to use it in response to a crisis.

### How the Nervous and Endocrine Systems Work Together

During stress, the sympathetic nervous system triggers the **endocrine system.** This system of glands, tissues, and cells helps control body functions by releasing **hormones** and other chemical messengers into the bloodstream to influence metabolism and other body processes. The nervous system handles very short-term stress, whereas the endocrine system deals with both short-term (*acute*) and long-term (*chronic*) stress. How do both systems work together in an emergency? Higher cognitive areas in your brain decide that you are facing a threat. The nervous and endocrine systems activate adrenal glands that release the hormones **cortisol** and **epinephrine** (adrenaline). These hormones then trigger a basic set of physical reactions to stressors (as shown in Figure 2.1).

These nearly instantaneous physiological changes have been known as the **fight-or-flight reaction** but currently are called **fight, flight, or freeze.** The rapid onset of fight-or-flight reactions and the autonomic nervous system are largely driven by the neurotransmitter adrenaline. The heart accelerates, pupils dilate, and muscle tone increases. In contrast, the freeze response is more of a behavior within our awareness, along with the parasympathetic division reactions, and is driven by a different neurotransmitter. The physiological changes of the fight, flight, or freeze reaction give you the heightened reflexes and strength you need to dodge a car accident.

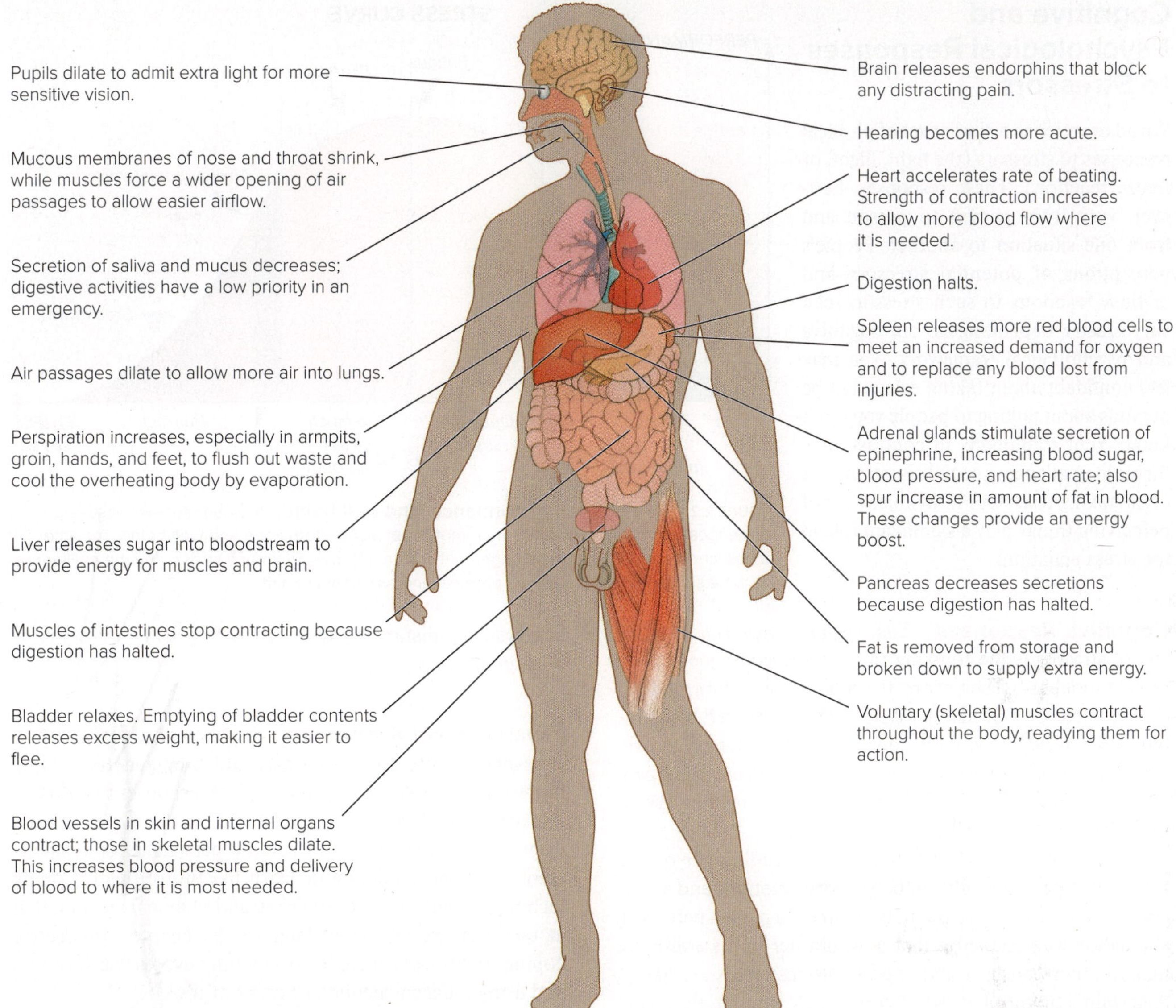


FIGURE 2.1 **Fight, flight, or freeze.** In response to a stressor, the autonomic nervous system and the endocrine system prepare the body to deal with an emergency.

**The Return to Homeostasis** A short time after your near miss with the car, you begin to feel normal again. Once a stressful situation ends, the autonomic nervous system regains its balance, usually as its parasympathetic division takes command and halts the stress response. It restores **homeostasis,** a state of balance in which blood pressure, heart rate, hormone levels, and other vital functions are maintained within a narrow range of normal. Your parasympathetic nervous system calms your body, slowing a rapid heartbeat, drying sweaty palms, and returning breathing to normal. Gradually your body resumes its normal "housekeeping" functions, such as digestion and temperature regulation. Damage that may have been sustained during the stress exposure is repaired (e.g., the extra blood sugar produced to give you more energy is reabsorbed into the bloodstream rather than increasing your risk for diabetes). The day after you narrowly dodge the car, you wake up feeling fine. In this way, your body can grow, repair itself, and acquire new reserves of energy. When the next crisis comes, you'll be ready to respond again instantly.

**The Fight, Flight, or Freeze Reaction in Modern Life** Fight, flight, or freeze is part of our biological heritage, a survival mechanism that has served humans well. In modern life, however, it is often absurdly inappropriate. Many of the stressors we face in everyday life—an exam, a mess left by a roommate, or a stoplight—do not require a physical response. The fight, flight, or freeze reaction prepares the body for physical action regardless of whether a particular stressor requires such a response.

**TERMS**

**homeostasis** A state of stability and consistency in an individual's physiological functioning.

## Cognitive and Psychological Responses to Stressors

We all experience a similar set of physical responses to stressors (the fight, flight, or freeze reaction). These responses, however, vary from person to person and from one situation to another. People's perceptions of potential stressors—and of their reactions to such stressors—can vary greatly, depending on our cognitive and psychological framework. You may feel confident about taking exams but be nervous about talking to people you don't know. Your roommate, in contrast, may thrive in challenging social situations but dread taking tests. Our individual ways of perceiving things play a significant role in the stress equation.

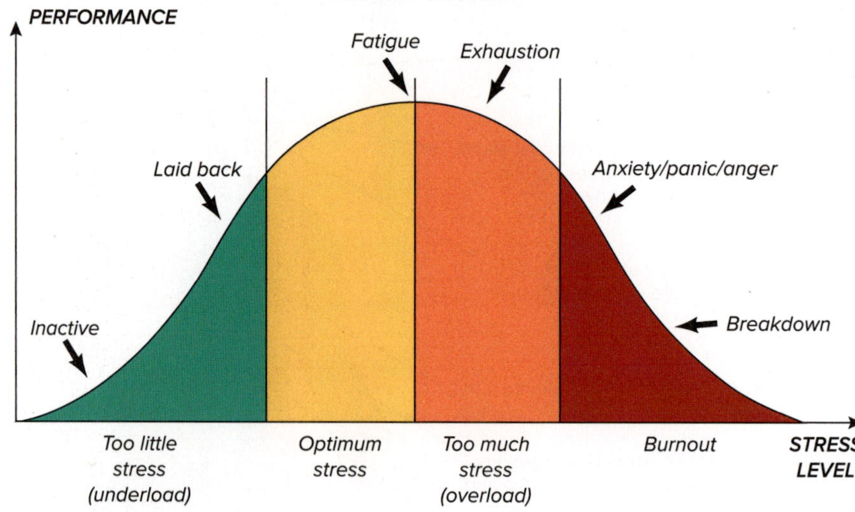


**FIGURE 2.2 Stress level, performance, and well-being.** A moderate level of stress challenges individuals in a way that promotes optimal performance and well-being. Too little stress, and people are not challenged enough to improve; too much stress, and the challenges become stressors that can impair physical and emotional health.

### Cognitive Responses

Your *cognitive appraisal* of a potential stressor is the thinking through the consequences of certain thoughts or behaviors, the processing of information.

The facts of a situation—Who? What? Where? When?—typically are evaluated fairly consistently from person to person. But evaluation with respect to personal outcome can vary: What does this mean for me? Can I do anything about it? Will it improve or worsen?

If a person perceives a situation as exceeding her or his ability to cope, the result can be negative emotions and an inappropriate stress response. If, by contrast, a person perceives a situation as a challenge that is within her or his ability to manage, more positive and appropriate responses are likely. A certain amount of stress, if coped with appropriately, can help promote optimal performance (Figure 2.2).

Two cognitive factors that can reduce the magnitude of the stress response are successful prediction and the perception of control. For instance, receiving a course syllabus at the beginning of the term allows you to predict the timing of major deadlines and exams. Having this predictive knowledge also allows you to exert some control over your study plans, which can help reduce the stress caused by exams.

Looking at responses to a widespread stressor such as the coronavirus outbreak, we see that people with too much anxiety may engage in socially disruptive behaviors such as panic buying or avoiding necessary health care at hospitals or doctors' offices for fear of contracting the virus. On the other hand, people who respond with too little anxiety may not take enough precautionary measures, such as physically distancing themselves or getting a vaccine or booster shot.

> **TERMS**
> **personality** The sum of behavioral, cognitive, and emotional tendencies.

### Psychological Responses

Psychological responses to stressors include cognitive ones, and they generally imply more emotion. Common psychological responses to stressors include anxiety, depression, and fear. Although emotional responses are determined in part by personality or temperament, we often moderate or learn to control them. Coping techniques that promote wellness and enable us to function at our best are discussed later in the chapter. Ineffective coping to stressors includes overeating; expressing hostility; and using tobacco, alcohol, or other drugs.

There are many factors that influence how each person responds to stress. Personality, cultural background, gender, and individual experience are important to consider when dealing with stressful situations.

**PERSONALITY** Some **personality** traits enable people to deal more effectively with stress. One such trait is *hardiness,* a particular form of optimism. People with a hardy personality view potential stressors as challenges and opportunities for growth and learning, rather than as burdens. They see fewer situations as stressful and react less intensely to stress than nonhardy people. Hardy people are committed to their activities, have a sense of inner purpose and an inner locus of control, and feel mostly in control of their lives.

Another psychological characteristic that prompts us to behave in a certain way is motivation. One type, *stressed power motivation,* is associated with people who are aggressive and argumentative and who need to have power over others. A study of college students found that persons with this personality trait tend to get sick when their need for power is blocked or threatened. In contrast, people with

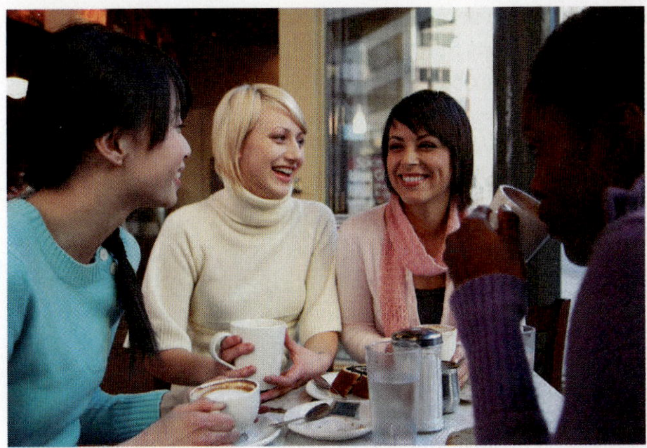

A person's emotional and behavioral responses to stressors depend on many factors, including personality, gender, and cultural background. Fancy/Alamy Stock Photo

*unstressed affiliation motivation* are drawn to others and want to be liked as friends. The same study of college students found that students with this trait reported the least illness. Another important personality trait—**resilience**—is especially associated with social and academic success in groups at risk for stress, such as people from low-income families and those with mental or physical disabilities. Resilient people tend to face adversity by accepting the reality of their situation, holding to a belief that life is meaningful, and being able to improvise.

Academic resilience helps college students flourish. Whether they need to bounce back from a poor grade or negative feedback, or master the art of juggling multiple academic pressures, students can learn techniques to stay and become resilient. One technique is to identify resources such as peers and counselors to lean on in times of crisis.

Contemporary research is repeatedly demonstrating that you can change some basic elements of your personality as well as your typical behaviors and patterns of thinking by using positive stress management techniques like those described later in this chapter.

**CULTURAL BACKGROUND** Young adults from around the world come to the United States for a higher education; most students finish college with a greater appreciation for other cultures and worldviews. The clash of cultures, however, can be a big source of stress for many students—especially when it leads to disrespectful treatment, harassment, or violence. It is important to consider that our reactions to stressful events are influenced by family and cultural background. Learning to appreciate the cultural backgrounds of other people can be both a mind-opening experience and a way to avoid stress over cultural differences.

**GENDER** Your **gender role**—the activities, abilities, and behaviors your culture expects of you based on your sex—can affect your experience of stress. Some behavioral responses to stressors, such as crying or openly expressing anger, may be deemed more appropriate for one gender than another.

### Ask Yourself

**QUESTIONS FOR CRITICAL THINKING AND REFLECTION**

Think of the last time you faced a significant stressor. How did you react? List the physical, cognitive, behavioral, and emotional reactions you experienced. Were the reactions appropriate to the circumstances? Did these reactions help you better deal with the stress, or did they interfere with your efforts to handle it?

Strict adherence to gender roles, however, can limit one's response to stress and can itself become a source of stress. Gender roles can also affect one's perception of a stressor. If a man derives most of his self-worth from his work, for example, retirement may be more stressful for him than for a woman whose self-image is based on several different roles.

In her book *Overwhelmed*, Brigid Schulte describes a continuing unequal gendered division of labor: Families work more hours than they used to, but American women spend even more childraising hours than they did in the 1960s, when fewer women worked outside jobs.

Today's girls deal with pressures to do well in school and extracurricular activities while also trying to be pretty, sexy, kind, and liked by everyone in the real and virtual worlds. Social media's visual platforms, such as Instagram and Snapchat, are dominated by adolescent girls. These platforms portray effortless perfection and reward conventionally feminine expected behaviors: pleasing, performing, and looking good. This narrowing ideal of success comes at the expense of self-worth and well-being.

**EXPERIENCE** Past experiences can profoundly influence the evaluation of a potential stressor. If you had a bad experience giving a speech in the past, you are much more likely to perceive an upcoming speech as stressful than someone who has had positive public-speaking experiences. Effective behavioral responses, such as preparing carefully and visualizing success, can help overcome the effects of negative past experiences.

## STRESS AND HEALTH

The American Psychological Association's *Stress in America* surveys have followed major trends in stress since 2007, focusing on stressors ranging from money, employment, health care, and social media to terrorism, the opioid epidemic, and discrimination, to name only a few. In 2020, self-reported

**TERMS**

**resilience** A personality trait associated with the ability to face adversity and recover quickly from difficulties.

**gender role** A culturally expected pattern of behavior and attitudes determined by a person's sex.

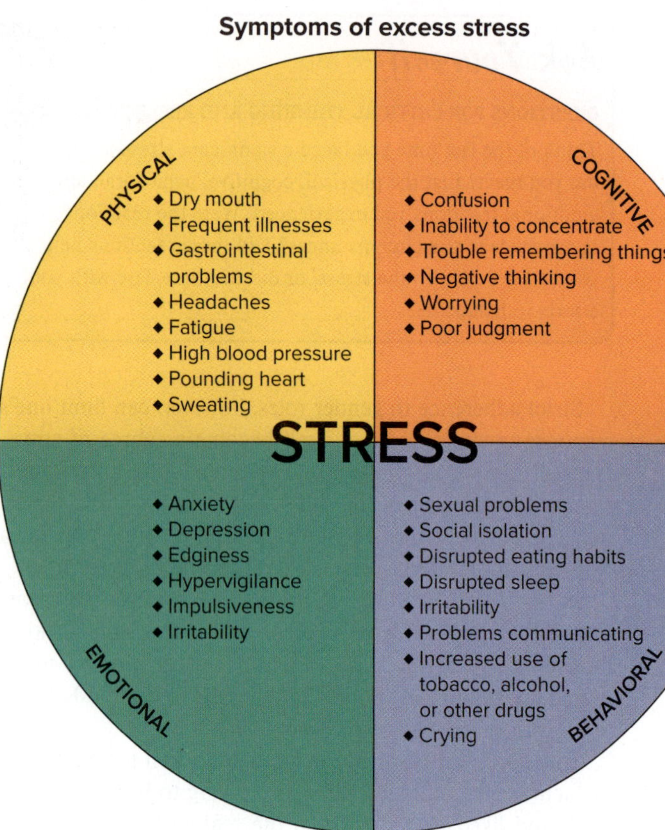


**FIGURE 2.3 Physical, cognitive, behavioral, and emotional symptoms of excess stress.**

stress levels increased significantly for the first time since the survey began; stress levels related to the coronavirus pandemic were even higher, particularly among parents of children under 18 and people of color. In 2022, the survey found that 87% of adults agreed that the last two years had been a constant stream of crises; 73% said they were feeling overwhelmed. The role of stress in health is complex, but evidence suggests that stress can increase vulnerability to many ailments. Figure 2.3 shows the physical, cognitive, behavioral, and emotional symptoms of excess negative stress. Some people feel nervous and anxious; some have headaches, fatigue, or irritability; others can't sleep or enter into mood swings and depression. Coupled with these symptoms are changes in behavior, like avoiding social situations or altering eating habits.

## The General Adaptation Syndrome

The concepts of homeostasis and adaptations to stressors came from the work of several scientists across the 20th century. The **general adaptation syndrome (GAS),** developed by biologist Hans Selye beginning in the 1930s and 1940s, is a theory that describes a universal and predictable response pattern to all stressors. It identifies an automatic self-regulation system of the mind and body that tries to return the body to a state of homeostasis after it is subjected to stress.

**TERMS**

**general adaptation syndrome (GAS)** A pattern of stress responses consisting of three stages: alarm, resistance, and exhaustion.

**eustress** Stress resulting from a stressor perceived to be pleasant.

**distress** Stress resulting from a stressor perceived to be unpleasant.

Some stressors, such as attending a party, are viewed as pleasant, while others, such as getting a bad grade, are viewed as unpleasant. In the GAS theory, stress triggered by a positive stressor is called **eustress;** stress triggered by a negative stressor is called **distress.** The sequence of physical responses associated with the GAS is the same for both eustress and distress and occurs in three stages (see Figure 2.4).

1. ***Alarm.*** The alarm stage includes the complex sequence of events brought on by the fight, flight, or freeze reaction. At this stage, the body is more susceptible to disease or injury because it is geared up to deal with a crisis. Someone in this phase may experience headaches, indigestion, anxiety, and disrupted sleeping and eating patterns.

2. ***Resistance.*** Under continued stress, the body develops a new level of homeostasis in which it is more resistant to disease and injury than usual. In this stage, a person can cope with normal life and added stress. However, at some point the body's resources will become depleted.

3. ***Exhaustion.*** The first two stages of GAS require a great deal of energy. If a stressor persists, or if several stressors occur in succession, general exhaustion sets in. This is not the sort of exhaustion you feel after a long, busy day. Rather, it's a life-threatening physiological exhaustion. The body's resources are depleted, and the body is unable to maintain normal function. If this stage is extended, long-term damage may result, manifesting itself in ulcers, digestive system trouble, depression, diabetes, cardiovascular problems, and/or mental illnesses.

## More Recent Ideas about Stress

Since the 1970s, researchers have developed instruments to measure brain waves, skin conduction, heart rates, and muscle tone (see discussion of biofeedback in the section "Managing Stress"). These tools allow the study of specific immediate and long-term impacts of the stress response.

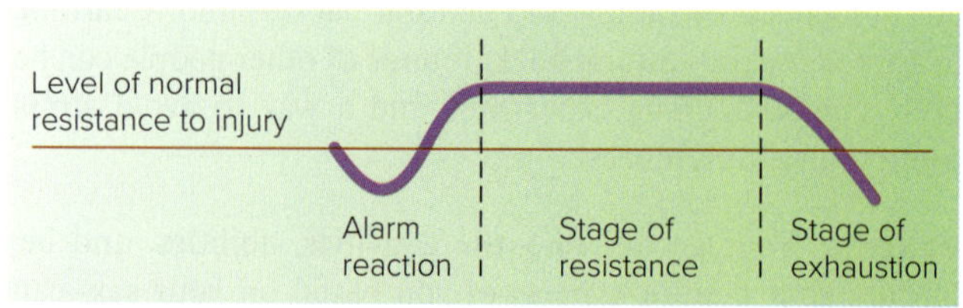


**FIGURE 2.4 The general adaptation syndrome.** During the alarm phase, the body's resistance to injury lowers. With continued stress, resistance to injury is enhanced. With prolonged exposure to repeated stressors, exhaustion sets in.

**Allostatic Load** The allostatic load is a system in which stability is achieved through changes to chemical messengers. By making internal changes to match external stressors (e.g., increasing heart rate and blood pressure during jogging), the body regains homeostasis. But over time, the wear and tear on the body that results from long-term exposure to repeated or chronic stress is called the **allostatic load.** A person's allostatic load depends on many factors, including genetics, life experiences, and emotional and behavioral responses to stressors.

The concept of allostatic load explains how frequent activation of the body's stress response, although essential for managing acute threats, can damage the body in the long run. For example, a student who experiences test anxiety manages a week of exams but collapses on the weekend with a severe cold. During the week, stress-related hormonal responses promote feelings of hunger and conversion of food to energy. Pizza and soda, which may be comforting in a time of stress, could also give the student diarrhea because their insulin level spiked and didn't properly promote glucose absorption. Over time, the student's allostatic load, along with a susceptibility to disease, can increase. The body's adaptations can be too much of a good thing, so that in a state of exhaustion, we're experiencing ill effects not just from the stressor, but from our bodies' response to it as well.

**Adaptive Calibration Model** A more recent model of stress takes an evolutionary perspective. Rather than focusing on risk factors for disease, we can view the calibrations made by the body to match current and future environments. The body can remember information about external threats and opportunities so that later it can adapt its parameters and more efficiently return to its needed equilibriums.

## Psychoneuroimmunology

One of the most fruitful areas of current research into the relationship between stress and disease is **psychoneuroimmunology (PNI).** PNI is the study of the interactions among the nervous system, the endocrine system, and the immune system. The underlying premise of PNI is that stress, through the actions of the nervous and endocrine systems, impairs the immune system and thereby affects health.

A complex network of nerve and chemical connections exists among the nervous and endocrine systems. In general, increased levels of cortisol are linked to a decreased number of immune system cells, or *lymphocytes*. Epinephrine appears to promote the release of lymphocytes but at the same time reduces their efficiency. Scientists have identified hormone-like substances called *neuropeptides* that appear to translate stressful emotions into biochemical events, some of which affect the immune system, providing a physical link between emotions and immune function.

Different types of stress may affect immunity in different ways. For instance, during **acute stress** (typically lasting between 5 and 100 minutes), white blood cells move into the skin, where they enhance the immune response. During a stressful event sequence, such as a personal trauma and the events that follow, however, there are typically no overall significant immune changes. Chronic (ongoing) stressors such as unemployment have negative effects on almost all functional measures of immunity. **Chronic stress** may cause prolonged secretion of cortisol (sometimes called the "antistress hormone" because it seeks to return the nervous system to homeostasis after a stress reaction) and may accelerate the course of diseases that involve inflammation, including multiple sclerosis, heart disease, type 2 diabetes, and clinical depression. In other words, this is one way that too many stress reactions over a prolonged length of time can have a negative impact on health.

Mood, personality, behavior, and immune functioning are intertwined. For example, people who are generally pessimistic may neglect the basics of health care, become passive when ill, and fail to engage in health-promoting behaviors. People who are depressed may reduce physical activity and social interaction, which may in turn affect the immune system and the cognitive appraisal of a stressor. Optimism, successful coping, and positive problem solving, by contrast, may positively influence immunity.

## Stress and Specific Conditions

Although much remains to be learned, it is clear that people who have unresolved chronic stress in their lives or who handle stressors poorly are at risk for a wide range of health problems.

**Cardiovascular Disease** During the stress response, heart rate increases and blood vessels constrict, causing blood pressure to rise. Chronic high blood pressure is a major cause of *atherosclerosis,* a disease in which blood vessels become damaged and caked with fatty deposits. These deposits can block arteries, causing heart attacks and strokes. The stress response can precipitate a heart attack in someone with atherosclerosis.

Certain emotional responses may increase a person's risk of CVD. As described earlier, people who tend to react to situations with anger and hostility are more likely to have heart attacks than are people with less explosive, more trusting personalities. Inflammation has been linked to stress and

**TERMS**

**allostatic load** The "wear and tear" on the body that results from long-term exposure to repeated or chronic stress.

**psychoneuroimmunology (PNI)** The study of the interactions among the nervous, endocrine, and immune systems.

**acute stress** Stress immediately following a stressor; may last only minutes or may turn into chronic stress.

**chronic stress** Stress that continues for days, weeks, or longer.

is a key component of the damage to blood vessels that leads to heart attacks (see Chapter 13 for more about CVD.)

**Psychological Disorders** Stress contributes to many psychological problems such as depression, panic attacks, anxiety, eating disorders, and posttraumatic stress disorder (PTSD). PTSD, which afflicts war veterans, rape victims, child abuse survivors, and others who have suffered or witnessed severe trauma, is characterized by nightmares, flashbacks, and a diminished capacity to experience or express emotion. (For information about psychological health, see Chapter 3.)

**Altered Immune Function** Some of the health problems linked to stress-related changes in immune function include vulnerability to colds and other infections, asthma and allergy attacks, and flare-ups of chronic sexually transmitted infections such as genital herpes and HIV infection.

**Headaches** More than 45 million Americans suffer from chronic, recurrent headaches. Headaches come in various types but are often grouped into the following three categories:

• ***Tension headaches.*** Approximately 90% of all headaches are tension headaches, characterized by a dull, steady pain, usually on both sides of the head. It may feel as though a band of pressure is tightening around the head, and the pain may extend to the neck and shoulders. Acute tension headaches may last from hours to days, whereas chronic tension headaches may occur almost every day for months or even years. Ineffective stress management skills, poor posture, and immobility are the leading causes of tension headaches. There is no cure, but the pain can sometimes be avoided and relieved with mindfulness skills (discussed later in the chapter), over-the-counter painkillers, and therapies such as massage, acupuncture, relaxation, hot or cold showers, and rest.

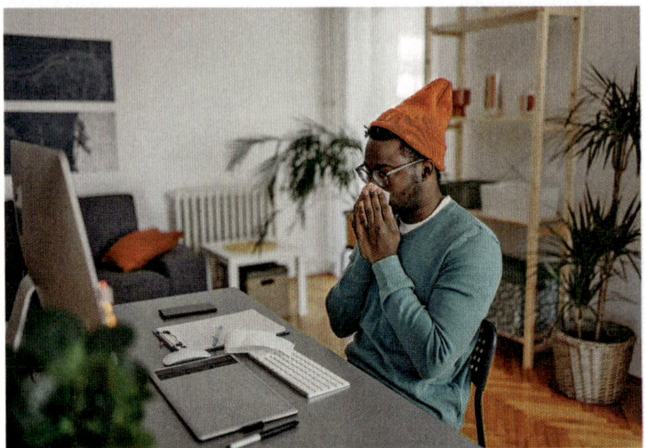

Ongoing stress has been shown to make people more vulnerable to everyday ailments, such as colds and allergies. supersizer/Getty Images

### Ask Yourself

**QUESTIONS FOR CRITICAL THINKING AND REFLECTION**

Have you ever been so stressed that you felt ill? If so, what were your symptoms? How did you handle them? Did the experience affect the way you reacted to other stressful events?

• ***Migraine headaches.*** Migraines typically progress through a series of stages lasting from several minutes to several days. They may produce a variety of symptoms, including throbbing pain that starts on one side of the head and may spread; heightened sensitivity to light; visual disturbances such as flashing lights or temporary blindness; nausea; dizziness; and fatigue. Women are more than twice as likely as men to suffer from migraines. Potential triggers include menstruation, stress, fatigue, atmospheric changes, bright light, specific sounds or odors, and certain foods. The frequency of attacks varies from a few in a lifetime to several per week. Treatment can help reduce the frequency, severity, and duration of migraines. Aerobic exercise is frequently recommended as a treatment for migraine headaches. However, whether exercise reliably reduces frequency and severity of migraine headaches is not entirely clear: Although some evidence indicates that exercise reduces stress levels, a known trigger for migraine headaches, researchers have not been able to replicate these findings consistently. Several studies have failed to show exercise as an effective treatment for migraine headaches. And for some people, exercise itself triggers migraines.

• ***Cluster headaches.*** Cluster headaches are severe headaches that cause intense pain in and around one eye. They usually occur in clusters of one to three headaches each day over a period of weeks or months, alternating with periods of remission in which no headaches occur. More than twice as many men as women suffer from cluster headaches. There is no known cause or cure for cluster headaches, but a number of treatments are available. During cluster periods, it is important to refrain from smoking cigarettes and drinking alcohol because these activities can trigger attacks. For more information on treating headaches and when a headache may signal a serious illness, see Appendix B.

**Other Health Problems** Many other health problems may be caused or worsened by excessive stress, including asthma, cancer, skin disorders, fibromyalgia, insomnia, digestive problems, injuries, and menstrual irregularities, impotence, and pregnancy complications.

## COMMON SOURCES OF STRESS

Recognizing potential sources of stress is an important step in successfully managing the stress in your life.

## Major Life Changes

Any major change in your life that requires adjustment and accommodation can be a source of stress. Early adulthood and the college years are associated with many significant changes, such as moving out of the family home. Even changes typically thought of as positive—graduation, job promotion, marriage—can be stressful.

Life changes that are traumatic, such as getting fired or divorced or experiencing the death of a loved one, may be linked to subsequent health problems in some people. Personality and coping skills, however, are important moderating influences. People with strong support networks and stress-resistant personalities are less likely to become ill in response to life changes than are people with fewer resources.

**QUICK STATS**

**Of students who seek treatment at college and university counseling centers, 65.5% report anxiety, 47% report depression, and 49% report stress.**

—Center for Collegiate Mental Health, 2021

## Daily Hassles

Although major life changes are stressful, they seldom occur regularly. Researchers have proposed that minor problems—life's daily hassles, such as losing your keys or driving in traffic—can be an even greater source of stress because they occur much more often.

People who perceive hassles negatively are likely to experience a moderate stress response every time they face one. Over time, this can take a significant toll on health. Studies indicate that, for some people, daily hassles contribute to a general decrease in overall wellness.

## College Stressors

College is a time of major changes. For many students, college means being away from home and family for the first time. Nearly all students share stresses like the following:

- ***Academic stress.*** Exams, grades, and an endless workload await every college student but can be especially troublesome for students just out of high school.
- ***Interpersonal stress.*** Most students are more than just students; they are also friends, children, employees, spouses, parents, and so on. Managing relationships while juggling the rigors of college life can be daunting, especially if some friends or family members are less than supportive.
- ***Time pressures.*** Class schedules, assignments, and deadlines are an inescapable part of college life. But these time pressures can be compounded drastically for students who also have job or family responsibilities.
- ***Financial concerns.*** The majority of college students need financial aid not just to cover the cost of tuition but also to survive from day to day while in school. For many, college life isn't possible without a job, and the pressure to stay afloat financially competes with academic and other stressors.
- ***Worries about anything but especially about the future.*** As college comes to an end, students face the next set of decisions: thinking about a career, choosing a place to live, and leaving the friends and routines of school behind.

## Job-Related Stressors

According to the *Stress in America* survey, work has been one of the highest-reported sources of stress for Americans. Tight schedules and overtime leave less time for exercising, socializing, and other stress-proofing activities. Worries about job performance, salary, job security, and interactions with others can contribute to stress. High levels of job stress are also common for people who are left out of important decisions relating to their jobs. When workers are given the opportunity to shape their job descriptions and responsibilities, job satisfaction goes up and stress levels go down.

If job-related (or college-related) stress is severe or chronic, the result can be *burnout,* a state of physical, mental, and emotional exhaustion. Burnout occurs most often in highly motivated and driven individuals who come to feel that their work is not recognized or that they are not accomplishing their goals. People in the helping professions—teachers, social workers, caregivers, police officers, and so on—are also prone to burnout. Healthcare workers and teachers were especially affected by burnout during the Covid-19 pandemic. For some people who suffer from burnout, a vacation or leave of absence may be appropriate. For others, a reduced work schedule, better communication with superiors, or a change in job goals may be necessary. Improving time management skills can also help.

## Social Stressors

Social networks can be real or virtual. Both types can help improve your ability to deal with stress, but any social network can also become a stressor in itself.

**Real Social Networks** The college years can be a time of great change in interpersonal relationships—becoming part of a new community, meeting people from different backgrounds, leaving old relationships behind. You may feel stress as you meet people of other ethnic, racial, or socioeconomic groups. You may feel torn between sticking with people who share your background and connecting with those you have not encountered before. If English is not

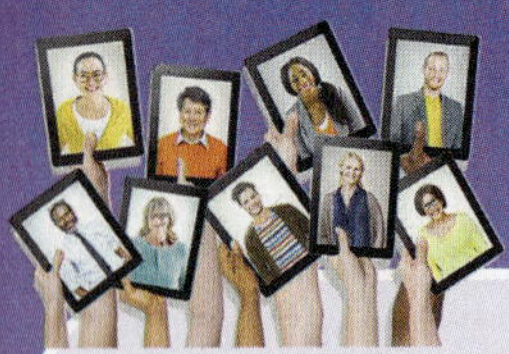

## DIVERSITY MATTERS
### Diverse Populations, Discrimination, and Stress

Stress is universal, but an individual's response to stress can vary depending on gender, cultural background, prior experience, and genetic factors. In diverse multiethnic and multicultural nations such as the United States, some groups face special stressors and have higher-than-average rates of stress-related physical and emotional problems. These groups include racial and ethnic minorities, people affected by poverty or physical or mental disabilities, and those who don't express mainstream gender roles.

Discrimination occurs when people speak or act according to their prejudices—biased, negative beliefs or attitudes toward some group. A blatant example, rising to the level of hate speech and criminal activity, is painting a swastika on a Jewish studies house or vandalizing a mosque. A more subtle example is when the police are called on a Black or Middle Eastern person by neighbors who see something suspicious in normal behavior, like having a barbecue or walking a dog.

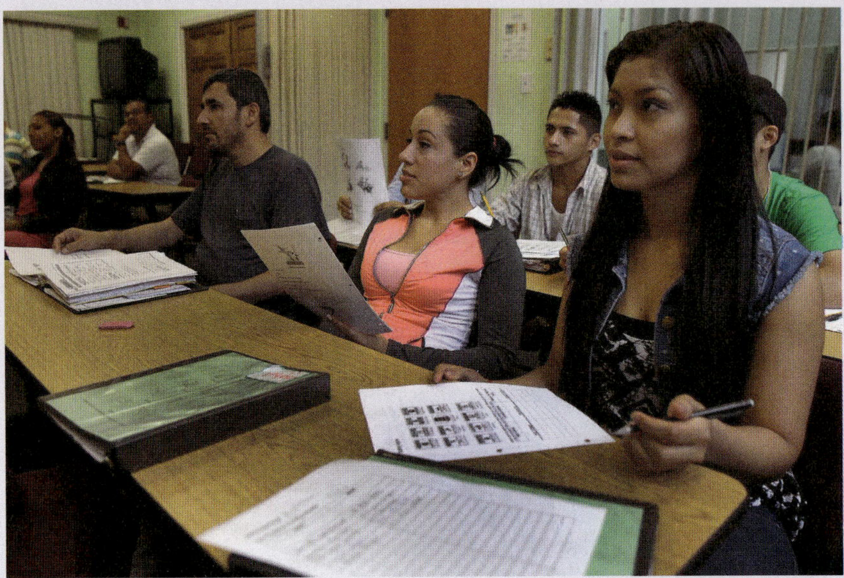

David L Ryan/The Boston Globe/Getty Images

Immigrants to the United States have to learn to live in a new society. Doing so requires a balance between assimilating and changing to be like the majority, and maintaining a connection to their own culture, language, and religion. The process of acculturation is generally stressful, especially when the person's background is radically different from that of the people he or she is now living among, or when people in the new community are suspicious or unwelcoming, as has recently been the case with immigrants from war-torn regions of the Middle East.

Both immigrants and minorities who have lived for generations in the United States can face job- and school-related stressors because of stereotypes and discrimination. They may make less money in comparable jobs with comparable levels of education and may find it more difficult to achieve leadership positions.

On a positive note, however, many who experience hardship, disability, or prejudice develop effective goal-directed coping skills and are successful at overcoming obstacles and managing the stress they face.

your first language, you may face the added burden of interacting in a language with which you are not completely comfortable. All these pressures can become significant sources of stress. (See the box "Diverse Populations, Discrimination, and Stress.")

**Digital Social Networks** Technology can connect you with people all over the world and make many tasks easier, but it can also increase stress. The 2018 *Stress in America* survey showed that social media provided a feeling of support for 55% of Generation Zs; 45% reported feeling judged, and 38% reported feeling bad about themselves. Being electronically connected to work, family, and friends all the time can impinge on your personal space, waste time, and distract you.

People who constantly check their phones and social media feeds report higher levels of overall stress than do those who do not engage with technology as often. They are also more likely to report feeling disconnected from their family as a result of technology and to report being stressed by political and cultural discussions on social media.

At the same time, social media can be beneficial when making meaningful connections with friends and family, learning a new skill, or accessing health care. Which activity the user chooses to do might be more important than the amount of time spent on the screen: studies have found that it's better for a person's well-being to actively engage, such as commenting on posts, than to passively scroll through them.

## Other Stressors

Have you tried to eat at a restaurant where the food was great, but the atmosphere was so noisy that it put you on edge? This is an example of a minor environmental stressor—a condition or event in the physical environment that causes stress.

## WELLNESS ON CAMPUS

### Coping with News of Traumatic Events

We are continually exposed to news of tragic events: shootings, natural disasters, war, pandemics, and poverty. Both experiencing trauma and observing it can result in extreme stress, requiring time and effort to recover. Such events can weaken your sense of security and create uncertainty about how the future may unfold. People react to such news in different ways, depending on their proximity to the event and how recent it was. People far from the site may suffer emotional reactions simply from watching endless coverage on television.

Responses to trauma include disbelief, shock, fear, anger, resentment, anxiety, mood swings, irritability, sadness, depression, panic, guilt, apathy, feelings of isolation or powerlessness, and many of the symptoms of excess stress. Some people affected by such violence develop PTSD, a more serious condition.

In the case of the 2022 Russian invasion of Ukraine, where thousands were killed, injured, and displaced, numerous videos appearing daily on television and online offer a grim view depicting the suffering. Communities mobilized quickly to respond to the expected surge in behavioral health needs generated by the attacks. Information sources and support groups were established for people grieving the loss of friends, family, neighbors, or colleagues.

Unfortunately these kinds of horrific events have been repeated numerous times in recent years. If you are becoming preoccupied with some recent disastrous event, such as war or a school shooting, take these steps:

- Be sure you have the best information about what happened and whether a continuing risk is present. That information may be available through websites or on local radio or TV stations; it's a good idea to check your facts through multiple sources.
- Don't expose yourself to so much media coverage that it overwhelms you.
- Take care of yourself. Use the stress-relief techniques discussed in this chapter.
- Share your feelings and concerns with others. Be a supportive listener.
- If you feel able, help others in any way you can, such as by volunteering to work with victims.
- If you feel emotionally distressed days or weeks after the event, consider asking for professional help.

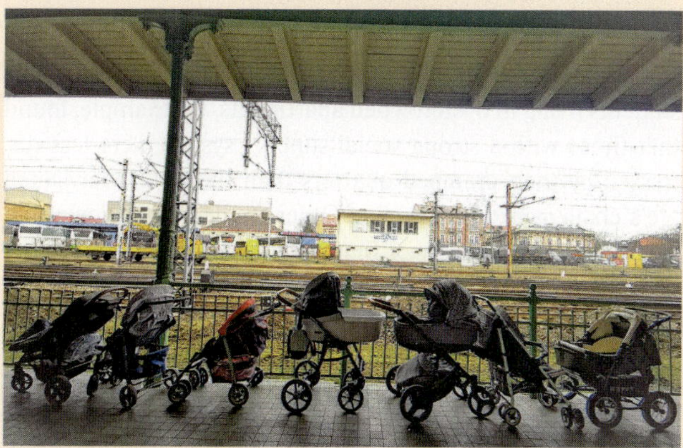

Communities mobilized: Here, volunteers offered strollers to Ukrainian refugee mothers arriving at a train station in Przemysl, Poland. Francesco Malavolta/ASSOCIATED PRESS

Examples of more disturbing and disruptive, even catastrophic, environmental stressors include pandemics, natural disasters, acts of violence, industrial accidents, and intrusive noises or smells. Many environmental stressors are mere inconveniences that are easy to avoid. Others, such as pollen, crime, or construction noise, may be unavoidable daily sources of stress. For those who live in poor or violent neighborhoods, the environment can contain major stressors, and in every corner of the country today, people are exposed to disturbing news and images via the media. According to the 2022 *Stress in America* survey, inflation and war are the biggest sources of stress for Americans at large.

Many stressors are found not in our environment but within ourselves, and often they are created by the ways we approach things. For example, striving to reach goals can enhance self-esteem if the goals are reasonable. Unrealistic expectations, however, can be a significant source of stress and can damage self-esteem. Other internal stressors are emotional states such as despair or hostility, and physical states, such as chronic illness and exhaustion; each can be both a cause and an effect of unmanaged stress.

Traumatic stressors are extreme stressors that result from exposure to events that are life threatening and that can cause bodily injury. For college-age people, the most common traumatic stressors are automobile accidents, assaults, and rape. Being the victim of or even witnessing such an event can result in posttraumatic stress disorder (PTSD). Symptoms can include obsessive thinking about what happened and going out of your way to avoid reminders of the event. This may be accompanied by anxiety, depression, and inability to sleep. PTSD is not something you can handle on your own. If symptoms are severe or persist, you should contact a counselor to help you (see the box "Coping with News of Traumatic Events").

### Ask Yourself

**QUESTIONS FOR CRITICAL THINKING AND REFLECTION**

What are the top two or three stressors in your life right now? Are they new to your life—as part of your college experience—or have you experienced them in the past? Do they include both positive and negative experiences (eustress and distress)?

## MANAGING STRESS

You can control most stress in your life by taking the following steps:

- Shore up your support system.
- Improve your communication skills.
- Develop healthy exercise and eating habits.
- Learn to identify and moderate individual stressors.
- Learn mindfulness skills.

The effort required for stress management is well worth the time. People who manage stress effectively not only are healthier but also have more time to enjoy life and accomplish goals.

### Social Support

Meaningful connections with others can play a key role in stress management and overall wellness. One study of college students living in overcrowded apartments, for example, found that those with a strong social support system were less distressed by their cramped quarters than those who navigated life's challenges on their own. Other studies have shown that married people live longer than single people and have lower death rates from a wide range of conditions, although some studies suggest that marriage benefits men more than women.

A sense of isolation can lead to chronic stress, which in turn can increase one's susceptibility to illnesses like colds and to chronic illnesses, such as heart disease. Although the mechanism isn't clear, social isolation can be as significant to mortality rates as factors like smoking, high blood pressure, and obesity.

There is no single best pattern of social support that works for everyone. However, research suggests that having a variety of types of relationships may be important for wellness. Here are some tips for strengthening your social ties:

- ***Foster friendships.*** Keep in regular contact with your friends. Offer respect, trust, and acceptance, and provide help and support in times of need. Build your communication skills, and express appreciation for your friends.

- ***Keep your family ties strong.*** Stay in touch with the family members you feel close to. If your family doesn't function well as a support system for its members, create a second "family" of people with whom you have built meaningful ties.

- ***Get involved with a group.*** Do volunteer work, take a class, attend a lecture series, or join a religious group. These types of activities can give you a sense of security, a place to talk about your feelings or concerns, and a way to build new friendships. Choose activities that are meaningful to you and that include direct involvement with other people.

**QUICK STATS**

**Before the pandemic, 73% of Americans reported exercising in the past month; in 2020, 83% in the past week, although the greatest increase occurred among male, white, university-educated, wealthier people.**

—Sher and Wu 2021

### Volunteering

Studies show that not all giving is the same—for example, donating money does not have the same beneficial health effects as volunteering that involves personal contact. A few simple guidelines can help you get the most out of giving:

- Choose a volunteer activity that puts you in contact with people.
- Volunteer with a group. Sharing your interests with other volunteers increases social support. Volunteering seems to have the most benefits for people who also have other close relationships and social interests.
- Know your limits. Helping that goes beyond what you can handle depletes your own resources and is detrimental to your health.

### Communication

Communicating in an assertive way that respects the rights of others—while protecting your own rights—can prevent stressful situations from getting out of control.

Some people have trouble either telling others what they need or saying no to the needs of others. They may suppress their feelings of anger, frustration, and resentment, and they may end up feeling taken advantage of or suffering in unhealthy relationships. At the other extreme are people who express anger openly and directly by being verbally or physically aggressive or indirectly by making critical, hurtful comments to others. Because their abusive behavior pushes away other people, they also have problems with relationships.

Better communication skills can help everyone form and maintain healthy relationships. Chapter 3 includes a discussion of anger and its impact on health and relationships. Chapter 5 discusses communication techniques for building healthy relationships.

### Exercise

Exercise helps maintain a healthy body and mind and even stimulates the birth of new brain cells. Regular physical activity can also reduce many of the negative effects of stress. Consider the following examples:

- Taking a long walk can decrease anxiety and blood pressure.
- A brisk 10-minute walk can leave you feeling more relaxed and energetic for up to two hours.
- People who exercise regularly react with milder physical stress responses before, during, and after exposure to stressors.
- In one study, people who took three brisk 45-minute walks each week for three months reported fewer daily hassles and an increased sense of wellness.

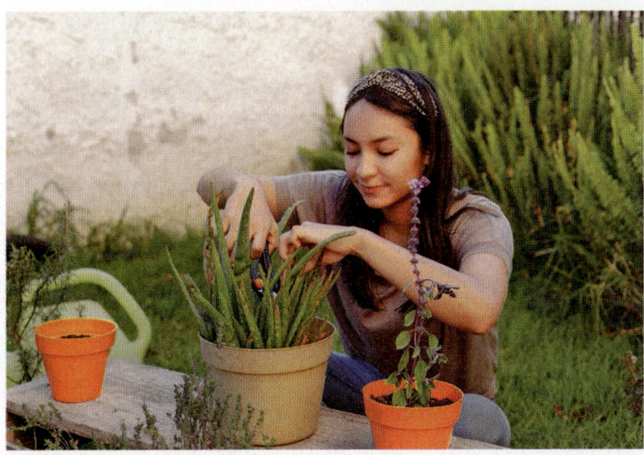

Exercise—even light activity—can be an antidote to stress. Fernanda_ Reyes/Shutterstock

## Nutrition

A healthful diet gives you an energy bank to draw from whenever you experience stress. Eating wisely also can enhance your feelings of self-control and self-esteem. Learning the principles of sound nutrition is easy, and sensible eating habits rapidly become second nature when practiced regularly. (For information about nutrition and healthy eating habits, see Chapter 10)

For managing stress, limit or avoid caffeine. Although one or two cups of coffee a day probably won't hurt you, caffeine is a mildly addictive stimulant that leaves some people jittery, irritable, and unable to sleep. Consuming caffeine during stressful situations can raise blood pressure and increase levels of cortisol.

Although your diet affects the way your body handles stress, the reverse is also true. Excess stress can negatively affect the way you eat. Many people, for example, respond to stress by overeating; other people skip meals or stop eating altogether during stressful periods. Not only are both responses ineffective (they don't address the causes of stress), but they are also potentially unhealthy.

## Time Management

Overcommitment, procrastination, and even boredom are significant stressors for many people. Try these strategies for improving your time management skills:

- ***Set priorities.*** Divide your tasks into three groups: essential, important, and trivial. Focus on the first two, and ignore the third.
- ***Schedule tasks for peak efficiency.*** You've probably noticed you're most productive at certain times of the day (or night). Schedule as many of your tasks for those hours as you can, and stick to your schedule.
- ***Set realistic goals and write them down.*** Attainable goals spur you on. Impossible goals, by definition, cause frustration and failure. Fully commit yourself to achieving your goals by putting them in writing.
- ***Budget enough time.*** For each project you undertake, calculate how long it will take to complete. Then tack on another 10–15%, or even 25%, as a buffer.
- ***Break up long-term goals into short-term ones.*** Instead of waiting for large blocks of time, use short amounts of time to start a project or keep it moving.
- ***Visualize the achievement of your goals.*** By mentally rehearsing your performance of a task, you will be able to reach your goal more smoothly.
- ***Keep track of the tasks you put off.*** Analyze why you procrastinate. If the task is difficult or unpleasant, look for ways to make it easier or more fun.
- ***Consider doing your least favorite tasks first.*** Once you have the most unpleasant ones out of the way, you can work on the tasks you enjoy more.
- ***Consolidate tasks when possible.*** For example, try walking to the store so that you run your errands and exercise in the same block of time.
- ***Identify quick transitional tasks.*** Keep a list of 5- to 10-minute tasks you can do while waiting or between other tasks, such as watering your plants, doing the dishes, or checking a homework assignment.
- ***Delegate responsibility.*** Asking for help when you have too much to do is no cop-out; it's good time management. Just don't delegate the jobs you know you should do yourself.
- ***Say no when necessary.*** If the demands made on you don't seem reasonable, say no—tactfully, but without guilt or apology.
- ***Give yourself a break.*** Allow time for play—free, unstructured time when you can ignore the clock. Don't consider this a waste of time. Play renews you and enables you to work more efficiently.
- ***Avoid your personal "time sinks."*** You can probably identify your own time sinks—activities that consistently use up more time than you anticipate and put you behind schedule, like binging Netflix, checking your social media notifications, or texting with friends. On particularly busy days, avoid these problematic activities altogether. For example, if you have a big paper due, don't sit down for a five-minute Instagram break if that's likely to turn into a two-hour break. Try a five-minute walk instead.
- ***Stop thinking or talking about what you're going to do, and just do it!*** Sometimes the best solution for procrastination is to stop waiting for the right moment and just get started. You will probably find that things are not as bad as you feared, and your momentum will keep you going.

## Cultivating Spiritual Wellness

Spirituality involves a sense or belief that there is more to being human than individual, bodily experience; spiritual people strive toward self-knowledge, personal growth, and a better, useful life. Researchers have linked spiritual wellness to longer life expectancy, reduced risk of disease, faster recovery, and improved emotional health. Although spirituality is difficult to study, and researchers aren't sure how or why spirituality seems to improve health, several explanations have been offered. To develop spiritual wellness, choose thoughtful activities that are meaningful to you, such as the following:

- Look inward. Spend quiet time alone with your thoughts and feelings.
- Spend time in nature, experiencing continuity with the natural world.
- Notice art, architecture, and music.
- Engage in a favorite activity that allows you to express your creative side.
- Engage in a personal spiritual practice, such as prayer, meditation, or yoga.

Reach out to others:

- Share writings that inspire you.
- Practice small acts of personal kindness for people you know as well as for strangers.
- Perform community service.

## Confiding in Yourself through Writing

Keeping a diary is analogous to confiding in others, except that you are confiding in and becoming more attuned to yourself. This form of coping with severe stress may be especially helpful for those who find it difficult to open up to others. Although writing about traumatic and stressful events may have a short-term negative effect on mood, over the long term, stress is reduced and positive changes in health occur. A key to promoting health and well-being through journaling is to write about your emotional responses to stressful events. Set aside a special time each day or week to write down your feelings about stressful events in your life.

## Thinking and Acting Constructively

Certain ideas, beliefs, perceptions, and patterns of thinking can add to your stress level. One way to address this is through **mindfulness,** the intentional cultivation of attention in a way that is nonjudging and nonstriving. This objectivity and openness makes mindfulness an ideal way to restore a sense of balance and manage stress. Each of the following techniques can help you change unhealthy thought patterns to ones that will help you manage stress. (also see the box "Mindfulness Meditation"). As with any skill, mastering these techniques takes practice and patience. Think back to the worries you had last week. How many of them were needless? By growing more aware of the ways you habitually think and feel, you can learn to recognize habits of mind that create distress and divest from them before they overwhelm you. Think about what you *can* control, particularly your way of looking at things. If you can successfully recognize that a stressor is occurring, you can better control your response to it. Invest energy in considering how you may better promote the things you want individually or socially. This may mean reflecting on how you may better deal with an unpleasant person or stay focused in a class you find boring.

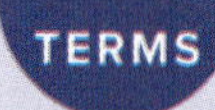


**mindfulness** The intentional cultivation of attention in a way that is nonjudging and nonstriving.

**Take Control** A situation often feels more stressful if you feel you're not in control of it. Time may seem to be slipping away before a big exam, for example. Unexpected obstacles may appear in your path, throwing you off course. When you feel your environment is controlling you instead of the other way around, take charge! Concentrate on what you can control rather than what you cannot, and set realistic goals. Be confident of your ability to succeed.

**Problem-Solve** Students with greater problem-solving abilities report easier adjustment to university life, higher motivation levels, lower stress levels, and higher grades. When you find yourself stewing over a problem, sit down with a piece of paper and try this approach:

1. Define the problem in one or two sentences.
2. Identify the causes of the problem.
3. Consider alternative solutions. Don't just stop with the most obvious one.
4. Weigh positive and negative consequences for each alternative.
5. Make a decision—choose a solution.
6. Make a list of tasks you must perform to act on your decision.
7. Carry out the tasks on your list.
8. Evaluate the outcome and revise your approach if necessary.

**Modify Your Expectations** Expectations are exhausting and restricting. The fewer expectations you have, the more possibilities for spontaneity and joy. The more you expect from others, the more often you will feel let down. And trying to meet the expectations others have of you is often futile.

**Stay Positive** If you tend to beat up on yourself—"Late for class again! You can't even cope with college! How do you expect to ever hold down a real job?"—try being kind to yourself instead. Talk to yourself as you would to a child you love: "You're a smart, capable person. You've solved other problems; you'll handle this one. Tomorrow you'll simply schedule things so you get to class with a few minutes to spare."

## TAKE CHARGE
### Mindfulness Meditation

Mindfulness meditation is a powerful way to manage stress and has been the topic of an enormous body of medical research since 1979. At the center of this research is mindfulness-based stress reduction (MBSR), which as a program continues to be the mindfulness intervention most intensively researched to this day. This research demonstrates that when it comes to stress and its influence on health, you can do far more for yourself than anyone else can.

MBSR was founded by Jon Kabat-Zinn in 1979 at the University of Massachusetts Medical Center and is now offered around the world.

Mindfulness is both a mental state and the practices that cultivate this mental state. We cultivate this mental state by paying attention in a kind and nonjudgmental way to our mental, physical, and behavioral activities as they happen. By investing this kind of attention in ourselves and our lives, we soon discover that we create most of our own stress, and that we can each do more than anyone else can to reduce that stress and take better care of ourselves. Here are two practices to use for stress reduction.

#### Mindful Breathing

You are always breathing, so this is a powerful and convenient way to become present wherever you go and in whatever you do. After you read these instructions, close your eyes and invest 5–15 minutes in being present with your breath.

Sitting comfortably where you are right now, bring your body into a posture that is upright and supported, with a sense of balance and dignity. Align your head, neck, and body in a way that is neither too rigid nor too relaxed, but somewhere in between. The intention is to be wakeful and alert, yet not tense; at ease, but not sleeping.

Bring attention to your breathing, wherever you feel it most prominently, and notice the sensations of your breath coming and going as it will, in its own way and with its own pace. If your mind wanders from your breath, return to it by feeling the sensations of the breath as they come and go. Use these sensations as your way to be present, here and now, in each successive moment for the time you have set aside. Research has repeatedly demonstrated that extending this practice to 30 or 45 minutes on a regular basis significantly reduces stress and stress-related illnesses and conditions.

#### Walking Meditation

Find a place where you can walk and be uninterrupted by other people or traffic—if possible, in natural surroundings, like in a park. You can adapt this practice to fit yourself, whatever your circumstances are with mobility—for example, it can become a mindful-rolling practice if you rely on a wheelchair. Once you're ready, begin walking—slowly at first (as slowly as possible for about 10 minutes)—paying close attention to each step and using the sensations of each foot touching the ground as your way to be present. When you are ready, accelerate your pace, broadening your attention to take in more of your experience as you walk. In this mindful-movement practice, you may walk any distance, anywhere, at any speed that feels right for you. In the beginning, however, give yourself about 30 minutes.

The principal instruction is to be fully present in each moment you are walking rather than consumed with mind chatter or destination. Be open to the experience of your environment and notice, for example, the way clouds move or how the sunlight glistens in the trees and foliage around you. Turn toward whatever calls your attention and be with it as long as you like, stopping if you want to take a close look at a bug or flowers or to listen to the rustling of leaves. Remember, the overarching intention is to be mindful, to be in this experience of the now.

As you become more skilled in mindful awareness practice, you will be able to do this anywhere, even on a bustling college campus.

**Practice Affirmations** One way of cultivating the positive is to systematically repeat positive thoughts, or *affirmations,* to yourself. For example, if you react to stress with low self-esteem, you might repeat sentences such as "I accept myself completely" and "It doesn't matter what others say, but what I believe." Say kinder and more loving things to yourself every day to promote more responding and less reacting.

**Cultivate Your Sense of Humor** When it comes to stress, laughter may be the best medicine. It is said, "He who can laugh at himself will never cease to be amused!" Even a fleeting smile produces changes in your autonomic nervous system that can lift your spirits. A few minutes of belly laughing can be as invigorating as brisk exercise. Hearty laughter elevates your heart rate, aids digestion, eases pain, and triggers the release of endorphins and other pleasurable and stimulating chemicals in the brain. After a good laugh, your muscles go slack; your pulse and blood pressure dip below normal. You are relaxed. Cultivate the ability to laugh at yourself, and you'll have a handy and instantly effective stress reliever.

**Progressive Muscle Relaxation** In this simple relaxation technique, you tense and then relax the muscles of the body one group at a time. Also known as deep muscle relaxation, this technique addresses the muscle tension that occurs when the body is experiencing stress. Consciously relaxing tensed muscles sends a message to other body systems to reduce the stress response.

Begin by inhaling as you contract your right fist. Then exhale as you release your fist. Repeat. Contract and relax your right bicep. Repeat. Do the same using your left arm. Then, working from forehead to feet, contract and relax other muscles. Repeat each contraction at least once, inhaling as you tense and exhaling as you relax. To speed up the process, tense and relax more muscles at one time—for example, both arms simultaneously. With practice, you'll be able to relax quickly just by clenching and releasing only your fists.

**Focus on What's Important** A major source of stress is trying to store too much data. Forget unimportant details (they will usually be self-evident) and organize important information. One technique you can try is to "chunk" important material into categories. If your next exam covers three chapters from your textbook, consider each chapter a chunk of information. Then break down each chunk into its three or four most important features. Create a mental outline that allows you to trace your way from the most general category down to the most specific details. This technique can be applied to managing daily responsibilities as well.

## Relaxation and Body Awareness Techniques

Practicing mindfulness promotes stronger connections between the prefrontal cortex and the amygdala. This connection has been demonstrated to facilitate greater problem-solving skills, emotional self-regulation, and resilience. Practicing mindfulness includes forms of meditation as well as more familiar forms of neuromuscular activities, such as yoga and tai chi.

**Yoga** Hatha yoga, the most common yoga style practiced in the United States, emphasizes physical balance and breath control. It integrates components of flexibility, muscular strength and endurance, and muscle relaxation; it also sometimes serves as a preliminary to meditation. A session of yoga typically involves a series of postures, each held for a few seconds to several minutes, which involve stretching and balance and coordinated breathing. Yoga can be a powerful way to cultivate body awareness, ease, and flexibility.

**Tai Chi** This martial art (in Chinese, *taijiquan*) is a system of self-defense that incorporates philosophical concepts from Taoism and Confucianism. In addition to self-defense, tai chi aims to bring the body into balance and harmony to promote health and spiritual growth. It teaches practitioners to remain calm and centered, to conserve and concentrate energy, and to manipulate force by becoming part of it—by "going with the flow." Tai chi is considered the gentlest of the martial arts. Instead of quick and powerful movements, tai chi consists of a series of slow, fluid, elegant movements, which reinforce the idea of moving *with* rather than *against* the stressors of everyday life.

**Biofeedback** Biofeedback helps people reduce their response to stress by enabling them to become more aware of their level of physiological arousal. In biofeedback, some measure of stress—perspiration, heart rate, skin temperature, or muscle tension—is electronically monitored, and feedback is given using sound (a tone or music), light, or a meter or dial. With practice, people begin to exercise conscious control over their physiological stress responses. The point of biofeedback training is to develop the ability to transfer the control skills to daily life without the use of electronic equipment.

**Sleep** Don't underestimate the value of a good night's sleep as a means of managing stress. Getting enough sleep isn't just good for you physically. Adequate sleep also improves mood, fosters feelings of competence and self-worth, enhances mental functioning, and supports emotional functioning. Chapter 4 will tell you more about the physiology of sleep and how you can sleep better.

## Counterproductive Coping Strategies

College is a time when you'll learn to adapt to new and challenging situations and gain skills that will last a lifetime. It is also a time when many people develop counterproductive and unhealthy habits in response to stress. Such habits can last well beyond graduation.

**Tobacco Use** Cigarettes and other tobacco products contain *nicotine,* a chemical that enhances the actions of neurotransmitters. Nicotine can make you feel relaxed and even increase your ability to concentrate, but it is highly addictive. In fact, nicotine dependence itself is considered a psychological disorder. Cigarette smoke also contains substances that cause heart disease, stroke, lung cancer, and emphysema. These negative consequences far outweigh any beneficial effects, and tobacco use should be avoided. The easiest way to avoid the habit is to not start. See Chapter 9 for more about the health effects of tobacco use and for tips on how to quit.

**Use of Alcohol and Other Drugs** Like nicotine, alcohol is addictive, and many alcoholics find it hard to relax without a drink. Having a few drinks might make you feel temporarily at ease, and drinking until you're intoxicated may help you forget your current stressors. However, using alcohol to deal with stress places you at risk for all the short- and long-term problems associated with alcohol abuse. It also does nothing to address the causes of stress in your life. For more about the responsible use of alcohol, refer to Chapter 9.

Using other psychoactive drugs to cope with stress is also usually counterproductive:

- ***Stimulants***, such as *amphetamines,* can activate the stress response. They also affect the same areas of the brain that are involved in regulating the stress response.

- Use of ***marijuana*** causes a brief period of euphoria and decreased short-term memory and attentional abilities. Physiological effects clearly show that marijuana use doesn't cause relaxation; in fact, some neurochemicals in marijuana act to enhance the stress response, and getting high on a regular basis can elicit panic attacks. To compound this, withdrawal from marijuana may also be associated with an increase in circulating stress hormones.

- ***Opioids*** such as morphine and heroin can mimic the effects of your body's natural painkillers and act to reduce anxiety. However, tolerance to opioids develops quickly, and many users become dependent.

- ***Tranquilizers*** such as Valium and Xanax mimic some of the functions of your body's parasympathetic nervous system, and as with opioids, tolerance develops quickly, causing increased dependency and toxicity.

QUICK STATS

**Alcohol-related deaths in the United States rose from 2019 to 2020 by 25% (99,000 deaths).**

—*JAMA*, 2022

For more information about the health effects of using psychoactive drugs, see Chapter 8.

**Unhealthy Eating Habits** The nutrients in the food you eat provide energy and substances needed to maintain your body. Eating is also psychologically rewarding. The feelings of satiation and sedation that follow eating produce a relaxed state. However, regular use of eating as a means of coping with stress may lead to unhealthy eating habits. In fact, the 2022 *Stress in America* survey found that since the Covid-19 pandemic began, almost three in five people had experienced unwanted weight changes.

Many dietary supplements are marketed for stress reduction, but supplements are not required to meet the same standards as medications in terms of safety, effectiveness, and manufacturing (see Chapters 10 and 16).

## Getting Help

What are the most important sources of stress in your life? Are you coping successfully with them? No single strategy or program for managing stress will work for everyone. The most important starting point for a successful stress management plan is to learn to listen to your body. When you recognize the stress response and the emotions and thoughts that accompany it, you'll be in a position to take charge of that crucial moment and handle it in a healthy way.

If the techniques discussed so far don't provide you with enough relief, you might need to look further. Excellent self-help guides can be found in bookstores or the library. Additional resources are listed in the For More Information section at the end of the chapter.

Your student health center or student affairs office can tell you whether your campus has a mindfulness-based stress-reduction program. If you are seeking social support, see if your campus offers a peer counseling program. Such programs are usually staffed by volunteer students with special training that emphasizes maintaining confidentiality. Peer counselors can guide you to other campus or community resources or can simply provide understanding.

Support groups are typically organized around a particular issue or problem. In your area, you might find a support group for first-year students; for reentering students; for single parents; for students of your race or ethnicity, religion, or national origin; for people with eating disorders; or for rape survivors. The number of such groups has increased in recent years as more and more people discover how therapeutic it can be to talk with others who share the same situation.

Short-term psychotherapy can also be tremendously helpful in dealing with stress-related problems. Your student health center may offer psychotherapy on a sliding-fee scale; the county mental health center in your area may do the same. If you belong to any type of religious organization, check to see whether pastoral counseling is available. Your physician can refer you to psychotherapists in your community. Not all therapists are right for all people, so be prepared to have initial sessions with several. Choose the one with whom you feel most comfortable.

### TIPS FOR TODAY AND THE FUTURE

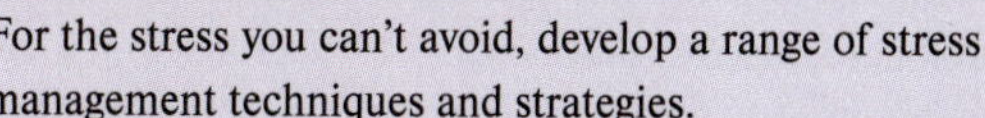

For the stress you can't avoid, develop a range of stress management techniques and strategies.

**RIGHT NOW YOU CAN:**

- Practice a mindfulness exercise for 5–45 minutes.
- Practice some aerobic exercise for 30–45 minutes.
- Get out your date book and schedule what you'll be doing the rest of today and tomorrow. Pencil in a short walk and a conversation with a friend.
- Reflect on your sleep habits and patterns.

**IN THE FUTURE YOU CAN:**

- Take a class or workshop, such as mindfulness-based stress reduction or one in assertiveness training or time management, to help you overcome a source of stress.
- Find a way to build relaxing time into every day. Just 15 minutes of meditation, stretching, or yoga can induce relaxation.
- Use your knowledge of factors that improve and detract from sleep to establish healthy patterns for yourself.

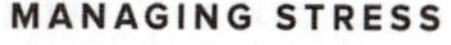

## SUMMARY

- When confronted with a stressor, the body undergoes a set of physical changes known as the fight, flight, or freeze reaction. The autonomic nervous system and endocrine system act on many targets in the body to prepare it for action.
- Emotional and behavioral responses to stressors vary among individuals. Ineffective responses increase stress but can be moderated or changed.
- Factors that influence emotional and behavioral responses to stressors include personality, cultural background, gender, and past experiences.
- The general adaptation syndrome (GAS) has three stages: alarm, resistance, and exhaustion.
- A high allostatic load characterized by prolonged or repeated exposure to stress hormones can increase a person's risk of health problems.
- Psychoneuroimmunology (PNI) looks at how the physiological changes of the stress response affect the immune system and thereby increase the risk of illness.
- Health problems linked to stress include cardiovascular disease, colds and other infections, asthma and allergies, flare-ups of chronic diseases, psychological problems, digestive problems, headaches, insomnia, and injuries.
- A cluster of major life events that require adjustment and accommodation can lead to increased stress and an increased risk of health problems. Minor daily hassles increase stress if they are perceived negatively.
- Sources of stress associated with college may be academic, interpersonal, time related, or financial pressures.
- Job-related stress is common, particularly for employees who have little control over decisions relating to their jobs. If stress is severe or prolonged, burnout may occur.
- New and changing relationships, prejudice, and discrimination are examples of interpersonal and social stressors.
- Social support systems help buffer people against the effects of stress and make illness less likely. Good communication skills foster healthy relationships.
- Exercise, nutrition, sleep, and time management are wellness behaviors that reduce stress and increase energy.
- Developing new and healthy patterns of thinking, such as practicing problem solving, monitoring self-talk, and cultivating a sense of humor, is important for coping with stress.
- Body awareness techniques, mindfulness exercises, and biofeedback are useful for some people.
- Along with exercise and good nutrition, good sleep is a critical pillar of good health.
- Additional help in dealing with stress is available from self-help books, peer counseling, support groups, and psychotherapy.

## FOR MORE INFORMATION

*American Headache Society.* Provides information for consumers and clinicians about different types of headaches, their causes, and their treatment.

http://www.americanheadachesociety.org

*American Psychiatric Association: Healthy Minds, Healthy Lives.* Provides information about mental wellness developed especially for college students.

http://www.psychiatry.org/news-room/apa-blogs

*American Psychological Association.* Provides information about stress management and psychological disorders.

http://www.apa.org

http://www.apa.org/helpcenter

*Association for Applied Psychophysiology and Biofeedback.* Provides information about biofeedback and referrals to certified biofeedback practitioners.

http://www.aapb.org

*Benson-Henry Institute for Mind Body Medicine.* Provides information about stress management and relaxation techniques.

https://bensonhenryinstitute.org/

*Center for Mindfulness in Medicine, Health Care, and Society (U Mass Medical School).* Provides information about mindfulness-based stress reduction (MBSR) professional training, research, and resources.

http://www.umassmed.edu/cfm/

*National Institute of Mental Health (NIMH).* Publishes brochures about stress and stress management as well as other aspects of mental health.

http://www.nimh.nih.gov

*Spirit Rock Meditation Center.* A resource for meditation retreats and education in mindfulness meditation.

http://www.spiritrock.org

## SELECTED BIBLIOGRAPHY


American Psychological Association. 2017. *Stress in America: Coping with Change.* Washington, DC: American Psychological Association.

American Psychological Association. 2017. *Stress in America: The State of Our Nation.* Washington, DC: American Psychological Association.

American Psychological Association. 2018. *Stress in America: Generation Z.* Washington, DC: American Psychological Association (https://www.apa.org/news/press/releases/stress/2018/stress-gen-z.pdf).

American Psychological Association. 2020. *Stress in America: Stress in the Time of COVID-19.* Volume 1. Washington, DC: American Psychological Association (https://www.apa.org/news/press/releases/stress/2020/stress-in-america-covid.pdf).

American College Health Association. 2021. *American College Health Association-National College Health Assessment III: Reference Group Executive Summary Fall 2021.* Hanover, MD: American College Health Association.

American Psychological Association. 2022. *Stress in America 2022.* Washington, DC: American Psychological Association (https://www.apa.org/news/press/releases/stress/2022/infographics-march).

Bellezza, S., N. Paharia, and A. Keinan. 2017. Conspicuous consumption of time: When busyness and lack of leisure time become a status symbol. *Journal of Consumer Research* 44(1): 118–138.

Caldwell, K., et al. 2010. Developing mindfulness in college students through movement-based courses: Effects on self-regulatory self-efficacy, mood, stress, and sleep quality. *Journal of American College Health* 58(5): 433–442.

Center for Collegiate Mental Health. 2022. *2021 Annual Report* STA: 22-132 (https://ccmh.psu.edu/annual-reports).

Centers for Disease Control and Prevention. 2018. *Coping with a Disaster or Traumatic Event* (http://emergency.cdc.gov/mentalhealth/general.asp).

Cohen, M. 2021. Tension Headache vs. Migraine: How to Tell the Difference. WebMD (https://www.webmd.com/migraines-headaches/migraine-vs-tension-headache).

Dallman, M. 2010. Stress-induced obesity and the emotional nervous system. *Trends in Endocrinology and Metabolism* 21(3): 159–165.

Darabaneanu, S. 2011. Aerobic exercise as a therapy option for migraine: A pilot study. *International Journal of Sports Medicine* 32(6): 455–460.

Davidson, R., and S. Begley. 2012. *The Emotional Life of Your Brain*. New York: Penguin.

Eisenberg, D., et al. 2016. Too distressed to learn? Mental health among community college students. *Wisconsin HOPE Lab*, March: 1–15.

Flory, E. S. 2019. Student stress surges: Community colleges strive to meet the increasing demand for mental health services nationwide. *Community College Journal*, August/September (https://www.ccjournal-digital.com/ccjournal/august_september_2019?pg=1#pg1).

Flugel Colle, K. F., et al. 2010. Measurement of quality of life and participant experience with the mindfulness-based stress reduction program. *Complementary Therapies in Clinical Practice* 16(1): 36–40.

Foureur, M., et al. 2013. Enhancing the resilience of nurses and midwives: Pilot of a mindfulness-based program for increased health, sense of coherence and decreased depression, anxiety and stress. *Contemporary Nurse* 45: 114–125.

Germer, C., R. Siegel, and P. Fulton. 2005. *Mindfulness and Psychotherapy.* New York: Guilford.

Hagenaars, M. A., M. Oitzl, and K. Roelofsa. 2014. Updating freeze: Aligning animal and human research. *Neuroscience & Biobehavioral Reviews* 47: 165–176.

Hensle, A. M., et al. 2015. Religious coping and psychological and behavioral adjustment after Hurricane Katrina. *Journal of Psychology* 149(6): 630–642.

Hinkelman, L. 2017. *The Girls' Index: New Insights Into the Complex World of Today's Girls.* Columbus, OH: Ruling Our Experiences, Inc.

Hölzel, B. K., et al. 2010. Stress reduction correlates with structural changes in the amygdala. *Social Cognitive and Affective Neuroscience* 5(1): 11–17.

Hook, J. N., et al. 2010. Empirically supported religious and spiritual therapies. *Journal of Clinical Psychology* 66(1): 46–72.

Jayson, S. 2013. Who's feeling stressed? *USA Today,* February 7.

Kabat-Zinn, J. 2011. *Mindfulness for Beginners: Reclaiming the Present Moment—and Your Life.* Louisville, CO: Sounds True.

Kemeny, M. 2012. Contemplative/emotion training reduces negative emotional behavior and promotes prosocial responses. *Emoticon* [1528-3542] (12): 338–350.

Kim, B. 2018. *Touch One Strand and the Entire Web Wavers.* (http://drbenkim.com/nervous-endocrine-system.htm).

Manzoni, G. C., et al. 2016. Age of onset of episodic and chronic cluster headache—a review of a large case series from a single headache centre. *Journal of Headache Pain* 17: 44.

Marsh, I. C., S. W. Y. Chan, and A. MacBeth. 2018. Self-compassion and psychological distress in adolescents—a meta-analysis. *Mindfulness* 9: 1011–1027.

McGonigal, K. 2015. *The Upside of Stress.* New York: Penguin Random House.

Neff, K. D., and C. K. Germer. 2013. A pilot study and randomized controlled trial of the mindful self-compassion program. *Journal of Clinical Psychology* 69: 28–44.

Roddenberry, A., and K. Renk. 2010. Locus of control and self-efficacy: Potential mediators of stress, illness, and utilization of health services in college students. *Child Psychiatry and Human Development* 41(4): 353–370.

Roelofs, K. 2017. Freeze for action: Neurobiological mechanisms in animal and human freezing. *Philosophical Transactions of the Royal Society of London. Series B, Biological Sciences,* 372(1718): 20160206.

Schulte, Brigid. 2014. *Overwhelmed: Work, Love, and Play When No One Has the Time.* New York: Sarah Crichton Books.

Schwartz, G. E. 1979. Biofeedback and the behavioral treatment of disorders of disregulation. *Yale Journal of Biology and Medicine* 52(6): 581–596.

Seaward, B. L. 2018. *Managing Stress: Principles and Strategies for Health and Well-Being.* 9th ed. Burlington, MA: Jones & Bartlett Learning.

Segerstrom, S., and D. Hodgson, (eds). 2019. Psychoneuroimmunology [Special Edition]. *Current Opinion in Behavioral Sciences* 28: 1–162.

Shapiro, S. L., and L. E. Carlson. 2009. *The Art and Science of Mindfulness: Integrating Mindfulness into Psychology and the Helping Professions.* Washington, DC: American Psychological Association.

Sher, C., and C. Wu. 2021. Who stays physically active during Covid-19? Inequality and exercise patterns in the United States. *Socius* 7: 1–3.

Simmons, R. 2018. *Enough As She Is: How to Help Girls Move Beyond Impossible Standards of Success and Live Healthy, Happy and Fulfilling Lives.* New York: HarperCollins.

Southwick, S. M., and D. S. Charney. 2012. *Resilience: The Science of Mastering Life's Greatest Challenges.* Cambridge, UK: Cambridge University Press.

Substance Abuse and Mental Health Services Administration. 2021. *Key Substance Use and Mental Health Indicators in the United States: Results from the 2020 National Survey on Drug Use and Health* (HHS Publication No. PEP21-07-01-003, NSDUH Series H-56). (http://www.samhsa.gov/data).

Taylor, S., et al. 2020. Development and initial validation of the COVID Stress Scales. *Journal of Anxiety Disorders* 72: 102232.

Telles, S., et al. 2009. Effect of a yoga practice session and a yoga theory session on state anxiety. *Perceptual and Motor Skills* 109(3): 924–930.

United Nations Human Rights. 2022. Bachelet urges respect for international humanitarian law amid growing evidence of war crimes in Ukraine. Office of the High Commissioner for Human Rights, April 22 (https://www.ohchr.org/en/press-releases/2022/04/bachelet-urges-respect-international-humanitarian-law-amid-growing-evidence).

U.S. Department of Health and Human Services. 2021. *Surgeon General's Advisory: Protecting Youth Mental Health.* Washington, DC: Office of the Surgeon General (https://www.hhs.gov/sites/default/files/surgeon-general-youth-mental-health-advisory.pdf).

White, A. M., et al. 2022. Alcohol-related deaths during the COVID-19 pandemic. *JAMA* 327(17): 1704–1706.

Yao, W., X. Zhang, and Q. Gong. 2020. The effect of exposure to the natural environment on stress reduction: A meta-analysis. *Urban Forestry & Urban Greenery* 57: 126932.

U.S. Department of Health and Human Services, National Institutes of Health. 2021. *Stress* (http://www.nlm.nih.gov/medlineplus/stress.html).

**Design Elements:** Assess Yourself icon: Aleksey Boldin/Alamy Stock Photo; Diversity Matters icon: Rawpixel Ltd/Getty Images; Wellness on Campus icon: Radius Images/Alamy Stock Photo; Take Charge icon: VisualCommunications/Getty Images; Critical Consumer icon: pagadesign/Getty Images.

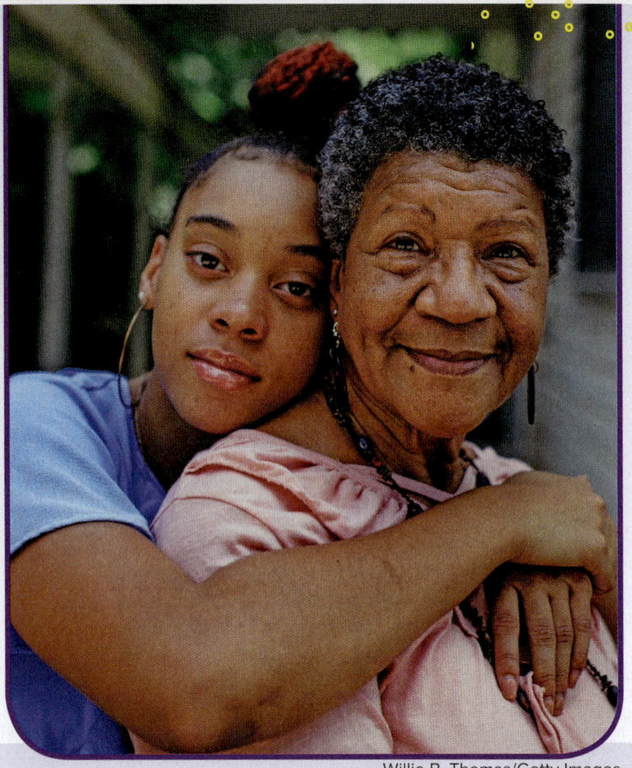

Willie B. Thomas/Getty Images

## CHAPTER OBJECTIVES

- Describe what it means to be psychologically healthy
- Discuss psychological approaches you can use to face life's challenges with a positive self-concept
- Describe common psychological disorders
- Recognize the warning signs, risk factors, and protective factors related to suicide
- Summarize the models of human nature on which therapies are based
- Describe the types of help available for psychological problems

CHAPTER 3

# Psychological Health

Psychological health contributes to every dimension of wellness. It can be difficult to maintain emotional, social, or even physical wellness if you are not psychologically healthy.

Psychological health, however, is a broad concept—one that is as difficult to define as it is important to understand. That is why we devote the first section of this chapter to explaining what psychological health is. In the rest of the chapter we discuss a number of common psychological problems (including mental illnesses), their symptoms, and their treatments.

## DEFINING PSYCHOLOGICAL HEALTH

**Psychological health** (or *mental health*) can be defined either negatively, as the absence of sickness, or positively, as the presence of wellness. The vast majority of people do not suffer from mental illness, yet all of us have to deal with stress, interpersonal conflicts, and difficult emotions. Psychological health refers to the extent to which we are able to function optimally in the face of these challenges, whether or not we have a mental illness.

### Positive Psychology

In his book *Toward a Psychology of Being,* psychologist Abraham Maslow adopted a perspective that he called "positive psychology." Maslow developed a *hierarchy of needs* (Figure 3.1): The most important kind is the satisfaction of physiological needs; following this is a feeling of safety, a state of being loved, maintenance of self-esteem, and finally, self-actualization.

When urgent (life-sustaining) needs—such as the need for food and water—are satisfied, less basic needs take priority. Maslow's conclusions were based on his study of a group of successful people who seemed to have lived, or to be living, at their fullest. He suggested that these people had fulfilled a

TERMS

**psychological health** Mental health, defined as the extent to which we are able to function optimally in the face of challenges, whether we have a mental illness or not.

◆ realism ◆ self-acceptance
◆ autonomy ◆ authenticity
◆ capable of intimacy ◆ creativity
Self-actualization
Self-esteem
◆ as a person ◆ as a doer
◆ in relationships
Love and Belongingness
◆ loved ◆ loving ◆ connected
Safety and Security
◆ safe surroundings ◆ protection by others
◆ knows to avoid risks
Physiological Needs
◆ food and water ◆ shelter ◆ sleep ◆ exercise ◆ sex

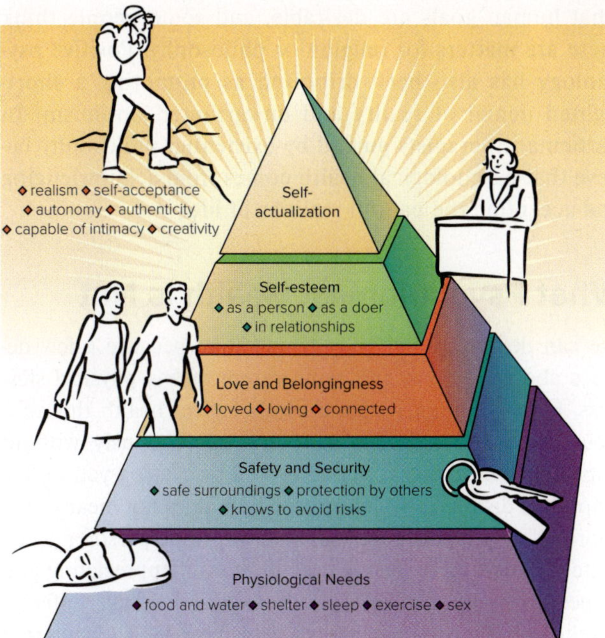

**FIGURE 3.1 Maslow's hierarchy of needs.**

SOURCE: Maslow, A. 1970. *Motivation and Personality,* 2nd ed. New York: Harper & Row.

good measure of their human potential and achieved **self-actualization.** Self-actualized people all share certain qualities:

QUICK STATS

**21% of U.S. adults experience mental illness.**

—National Alliance on Mental Illness, 2021

- ***Realism.*** Self-actualized people know the difference between what they want and what is real. As a result, they can cope with the world as it exists without demanding that it be different; they know what they can and cannot change. Just as important, realistic people accept evidence that contradicts what they want to believe.

- ***Acceptance.*** Self-accepting people have a positive but realistic **self-concept,** or *self-image*. They typically feel satisfaction and confidence in themselves, and thus they have healthy **self-esteem.** Self-acceptance also means being tolerant of your own imperfections—an ability that makes it easier to accept the imperfections of others.

- ***Autonomy.*** *Autonomous* people can direct themselves, acting independently of their social environment. **Autonomy** is more than physical independence. It is social, emotional, and intellectual independence, as well.

- ***Authenticity.*** Self-actualized people are not afraid to be themselves. Sometimes, in fact, their capacity for being "real" may give them a certain childlike quality. They respond in a genuine, or *authentic,* spontaneous way to whatever happens, without pretense or self-consciousness.

- ***Capacity for intimacy.*** People capable of intimacy can share their feelings and thoughts without fear of rejection. They are open to the pleasure of physical contact and the satisfaction of being close to others—but without being afraid of the risks involved in intimacy, such as the possibility of rejection. (Chapters 5 and 6 discuss intimacy in more detail.)

- ***Creativity.*** Creative people continually look at the world with renewed appreciation and curiosity. Such buoyancy can enhance creativity.

Self-actualization is an ideal to strive for rather than something most people can reasonably hope to achieve. Maslow believed it was rarely achieved. An additional adjustment we might make to Maslow's model is that it is more fluid than originally conceived: Studies have found that social reputation is so important that people will risk their safety and instead prioritize their sense of belonging when they choose to perform a disgusting or painful task rather than have negative information about them made public. For example, in one study, participants took a test that (falsely) identified them as racist. Most people opted to fully submerge their hands in a bucket of live worms or near-freezing water to stop their scores from being published. Still, Maslow's pyramid offers a model for goals to work for, whether we strive for a personal target or consider welfare policies that protect others' needs.

Influenced by the work of Maslow, psychologist Martin Seligman suggests that the goal of **positive psychology** is "to find and nurture one's own genius and talent" and "to make normal life more fulfilling" rather than just to identify and treat illness. In other words, it means being able to define positive goals and identify concrete, measurable ways of achieving them.

According to Seligman, happiness can be cultivated through three equally valid dimensions:

- ***The pleasant life.*** This life is dedicated to maximizing positive **emotions** about the past, present, and future, and to minimizing pain and negative emotions.

- ***The engaged life.*** This life involves cultivating positive personality traits (such as courage, leadership, kindness, and integrity) and actively using your talents. "Engagement" also

TERMS

**self-actualization** The highest level of growth in Maslow's hierarchy of needs.

**self-concept** The ideas, feelings, and perceptions a person has about himself or herself; also called *self-image.*

**self-esteem** Satisfaction and confidence in yourself; the valuing of yourself as a person.

**autonomy** Independence; the sense of being self-directed.

**positive psychology** The ability to define positive goals and to identify concrete, measurable ways of achieving them.

**emotion** A feeling state involving some combination of thoughts, physiological changes, and an outward expression or behavior.

**Ask Yourself**

**QUESTIONS FOR CRITICAL THINKING AND REFLECTION**

Have you ever had a reason to feel concerned about your own psychological health? If so, what was the reason? Did your concern lead you to talk to someone about the issue, or to seek professional help? If you did, what was the outcome, and how do you feel about it now?

involves cultivating a capacity to live in the moment and immerse yourself fully in your activities.

A key to being engaged and successful in life is the positive personality trait of **emotional intelligence.** Emotionally intelligent people can identify and manage their own emotions and respond to the emotions of others. Psychologists and educators believe that emotional intelligence is not as rooted as abstract intelligence and that it can be learned.

- ***The meaningful life.*** Another road to happiness entails working with others toward a meaningful end. Many people find meaning in their connections with and service to families, friends, religious institutions, social causes, and/or work. The happiness to be found by following this path is strongest when meaning comes from more than one source.

Not everyone accepts the ideas of positive psychology—or even the concept of psychological health—because they involve value judgments that are inconsistent with psychology's scientific status. Defining psychological health requires making assumptions and value judgments about what human goals are desirable, and some people think these are matters for religion or philosophy. Positive psychology has also been criticized as promoting a shortsighted denial of reality and unwarranted optimism. In particular, therapists guided by existential philosophy believe that psychological health comes from acknowledging and accepting the painful realities of life.

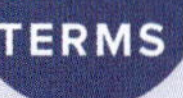

**emotional intelligence** The capacity to identify and manage your own emotions and, where possible, the emotions of others.

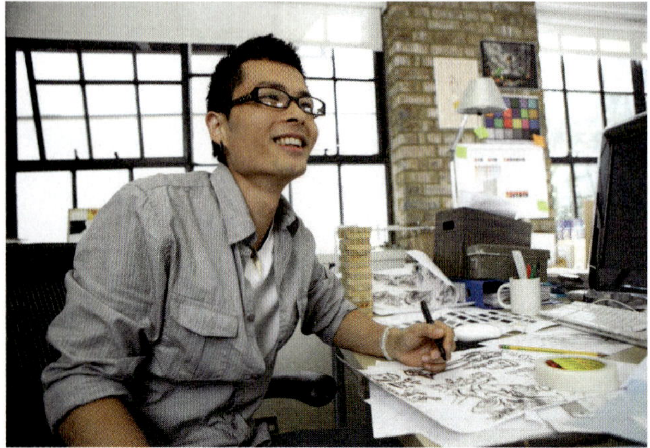

You can develop happiness in any number of ways. The keys are to focus on work and activities you enjoy and to develop a supportive network of friends and family. Ciaran Griffin/Lifesize/Getty Images

## What Psychological Health Is Not

We can define normal body temperature because a few degrees above or below this temperature means physical sickness, but we cannot measure psychological health this way. Your ideas and attitudes can vary tremendously without impeding your ability to function well or causing you to feel emotional distress. Psychological health does not mean being "normal": What is considered healthy for one person may be quite different for someone else. Moreover, appreciating and respecting psychological diversity—how individuals differ in psychological terms—is actually a valuable asset; encountering a wide range of ideas, lifestyles, and attitudes broadens our perspectives and helps us solve problems of the social world.

Seeking help for personal problems does not mean someone is psychologically unhealthy or mentally ill. On the other hand, unhappy and unhealthy people may avoid seeking help for many reasons, and severely disturbed people may not even realize they need help.

Further, we can't say people are "mentally ill" or "mentally healthy" based solely on the presence or absence of symptoms. Consider the symptom of anxiety, for example. Anxiety can help you face a problem and solve it before it becomes too big. Someone who shows no anxiety may be refusing to recognize problems or to do anything about them. A person who is anxious for good reason may be more psychologically healthy in the long run than someone who is inappropriately calm.

Finally, we cannot judge psychological health from the way people look. All too often, a person who seems to be okay and even happy suddenly takes their own life. At an early age, we learn to conceal our feelings and even to lie about them. We may believe that our complaints put unfair demands on others. Although maintaining privacy about emotional pain may seem to be a virtue, it can also be an impediment to getting help.

# MEETING LIFE'S CHALLENGES WITH A POSITIVE SELF-CONCEPT

Life is full of challenges—large and small. For emotional and mental wellness, each of us must continue to cultivate an adult identity that enhances our self-esteem and autonomy.

## Growing Up Psychologically

Our responses to life's challenges influence the development of our personality and identity. Psychologist Erik Erikson proposed that development proceeds through a series of eight stages that extend throughout life. Each stage is characterized by a conflict or turning point—a time of increased vulnerability as well as increased potential for psychological growth.

The successful mastery of one stage is a basis for mastering the next, so early failures can have repercussions in later life. Fortunately, life provides ongoing opportunities for mastering these tasks. For example, although the development of trust begins in infancy, it is refined as we grow older. We learn to trust some people outside our immediate family and to identify others as untrustworthy.

**Developing a Unified Sense of Self** The development of an adult identity begins in adolescence; this unified sense of self can be seen in the attitudes, beliefs, and ways of acting that are genuinely your own. To know who you are, what you are capable of, what roles you play, and your place among your peers gives you a voice to respond to ambiguous situations. This self-identification gives a sense of your uniqueness but also appreciation for what you have in common with others. It lets you view yourself realistically and be able to assess your strengths and weaknesses without relying on the opinions of others. Identifying with some core traits also means that you can form intimate relationships with others while maintaining a strong sense of self.

Identity does not develop in isolation. Our identities evolve as we interact with the world and make choices about what we'd like to do and whom we'd like to model ourselves after. We all experiment with different self-representations as we proceed through adolescence. We show different sides of ourselves, not just as we pass through different ages, but also from one day to the next, depending on whom we're with or the environment we're in.

Early identities are often modeled after parents and adult caregivers—or they are modeled after the opposite of parents, in rebellion against what they represent. Over time, peers, celebrities, athletes, and religious figures are added to the list of possible role models. In high school and college, people often join cliques that assert a certain identity, such as "jocks," "nerds," or "hipsters." Although much of our identity is internal—a way of viewing ourselves and the world—certain aspects of it can be external, in terms of the way we express ourselves through styles of talking and dressing, and in terms of the names given to us by other people.

Early identities are rarely permanent. A hardworking student seeking approval one year can turn into a dropout devoted to sleeping all day and partying all night the next year. At some point, however, most of us adopt a more stable, individual set of identities that ties together the experiences of childhood and the expectations and aspirations of adulthood. A unified sense of self reflects a lifelong process, and it changes as a person develops new relationships and roles.

**Developing Values and Purpose in Your Life** **Values** are criteria for judging what is good and bad, and they underlie our moral decisions and behavior. The first morality of the young child is to consider "good" to mean what brings immediate and tangible rewards, and "bad" to mean whatever results in punishment. An older child will explain right and wrong in terms of authority figures and rules. But the final stage of moral development, one that not everyone attains, is being able to conceive of right and wrong in more abstract terms such as justice and virtue.

As adults we need to assess how far we have evolved morally and what values we have adopted. Without an awareness of our personal values, our lives may be hurriedly driven forward by immediate desires and the passing demands of others. Living according to values means considering your options carefully before making a choice, choosing among options without succumbing to outside pressures that conflict with your values, and making a choice and acting on it rather than doing nothing.

Your actions and how you justify them proclaim to others what you stand for.

## Achieving Healthy Self-Esteem

Having a healthy level of self-esteem means regarding your self—which includes all aspects of your identity—as good, competent, and worthy of love. It is a critical component of wellness.

**Developing a Positive Self-Concept** Ideally, a positive self-concept begins in childhood, based on experiences both within the family and outside it. Children need to develop a sense of being loved and being able to give love and to accomplish their goals. If they feel rejected or neglected by their parents, they may fail to develop feelings of self-worth. They may grow to have a negative concept of themselves.

### Ask Yourself

?

**QUESTIONS FOR CRITICAL THINKING AND REFLECTION**

Write down times when you felt

- Free
- Aloof
- Angry
- Generous
- Happy
- Talkative

For each moment you recall, whom were you with when you felt those ways? What had recently happened in your life? Where were you? Did you feel most "yourself" in any of those moments? Which?

**TERMS**

**values** Criteria for judging what is good and bad, which underlie an individual's moral decisions and behavior.

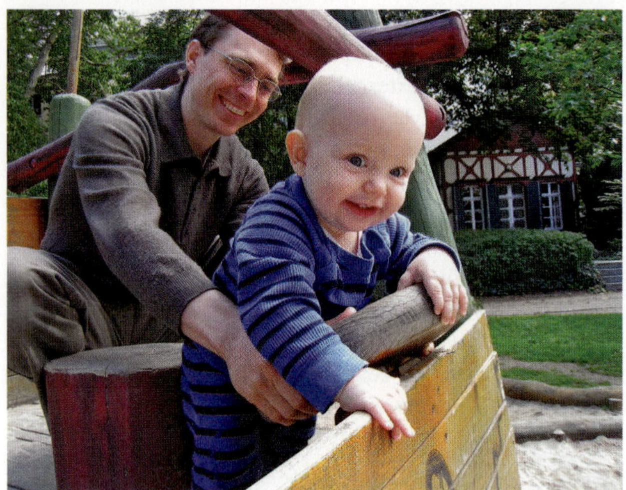

A positive self-concept begins early. Feeling loved and valued gives this infant a solid basis for lifelong psychological health.
Jeff Klingner

Another component of self-concept is *integration*. An integrated self-concept is one that you have made for yourself—not someone else's image of you or a mask that doesn't quite fit. Important building blocks of self-concept are the personality characteristics and mannerisms of parents, which children may adopt without realizing it. Later they may be surprised to find themselves acting like one of their parents. Eventually such building blocks may be reshaped and integrated into a new, individual personality.

Another aspect of self-concept is *stability*. Stability depends on the integration of the self and its freedom from contradictions. People who have gotten mixed messages about themselves from parents and friends may have contradictory self-images, which defy integration and make them vulnerable to shifting levels of self-esteem. At times they regard themselves as entirely good, capable, and lovable—an ideal self—and at other times they see themselves as entirely bad, incompetent, and unworthy of love. Neither of these extreme self-concepts allows people to see themselves or others realistically, and their relationships with other people are filled with misunderstandings and ultimately with conflict.

**Meeting Challenges to Self-Esteem** As an adult, you sometimes run into situations that challenge your self-concept. People you care about may tell you they don't love you or feel loved by you, for example, or your attempts to accomplish a goal may end in failure.

You can react to such challenges in several ways. The best approach is to acknowledge that something has gone wrong and try again, adjusting your goals to your abilities without radically revising your self-concept. Less productive responses are denying that anything went wrong and blaming someone else. These attitudes may preserve your self-concept temporarily, but in the long run they keep you from meeting the challenge.

The worst reaction is to develop a lasting negative self-concept in which you feel bad, unloved, and ineffective—in other words, to become demoralized. Instead of coping, the demoralized person gives up (at least temporarily), reinforcing the negative self-concept and setting in motion a cycle of bad self-concept and failure. In people who are genetically predisposed to depression, demoralization can progress to additional symptoms, which are discussed later in the chapter.

**NOTICE YOUR PATTERNS OF THINKING** One method for fighting demoralization is to recognize and test the negative thoughts and assumptions you may have about yourself and others. Note exactly when an unpleasant emotion—feeling worthless, wanting to give up, feeling depressed—occurs or gets worse, so that you can identify the events or daydreams that trigger that emotion, and observe whatever thoughts arise just before or during the emotional experience. Keep a daily journal about such events.

**AVOID FOCUSING ON THE NEGATIVE** Imagine that you are waiting for a friend to meet you for dinner, but he's 30 minutes late. What kinds of thoughts go through your head? You might wonder what caused the delay: Perhaps he is stuck in traffic, you think, or needs to help a roommate who has the flu. This kind of reaction is healthy.

By contrast, people who are demoralized tend to use all-or-nothing thinking. They overgeneralize from negative events. They overlook the positive and make negative assumptions, minimizing their own successes and magnifying the successes of others. They take responsibility for unfortunate situations that are not their fault, then jump to more negative conclusions and more unfounded overgeneralizations. Patterns of thinking that make events seem worse than they are in reality are called **cognitive distortions.**

**DEVELOP REALISTIC SELF-TALK** When you react to a situation, an important piece of that reaction is your **self-talk**—the statements or chatter you hear your mind making. To pick up on our earlier example, suppose your friend is late for a dinner date.

Someone who is demoralized or wrestling with a poor self-concept might immediately react with negative self-talk: "He isn't coming. It's my fault; he probably doesn't like me because I'm boring. I bet he's with someone else." In your own fight against demoralization, you may find it hard to think of a rational response until hours or days after the event that upset you.

Once you get used to noticing the way your mind works, however, you may be able to catch yourself thinking negatively and change the process before it goes too far. This approach to controlling your reactions is not the same as positive thinking—which means substituting a positive

**TERMS**

**cognitive distortion** A pattern of negative thinking that makes events seem worse than they are.

**self-talk** The statements a person makes to himself or herself.

## TAKE CHARGE
### Realistic Self-Talk

Do your patterns of thinking make events seem worse than they truly are? Substituting realistic self-talk for negative self-talk can help you build and maintain self-esteem and cope better with the challenges in your life. Below are examples of common types of distorted, negative self-talk, along with suggestions for more accurate and rational responses.

| COGNITIVE DISTORTION | NEGATIVE SELF-TALK | REALISTIC SELF-TALK |
|---|---|---|
| Focusing on negatives | Babysitting is such a pain in the neck; I wish I didn't need the extra money so badly. | This is a tough job, but at least the money's decent and I can study once the kids go to bed. |
| Expecting the worst | I know I'm going to get an F in this course. I should just drop out of school now. | I'm not doing too well in this course. I should talk to my professor to see what kind of help I can get. |
| Overgeneralizing | My hair is a mess and I'm gaining weight. I'm so ugly. No one would ever want to date me. | I could use a haircut and should try to eat better. This way I'll start feeling better about myself and will be more confident when I meet people. |
| Minimizing | It was nice of everyone to eat the dinner I cooked, even though I ruined it. I'm such a rotten cook. | Well, the roast was a little dry, but they ate every bite. The veggies and rolls made up for it. I'm finally getting the hang of cooking! |
| Blaming others | Everyone I meet is such a jerk. Why aren't people friendlier? | I am going to make more of an effort to meet people who share my interests. |
| Expecting perfection | I cannot believe I flubbed that solo. They probably won't even let me audition for the orchestra next year. | It's a good thing I didn't stop playing when I hit that sour note. It didn't seem like anyone noticed it as much as I did. |
| Believing you're the cause of everything | Jamar and Luke broke up, and it's my fault. I shouldn't have insisted that Jamar spend so much time with me and the guys. | It's a shame Jamar and Luke broke up. I wish I knew what happened between them. Maybe Jamar will tell me at soccer practice. At any rate, it isn't my fault; I've been a good friend to both of them. |
| Thinking in either-or terms | I thought that Remy was really cool, but after what they said today, I realize we have nothing in common. | I was really surprised that Remy disagreed with me today. I guess there are still things I don't know about them. |
| Magnifying events | I stuttered when I was giving my speech today in class. I must have sounded like a complete idiot. I'm sure everyone is talking about it. | My speech went really well, except for that one stutter. I'll bet most people didn't even notice it, though. |

thought for a negative one. Instead you simply try to make your thoughts as logical and accurate as possible, based on the facts of the situation as you know them, and not on snap judgments or conclusions that may turn out to be false.

Demoralized people can be tenacious about their negative beliefs, making them come true in a self-fulfilling prophecy. For example, if you conclude that you are so boring that no one will like you anyway, you may decide not to bother socializing. This behavior could make the negative belief become a reality because you limit your opportunities to meet people and develop new relationships.

For additional tips on changing distorted, negative ways of thinking, see the box "Realistic Self-Talk."

## Psychological Defense Mechanisms—Healthy and Unhealthy

We are always trying to manage our feelings, even if we aren't aware we are doing it. We try to manage uncomfortable feelings through what are called psychological defenses. By using defense mechanisms, we change unacceptable feelings (like shame or anger or anxiety) into ones with which we are more comfortable. Table 3.1 lists some standard **defense mechanisms.** Defense mechanisms can be healthy and adaptive—such as humor and altruism—but they can also be maladaptive. For example, it would be maladaptive to displace your anger at your teacher by yelling at your roommates because doing so doesn't help your relationship with your teacher or your roommates. The drawback of many defenses is that they make you feel better temporarily but don't address underlying causes.

Recognizing our own defense mechanisms can be difficult because they occur unconsciously. But we all have some inkling about how our minds operate. By remembering the details of conflict situations, a person may be able to figure out which defense mechanisms they used in successful or unsuccessful attempts to cope. Recall a psychologically stressful situation and view yourself as an objective outside observer would; now analyze your thoughts and behavior in that situation. Having insight into what strategies you typically use can lead to new, more rewarding and effective ways of coping.

TERMS

**defense mechanism** A mental strategy that uses techniques such as humor or denial to cope with conflict or anxiety.

**pessimism** The tendency to expect an unfavorable outcome.

**optimism** The tendency to expect a favorable outcome.

## Being Optimistic

Most of us have a predisposition toward optimism or pessimism. **Pessimism** is a tendency to focus on the negative and expect an unfavorable outcome; **optimism** is a tendency to emphasize the hopeful and expect a favorable outcome. Pessimists not only expect repeated failure and rejection but also accept it as deserved. They do not see themselves as capable of success and irrationally dismiss any evidence of their own accomplishments. This negative point of view is learned, typically at a young age from parents and other authority figures. Optimists, by contrast, consider bad events to be temporary and consider failure to be limited and look forward to new pursuits.

You can learn to be optimistic by recording adverse events in a diary, along with the reactions and beliefs with which you met those events. By doing so, you learn to recognize and dispute the false, negative predictions you generate about yourself.

## Maintaining Honest Communication

Communicating your feelings appropriately and clearly is important. It can be very frustrating for us and for people around us if we cannot express what we want and feel.

Some people know what they want others to do but don't state it clearly because their request may be denied, which they interpret as personal rejection. Such people

**Table 3.1** Defense and Coping Mechanisms

| MECHANISM | DESCRIPTION | EXAMPLE |
|---|---|---|
| Projection | Reacting to unacceptable impulses by denying their existence in yourself and attributing them to others | A student who dislikes his roommate feels that the roommate dislikes him. |
| Repression | Keeping an unpleasant feeling, idea, or memory out of awareness | The child of an alcoholic, neglectful father remembers only when her father showed consideration and love. |
| Denial | Refusing to acknowledge to yourself what you really know to be true | A person believes that smoking cigarettes won't harm her because she's young and healthy. |
| Displacement | Shifting your feelings about a person to another person | A student who is angry with one of his professors returns home and yells at one of his housemates. |
| Dissociation | Detaching from a current experience to avoid emotional distress | Rather than listen to his angry father, Beethoven composes a piece in his mind. |
| Rationalization | Giving a false, acceptable reason when the real reason is unacceptable | A shy young man decides not to attend a dorm party, telling himself he'd be bored. |
| Reaction formation | Concealing emotions or impulses by exaggerating the opposite ones | A person who dislikes children frequently buys expensive gifts for, and speaks with enthusiasm about, the children of her friends. |
| Substitution | Replacing an unacceptable or unobtainable goal with an acceptable one | A person in love with an unavailable partner becomes active in training for a marathon. |
| Acting out | Engaging in an action that makes an unacceptable feeling go away | A person who feels disrespected and devalued gets into a fight at a bar with a stranger. |
| Humor | Finding something funny in unpleasant situations | A student whose bicycle has been stolen thinks how surprised the thief will be when he or she starts downhill and discovers the brakes don't work. |
| Altruism | Serving others without expecting anything in return | A person with little money to spare volunteers at a foundation that helps people get out of poverty. |

might benefit from assertiveness training: learning to insist on their rights and to bargain for what they want. **Assertiveness** includes being able to say no or yes depending on the situation.

## Finding a Social Media Balance

For many (if not most) young adults, social media platforms are an important part of their social and intellectual lives. More nuanced information about social media, such as when to use them, is needed. A study of more than 84,000 people of all ages in Britain revealed two distinct times in adolescence when heavy use of social media corresponded with more depression and anxiety: for girls, ages 11–13; for boys, ages 14–15. Then, for all genders, around age 19.

Some people believe that social media use can lead to more social interaction and less loneliness, while others believe it can lead to social isolation and psychological harm. Use your own judgment when looking at how much time you spend on the internet. Is social media helping you feel connected? Or left out? Is it widening your community or keeping you from things (like getting together with people—or doing your classwork!)? Everyone needs to find a balance in their social media use for it to be healthy for them.

## Dealing with Loneliness

It can be hard to strike the right balance between being alone and being with others. Some people are motivated to socialize out of a fear of being alone. If you discover how to enjoy being by yourself, you'll be better able to cope with periods when you're forced to be alone. For many of us, the Covid pandemic has been a time that increased loneliness, as our usual avenues for connection may have been cut off. Sometimes there are external reasons for our loneliness—for example, when we are in fact physically cut off by people. But sometimes our loneliness is a feeling that we have in spite of our circumstances.

Loneliness may come from feelings of rejection—that others are not interested in spending time with you. Before you reach such a conclusion, be sure that you give others a real chance to get to know you.

Examine your patterns of thinking: You may harbor unrealistic expectations about other people. Not everyone you meet is suitable and willing to have a close or intimate relationship.

Loneliness is a passive feeling state. If you decide that you're not spending enough time with people, change the situation. Decide whether scrolling through your social media feed is a way of avoiding contact with others or enhances your social life. College life provides many opportunities to meet people. If you're shy or introverted, you may have to push yourself to join a group. Look for something you've enjoyed in the past or in which you have a genuine interest.

## Dealing with Anger

Anger is a part of the array of normal emotions, yet it is often confusing and difficult to deal with. Some people feel that expressing anger is beneficial for psychological and physical health. However, if angry words or actions damage relationships or produce feelings of guilt or loss of control, they do not contribute to psychological wellness. It is important to distinguish between a destructive expression of anger and a reasonable level of self-assertiveness—standing up for yourself firmly but without aggression.

At one extreme are people who never express anger or any opinion that might offend others, even when their own rights and needs are being jeopardized. They may be trapped in unhealthy relationships or chronically deprived of satisfaction at work and at home. If you have trouble expressing your anger, consider training in assertiveness and appropriate expressions of anger to help you learn to express yourself constructively.

At the other extreme are people whose anger is explosive or misdirected; such expressions of anger can signal a condition called *intermittent explosive disorder (IED)*. It may also be a symptom of a more serious problem—angry outbursts, for instance, are associated with posttraumatic stress disorder. Explosive anger may also happen during periods of intoxication with alcohol or drugs such as amphetamines or cocaine. Explosive anger or rage, like a child's tantrum, renders an individual temporarily unable to think straight or to act in their own best interest. During an IED episode, a person may lash out uncontrollably, hurting someone else physically or verbally, or destroying property. Anyone who expresses anger this way should seek professional help. Some studies have suggested that overtly hostile people are at higher risk for heart attacks.

**Managing Your Anger** If you feel explosive anger coming on, consider the following two strategies to head it off. First, try to *reframe* what you're thinking at that moment. You'll be less angry at another person if there is a possibility that their behavior was not intentionally directed against you. Imagine that another driver suddenly cuts in front of you. You would certainly be angry if you knew the other driver did it on purpose, but you probably would be less angry if you knew they simply did not see you. If you're angry because you've just been criticized, avoid mentally replaying scenes from the past when you received other unjust criticisms. Think about what is happening now, and try to act differently from how you would have in the past—less defensively and more analytically.

Second, until you're able to change your thinking, try to *distract* yourself. Use the old trick of counting to 10 before you respond, or start concentrating on your breathing. If

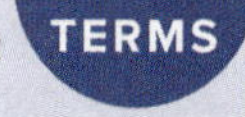


**assertiveness** Expression that is forceful but not hostile.

## Ask Yourself

**QUESTIONS FOR CRITICAL THINKING AND REFLECTION**

Think about the last time you were truly angry. What triggered your anger? How did you express it? Do you typically handle your anger in the same manner? How appropriate does your anger-management technique seem?

necessary, cool off by leaving the situation until your anger has subsided. This does not mean that you should permanently avoid the sensitive topics. Return to the matter after you've had a chance to think clearly about it.

### Dealing with Anger in Other People

Anger can be infectious, and it disrupts cooperation and communication. If someone you're with becomes very angry, respond "asymmetrically" by reacting not with anger but with calm. Try to validate the other person by acknowledging that they have some reason to be angry: "I totally get that this is making you mad," or "If I were you, I'd be upset, too." This does not mean apologizing if you don't think you're to blame, or accepting verbal abuse. It means that you have considered the other's perspective and that you understand why they might be angry. Finally, if the person cannot be calmed, it may be best to disengage, at least temporarily. After a time-out, you may have better luck trying to solve the problem rationally.

QUICK
STATS
Only 46% of U.S. adults with mental illness receive treatment in a given year.
—SAMHSA, 2021

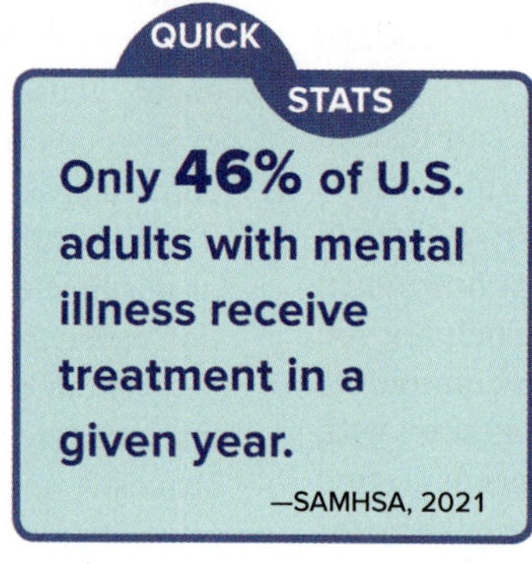

## PSYCHOLOGICAL DISORDERS

When emotions or irrational thoughts interfere with daily activities and rob us of peace of mind, they can be considered symptoms of a psychological disorder. Psychological disorders are generally the result of many factors. Genetics, which underlies differences in how the brain processes information and experiences, are known to play an important role, especially in certain disorders such as autism, schizophrenia, and bipolar disorder. However, exactly which genes are involved, and how they alter the structure and chemistry of the brain, is still under study. A dysfunctional interaction between neurotransmitters and their receptors is associated with some psychiatric disorders (Figure 3.2). The trouble may begin when neurotransmitters (chemicals that transmit messages between nerve cells) misfire and the nerve cells do not communicate properly.

Learning and life events are important, too: Although one identical twin is often at higher risk of having a disorder if the other has it, the two may not necessarily have the same psychological disorders despite having identical genes.

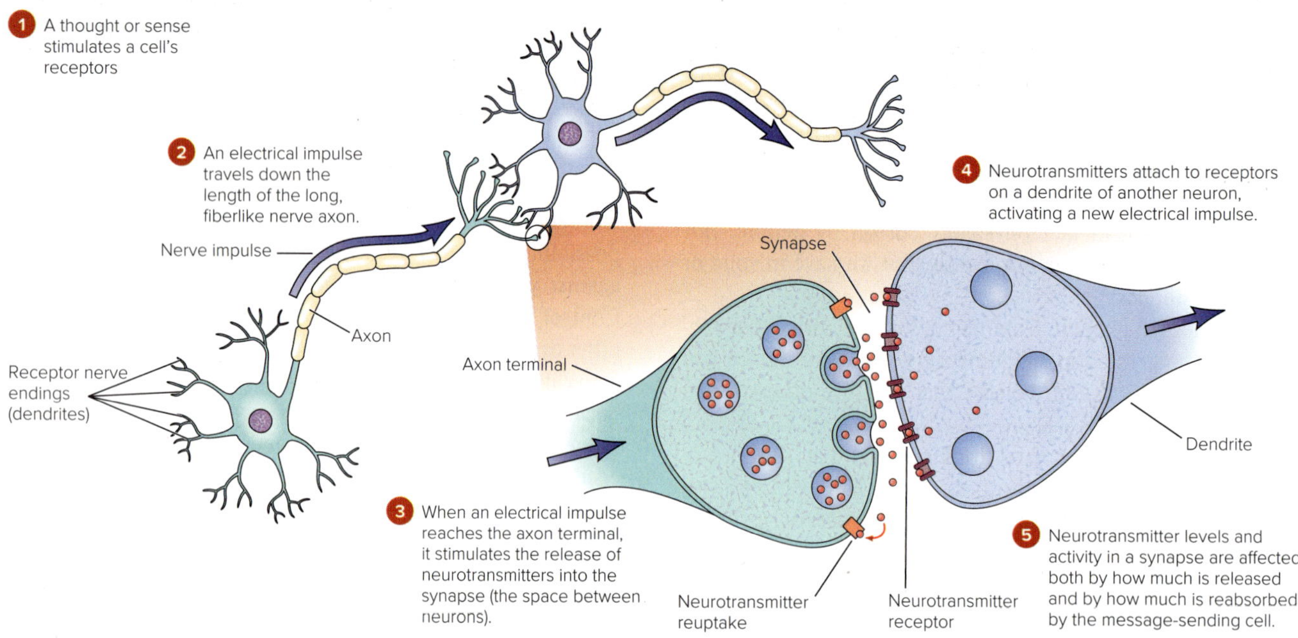


FIGURE 3.2 **Nerve cell communication.** Nerve cells (neurons) communicate through a combination of electrical impulses and chemical messages. Neurotransmitters such as serotonin and norepinephrine alter the overall responsiveness of the brain and are responsible for mood, levels of attentiveness, and other psychological states. Many psychological issues are related to problems with neurotransmitters and their receptors, and drug treatments frequently target them. For example, some antidepressant drugs increase levels of serotonin by slowing the resorption (reuptake) of serotonin.

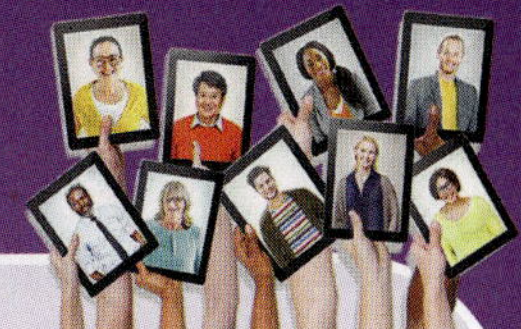

## DIVERSITY MATTERS

# Ethnicity, Race, Culture, and Psychological Health

Cultures develop unique ideas about mental health—about what is normal and what is problematic, how symptoms should be interpreted and communicated, whether treatment should be sought, and whether a social stigma is attached to a particular symptom or disorder. What happens to these culturally distinct ideas when the group comes into contact with other groups? The United States is the leading destination of international migration, but the politics of immigration can have their own impact on psychological health and well-being. What specific stressors do immigrants face, having left one home for another and having now become minorities?

Asian immigrants to the United States have often come from *collectivist* cultures that anticipate and care for the needs of each other, so that individuals don't need to request support. In U.S. cultures, usually no group is expected to look after the needs of an individual; rather, individuals or their close families are responsible for seeking help for themselves. For this reason Asian immigrants appear to have more trouble than European Americans asking for explicit social support.

A hybrid identity can be greater than the sum of its parts—for example, a Mexican American is now both Mexican and American, and may now be both English and Spanish speaking—and this biculturalism can provide more options for healthy living. There is evidence that immigrants who arrive after adolescence tend to experience better mental health than adults who were born in the United States.

Although biculturalism helps bring about better mental health, sometimes younger immigrants and second-generation immigrants may be particularly vulnerable to the effects of *acculturation*, the process by which individuals and groups adapt to each other's cultures. The children of immigrants respond positively when parents pass along ideas about heritage and customs that promote ethnic pride. Children may also respond well to teachings about how to cope with discrimination and racial bias; however, too much focus on negative cultural identities has resulted in depressive symptoms, according to studies of both Asian and Latino children of immigrants.

Children of Asian and Latino immigrants, who collectively make up 77% of all immigrant children in the United States, can face common transcultural stressors, such as economic hardships and living in neighborhoods with fewer resources. Studies have found differences, however, in the ways these groups react to such stressors: Adolescent children of Chinese immigrants tended to internalize their parents' economic hardships by expressing depressive symptoms. The ones who lived in worse neighborhoods externalized, or acted outwardly toward others, through behaviors like bullying and vandalism. These behaviors then eroded positive parenting practices, including spending enough time monitoring the children.

Reasons for the negative psychological effects of acculturation may be the stresses of cultural disparities concerning concepts of individuality, interpersonal relationships, and what it means to succeed. Despite these problems, second-generation Americans nevertheless tend to have higher rates of insurance coverage and access to health care. Their greater facility with English is correlated with higher frequencies of general physical, vision, and dental checkups. Regardless of one's generation, other factors affect immigrants' health outcomes living in the United States: education, wealth, and occupational and language skills all influence their lifestyles, as well as the policies of the government and attitudes of Americans already here.

Race and immigrant status can be difficult to disentangle, and both demographics have a clear impact on psychological health and well-being. Many immigrant groups have been viewed negatively (like Italian, Irish, German, Polish, Jewish, Black, Hispanic, Asian, and others); those with physical features or a language different from those in the dominant culture have had specific difficulties and challenges when coming to the United States.

SOURCES: Enriquez, L. E., et al. 2022. Mental health and COVID-19 pandemic stressors among Latina/o/x college students with varying self and parental immigration status. *Journal of Racial and Ethnic Health Disparities* (https://doi.org/10.1007/s40615-021-01218-x); McDermott, M., and A. Ferguson. 2022. Sociology of whiteness. *Annual Review of Sociology* 48: 257–276; Kim, S. Y., et al. 2018. Culture's influence on stressors, parental socialization, and developmental processes in the mental health of children of immigrants. *Annual Review of Clinical Psychology* 14: 343–370; Leyse-Wallace, R. 2013. *Nutrition and Mental Health*. Boca Raton, FL: CRC Press; Lara, M., et al. 2005. Acculturation and Latino health in the United States: A review of the literature and its sociopolitical context. *Annual Review of Public Health* 26: 367–397.

Some people have been exposed to more traumatic events than others, leading them to develop either better coping skills or greater vulnerability to future traumas. Historically, people who identify as lesbian, gay, bisexual, transgender, questioning, intersex, and asexual (LGBTQIA+) have faced higher rates of mental illness than non-LGBTQIA+ peers. This disparity has been associated with their different work, life, and health care experiences, including stigma and discrimination. What your parents, peers, and others have taught you strongly influences your level of self-esteem and how you deal with frightening or depressing life events (see the box "Ethnicity, Race, Culture, and Psychological Health").

This section examines some of the more common psychological disorders, including anxiety disorders, mood disorders, and schizophrenia. Table 3.2 shows the likelihood of these disorders occurring during a lifetime.

VITAL STATISTICS

**Table 3.2** Prevalence of Selected Psychological Disorders among Americans

| | MEN | WOMEN |
|---|---|---|
| DISORDER | LIFETIME PREVALENCE (%) | LIFETIME PREVALENCE (%) |
| Anxiety disorders* | | |
| Specific phobia | 9.9 | 17.5 |
| Social anxiety disorder | 11.8 | 14.2 |
| Panic disorder | 3.3 | 7.0 |
| Generalized anxiety disorder | 4.6 | 7.7 |
| Obsessive-compulsive disorder | 1.8 | 3.6 |
| Posttraumatic stress disorder | 4.0 | 11.7 |
| Mood disorders | | |
| Major depressive episode | 14.7 | 26.1 |
| Bipolar disorder | 2.5 | 2.5 |
| Manic episode | 1.0 | 1.0 |
| Schizophrenia | 3.7 | 3.4 |

*Anxiety disorders from the National Comorbidity Survey Replication, based on DSM-IV-TR/CIDI. OCD and PTSD are no longer categorized as anxiety disorders in the DSM-5.

SOURCES: Hasin, D. S., et al. 2018. Epidemiology of adult DSM-5 major depressive disorder and its specifiers in the United States. *JAMA Psychiatry* 75(4): 336–346; Kessler, R. C., et al. Twelve-month and lifetime prevalence and lifetime morbid risk of anxiety and mood disorders in the United States. *International Journal of Methods in Psychiatric Research* 21(3): 169–184; Lee, J., et al. 2017. Bipolar I disorder. Johns Hopkins Psychiatry Guide (https://www.hopkinsguides.com/hopkins/view/Johns_Hopkins_Psychiatry_Guide/787045/all/Bipolar_I_Disorder); McGrath, J., et al. 2008. Schizophrenia: A concise overview of incidence, prevalence, and mortality. *Epidemiologic Reviews* 30: 67–76.

## Anxiety Disorders

Fear is a basic and useful emotion. Its value for our ancestors' survival cannot be overestimated. For modern humans, too, fear motivates us to protect ourselves and to learn how to cope with new or potentially dangerous situations. We consider fear to be a problem only when it is out of proportion to real danger. **Anxiety** is another word for fear, in particular, fear that is not in response to any definite threat. It becomes a disorder when it occurs almost daily or in life situations that recur and cannot be avoided, interfering with your relationships and the ability to function in social and professional situations.

### Specific Phobia

The most common and understandable anxiety disorder, called **specific phobia,** is a fear of something definite like lightning, a particular type of animal, or a place. Snakes, spiders, and dogs are commonly feared animals; high or enclosed spaces are often frightening places. Sometimes, but not always, these fears originate in bad experiences, such as being bitten by a dog.

TERMS

**anxiety** Fear that is not a response to any definite threat.

**specific phobia** A persistent and excessive fear of a specific object, activity, or situation.

**social anxiety disorder (social phobia)** An excessive fear of being observed by others; speaking in public is the most common example.

**panic disorder** A syndrome of severe anxiety attacks accompanied by physical symptoms.

### Social Anxiety Disorder

The 15 million Americans with **social anxiety disorder** (previously called **social phobia**) fear humiliation or embarrassment. Fear of speaking in public is perhaps the most common phobia of this kind. Extremely shy people can have social fears in almost all social situations; this is in contrast to being introverted, which is not a psychological problem. People with these kinds of fears may not continue in school as far as they could and may restrict themselves to lower-paying jobs in which they do not have to come into contact with new people.

### Panic Disorder

People with **panic disorder** experience sudden unexpected surges in anxiety, accompanied by symptoms such as rapid and strong heartbeat, shortness of breath, loss of physical equilibrium, and a feeling of losing mental control. Such attacks usually begin in a person's early twenties and can lead to a fear of being in crowds or closed places or of driving or flying. Sufferers fear that a panic attack will occur in a situation from which escape is difficult (in an elevator), where the attack could be incapacitating and result in a dangerous or embarrassing loss of control (while driving a car), or where no medical help would be available if needed (alone away from home). These fears can drive avoidance of potentially problematic situations, which may spread until a person is virtually housebound, a condition called **agoraphobia.** People with panic disorder can often function normally in feared situations if they are with someone they trust. Panic disorder is different from an occasional **panic attack,** which affects about 40 million American adults aged 18 and older every year. This occasional attack of overwhelming anxiety may have no obvious cause and usually resolves in an hour or less.

QUICK STATS

**In the USA, about 10% of women compared with 4% of men develop PTSD sometime in their lives.**

—U.S. Department of Veterans Affairs, 2021

### Generalized Anxiety Disorder

A basic reaction to future threats is to worry about them. **Generalized anxiety disorder (GAD)** is a diagnosis given to people whose worries about multiple issues linger more than six months. Worries may involve family, other relationships, work, school, money, and health.

The GAD sufferer's worrying is not completely unjustified—after all, thinking about problems can result in solutions. But this kind of thinking often goes around in circles, and the more you try to stop it, the more you feel at its mercy. The end result is a persistent feeling of nervousness, often accompanied by depression.

### Obsessive-Compulsive Disorder

Someone diagnosed with **obsessive-compulsive disorder (OCD)** struggles with obsessions, compulsions, or both. **Obsessions** are recurrent, unwanted thoughts or impulses. Unlike the worries of GAD, they are not ordinary concerns but improbable fears, like suddenly committing an antisocial act or of having been contaminated by germs.

**Compulsions** are repetitive, difficult-to-resist urges to act in a certain way, usually associated with obsessions and against one's own wishes. A common compulsion is hand washing, associated with an obsessive fear of contamination by dirt. Other compulsions are counting and repeatedly checking whether something has been done—for example, whether a door has been locked or a stove turned off.

People with OCD feel anxious, out of control, and embarrassed. Their rituals can occupy much of their time and make them inefficient at work and difficult to live with.

### Posttraumatic Stress Disorder

People who suffer from **posttraumatic stress disorder (PTSD)** are reacting to severely traumatic events (defined as exposure to actual or threatened death, serious injury, or sexual violence). Trauma occurs in personal assaults (sexual assault, interpersonal violence, military combat), natural disasters (floods, hurricanes), and accidents (fires, airplane or car crashes).

Symptoms include reexperiencing the trauma in dreams and in intrusive memories, trying to avoid anything associated with the trauma, and numbing of feelings. Hyperarousal (being on edge or easily startled), sleep disturbances, and other symptoms of anxiety and depression also commonly occur. Such symptoms can last months or even years. Those whose symptoms have lasted only a month before resolving are considered to have **acute stress disorder.** PTSD symptoms often decrease over time, but up to one-third of PTSD sufferers do not fully recover. Recovery may be slower in those who have previously experienced trauma or who suffer from other ongoing psychological problems.

### Treating Anxiety Disorders

Therapies for anxiety disorders range from medication to psychological interventions concentrating on a person's thoughts and behavior. Both drug treatments and cognitive-behavioral therapies are effective in panic disorder, OCD, and GAD. Specific phobias are best treated without drugs.

## Attention-Deficit/Hyperactivity Disorder

**Attention-deficit/hyperactivity disorder (ADHD)** is one of the most common disorders of childhood and adolescence. About 4% of adults also have ADHD. The main features of ADHD are inattention, hyperactivity, and/or impulsivity. *Inattention* includes failure to pay close attention to details; tendency to make careless mistakes; trouble holding attention; failure to listen when spoken to directly; inability to follow through on or complete a task; avoidance of activities that

TERMS

**agoraphobia** An anxiety disorder characterized by fear of being alone away from help and by avoidance of many different places and situations; in extreme cases, a fear of leaving home.

**panic attack** A brief surge of overwhelming anxiety that usually resolves in an hour or less.

**generalized anxiety disorder (GAD)** An anxiety disorder characterized by excessive, uncontrollable worry and anxiety in many situations.

**obsessive-compulsive disorder (OCD)** An anxiety disorder characterized by uncontrollable, recurring thoughts and the performing of senseless rituals.

**obsession** A recurrent, irrational, unwanted thought or impulse.

**compulsion** An irrational, repetitive, forced action, usually associated with an obsession.

**posttraumatic stress disorder (PTSD)** An anxiety disorder characterized by reliving traumatic events through dreams, flashbacks, and hallucinations.

**acute stress disorder** An anxiety disorder that resolves in a month or less.

**attention-deficit/hyperactivity disorder (ADHD)** A disorder characterized by persistent, pervasive problems with inattention and/or hyperactivity to a degree that is not considered appropriate for a child's developmental stage and that causes significant difficulties in school, work, or relationships.

require sustained effort; and tendency to get easily distracted. *Hyperactivity* and *impulsivity* include a tendency to fidget or squirm; inability to stay seated when expected; inability to play quietly; tendency to be high energy, to talk excessively, and to interrupt others; and inability to wait their turn.

To be diagnosed with ADHD, a person must have inattentive or hyperactive-impulsive symptoms of ADHD before age 12 (even if an adult at first diagnosis). There must also be evidence that the ADHD behaviors are present in two or more settings—for example, at home, school or work; with friends and family; and in other activities. Someone who can pay attention at work but is inattentive only at home usually wouldn't qualify for a diagnosis of ADHD. Additionally, it must be clear that the symptoms interfere with or reduce the quality of functioning in social, school, or work settings.

ADHD has no cure, and scientists are still working on treatments. They are using tools such as brain imaging to find ways to prevent it. The use of medications is standard for people who have ADHD and whose functioning is clearly impaired by it; however, medications are considered controversial by some who feel that ADHD is overdiagnosed in people who do not actually have it. Other important treatments include psychotherapy, education and training, and a combination of treatments.

## Mood Disorders

We've all experienced sadness and feeling "down" or irritable, but sometimes these feelings can be persistent or severe and interfere with life functioning. The two main types of **mood disorder,** major depressive disorder and bipolar disorder (what used to be called manic-depression), are together the most common mental disorders in the United States.

**Depression** Depression differs from person to person but includes the following symptoms that persist most of the day and last more than two consecutive weeks:

- A feeling of sadness and hopelessness or loss of pleasure in doing usual activities (anhedonia)
- Poor appetite and weight loss or, alternatively, increased eating compared to usual
- Insomnia or disturbed sleep, including sleeping more than normal
- Decreased energy
- Restlessness or, alternatively, slowed thinking or activity
- Thoughts of worthlessness and guilt
- Trouble concentrating or making decisions
- Thoughts of death or suicide

A person experiencing depression may not have all of the symptoms listed here but must have depressed mood or anhedonia (inability to experience pleasure) and at least four other symptoms. People can have multiple symptoms of depression without feeling depressed, although they usually experience a loss of interest or pleasure.

In some cases, depression is a clear-cut reaction to a specific event, such as the loss of a loved one or a failure in school or work, whereas in other cases no trigger event is obvious. Regardless of the reason, severe symptoms should be taken seriously. Someone who has symptoms of major depression for more than two weeks, even if it is in reaction to a specific event, should consider treatment. One danger of severe depression is suicide, which is discussed later in this chapter, but the overall impact of depression on general health and ability to function, with or without suicidal thoughts, can be devastating.

The National Institutes of Health estimates that **depression** strikes nearly 8.4% of Americans annually—20% of people have it in their lifetime—making depression the most common mood disorder. Depression affects youths as well as adults; about 17% of adolescents ages 12–17 suffer a major depressive episode each year. Depression tends to be more severe and persistent in Black people than in those of other races. Despite this, only about 60% of Black people affected by depression receive treatment for it. Almost twice as many women as men have serious depression. Overall, about three times as many women as men attempt suicide, but women's attempts are less likely to be lethal.

Why more women than men have depression is a matter of debate. Some experts think much of the difference is the result of reporting bias: Women are more willing to admit experiencing negative emotions, being stressed, or having difficulty coping. Women may also be more likely to seek treatment. Other experts point to biologically based sex differences, particularly in the level and action of hormones. It may also be that men are more likely than women to have symptoms such as anger or irritability when they are depressed, leading them to be misdiagnosed or for the diagnosis to be missed. In addition, women's social roles and expectations often differ from those of men. Women may put more emphasis on relationships in determining self-esteem, so the deterioration of a relationship is a cause of depression that can hit women harder than men. Culturally determined gender roles are more likely to place women in situations where they have less control over key life decisions, and lack of autonomy is associated with depression.

The best initial treatment for moderate to severe depression is probably a combination of drug therapy and psychotherapy. Newer prescription antidepressants work well, although they may need several weeks to take effect, and patients may need to try multiple medications before finding one that works well. If someone is severely depressed and at

TERMS

**mood disorder** An emotional disturbance that is intense and persistent enough to affect normal function; two common mood disorders are depression and bipolar disorder.

**depression** A mood disorder characterized by loss of interest, sadness, hopelessness, loss of appetite, disturbed sleep, and other physical symptoms.

risk of suicide, hospitalization for more intensive treatment to ensure the patient's safety is sometimes necessary.

Antidepressants work by targeting key neurotransmitters in the brain, including serotonin. When you take an antidepressant, your levels of serotonin increase. This increase has been revealed to help depression and other body conditions that serotonin influences, including mood, sexual desire and function, appetite, sleep, memory and learning, temperature regulation, and some social behavior.

When women take antidepressants, they may need a lower dose than men; at the same dosage, blood levels of medication tend to be higher in women. An issue for women who may become pregnant is whether antidepressants can harm a fetus or newborn. The best evidence indicates that the most frequently prescribed types of antidepressants do not cause birth defects, although some studies have reported withdrawal symptoms in some newborns whose mothers used certain antidepressants.

Repetitive transcranial magnetic stimulation (rTMS) is a new treatment that targets specific areas of the brain with electromagnetic pulses. rTMS treatments are usually done in 30- to 60-minute sessions five to six times per week for several weeks. It may help some patients whose depression has not responded to other medications.

**Electroconvulsive therapy (ECT)** is effective for severe depression when other approaches have failed, including medications and other electronic therapies. In ECT, an epileptic-like seizure is induced by an electrical impulse transmitted through electrodes placed on the head. Patients are given an anesthetic and a muscle relaxant to reduce anxiety and prevent injuries associated with seizures. ECT usually includes three treatments per week for two to four weeks.

QUICK STATS

**Suicide was among the 9 leading causes of death in the United States for people ages 10–64 in 2020.**

—Centers for Disease Control and Prevention, 2022

For patients with **seasonal affective disorder (SAD)**—a type of depression—the treatment involves sitting with eyes open in front of a bright light source every morning. For patients with SAD, depression worsens during winter months as daylight hours diminish. Light therapy may work by extending the perceived length of the day and thus convincing the brain that it is summertime even during the winter months. The American Psychiatric Association estimates that 10–20% of Americans suffer symptoms that may be linked to the disorder. SAD is more common among people who live at higher latitudes, where there are fewer hours of light in winter.

### Bipolar Disorder

People who experience **mania,** characteristic of a severe mood disorder called **bipolar disorder,** undergo discrete periods of time when they may be restless, have excess energy or activity, feel rested with less sleep than usual, and speak rapidly. They may feel elevated (that is, much better than normal) or abnormally irritable. These feelings are often accompanied by impulsive behavior without regard for the consequences—for example, spending too much money or engaging in risky sexual activity. When such episodes are severe (requiring hospitalization, for example, or producing severe consequences), they are known as manic episodes, and the person who experiences them has what is known as *bipolar I disorder.* If such episodes of elevation or irritability are not so severe as to significantly impair functioning, they are known as *hypomanic episodes.* If hypomania alternates with periods of depression, that person is diagnosed with what is known as *bipolar II disorder.*

People with bipolar disorder typically have periods of both mania or hypomania and depression, and the periods of depression can be persistent and severe. Bipolar disorder typically begins in the late teens through the twenties. Many people with bipolar disorder also struggle with substance and alcohol abuse and anxiety. Suicide rates are high in bipolar disorders, especially early in life. This syndrome affects men and women equally.

Antimanic drugs include lithium (a salt that treats manic episodes), mood stabilizers, and antipsychotic medications. For people who have recurrent episodes of mania or depression, continued, lifelong medication treatment is recommended. Specific medications to treat bipolar depression may also be prescribed.

## Schizophrenia

**Schizophrenia** is a devastating mental disorder that affects a person's thinking and perceptions of reality. People with schizophrenia frequently develop paranoid ideas, false beliefs (delusions), or hallucinations that they believe to be real. The disease can be severe and debilitating or so mild that it's hardly noticeable. Although people are capable of diagnosing their own depression, they usually don't diagnose their own schizophrenia because they often can't see that anything is wrong. This disorder is not rare; in fact, 1 in every 100 people has schizophrenia, most commonly starting in adolescence, which is perhaps what is most tragic and disturbing about the disease—that it starts to affect people in the prime of their lives.

Schizophrenia is likely caused by a combination of genetic and environmental factors that occur during pregnancy and development. For example, children born to older fathers

TERMS

**electroconvulsive therapy (ECT)** The use of electric shock to induce brief, generalized seizures; used in the treatment of selected psychological disorders.

**seasonal affective disorder (SAD)** A mood disorder characterized by seasonal depression, usually occurring in winter, when there is less daylight.

**mania** A mood disorder characterized by excessive elation, irritability, talkativeness, inflated self-esteem, and expansiveness.

**bipolar disorder** A mental illness characterized by alternating periods of depression and mania.

**schizophrenia** A psychological disorder that involves a disturbance in thinking and in perceiving reality.

> ## Ask Yourself
> **QUESTIONS FOR CRITICAL THINKING AND REFLECTION**
>
> Have you ever wondered if you were depressed? Try to recall your situation at the time. How did you feel, and what do you think brought about those feelings? What, if anything, did you do to bring about change and to feel better?

have higher rates of schizophrenia, as do children with prenatal exposure to certain infections or medications. Some general characteristics of schizophrenia include the following:

- ***Disorganized thoughts.*** Thoughts may be expressed in a vague or confusing way.
- ***Disorganized or abnormal motor behavior.*** There may be unexplained agitation, catatonic behavior (not moving or odd postures), or "silly," childlike behavior.
- ***Delusions.*** People with delusions—firmly held false beliefs—may think that their minds are controlled by outside forces, that people can read their minds, that they are great personages like Jesus Christ or the queen of England, or that they are being persecuted by a group such as the CIA.
- ***Auditory hallucinations.*** People with schizophrenia may hear voices when no one is present. Sometimes these voices tell them to do things (like harm themselves or others), belittle and criticize them, or give them a running commentary on their thoughts and behaviors. These voices can seem very real to the person hearing them and therefore are quite terrifying.
- ***Deteriorating social and work functioning.*** Social withdrawal and increasingly poor performance at school or work may be so gradual that they are hardly noticed at first, but over time people suffering from the disease fall far behind their peers—and far behind others' earlier expectations.

None of these characteristics is invariably present. Some schizophrenic people are quite logical except on the subject of their delusions. Others show disorganized thoughts but no delusions or hallucinations.

A schizophrenic person needs help from a mental health professional. Suicide is a risk in schizophrenia, and expert treatment can reduce that risk and minimize the social consequences of the illness by shortening the period when symptoms are active. The key element in treatment is regular medication. Sometimes hospitalization is required temporarily to relieve family and friends.

## SUICIDE

In the United States, suicide is the second leading cause of death for young people ages 10–14 and 25–34. In 2020, an estimated 5% of adults seriously considered suicide; 1% planned suicide, and 0.5% attempted it (see Figure 3.3 for data on suicidal thoughts). Suicide rates vary by race or ethnicity and gender: The suicide rate is highest among American Indians or Alaska Natives and second highest among European Americans. The suicide rate among men is about four times higher than that among women.

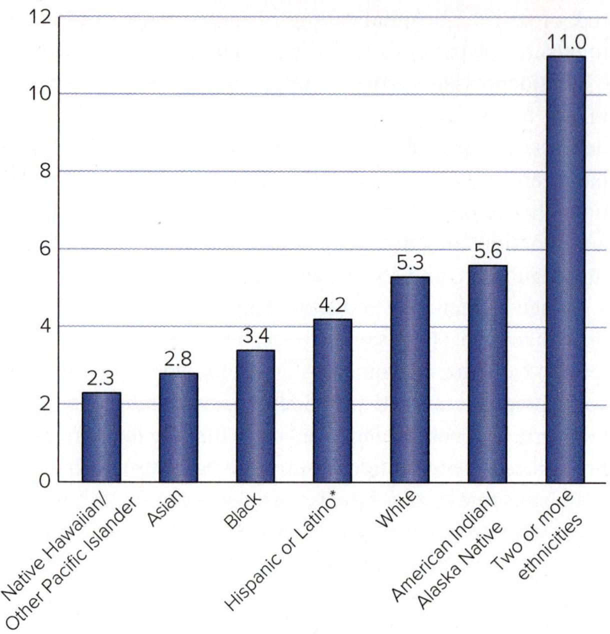


**FIGURE 3.3 Percentages of American adults having suicidal thoughts in 2020, by ethnicity.**

SOURCE: National Institute of Mental Health, 2021.

Of those who had seriously considered suicide, made a suicide plan, or made a suicide attempt, the rate was highest among those ages 18–25. LGBTQ youth were 2–3 times more likely to attempt suicide than straight youth.

Suicide rarely occurs without warning signs (see Table 3.3). About 60% of people who kill themselves are depressed. The more symptoms of depression a person has, the greater the risk. A threat of suicide should be taken not only as a cry for help but also as a possible future occurrence. Here are specific warning signs:

- Any mention of dying, disappearing, jumping, shooting oneself, or other types of self-harm
- Changes in personality, including sadness, withdrawal, irritability, anxiety, fatigue, indecisiveness, or apathy
- A sudden, inexplicable brightening of mood (which can mean the person has decided to attempt suicide)
- A sudden move to give away important possessions, accompanied by statements, such as "I won't be needing these anymore"
- An increase in reckless behaviors

In addition to warning signs, certain risk factors increase the likelihood that someone will attempt suicide (see the box "Deliberate Self-Harm"). Protective factors decrease the likelihood. Risk factors and protective factors can be *intrapersonal, social/situational,* or *cultural.*

## WELLNESS ON CAMPUS
### Deliberate Self-Harm

In general, people want to be well and healthy and to protect themselves from harm. But many individuals—predominantly in their teens and adolescence—do deliberately harm themselves, although in a nonfatal way. A common method of self-harm involves people cutting or burning their own skin, leaving scars that they hide beneath their clothes.

Self-cutting and other self-injurious behaviors are not aesthetically motivated. Many people who engage in these behaviors report seeking the physical sensations (including pain) produced by a self-inflicted injury, which may temporarily relieve feelings of tension, perhaps through a release of endorphins.

The Center for Collegiate Mental Health found that after rising nine consecutive years, self-injury among college students receiving counseling services significantly decreased in 2021, to 26.7%. In examining differences between self-injurers and noninjurers, individuals who had recently engaged in self-harm were significantly more depressed, anxious, and disgusted with themselves. Compared to noninjurers, self-injurers were roughly 4 times more likely to report a history of physical abuse and 11 times more likely to report a history of sexual abuse.

Self-injury is not the same as a suicide attempt, but individuals who repeatedly hurt themselves are more likely than the general population to kill themselves. In any case, self-injury should be taken seriously. Treatment usually includes group therapy, individual therapy, medication (e.g., antidepressants), or stress reduction and management skills. Pharmacological therapy (medication) is a common form of treatment for many psychological disorders. Medications can be very effective, but they have risks and side effects, and they do not work for all patients.

The following are key risk factors:

- A history of previous attempts
- A sense of hopelessness, helplessness, guilt, or worthlessness
- Alcohol or other substance use disorders
- Serious medical problems
- Mental disorders, particularly mood disorders such as depression and bipolar disorder
- Availability of a weapon
- Family history of suicide
- Social isolation
- A history of having been abused or neglected

**Table 3.3** Myths about Suicide: Don't Be Misled

| MYTH | FACT |
|---|---|
| People who really intend to kill themselves do not let anyone know about it. | This belief can be an excuse for doing nothing when someone says they might attempt suicide. In fact, most people who eventually follow through with suicide *have* talked about doing it. |
| People who made a suicide attempt but survived did not really intend to die. | This belief may be true for certain people, but people who seriously want to end their lives may fail because they misjudge what it takes. Even a pharmacist may misjudge the lethal dose of a drug. |
| People who succeed in suicide really wanted to die. | We cannot be sure of that either. Some people are only trying to make a dramatic gesture or plea for help but miscalculate. |
| People who really want to kill themselves will do it regardless of any attempts to prevent them. | Few people are single-minded about suicide even at the moment of attempting it. People who are quite determined to take their lives today may completely change their minds tomorrow. |
| Suicide is proof of mental illness. | Many suicides are carried out by people who do not meet ordinary criteria for mental illness, although people with depression, schizophrenia, and other psychological disorders (including substance use disorders) have a much higher than average suicide rate. |
| People inherit suicidal tendencies. | Certain kinds of depression that lead to suicide do have a genetic component. But many examples of suicide running in a family can be explained by factors such as psychologically identifying with family members who kill themselves, often a parent. |
| All suicides are irrational. | By some standards, all suicides may seem "irrational." But many people find it at least understandable that someone might want to attempt suicide–for example, when approaching the end of a terminal illness or when facing a long prison term. |

- A current or past experience of being a victim of bullying, in person or online

The following are key protective factors:

- Strong religious faith or other cultural prohibition on suicide
- Connection to other people, including family that is supportive
- Engagement in treatment in which the person is getting help
- Connection with one's own children (or even pets)
- Lack of access to lethal means (guns, pills, railroad tracks)

If you are severely depressed or know someone who is, expert help from a mental health professional is essential. Don't be afraid to discuss the possibility of suicide with someone you fear is suicidal. Ask direct questions to determine whether someone seriously intends to kill themself. Encourage them to talk and to take positive steps to improve their situation. You can call the National Suicide Prevention Lifeline at 800-273-TALK (8255). Trained crisis workers are available to talk 24 hours a day, 7 days a week. As of July 2022, dialing, texting, or chatting 988 also connects people to trained counselors. If you think someone is in immediate danger, do not leave them alone. Call for help or take them to an emergency room.

Firearms are used in more suicides than homicides. Among gun-related deaths in the home, 83% are the result of suicide, often by someone other than the gun owner. If you learn someone at high risk for suicide has access to a gun, try to convince him or her to put it in safekeeping.

## MODELS OF HUMAN NATURE AND THERAPEUTIC CHANGE

The psychological disorders discussed in this chapter can be evaluated from at least four perspectives: biological, behavioral, cognitive, and psychodynamic.

### The Biological Model

The *biological model* emphasizes that the mind's activity depends entirely on an organic structure, the brain, whose composition is genetically determined. The activity of neurons, mediated by complex chemical reactions, gives rise to our most sophisticated thoughts, our most ardent desires, and our most pathological behaviors. As an organ, the brain responds well to healthy lifestyle behaviors. When severe mental health issues arise, however, drug therapies can help.

**TERMS**

**stimulus** Anything that causes a response.

**response** A reaction to a stimulus.

**reinforcement** Increasing the future probability of a response by following it with a reward.

**Pharmacological Therapy** The most important kind of therapy inspired by the biological model is pharmacological, or medication treatment. All medications require a prescription from a psychiatrist or other medical doctor. All have received U.S. Food and Drug Administration approval as being safe and more effective than a placebo. However, as with all pharmacological therapies, these drugs may cause side effects. For example, the side effects of widely used antidepressants range from diminished appetite to loss of sexual pleasure. In addition, a patient may have to try several drugs before finding one that is effective and has acceptable side effects. Some of the popular medications currently used for treating psychological disorders are antidepressants, mood stabilizers, antipsychotics, anxiolytics, hypnotics, and stimulants. Neurostimulation is also becoming increasingly available due to its safety and effectiveness.

**Issues in Drug Therapy** The discovery that many psychological disorders have a biological basis in disordered brain functioning has led to a revolution in the treatment of many disorders, particularly depression. The new view of depression as based in brain function may have also lessened the stigma attached to the condition, leading more people to seek treatment. Antidepressants are now among the most widely prescribed drugs in the United States. The development of effective drugs has provided relief for many people, but the wide use of antidepressants has also raised many questions. Critics of drug therapy ask whether the efficacy of antidepressants has been exaggerated by drug company-sponsored research, and they claim that psychological treatments of depression are usually just as good.

Research indicates that, for mild cases of depression, psychotherapy may be more effective than antidepressants. For moderate to severe depression, combined therapy appears to be significantly more effective than either type of treatment alone. Psychotherapy can provide help in managing symptoms and putting them in perspective. A therapist can provide guidance in changing patterns of thinking and behavior that contribute to the problem.

### The Behavioral Model

The *behavioral model* focuses on what people do—their overt behavior—rather than on brain structures and chemistry or on thoughts and consciousness. This model regards psychological problems as "maladaptive behavior" or bad habits. When and how a person learned maladaptive behavior is less important than what makes it continue in the present.

Behaviorists analyze behavior in terms of **stimulus, response,** and **reinforcement.** The essence of behavior therapy is to discover what reinforcements keep an undesirable behavior going and then to try to alter those reinforcements. For example, if people who fear speaking in class (the stimulus) remove themselves from that situation (the response), they experience immediate relief, which acts as reinforcement for future avoidance and escape.

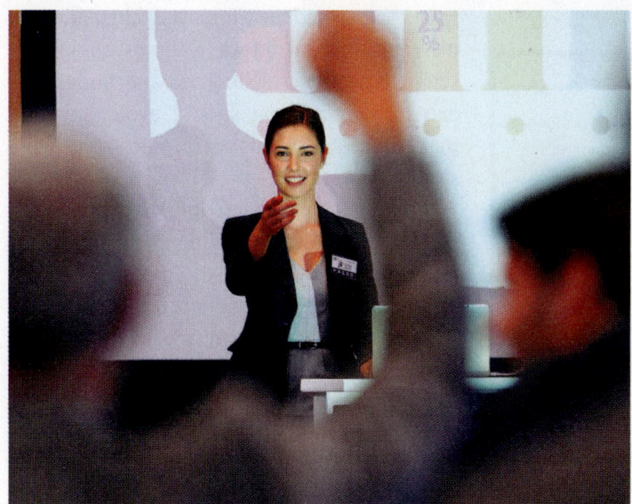

Behavioral therapy can help people overcome many kinds of fears, including that of public speaking. PeopleImages/Digital Vision/Getty Images

To change their behavior, fearful people are taught to practice **exposure**—to deliberately and repeatedly enter the feared situation and remain in it until their fear begins to abate. A student who is afraid to speak in class might begin his behavioral therapy program by keeping a diary listing each time he makes a contribution to a classroom discussion, how long he speaks, and his anxiety levels before, during, and after speaking. He would then develop concrete but realistic goals for increasing his speaking frequency and contract with himself to reward his successes by spending more time in activities he finds enjoyable.

Although exposure to the real situation works best, exposure in your imagination or through the virtual reality of computer simulation can also be effective. For example, in the case of someone who is afraid of flying, a simulated scenario would likely be vivid enough to elicit the fear necessary to practice exposure techniques.

## The Cognitive Model

The *cognitive model* emphasizes the effect of ideas on behavior and feeling. According to this model, behavior results from complicated attitudes, expectations, and motives rather than from simple, immediate reinforcements.

Cognitive therapy tries to expose and identify false ideas that produce feelings such as anxiety and depression. For example, a student afraid of speaking in class may harbor thoughts such as "If I begin to speak, I'll say something stupid; if I say something stupid, the teacher and my classmates will lose respect for me; then I'll get a low grade, my classmates will avoid me, and life will be hell." In cognitive therapy, these ideas will be examined critically. If the student prepares, will they really sound stupid? Does every sentence said have to be exactly correct and beautifully delivered, or is that an unrealistic expectation? Will classmates' opinions be completely transformed by one presentation? Do classmates even care that much? And why does the student care so much about what *they* think? People in cognitive therapy are taught to notice their unrealistic thoughts and to substitute more realistic ones, and they are advised to repeatedly test their assumptions.

## The Psychodynamic Model

The *psychodynamic model* also emphasizes thoughts. Proponents of this model, however, do not believe thoughts can be changed directly because they are fed by other unconscious ideas and impulses. Symptoms are not isolated pieces of behavior but the result of a complex set of wishes and emotions hidden by active defenses (see Table 3.2). In psychodynamic therapy, patients are strongly encouraged to speak and try to gain an understanding of the basis of their feelings toward the therapist and others. Through this process, patients gain insights that help them overcome their maladaptive patterns. Current therapies of this type tend to focus more on the present (the here and now) than on the past, and the therapist tries to facilitate self-exploration rather than providing explanations.

## Evaluating the Models

Most clinicians do not subscribe to a single model but understand mental illness through a *biopsychosocial model.* This model combines many aspects of understanding the mind, recognizing that people are vulnerable to their own genetic history in an environment that includes relationships, culture, and personal idiosyncrasies. Ignoring theoretical conflicts among psychological models, therapists have recently developed pragmatic *cognitive-behavioral therapies* (CBTs) that combine effective elements of both models in a single package. For example, the package for treating social anxiety emphasizes exposure as well as changing problematic patterns of thinking (see the Behavior Change Strategy "Dealing with Social Anxiety" at the end of the chapter). Combined therapies have also been developed for panic disorder, obsessive-compulsive disorder, generalized anxiety disorder, and depression. These packages, involving 10 or more individual or group sessions with a therapist and homework between sessions, have been shown to produce significant improvement.

Drug therapy and CBTs are also sometimes combined, especially in the case of depression. For anxiety disorders, both kinds of therapy are equally effective, but the effects of drug therapy last only as long as the drug is being taken, whereas CBTs produce longer-term improvement. For schizophrenia, drug therapy is a must, but a continuing relationship with therapists who give support and advice is also indispensable.

Psychodynamic therapies have been criticized as ineffective and endless. Of course, effectiveness is hard to demonstrate for therapies that do not focus on specific symptoms. But common sense tells us that being able to open yourself up and

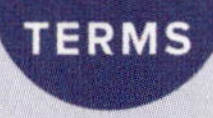


**exposure** A therapeutic technique for treating fear; the subject learns to come into direct contact with a feared situation.

discuss your problems with a supportive but objective person who focuses on you and lets you speak freely can enhance your sense of self and reduce feelings of confusion and despair.

## Other Psychotherapies

In addition to existing forms of treatment, newer psychotherapies such as *dialectical behavior therapy* (DBT) have become available. Developed by psychologist Marsha Linehan, DBT is used to treat borderline personality disorder and chronic suicidal behavior, but it has since been expanded to treat other disorders, such as drug addiction and eating disorders. This therapy uses the principles of standard CBT by encouraging distress tolerance and acceptance of painful feelings and emotions through *mindfulness* (see Chapter 2), originally derived from Buddhist meditation and other Eastern practices. Mindfulness encourages a person to be aware of feelings rather than react to them, and to learn techniques to regulate emotions, by decreasing the intensity of emotional reactions. Mindfulness is practiced in group and individual therapy, often involving the use of workbooks and homework between sessions.

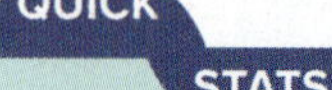


**Since the start of the Covid pandemic, 4 in 10 psychologists said they had been unable to meet the demand for treatment.**

–American Psychological Association, 2021

# GETTING HELP

Understanding the different therapeutic models can help you decide which option might be the best fit for you. When you know you need help, it can seem overwhelming to decide where to turn. Options include self-help, peer counseling, support groups, online help, and professional help—and all of them offer distinct advantages.

## Self-Help

A smart way to begin helping yourself is by finding out what you can do on your own. For example, certain behavioral and cognitive approaches can be effective because they involve developing an awareness of self-defeating actions and ideas for combating them. Start with a self-help list: being more assertive or less aggressive, depending on what's appropriate; communicating honestly; raising your self-esteem by avoiding negative thoughts, people, and actions that undermine it. Confront rather than avoid the things you fear. Although information from books in the psychology or self-help sections of libraries and bookstores can be helpful, you should avoid any that make fantastic claims or deviate from mainstream approaches.

Some people find it helpful to express their feelings in a journal. Writing about painful experiences may provide an emotional release and can help you develop more constructive ways of dealing with similar situations in the future. Research indicates that using a journal in this way can improve physical as well as emotional wellness.

For some people, religious belief and practice may promote psychological health. Religious organizations provide a social network and a supportive community, and religious practices, such as prayer and meditation, offer a path for personal change and transformation.

### Ask Yourself

**QUESTIONS FOR CRITICAL THINKING AND REFLECTION**

Does using computer technology and social media affect you negatively or positively? Do you fear missing out? Do you compare yourself negatively to peers? Are you more engaged with your peers than you otherwise would be? Have you accessed mental health resources or support this way?

## Peer Counseling and Support Groups

Sharing your concerns with others is another helpful way of dealing with psychological health challenges. Just being able to share what's troubling you with an accepting, empathetic person can bring relief. Comparing notes with people who have problems similar to yours can give you new ideas about coping.

Many colleges offer peer counseling through a health center or through the psychology or education department. Volunteer students specially trained in maintaining confidentiality are usually those who offer counsel. They may steer you toward an appropriate campus or community resource or simply offer a sympathetic ear. Support groups are typically organized around a specific problem, such as eating disorders or substance abuse. There are self-help groups through online social media such as Facebook and Twitter (among many platforms), but it is sometimes hard to be certain of their legitimacy. National organizations such as the National Alliance on Mental Illness (NAMI; nami.org) and the Depression and Bipolar Support Alliance (DBSA; dbsalliance.org) can direct you to such support.

## Online Help and Apps

With advances in technology, there are more ways to access help both online and through mobile apps, but these are still very new and are not well tested or studied. The Department of Veterans Affairs has developed a series of free mobile apps, available to the general public, to help with PTSD, insomnia, and other problems.

The Covid pandemic accelerated the development of treatments available through video conferencing, over the phone or on video chat, by exchanging messages or files through secure messaging services; and using remote monitoring technology that allows medical staff to gather and monitor important health

## CRITICAL CONSUMER
### Choosing and Evaluating Mental Health Professionals

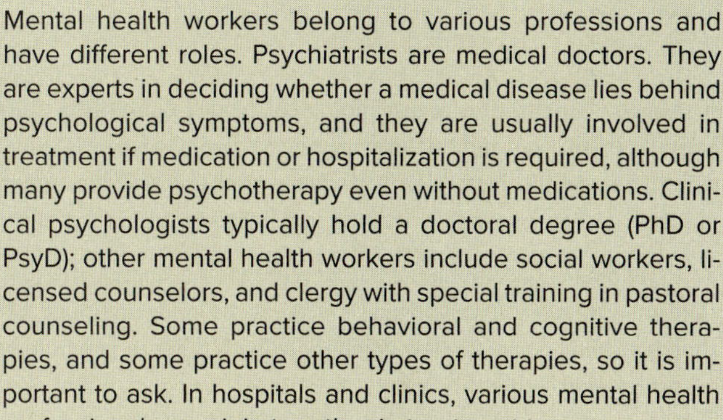

Mental health workers belong to various professions and have different roles. Psychiatrists are medical doctors. They are experts in deciding whether a medical disease lies behind psychological symptoms, and they are usually involved in treatment if medication or hospitalization is required, although many provide psychotherapy even without medications. Clinical psychologists typically hold a doctoral degree (PhD or PsyD); other mental health workers include social workers, licensed counselors, and clergy with special training in pastoral counseling. Some practice behavioral and cognitive therapies, and some practice other types of therapies, so it is important to ask. In hospitals and clinics, various mental health professionals may join together in treatment teams.

In choosing a mental health professional, financial considerations are important. Research the costs and what your health insurance will cover. City, county, and state governments may support mental health clinics for those with few financial resources. Some on-campus services may be free or offered at very little cost.

The cost of treatment is linked to how many therapy sessions will be needed, which in turn depends on the type of therapy and the nature of the problem. Getting this information before you start treatment is important. Many mental health professionals do not accept health insurance payments and only accept direct payments from patients. Psychological therapies focusing on specific problems may require weekly visits for a period of 8–24 sessions, depending on the type of therapy. Therapies based on CBT and DBT are often time limited, and your therapist can tell you how many sessions to expect. Therapies aiming for psychological awareness and personality change, such as psychodynamic therapies, can last months or years.

Deciding whether a therapist is right for you will require meeting the therapist in person. More recently, psychotherapies are offered remotely by video (by computer, tablet, or smartphone), which don't require visiting a physical office. Before or during your first meeting, find out about the therapist's background and training:

- Do they have a degree from an appropriate professional school and a state license to practice?
- Have they had experience treating problems similar to yours?
- How much will therapy cost?

You have a right to know the answers to these questions and should not hesitate to ask them. After your initial meeting, evaluate your impressions:

- Does the therapist seem like a warm, attentive person who would be able to help you and seems interested in doing so?
- Are you comfortable with the therapist's personality, values, and beliefs?
- Are they willing to talk about the techniques in use? Do these techniques make sense to you?

If you answer yes to these questions, this therapist may be satisfactory for you. If you feel uncomfortable—and you're not in need of emergency care—it's worthwhile to set up one-time consultations with one or two others before you make up your mind. Take the time to find someone who feels right for you.

Later in your treatment, evaluate your progress:

- Are you being helped by the treatment?
- If you are displeased, is it because you aren't making progress, or because therapy is raising difficult, painful issues you don't want to deal with?
- Can you express dissatisfaction to your therapist? Such feedback can improve your treatment.

The most important predictor of whether your therapy will be helpful is how much rapport you feel with your therapist *at the first session.* This has been shown to be true no matter what model of psychotherapy the therapist is practicing. You have to like your therapist and feel that they will be able to help you—if you do, there's a good chance that it will be helpful. If you sense that your therapy isn't working or is actually harmful, thank your therapist for their efforts, and find another. It's extra work for you, but it's important for your health.

information, like vital signs. Mental health treatment is particularly amenable to treatment by video, and many people find it as effective and helpful as in-person, face-to-face meetings.

## Professional Help

Sometimes trying self-help or talking to nonprofessionals is not enough, especially if you might have a mental illness. Professional help is appropriate in any of the following situations:

- Depression, anxiety, or other emotional problems interfere seriously with school or work performance or in getting along with others.
- Suicide is attempted or is seriously considered.
- Symptoms such as hallucinations, delusions, incoherent speech, or loss of memory occur.
- Alcohol or drugs are used to the extent that they impair normal functioning much of the time or reducing their dosage leads to psychological or physiological withdrawal symptoms.

Widespread education efforts seem to be reducing the stigma of getting help for psychological symptoms. The rate of college students in treatment increased from 19% in 2007 to 34% by 2017. This number has continued to rise to

## TIPS FOR TODAY AND THE FUTURE

Most of life's psychological challenges can be met with self-help and everyday skills. You can take many steps to maintain your mental health.

**RIGHT NOW YOU CAN:**

- Take a serious look at how you've felt recently. If you have any feelings that are especially hard to handle, consider how you can get help with them.
- Think of the way in which you are most creative (an important part of self-actualization), whether it's in music, art, or whatever you enjoy. Try to focus at least an hour each week on this activity.
- Review the list of defense mechanisms in Table 3.2. Have you used any of them recently or consistently over time? Think of a situation in which you used one of those mechanisms, and determine how you could have coped with it differently.

**IN THE FUTURE YOU CAN:**

- Write 100 positive adjectives that describe you. This exercise may take several days to complete. Post your list in a place where you will see it often.
- Record your reactions to upsetting events in your life. Are your reactions and self-talk typically negative or neutral? Decide whether you are satisfied with your reactions and if they are healthy.

the present. This does not necessarily mean that more students have mental illnesses, but perhaps that the stigma surrounding mental illness (such as depression) or psychological distress may have decreased. Surveys of college presidents reveal that more than 8 in 10 of them reported that improved student mental health was a priority on their campuses.

Despite these gains, it was widely reported that during the Covid-19 pandemic mental health challenges among certain demographics, including younger adults, have been disproportionately troubling; in one survey conducted by the CDC, a quarter of respondents ages 18–24 said they had seriously considered suicide in the past month.

A person has many options when seeking professional help (see the box "Choosing and Evaluating Mental Health Professionals"). Many kinds of professionals are trained to evaluate people's psychological and psychiatric needs and to provide treatment. Psychotherapists come from a variety of backgrounds, including licensed social workers and family and marital therapists (with master's degrees); specially trained nurses with advanced degrees; psychologists (with doctorates); and psychiatrists, who have medical degrees and thus can prescribe medication.

## SUMMARY

- Psychological health refers to the extent to which we are able to function optimally in the face of challenges, whether we have a mental illness or not.
- Maslow's definition of psychological health centers on self-actualization, the highest level in his hierarchy of needs. Self-actualized people have high self-esteem and are realistic, inner directed, authentic, capable of emotional intimacy, and creative.
- Psychological health encompasses more than a single particular state of normality. Psychological diversity—the understanding, acceptance, and respect for how much individuals differ in psychological terms—is valuable.
- Crucial parts of psychological wellness include developing an adult identity, establishing intimate relationships, and developing values and purpose in life.
- A sense of self-esteem develops during childhood as a result of giving and receiving love and learning to accomplish goals. Self-concept is challenged every day; healthy people adjust their goals to their abilities.
- Using defense mechanisms to cope with problems can make finding solutions harder. Analyzing thoughts and behavior can help people develop less defensive and more effective ways of coping.
- A pessimistic outlook can be damaging; it can be overcome by developing more realistic self-talk.
- Honest communication requires recognizing what needs to be said and saying it clearly. Assertiveness enables people to insist on their rights and to participate in the give-and-take of good communication.
- People may be lonely if they haven't developed ways to be happy on their own or if they interpret being alone as a sign of rejection. People who are lonely can take action to expand their social contacts.
- Dealing successfully with anger involves distinguishing between a reasonable level of assertiveness and gratuitous expressions of anger; heading off rage by reframing thoughts and distracting yourself; and responding to the anger of others with an asymmetrical, problem-solving orientation.
- Some people with psychological disorders have symptoms severe enough to interfere with daily living.
- Anxiety is a fear that is not directed toward any definite threat. Anxiety disorders include simple phobias, social anxiety disorders, panic disorder, generalized anxiety disorder, obsessive-compulsive disorder, and posttraumatic stress disorder.
- Depression is a common mood disorder in which a person experiences loss of interest or pleasure in things (anhedonia) in combination with at least four other symptoms. Severe depression carries a high risk of suicide, and suicidal depressed people need professional help.
- Symptoms of mania include abnormally elevated moods or abnormal irritability with unrealistically high self-esteem, little need for sleep, and rapid speech. Mood swings between mania and depression characterize bipolar disorder.

## BEHAVIOR CHANGE STRATEGY
### Dealing with Social Anxiety

Shyness is often the result of both high anxiety levels and lack of key social skills. To help overcome shyness, you need to learn to manage your fear of social situations and to develop social skills such as making appropriate eye contact, initiating topics in conversations, and maintaining the flow of conversations by asking questions and making appropriate responses.

As described in the chapter, repeated *exposure* to the source of your fear—in this case, social situations—is the best method for reducing anxiety. When you practice new behaviors, they gradually become easier and you experience less anxiety.

A counterproductive strategy is avoiding situations that make you anxious. Although this approach works in the short term—you eliminate your anxiety because you escape the situation—it keeps you from meeting new people and having new experiences. Another counterproductive strategy is to self-medicate with alcohol or drugs. Being under their influence actually prevents you from learning new social skills and new ways to handle your anxiety.

To reduce your anxiety in social situations, try some of the following strategies:

- Remember that physical stress reactions are short-term responses to fear. Don't dwell on them. Remind yourself that they will pass, and they will.
- Refocus your attention away from the stress reaction you're experiencing and toward the social task at hand. Your nervousness is much less visible than you think.
- Allow a warm-up period for new situations. Realize that you will feel more nervous at first, and take steps to relax and become more comfortable. Refer to the suggestions for deep breathing and other relaxation techniques in Chapter 2.
- If possible, take breaks during anxiety-producing situations. For example, if you're at a party, take a moment to visit the restroom or step outside. Alternate between speaking with good friends and striking up conversations with new acquaintances.
- Watch your interpretations. Having a stress reaction doesn't mean that you don't belong in the group, that you're unattractive or unworthy, or that the situation is too much for you. Think of yourself as excited or highly alert instead of anxious.
- Avoid cognitive distortions and practice realistic self-talk. Replace your self-critical thoughts with more supportive ones, such as "No one else is perfect, and I don't have to be either" or "It would have been good if I had a funny story to tell, but the conversation was interesting anyway."
- Give yourself a reality check: Ask if you're really in a life-threatening situation (or just at a party), if the outcome you're imagining is really likely (or the worst thing that could possibly happen), or if you're the only one who feels nervous (or if many other people might feel the same way).
- Don't think of conversations as evaluations. Remind yourself that you don't have to prove yourself with every social interaction. And remember that most people are thinking more about themselves than they are about you.

Starting and maintaining conversations can be difficult for shy people, who may feel overwhelmed by their physical stress reactions. If small talk is a problem for you, try the following strategies:

- Introduce yourself early in the conversation. If you tend to forget names, repeat your new acquaintance's name to help fix it in your mind ("Nice to meet you, Amelia").
- Ask questions and look for shared topics of interest. Simple, open-ended questions like "How's your presentation coming along?" or "How do you know our host?" encourage others to carry the conversation for a while and help bring up a variety of subjects.
- Take turns talking, and elaborate on your answers. Simple yes and no answers don't move the conversation along. Try to relate something in your life—a course you're taking or a hobby you have—to something in the other person's life. Match self-disclosure with self-disclosure.
- Have something to say. Expand your mind and become knowledgeable about current events and local or campus news. If you have specialized knowledge about a topic, practice discussing it in ways that both beginners and experts can understand and appreciate.
- If you get stuck for something to say, try giving a compliment ("Great presentation!" or "I love your earrings.") or performing a social grace (pass the chips or get someone a drink).
- Be an attentive listener. Reward the other person with your full attention and with regular responses. Make frequent eye contact and maintain a relaxed but alert posture. (See Chapter 5 for more on being an effective listener.)
- At first, your new behaviors will likely make you anxious. Don't give up—things *will* get easier.

SOURCES: Aron, E. 2010. *The Undervalued Self.* New York: Little, Brown and Co.; Brown, B. 2010. *The Gifts of Imperfection: Let Go of Who You Think You're Supposed to Be and Embrace Who You Are. Your Guide to a Wholehearted Life.* Center City, MN: Hazelden.

• Schizophrenia is characterized by disorganized thoughts, inappropriate emotions, delusions, auditory hallucinations, and deteriorating social and work performance.

• The biological model of understanding human nature and behavior emphasizes that the mind's activity depends on the brain, whose composition is genetically determined. Therapy based on the biological model is primarily pharmacological.

• The behavioral model focuses on overt behavior and treats psychological problems as bad habits. Behavior change is the focus of therapy.

• The cognitive model considers how ideas affect behavior and feelings; behavior results from complicated attitudes, expectations, and motives, not just from simple reinforcements. Cognitive therapy focuses on changing a person's thinking.

• The psychodynamic model asserts that false ideas are fed by unconscious ideas and cannot be addressed directly. In psychodynamic therapy, patients speak as freely as possible in front of the therapist and try to gain an understanding of the basis of their feelings toward the therapist and others.

• Help is available in a variety of forms, including self-help, peer counseling, support groups, and therapy with a mental health professional.

## FOR MORE INFORMATION

*American Association of Suicidology.* Provides information about suicide and resources for people in crisis.

http://www.suicidology.org

*The Annenberg Health and Risk Communication Institute.* Offers information on mental health issues specifically for adolescents and young adults.

http://www.annenbergpublicpolicycenter.org/ahrci/adolescent-mental-health-initiative-book-series/

*Anxiety and Depression Association of America (ADAA).* Provides information and resources related to anxiety disorders and depression.

http://www.adaa.org

*Depression and Bipolar Support Alliance (DBSA).* Provides educational materials and information about support groups.

http://www.dbsalliance.org

*Mental Health America.* Promotes mental health as a critical part of overall wellness, with specific resources for anti-racism and for help during the Covid-19 pandemic.

https://www.mhanational.org/

*NAMI (National Alliance on Mental Illness).* Provides information and support for people affected by mental illness.

800-950-NAMI (help line)

http://www.nami.org

*National Hopeline Network.* An organization devoted to suicide intervention, prevention, awareness, and education. Resources include a 24-hour hotline for people who are thinking about suicide or know someone who is; calls are routed to local crisis centers.

https://www.thehopeline.com

*National Institute of Mental Health (NIMH).* Provides helpful information about anxiety, depression, eating disorders, and other challenges to psychological health.

http://www.nimh.nih.gov

*Substance Abuse and Mental Health Services Administration.* A one-stop source for information and resources relating to mental health.

http://www.samhsa.gov

*U.S. Food and Drug Administration.* Provides access to Medication Guides, which are paper handouts that come with many prescription drugs.

https://www.fda.gov/drugs/drug-safety-and-availability/medication-guides

## SELECTED BIBLIOGRAPHY


Ahmedani, Brian K. 2015. "Racial/Ethnic Differences in Health Care Visits Made Before Suicide Attempt across the United States." *Medical Care* 53(5): 430–435.

American Psychiatric Association. 2013. *Diagnostic and Statistical Manual of Mental Disorders (DSM-5),* 5th ed. Washington, DC: American Psychiatric Publishing.

American Psychiatric Association. 2018. *What Is Mental Health?* (http://www.psychiatry.org/patients-families/what-is-mental-illness).

American Psychological Association. 2021. Demand for mental health treatment continues to increase, say psychologists. *News & Advocacy Press Release* (https://www.apa.org/news/press/releases/2021/10/mental-health-treatment-demand).

Anxiety and Depression Association of America. 2022. Social anxiety disorder (https://adaa.org/understanding-anxiety/social-anxiety-disorder).

Asselmann, E., et al. 2016. Risk factors for fearful spells, panic attacks and panic disorder in a community cohort of adolescents and young adults. *Journal of Affective Disorders* 193: 305–308.

The Association for University and College Counseling Center Directors. 2019. *The Association for University and College Counseling Center Directors Annual Survey: 2019* (https://www.aucccd.org/assets/documents/Survey/2019%20AUCCCD%20Survey-2020-05-31-PUBLIC.pdf).

Carver, C. S., M. F. Scheier, and S. C. Segerstrom. 2010. Optimism. *Clinical Psychology Review* 30(7): 879–889.

Center for Behavioral Health Statistics and Quality. 2021. *Results from the 2020 National Survey on Drug Use and Health: Detailed tables.* Rockville, MD: Substance Abuse and Mental Health Services Administration (https://www.samhsa.gov/data/).

Center for Collegiate Mental Health. 2022. *2021 Annual Report.* Publication No. STA 22-132 (https://ccmh.psu.edu/annual-reports).

Centers for Disease Control and Prevention. 2022. *Facts About Suicide* (https://www.cdc.gov/suicide/facts/index.html).

Czeisler M. É., et al. 2020. Mental health, substance use, and suicidal ideation during the COVID-19 pandemic – United States, June 24–30, 2020. *Morbidity and Mortality Weekly Report* 69: 1049–1057.

Dawson, L., et al. 2021. The impact of the Covid-19 pandemic on LGBT+ people's mental health. Kaiser Family Foundation (https://www.kff.org/other/issue-brief/the-impact-of-the-covid-19-pandemic-on-lgbt-peoples-mental-health/).

Depression Association of America. 2021. Adult ADHD (attention deficit hyperactive disorder) (https://adaa.org/understanding-anxiety/related-illnesses/other-related-conditions/adult-adhd).

Eder, S. 2022. As a crisis hotline grows, so do fears it won't be ready. *The New York Times,* March 13 (https://www.nytimes.com/2022/03/13/us/suicide-hotline-mental-health-988.html).

Gaynes, B. N., et al. 2014. Repetitive transcranial magnetic stimulation for treatment-resistant depression: A systematic review and meta-analysis. *Journal of Clinical Psychiatry* 75(5): 477–489.

Greenhoot, A. F., et al. 2013. Making sense of traumatic memories: Memory qualities and psychological symptoms in emerging adults with and without abuse histories. *Memory* 21(1): 125–142.

Harvard Health Publishing. 2017. What causes depression? Onset of depression more complex than a brain chemical imbalance. Harvard Medical School (https://www.health.harvard.edu/mind-and-mood/what-causes-depression).

Kirov, G. G., et al. 2016. Evaluation of cumulative cognitive deficits from electroconvulsive therapy. *British Journal of Psychiatry* 208(3): 266–270.

Klein, D. N., et al. 2013. Predictors of first lifetime onset of major depressive disorder in young adulthood. *Journal of Abnormal Psychology* 122(1): 1–6.

Kochanek, K. D., et al. 2016. Deaths: Final data for 2014. *National Vital Statistics Reports* 65(4).

Lattie, E. G., S. K. Lipson, and D. Eisenberg. 2019. Technology and college student mental health: Challenges and opportunities. *Frontiers in Psychiatry* 10: 246.

Lin, Y. R., et al. 2008. Evaluation of assertiveness training for psychiatric patients. *Journal of Clinical Nursing* 17(21): 2875–2883.

Linehan, M. M. 1993. *Cognitive-Behavioral Treatment of Borderline Personality Disorder*. New York: Guilford.

Lipson, S. K., E. G. Lattie, and D. Eisenberg. 2019. Increased rates of mental health service utilization by U.S. college students: 10-year population-level trends (2007–2017). *Psychiatric Services* 70(1): 60–63.

Mayo Clinic. 2020. *Schizophrenia* (https://www.mayoclinic.org/diseases-conditions/schizophrenia/symptoms-causes/syc-20354443).

Merritt Hawkins. 2017. *2017 Review of Physician and Advanced Practitioner Recruiting Incentives: An Overview of the Salaries, Bonuses, and Other Incentives Customarily Used to Recruit Physicians, Physician Assistants and Nurse Practitioners*. 24th ed. Dallas, TX: Merritt Hawkins.

Molouki, S., and D. M. Bartels. 2017. Personal change and the continuity of the self. *Cognitive Psychology* 93: 1–17.

Muppala, V., et al. 2021. Alarming trends in suicide by firearms in young Americans. *Annals of Public Health and Research* (https://www.jscimedcentral.com/PublicHealth/publichealth-8-1106.pdf).

National Alliance on Mental Health. 2022. *About Mental Illness* (https://namiofdel-mor.org/resources/about-mental-illness/).

National Institute of Mental Health. 2018. *Anxiety Disorders* (https://www.nimh.nih.gov/health/topics/anxiety-disorders).

National Institute of Mental Health. 2022. *Major Depression* (http://www.nimh.nih.gov/health/statistics/major-depression).

National Institute of Mental Health. 2022. *Prevalence: Any Mental Illness (AMI) among U.S. Adults* (https://www.nimh.nih.gov/health/statistics/mental-illness.

Oldis, M., et al. 2016. Trajectory and predictors of quality of life in first episode psychotic mania. *Journal of Affective Disorders* 195: 148–155.

Orben, A., et al. 2022. Windows of developmental sensitivity to social media. *Nature Communications* 13(1649) (https://doi.org/10.1038/s41467-022-29296-3).

Penn State Center for Collegiate Mental Health. 2016. *2015 Annual Report on Student Counseling Centers* (Publication No. STA 15-108).

Pozzi, M., et al. 2016. Antidepressants and, suicide and self-injury: Causal or casual association? *International Journal of Psychiatry in Clinical Practice* 20(1): 47–51.

Rickwood, D., and S. Bradford. 2012. The role of self-help in the treatment of mild anxiety disorders in young people: An evidence-based review. *Psychology Research and Behavior Management* 5: 25–36.

Rico, A., et al. 2022. Adolescent behaviors and experiences survey—United States, January–June 2021. *Morbidity and Mortality Weekly Report* 71(3).

Rosenthal, B. S., and W. C. Wilson. 2012. Race/ethnicity and mental health in the first decade of the 21st century. *Psychological Reports* 110(2): 645–662.

Rothwell, J. D. 2009. *In the Company of Others: An Introduction to Communication,* 3rd ed. New York: McGraw Hill.

Schatzberg, A. F., and C. DeBattista. 2019. *Manual of Clinical Psychopharmacology,* 9th ed. Washington, DC: American Psychiatric Publishing.

Seligman, M. E. P. 2008. Positive health. *Applied Psychology: An International Review* 57, 3–18.

Simon, G. 2009. Collaborative care for mood disorders. *Current Opinion in Psychiatry* 22(1): 37–41.

Singh, N. N., et al. 2007. Individuals with mental illness can control their aggressive behavior through mindfulness training. *Behavior Modification* 31(3): 313–328.

Soeteman, D., M. Miller, and J. J. Kim. 2012. Modeling the risks and benefits of depression treatment for children and young adults. *Value in Health* 15(5): 724–729.

Substance Abuse and Mental Health Services Administration. 2021. *Key Substance Use and Mental Health Indicators in the United States: Results from the 2020 National Survey on Drug Use and Health* (HHS Publication No. PEP21-07-01-003, NSDUH Series H-56). Rockville, MD: Center for Behavioral Health Statistics and Quality, Substance Abuse and Mental Health Services Administration (https://www.samhsa.gov/data/).

Thurber, C. A., and E. A. Walton. 2012. Homesickness and adjustment in university students. *Journal of American College Health* 60(5): 415–419.

Turner, B. J., A. L. Chapman, and B. K. Layden. 2012. Intrapersonal and interpersonal functions of nonsuicidal self-injury: Associations with emotional and social functioning. *Suicide & Life-Threatening Behavior* 42(1): 36–55.

U.S. Department of Veterans Affairs. 2019. *How Common Is PTSD in Adults?* (https://www.ptsd.va.gov/understand/common/common_adults.asp).

Verhaak, P. F., et al. 2009. Receiving treatment for common mental disorders. *General Hospital Psychiatry* 31(1): 46–55.

Vonasch, A. J., et al. 2017. Death before dishonor: Incurring costs to protect moral reputation. *Social Psychological and Personality Science* (https://doi.org/10.1177/1948550617720271).

Williams, D., et al. 2007. Prevalence and distribution of major depressive disorder in African Americans, Caribbean blacks, and non-Hispanic whites. *Archives of General Psychiatry* 64: 305–315.

Williams, J. 2014. Inside the *New York Times Book Review* "My Age of Anxiety." *New York Times,* January 24, 2014.

**Design Elements:** Assess Yourself icon: Aleksey Boldin/Alamy Stock Photo; Diversity Matters icon: Rawpixel Ltd/Getty Images; Wellness on Campus icon: Radius Images/Alamy Stock Photo; Take Charge icon: VisualCommunications/Getty Images; Critical Consumer icon: pagadesign/Getty Images.

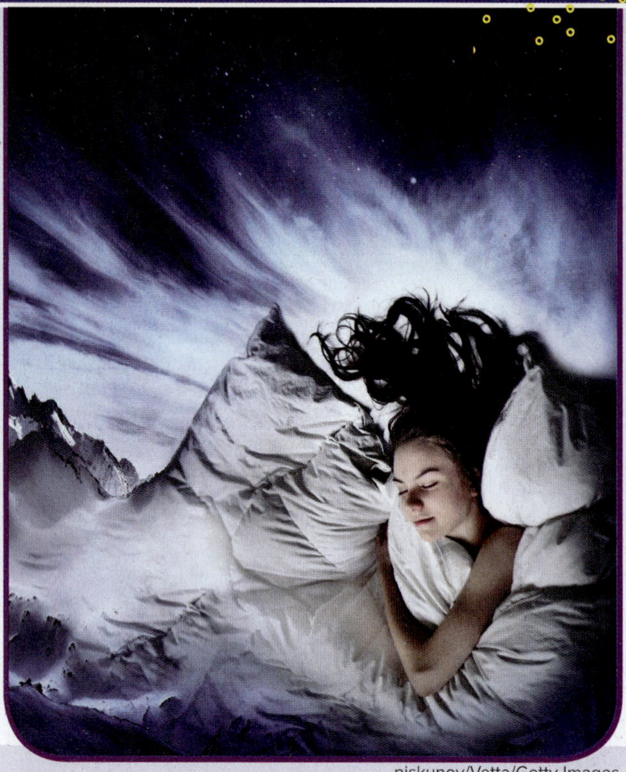

piskunov/Vetta/Getty Images

## CHAPTER OBJECTIVES

- Identify the three stages of sleep
- Understand how to apply good sleep habits
- Explain the health-related benefits of sleep and the consequences of disrupted sleep
- Understand changing sleep needs throughout the life span
- List common sleep disorders, their symptoms, and their treatments
- Understand your patterns of sleepiness and alertness throughout the day
- Understand sleep disrupters and how to reduce their effects

CHAPTER 4

# Sleep

We spend almost one-third of our lives asleep, but few of us understand what sleep is for and why it is necessary for our health. Since we are mostly unconscious during sleep, it is not uncommon to feel that we could be better off if we did not need sleep, and it can be tempting to cut back on sleep to make more time for entertainment or work. As we learn more about how sleep promotes all aspects of our health, however, we see that sleep is as vital as nutrition and physical fitness.

## SLEEP BIOLOGY

Sleep affects almost all systems of the body, including the respiratory, cardiovascular, endocrine, gastrointestinal, urinary, and nervous systems. When we fall asleep, our heart rate and respiratory rates slow, our blood pressure drops, and our body temperature declines. Our consciousness is also profoundly changed during sleep.

### Sleep Stages

Even though we are not conscious when we are sleeping, our brains are still active. Sleep is divided into distinct stages characterized by different patterns of electrical brain activity. The way these patterns come together is called *sleep architecture*, and it changes over the course of the life span.

Brain activity during sleep is typically measured by a monitoring device called an **electroencephalogram (EEG).** During wakefulness, when a person is quietly resting with eyes closed, the EEG shows a pattern called the alpha rhythm. This pattern is characterized by regular brain waves that occur 8–10 times per second. These brain waves change, and different parts of the brain are activated or suppressed as a person progresses through the three stages of sleep.

> **TERMS**
> **electroencephalogram (EEG)** A monitoring device that records brain activity.

**NREM Sleep** The first three stages of sleep are grouped together as **non-rapid eye movement (NREM) sleep.** The purpose of NREM sleep remains mysterious, but theories suggest that it improves neural connections; it also facilitates information processing, cell repair, and removal of waste from the brain. As we move through the stages of NREM sleep, brain waves grow larger and slower. Resting with eyes closed produces an EEG pattern called the alpha rhythm. Stage I and II sleep produce theta waves. In the deepest stage of sleep, Stage III, delta waves are even slower, like large waves in the ocean (see Figure 4.1).

**STAGE I** Stage I is a brief transitional phase from wakefulness to sleep. It is light sleep, easily disturbed by outside stimuli. Sometimes it is hard to differentiate between a person's awake state and Stage I. Someone who wakes from this stage may not even be aware they had fallen asleep. In Stage I, the eyes may move slowly back and forth (not to be confused with rapid eye movement sleep, described below); respiration grows more regular than during wakefulness; and muscles relax and may twitch.

**STAGE II** In most adults, about 50% of nightly sleep will consist of Stage II sleep. In Stage II sleep, the heart rate slows and body temperature drops. The EEG shows bursts of brain activity called *sleep spindles* and *k-complexes.* Lasting one or two seconds, these waves appear only during NREM sleep, and they occur most often in Stage II. These bursts represent the brain working to remain asleep during occurrences of external stimuli, such as a noise in the room. They are also thought to be involved in memory processing. In this stage of sleep, sensory stimuli from the environment can no longer reach the higher-level brain centers, meaning people are not as responsive. If awakened, people in Stage II are more likely to know they have been asleep.

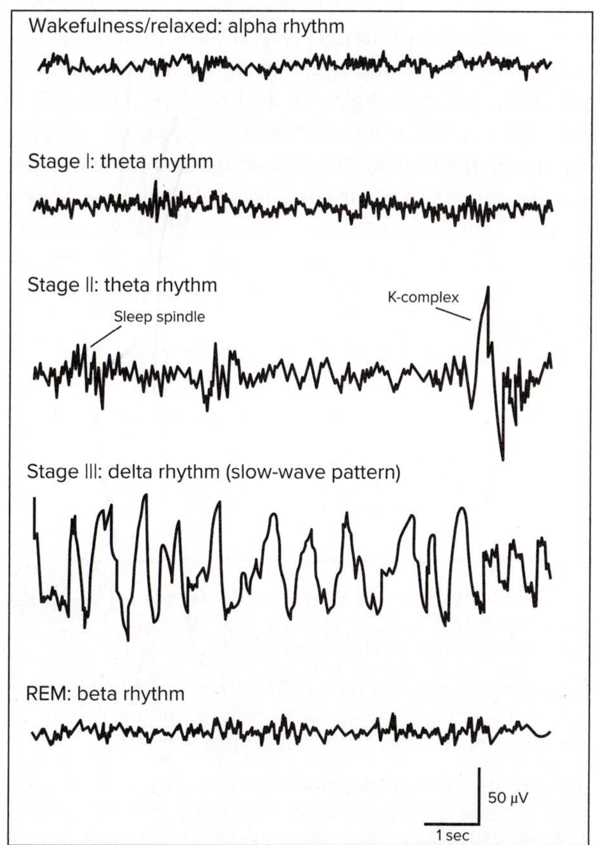


**FIGURE 4.1 EEG patterns change with each stage of sleep.**

**STAGE III** Stage III is the deepest stage of sleep and the one most necessary for feeling well rested upon waking. It is also believed to be the stage that supports the most restorative functions, such as rejuvenating actions like synthesizing proteins or managing stress. The length of this stage increases after physical exercise or extended periods without sleep.

In this **slow-wave sleep,** or deep sleep, it is difficult for us to wake up quickly and, if awakened, we may at first be confused for several minutes. Parts of the brain associated with memory, learning, and other cognitive functions can become active during Stages II and III.

**REM Sleep** The final stage of sleep is **rapid eye movement (REM) sleep.** REM sleep is named for periods during which the eyes under closed lids move quickly, similar to a person who is awake. This is when most vivid dreaming occurs. Although it can be difficult to wake people from REM sleep, once awake they are usually oriented to their surroundings and not confused.

Unlike the synchronized brain waves of NREM sleep, in REM sleep the brain exhibits electrical activity that is indistinguishable from that of a person who is awake and engaged in complex thinking. Some regions of the brain are up to 30% more active during REM sleep than during wakefulness. This is especially evident in parts of the brain that are related to emotions. Blood pressure, respiration, and heart rate also rise in REM sleep. Muscles in the limbs, however, are actively inhibited by the brain so that the body is prevented from moving during dreaming, a form of paralysis.

**Sleep Cycles** When people fall asleep, they first cycle through the three stages of NREM sleep (N1–N3), possibly repeating N2 after completing N3 (Figure 4.2). This is followed by a period of REM sleep, which is always a final stage

**TERMS**

**non–rapid eye movement (NREM) sleep** Of two main sleep phases, the phase that constitutes three substages, including one with the deepest sleep and with slow-wave brain activity.

**slow-wave sleep** Characteristic patterns of electrical brain activity measured by the electroencephalogram (EEG) during the deepest stage of sleep, Stage III.

**rapid eye movement (REM) sleep** One of two main phases of sleep, the final phase of a sleep cycle, when most dreaming occurs and eyes rapidly move under closed eyelids. Brain activity increases to levels equal to or greater than those during waking hours, and blood pressure, respiration, and heart rates rise.

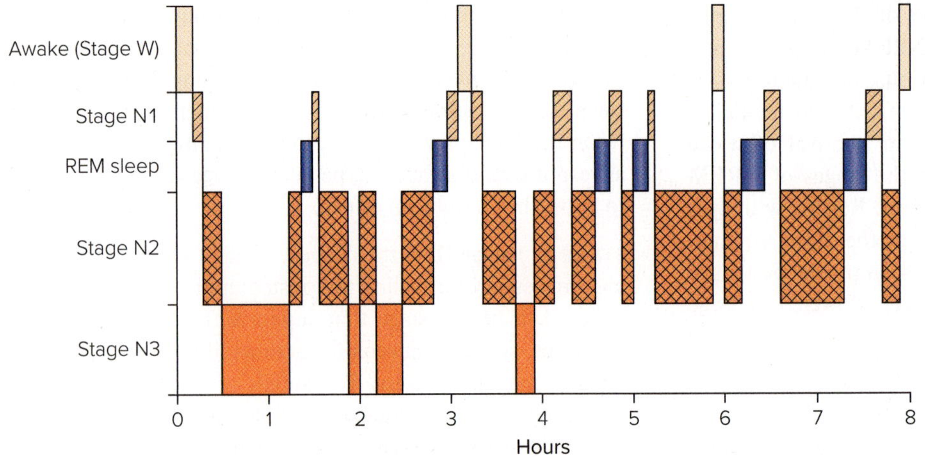


**FIGURE 4.2 Sleep stages and cycles. During one night of sleep, the sleeper typically goes through four or five cycles of NREM sleep (three stages) followed by REM sleep.**

SOURCE: Schwab, R. J. 2020. *Overview of Sleep.* Merck Manual: Consumer Version (https://www.merckmanuals.com/home/brain,-spinal-cord,-and-nerve-disorders/sleep-disorders/overview-of-sleep).

in the sleep cycle. From beginning to end, the sequence lasts about 90 minutes, and then the cycle repeats. During one night of sleep, a person may go through four to five cycles, but the cycles differ somewhat over the course of the night. The periods of slow-wave sleep are longer earlier in the night, and the periods of REM are longer in the last part of the night. Because people have more REM sleep in the last part of the night, that is when dreaming most often occurs.

## Natural Sleep Drives

One key for understanding both how sleep can be disrupted and how it can be improved is to understand the natural biological sleep drives. There are two major biological processes that regulate the drive to sleep: the circadian rhythm and the homeostatic sleep drive.

### Circadian Rhythm

The **circadian rhythm** is the typically 24-hour sleep-and-wake pattern coordinated by the brain's master internal clock, the **suprachiasmatic nucleus (SCN).** The SCN controls the sleep-wake cycle not only of the brain but also of the entire body. Every cell in every organ has DNA machinery that produces an internal clock, and these cellular clocks are synchronized by the SCN. The SCN also regulates the timing of hundreds of other biological processes, including hunger and thirst, sexual behavior, body temperature, and emotions. The power of the circadian system for many different aspects of biology is being increasingly recognized, and the 2017 Nobel Prize in Physiology was awarded to Jeffrey Hall, Michael Rosbash, and Michael Young, scientists who helped explain the genetic mechanisms underlying clock timing on the cellular level (see Figure 4.3).

Night is our circadian rest phase, and though we are physically inactive during sleep, our bodies are repairing cells, removing toxins, and consolidating memory. Insufficient sleep at night greatly hinders the body from accomplishing these life-sustaining tasks.

#### CIRCADIAN RHYTHM VARIATION

Are you a "night owl" or a "morning lark"? Genetics plays a role. Larks perform better in the morning, but tire earlier in the day and are more sensitive to sleep loss. Owls perform better in the evening and handle sleep loss better. But because they don't grow sleepy until later in the evening, and social obligations often come early in the day, the sleep needs of night owls are often difficult to attain. Many of us fall somewhere in between these two types.

Throughout the day, we also encounter external stimuli that can influence our master clock. Some of us are more sensitive to these "time-givers," called **zeitgebers,** so it is important to be aware of how they can affect sleep quality, needs, and behavior. There are many zeitgebers, including activity, exercise, and eating, but the strongest and most important is light.

**LIGHT** Light has a direct connection to the SCN master clock via specific cells in the eye. Instead of processing vision, these cells send impulses directly to the SCN to allow it to measure light. If we are exposed to light in the morning at a certain time on a regular basis, this exposure signals the SCN that it should set the internal clock to wake around that time. This allows us to develop sleep habits that are naturally regulated. But exposure to light can also reinforce unhealthy behavior. For example, if we are regularly exposed to bright light late at night, then the SCN will reset itself, shifting our sleep and wake periods to occur later. This is because the body responds to light in the evening by delaying the sleep phase. In contrast, when we are exposed to light in the morning, our body resets to an earlier clock time and earlier wake time, advancing the sleep phase.

If your goal is advancing the sleep phase, the early-morning light exposure needs to occur about two hours prior to your usual wake time, and not before. For example, let's say you usually get up at 10:00 a.m. You stay up late with the light on, and even though a 6:00 a.m. light gets you out of bed,

**TERMS**

**circadian rhythm** The body's sleep-and-wake pattern coordinated by the brain's master internal clock, the suprachiasmatic nucleus (SCN).

**suprachiasmatic nucleus (SCN)** Master clock that sets and controls the sleep–wake cycle, sending signals to the brain and to every cell in every organ of the body.

**zeitgebers** Phenomena that can influence and reset the body's master clock, such as light, activity, exercise, and eating. Light directly affects cells in the eye to send signals directly to the SCN to measure outside light.

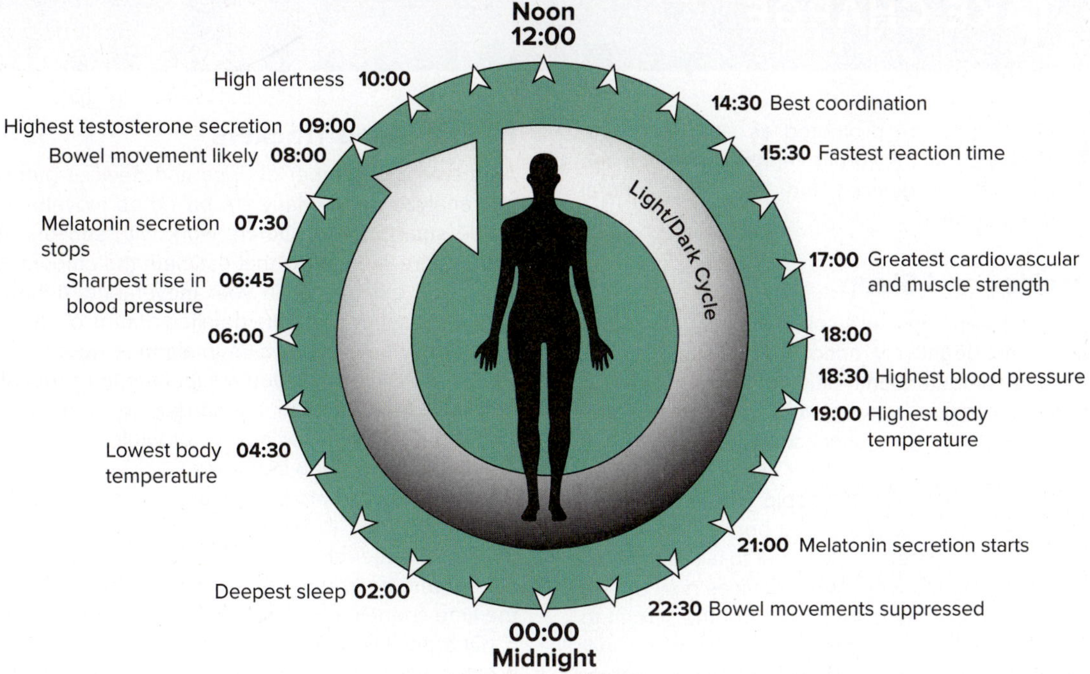


**FIGURE 4.3 The circadian clock of a person who wakes up in the morning and sleeps at night.**

SOURCE: School of Biological Sciences, Royal Holloway University of London, Matthew Ray/EHP

> **Ask Yourself**
>
> **QUESTIONS FOR CRITICAL THINKING AND REFLECTION**
>
> Do you ever use a device right before going to sleep? Do you ever wake up at night to check your phone? How could you change your digital behavior to improve your sleep?

your sleep phase the following evening is still delayed. That 6:00 a.m. light hit you too early, and you will still not feel like sleeping at an early bedtime.

A light exposure that would cause a morning reset of sleep time would be between 8:00 and 9:00. This exposure would advance your sleep phase, so that you feel like waking up a little earlier the next day. Interestingly, the reversal point at which the effect of light changes the SCN coincides with the time when body temperature is lowest.

Another mechanism involving the SCN detects the loss of light at the end of the day. When natural light fades at dusk, an impulse is conveyed via the SCN to the pineal gland in the brain to produce **melatonin,** which signals to systems that are involved in preparation for sleep (see Figure 4.4). People who are blind often have problems with sleep because they lack the visual light signals that help synchronize circadian rhythms.

> **TERMS**
>
> **melatonin** A hormone secreted by the pineal gland, especially in response to darkness and in inverse proportion to the amount of light received by the retina. It helps control sleep-and-wake cycles and circadian rhythms.

To strengthen the circadian rhythm, it can help to get good light exposure in the morning and throughout the day and to reduce exposure to light at night. The challenge is that, day and night, we are exposed to abundant sources of artificial light, which undermine our reliance on the sun's natural 24-hour cycle. Electronics compound our unnatural light exposure, especially by introducing blue light. We commonly use backlit electronic devices at night, which can affect our sleep, as well as sleep on the following nights. See the box "Digital Devices: Help or Harm for a Good Night's Sleep?"

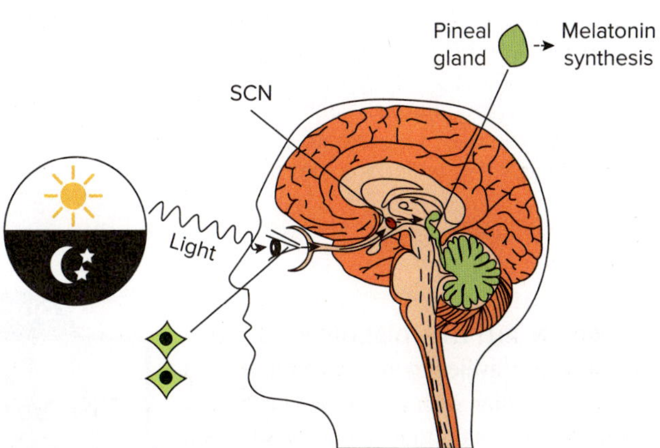


**FIGURE 4.4 Light coming into the eye is conveyed via the SCN to the pineal gland, which produces melatonin.**

SOURCE: Tan, D-X., et al. 2011. Significance and application of melatonin in the regulation of brown adipose tissue metabolism: Relation to human obesity. *Obesity Review* 12(3): 167–188.

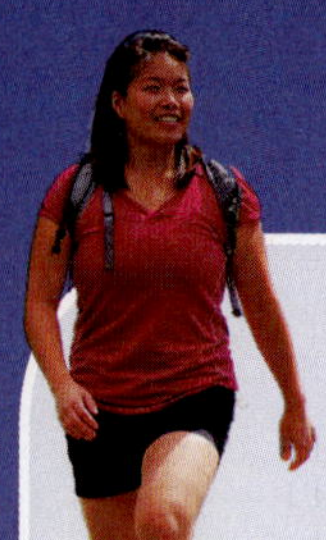

## TAKE CHARGE
## Digital Devices: Help or Harm for a Good Night's Sleep?

Many apps are promoted as sleep aids and trackers. Can they really improve sleep? Or can using digital devices hurt the body's natural sleep cycles?

### Digital Devices and Sleep

Before we look at sleep apps, let's consider how your use of digital devices can negatively affect your sleep. Tablets, smartphones, and computers emit blue light, which impedes the release of melatonin, a hormone that affects sleep-and-wake cycles. In one study, researchers compared the sleep of people who read an e-book on a backlit digital device in the hours before bedtime with that of people who read a print book. Those who read the backlit digital book had reduced melatonin release and therefore took longer to fall asleep and were less alert the next morning. Many devices now offer a "night mode," which shifts the color balance of the screen to reduce blue light. However, several studies found no evidence that enabling this feature actually benefits melatonin release or sleep.

Does heavy texting affect sleep? Psychologist Karla Murdock reported that texting was a direct predictor of sleep problems among first-year students in a study that examined links among interpersonal stress, text-messaging behavior, and three indicators of college students' health: burnout, sleep problems, and emotional well-being.

To best avoid the impacts of light and psychological stress, Murdock and other sleep experts suggest turning off your screens. Use them less during the day and also when preparing to sleep at night. If you have trouble relaxing and transitioning to sleep in the evenings, shut down all your devices an hour or more before you intend to sleep.

### Digital Aids for Relaxation

Now that you are resting in the dark, why would you consider using a sleep app or digital tracker? Ironically, a smartphone may help you get to sleep.

Many free and low-cost apps provide aids for relaxation and for improving sleep. Some include music, white noise, or nature sounds (e.g., wind, rain, waves, or songbirds). Others offer specific techniques, such as guided meditation or breathing exercises, to promote relaxation to aid in falling asleep. Experiment to find the aids that work best for you.

### Digital Sleep Trackers

An increasing number of apps and devices purport to track and analyze sleep. Many are based on movement detectors inside smartphones. Others work with sensors attached to your mattress or pillow that estimate the amount and type of sleep you get based on your movements during the night. These apps may generate detailed graphs of your sleep quality and may time your wake-up alarm to go off at the point in your sleep cycle when you will feel the most refreshed. Some apps also include a sound recorder, which detects sleep talking, snoring, and other noises, providing further information about nighttime sleep behavior.

In addition to smartphone apps, specialized fitness wristbands designed to be worn 24 hours a day include sleep trackers. These rely on wearable movement detectors. Some incorporate heart-rate data as well, which is used to estimate the time spent in each stage of sleep throughout the night.

One positive effect of using a sleep tracker is simply the greater focus it places on sleep. But these devices should be used with caution, since constantly monitoring our sleep and activity can also increase our anxiety toward sleep and exacerbate insomnia symptoms in some people.

Apps and devices may be popular, but no current consumer technology can match a sleep lab when it comes to detecting sleep stages or diagnosing specific sleep disorders such as sleep apnea. If you enjoy the features of an app or wearable tracker, go ahead and use them, but don't rely on an app to diagnose the presence or absence of a serious sleep problem.

SOURCES: Baron, K. G., et al. 2017. Orthosomnia: Are some patients taking the quantified self too far? *Journal of Clinical Sleep Medicine* 13(2): 351–354; Chang, A. M., et al. 2015. Evening use of light-emitting eReaders negatively affects sleep, circadian timing, and next-morning alertness. *Proceedings of the National Academy of Sciences* 112(4): 1232–1237; Bhat, S., et al. 2015. Is there a clinical role for smartphone sleep apps? Comparison of sleep cycle detection by a smartphone application to polysomnography. *Journal of Clinical Sleep Medicine,* February 3; Duraccio K. M., et al. 2021. Does iPhone night shift mitigate negative effects of smartphone use on sleep outcomes in emerging adults? *Sleep Health* 7(4): 478–484; Gradisar, M., et al. 2013. The sleep and technology use of Americans. *Journal of Clinical Sleep Medicine* 9(12): 1291–1299; Behar, J., et al. 2013. A review of current sleep screening applications for smartphones. *Physiological Measurement* 34(7): R29–R46; Ritterband, L. M., et al. 2009. Efficacy of an Internet-based behavioral intervention for adults with insomnia. *Archives of General Psychiatry* 66: 692–698.

**CIRCADIAN RHYTHM DISRUPTIONS** Anyone who has traveled to another time zone is probably familiar with jet lag, which occurs when the internal body clock is set to a different time from that of a new environment. People with jet lag commonly experience difficulty falling asleep and waking up at appropriate times. It can also cause nausea and loss of appetite, which is related to the gastrointestinal system's being out of sync with the new time zone.

> **QUICK STATS**
>
> **The best time to start a nap is between 12:30 and 2 pm.**
>
> —Sleep.org, 2021

Habits can also cause people's internal body clocks to be set at a time that is different from the time zone where they live. An example is a person who stays up regularly until 4:00 a.m. and sleeps until noon, a pattern called *delayed sleep phase*. If this person occasionally has to wake up earlier—say, to attend a morning lecture or appointment—the switch can be difficult, and the person may feel unwell, just like a person with jet lag.

**Homeostatic Sleep Drive** The homeostatic sleep drive and circadian system work independently of each other, although they are broadly aligned to promote sleep and wakefulness. The **homeostatic sleep drive** is the pressure to sleep that builds in relation to the amount of sleep you've had and your duration of wakefulness. The homeostatic sleep drive is like an hourglass that turns over the moment you wake in the morning: the pressure for sleep builds up steadily throughout the day. The homeostatic sleep drive is thought to be mediated biologically by the accumulation of the neurochemical **adenosine** in the brain. This is a by-product of energy metabolism in the brain and promotes sleep onset. When one falls asleep, this by-product is cleared, and the pressure to sleep is reduced. Naps in the afternoon will clear adenosine and reduce feelings of sleepiness during the day, but they may also reduce the pressure to sleep at night.

Someone with insomnia, who has a problem falling asleep or staying asleep, might benefit from trying to increase sleep pressure and strengthen the homeostatic sleep drive. This can be done by setting a reasonably early wake time every morning and avoiding naps during the day, allowing enough wake time for the sleep drive to increase. Caffeine blocks the homeostatic sleep drive by blocking adenosine receptors in the brain. It is important to know that caffeine can have effects for up to 24 hours.

## CHANGES IN SLEEP BIOLOGY ACROSS THE LIFE SPAN

Sleep rhythms and needs change throughout our lives. Babies need the most sleep and may sleep up to 19 hours per day. As you can see from Figure 4.5, the number of sleep hours we need generally declines until adulthood, at which point most people need between 7 and 9 hours of sleep. Teenagers typically need 8–10 hours of sleep nightly, but surveys of adolescents across the world make it clear that most teenagers get much less than the recommended amount, which can have consequences for emotional and cognitive health.

It is important to realize that the requirement for sleep depends on the individual. Genetics plays a role in how much sleep we need. Carriers of specific rare genes may be so-called short sleepers, who need only 4 to 6 hours of sleep per night to prevent sleep deprivation. Other individuals need 9 or 10 hours of sleep to feel their best.

**TERMS**

**homeostatic sleep drive** Pressure to sleep that builds the longer one is awake, mainly driven by adenosine, a neurochemical that accumulates in the brain. Sleep clears the adenosine, thereby reducing the pressure to sleep.

**adenosine** An important neurochemical that accumulates during wakefulness, and after a prolonged period will mediate sleepiness.

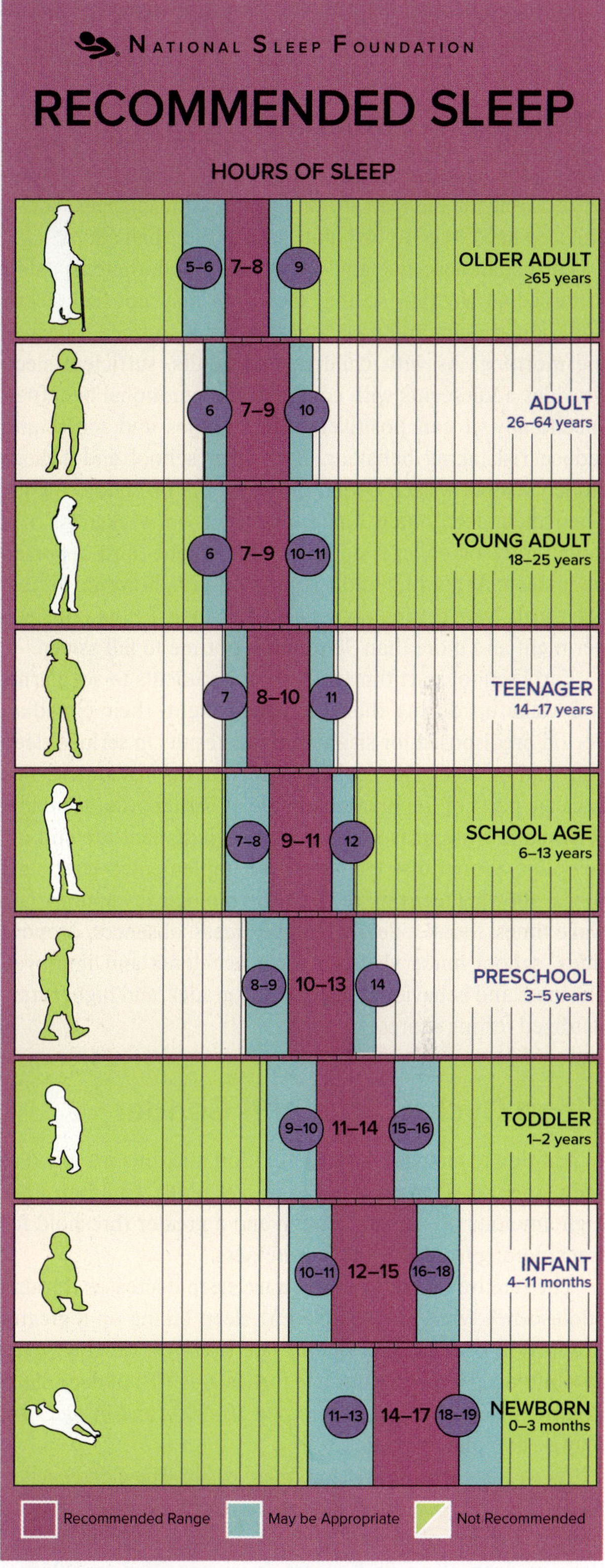


**FIGURE 4.5 Sleep needs change over the course of the life span.**

SOURCE: National Sleep Foundation

For most people, the optimal amount of sleep fall within the ranges recommended by research.

## Changes in Circadian Rhythm

Among the most prominent changes with respect to sleep patterns during the life span are circadian rhythm changes. Young children need to go to bed quite a bit earlier than adults.

During adolescence and young adulthood, there is a shift in circadian rhythm, so that teenagers may not feel sleepy until late at night and have a natural drive to sleep longer in the morning. As with children and adults, sufficient sleep provides adolescents with cognitive and emotional benefits—specifically, it can positively affect grades and mood and reduce risk-taking behavior. Both high school and college students show a sleep deficit of 1–3 hours on school nights. Then they sleep much longer and later on weekends. In a large study of college students, almost one-third reported poor sleep. According to the study's criteria, however, almost two-thirds were getting poor sleep—less than 7 hours of sleep per night and more than 30 minutes of time to fall asleep.

Early school start times often force students to set alarms and wake up during their biological night—their circadian period predisposed for sleep—and this results in serious sleep deprivation. Sleep is especially important during adolescence because parts of the brain in charge of higher-order thinking, problem solving, reasoning, and good judgment are still developing. School districts that have implemented later start times, allowing teens more sleep and biologically appropriate wake times, found a decrease in tardiness, absences, dropout rates, school nurse visits, and car accidents and improved alertness and behavior in class, better grades, and higher standardized testing scores.

## Sleep Cycles, Age, and Gender

In addition to changes in sleep duration, the time we spend in each stage of sleep changes as we get older. Children have high amounts of slow-wave sleep and a greater threshold for transitioning from sleep to wakefulness.

The relative amount of slow-wave sleep decreases through adolescence, with Stage II NREM sleep taking up a greater proportion of the night. By our late twenties, we enter even less into deep sleep. By our late forties, 60–70% of deep sleep is gone. By age 70, it has decreased 80–90%, and by age 74 it may be completely absent.

As we get older, we wake up more easily. The elderly generally wake up more often during the night because they are in lighter stages of sleep. They spend only a short amount of time in deep sleep and so are more sensitive to external stimuli. The shift to earlier sleep and wake times, combined with reduced deep sleep, can cause inadvertent napping late in the day, which can in turn prevent sleep when it is attempted at bedtime. Their advanced circadian rhythm prevents catch-up sleep in the morning and leads to more sleepiness during the day.

Age not only reduces the time spent in restorative sleep, it also diminishes the number and the intensity of deep-sleep brain waves. Scientists don't yet know if reduced slow-wave sleep may be a response to lifestyle changes, such as less physical activity and learning, or an indication that the brains of older adults lose the ability to sustain the slow, coordinated brain activity of deep sleep. Reduced or absent slow-wave sleep may also increase the risk of neurodegeneration.

Women in general report more symptoms of sleeplessness and are more likely to be diagnosed with insomnia; men report more snoring and are more likely to be diagnosed with **sleep apnea,** repeated involuntary breathing pauses during sleep. One reason women may notice changes in their sleep patterns is hormones. During the menstrual cycle, some women may experience increased sleepiness or disrupted sleep. Progesterone levels rise during the second half of the menstrual cycle, promoting sleep, but drop just before the cycle begins, causing sleep difficulty. During pregnancy, extra weight and the position of the fetus can make sleep difficult. During menopause, many women have additional sleep problems, such as hot flashes. Awareness of these changes in sleep can help women cultivate strategies to ensure that they meet their sleep needs.

**TERMS**

**sleep apnea** The involuntary, repeated interruption of normal breathing during sleep, caused by blocked airways (for example, throat or trachea) or faulty brain signaling to muscles that support breathing.

### Ask Yourself

**QUESTIONS FOR CRITICAL THINKING AND REFLECTION**

Can you think of a time you had an early class and had difficulty focusing? Did you make adjustments to your schedule? What other actions improved the way you felt?

# SLEEP AND ITS RELATION TO HEALTH

Sleep directly influences our moods, creativity, and ability to learn, and it has an impact on immune function and longevity. College students who sleep enough hours and sleep efficiently have faster reaction times, higher grades, more optimism, and higher energy levels. They suffer less daytime sleepiness, and have a lower risk of traffic accidents and fewer mental health complaints.

## Mood and Depression

Depression and anxiety are common; most people will experience them at some point in their lives. Sleeping difficulty, especially insomnia, is often also present in people struggling with depression or mood disorders. Research shows that the risk for depression rises with insomnia, even when people were not depressed when sleep troubles began. Studies have also shown that when patients with depression specifically treat sleep problems, their depression also improves, even if the treatments are not medicinal. One explanation for this link is that the neurochemical changes associated with sleep problems make people more vulnerable to depression.

Studies conducted during the Covid-19 pandemic highlighted the link among depression, anxiety, and insomnia. An international survey of more than 22,000 adults found that rates of insomnia at the beginning of the pandemic were twice as high in many countries as pre-pandemic rates, with anxiety and depression significantly elevated as well.

It is probably apparent to most people that a night of poor sleep can make them irritable the next day. This effect can compound over the course of many days or weeks. Lack of sleep can also make people more volatile and disinhibited, which can lead to behaviors people might regret or decisions that are not carefully thought out. In adolescence and young adulthood, risk-taking behaviors have been shown to increase with insufficient sleep.

Sometimes sleep problems are correlated with suicide risk, especially among young adults. A study of 438 female college students reports an important association between insomnia and suicidal thoughts. Other studies of college students found an association between nightmares and suicidal thoughts. Some students classified as suicidal also reported taking sleep medications and often feeling too cold while sleeping. Being aware of the connections between mood and sleep, and prioritizing sleep health, can contribute to better mental health.

## Dementia

One major disease that can affect memory as we get older is dementia. Dementia is so common that up to 20% of us are likely to develop memory problems as we age. This is a devastating disease, but it turns out that better sleep may help prevent us from developing mild cognitive impairment and dementia. Studies in mice have revealed that there are changes in the fluid that surrounds the brain during sleep, such that the flow around the nerve cells or the cerebrospinal fluid increases by 90% in the tissues of the brain while we sleep. It appears that this increase in flow allows for by-products of nerve metabolism to clear out. These by-products include proteins such as amyloid, which can accumulate in the brain during the day and have been associated with the development of Alzheimer's disease, a form of dementia. The fluid-clearance system in the brain, called the glymphatic system, processes the waste from the brain. Without sleep, this system does not clear as efficiently. Epidemiological studies and cohort studies in humans provide further evidence that poor sleep, and particularly sleep disruption at night, increases the risk for dementia or causes it to develop earlier.

> **Ask Yourself** ?
>
> **QUESTIONS FOR CRITICAL THINKING AND REFLECTION**
>
> Can you remember a time when you were sleep deprived and did something you regretted? How did you feel that day?

## Athletic Performance

Because performance can be improved by changing our sleep habits, professional sports teams and athletes have started hiring sleep consultants. One researcher studying competitive college swimmers observed that after adhering to a more rigid sleep schedule, students performed their personal bests. The research was more formally developed to evaluate college basketball players, and it showed that shooting accuracy and sprint times improved after several weeks of instituting a 10-hour sleep schedule.

The amount of sleep is not the only influential factor: Circadian rhythms also affect performance. A study of 40 years of NFL games compared West Coast versus East Coast teams who were playing on the opposite coast. Crossing time zones, especially with longer flights, increases fatigue and jet lag for most athletes. But the real disadvantage hits the East Coast teams playing night games on the West Coast. They consistently performed poorly due to circadian factors that kick in by the game's end, around 2:00 a.m. on their body clocks. In a study of 909 college students, nighttime exercise was associated with later bedtimes and worse sleep quality compared to morning exercise.

Among a number of other sleep-related physiological factors that affect performance are hormones. Growth hormones and testosterone, for example, are released during sleep, and their levels are reduced with sleep loss.

Finally, sleep is vitally important for intense skills training. Sleep can help consolidate the motor learning required to make new techniques more efficient and automated. For example, getting a night's sleep after learning to press a sequence on the keyboard enhanced study participants' speed and accuracy on the computer. Some studies have shown that there is only one opportunity to take advantage of this. If you do not get enough sleep the first night after learning, getting extra sleep on subsequent nights will not result in skills improvement.

## Musculoskeletal Pain

Poor sleep can increase our risk for developing body pain and create a lower pain threshold. If someone is suffering from body pain, it is especially worthwhile to screen for sleep disorders. Improving a patient's sleep can improve pain symptoms. One challenge to this approach is that pain can interfere with sleep, creating a feedback loop; however, in some patients it may be easier to address sleep problems, which can ease pain symptoms and, in turn, lead to better sleep.

## Obesity and Weight Management

We eat more and gain more weight when we don't get enough sleep. Obesity is a big public health problem in the United States, and many more people who are not obese are overweight (see Chapter 12). Healthy eating habits and exercise are necessary for maintaining a healthy weight, and attention to sleep is also helpful. Ghrelin and leptin, hormones that regulate appetite, are affected by sleep. Ghrelin rises when we have not eaten, increasing appetite. Leptin rises after we eat, reducing hunger and making us feel full. When people are sleep deprived, leptin levels are 20–30% lower, while ghrelin levels can increase 20–30%. One study found that teens sleeping less than 8 hours per night were more likely to eat unhealthy food, putting them at risk for weight gain and worse cardiometabolic outcomes.

## Cardiovascular Disease

The connection between sleep and cardiovascular disease has been studied extensively. The strongest connection is between sleep apnea, which is prevalent in people who snore, and hypertension (abnormally high blood pressure). One of the largest studies showed that people with mild sleep apnea had twice the risk of developing hypertension in the next four years, while those with moderate or severe apnea had three times the risk.

Hypertension is particularly worrisome because it is directly related to risks of other cardiac disorders, such as coronary artery disease, heart attacks, and strokes. In addition to causing hypertension, sleep apnea directly promotes inflammatory pathways that are thought to further contribute to the buildup of plaques that narrow the arteries of the heart and brain. Cardiac arrhythmias, including atrial fibrillation, which is a major risk factor for stroke, can also be promoted by sleep apnea.

People who sleep less or who have insomnia also appear to have increased cardiovascular risk. In men with insomnia and sleep duration of less than six hours, there was an increased risk of mortality over 14 years of 400%. If these men also had hypertension, the risk rose to 700%. A study of more than 6000 people showed that insomnia in midlife led to a threefold greater risk of mortality over 13–15 years. How helpful are sleep medications? Because sleeping pills generally inhibit neural activity and do not produce natural sleep, it is best to avoid them if possible. Several large studies suggest that the use of sleep medications is associated with a higher mortality risk.

## Diabetes

Diabetes is also a common condition, and it increases the risk for other disorders, including cardiovascular diseases. According to the Centers for Disease Control and Prevention (CDC), prediabetes is present in over one-third of people aged 18 or older and in nearly half of people 65 or older. Diabetes mellitus is also listed as the seventh most common cause of death in the United States. While obesity is by far the major risk factor for the development of diabetes after childhood, sleep can affect the risk of diabetes as well. In studies of short sleep duration, the risk for type 2 diabetes was shown to rise, especially in men. Men with short sleep durations had twice the risk for developing diabetes. In another series of studies in which people were asked about their sleep quality, those who reported problems falling asleep or staying asleep had a 50% increased risk for developing diabetes.

When sleep apnea goes untreated, people appear to have problems with glucose regulation also seen in diabetes. In young, healthy people, when slow-wave sleep was disrupted by low-grade noise, even when the total sleep time remained the same, the ability of insulin to regulate glucose was impaired.

## Public Health Impact

Because we consistently underestimate how sleep deprived we are, we risk our own and others' lives without realizing it. One misconception is that we can recover from missed sleep with one or two good nights' rest. But even three nights of recovery sleep does not bring us back to full functioning. How many errors are committed on the road, in the skies, or while controlling hazardous materials because the operator falls asleep? What can we do about this?

You can notice a sleep deficit with the following signs: difficulty getting out of bed in the morning and missed alarm clocks, an ability to fall back asleep at 10:00 or 11:00 a.m., an inability to feel alert before noon without caffeine, grogginess that lasts more than a half hour after waking or continues after the natural circadian post-lunch dip, and a tendency to fall asleep while reading or watching a movie.

**Auto Accidents** Do not get behind the wheel without enough sleep. In driving simulations, study participants who slept only four hours a night drove off the road six times more often than people who had slept eight hours. The number of errors committed by the sleep-deprived matched the number committed by another group of participants who had slept eight hours but were legally drunk. A fourth group, both sleep-deprived and drunk, drove off the road almost 30 times more than the rested, sober group. This means that the combination of alcohol and sleep deprivation are exponentially lethal; unfortunately, people tend to drink alcohol at nighttime, when sleep pressure is greatest.

In many states, driving while sleepy is considered driving while impaired, and people can be fully liable for the consequences (see Chapter 17). The National Highway Traffic Safety Administration estimates that sleepiness accounts for more than 100,000 traffic accidents per year. The CDC, which believes much drowsy driving is under-reported, estimates sleep-deprived drivers are responsible for nearly 6000 fatal crashes each year.

QUICK
STATS
24% of drivers, at least once in the past month, were so tired they could barely keep their eyes open.
— AAA Foundation, 2020

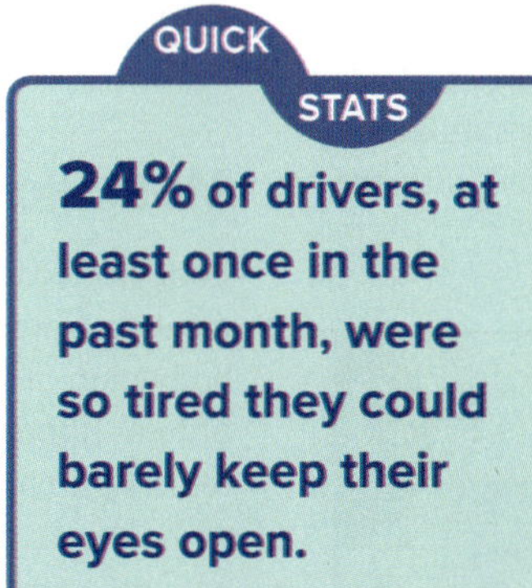

A **microsleep,** or momentary lapse in concentration, can last just a few seconds. That brief moment, however, is time enough to fatally crash your vehicle. During a microsleep, your brain loses perception of the outside world. You lose sight, your eyelids closing partially or all the way, and you lose control of your motor skills. Most of the time you don't even realize you've had a microsleep.

People who are most at risk for falling asleep driving are those who regularly get less than seven hours of sleep. They include young people aged 18–29 and men slightly more often than women. Other candidates are parents with small children, shift workers, people who have accumulated sleep debt, or those who have other untreated sleep disorders such as sleep apnea or insomnia. Although they can occur at any time, the peak period for drowsiness-related accidents is 4:00 to 6:00 a.m. Sleepiness can increase when people take substances such as muscle relaxants, antihistamines, cold medicines, or alcohol.

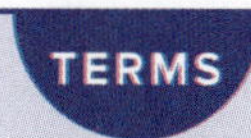


**microsleep** A momentary lapse in which some parts of the brain lose consciousness.

The good news is that accidents due to sleepiness can be prevented. First and foremost, it is important to ensure adequate sleep time and avoid extremes of sleep deprivation and ensure that any disorder of sleep, like sleep apnea, is properly treated. If you feel drowsy while driving, it is best to immediately pull over and stop driving.

## GETTING STARTED ON A HEALTHY SLEEP PROGRAM

By analyzing your sleep, eating, and exercise habits, and identifying obstacles to sleeping such as medical conditions, you can devise strategies to improve your sleep behaviors. Use the suggestions below to guide you.

### Step I: Take an Inventory

Use the sleep questionnaire in the Assess Yourself box to get a general idea of whether you are getting enough sleep. You can then use the sleep diary (Figure 4.6) for a closer look at your sleep habits.

**Sleep Diary**

| | Name | | | | | | | |
|---|---|---|---|---|---|---|---|---|
| Complete in the Morning | Today's date (include month/day/year): | Mon | Tues | Wed | Thurs | Fri | Sat | Sun |
| | Time I went to bed last night:<br>Time I woke up this morning:<br>No. of hours slept last night: | | | | | | | |
| | Number of awakenings and total time awake last night: | | | | | | | |
| | How long I took to fall asleep last night: | | | | | | | |
| | How awake did I feel when I got up this morning?<br>1—Wide awake<br>2—Awake but a little tired<br>3—Sleepy | | | | | | | |
| Complete in the Evening | Number of caffeinated drinks (coffee, tea, cola) and time when I had them today: | | | | | | | |
| | Number of alcoholic drinks (beer, wine, liquor) and time when I had them today: | | | | | | | |
| | Naptimes and lengths today: | | | | | | | |
| | Exercise times and lengths today: | | | | | | | |
| | How sleepy did I feel during the day today?<br>1—So sleepy had to struggle to stay awake during much of the day<br>2—Somewhat tired<br>3—Fairly alert<br>4—Wide awake | | | | | | | |

**FIGURE 4.6 A sleep diary can help you discover your sleep pattern.**

SOURCE: National Heart, Lung, and Blood Institute (NHLBI)

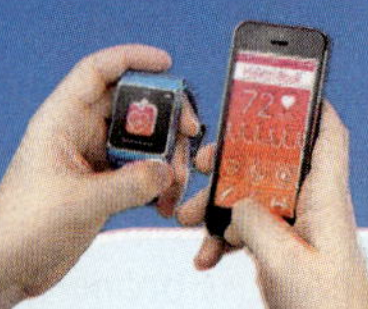

## ASSESS YOURSELF

### Questionnaire: Do I Get Enough Sleep?

Here is a brief questionnaire to help you reflect on your sleep habits and patterns.

Directions: For each description, choose the number under the heading (Usually, Sometimes, Rarely, Never) that corresponds most closely to your experience. Notice that the numbers vary in each column.

| | USUALLY | SOMETIMES | RARELY | NEVER |
|---|---|---|---|---|
| 1. I sleep soundly. | 1 | 2 | 3 | 4 |
| 2. I feel that I get enough sleep. | 1 | 2 | 3 | 4 |
| 3. I go to bed at about the same time each night. | 1 | 2 | 3 | 4 |
| 4. I engage in a stimulating activity just before bedtime. | 4 | 3 | 2 | 1 |
| 5. I drink coffee a few hours before bedtime. | 4 | 3 | 2 | 1 |
| 6. My snoring wakes me up. | 4 | 3 | 2 | 1 |
| 7. I take a nap during the day. | 4 | 3 | 2 | 1 |
| 8. I feel sleepy during the day. | 4 | 3 | 2 | 1 |
| 9. I fall asleep reading or watching TV. | 4 | 3 | 2 | 1 |
| 10. I wake up more than once during the night. | 4 | 3 | 2 | 1 |
| 11. I have difficulty falling asleep. | 4 | 3 | 2 | 1 |
| 12. I wake up feeling rested. | 1 | 2 | 3 | 4 |
| 13. I remember that I had dreams when I wake up. | 1 | 2 | 3 | 4 |
| 14. I have a problem waking in the morning. | 4 | 3 | 2 | 1 |
| 15. I drink alcohol a few hours before or near to bedtime. | 4 | 3 | 2 | 1 |
| 16. I look at the clock several times before getting up. | 4 | 3 | 2 | 1 |
| 17. I have to get up to use the bathroom. | 4 | 3 | 2 | 1 |
| 18. I take medication to sleep. | 4 | 3 | 2 | 1 |
| 19. If I wake up during the night, I have trouble going back to sleep. | 4 | 3 | 2 | 1 |
| 20. I feel sleep deprived. | 4 | 3 | 2 | 1 |

#### Scoring

**To calculate your score,** total the numbers you selected. The result is your total score.

If your score is above 40, you should track your sleep in Figure 4.6. This chapter describes many coping strategies that can help you improve the quality of your sleep. Your school's counseling center can also provide valuable support.

## Step II: Identify Sleep Disrupters

**Sleep disrupters** are factors that interfere with the ability to fall asleep or stay asleep that can usually be corrected if they are targeted specifically.

SLEEP DISRUPTER CHECKLIST

- Do I have symptoms of apnea or risk for apnea (snoring or gasping even if healthy weight)?
- Do I have symptoms of restless leg syndrome, or do I kick in my sleep frequently?
- Do I have frequent rhinitis or nasal congestion?
- Do I have reflux?
- Do I often have to get up to use the bathroom at night?
- Do I have discomfort or pain at night?
- Is there something in the bedroom that wakes me up at night?

**Disrupters** There are certain medical and health conditions that can physiologically affect sleep.

**REFLUX** Reflux, a common hidden sleep disrupter, occurs when a small amount of fluid from the acidic contents of the

> **TERMS**
> **sleep disrupters** Factors that interfere with the ability to fall asleep or stay asleep that can usually be corrected if they are targeted specifically. Examples are caffeine, reflux, nasal congestion, cough, urination, anxiety or stress, pain, and environmental factors, among others.

stomach rises into the esophagus, irritating the upper airway. This can cause impaired sleep quality and awakenings. Reflux is worsened by caffeine, chocolate, and mint, which cause the muscle that closes the stomach opening (the gastroesophageal sphincter) to relax. Most people have experienced reflux symptoms, which can also be more common at night when lying down.

Even babies and small children can have reflux that pauses their breathing and disrupts sleep. One sign of reflux can be a dry cough at night or a hoarse voice during the day, even when there is no sensation of acid. For anyone suffering disrupted sleep, it is worthwhile to consider avoiding food and fluid for at least three hours before bedtime. Take vitamins, medicines, or supplements during the day so they do not aggravate reflux problems at night.

**NASAL CONGESTION AND COUGH** Many people suffer from allergies that cause a runny or stuffy nose. Even when mild, this can lead to changes in breathing at night and cause sleep disruption. Measures that can be taken to reduce this problem include using anti-allergy pillow covers and clean bedsheets. There are also nasal saline sprays, and if needed, over-the-counter nasal anti-inflammatory steroid types of medications. It is important not to take medications that have ephedrine on a long-term basis since these can worsen nasal congestion. Nasal saline and nasal steroid sprays do not cause these problems. If nasal obstruction is more severe, it can sometimes be beneficial to discuss this with an ear, nose, and throat specialist. Coughing can cause sleep disruption at night. Common causes of coughing at night are postnasal drip, asthma, and reflux. It is best to avoid using cough suppressants if possible. It is generally better to find and treat the cause of the cough.

**URINATION** People can be awakened by needing to use the bathroom at night. One simple remedy can be to avoid all fluids in the three hours prior to bedtime.

**ANXIETY AND STRESS** Stress and worry can make sleeping more difficult. (See Chapter 2 to learn about how to manage stress.) Daytime exercise can be helpful for reducing stress and may reduce anxiety at night. It is important not to engage in stimulating or stressful activities right before bed. Students are often studying and working in the evening, and it can be better to stop these activities about an hour before bedtime to have a "wind-down" period. To avoid having to deal with problems left until nighttime, set aside some time during the day to allow for planning. Meditation and other relaxation strategies in the evening can also help to clear one's mind before bedtime.

**PAIN** Pain can be a significant sleep disrupter. Lack of sleep can worsen pain symptoms. There are some commonsense interventions that may be helpful in alleviating pain at night. Replace the mattress if it promotes pain. Pillows should be of appropriate thickness for optimal neck positioning. Mattress toppers, including the memory foam type, may be beneficial for joint pain. Be cautious with pain medications (see the box "Sleep-Improving and Sleep-Disrupting Medications").

**THE BEDROOM** To sleep well, you need a physical environment that is comfortable and does not interfere with normal physiological sleep processes. Ideal room temperature is warm enough for a person to be comfortable but cool enough to allow body temperature to decline as a person falls asleep. Some people tend to have cold feet or hands before going to bed, and for those people it may be beneficial to take a bath or be adequately warmed before getting into bed. A bedroom should also be quiet and dark, without television and pets. Pets should generally be trained to stay off the bed, though good sleepers may like to have them in the bedroom.

**TOO MUCH CAFFEINE** If you have problems falling or staying asleep, you should consider the possibility that caffeine is interfering with sleep. When you try to fall asleep at night, you may have enough sleep pressure to do so quickly; however, as your sleep pressure is relieved, the effects of caffeine consumed earlier in the day may grow more pronounced. It is important to be aware of the many hidden sources of caffeine and the variability in caffeine content in these sources (Table 4.1).

## NEXT STEPS

- Sleep log–keep a sleep diary to discover your sleep pattern. It is best when doing the sleep diary to fill it out just once per day following the night of sleep. The sleep time should be an estimate and does not have to be exact, since it is best not to have any clocks visible at night in the bedroom.
- Choose some principles to implement or sleep disrupters to target.
- Which sleep disrupters did you identify as potential problems?

**Table 4.1** Caffeine Content of Common Beverages and Chocolate

| FOOD | SERVING SIZE | CAFFEINE (MG) |
|---|---|---|
| Coffee, Starbucks, brewed | 8 fl. oz | 160 |
| Coffee, regular, brewed | 8 fl. oz | 130 |
| Frappuccino beverage, Starbucks | 9.5 fl. oz | 115 |
| Red Bull | 8.3 fl. oz | 80 |
| Ice cream, coffee | 8 fl. oz | 50–80 |
| Espresso, Starbucks | 1 fl. oz | 75 |
| Vault | 12 fl. oz | 70 |
| Mountain Dew | 12 fl. oz | 55 |
| Tea, regular, brewed | 8 fl. oz | 50 |
| Tea, latte, Starbucks Tazo Chai | 8 fl. oz | 50 |
| Espresso, regular | 1 fl. oz | 40 |
| Coca-Cola/Pepsi, regular, flavored, diet | 12 fl. oz | 35–40 |
| Tea, fruited, Snapple | 8 fl. oz | 20 |
| Dark chocolate, Hershey's | 1.45 oz | 20 |
| Milk chocolate, Hershey's | 1.55 oz | 10 |
| Sprite/7-Up | 12 fl. oz | 0 |

SOURCE: Insel, Paul, Don Ross, Kimberley McMahon, and Melissa Bernstein. 2021. *Nutrition*. 7th ed. Burlington, MA: Jones & Bartlett Learning.

## WELLNESS ON CAMPUS: Sleep-Improving and Sleep-Disrupting Medications

*Should I take a sleeping aid?*

Most sleep medications sold over the counter contain diphenhydramine (the active ingredient in Benadryl) or a similar antihistamine product. Histamine is a normal wake-promoting neurochemical in the brain, so antihistamines will tend to induce sleepiness. Over-the-counter sleep aids (Tylenol PM, Advil PM) contain twice the amount of diphenhydramine found in most allergy medications. These can slow down cognitive function and cause forgetfulness—they should rarely be taken on a regular basis. Melatonin is an over-the-counter medicine with relatively few side effects, making it a better choice than diphenhydramine and cetirizine. Taking a low dose several hours before bedtime mimics the natural release of the melatonin that occurs at dusk. If possible, prescription sleep medications should be avoided. They have been associated with a variety of problems, including sleepwalking, incoordination and falls, sleep-eating, car accidents, and in some studies, dementia and earlier mortality. These are generally not intended for long-term use, and studies have shown that nonmedicinal interventions are as effective and have longer-term benefits without the side effects of prescription medications.

### Alcohol and Tobacco

Some people think that an alcoholic drink at night helps with sleep. Although alcohol may help with sleep onset in some people, most find that it has a negative effect later in the night, resulting in nighttime awakenings and poor-quality sleep. Even if people are not aware of this overnight, they will feel the effects the next day. Alcohol also worsens sleep-related breathing disorders.

Tobacco also has adverse effects on sleep. Tobacco is a stimulant and can directly interfere with sleep. In heavier users, it also has withdrawal effects that can wake them up.

### Medications

Many medications cause insomnia or interfere with sleep, and other medications cause sleepiness. If you are having trouble sleeping and are taking medications prescribed by a doctor, it may be important to review these medications to ensure that none is responsible for the sleep difficulty or increased sleepiness. For medications that can promote insomnia, it might be helpful to discuss alternative medications that cause less sleep disruption or to discuss dosing these at earlier times of the day. Medications that cause sleepiness should be taken later in the day.

Common medications that may cause insomnia include many antidepressants, beta-blockers for high blood pressure, steroid medications, and over-the-counter medications labeled for daytime use. In susceptible people, medications for thyroid disorders or attention disorders can reduce sleep quality if these are taken in the afternoon or evenings.

Pain medications can also be bad for sleep. Opioids, in particular, cause a large number of problems, including addiction and sleep disruption. These medications negatively affect breathing and cause sleep apnea.

Opioids also directly cause sleepiness in almost 75% of people. Muscle relaxants can also affect respiration at night and can cause considerable sleepiness. While these may be prescribed for short periods, there are almost always alternatives.

## Step III: Improve Sleep Fitness

In general, once sleep disrupters have been addressed, improving sleep often comes down to consolidating sleep or identifying the best sleep window for your biological rhythms, and as much as possible trying to adhere to that optimal frame for obtaining good sleep.

**Lack of Sleep** Daytime sleepiness is a major problem for college students. It can act as a roadblock to good grades, wellness, and achieving the optimal college experience, which is a foundation for later independence, employment, and social well-being.

It's important to understand that the physiological tendency to sleep has only one primary cause, which is the ever-building pressure to sleep exerted by the homeostatic sleep drive. Knowing this, we won't be tempted to blame our sleepiness on dull sedentary situations, such as warm rooms, boring classes, long drives, or alcohol. With adequate and quality sleep, and little sleep debt, alertness, energy, motivation, and optimal functioning should continue throughout the day.

If your drowsiness is related to insufficient sleep, start by thinking about your baseline sleep needs. People are different in terms of how much sleep they need. Start with a trial of simply increasing the time that is allowed for sleep to see what amount provides you with optimal functioning. This is the type of exercise that was instituted in some of the studies of athletes that led to better athletic performance, but increasing sleep time has also been shown to enhance school performance. To implement a 9- or 10-hour sleep opportunity, first identify a consistent time to wake up that would allow enough time to meet obligations in the morning. Depending on your sleep needs, even trying to ensure an 8-hour sleep opportunity might change your life.

**Social Jet Lag** If you are someone who regularly sleeps until noon on the weekends, it may be difficult to sleep when you are trying to get up and ready for the work or school week, which for most people is on Sunday night.

## TAKE CHARGE
### Delayed Sleep Phase

Common to young adults and college students is the delayed sleep phase. As teenagers, our circadian rhythm shifts forward, so we naturally stay up later than our parents. As we age into young adults, or even middle-aged adults, our schedule gradually slides back to bedtimes somewhere around 10:00 or 11:00 p.m. In this transition time, we can nevertheless get into the habit of staying up too late—and have great difficulty getting up in the morning. People who have a biologically based night-owl tendency are more likely to fall into this pattern. A variety of tactics can be used to get us our optimal amounts of sleep.

#### 1. Bedtime Goal

A bedtime goal can be calculated by figuring out what your individual sleep need is. It may be helpful to identify a time in your life when you felt you were sleeping well and were able to function and engage well during the day with less difficulty getting up. Once you consider how many hours of sleep you were getting at that time, you can set up a goal sleep time frame. If you function best with 8.5 hours of sleep and have to get up at 7:00 a.m., then the goal bedtime might be 10:30. People with delayed tendencies should be realistic about setting an attainable schedule.

No matter your schedule, think about how to strengthen your circadian rhythm to help you get sleepy around the goal bedtime. Delayed-type people tend to eat late at night, so it is important to count back three hours before your intended bedtime to try to finish eating. Similarly, physical activity should occur during the day and not in the evening.

#### 2. Winding Down

You should give yourself a wind-down time of about an hour before bedtime. During this time, avoid engaging with work, electronic devices, or any negative mental activity; instead this time might be spent arranging things in the house or setting things up to make yourself ready for the next morning when people are typically less alert. Some people find that taking a low dose of melatonin a few hours before their wind-down time is helpful.

#### 3. Getting an Early Start

It is helpful to get good sunlight in the early part of the day, to start the circadian period. Also, it may be helpful to eat a snack or a light breakfast to start the circadian clock.

Strengthening the circadian rhythm will not be effective if a reasonably consistent wake time is not also adhered to. In a person with delayed sleep phase tendencies it can be especially important not to let the wake time drift later, since that will also make it harder to fall asleep that night. Keeping the wake times in a set range will help reinforce the realignment of the circadian rhythm.

#### 4. Limit Caffeine and Napping

A few things can sabotage progress on counteracting delayed sleep phase tendencies. These include caffeine—people with delayed sleep phase can be sensitive to caffeine because it will block the buildup of sleep pressure, and if keeping a set bedtime continues to be a problem, it is worth trying to taper off the use of caffeine, including in the morning.

As discussed earlier, if delayed sleep phase continues to be a problem, consider the potential negative effect of napping. Naps absorb the sleep pressure that accumulates during the day, in the natural homeostatic sleep drive. If a nap is necessary, it is better to take it before 2:00 p.m. and limit it to 20 minutes.

When a circadian rhythm is out of sync between the weekdays and weekends, the effects can be profound. Remember that every cell in the body and every organ has a circadian rhythm, and when these are not in sync, people can experience not only sleepiness but also nausea, changes in mood, and changes in alertness and in their ability to learn, think, and work. In general, it may be better to avoid sleeping late two days in a row or sleeping much later than usual. For those people with insomnia or delayed sleep phase tendencies, it may be especially important to avoid changing your wake time too much on the weekends, even if you stay up a little later in the evening.

## SLEEP DISORDERS

As many as 70 million Americans suffer from chronic sleep disorders—medical conditions that prevent them from sleeping well.

### Chronic Insomnia

Many people have trouble falling asleep or staying asleep—a condition called **insomnia.** About 30% of U.S. adults have some symptoms of insomnia, and as many as 10% suffer from pure insomnia.

**Insomnia Symptoms** People with insomnia who do not have circadian rhythm issues or a sleep disrupter typically do not feel sleepy in the daytime because they tend to have a higher arousal tendency. That is, they have trouble sleeping not only at night, but also in the day (even though they may feel fatigued). A person is considered to have chronic insomnia if sleep disruption occurs at least three nights per week and lasts at least three months.

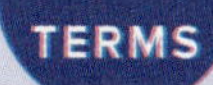


**insomnia** A sleep problem involving the inability to fall or stay asleep.

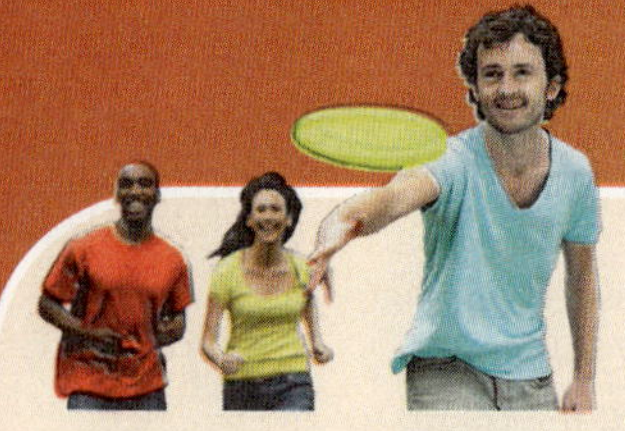

## WELLNESS ON CAMPUS: Learning While Sleeping

The connection of sleep to memory and learning is an exciting and relatively recent area of sleep science research. Around 100 years ago, the first sleep-memory experiments asked their subjects to learn a list of nonsense syllables. The researchers found that when the subjects slept after learning the list, they could recall more syllables than if they stayed awake. In a Harvard study, students learned to navigate a complex maze. Some napped for 90 minutes; others stayed awake. When the students tried to solve the maze again, only the few who dreamed about it during their naps did better. These results suggest that dreaming may reactivate and reorganize recently learned material, which would help memory and boost performance.

How does sleeping help us learn? Our memories develop in three stages: encoding, consolidating, and retrieving. When we first experience information, it is encoded, or converted from sensory stimuli into a representation stored in the area of the brain called the hippocampus. When we then sleep, some of the newly encoded memories are consolidated, or stabilized in the cerebral cortex, where they become more permanent. The information we recently learned is selected to be rehearsed and becomes more ingrained and available for later retrieval, or reactivation.

Some studies indicate that NREM sleep is especially important for learning of certain types, like learning a new motor sequencing task or learning new word associations. But REM sleep might be better for other types of learning consolidation and problem solving. Researchers gave 77 participants a list of creative problems in the morning. Everyone was asked to think about solutions, and half of the participants took a nap before being tested.

All the nappers were monitored during sleep. Only those who took longer naps entered REM sleep, which occupied about 14 minutes of the 73-minute naps. NREM napping did not boost creative problem solving, but people who entered REM sleep enhanced their performance by nearly 40%, as compared with both non-nappers and NREM nappers. The improvement was specific for problems that were introduced before napping; rather than simply boosting alertness and attention, REM sleep allowed the brain to work creatively on problems posed before sleep.

When sleep is disrupted, we can develop problems with attention, which can interfere with learning. Children and young adults who have trouble sleeping at night are especially prone to developing problems during the day—not so much that they are sleepy, but that they have trouble focusing their attention. One study looked at sleep apnea in first graders who were performing at or below the 10th percentile. Among the group who screened positive for sleep apnea, some followed a treatment plan. In the next grade, those children who were treated increased their performance to the 50th percentile; those who did not receive treatment remained at or below the 10th percentile.

Pulling all-nighters does not help grades and learning. Subjects who stayed awake 35 hours managed performances on memory tests that would earn them the equivalent of two letter grades lower than subjects who had slept.

SOURCES: Puller, K. A., and D. Oudielle. 2018. Sleep learning gets real. *Scientific American* 319(5): 27–31; Harvard Men's Health Watch. 2012. Learning while you sleep: Dream or reality. Harvard Health Publishing, Harvard Medical School (https://www.health.harvard.edu/staying-healthy/learning-while-you-sleep-dream-or-reality); Hershner, S. D., and R. D. Chervin. 2014. Causes and consequences of sleepiness among college students. *Nature and Science of Sleep* 6: 73–84; Vorster, A. P., and J. Borna. 2015. Sleep and memory in mammals, birds and invertebrates. *Neuroscience & Biobehavioral Reviews* 50: 103–119.

**Insomnia Treatment** Behavioral intervention and treatment of insomnia rely on addressing sleep disrupters or circadian rhythm factors. Examples of sleep disrupters are caffeine, reflux, congestion, cough, urination, anxiety or stress, pain, and environmental factors, among others. Even if those are not the sole reason for sleeplessness, it is helpful to treat those first or at least simultaneously; otherwise an insomnia treatment is unlikely to succeed. Most people can overcome insomnia by discovering the cause of poor sleep and taking steps to remedy it. If your insomnia lasts more than six months and interferes with daytime functioning, you should probably talk to a sleep specialist in a medical center. Sleeping pills are not recommended for chronic insomnia because they can be habit-forming; they also lose their effectiveness over time.

**SLEEP ROUTINE** If you suffer from insomnia, changing your sleep schedule can bring relief. Counterintuitively, the core behavioral approach for treating insomnia is based on shortening the sleep period slightly and setting a very strict sleep window. Go to bed at the same time every night and, more important, get up at the same time every morning, seven days a week, regardless of how well you slept. This increases the homeostatic pressure to drive sleep onset (a longer time to build up sleepiness in the day) and also sets a consistent wake time and sleep time to establish circadian synchrony. When the sleep-window approach fails, it's usually because people tend to go to bed earlier than their sleep frame bedtime, or they sleep later in the morning. Sleep restriction or consolidation approaches to treating insomnia are very effective.

Another important component of a sleep routine is that naps during the day need to be limited. Typically naps should be limited to 20 minutes and taken before 2:00 p.m. Because the sleep-window treatment is meant to produce sleepiness, naps should be taken only if absolutely necessary. Daytime sleepiness means the treatment is working! It can be tempting to try to stock up on sleep, but there are no biological benefits to oversleeping. In fact, it can extend your homeostatic sleep drive and delay your sleep phase, leading to another bout of insomnia.

Some mindset tips are useful. If you find yourself lying in bed, unable to fall asleep, that is okay. Disregard occasional setbacks and remember that light dozing or daydreaming have restorative value. You do not need to be completely unconscious, as long as you are relaxed. If you get anxious and start to worry, you might need to leave the bedroom and engage in a quiet activity to relax again. It is better to return to the bedroom when you feel sleepy again. Finally, it is important not to look at the clock. Try to forget about time once you are in bed.

QUICK STATS

**Nearly three-quarters of U.S. adults report stress during the pandemic, and of those, one-third report changes in sleeping habits.**

—American Psychological Association, 2021

**ENVIRONMENTAL AND OTHER FACTORS** After addressing your sleep patterns, turn your attention to other factors that influence your sleep. First, create a healthy sleep environment. While sleeping, keep your space quiet, dark, and at a comfortable temperature. Use your bed only for sleep; don't eat, read, study, or watch television there. This helps you associate your bed with sleep, which can support your routine.

Exercise every day, but not too close to bedtime. Your metabolism takes up to six hours to slow down after exercise, so you may feel more awake during that time.

Everyone is different with respect to how they respond to caffeine, but people who are light sleepers can be much more sensitive. As bedtime approaches, relax with a bath, a book, music, or relaxation exercises. Try to avoid screen-based technology to limit your exposure to blue light.

**PROFESSIONAL HELP** If sleep problems persist, visit your physician for help. If you take any medications (prescription or not), ask if they interfere with sleep. If you and your physician cannot identify potential problems, ask for a referral to a sleep specialist. You may be a candidate for a sleep study—an overnight evaluation of your sleep pattern that can uncover sleep-related disorders.

## Restless Leg Syndrome

**Restless leg syndrome (RLS)** is an important sleep disrupter to identify because it is common and may be treatable with some simple interventions. RLS affects about 5% of the adult population and can affect as many as 25% of pregnant women. People are more susceptible to developing it if they have a family member who has it, and as many as 50% of people with RLS can identify another family member who has similar symptoms. RLS is characterized by a feeling of discomfort or body tension, often affecting the legs (the exact kind of discomfort can vary from person to person; it is often a feeling of something crawling under the skin, but it can be an ache, a tingling feeling, or a deep or sharp pain). The symptoms are related to the time of day, and they happen more in the evening or when lying down at night. Symptoms are helped by walking around or moving the legs, and they are worsened by sitting still, like during long airplane or car rides. RLS can be associated with small kicking movements during the night while sleeping that can cause arousals, even if one is not aware of them. If the person is awakened, the symptoms can make it harder to fall back to sleep.

TERMS

**restless leg syndrome (RLS)** A sleep disrupter characterized by a feeling of discomfort or body tension, often affecting the legs.

**Restless Leg Syndrome Treatment** Simple measures that help RLS include getting more exercise during the day, avoiding all caffeine, stretching legs and muscles before bedtime, and ensuring that iron levels are in the middle range. Certain substances such as diphenhydramine (Benadryl), a common ingredient in over-the-counter sleeping pills (e.g., Tylenol PM, Advil PM), paradoxically worsen this symptom and can worsen sleep. Medications can sometimes be needed to treat RLS when the behavioral interventions and elimination of triggers have not been successful. In cases that are resistant to these types of interventions, a health care provider may need to offer specialized expertise for treatment.

## Sleep Apnea

Sleep apnea is probably the most common disrupter of sleep. The risk for sleep apnea increases with age, and up to 50% of people may have sleep apnea after age 65. In younger and middle-aged groups, the rate is approximately 10–15%. If a person is a loud snorer with sleep problems, or has a primary relative with these symptoms, that person should probably seek evaluation. Covid-19 infection may increase the risk of developing sleep apnea, due to the disease's negative impact on lung health.

The disorder is usually caused by a narrowed airway that gets more obstructed when sleeping, causing short, repeated breathing pauses (see Figure 4.7). Major medical problems,

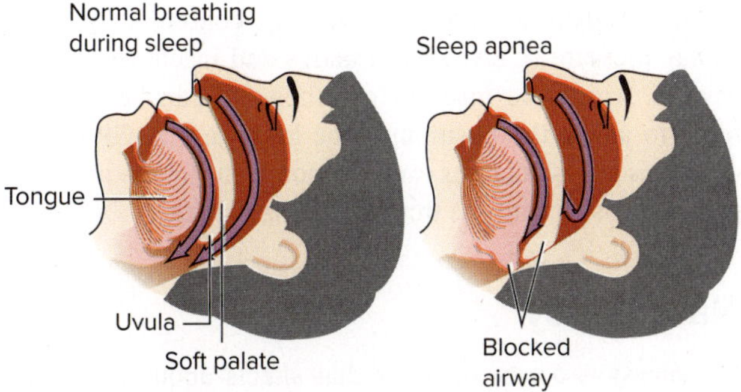


**FIGURE 4.7** **Sleep apnea.** Sleep apnea occurs when soft tissues surrounding the airway relax, "collapsing" the airway and restricting airflow.

## Ask Yourself

**QUESTIONS FOR CRITICAL THINKING AND REFLECTION**

You or someone you know has insomnia, but the sleep window is not working. Are you:

- Sleeping late—past the end of the sleep window time frame in the morning?
- Drinking a coffee in the morning?
- Having an alcoholic drink at night?
- Going to bed too early—before the sleep time frame starts at night?
- Making sure you don't have RLS, or sleep apnea, or another sleep disrupter you have not addressed? If you suspect sleep apnea could be a possibility, definitely have this checked. Remember even thin people can have apnea. If you have a snoring tendency or there is a family snoring tendency, you should be even more suspicious.

including high blood pressure, heart attack, and stroke, are associated with sleep apnea. It also has a negative impact on diabetes and increases the risk of work-related and automobile accidents. In children, if untreated, it can lead to poorer school performance and attention problems. Although sleep apnea is most common when people are overweight, it can affect people of any weight.

Not all people with sleep apnea are sleepy during the day, nor do all people realize that their sleep is disrupted, because they have become accustomed to it. Moderate to loud snoring and a family history for sleep apnea should make one consider checking for this possibility even in the absence of symptoms.

**Sleep Apnea Treatment** Sleep apnea is treatable, and treatment can have a major impact on quality of life and daytime function while also reducing associated risks. There are a number of treatments for sleep apnea, ranging from lifestyle adjustments to medical devices. Lifestyle changes include weight loss, sleeping on your side, quitting smoking, and using nasal sprays or allergy medicines to keep nasal passages open at night. Medical interventions include removal of the tonsils or adenoids, oral appliances, or continuous positive airway pressure (CPAP) nasal masks and machines. Dental devices, which are inserted mouthpieces, can be worn at night to adjust the position of the lower jaw. A CPAP machine has a mask that fits over the mouth and/or the nose and gently blows air into the throat, keeping it open.

## Narcolepsy

**Narcolepsy** is a rare disorder that affects about 1 in 2000 people and appears between the ages of 10 and 20. The condition comes from a gene mutation in the brain and cannot be passed down from parent to child. Its symptoms include excessive daytime sleepiness, sleep paralysis, and sudden loss of muscle control.

When narcoleptic people feel sleepy in the daytime, it can come as an overwhelming urge to sleep while driving, working, or eating—very inconvenient times. At nighttime, they do not sleep well. And in the transition to waking, the paralysis that we all experience during REM lingers for people with narcolepsy: Instead of the brain releasing them from paralysis at just the right time, they may have difficulty talking or moving. Gradually the paralysis wears off. The third symptom, called *cataplexy*, is a sudden loss of muscle control that might be noticeable in slurred speech, a jaw dropping, or legs buckling. The cataplexy can be triggered by strong emotions like laughing hard or getting startled. In these moments, a narcoleptic person may collapse into a body paralysis.

**Narcolepsy Treatment** Unfortunately, treatments for narcolepsy are few and ineffective. The disorder is rare enough that drug companies have not found it profitable to invest much research in drug therapies. But patients can take a drug called Provigil to help them stay awake during the day and antidepressants to help suppress REM sleep and thus the paralysis characteristic of the other two symptoms.

## TIPS FOR TODAY AND THE FUTURE

**RIGHT NOW YOU CAN:**

- Identify sleep disrupters using the "Sleep Disrupter Checklist" (page 76).
- Be aware of sleep-disrupting substances such as caffeine, performance protein supplements, alcohol, and stimulants.
- Determine your natural sleep rhythm (night owl or morning lark) and overall individual sleep need (short sleeper, long sleeper).
- Evaluate your sleep environment and bedtime activities: How are the temperature, darkness, and noise in your bedroom? Is there a problem disengaging from distractors and electronics at night?

**IN THE FUTURE YOU CAN:**

- Design your optimal sleep period.
- Avoid going to bed too early or getting up too late (if you didn't have a good night's sleep). Keep to a specific time frame, and set clear sleep and wake times. Avoid lying down to rest or nap for more than 20 minutes.
- Exercise during the day, but not at night.

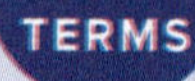


**narcolepsy** A rare neurological disorder characterized by excessive daytime sleepiness, sleep paralysis, and sudden loss of muscle control.

# LAB EXERCISES
## Sleep Case Scenarios

These cases by no means exhaust the many patterns of sleep issues people may face, and most people can encounter some of these various problems at different times. Being aware of how to troubleshoot sleep problems can help you take charge of your sleep-related health and know when to seek further help when a problem becomes more persistent.

**Case 1.** I have trouble falling asleep at night.

Some potential remedies: (1) Cut down and eliminate all sources of caffeine—even in the morning. (2) Avoid all daytime naps or at least limit these to 20 minutes before 2:00 p.m. (may set an alarm). (3) Avoid bright lights and electronic activities in the hour before bedtime, and remove clocks or devices that tell the time from the bedroom. It is best if cell phones are charged outside of the bedroom. (4) Increase bright light exposure in the morning. (5) Avoid exercising in the evening. (6) Set bedtime late enough to allow for sleep drive to accumulate (an appropriate bedtime might be 11:00 p.m. or later for some people). (7) Set wake time early enough so that there is enough time to develop sleep need over the day. (8) Ensure that you are not accidentally dozing before bedtime and using up the sleep drive that helps you fall asleep (you can try to sit in less comfortable chairs or be more active in the evenings if this is the case).

**Case 2.** I have several episodes of waking up during the night.

(1) Ensure that you are not drinking or eating in the three hours before bedtime. (2) Do you have any nasal allergies? Treatment of these may improve sleep continuity. (3) Have you been drinking any caffeine during the day? Caffeine can cause wake-ups during the night after the sleep drive has worn off, and eliminating caffeine can help. (4) Do you have a family history of apnea, or are you a snorer? Is there a possibility you might have apnea? (5) Are there factors in the environment waking you up? Noise? Is the temperature too hot? Are there pets in the bedroom? (6) Did you drink alcohol before going to bed?

**Case 3.** I have trouble waking up in the morning.

(1) Do you have different times that you wake up on different days—for example, do you wake up much later on the weekend and much earlier on certain days of the week? If so, you may be putting your body through a frequent jet-lag experience, and keeping your wake times closer to one another from day to day may be helpful to keep your circadian rhythm in sync. (2) Are you getting enough sleep? Do you need to wind down earlier? (3) Do your bedtimes tend to get later and later? You may need to anchor your circadian rhythm with more light in the morning. (4) Are there sleep disrupters at night that are disturbing your sleep (see Case 2)?

**Case 4.** I am too sleepy in the daytime.

(1) Are you getting enough sleep at night? This problem may be helped by increasing your sleep time. You may be a naturally long sleeper and need more sleep time. (2) Is nighttime sleep disrupted by snoring, possible apnea, reflux, nasal congestion, noise, or other factors so that you are not getting enough continuous sleep at night even though you are in bed? (3) Are you taking medications that can worsen sleepiness? (4) Do most of your problems with sleepiness occur in the morning, and might you have problems outlined in Case 3?

## SUMMARY

- Sleep affects almost all systems of the body, including respiratory, cardiovascular, endocrine, gastrointestinal, urinary, and nervous systems.
- Sleep occurs in two main phases: rapid eye movement (REM) sleep and non-rapid eye movement (NREM) sleep, which constitutes three stages. A sleeper goes through several cycles of NREM and REM sleep each night. Each stage is characterized by different patterns of electrical brain activity as measured by the electroencephalogram (EEG) and accomplishes different functions.
- Two main natural forces drive us toward sleep–the homeostatic sleep drive and the circadian rhythm. Homeostatic sleep drive is driven by a neurochemical that promotes sleep onset, adenosine, which accumulates in the brain as a by-product of energy the brain uses. The drive is strengthened by a reasonable wake-sleep schedule without naps and caffeine.
- Circadian rhythm is the sleep-and-wake pattern coordinated by the brain's master internal clock, the suprachiasmatic nucleus (SCN). The SCN sets and controls, or synchronizes, the wake-sleep cycle of the brain and of every cell in every organ of the body. The rhythm can be disrupted by jet lag and irregular sleep practices, as well as by substances such as caffeine and alcohol. Our circadian rhythm is most strongly influenced by light exposure, as well as by activity, exercise, and eating–zeitgebers that can reset our wake-sleep clocks. Good light exposure in the morning and daytime and reduced exposure to light at night strengthen the rhythmic effects.
- Sleep rhythms and needs change with aging. In the teen years, a delayed sleep phase develops, and other circadian rhythms change. Adults consistently need 7–9 hours of sleep per night. As we age, however, the amount of overall sleep and the amount of deep sleep we get diminish. Differences in sleep arousal evolve throughout life.

• Sleep is important for mental health, mood, creativity and learning, and physical health. It promotes longevity and diminishes the risk for the emergence of major diseases. Poor-quality or insufficient sleep has been associated with a number of health problems and impairments—heart disease, high blood pressure, depression, earlier death, increased risk for dementia, weight gain, poorer glucose control, increased risk for accidents, reduced motivation and attention, and increased irritability or hyperactivity. Improving your sleep can combat our national public epidemic of sleep deprivation.

• Lack of sleep has a great impact on stress. In someone who is suffering from sleep deprivation (not getting enough sleep over time), mental and physical processes deteriorate steadily. A sleep-deprived person experiences headaches, feels irritable, cannot concentrate, and is prone to forgetfulness. Poor-quality sleep has long been associated with stress and depression.

• Drowsiness slows your reaction time and lessens your ability to pay attention and make good decisions. People who are most at risk for falling asleep while driving include young adults aged 18–29. Researchers estimate that drowsy driving is responsible for more than 70,000 crashes, 40,000 injuries, and as many as 7500 deaths per year. Accidents due to sleepiness are preventable.

• As many as 70 million Americans suffer from chronic sleep disorders—medical conditions that prevent them from sleeping well. Very common sleep disorders are chronic insomnia, trouble falling asleep or staying asleep; restless leg syndrome, and sleep apnea, repeated stops in breathing for short periods—frequently 20 to 40 seconds—while asleep. They can all be treated, some through lifestyle changes.

• Sleep disrupters are specific factors that interfere with the ability to fall or stay asleep that can usually be corrected if they are targeted specifically. These include caffeine, reflux, nasal congestion, cough, urination, anxiety or stress, pain, environmental factors such as room temperature and lighting, electronic devices, alcohol, tobacco, and medications, among others.

• Sleep time has to be tailored to the individual, and then reasonable practices can be developed that improve quality of sleep: supporting natural sleep rhythms and drives, creating a good sleep environment, and avoiding substances and events that disrupt sleep.

• You can take control of your sleep by monitoring your sleep habits (keeping a sleep diary to identify your schedule and the best hours for adequate sleep), tracking your eating and exercise behaviors, and noting any medical conditions that might interfere, and then setting goals and identifying strategies for improving sleep behaviors.

• Chronic insomnia, repeated disrupted sleep that lasts for months, is very common and affects an estimated 10% of the population. Behavioral intervention and treatment is based on shortening the sleep period slightly and setting a very strict sleep window—denying sleep outside that time constraint—to slightly sleep-deprive the person. That in turn has the effect of "kickstarting" the natural physiological sleep rhythms.

• While a good effect of using a digital sleep tracker is the greater focus it places on sleep, no consumer technology can equal the ability of a sleep lab to detect sleep stages or diagnose specific sleep disorders.

• General benefits of adequate sleep:

  Improves memory of recently learned information

  Washes waste from the brain that can contribute to mild cognitive impairment

  Addressing a sleep disorder may improve inattention symptoms and learning capacity

  Helps optimize athletic performance

  Positively affects appetite regulation factors ghrelin and leptin

  Improves mood and stamina against depression

• The good news is that with more knowledge about sleep and the factors that affect it, people can improve their sleep and, in turn, their health. Along with exercise and good nutrition, good sleep is a critical pillar of good health.

## FOR MORE INFORMATION

*American Academy of Sleep Medicine*. Advocates research and advocacy to improve sleep health.

https://aasm.org/

*American Sleep Association*. Advances the medical specialty of sleep medicine.

https://www.sleepassociation.org

*Centers for Disease Control and Prevention*. Seeks to raise awareness about the problems connected to insufficient sleep and related disorders.

https://www.cdc.gov/sleep/index.html

*Healthy Sleep*. An education resource offered by Harvard Medical School Division of Sleep Medicine.

https://sleep.hms.harvard.edu/education-training/public-education/sleep-and-health-education-program/sleep-health-education

*National Institutes of Health*. Supports research about key health topics, including sleep.

http://www.nih.gov

*National Sleep Foundation*. Provides information about sleep and how to overcome sleep problems such as insomnia and jet lag.

https://www.sleepfoundation.org/

## SELECTED BIBLIOGRAPHY

AAA Foundation for Traffic Safety. 2018. *Prevalence of Drowsy Driving Crashes: Estimates from a Large-Scale Naturalistic Driving Study*. AAA Foundation for Traffic Safety.

American Psychological Association. 2021. Stress in America™ 2021: Pandemic impedes basic decision-making ability. (https://www.apa.org/news/press/releases/2021/10/stress-pandemic-decision-making).

Baroni, A., et al. 2018. Impact of a sleep course on sleep, mood and anxiety symptoms in college students: A pilot study. *Journal of American College Health* 66(1): 41–50.

Becker, S. P., et al. 2018. Sleep in a large, multi-university sample of college students: Sleep problem prevalence, sex differences, and mental health correlates. *Sleep Health* 4(2): 174–181.

Becker, S. P., et al. 2018. Sleep problems and suicidal behaviors in college students. *Journal of Psychiatric Research* 99: 122–128.

Berry, J. D., et al. 2012. Lifetime risks of cardiovascular disease. *New England Journal of Medicine* 366: 321–329.

Cappuccio, F. P., et al. 2010. Quantity and quality of sleep and incidence of type 2 diabetes: A systematic review and meta-analysis. *Diabetes Care* 33(2): 414–420.

Centers for Disease Control and Prevention. 2020. *Diabetes Home* (www.cdc.gov/diabetes/data/statistics/statistics-report.html).

Centers for Disease Control and Prevention. 2019. *Drowsy Driving: Asleep at the Wheel.* CDC Features (www.cdc.gov/features/dsdrowsydriving/index.html).

Chaput, J-P., C. Dutil, and H. Sampasa-Kanyinga. 2018. Sleeping hours: What is the ideal number and how does age impact this? *Nature and Science of Sleep* 10: 421–430.

Dement, W. 2006. *The Stanford Sleep Book*. Stanford, CA: Author.

Duraccio, K. M., et al. 2021. Losing sleep by staying up late leads adolescents to consume more carbohydrates and a higher glycemic load. *Sleep* 45(3): zsab269.

Fuentes, G. 2021. "Latest Surface Navy Sleep Policy Aims for Better-Rested, More Alert, Healthier Crews." *USNI News,* 28 January (https://news.usni.org/2021/01/28/latest-surface-navy-sleep-policy-aims-for-better-rested-more-alert-healthier-crews).

Glavin, E. E., et al. 2021. Relationships between sleep, exercise timing, and chronotype in young adults. *Journal of Health Psychology* 26(13): 2636–2647.

Gozal, D. 1998. Sleep-disordered breathing and school performance in children. *Pediatrics*. 102: 616–620.

Greer, S. M., A. N. Goldstein, and M. P. Walker. 2013. The impact of sleep deprivation on food desire in the human brain. *Nature Communications* 4: 2259.

Hauser, C., and I. Kwai. 2019. California tells schools to start later, giving teenagers more sleep. *The New York Times*, 14 October (https://www.nytimes.com/2019/10/14/us/school-sleep-start.html).

Karni, A., et al. 1994. Dependence on REM sleep of overnight improvement of a perceptual skill. *Science* 265: 679–682.

Kripke, D. F. 2016. Mortality risk of hypnotics: Strengths and limits of evidence. *Drug Safety* 39: 93–107.

Lewis, P. 2013. *The Secret World of Sleep*. New York: St. Martin's Press.

Luckhaupt, S. E. 2012. Short sleep duration among workers—United States, 2010. *Morbidity and Mortality Weekly Report* 61(6): 281–285.

Mander, B. A., et al. 2017. Sleep and human aging. *Neuron* 94(1): 19–36.

Marin, J., et al. 2005. Long-term cardiovascular outcomes in men with obstructive sleep apnoea-hypopnoea with or without treatment with continuous positive airway pressure: An observational study. *Lancet* 365: 1046–1053.

Meltzer, L. J., et al. 2022. Impact of changing school start times on parent sleep. *Sleep Health* 8(1): 130–134.

Miller, M. A., and F. P. Cappuccio. 2021. A systematic review of COVID-19 and obstructive sleep apnoea. *Sleep Medicine Reviews* 55: 101382.

Morin, C. M., et al. 2021. Insomnia, anxiety, and depression during the COVID-19 pandemic: An international collaborative study. *Sleep Medicine* 87: 38–45.

Nagare, R., B. Plitnick, and M. G. Figueiro. 2019. Does the iPad Night Shift mode reduce melatonin suppression? *Lighting Research & Technology* 51(3): 373–383.

National Institute of Neurological Disorders and Stroke. 2017. *Brain Basics: Understanding Sleep*. Patient & Caregiver Education (www.ninds.nih.gov/Disorders/Patient-Caregiver-Education/Understanding-Sleep).

National Sleep Foundation. 2020. *Sleep in America Poll 2020* (https://www.sleepfoundation.org/wp-content/uploads/2020/03/SIA-2020-Q1-Report.pdf).

Newsome, R. 2022. The link between sleep and job performance. *Sleep Foundation* (https://www.sleepfoundation.org/sleep-hygiene/good-sleep-and-job-performance).

Nielsen, L. S., et al. 2011. Short sleep duration as a possible cause of obesity: Critical analysis of the epidemiological evidence. *Obesity Reviews* 12: 78–92.

Peppard, P. E., et al. 2000. Prospective study of the association between sleep-disordered breathing and hypertension. *New England Journal of Medicine* 342: 1378–1384.

Sivertsen, B., et al. 2014. Midlife insomnia and subsequent mortality: The Hordaland health study. *BMC Public Health* 14: 720.

Steiner, S., et al. 2008. Impact of obstructive sleep apnea on the occurrence of restenosis after elective percutaneous coronary intervention in ischemic heart disease. *Respiratory Research* 9: 50.

Stickgold, R. 2005. Sleep-dependent memory consolidation. *Nature* 437(27): 1272–1278.

Stickgold, R., L. James, and J. A. Hobson. 2000. Visual discrimination learning requires sleep after training. *Nature Neuroscience* 3(12): 1237–1238.

Tasali E., et al. 2022. Effect of sleep extension on objectively assessed energy intake among adults with overweight in real-life settings: A randomized clinical trial. *JAMA Internal Medicine* 182(4): 365–374.

Taylor, D. J., et al. 2013. Epidemiology of insomnia in college students: Relationship with mental health, quality of life, and substance use difficulties. *Behavior Therapy* 44(3): 339–348.

Vgontzas, A. N., et al. 2009. Insomnia with objective short sleep duration is associated with type 2 diabetes: A population-based study. *Diabetes Care* 32(11): 1980–1985.

Vgontzas, A. N., et al. 2010. Insomnia with short sleep duration and mortality: The Penn State cohort. *Sleep* 33: 1159–1164.

Vgontzas, A. N., et al. 2013. Insomnia with objective short sleep duration: The most biologically severe phenotype of the disorder. *Sleep Medicine Reviews* 17: 241–254.

Vitale, K. C., et al. 2019. Sleep hygiene for optimizing recovery in athletes: Review and recommendations. *International Journal of Sports Medicine* 40(08): 535–543.

Vyazovskiy, V. V., and A. Delogu. 2014. NREM and REM sleep: Complementary roles in recovery after wakefulness. *The Neuroscientist* 20(3): 203–219.

Walker, M. 2017. *Why We Sleep: Unlocking the Power of Sleep and Dreams.* New York: Scribner.

Williamson, A. M., and A.-M. Feyer. 2000. Moderate sleep deprivation produces impairments in cognitive and motor performance equivalent to legally prescribed levels of alcohol intoxication. *Occupational and Environmental Medicine* 57(10): 649–655.

Wolfson, A. R., and M. A. Carskadon. 1998. Sleep schedules and daytime functioning in adolescents. *Child Development* 69(4): 875–887.

**Design Elements:** Assess Yourself icon: Aleksey Boldin/Alamy Stock Photo; Diversity Matters icon: Rawpixel Ltd/Getty Images; Wellness on Campus icon: Radius Images/Alamy Stock Photo; Take Charge icon: VisualCommunications/Getty Images; Critical Consumer icon: pagadesign/Getty Images.

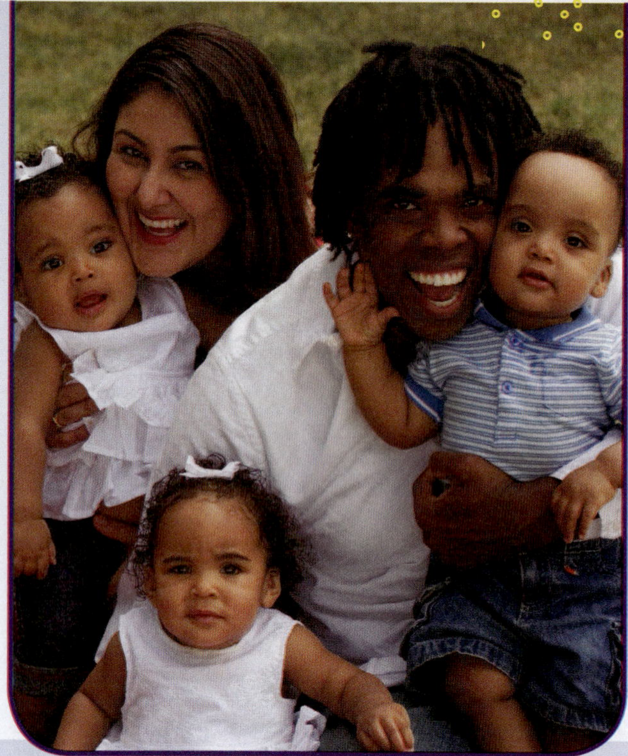
digitalskillet/Shutterstock

## CHAPTER OBJECTIVES

- Explain the qualities that help people develop and maintain intimate relationships
- Explain elements of healthy and productive communication
- Describe types of love relationships as well as singlehood
- Discuss the benefits and challenges of marriage
- Describe challenges and rewards of family life

CHAPTER 5

# Intimate Relationships and Communication

We are born needing others. Our survival as a species has always relied on our ability to form strong mutual attachments, cherish each other, provide mutual economic, social, and emotional support, and create social groups, like families or villages, to raise children and produce the next generation of humans. Relationships are held together by a variety of factors. Those relationships we consider closest–family, friends, spouses, sexual partners–are healthiest when we can both give and receive love. Love in its many forms is the wellspring from which much of life's meaning and delight flow.

## DEVELOPING INTERPERSONAL RELATIONSHIPS

Psychologist Carl Rogers described three conditions that characterize healthy relationships: genuineness, empathy, and unconditional positive regard. *Genuineness* refers to honest and accurate communication of thoughts and feelings. *Empathy* refers to stepping into another's shoes and trying to understand someone else's position regardless of personal feeling. *Unconditional positive regard* is the ability to experience another person without judgment and negative feelings. We must be willing to share our ideas, feelings, time, and needs and to recognize what others want to give us in return. Just as important is the relationship we develop with ourselves–that is, how we generally feel about ourselves.

### Self-Concept, Developing from Childhood

Building successful relationships with others requires having a healthy relationship with yourself. This means being able to soothe yourself, manage your emotions, and feel comfortable with your own company. These factors allow us to love and respect others.

Our identity and sense of self begins to form in childhood, through the relationships we have with our caregivers. As adults, we are more likely to feel that we are basically lovable, and to view ourselves as worthwhile people who can trust others, if we had the following experiences as babies and children:

- We felt loved, valued, accepted, and respected.
- Adults responded to our needs in appropriate ways.
- Adults gave us the freedom to play, explore, and develop a sense of being separate individuals.

These conditions encourage us to develop a positive self-concept and healthy self-acceptance, and they contribute to a basic self-confidence that helps us navigate life's inevitable challenges.

**Gender Role and Communication** In early childhood we learn to take on a **gender role**—the activities, abilities, and other characteristics our culture considers appropriate for our biological sex. Gender roles are cultural creations rather than biological facts, so an individual's natural abilities, preferences, likes and dislikes, personality characteristics, or internal sense of self (gender identity) may not match their assigned gender role. This can cause problems in societies, like our own, which traditionally discouraged gender role crossing or have powerful cultural or religious beliefs that gender roles are ordained by God or deeply rooted in nature (biology).

Over the past decades, in the United States and elsewhere, traditional cultural expectations about gender have been changing. For example, the so-called traditional division of labor, with the male provider role and mother at home caring for the children, is a relatively recent invention found in large, hierarchical societies. Even in the United States, some women, especially single and poorer married women, have always worked outside the home. Today, however, women make up almost half of the total labor force and, like men, consider job/career a central part of their lives.

The enormous growth of research on gender has challenged other cultural beliefs. We now know that U.S. gender stereotypes, such as males being more "logical" and females more "emotional," are neither universal nor biologically real.

Studies have shown that girls do not necessarily play more cooperatively or less competitively than boys and that gender behaviors that previously seemed so ingrained can be changed depending on the messages children receive from caregivers, mass media, and other **socializing** influences.

You may have heard that men and women in the United States speak different languages or have different communicative styles that can lead to misinterpretation and even conflict. But while we can find variations in speech styles of some men and women, the research on gendered communication reveals a more complex reality.

For example, girls in early adolescence often start using their voices so that in one moment they speak in a low pitch and in the next a high one. Boys, by contrast, decrease their range in pitch, sounding relatively monotone. These represent cultural ways that adolescents differentiate their genders, preparing to participate in what sociolinguist Penelope Eckert calls a heterosexual market. They speak differently in order to fit in socially and eventually find a mate. So there is no gene for gendered language. We learn how to communicate in gendered ways, just as we learn other aspects of our culture's gender roles. But we can decide how we want to communicate based on any particular situation.

**Attachment** Where do we learn how to relate to others? Psychologists have suggested that our adult styles of affection and loving are based on the type of **attachment** we established in infancy with our mother, father, siblings, or other primary caregivers. According to this view, people who are secure in their intimate relationships as adults probably had a secure, trusting, mutually satisfying attachment to their parents or caregivers. Securely attached people find it relatively easy to get close to others, and they don't worry excessively about being abandoned or others' getting too close. They feel that other people accept them and are generally well intentioned.

People who run from relationships may have experienced an "anxious/avoidant" attachment as children. In this type of attachment, a parent's responses were either engulfing or abandoning. Anxious/avoidant adults feel uncomfortable being close to others and seek escape from another's control. They're distrustful and fearful of becoming dependent on and intimate with their partners.

Individuals who endured distant and aloof attachments as children can still establish satisfying relationships later in life. Human beings can be resilient and flexible. And cultures vary in their ways of expressing attachment and intimacy. We have the capacity to change our ideas, beliefs, and behaviors. We can learn ways to raise our self-esteem and become more trusting, accepting, and appreciative of others and ourselves. We can acquire the communication and conflict resolution skills needed to maintain successful relationships. Although it helps to have a good start in life, it may be even more important to begin again, right from where you are.

## Nonsexual Intimate Relationships: Family, Friends, Peers

In childhood, we often develop close relationships with people outside our immediate family, such as adult caregivers in our home or at a child care center or teachers at our school. Extended family—grandparents, aunts, uncles, cousins—play an important role in many people's lives, not just as caregivers but also in social and emotional ways. Peer relationships also are influential in our growth. Through these encounters,

**TERMS**

**gender role** The activities, abilities, and characteristics deemed culturally appropriate for us based on our sex.

**socialization** The process of learning to behave in a way that is acceptable to society.

**attachment** The emotional tie between an infant and their caregiver or between two people in an intimate relationship.

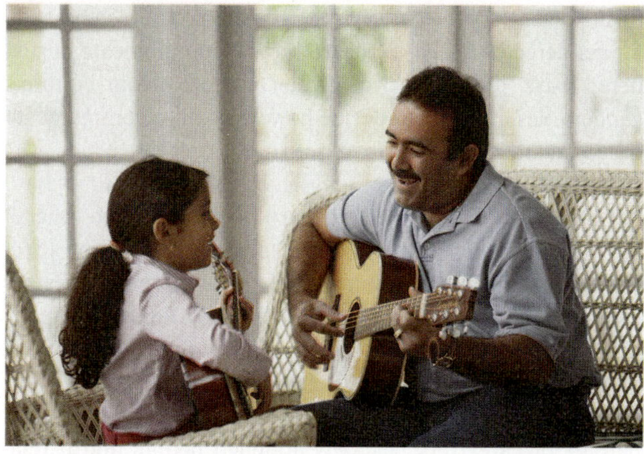

The type and strength of our attachment to our caregivers can affect other relationships throughout our lives. Ariel Skelley/Blend Images

we learn about the complexities of human relationships, positive and negative. But we also learn about tolerance, sharing, trust, and other aspects of successful intimate peer relationships, including friendships. Healthy friendships usually include the following characteristics:

- ***Companionship*** is the good feeling you have when you're with someone else. Friends are usually relaxed and happy when together. They typically share common values and interests. Friends can also be tense and unhappy with each other, but even on bad days, they support one another.
- ***Respect.*** Friends respect each other's feelings and opinions and work to resolve their differences without demeaning or insulting each other.
- ***Acceptance.*** Friends accept each other "warts and all." They feel free to be themselves and express their feelings honestly without fear of ridicule or criticism.
- ***Help.*** Friends know they can rely on each other in times of need. Help may include sharing time, energy, and material goods.
- ***Trust.*** Friends will not intentionally hurt each other. They feel safe confiding in one another.
- ***Loyalty.*** Friends can count on one another. In conflicts, friends will stand up for one another rather than join the opposition.
- ***Mutuality.*** Friends retain their individual identities, but close friendships are characterized by a sense of mutuality—"what affects you affects me." Friends share the ups and downs in each other's lives.
- ***Reciprocity.*** Friendships are reciprocal. There is give-and-take between friends and mutual exchange of joys and burdens.

Intimate sexual partnerships are like friendships in many ways. But in addition to sexual desire and expression, there is often a greater demand for exclusiveness and deeper levels of caring. Friends are often more accepting and less critical than lovers, perhaps because their expectations differ. Friendships may be more stable and longer lasting. Like other intimate relationships, friendships bind society together, providing people with emotional support and buffering them from stress.

## Love, Sex, and Intimacy

Love is one of the most basic and profound human emotions. Most of us first experience intense love in our families. As we grow older, we expand our love circle, even to people we don't know, like celebrities. We seem to love to love. Love can encompass opposites: affection and anger, excitement and boredom, stability and change, bonds and freedom. Love cannot give us complete happiness, but it can give our lives more meaning.

As adults, our love relationships may be intertwined with sexuality. Most religious traditions have considered marriage the only acceptable context for sexual activity, particularly for females. Many religions also traditionally viewed having children as the goal of marriage rather than love or sexual pleasure. Today, in the United States and elsewhere, many people reject these ideas and rely on other norms and values to make sexuality-related decisions. According to Pew research, about two-thirds of U.S. adults say sex between unmarried adults in a committed relationship can be acceptable; 62% accept, at least sometimes, casual sex between consenting adults not in a committed relationship. Guttmacher Institute reports the average age in the United States for first sex is now 18. At the same time, the age at which we first marry keeps rising, currently around 28 for females, 30 for males. Clearly, for more and more people, engaging in a sexual relationship and getting married are separate decisions.

Almost half of young people experience a romantic or dating relationship before age 18. Scholars have found that the quality of these early relationships strongly predicts our well-being as adults, including the likelihood of experiencing major depression, low self-esteem, and suicide attempts. Schools are starting to incorporate relationship issues, including how to negotiate safe sex practices or say no to sex, into their comprehensive sex education programs. Interestingly, among high school students, the percentage having had sexual intercourse has declined for three decades, from 54% in 1991 to 38% in 2019. Most Americans see love, sex, and commitment as closely linked. Love reflects the positive factors that draw people together and sustain their relationship. It includes trust, caring, respect, loyalty, interest in the other, and concern for their well-being. Sex intensifies the relationship, bringing excitement, passion, fascination, and pleasure. Commitment contributes stability, which helps maintain an honest, long-term relationship. According to psychologist Robert Sternberg, different stages and types of love reflect different combinations of *intimacy*, *passion*, and *commitment* (Figure 5.1). Relationships based on two or three of these values are more likely to survive than those based on only one.

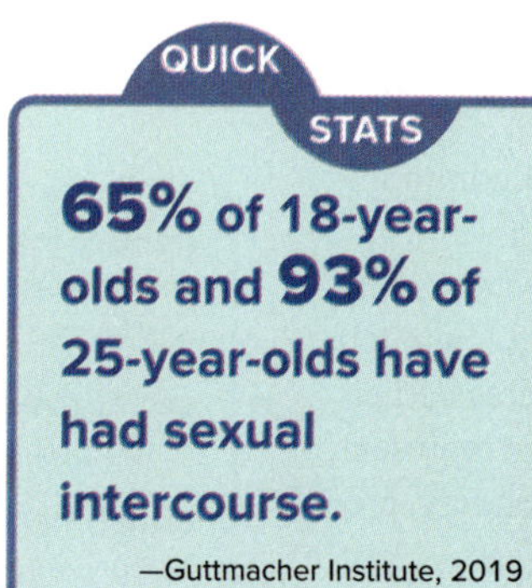

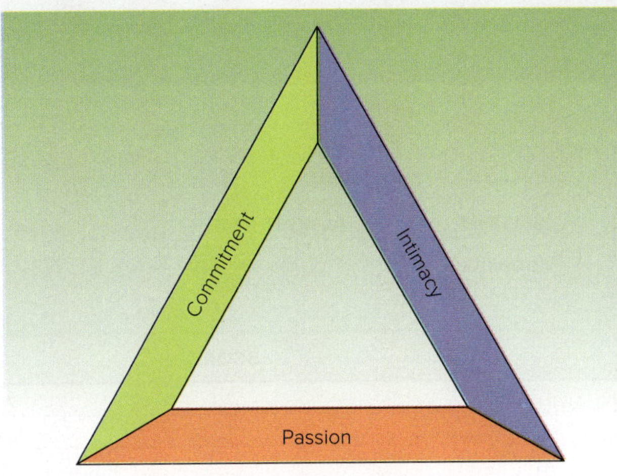


**FIGURE 5.1 The triangular theory of love.**

Other elements can be identified as features of intimate-sexual-romantic love, such as euphoria, preoccupation, idealization or devaluation of the loved one, and so on, but these elements tend to be temporary. They often fade or deepen into something more substantial. As relationships progress, the central aspects of love and commitment increase in importance.

Researchers suggest that gender plays a role in attitudes toward sexual intimacy. Although many men report that their most erotic sexual experiences occur in the context of a love relationship, studies find that men separate love from sex more easily than women do. Women more often view sex as an expression of an intimate relationship. This probably reflects deeply internalized cultural gender roles and our history of shaming females who pursue sex purely for pleasure. Yet more females as well as males now believe you can have satisfying sex without love, whether with friends, acquaintances, or strangers, unpaid or paid.

**The Pleasure and Pain of Love** Intense love has confused and tormented lovers throughout history. Artists, writers, and popular culture all describe a tumultuous state of excitement, subject to wildly fluctuating feelings of joy and despair. Lovers lose their appetite, can't sleep, and think of nothing but the loved one. Is this happiness? Misery? Both?

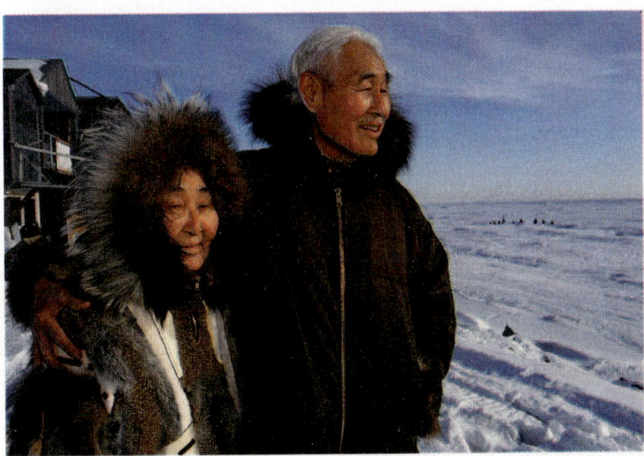

Although passion and physical intimacy often decline with time, other aspects of a relationship—such as commitment—tend to grow as the relationship matures. Jeff Schultz/Design Pics Inc/Alamy Stock Photo

The contradictory nature of passionate love can be understood by recognizing that human emotions have two components: physiological arousal and an emotional impetus for the arousal. Although experiences like attraction and sexual desire are pleasant, extreme excitement can be disturbing. For this reason, passionate love may be too intense for some people to enjoy. Over time, the physical intensity and excitement tend to diminish. When this happens, pleasure may actually increase.

**The Transformation of Love** Human relationships change over time, and love relationships are no exception. At first, love is likely to be characterized by high levels of passion and rapidly increasing intimacy. Passion decreases as we become habituated to it and to the person. The diminishing of romance or passionate love can be experienced as a crisis in a relationship. If a more lasting love fails to emerge, the relationship will likely break up.

Unlike passion, commitment does not necessarily diminish over time. Commitment brings stability to a relationship but also helps partners overcome its inevitable ups and downs. Committed partners put effort and energy into their relationship. They make time to indulge their partners, give compliments, and resolve conflict when it arises. To many people, commitment is the most important part of a relationship. When intensity diminishes, partners often discover a more enduring love. They can now move from absorption in each other to a relationship that includes external goals and projects, family, and friends. Successful relationships are based on closeness, caring, and the promise of a shared future.

## Challenges in Relationships

Although love makes an intimate relationship easier to begin and maintain, obstacles and challenges inevitably arise. Even in the best of circumstances, a loving relationship will be tested. Partners enter a relationship with diverse needs, desires, backgrounds, and ways of handling inter personal problems. These differences may emerge only at times of change or stress. Relationship challenges can relate to commitment, expectations, competitiveness, jealousy, and self-disclosure.

**Honesty and Openness** At the beginning of a relationship most of us prefer to present ourselves in the most favorable light. Although sharing thoughts and feelings can be emotionally risky, honesty is necessary in an intimate relationship. Over time, you and your partner will learn more about each other and feel more comfortable sharing. In fact, intimate familiarity with your partner's life is a key characteristic of successful long-term relationships.

**Emotional Intelligence** Recent research shows that classical IQ measures only a few, rather narrow, components

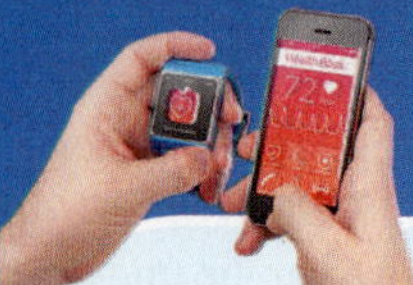

## ASSESS YOURSELF
### Are You Emotionally Intelligent?

In the statements below, give a rating for how often they hold true for you:

| ALWAYS | USUALLY | SOMETIMES | SELDOM | ALMOST NEVER |
|---|---|---|---|---|
| 5 points | 4 points | 3 points | 2 points | 1 point |

| | BEHAVIORAL HABIT | SCORE |
|---|---|---|
| 1. | I respect other people and their feelings | |
| 2. | I can easily identify my feelings | |
| 3. | I take responsibility for own emotions | |
| 4. | I feel that my life is spent doing things that are meaningful | |
| 5. | I find it easy to validate others' feelings and values | |
| 6. | I do not rush to judge or label other people and situations | |
| 7. | I have overcome setbacks to conquer an important challenge | |
| 8. | I challenge my habitual responses and am willing to try considered alternatives | |
| 9. | I live in the present, learn from experiences, and do not carry negative feelings forward | |

**Scoring:**

40–45 = You have a high level of emotional maturity, awareness, and control. You have a positive and inspiring impact on others.

35–39 = You have a higher than average level of emotional intelligence. Concentrate on self-awareness and control, and developing increased empathy for others.

27–34 = You have a baseline awareness of what emotional intelligence is. Be alert for opportunities to increase levels of self-awareness and empathy toward others, and to refine responses.

9–26 = Now that you're aware of emotional intelligence, monitor your emotions and their impact on you and others. Notice how your behavior affects others, and get feedback on how to modify behavior that provokes a defensive response.

SOURCE: Blanchard, C., et al. 2021. Emotional intelligence, burnout, and professional fulfillment in clinical year medical students. Medical Teacher 43(9): 1063–1069; Earl, D. 2022. *Emotional Intelligence Quiz* (https://www.donnaearltraining.com/articles-quizzes/emotional-intelligence-quiz/).

of what we call human intelligence. To function well in life requires a wide range of abilities, including self-awareness, self-discipline, empathy, the ability to understand others' perspectives, and to communicate effectively—in short, what some have called *social* or *emotional* intelligence.

The key to developing emotional intelligence lies in cultivating *mindfulness*—the ability to dispassionately observe thoughts and feelings as they occur (see Chapter 2). When we observe emotions without judging or immediately acting on them, we can make more measured, wise, and skillful responses. These skills can be particularly helpful when we are in an argument or a conflict with someone with whom we have a close relationship.

Recent studies of emotional intelligence find a connection between empathy and prejudice. Participants who were better at managing and regulating their emotions showed higher levels of empathy, especially in taking on new perspectives, and lower levels of bias related to ethnicity, sex, or gender identity. Lower levels of emotional intelligence were related to higher acceptance of right-wing authoritarianism, social dominance orientation, and racial prejudice. In caregiving professions such as the medical profession, a lack of empathy also leads to a higher risk of burnout for the doctor, nurse, or medical student.

**Unequal or Premature Commitment** When one person in an intimate partnership becomes more serious about the relationship than the other, feelings are bound to be hurt. Sometimes a couple makes a premature commitment, and then one partner has second thoughts. Eventually both partners recognize that something is wrong, but each is afraid to tell the other. It may be painful but necessary to resolve this conflict by stepping up and saying, "We have a problem. Can we have an honest talk about it?" Such problems usually can be resolved only by honest and sensitive communication.

**Unrealistic Expectations** Each partner brings hopes and expectations to a relationship. Some may be unrealistic,

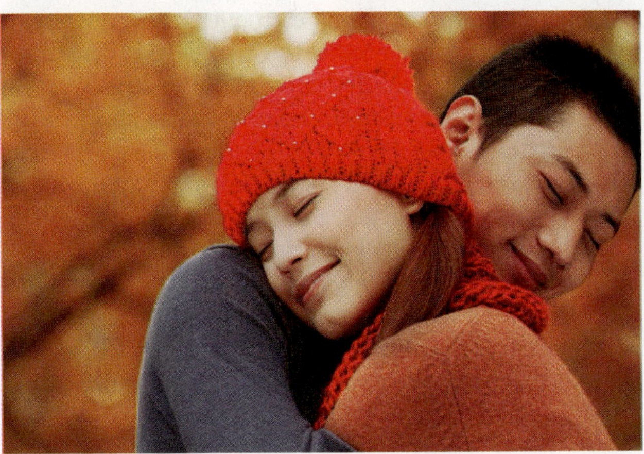

Supportiveness is a sign of commitment and compassion and is an important part of any healthy relationship. Jade/Blend Images/ Getty Images

unfair, and ultimately damaging to the relationship. These include the following:

- Expecting your partner to change.
- Assuming that your partner has all the same opinions, priorities, interests, and goals as you.
- Believing a relationship will fulfill all your personal, financial, intellectual, and social needs.

**Competitiveness** If one partner feels compelled or entitled to compete and win—traditionally the male over the female in a patriarchal culture—it can detract from the sense of connectedness, equality, and mutuality between partners. The same can be said for a perfectionistic need to always be right and win every argument.

If competitiveness is a problem for you, ask yourself if your need to win is more important than your partner's feelings or the future of your relationship. Try noncompetitive activities or an activity where you are a beginner and your partner excels. Accept that your partner's views may be just as valid and important to them as your own views are to you.

**Balancing Time Together and Apart** You may enjoy time together with your partner, but it is healthy to also spend time alone or with family and friends. Interpreting this as rejection or a lack of commitment can damage the relationship. Talk with your partner about your expectations and what time apart and together means to you. Consider your partner's feelings carefully, and try to reach a compromise that satisfies both of you.

Differences in expectations can mirror differences in ideas about emotional closeness. Any romantic relationship requires giving up some autonomy in order to develop as a couple. But remember that people are not all the same in their needs for distance and closeness in a relationship.

**Jealousy** Jealousy is the angry, painful response to a partner's real, imagined, or possible involvement with something outside the relationship, like a person or activity. Some people (and cultures) believe that the existence of jealousy proves the existence of love, but jealousy is often a sign of insecurity or possessiveness.

In its extreme forms, jealousy can destroy a relationship by its attempts at control. Jealousy is a factor in the violence in dating relationships among both high school and college students. An abusive spouse often uses jealousy to justify violence.

When jealousy occurs in a relationship, it's important for the partners to communicate clearly with each other. In this sense, jealousy can offer partners the chance to look closely at issues like possessiveness; insecurity; low self-esteem; and feelings of entitlement, control, and dominance. This can strengthen the relationship.

**Supportiveness** Another key to successful relationships is the ability to ask for and give support. Partners need to know that they can count on each other during difficult times.

## Unhealthy Intimate Relationships

Interactions between individuals of very unequal status often differ significantly from those between equals. Those with authority and power can enforce their will on others, with or without discussion or agreement. Criticism can be one means to prevail. They can choose to abuse, verbally and even physically, those in subordinate positions.

Hierarchical relationships have traditionally characterized families in the United States and elsewhere, with status based on generation, age, kinship relationship, and gender. In its patriarchal form, the oldest male is the head of the family with legal authority over other members. By today's standards, however, healthy intimate relationships are characterized by mutual respect, reciprocity, collaboration, and consensus building.

Examples of unhealthy relationships are those that are physically or emotionally abusive or that involve extreme dependency by one or both partners. According to the Centers for Disease Control and Prevention, almost 1 in 11 female and 1 in 14 male high school students report that their romantic relationship involved physical violence in the past year. Intimate partner violence is also a problem on college campuses.

There are physical and mental consequences of being in an unhappy relationship. Although breaking up is painful, it is ultimately better than living in a toxic relationship.

## Ending a Relationship

Even when a couple starts out with the best of intentions, an intimate relationship may not last. Some breakups happen quickly following direct action by one or both partners, but many occur over an extended period as the couple goes through cycles of separation and reconciliation.

If you are involved in a breakup, the following suggestions may help make the ending easier:

- Give the relationship a fair chance before breaking up.
- Be fair and honest.

- Be tactful and compassionate.
- If you feel rejected, give yourself time to resolve your anger and pain.
- Recognize the value in the experience.

Use the recovery period following a breakup for self-renewal. Redirect more attention to yourself, and reconnect with people and areas of your life that were neglected during your relationship. Time will help heal the pain of the loss.

Finally, be aware of the impulse to "rebound" quickly into another relationship. Although it may mute the pain of a breakup, forming a relationship in order to avoid feeling pain is not a good strategy. Too often, rebound relationships fail because they were designed to be "lifeboats" or because one or both partners is not truly ready for another intimate relationship.

# COMMUNICATION

A key to developing and maintaining healthy intimate relationships is good communication. Most of the time we don't think about communicating; we simply talk and behave normally. But when problems arise–when we feel others don't understand us or when someone accuses us of not listening–we become aware of our limitations or, more commonly, what we think are other people's limitations.

## Nonverbal Communication

Even when we're silent, we're communicating. We send messages when we look at someone or look away, lean forward or sit back, smile or frown. Especially important forms of nonverbal communication in the United States are touch, eye contact, and proximity. If someone we're talking to touches our hand or arm, looks into our eyes, and leans toward us when we talk, we get the message that the person is interested in us and cares about what we're saying. If a person keeps looking around the room while we're talking or takes a step backward, we get the impression the person is uninterested or wants to end the conversation.

The ability to interpret nonverbal messages correctly is important to the success of relationships. It's also important, when sending messages, to make sure our body language agrees with our words. When our verbal and nonverbal messages don't correspond, we send a mixed message.

**Ask Yourself**

**QUESTIONS FOR CRITICAL THINKING AND REFLECTION**

Have you ever ended an intimate relationship? If so, how did you handle it? How did you feel after the breakup? How do you think the breakup affected your former partner? Did the experience help you in other relationships?

Attunement, or tuning in to each other's tone of voice, is important. More than any other cue, tone of voice can convey most accurately a person's emotional state. Our effectiveness at connecting or reconnecting emotionally with another depends on the accuracy of our attunement. Effective attunement recreates a healthy child-caregiver connection, or it provides a connection that was lacking during childhood.

How we feel when communicating with another can give the listener important data about the speaker. If "out of nowhere" we begin to feel sad, anxious, or angry, these may be emotional states the other person is communicating. An example would be feeling sad when communicating with a grieving friend.

## Digital Communication and Our Social Networks

Social media enable us to communicate more rapidly, but some experts question whether this capability is undermining interpersonal relations and our ability to relate to others in person. Some evidence suggests the opposite is true: 2018 surveys by the Pew Internet and American Life Project found that technology users had larger and more diverse discussion networks and were just as involved in their communities as people who communicate face-to-face. Many young adults (aged 18–29 years) who were in a serious relationship reported feeling closer to their spouse or partner due to online or text-message conversations. Some said they were able to resolve arguments that they couldn't face-to-face. The critical question is really what users are doing on social media, and the content to which they are being exposed, not the amount of time spent.

Social media create diverse forms of communication. The brief immediacy of a tweet is very different from an extended conversation over a video chat. But people often use a tweet to communicate something too complicated for anything other than Skype.

Some observers worry that technologies alter the nature of the social environment and the size and makeup of social networks. Facebook, for example, facilitates relationships with people we have shared interests with but may never meet in person. As it becomes more common for family members to live apart and as online communication evolves, the face-to-face aspects of relationships may become less significant, but perhaps more valued.

Social media do provide some advantages. They allow for instant and easy communication with others across the globe. They enable long-distance connections; reconnections with important people from our past; and affiliations with others who share similar, sometimes rare, identities, interests, and experiences.

But they also make it easier to communicate impulsively, such as sending angry or threatening messages, stalking, posting embarrassing pictures of peers or ex-partners, or pursuing new partners while in a supposedly monogamous relationship. Some people even end intimate relationships online. Electronic bullying (and "shaming") is a significant problem among pre-college students and has led to several suicides. According to a 2021 report, 23% of teenagers reported having been cyberbullied in the past month. LGBTQ youth experienced 50% more bullying than non-LGBTQ youth, and whites and multiracial students reported being the victims of cyberbullying more often than students of other races.

QUICK STATS

**Female, trans, queer, nonbinary, and questioning college students reported experiencing sexual contact without their consent four times as often as straight, cisgender men.**

—Association of American Universities, 2020

Here are other problem areas online:

- ***Missing nonverbal cues such as body language and tone of voice.*** A comment or joke intended as playful may instead come off as critical or harsh.
- ***Promoting an idealized version of oneself.*** Many of us promote a version that involves only the most flattering photos and happiest moments. Doing so can have a serious downside if the gap between one's "real" and online lives becomes too large.
- ***Spying.*** In the past, people who suspected their partners of cheating had to follow them or hire detectives to see what they were doing. These days, it is as easy as checking statuses and messages, which makes it more tempting to invade a partner's privacy when feeling suspicious or insecure.
- ***Checking one's phone rather than staying present.*** How often have you seen a couple at a restaurant, and both of them are checking their phones rather than engaging in conversation? Social media can be great tools, but only when they don't replace experiencing life in the moment.
- ***Publicizing more areas of one's life.*** Sometimes people in a relationship differ dramatically in their ideas about what should be public versus private, so discuss before uploading information to social media.

## Communication Skills

Three skills essential to good communication in relationships are self-disclosure, listening, and feedback:

- ***Self-disclosure*** involves revealing personal information that we ordinarily wouldn't reveal due to the risk involved. It usually increases feelings of closeness and moves the relationship to a deeper level of intimacy. Friends often confide in each other, sharing feelings, experiences, hopes, and disappointments. Married couples sometimes feel less need to share, making unwarranted assumptions because they think that they already know everything about each other.
- ***Listening*** requires that we spend more time and energy trying to fully understand another person's "story" and less time judging, evaluating, blaming, advising, analyzing, or trying to control. Empathy, warmth, respect, and genuineness are qualities of skillful listeners. Attentive listening encourages friends or partners to share more and, in turn, to be attentive listeners. To connect with other people and develop real emotional intimacy, listening is essential.
- ***Feedback,*** a constructive response to another's self-disclosure, is the third key to good communication. Giving positive feedback means acknowledging that the friend's or partner's feelings are valid—no matter how upsetting or troubling—and offering self-disclosure in response. If, for example, your partner discloses unhappiness about your relationship, it is more constructive to say that you're concerned or saddened by that and want to hear more about it than to get angry, blame, try to inflict pain, or withdraw. Self-disclosure and feedback can open the door to change, whereas other responses block communication and change. (For tips on improving your skills, see the box "Guidelines for Effective Communication.")

## Conflict and Conflict Resolution

Conflict is normal in intimate relationships. No matter how close two people become, they remain separate individuals with their own needs, desires, past experiences, and ways of seeing the world. In fact, the closer the relationship, the more differences and the more opportunities for conflict.

Although conflict may suggest that the relationship is deepening, if it is not handled constructively, conflict can damage—and ultimately destroy—the relationship. Consider the guidelines discussed here, but remember that different couples communicate in different ways around conflict. Gender, family and cultural background, education, and income level are among factors that influence how we experience and deal with conflict.

Conflict is often accompanied by anger—a natural emotion—but one that can be difficult to handle, especially for those who haven't learned to channel it in a constructive way. If we express anger aggressively, we risk creating

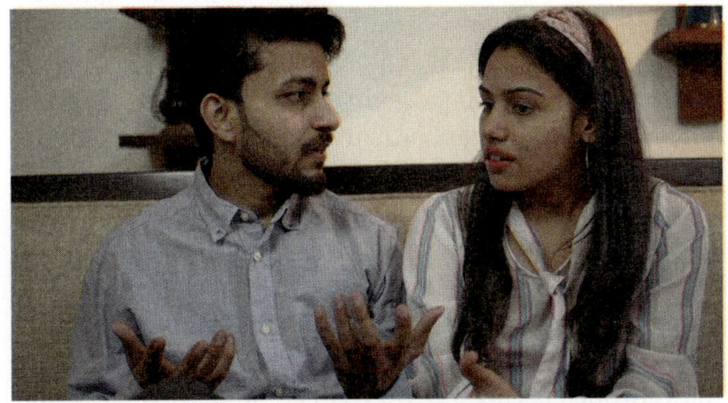

Conflict is an inevitable part of any intimate relationship. How can we resolve our conflicts in constructive ways? Wirestock Creators/Shutterstock

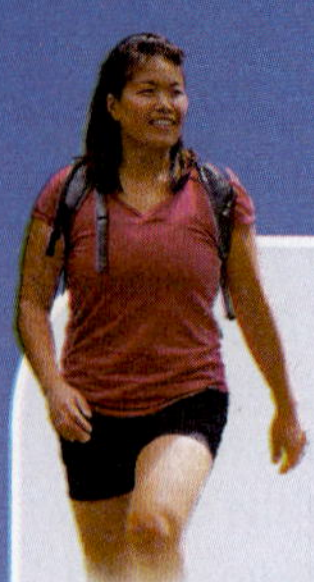

## TAKE CHARGE
## Guidelines for Effective Communication

### Getting Started

- When you want to have a serious discussion with your partner, choose a private place and a time when you won't be interrupted or rushed. Avoid having important conversations via text or other media.
- Face your partner and maintain eye contact. Use nonverbal feedback to show that you are interested and involved.

### Being an Effective Speaker

- State your concern or issue as clearly as you can.
- Use "I" statements rather than statements beginning with "you." When you use "I" statements, you take responsibility for your feelings. "You" statements are often blaming or accusatory and will probably get a defensive or resentful response. The statement "I feel unloved," for example, sends a clearer, less blaming message than the statement "You don't love me."
- Focus on a behavior, not the whole person. Be specific about the behavior you like or don't like. Avoid generalizations beginning with "you always" or "you never." Such statements make people feel defensive.
- Make constructive requests. Opening your request with "I would like" keeps the focus on your needs rather than your partner's supposed deficiencies.
- Avoid blaming, accusing, and belittling. Even if you are right, you have little to gain by putting your partner down. When people feel criticized or attacked, they are less able to think rationally or solve problems constructively.
- Set up your partner for success. Tell your partner what you would like to have happen in the future; don't wait for him or her to blow it and then express anger or disappointment.

### Being an Effective Listener

- Provide appropriate nonverbal feedback (nodding, smiling, making eye contact, and so on).
- Don't interrupt.
- Listen reflectively. Don't judge, evaluate, analyze, or offer solutions (unless asked to do so). Your partner may just need to sort out their feelings. By jumping in to "fix" the problem, you may cut off communication.
- Don't offer unsolicited advice. Giving advice implies that you know more about what a person needs to do than they do; therefore, it often evokes anger or resentment.
- Clarify your understanding of what your partner is saying by restating it in your own words and asking if your understanding is correct. "I think you're saying that you would feel uncomfortable having dinner with my parents and that you'd prefer to meet them in a more casual setting. Is that right?" This type of specific feedback prevents misunderstandings and helps validate the speaker's feelings and message.
- Be sure you are really listening, not off somewhere in your mind rehearsing your reply. Try to tune in to your partner's feelings and needs as well as the words. Accurately reflecting the other person's feelings and needs is often a more powerful way of connecting than just reframing their thoughts.
- Let your partner know that you value what they are saying and want to understand. Respect for the other person is the cornerstone of effective communication.

distrust, fear, and distance. If we act out our anger, we can cause the conflict to escalate. If we suppress anger, it may turn into resentment and hostility. The best way to handle anger in a relationship is to recognize it as a symptom of something that requires attention and needs to be addressed. When angry, partners should exercise restraint so as not to become abusive. It is important to express anger skillfully and not in a way that is out of proportion to the issue at hand. The best time to express yourself is when you are not boiling over with strong emotions.

The sources of conflict for couples change over time but revolve, at least on the surface, primarily around issues of finances, sex, children, in-laws, and household responsibilities. Issues of power, authority, and challenges to traditional gender roles are often deeper roots of conflict. Although there are numerous theories on and approaches to conflict resolution, these fundamental strategies can be helpful:

1. ***Clarify the issue.*** Take responsibility for thinking through your feelings and discovering what's really bothering you. Agree that one partner will speak first and have the chance to speak fully while the other listens. Then reverse the roles. Try to understand your partner's position fully by repeating what you've heard and asking questions to clarify or elicit more information. Agree to talk only about the topic at hand and not get distracted by other issues. Sum up what your partner has said.
2. ***Find out what each person wants.*** Ask your partner to express their desires. Don't assume you know what your partner wants, and don't speak for them.
3. ***Determine how you both can get what you want.*** Brainstorm to come up with a variety of options.
4. ***Decide how to negotiate.*** Work out a plan for change. Be willing to compromise, and avoid trying to "win."

5. ***Solidify the agreements.*** If necessary, go over the plan and write it down, to ensure that you both understand and agree to it.
6. ***Review and renegotiate.*** Decide on a time frame for trying out your plan, and set a time to discuss how it's working. Make adjustments as needed.

To resolve conflicts, partners must feel safe in voicing disagreements. They have to trust that the discussion won't get out of control, that they won't be abandoned, and that their vulnerability won't be taken advantage of. Partners should follow some basic ground rules when they argue, such as avoiding ultimatums, resisting the urge to give the silent treatment, refusing to "hit below the belt," and not using sex to smooth over disagreements.

When you argue, maintain a spirit of goodwill and avoid being harshly critical or contemptuous. Remember–you care about your partner and want things to work out. See the disagreement as a difficulty that the two of you have together rather than as something your partner does to you. Finish serious discussions on a positive note by expressing your respect and affection for your partner and your appreciation for having been listened to. If you and your partner find that you argue again and again over the same issue, it may be better to stop trying to resolve that problem and instead come to accept the differences between you, or part ways if the differences are intolerable.

# PAIRING AND SINGLEHOOD

Alternatives to the old model of marriage are increasingly popular. Cohabitation, divorce, and singlehood have become common. Same-sex marriage is now legal in all 50 states, and the concept of family is expanding. Multiple marriages, polymorphy (three-or-more-person relationships), blended families, and nonkinship-based families are examples of new creative intimate social arrangements.

## Choosing a Partner

Studies have shown that most people pair with someone who lives in the same geographic area; comes from a similar racial, ethnic, and socioeconomic background; has a similar educational status; leads a lifestyle like theirs; and has (what they think is) the same level of physical attractiveness.

Once the euphoria of romantic love winds down, personality traits, behaviors, and socioeconomic status become more significant in how partners view each other. The emphasis shifts to basic values and future aspirations regarding career, family, and children. At some point, they decide whether the relationship feels viable and is worthy of their continued commitment.

Perhaps the most important question for potential mates to ask is, "How much do we have in common?" Although differences add interest to a relationship, similarities increase its chance of success. Differences in values, religion, race, ethnicity, cultural background, socioeconomic status, and beliefs about gender and sexuality can produce strains. But acceptance and communication skills go a long way toward making a relationship work, no matter how different the partners.

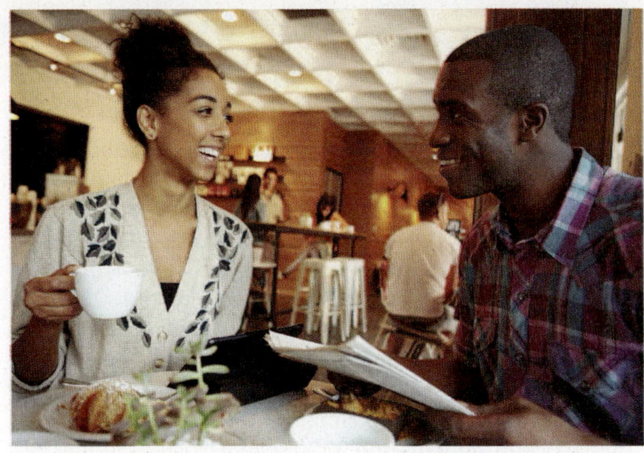

Physical attraction plays a strong role in the initial choosing of a partner. People tend to gravitate toward others who share similar characteristics, such as appearance, race, ethnicity, education, and socioeconomic background. iStockphoto/Getty Images

## Dating

Every culture has certain criteria and rituals for finding and choosing mates. American cultural norms of romantic love and personal choice in courtship and mate selection have an enormous appeal globally. Themes of romantic love and finding one's soul mate permeate popular culture (movies, music, videos, TV) and consumer marketing around the world. But in the United States, as elsewhere, the popularity of dating services and online matchmaking suggests that people want help finding a suitable partner.

Dating is still a common way to find a romantic partner. If sexual involvement develops, it is more likely to be based on friendship, respect, and common interests than on gender role expectations. Such relationships may lead to marriage. In contrast, some teenagers and young adults are turning to *hooking up*–casual sexual activity without any relationship commitment.

## Online Dating and Relationships

Until 2013, probably since the earliest days of mating, the most popular way to meet a potential mate was through family and friends. Over the past few years, online dating has continued to grow, and it has now surpassed all other ways to date. For one, the sets of people available to meet are larger than friend connections. These numbers are especially valuable for people searching for particular qualities or orientations. Since the start of the Covid-19 pandemic, researchers are noting new online dating trends (see the box "Love in the Time of Pandemic").

## WELLNESS ON CAMPUS

## Love in the Time of Pandemic: What Has Happened to the Dating Scene

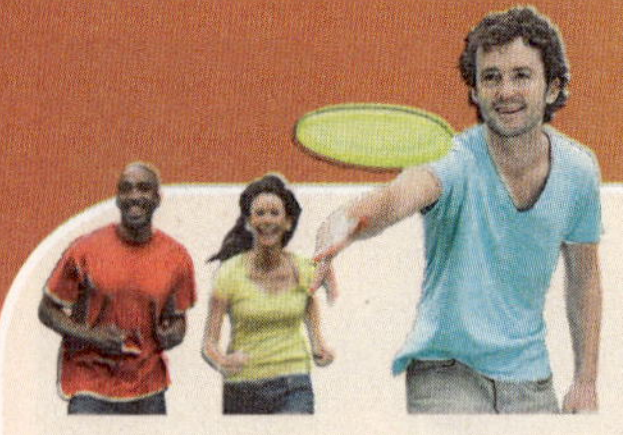

The Covid-19 pandemic has disrupted relationships of almost every kind, and notably complicated those with romantic and sexual aspects. The truth is, a decline in sexual activity began a decade earlier. Compared to reports of adult sexual activity in 2009, study respondents in the U.S., U.K., Australia, Germany, and Japan reported less penile-vaginal penetration, partnered masturbation, oral sex, and anal intercourse in 2018. Adolescents also reported less solo masturbation.

For college students, the 2020 school closures further disrupted romantic and sexual activity. About 15% of students reported breaking up with their partners; many existing relationships became long-distance; and everyone lost opportunities to meet new people. Before campuses closed, 2.6% of U.S. students lived at home; by April 2020, 71.0% did. Living at home can limit the sexual exploration that happens for many young adults in college.

Research shows that sex can contribute to students' well-being: both casual and committed relationships can bring sexual pleasure and social support. Sex can help people relax, fall asleep, reduce stress, and feel more intimate with their partners. The freedom to explore also keys us into who we are and what we prefer, including the choice to call ourselves asexual.

*Hooking up*—having casual sexual encounters with acquaintances or strangers with no commitment or investment in an emotionally intimate relationship—is said to have its roots in the changing social and sexual patterns of the 1960s. Since then, changes in college policies (e.g., the trend toward coed dorms) and wider social trends (e.g., getting married at a later age, effective contraception, the availability of dating apps) have contributed to an increase in hooking up. Hooking up addresses the desire for "instant intimacy" but also protects the participants from the risk or responsibility of emotional involvement.

Concerns about alcohol-fueled risk taking and negative health effects, including Covid transmission, unintended pregnancies, and sexually transmitted infections, may, however, have contributed to the more recent decline in sex. Other possible factors include increasing media consumption, which can replace time spent seeking and developing sexual relationships. Whether we've lost jobs, child care, or loved ones to Covid-19, the pandemic has brought a lot of stress and destabilization. Lower income, anxiety, and depression all influence sexual interest and drives.

Single people these days appear to be looking for more committed relationships. Online dating was already becoming the most popular way to meet new people. Now, with increased physical social distancing, singles are forced to return to more traditional courting tactics. With an enormous rise in video chatting, potential partners have more time to talk and get to know one another before the kissing starts. Clear communication and emotional intelligence become important areas to develop, skills that help us in all our relationships. Each person must assess and communicate their own comfort levels with safety and risk during this disruptive time.

SOURCES: Fisher, H. 2020. How coronavirus is changing the dating game for the better, *The New York Times,* May 7; Wade, L. 2017. *American Hookup: The New Culture of Sex on Campus.* New York: W. W. Norton; Herbenick, D., et al. 2021. Changes in penile-vaginal intercourse frequency and sexual repertoire from 2009 to 2018: Findings from the National Survey of Sexual Health and Behavior. *Archives of Sexual Behavior* (https://doi.org/10.1007/s10508-021-02125-2); Willingham, E. 2022. People have been having less sex—whether they're teenagers or 40-somethings. *Scientific American* (https://www.scientificamerican.com/article/people-have-been-having-less-sex-whether-theyre-teenagers-or-40-somethings/).

Another benefit of connecting online is freedom from your family, friends, and even candidate dating partners. Connecting with others online allows people to communicate in a relaxed way, try out different personas, and share things they normally would not reveal face-to-face. You can set your own pace and start and end relationships at any time.

Some people, however, misrepresent themselves, pretending to be older or younger or even of a different sex than they really are. Investing time and emotional resources in such relationships can be painful. In rare cases, online romances become dangerous or even deadly.

Because people online reveal only what they want to, users may see idealized versions of online partners. If your online friend seems perfect, take that as a warning sign. You may search for perfection, find fault quickly, and not give people a chance; conversely, you may act on impulse with insufficient information.

QUICK
STATS
40% of Gen Z Tinder members say they will continue to go on digital dates, even after Covid-19 restrictions end.
—Wiederhold, B., *Cyberpsychology, Behavior, and Social Networking,* 2021

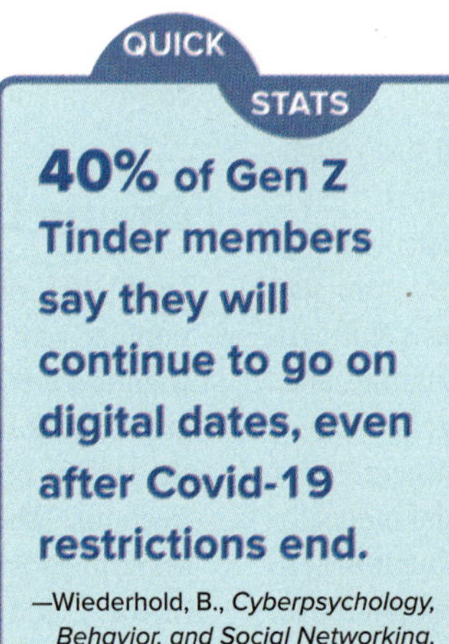

Relationship sites also remove an important and powerful element from the process: chemistry and in-person intuition. Much of our communication is transmitted through body language, tone, and even scent. Consider these questions. Are you comfortable disclosing personal information about yourself? Is there a balance in the amount of time spent talking by each of you? Is the other person respecting your boundaries? Just as in face-to-face dating, online relationships require you to use common sense and to trust your instincts.

If you pursue an online relationship, these guidelines may help you have a positive experience and stay safe:

- Choose a site that fits with your own relationship goals. Some sites are primarily geared for hookups—that is, arranging meetings for casual sex—whereas others aim to facilitate classic dating relationships. Inspect each site thoroughly before registering or providing any information about yourself. If you aren't comfortable with a site's content or purpose, close your web browser and clear out its cache and its store of cookies.

- Know what you are looking for as well as what you can offer someone else. If you are looking for a relationship that is not just physical, make that clear. Find out the other person's intentions, and maybe vaccination status.

- Don't post photos unless you are completely comfortable with potential consequences (e.g., they might be downloaded by others).

- Don't give out personal information, including your real full name, school, or place of employment, until you feel sure that you are giving the information to someone who is trustworthy.

- Set up a second email account for sending and receiving dating-related emails.

- If someone does not respond to a message, don't take it personally. There are many reasons why a person may not pursue the connection. Don't continue to send messages to an unresponsive person; doing so could lead to an accusation of stalking.

- Before deciding whether to meet an online contact in person, consider talking by video or over the phone.

- Don't agree to meet someone face-to-face unless you feel comfortable about it. Always meet initially in a public place—a museum, a coffee shop, or a restaurant. Consider bringing along a friend to increase your safety, and let others know where you will be.

- At the same time, don't let too much time pass exchanging messages: It's important to discover your compatibility in person.

If you pursue online relationships, don't let them interfere with your other personal relationships and social activities. To support your emotional and personal wellness, use the internet to widen your circle of friends, not shrink it.

## Sexual Orientation and Gender Identity in Society

People demonstrate great diversity in their emotional and sexual attractions (see Chapter 6). **Sexual orientation** refers to a pattern of emotional and sexual attraction to persons of the same sex or gender, a different sex or gender, or more than one sex or gender. The term **queer** has emerged to describe sexual orientations other than **straight (heterosexual).**

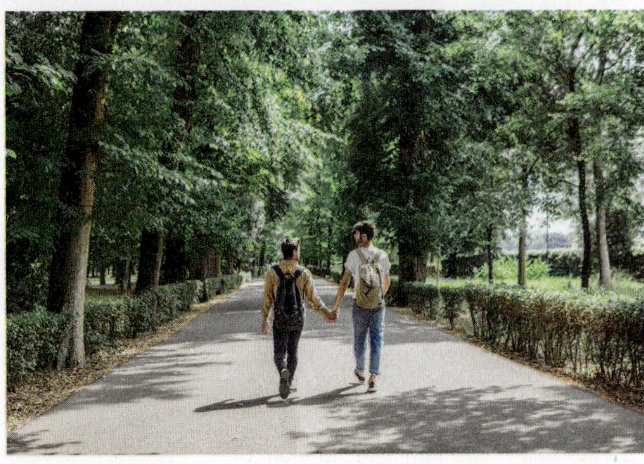

Same-sex partnerships constitute a minority of the population; growing social acceptance has allowed them to be more visible than in the past. Westend61/Getty Images

People identify as gay or lesbian, bisexual, nonbinary, transgender, or with a sexual or gender identity that does not conform to dominant societal norms. They may all be considered as gender nonconforming. Categories are human inventions and can be disrupted, as we see happening today with sexual orientation and gender categories. The terminology of sex-gender is complex and constantly changing. Sometimes we're not sure what terms to use for ourselves or for other people. The best approach is usually to respect and use, when possible, the identity or label people choose for themselves.

Regardless of sexual orientation, most people look for love in a committed relationship. Like any intimate relationship, queer partnerships provide intimacy, passion, and security. However, there are some significant differences. Same-sex partnerships tend to be more egalitarian (equal) than heterosexual partnerships, probably because they are not bound by traditional gender roles. Same-sex couples put greater emphasis on partnership. Most reject the traditional roles common in the division of labor. Domestic responsibilities are shared or divided, and both partners contribute financially or are self-supporting. Having children, however, often disrupts this equality; between career demands and lack of affordable child care options, same-sex partnerships can become divided along more heteronormative lines, with one partner having a higher income and the other partner having more child-rearing and domestic duties.

Same-sex couples also experience challenges related to their sexual orientation, especially if they come from families, religions, or communities that do not accept alternatives to

**TERMS**

**sexual orientation** A consistent pattern of emotional and sexual attraction based on biological sex; it exists in many forms, including attraction to people of another sex, of the same sex, of a range of sexes/genders, or to no one at all.

**queer** Sexual orientations other than heterosexual/straight.

**heterosexual/straight** Attraction to people of the other sex.

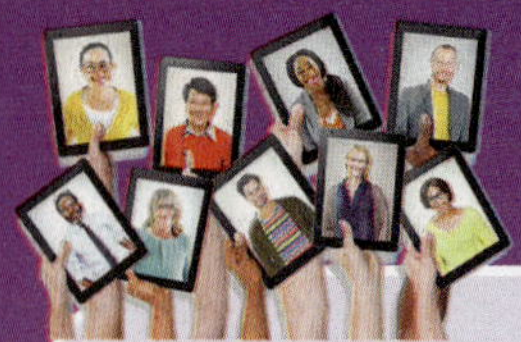

## DIVERSITY MATTERS
### Marriage Equality

In its legal definitions, marriage is an institution in which couples derive legal and economic rights and responsibilities from state and federal statutes. The U.S. Government Accountability Office says more than 1000 federal laws make distinctions based on marriage. Marital status affects many aspects of life, such as Social Security benefits, federal tax status, inheritance, and medical decision making.

The push for legal recognition of same-sex partnerships has gone on for decades. Supporters of same-sex marriage rights have met opposition at the local, state, and federal levels, in both the public and private sectors. However, support for marriage equality has increased rapidly in the past several years. Gallup polls tracking support for marriage equality show a steady climb, from 27% support in 1996, the first year Gallup asked the question, to a record-high 70% in 2021. In 2013, the U.S. Supreme Court ruled that the federal government must recognize same-sex marriages performed by states that allow them, and in 2015, it declared all state bans on same-sex marriage unconstitutional.

Couples in which one or both partners are transgender are affected by this ruling as well, but only if their legal gender classifies them as a same-sex couple at the time of their marriage. Heterosexual transgender couples were generally able to marry previous to this ruling, so long as they were legally man-and-woman at the time of the marriage.

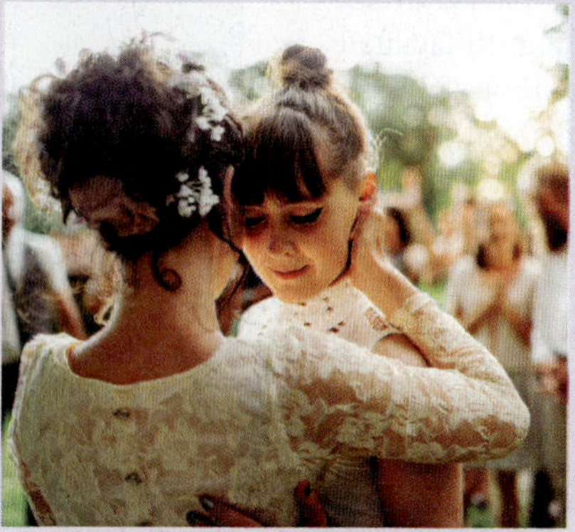

Hinterhaus Productions/Getty Images

What are benefits of marriage for same-sex couples?

- Health insurance and retirement benefits for employees' spouses
- Social Security benefits for spouses, widows, and widowers
- Support and benefits for military spouses, widows, and widowers
- Joint income tax filing and exemption from federal estate taxes
- Immigration protections for binational couples
- Rights to creative and intellectual property
- Protection from some types of employment discrimination (e.g., getting fired for marrying a same-sex spouse)

Marriage also matters in terms of child rearing. Children who grow up with married parents benefit because their parents' relationship is recognized by law and receives legal protections. Additionally, spouses are generally entitled to joint child custody and visitation should the marriage end in divorce. They also bear an obligation to pay child support.

Finally, marriage can have an impact on emotional well-being. Research shows that married people tend to live longer, have higher incomes, engage less frequently in risky behaviors, have a healthier diet, and have fewer psychological problems than unmarried people. Finally, studies show that denying same-sex couples the right to marry has a negative impact on their mental health. The long-term impact of marriage equality is not yet known, but it is likely to benefit the legal, economic, and emotional well-being of millions of Americans.

SOURCES: Shah, Dayna K. 2004. Letter to Senator Bill Frist (http://www.gao.gov/new.items/d04353r.pdf); Marriage Equality FAQ: Frequently Asked Questions about the Supreme Court's Marriage Ruling (https://marriageequalityfacts.org/); McCarthy, J. 2021. Record-high 70% in U.S. support same-sex marriage. *Gallup* (https://news.gallup.com/poll/350486/record-high-support-same-sex-marriage.aspx); Gonzales, G. 2014. Same-sex marriage—A prescription for better health. *New England Journal of Medicine* 370: 1373–1376; Wight, R. G. 2013. Same-sex legal marriage and psychological well-being: Findings from the California Health Interview Survey. *American Journal of Public Health* 103(2): 339–346.

heterosexuality. Sexual minorities often deal with social hostility, ambivalence, or simple discomfort with their relationships, in contrast to the social approval and rights given to straight couples (see the box "Marriage Equality"). Such discrimination can be obvious, as in the case of violence or unequitable laws, or it can be subtler, as in stereotypical portrayals of same-sex couples in the media. Societal and personal sources of rejection often take their toll, especially among young people, and easily accessible sources of support are essential. Many communities offer support groups for same-sex partners and families to help them build social networks.

See Chapter 6 for more information about sexual orientation, gender identity, and sexual behavior.

## Singlehood

Research shows that a growing percentage of American adults are single. In 2020, according to the U.S. Census, approximately half of all adults over age 15 were married. The remaining 50%, or about 130 million people, were single. Of course, not all singlehood is voluntary. Being single includes people who are no longer married, are divorced or widowed, or have never married.

Several factors contribute to the growing number of singles. One is a much more positive view toward singlehood. Education and careers are delaying the age at which young people marry. More young people are living with their parents as they complete their education, seek jobs, pay off debts, and strive for financial independence. As cohabitation has gained acceptance, many singles simply live with partners rather than marry. High divorce rates also create more singles.

Being single, however, does not mean living without intimate relationships. Single people date, enjoy active and fulfilling social lives, and have a variety of sexual experiences and relationships. Other advantages of being single, especially for those without children, include more opportunities for personal and career development, fewer family obligations, and more freedom and control over life choices. Disadvantages include less companionship, potential loneliness, and sole responsibility for one's life (home, health, economic situation, recreation, etc.). Living on one income, especially in today's economy and housing market, can be a challenge for anyone, but particularly for lower-income workers and for women who, on average, earn less than men. Singles may experience discrimination because of their marital status and social pressure to get married.

How enjoyable and valuable single life is depends on several factors. These include whether it is by choice; the quality of one's social relationships, standard of living, and job; how comfortable one is with being alone; and how resourceful and energetic the person is about creating an interesting and fulfilling life.

**QUICK STATS**

**Almost half of young adults said the relationship with their spouse or partner improved during the past year when they worked remotely and spent more time together.**

—*Forbes*, 2021

## Living Together

Living together, or cohabitation, is one of the most dramatic social changes of the past few decades. Both attitudes and behavior have changed. A 2019 Pew Research Center study, "Marriage and Cohabitation in the United States," found that more adults (ages 18–44) have now lived with a romantic partner than have ever been married (Figure 5.2). Several factors are involved in this change, including greater acceptance of sex outside of marriage, the availability of contraceptives, more emphasis on career development, and a desire to delay marriage and children. Financial concerns, such as student debt burden and skyrocketing housing costs, also play a role. In the Pew Study, about 40% of those who were cohabiting (versus married) cited financial considerations and "convenience" as important reasons for moving in with their partners. In addition, many people have experienced divorce in their own families or marriages. They may be wary of making a marriage commitment without living together first.

Cohabitation provides many of the benefits of marriage: a steady intimate, romantic, and sexual partner; companionship; and an opportunity to develop greater intimacy through learning, compromising, and sharing. In the Pew study, love and companionship were the two major reasons couples gave for cohabiting, as well as for marrying.

Are there advantages to living together and not marrying? For one thing, it may give both partners a greater sense of autonomy. Not bound by the social rules and expectations of marriage, partners may find it easier to experiment with living arrangements that match their identities, interests, and abilities. For some couples, cohabitation is a chance to try out the relationship before assuming legal entanglements. If things don't work out, it may be easier to leave. Researchers previously believed that cohabiting before marriage led to higher divorce rates, but a 2014 study by the Council on Contemporary Families found that what has a greater impact on relationship longevity is the age at which couples first cohabit or marry. Those who wait until at least age 23 to marry or cohabit have the best relationship outcomes.

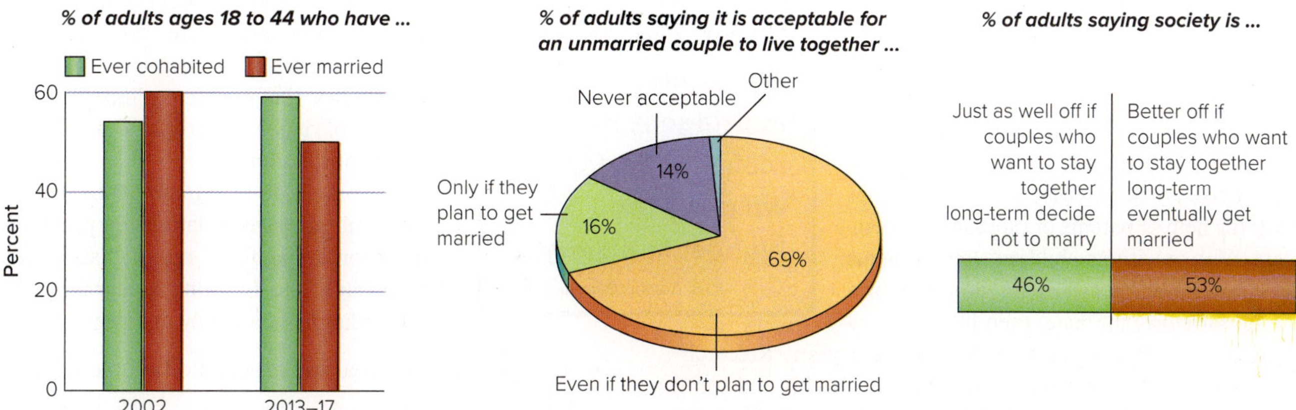


**FIGURE 5.2** **Wide acceptance of cohabitation, even as many Americans see societal benefits in marriage.**

**SOURCE:** Pew Research Center, 2019 (https://www.pewsocialtrends.org/2019/11/06/marriage-and-cohabitation-in-the-u-s/psdt_11-06-19_cohabitation-00-010/).

According to the Pew study, almost half of U.S. adults say that living together before marriage increases the chance of its success. Among married couples in the study who had lived with their spouses before marriage, 66% said they initially viewed cohabitation as a step toward marriage. Younger people are much more likely than older people to view cohabitation as increasing the chances of a successful marriage.

Of course, living together unmarried has drawbacks. The legal protections of marriage are often absent, such as health insurance benefits and property and inheritance rights. These can be serious if the couple has children or if partners become ill or are aging. Married couples, especially with only one earner, receive substantial tax benefits from filing jointly. Couples may feel social or family pressure to marry or otherwise change their living arrangements. The general trend, however, is toward legitimizing nonmarital partnerships; for example, some employers, communities, and states now extend benefits and legal rights to registered unmarried domestic partners.

> **Ask Yourself**
>
> **QUESTIONS FOR CRITICAL THINKING AND REFLECTION**
>
> How do you define "commitment" in a relationship? Is it simply a matter of staying faithful to a partner, or is there more? In your own relationships, what signs of commitment do you look for from your partner? What signs of commitment does your partner see in you?

## MARRIAGE

Marriage has been both challenged and transformed over the past decades. At the same time, it remains very popular, even among those who choose to cohabit. For many same-sex couples, marriage has a connotation and symbolism that is not attainable through cohabitation or *domestic partnership*. Marriage, though it varies enormously across cultures, seems to be universal in human societies. It addresses many basic human and societal needs. Social, political, economic, reproductive, sexual, and other considerations often guided marriage choices in the past, such as raising children or forming an economic unit. Today people in the United States marry more for personal, emotional, and companionship reasons.

### The Benefits of Marriage

The primary functions and benefits of marriage are those of any intimate relationship: affection, personal affirmation, companionship, sexual fulfillment, and emotional growth. Marriage also provides a setting in which to raise children, although an increasing number of couples choose not to have children. For those with children, more are choosing to raise them without being married, either by themselves, with a partner, or with the help of parents or other family members. With or without children, commitments to long-term relationships are motivated by a desire for close, intimate, even lifelong companions as well as some insurance for later years. Research also indicates that marriage contributes to health and well-being, particularly for men but for women as well. Married couples tend to have more daily social interactions, which are associated with reduced risk for dementia and harmful lifestyle behaviors. Research from Harvard Medical School and other sources finds that married people live longer and survive cancer and other diseases more often.

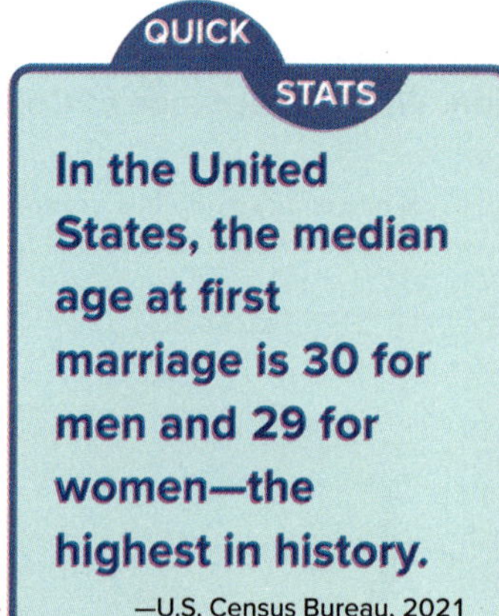


### Issues and Trends in Marriage

Traditional marriage roles have undergone profound changes. Most married couples today have two working spouses. A 2021 Pew Research study reported that women in same-sex marriages, compared to those in different-sex marriages, were more likely to be employed. Compared with men married to women, men married to men were more likely to have a higher educational level and income. Both men and women in same-sex marriages were more likely to be married to someone of a different race or ethnicity. The vast majority of married heterosexual families (over 80%) no longer follow a traditional "male as the provider" model.

Today's husbands participate more in domestic and child-rearing activities, particularly when wives are employed. Somethere is no choice, as when a mother's work schedule makes it impossible to drive her children to school or to pre-meals. But many men have been exposed to new, shared models of family responsibilities and are willing to help out, especially when asked explicitly.

At the same time, old patterns die slowly when it comes to boring, tedious, unrewarding household tasks. A recent Pew study found that few married (or cohabiting) couples report equal sharing of child-related or household responsibilities. Wives are more likely to say they do more than their spouse in many areas. The Pew study also finds that married couples who report more equally shared responsibilities are more satisfied with their arrangements. This suggests, as do other studies, that a more egalitarian sexual division of labor contributes to greater marital satisfaction.

For some, love is not enough to make a successful marriage. Relationship problems can become magnified rather than solved by marriage. The following appear to be the best predictors of a happy marriage:

- The partners have realistic expectations about their relationship.
- Each feels good about the personality of the other.
- Partners develop friendships with other couples.

- They communicate well.
- They have effective ways of resolving conflicts.
- They agree on religious/ethical values.
- They have an egalitarian role relationship.
- They have a good balance of individual versus joint interests and leisure activities.

Once married, couples must provide each other with emotional support, negotiate and establish marital roles, establish domestic and career priorities, handle their finances, make sexual adjustments, manage boundaries and relationships with their extended family, and participate in the larger community.

## Separation and Divorce

Divorce has become quite common in the United States, a dramatic change from 60 years ago, when both religious and civil society strongly discouraged or even prohibited divorce. Current estimates are that about 40 to 50% of first marriages will end in divorce. For those who remarry, divorce rates are higher for subsequent marriage.

High divorce rates in the United States may partially reflect our high expectations for emotional fulfillment and satisfaction in marriage. Young people often receive harmful and unrealistic messages about marriage through movies and other media. But we also may no longer embrace the concept of marriage as permanent, regardless of the quality of the relationship. This may partially explain why divorce rates are rising among older couples, many married for decades.

The process of divorce usually begins with an emotional separation. Often one partner is unhappy and looks for a more satisfying relationship. Dissatisfaction increases until the unhappy partner decides they can no longer stay. Physical separation follows, although it may take longer for the relationship to be over legally and then emotionally.

Divorce can be one of the greatest stress-producing events in life. Many people experience turmoil, depression, and lowered self-esteem during and after divorce. People may experience separation distress and loneliness for about a year and then begin a recovery period of one to three years. During this time they gradually construct a postdivorce identity, along with a new pattern of life. Most people are surprised at how long it takes to recover from divorce.

Children are especially vulnerable to the trauma of divorce, and counseling can help them adjust to the change. However, recent research finds that children who spend substantial time with both parents are usually better adjusted than those in sole custody and are as well adjusted as their peers from intact families. Coping with divorce is difficult for children at any age, including adult children.

Despite the distress of separation and divorce, the negative effects are usually balanced sooner or later by the possibility of finding a more suitable partner, constructing a new life, and developing new aspects of one's self. One result of the high divorce and remarriage rate is a growing number of merged families, either informally or legally, as stepfamilies.

# FAMILY LIFE

American families are very different today from families decades ago. In the 1960s, 88% of children under the age of 18 lived with both parents; in 2020, it was 70%. Over the same time period, the proportion of children living with a single mother nearly tripled, from 8% to 21%, and the percentage living with only their father increased from 1% to 4.5%. An additional 4% of children currently live without a parent; over half of these children live with a grandparent.

## Becoming a Parent

Few new parents are prepared for the job of parenting. Both mothers and fathers learn and become more confident in their parenting skills. This lays the groundwork for shared parenting and eliminates the typical gender gap in parenting "skills" that arises because only one parent is doing the initial parenting. Ideally, if both parents have jobs with paid parental leave, or are able to work part-time, they could participate equally, or nearly equally, in caring for the new infant. The U.S. is far behind other wealthy, industrialized countries when it comes to parental leave, especially paid parental leave, and especially for fathers. Bureau of Labor Statistics data show that in 2021, only 23% of civilian workers had access to paid family leave.

Most research indicates that mothers have to make greater changes in their lives than fathers do. Women are usually the ones who make job changes, either quitting work or reducing work hours to stay home with the baby. Many mothers juggle the multiple roles of mother, homemaker, and employer/employee and feel guilty that they never have enough time to do justice to any of these roles.

Not surprisingly, marital satisfaction often declines after the birth of the first child. Parents, employed or not, are often stressed. Working and parenting means double obligations. Mothers who stay at home may feel cut off from the world and their careers. Employed fathers can experience additional stress from becoming the sole earner.

But marital dissatisfaction after the baby is born is not inevitable. Couples who successfully weather the stresses of a new baby are reported to have:

- developed a strong relationship before the baby was born.
- planned to have the child.
- good communication about their feelings and expectations.
- an understanding about the need to share household and child care responsibilities and concrete strategies for doing so.

## Parenting

No one action or decision (within limits) will determine a child's personality or development. Instead, the *parenting style,* or overall approach to parenting, is most important.

Parenting styles vary according to how parents approach each of the following:

- *Demandingness* encompasses the use of discipline and supervision, the expectation that children act responsibly and maturely, and the direct reaction to disobedience.
- *Responsiveness* refers to the parents' warmth and intent to facilitate independence and self-confidence in their child by being supportive, connected, and understanding of their child's needs.

Several parenting styles have been identified. Each style emerges according to the parents' balance of demandingness and responsiveness. Here are some examples:

- *Authoritarian* parents are high in demandingness and low in responsiveness. They give orders and expect obedience, giving little warmth or consideration to their children's needs.
- *Authoritative* parents are high in both demandingness and responsiveness. They set clear boundaries and expectations, but they are also loving, supportive, and attuned to their children's needs.
- *Permissive* parents are high in responsiveness and low in demandingness. They do not expect their children to act maturely but instead allow them to follow their own impulses. They are very warm, patient, and accepting, and they are focused on not stifling their child's innate creativity.
- *Uninvolved* parents are low in both demandingness and responsiveness. They require little from their children and respond with little attention, frequency, or effort. In extreme cases, this style of parenting might reach the level of child neglect.

**QUICK STATS**

**4% of American children live in a home where neither parent is present.**

—U. S. Census Bureau, 2020

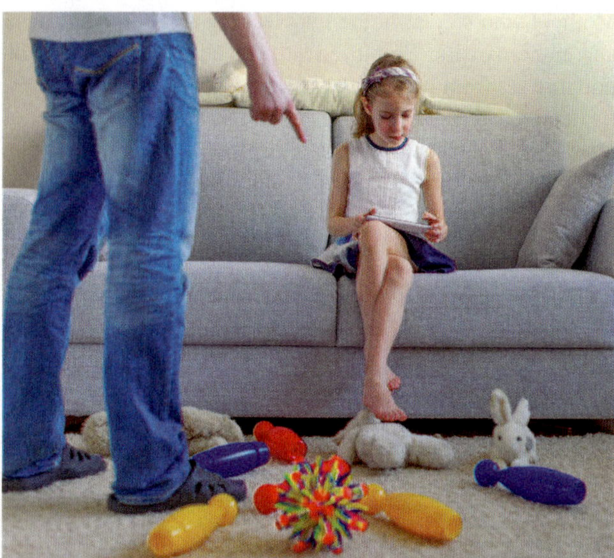

Setting clear boundaries, holding children to high expectations, and responding with warmth to children's needs are all positive parenting strategies. Dmitri Ma/Shutterstock

At each stage of the family life cycle, the relationship between parents and children changes. And with those changes come new challenges. The parents' initial responsibility to a baby is to ensure its physical well-being around the clock. As babies grow into toddlers and begin to walk and talk, they begin to take care of some of their own physical needs. For parents, the challenge at this stage is to strike a balance between giving children the freedom to explore and setting limits that will keep them safe and secure. As children grow into adolescents, parents need to give them increasing independence and be willing to let them risk success or failure on their own.

Marital satisfaction for most couples tends to decline during their children's school years. Reasons include the financial and emotional pressures of a growing family and the increased job and community responsibilities of parents in their thirties, forties, fifties, and even sixties. Many parents also start assuming greater responsibility for their own aging parents, producing the so-called Sandwich Generation.

## Single Parents

Single parenthood, like singlehood, is becoming increasingly common. According to the 2020 data from the U.S. Census Bureau, there are nearly 18.6 million children living with only one parent (Figure 5.3). Economic difficulties can be substantial, especially for those with little education or job skills or from poorer families. On the other hand, some single parents are well-established in their careers and in a solid financial position, so they can find nannies or other child care arrangements while they continue in their professions.

Single parents, especially those without partners, may experience conflicting demands of being both father and mother and the difficulty of satisfying their own needs for

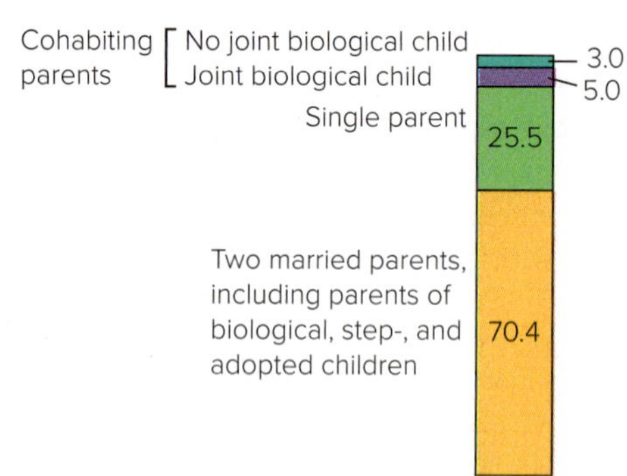


**FIGURE 5.3 Living arrangements for American families with children under age 18.**

SOURCE: U.S. Census Bureau. 2020. America's Families and Living Arrangements: 2020

adult companionship and affection. Having strong family or other social networks, however, can greatly ease the demands of single parenting.

Research about the effect on children of growing up in a single-parent family is inconclusive. Evidence suggests that educational level and financial resources of parents, whether one or two, and the quality of the relationships among children, parents, and other caretakers are the most important factors in children's well-being. Two-parent families are not necessarily better if one of the parents spends little time relating to the children or is physically or emotionally abusive. Extended families have traditionally played a significant role in child rearing cross-culturally and within some U.S. communities. They can offer enormous support for single parents.

## Stepfamilies/Blended Families

Single parenthood is often a transitional stage: About three of four divorced women and about four of five divorced men will remarry. If either partner brings children into the new family unit, a stepfamily (or *blended family*) is formed. The American Psychological Association recommends three key issues to consider.

1. **Financial and living arrangements.** Couples who share most of their finances have reported greater family satisfaction than those working from individual accounts. Moving to a home that is new for everyone can create a feeling of a shared, level playing field.
2. **Resolving feelings and issues from the previous marriage.** Old hurts and patterns can resurface, for both adults and children, if not worked out. Hearing that a parent plans to remarry can sadden a child who hoped their parents might reconcile.
3. **Parenthood.** Couples should discuss the role that the stepparent will take with the new spouse's children. Stepparents should first take on a role more akin to friend or "camp counselor," rather than disciplinarian. Younger children, those under age 10, are usually more accepting of a new adult in the family than are adolescents.

Stepfamilies can be very different from primary families, although a lot depends on the age of children and the nature of their relationships with prior and new family members. It's important for the other parent, outside the stepfamily, to continue regular visits and maintain a good relationship with the children so that they don't feel abandoned. Seeing a psychologist can help everyone in the family. It may take two to four years for a new stepfamily to adjust to living together.

Stepfamilies may find it difficult to duplicate the emotions and relationships of a primary family. Research has shown that healthy stepfamilies are less cohesive but more adaptable than healthy primary families; they have a greater capacity to allow for individual differences and accept that biologically related family members will have emotionally closer relationships. Stepfamilies gradually gain a sense of being a family as they build a history of shared daily experiences and major life events.

## Successful Families

Family life can be extremely challenging. A strong family is not a family without problems; it's a family that copes successfully with stress and crisis.

An excellent way to build strong family ties is to develop family rituals and routines, repeated activities that have meaning for family members. Some common routines identified in research studies are dinnertime, a regular bedtime, and household chores; common rituals include birthdays, holidays, and weekend activities. Family routines may even serve as protective factors, balancing out potential risk factors associated with single-parent families and families with divorce and remarriage. Incorporating a regular family mealtime into a family's routine allows parents and children to develop closer relationships and leads to better parenting, healthier children, and better school performance.

Experts have proposed seven major characteristics of strong American families:

1. ***Commitment.*** The family is very important to its members, and members take their responsibilities seriously. Everyone knows they are loved, valued, and special to each other.
2. ***Appreciation.*** Family members care about one another and express their appreciation. They don't wait for special occasions to celebrate each other.
3. ***Communication.*** Family members spend time listening to one another and enjoying each other's company. They talk through disagreements and attempt to solve problems.
4. ***Time together.*** Family members do things together—often simple activities that don't cost money. They put down their devices and their work, and they focus on each other.
5. ***Spiritual wellness.*** The family promotes sharing, love, and compassion for other human beings.
6. ***Stress and crisis management.*** When faced with illness, death, marital conflict, or other crises, family members pull together, seek help, and use other coping strategies to meet challenges.
7. ***Affectionate physical contact.*** People of all ages need hugs, cuddles, and caresses for their emotional health and to demonstrate caring and love for one another.

It may surprise some people that members of strong families are often seen at counseling centers. They know that the smartest thing to do in some situations is to get help.

### Ask Yourself

**QUESTIONS FOR CRITICAL THINKING AND REFLECTION**

Do you think of your own family as successful? In what ways could your family relationships improve? Are you comfortable talking to your family about these issues?

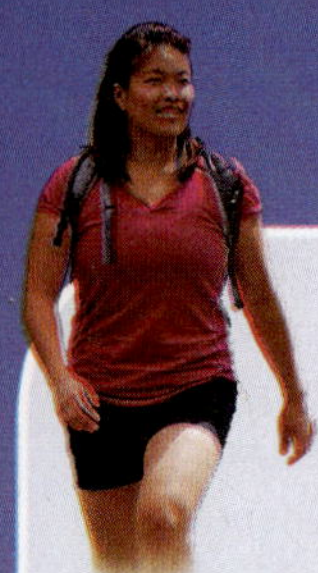

## TAKE CHARGE
### Strategies of Strong Families

Life is full of challenges, but strong families work together to meet those challenges. Strong families use the following strategies to deal with life's difficulties:

- ***Look for something positive in difficult situations.*** No matter how difficult, most problems teach us lessons that we can draw on in future situations.
- ***Pull together.*** Think of the problem not as one family member's difficulty but as a challenge for the family as a whole.
- ***Get help outside the family.*** Call on extended family members, supportive friends, neighbors, colleagues, members of your religious community, and health care and community professionals.
- ***Listen and empathize.*** Offer each other nonjudgmental support.
- ***Use rituals for bonding and healing.*** A ritual could include a memorial event, a tradition that the family repeats each year on a significant date or for a holiday, or a shared daily meal or time for conversation.
- ***Be flexible.*** Crises often force family members to learn new approaches to life or take on different responsibilities. Each person needs time to heal from challenges at their own pace.
- ***Give each other space.*** Respect family members' need for privacy and alone time.
- ***Focus on the big picture and set priorities.*** Getting caught up in details rather than the essentials can make people edgy, even hysterical.
- ***Take care of each other.*** We often forget that we are biological beings. Like kindergartners, we need a good lunch and time to play. We need to have our hair stroked, a hug, or a nap.
- ***Validate each other.*** Offer appreciation and praise.
- ***Create a life full of meaning and purpose.*** We all face severe crises in life; they're unavoidable. Sometimes it helps to focus on others, to offer service to the community. Giving of ourselves brings richness and dignity to our lives despite the troubles we endure.
- ***Actively meet challenges head-on.*** Life's disasters do not go away when we look in another direction.
- ***Go with the flow to some degree.*** Sometimes we are relatively powerless in the face of a crisis. Simply saying to ourselves that things will get better with time can be useful.
- ***Be prepared in advance for life's challenges.*** Healthy family relationships are like an ample bank balance: If our relational accounts are in order, we will be able to weather life's most difficult storms—together.

SOURCES: Binghamton University Counseling Center. n.d. Dealing with crisis and trauma events. American Academy of Experts in Traumatic Stress (http://www.aaets.org/article164.htm); Olson, D. H., and J. DeFrain. 2007. *Marriages and Families: Intimacy, Diversity, and Strengths*, 6th ed. New York: McGraw Hill Education. Copyright © 2007.

## TIPS FOR TODAY AND THE FUTURE

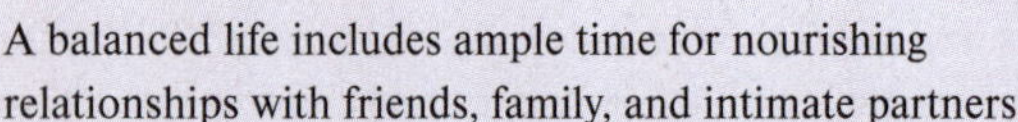

A balanced life includes ample time for nourishing relationships with friends, family, and intimate partners.

**RIGHT NOW YOU CAN:**

- Seek out an acquaintance or a new friend and arrange a coffee date to get to know the person better.
- Call someone you love and tell them how important the relationship is to you. Don't wait for a crisis.

**IN THE FUTURE YOU CAN:**

- Think about the conflicts you have had in the past with your close friends or loved ones and consider how you handled them. Decide whether your conflict management methods were helpful. Using the suggestions in this chapter and Chapter 3, determine how you could better handle similar conflicts in the future.
- Think about your prospects as a parent. What kind of example have your parents set? If you don't already have children, how do you feel about having them in the future? What can you do to prepare yourself to be a good parent?

## SUMMARY

- Healthy intimate relationships are an important component of the well-being of both individuals and society. Many intimate relationships are held together by love.
- Successful relationships begin with a positive sense of self and reasonably high self-esteem. Personal identity, gender roles, and attachment styles, all rooted in childhood experiences, contribute to this sense of self.
- Characteristics of friendship include companionship, respect, acceptance, help, trust, loyalty, mutuality, and reciprocity.
- Love, sex, and commitment are closely linked ideals in intimate relationships. Love includes trust, caring, respect, and loyalty. Sex brings excitement, fascination, and passion to the relationship. Commitment contributes stability, which helps maintain a relationship.
- Common challenges in relationships relate to issues of self-disclosure, commitment, expectations, competitiveness, balance of time together and apart, and jealousy. Gender roles, especially traditional gender roles, influence each of these.

- Partners in successful relationships have strong communication skills and support each other during difficult times. Social media can both ease and undermine communication in relationships.

- The keys to good communication in relationships are self-disclosure, listening, and feedback.

- Conflict is inevitable in intimate relationships; partners need to find ways to negotiate their differences. Conflict is often accompanied by anger, and the best way to handle anger in a relationship is to recognize it as a symptom of something that needs to be addressed.

- People usually choose partners like themselves (except on gender). If partners are very different, acceptance and good communication skills are especially necessary to maintain the relationship.

- Most Americans find partners through dating or getting together in groups. Internet sites that match people can expand dating options and create positive experiences as long as safety precautions are taken. Cohabitation is a growing social pattern that allows partners to get to know each other intimately without being married.

- Same-sex partnerships are similar to heterosexual partnerships, with some differences. Same-sex couples put greater emphasis on partnership than on role assignment, and they may experience social hostility or ambivalence rather than approval of their partnerships.

- Singlehood is a growing lifestyle in our society. Advantages include autonomy, greater variety in intimate partners, and more freedom to make and pursue life choices; disadvantages include greater possibility of economic hardship, sole responsibility for a household, and lack of companionship.

- Marriage fulfills many functions for individuals and society. It can provide people with affection, affirmation, and sexual fulfillment; a context for child rearing; and the promise of lifelong companionship.

- Love isn't enough to ensure a successful marriage. Partners must be realistic, feel good about each other, have communication and conflict resolution skills, share values, and balance their individual and joint interests.

- When problems can't be worked out, people often separate and divorce. Divorce can be traumatic for all involved, especially children, but the negative effects are usually balanced in time by positive ones.

- At each stage of the family life cycle, relationships change. Marital satisfaction may be lower during the child-rearing years and higher later.

- Many families today are single-parent families. The quality of the caretaker relationships and the parents' education level and financial resources are the most important factors in children's well-being.

- Stepfamilies, also referred to as blended families, are formed when single, divorced, or widowed people remarry and create new family units. Stepfamilies gradually gain more of a sense of being a family as they build a history of shared experiences.

- Important qualities of successful families include commitment to the family, appreciation of family members, communication, physical affection, time spent together, spiritual wellness, sharing of responsibilities, and effective methods of dealing with stress.

## FOR MORE INFORMATION

For resources in your area, check your campus directory for a counseling center or peer counseling program, or search online.

*American Association for Marriage and Family Therapy.* Provides information about a variety of relationship issues and referrals to therapists.

http://www.aamft.org

*American Psychological Association.* Offers general and specific advice about how to navigate marriage, divorce, and family life.

https://www.apa.org

*Association for Couples in Marriage Enrichment (ACME).* Promotes activities to strengthen marriage; a resource for books, tapes, and other materials.

http://www.bettermarriages.org

*The Blended Family Podcast.* Conversations with real parents in blended families about their strategies for making things work.

http://www.blendedfamilypodcast.com

*Conflict Resolution Information Source.* Provides links to a broad range of internet resources for conflict resolution. Information covers interpersonal, marital, family, and other types of conflicts.

http://www.crinfo.org

*Family Education Network.* Provides information about education, safety, health, and other family-related issues.

http://www.familyeducation.com

*The Gottman Institute.* Includes tips and suggestions for relationships and parenting, including an online relationships quiz.

http://www.gottman.com

*Parents Without Partners (PWP).* Provides educational programs, literature, and support groups for single parents and their children. Search the online directory for a referral to a local chapter.

https://www.parentswithoutpartners.org/

*Pew Research Center.* Surveys Americans about issues and attitudes and analyzes publications in mass media and social science research.

http://www.pewresearch.org

*Robert J. Sternberg.* Sternberg includes in his homepage links to his theories of love and an interactive website that helps you learn about your own relationships.

http://www.robertjsternberg.com/love

*U.S. Census Bureau.* Provides current statistics on births, marriages, and living arrangements.

http://www.census.gov

See also the listings for Chapters 3 and 8.

## SELECTED BIBLIOGRAPHY

American College Health Association. 2021. *American College Health Association-National College Health Assessment III Spring 2021 Reference Group Data Report.* Hanover, MD: American College Health Association.

Association of American Universities. 2020. *Report on the AAU Climate Survey on Sexual Assault and Sexual Misconduct* (https://www.aau.edu/key-issues/campus-climate-and-safety/aau-campus-climate-survey-2019).

Auxier, B. 2020. 64% of Americans say social media have a mostly negative effect on the way things are going in the U.S. today. *Pew Research Center* (https://www.pewresearch.org/fact-tank/2020/10/15/64-of-americans-say-social-media-have-a-mostly-negative-effect-on-the-way-things-are-going-in-the-u-s-today/).

Barroso, A. 2020. Key takeaways on Americans' views of and experiences with dating and relationships. *Pew Research Center* (https://www.pewresearch.org/fact-tank/2020/08/20/key-takeaways-on-americans-views-of-and-experiences-with-dating-and-relationships/).

Barroso, A. 2021. For American couples, gender gaps in sharing household responsibilities persist amid pandemic. *Pew Research Center* (https://www.pewresearch.org/fact-tank/2021/01/25/for-american-couples-gender-gaps-in-sharing-household-responsibilities-persist-amid-pandemic/).

Barroso, A., and R. Fry. 2021. On some demographic measures, people in same-sex marriages differ from those in opposite-sex marriages. *Pew Research Center* (https://www.pewresearch.org/fact-tank/2021/07/07/on-some-demographic-measures-people-in-same-sex-marriages-differ-from-those-in-opposite-sex-marriages/).

Boyce, W. T. 2019. *The Orchid and the Dandelion*. New York: Alfred A. Knopf.

Centers for Disease Control and Prevention. 2020. Youth Risk Behavior Surveillance–United States, 2019. *MMWR Surveillance Report* 69(SS-01) (https://www.cdc.gov/healthyyouth/data/yrbs/pdf/trendsreport.pdf).

Centers for Disease Control and Prevention. 2021. *Preventing Child Abuse & Neglect* (https://www.cdc.gov/violenceprevention/childabuseandneglect/fastfact.html).

Centers for Disease Control and Prevention. 2021. *Preventing Teen Dating Violence* (https://www.cdc.gov/violenceprevention/intimatepartnerviolence/teendatingviolence/fastfact.html).

Centers for Disease Control and Prevention. 2021. *Teen Dating Violence* (https://www.cdc.gov/violenceprevention/intimatepartnerviolence/teendatingviolence/fastfact.html).

Chin, B., et al. 2017. Marital status as a predictor of diurnal salivary cortisol levels and slopes in a community sample of healthy adults. *Psychoneuroendocrinology*, Apr 78: 68–75 (https://www.ncbi.nlm.nih.gov/pmc/articles/PMC5365082/).

Davis, E. M., K. Kim, and K. L. Fingerman. 2018. Is an empty nest best? Coresidence with adult children and parental marital quality before and after the Great Recession. *The Journals of Gerontology: Series B* 73(3): 372–381.

DePaulo, B. 2017. Is it true that single women and married men do best? Sex differences in marriage and single life: Still debating after 50 years. *Psychology Today* (https://www.psychologytoday.com/us/blog/living-single/201701/is-it-true-single-women-and-married-men-do-best).

DePaulo, B. 2020. A darker side of singlism: Discrimination in the legal code. *Psychology Today* (https://www.psychologytoday.com/us/blog/living-single/202005/darker-side-singlism-discrimination-in-the-legal-code).

Denworth, L. 2019. Social media has not destroyed a generation. *Scientific American*, November, 46–49 (https://www.scientificamerican.com/article/social-media-has-not-destroyed-a-generation/).

Eckert, P., and S. McConnell-Ginet. 2013. *Language and Gender*, 2nd ed. New York: Cambridge University Press.

Federal Interagency Forum on Child and Family Statistics. 2015. *America's Children: Key National Indicators of Well-Being, 2015*. Washington, DC: U.S. Government Printing Office.

Federal Interagency Forum on Child and Family Statistics (Forum). 2021. *America's Children: Key National Indicators of Well-Being, 2021* (https://www.childstats.gov/americaschildren/family1.asp).

Fry, R., and K. Parker. 2021. Rising Share of U.S. Adults Are Living Without a Spouse or Partner. Pew Research Center (https://www.pewresearch.org/social-trends/2021/10/05/rising-share-of-u-s-adults-are-living-without-a-spouse-or-partner/).

Goleman, D. 1995. *Emotional Intelligence: Why It Can Matter More Than IQ*. New York: Bantam Books.

Goodwin, M. H. 2006. *The Hidden Life of Girls: Games of Stance, Status, and Exclusion*. Oxford, UK: Blackwell.

Guttmacher Institute. 2019. Fact Sheet: Adolescent Sexual and Reproductive Health in the United States (https://www.guttmacher.org/fact-sheet/american-teens-sexual-and-reproductive-health).

Hancock, J. T., et al. 2019. Social Media Use and Well-Being: A Meta-Analysis, *69th Annual International Communication Association Conference*, Washington, D.C.

Haseltine, W. A. 2021. One fifth of adults report a relationship breakdown during the pandemic. *Forbes* (https://www.forbes.com/sites/williamhaseltine/2021/08/31/one-fifth-of-adults-report-a-relationship-breakdown-during-the-pandemic/?sh=4290884e5a42).

Hazan, C, and P. Shaver. 1987. Romantic love conceptualized as an attachment process. *Journal of Personality and Social Psychology* 52(3): 511–524.

Heggeness, M. 2021. Tracking job losses for mothers of school-age children during a health crisis. *United States Census Bureau* (https://www.census.gov/library/stories/2021/03/moms-work-and-the-pandemic.html).

Hemez, P., and C. Washington. 2021. Percentage and number of children living with two parents has dropped since 1968. U.S. Census Bureau (https://www.census.gov/library/stories/2021/04/number-of-children-living-only-with-their-mothers-has-doubled-in-past-50-years.html).

Herbenick, D., et al. 2021. Sex and relationships pre- and early-COVID-19 pandemic: findings from a probability sample of U.S. undergraduate students. *Archives of Sexual Behavior* (https://doi.org/10.1007/s10508-021-02265-5).

Hinduja, S. 2021. *Cyberbullying in 2021 by Age, Gender, Sexual Orientation, and Race* (https://cyberbullying.org/cyberbullying-statistics-age-gender-sexual-orientation-race).

Kamer, F. 2021. Are you anxious, avoidant, or secure? *The New York Times*, 6 November (https://www.nytimes.com/2021/11/06/style/anxious-avoidant-secure-attached-book.html).

Kirschenbaum, H., and V. Henderson. 1989. *The Carl Rogers Reader*. Boston: Houghton Mifflin.

Lehman, C. 2020. Fewer America high schoolers having sex than ever before. *Institute for Family Studies* (https://ifstudies.org/blog/fewer-american-high-schoolers-having-sex-than-ever-before).

Mead, M. 1928. *Coming of Age in Samoa*. New York: William Morrow & Co.

Mernitz, S. E., and C. Kamp Dush. 2016. Emotional health across the transition to first and second unions among emerging adults. *Journal of Family Psychology* 30(2): 233–244.

Miller, C. 2018. How same-sex couples divide chores, and what it reveals about modern parenting. *The New York Times*, 16 May (https://www.nytimes.com/2018/05/16/upshot/same-sex-couples-divide-chores-much-more-evenly-until-they-become-parents.html).

Mukhopadhyay, C. C., and T. Blumenthal. 2020. "Gender and Sexuality." *In Perspectives: An Open Invitation to Cultural Anthropology*, 2nd ed., ed. N. Brown, T. McIlwraith, and L. Tubelle de González. *The Society for Anthropology in Community Colleges* (http://perspectives.americananthro.org/).

National Center for Health Statistics. 2019. National Survey of Family Growth (https://www.cdc.gov/nchs/data/factsheets/factsheet_nsfg.pdf).

Onraet, E., et al. 2017. The relationship of trait emotional intelligence with right-wing attitudes and subtle racial prejudice. *Personality and Individual Differences* 110: 27–30.

Pew Research Center. 2018. *Teens' Social Media Habits and Experiences* (https://www.pewresearch.org/internet/2018/11/28/teens-and-their-experiences-on-social-media/).

Pew Research Center. 2019. *Marriage and Cohabitation in the U.S.* (https://www.pewsocialtrends.org/2019/11/06/marriage-and-cohabitation-in-the-u-s/psdt_11-06-19_cohabitation-00-010/).

Rogers, C. R. 1961. *On Becoming a Person*. Boston: Houghton Mifflin.

Rosenfeld, M. J., R. J. Thomas, and S. Hausen. 2019. Disintermediating your friends: How online dating in the United States displaces other ways of meeting. *Proceedings of the National Academy of Sciences of the United States of America* 116 (36): 17753–17758.

Salovey, P., et al., eds. 2004. *Emotional Intelligence: Key Readings on the Mayer and Salovey Model*. Port Chester, NY: Dude Publishing.

Schlagel, D. 2019. *Our Modern Blended Family: A Practical Guide*. Emeryville, CA: Rockridge Press.

Schmerling, R. H. 2016. The health advantages of marriage. Harvard Health Publishing blog (https://www.health.harvard.edu/blog/the-health-advantages-of-marriage-2016113010667).

Schoen, R., et al. 2007. Family transitions in young adulthood. *Demography* 44(4): 807–820.

Simpson, D. M., N. D. Leonhardt, and A. J. Hawkins. 2018. Learning about love: A meta-analytic study of individually-oriented relationship education programs for adolescents and emerging adults. *Journal of Youth and Adolescence* 47(3): 477–489.

Sommerlad, A., et al. 2018. Marriage and risk of dementia: Systematic review and meta-analysis of observational studies. *Journal of Neurology, Neurosurgery, and Psychiatry* 89: 231–238.

Tannen, D. 1994. *Gender and Discourse*. New York: Oxford University Press.

Taylor, D. 2020. Same-sex couples are more likely to adopt or foster children. United States Census Bureau (https://www.census.gov/library/stories/2020/09/fifteen-percent-of-same-sex-couples-have-children-in-their-household.html).

Twenge, J. M., R. A. Sherman, and B. E. Wells. 2015. Changes in American adults' sexual behavior and attitudes. *Archives of Sexual Behavior* 44: 2273.

U.S. Bureau of the Census. 2021. Number, timing, and duration of marriages and divorces (https://www.census.gov/newsroom/press-releases/2021/marriages-and-divorces.html).

U. S. Bureau of Labor Statistics. 2021. Employment Characteristics of Families Summary (https://www.bls.gov/news.release/famee.nr0.htm).

U.S. Department of Health & Human Services, Administration for Community Living, Administration on Aging. 2021. *2020 Profile of Older Americans* (https://acl.gov/sites/default/files/Aging%20and%20Disability%20in%20America/2020ProfileOlderAmericans.Final_.pdf).

U.S. Department of the Treasury. 2021. *The Economics of Child Care Supply in the United States* (https://home.treasury.gov/system/files/136/The-Economics-of-Childcare-Supply-09-14-final.pdf).

Wiederhold, B. 2021. How COVID has changed online dating–and what lies ahead. *Cyberpsychology, Behavior, and Social Networking* 24(7) (https://doi.org/10.1089/cyber.2021.29219.editorial).

Zhong, B. 2021. *Social Media Communication: Trends and Theories*. Malden, MA: Wiley-Blackwell.

**Design Elements:** Assess Yourself icon: Aleksey Boldin/Alamy Stock Photo; Diversity Matters icon: Rawpixel Ltd/Getty Images; Wellness on Campus icon: Radius Images/Alamy Stock Photo; Take Charge icon: VisualCommunications/Getty Images; Critical Consumer icon: pagadesign/Getty Images.

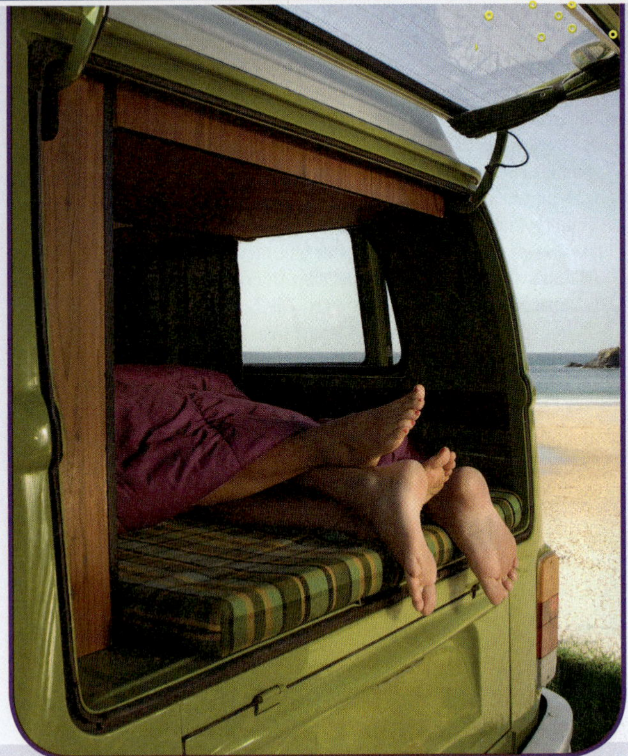

Chris Whitehead/Getty Images

## CHAPTER OBJECTIVES

- Describe the parts and functions of human genital-sexual anatomy
- Explain the role of hormones in sexual and genital development
- Describe how the body works during sexual activity
- Explain the range of gender roles and sexual orientations
- Explain the development and varieties of sexual behavior
- Explain the principles of fertility and infertility
- Describe the physical and emotional changes related to pregnancy
- Identify the stages of fetal development

CHAPTER 6

# Sexuality, Pregnancy, and Childbirth

The phrase human **sexuality** refers to a complex and interconnected group of *physical-biological* characteristics and capacities. Understanding our sexuality requires science-based knowledge of sexual anatomy (body parts), physiology (how the body moves and works), and sexual functioning. But human sexuality is not just biological; it is deeply shaped by society, cultural norms, and beliefs about gender and sex. Achieving sexual wellness involves critical awareness of messages we've learned and continue to receive about our sexuality.

## SEXUALITY, HUMAN STYLE

Human sexuality is generally viewed as natural, rooted in biological capacities and motivations that we share with other animals. But what is purely natural about how we experience human bodies, our desires, capacities; what and who is sexy, arousing, or repulsive; and what do we even mean by *sex*?

Human sexuality is one of the most culturally significant, socially regulated, and profoundly symbolic areas of human life. Society, the larger set of institutions and rules that govern how we all live together, moves us to have sex or get married or do neither in certain ways. Violating norms has consequences, psychologically, emotionally, and socially. Families and communities also influence our behaviors, and in more daily, mundane ways. The idea of romantic love may be widespread across cultures. But love-based sexual relationships are not universally valued or even typical of human sexual encounters.

### Opposites? Hardly

This chapter tries to separate biological fact from cultural-social fiction, including some deeply held beliefs about sexuality and about males and females. One example is the opposite-sex approach to gender and biological sex. This idea assumes that the human species neatly divides into two distinct groups, males and females, what some call a **binary** view of sex and gender.

TERMS

**sexuality** A dimension of personality shaped by biological, psychosocial, and cultural forces and concerning all aspects of sexual behavior and feelings.

**binary** A division into two groups often considered opposites.

It also implies that males and females are profoundly different from each other, at opposite ends of a spectrum. This cultural model has influenced how scientists study and describe human sexuality, focusing on reproductive aspects, emphasizing male-female differences in anatomy and physiological processes, even creating different names for the same hormones or body parts.

## When Sex Became Gender

Contemporary science challenges these old views and the language associated with them. A good example is the term sex. In the past, *sex* referred both to sexuality and to the different sexes. Today, we generally use *gender* for aspects of sexuality that may not be strongly linked to physicality (e.g., sex organs and characteristics).

The change reflects profound alterations in **gender ideology,** ideas about gender that institutions and individuals use to make sense of our world and assert power relations. Two distinct phenomena—sexual preference and gender role—were conflated because of beliefs that both were rooted in biology. Differences in sexual preference were linked to differences in gender role behavior. Adult sexual preference—the sex to whom one was attracted—was assumed to be heterosexual.

Conventionally masculine men were assumed to be attracted to "feminine" women and vice versa. People attracted to their own sex were believed to have a gender identity problem. But scientists now understand that human cultures, not nature, create the gender roles and ideologies that go along with being born biologically male or female, and the ideologies vary widely across cultures. Not all societies are gender-binary. Some recognize three or even four genders. Sexual behavior and orientation are complex, fluid, often situationally specific, distinct phenomena.

## Cultural Norms and Biological Variations

Culture and society profoundly shape our experiences as individuals, altering our bodies, our brains, our emotions. Neuroscience research in the past 30 years has shown that human brains are not fixed at birth but are highly plastic and change in response to learning and the environment.

In her book *Gender and Our Brains,* neuroscientist Gina Rippon discusses the plasticity and constant alteration of the brain, and how socializing girls and boys into different activities can affect their brains. Boys are more likely to have construction-type toys or play target sports, which gives them spatial experience that then shows up in their brains. A group of 26 girls, after playing Tetris weekly for three months, showed enlargement in cortical areas associated with visuospatial processing. Starting at birth (if not before), our brains are changing in response to what we experience, especially socially. Brains continue to change in neurologically identifiable ways throughout life as we live in gendered ways.

Research also demonstrates how much variability exists among human beings, biologically and behaviorally.

### Ask Yourself

**QUESTIONS FOR CRITICAL THINKING AND REFLECTION**

Reflect on how you learned about sexuality, including your own body, starting with when you were a child. What messages, direct and indirect, did you get from your family, school, religious institutions, and from popular culture, like music videos and games you played?

Unfortunately, the current language of gender and sexuality, such as that used for biologic sex, gender, or sexual orientation, can mask that variation. Readers should recognize that the categories and labels used in the chapter do not describe everyone and every situation. The categories are always evolving.

For purposes of this chapter, the term *sex* (male, female) refers to **biological sex**—that is, biological traits associated with typical male and female chromosomal patterns and sexual differentiation processes. *Gender* refers to nonbiologically rooted aspects of being male or female. It includes **gender roles,** the meanings and behaviors attached to being male and female, and individual identities.

How we see ourselves along a spectrum of possibilities can be called our gender identity. It may include **sexual orientation,** to which gender/s we are attracted sexually. Sometimes these align along a typical binary, reproductively oriented pattern: Our biologic sex, gender role, gender identity, and sexual orientation all in alignment can be called **cisgender.** Although cisgender is the most common pattern, there are others. The term *gender nonconforming* refers to these alternatives.

# SEXUAL ANATOMY: VARIATIONS ON A COMMON THEME

Despite surface differences in males and females, most sex organs develop from **homologous** (the same) tissues. Most fulfill similar functions, including in reproduction and sexual pleasure. This view—of typical female and male sexual

**TERMS**

**gender ideology** Complex sets of ideas about gender capacities, preferences, identities, social roles and power relationships.

**biological sex** Biological traits associated with typical male and female chromosomal patterns and sexual differentiation processes.

**gender roles** Behaviors that society, religion, and culture attach to being male and female

**sexual orientation** Who you are drawn to emotionally, romantically, and sexually.

**cisgender** A term for individuals whose sex and gender assignment align with their personal gender identity.

**homologous** Having a similar structure.

anatomy and physiology as variations on a common theme—needs emphasizing because so often popular culture and media messages focus on biological differences.

If we consider the human body as a whole, males and females are nearly identical, biologically speaking. Human cells (except **germ cells**—egg and sperm) typically have 46 chromosomes in 23 pairs, one of each pair inherited from the mother, one from the father. Of these 23 pairs, 22 pairs are *autosomes* (i.e., chromosomes that are not **sex chromosomes**) and are the same for males and females. It is only the 23rd pair of chromosomes that defines our biologic sex. Typically we have either two X chromosomes (female) or one X and one Y chromosome (male).

Some differences in our sexual anatomy have virtually no impact, especially on sexual pleasure. But others have enormous consequences concerning reproduction. Populations cannot survive without reproducing and, specifically, without women reproducing. Perhaps that is why historically, so many cultural models of sex and gender seem obsessed with reproduction and with controlling sexuality, especially female sexuality.

## Human Sexual Anatomy: The Basic Plan

Many of us have been taught to think of our sexual anatomy and hormones as binary and opposite. Males have a penis, scrotum, and testes; females have breasts, a vagina, a uterus, and ovaries. Yet at the beginning, when a **sperm** and an egg merge into a single cell, and as the fertilized egg divides repeatedly into a larger-celled organism, males and females possess the same basic reproductive and sexual system.

**Gonads (Ovaries and Testes)** Around the fifth week, a normal embryo, whether XX or XY, has a pair of **gonads,** which are the primary organs that produce germ cells and sex hormones. The embryo also has two sets of ducts (Wolffian and Mullerian) and a set of tissues that will eventually become the external genitals. The sex chromosomes then start to direct the gonads to differentiate along either male or female lines.

**Hormones** Testes and ovaries start producing hormones that further differentiate the genital system along sex lines. In females, the Mullerian ducts turn into fallopian tubes, the uterus, and the upper section of the vagina. The Wolffian ducts degenerate and eventually disappear. But all other genital tissue remains, becoming the clitoris and other parts of the vulva.

In males, the testes secrete a substance that causes the Mullerian system to atrophy. **Testosterone** produced by the testes interacts with receptors on the Wolffian ducts to develop into the epididymis, the vas deferens, and the ejaculatory duct. The remaining tissue becomes sex differentiated, but along male lines, into the penis and the scrotum.

The ovaries and testes gradually change in shape and position, moving closer to the pelvis. Eventually the testes descend into the scrotum. By the time of birth, males and females possess a sexual anatomy primarily derived from the same embryonic tissues. The only exception is the duct system, either Mullerian or Wolffian. Yet even these structures have similar reproductive functions. Male and female gonads have the same two basic functions: nurturing germ cells and producing sex hormones. Both ovaries and testes manufacture and secrete three kinds of sex steroid hormones: **androgens** (mainly *testosterone*), **progesterone,** and **estrogens** (mainly *estradiol*). What varies is the amounts produced, particularly testosterone and estrogens, although this gap fluctuates throughout the life cycle. Sex hormones are also produced by the adrenal glands.

This is a simplified version of what occurs. Biological development, and the processes through which our bodies become sex differentiated, are very complex. Even when the process goes smoothly, there is tremendous variability within each sex. But there are also opportunities for errors. Most babies can be classified at birth as either biologically male or female, based on their genitals, which usually match their chromosomes (XY, XX). Yet a surprisingly large number of individuals don't fit these simple categories: their chromosomes or genitals are atypical. When this occurs, the person is said to have an **intersex** condition. Their biological ambiguity makes it difficult to assign them a gender, especially in binary, two-category gender systems like in the United States.

## Female Sex Organs

The external sex organs (genitals) of people assigned female at birth are collectively called the **vulva.** The internal sexual organs consist of the vagina, vestibular bulbs, Skene's glands, uterus, ovaries, and fallopian tubes.

**TERMS**

**germ cells** Sperm and ova (eggs).

**sex chromosomes** The X and Y chromosomes, which contribute to genital development, hormone secretion and, thus, the sex that we are assigned at birth.

**sperm** A germ cell produced by a testis; if combined with an ovum, it can produce what will become an embryo.

**gonads** The primary organs that produce germ cells and sex hormones; the ovaries and testes.

**testosterone** The hormone responsible for male prenatal sexual differentiation and later at puberty, for secondary sex characteristics such as facial and body hair; also affects sexual desire.

**androgens** Sex hormones that are produced by the testes, ovaries, and adrenal glands. The most prominent is testosterone.

**progesterone** A sex hormone produced by the ovaries and testes, that sustains reproductive and other sexual functions, especially menstruation and pregnancy. The active ingredient in many long-acting forms of contraception.

**estrogens** Sex hormones that are produced by the ovaries, testes and adrenal glands.

**intersex** A condition in which a person with atypical chromosomes, gonads, genitals and/or hormones cannot be classified as either male or female.

**vulva** The external female genitals, or sex organs.

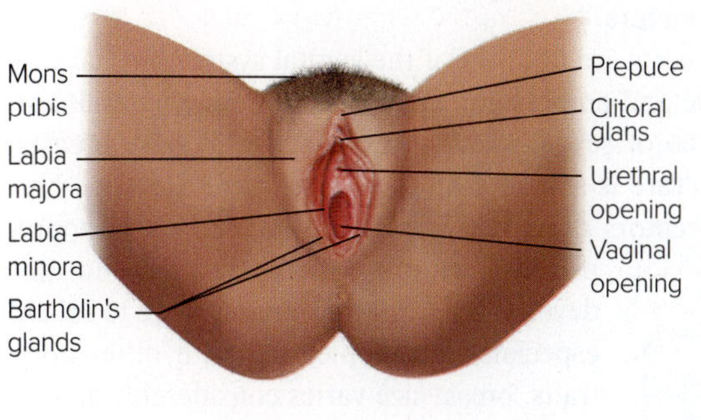


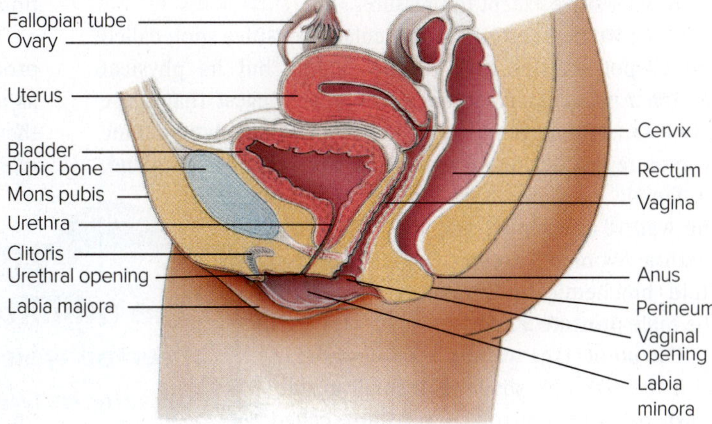


**FIGURE 6.1 (a) An external view of the vulva. (b) An internal view of the pelvis.**

Commonly confused with the vagina, the vulva includes the *mons pubis*, *labia majora* and *minora*, clitoris, and urethral and vaginal openings (Figure 6.1a). The *mons pubis,* a rounded mass of fatty tissue over the pubic bone, becomes covered with hair during puberty. Below it are two paired folds of skin called the *labia majora* (outer lips) and the *labia minora* (inner lips). Enclosed within these folds are the clitoris, the opening of the urethra, and the opening of the vagina. Vulvas vary widely in size, color, shape, and overall appearance.

The **clitoris** is highly sensitive and, plays an important role in sexual arousal and orgasm. The clitoris is homologous to the penis. The clitoris consists of the glans, or head, a knob of spongy erectile tissue in front of the vaginal opening, and a shaft that extends internally into the wall of the vagina (Figure 6.1b). Both the glans and the shaft fill with blood during sexual excitement.

Like the penis, the clitoris is richly supplied with nerve endings and responds to touch. Most women find it more sensitive to erotic stimulation than other parts of the body. Erection of the clitoris is a sign of sexual arousal. The shaft becomes firmer because it is surrounded by tough tissue that restricts its expansion, as with the penis. The *vestibular bulbs* are erectile tissues that lie beneath the minor lips. These become erect during sexual arousal and help lengthen and stiffen the vagina. Muscles associated with the clitoris can contract during sexual arousal, tightening the vaginal opening.

The outer lips (*labia majora*) are fatty tissues along both sides of the vaginal opening covered with pubic hair. The inner lips (*labia minora)* are hairless skinfolds between the outer lips and the edge of the vaginal opening. The lips are well supplied with glands, blood vessels, and nerve endings, making them erotically sensitive and important in sexual stimulation and arousal. Inside the inner lips, on either side of the vaginal opening, are the *Bartholin glands*. Their function remains unknown.

The clitoral hood, or **prepuce** (foreskin), which covers the glans of the clitoris, is formed from the upper portion of the inner lips. Ointment-like secretions (*smegma*) lubricate the movement of the hood over the clitoris. When dry, they can collect under the hood and cause itching. They can be removed through washing the foreskin.

The vulva also includes the **perineum,** a sensitive area between the vaginal opening and the anus (between the scrotum and anus in males) and the **urethra,** which transports urine from the urinary bladder. Females have a separate urinary opening that lies about halfway between the clitoris and the vaginal opening. For males, the urethra passes through the penis. Since most women have a much shorter urethra than men, they are more susceptible to urinary tract or bladder infections (UTIs). It is a good habit to urinate after sexual activity. The **hymen** is a thin membrane that may partially cover the vaginal opening. It has been the subject of a surprising amount of medical research given that it has no biological function.

The vagina has both sexual and reproductive functions. It can be used for **sexual intercourse,** or coitus. It is also the canal (birth canal) through which a baby travels during vaginal delivery and through which menstrual fluid is expelled. It is a tube-shaped organ about 3 to 4 inches long but capable of expanding during arousal or when giving birth. The vagina's nerve supply is mainly in the lower third, near the entrance, and is most sensitive to erotic stimulation. The remaining

**TERMS**

**clitoris** A highly sensitive genital structure located on the vulva; its only known function is to contribute to sexual pleasure.

**prepuce** The foreskin of the clitoris or penis.

**perineum** A sensitive area between the vaginal opening or scrotum and the anus.

**urethra** The duct that carries urine from the bladder to the outside of the body.

**hymen** A thin membrane that may partially cover the vaginal opening.

**sexual intercourse** Sexual relations involving penis and vagina, also called *coitus*.

two-thirds contain almost no nerve endings, making it relatively insensitive except to pressure.

Some women describe a particularly sensitive spot, called the G-spot, in this area of the vagina, but its physical existence is debated. Some researchers suggest that these erotic sensations, along with the feeling of ejaculation some women report during orgasm, come from the **Skene's gland,** or female prostate. It is located between the wall of the vagina and the wall of the urethra. Women who secrete fluid produce fluid biochemically similar to that from the male prostate gland.

QUICK
STATS
One milliliter
of semen typically
contains between
20 million and
150 million sperm.
—U.S. National Library
of Medicine, 2018

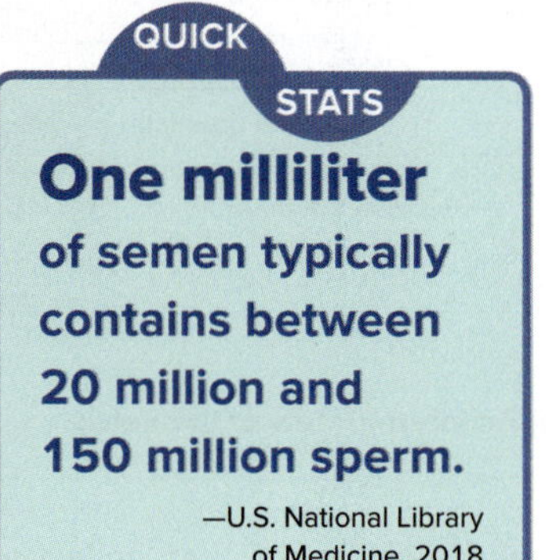

The **uterus** (the womb) is a hollow organ with the size and shape of a small upside-down pear. The narrow, lower third, called the cervix, opens into the upper part of the vagina. The major functions of the uterus are to hold and nourish the developing fetus. Like the vagina, it consists of three layers. The middle layer, the *myometrium*, is muscular, highly elastic, and involved in the contractions of labor and orgasm. The *fallopian tubes* (or *oviducts*) surround an **ovary** and guide the mature egg into the uterus. Ovaries are about the size and shape of an unshelled almond (similar to male testes) and contain numerous follicles. Each follicle holds a developing egg cell. Females, unlike males, are born with all their germ cells, several million eggs. Only a tiny portion ever mature.

The breasts are not part of the genital system but have reproductive and erotic significance, both producing milk and as a source of sexual stimulation. Males also have breasts; their structure is similar, and the tissues have the same hormonal receptors as female breasts. In the absence of appropriate hormones, they typically do not develop fully. Yet they are sensitive to touch, especially the nipples. As with other body traits, breast size varies considerably among females (and males), especially across different populations.

Many girls grow up knowing little about their sexual anatomy, but sexual health and pleasure benefit from knowing about one's own body. The vagina does not need special cleansing, and douching can be harmful. More females (and males) are being taught how to use a mirror and a flashlight, or even a speculum, to familiarize themselves (and others) with their "private parts." There are now detailed diagrams, TED talks, and organizations whose goal is to demystify and destigmatize discussion of the clitoris.

TERMS

**Skene's gland** The female prostate that can cause some women to ejaculate during orgasm.

**uterus** The hollow, thick-walled, muscular organ in which a fertilized egg might develop and where menstrual blood collects each month.

**ovaries** Paired glands that produce ova (eggs) and sex hormones; one of two types of gonads. Male equivalent is testes.

**penis** The genital structure consisting of a glans, shaft, and spongy tissue that often becomes engorged with blood during sexual excitement. The basis for assigning a male sex at birth.

## Male Sex Organs

The most noticeable male sex organs are called the penis and scrotum (Figure 6.2a). The **penis** serves important roles in reproduction, sexual pleasure, and the elimination of body wastes through urination. Males are generally comfortable exploring their own genitals and need to be familiar with them, with proper hygiene, and with potential health problems, whether STIs or cancer. Testicular cancer tends to be relatively rare but is mainly found in younger men; prostate cancer is more common but occurs later in life.

The penis comprises a glans and a shaft. Also known as the head, the glans is typically the most sensitive part of the penis. The tip has an opening (*urethral opening*) through

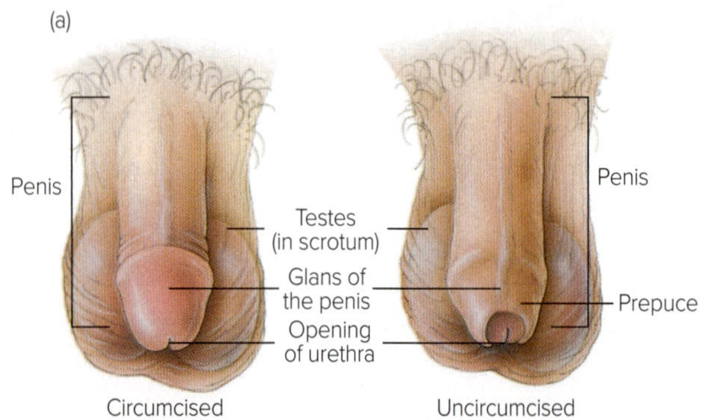


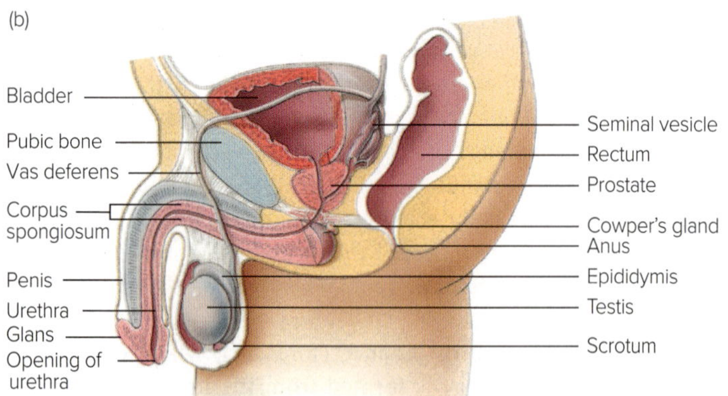


FIGURE 6.2 **(a) An external view of the penis and scrotum. (b) An internal view of the pelvis.**

which urine and semen pass. The shaft extends from the head to the body of the penis and is made up of spongy tissue that can become engorged with blood during sexual excitement, causing the organ to enlarge and become erect.

The raised ridge at the edge of the glans (or head) is called the corona. While the entire penis is sensitive to sexual stimulation, the glans and the corona are most richly endowed with nerve endings.

Internally, the penis consists of three cylinders of spongy erectile tissue that run parallel to the urethra (Figure 6.2b). Two spongy bodies lie on top of the penis and are called the *corpora cavernosa;* the one on the bottom is called the *corpus spongiosum* (through which the urethra runs). These tissues are richly supplied with blood vessels and nerves. During arousal, the tissues become filled with blood, causing the organ to enlarge and become stiff (*erection*). The skin of the penis typically is hairless, with loose folds that allow for expansion during erection. Penis size, flaccid, seems to bear little relationship to erect penis size. Flaccid, the average range is 2.5 to 4 inches; the erect average is 6 inches. Penis size varies among individuals, but there is no evidence that larger penis size is correlated with greater sexual pleasure, for either the male or his partner.

The foreskin, or prepuce, of the penis forms a hood or sheath-like covering over the glans. The **scrotum** is a pouch that contains a pair of sperm-producing gonads, called **testes.** It is made of tissue homologous to the female labia. During prenatal sex differentiation, this tissue fuses and becomes the scrotum into which the testes descend. The testes resemble the ovaries in shape and size. Because sperm production is an extremely heat-sensitive process, the scrotum's ability to regulate the temperature of the testes is important. The scrotum maintains the testes at a temperature approximately 5°F below that of the rest of the body—that is, at about 93.6°F. In hot temperatures, the muscles in the scrotum relax and the testes move away from the heat of the body.

The penile urethra is a tube that runs through the entire length of the penis and carries both urine and **semen** (sperm-carrying fluid) to the opening at the tip of the penis. The **Cowper's glands** are two small structures flanking the urethra. During sexual arousal, these glands excrete a clear, mucous-like fluid that appears at the tip of the penis. This preejaculatory fluid is thought to help lubricate the urethra to facilitate the passage of sperm and flush out any urine remaining in the tube. The release of preejaculatory fluid is an involuntary reflex and may contain sperm. This means that, for penile-vaginal coitus, withdrawal of the penis before ejaculation is not a reliable form of contraception. It is also possible to contract a sexually transmitted infection (STI)—in the mouth, anus, or vagina—from preejaculatory fluid.

Sperm production—at a rate of approximately 400 million per day—begins at about age 14. Sperm then take the following journey:

1. Sperm are produced inside a maze of tiny, tightly packed tubules within the testes. As they begin to mature, sperm flow into a single storage tube called the **epididymis,** which lies on the surface of each testis.
2. Upon ejaculation, sperm move from each epididymis into another tube—called the **vas deferens.** It is the vas that is cut in a vasectomy.
3. The two *vasa deferentia* eventually merge into a pair of **seminal vesicles,** whose secretions provide nutrients for the sperm. The sperm then pass through an organ called the **prostate gland,** where they pick up a milky fluid and become semen.
4. On the final stage of their journey, sperm flow into the ejaculatory ducts. Although urine and semen share a common passage, they are prevented from mixing together by muscles that control their entry into the urethra.

QUICK STATS

**Almost three times as many women (17.4%) as men (6.2%) aged 18–44 reported any same-gender sexual contact in their lifetime.**

—National Health Statistics Report, 2016

## Ask Yourself

**QUESTIONS FOR CRITICAL THINKING AND REFLECTION**

What are your personal views on circumcision? What are your views about other forms of genital cutting? Who or what has influenced those opinions? Are the bases of your views cultural, moral, or medical? If you had a child, would you want their genitals altered?

TERMS

**scrotum** The loose sac of skin and muscle fibers that contains the testes.

**testis** The site of sperm production; plural, *testes.* Also called *testicle.*

**semen** The fluid that carries sperm out of the penis during ejaculation.

**Cowper's gland** A small organ that produces preejaculatory fluid from the penis.

**epididymis** A storage duct for maturing sperm, located on the surface of each testis.

**vas deferens** A tube that carries sperm from the epididymis through the prostate gland to the seminal vesicles; plural, *vasa deferentia.*

**seminal vesicle** A tube leading from the vas deferens to the ejaculatory duct; secretes nutrients for the sperm.

**prostate gland** A reproductive organ that produces some of the fluid in semen, which helps to transport and nourish sperm.

# HUMAN SEXUAL DEVELOPMENT: PUBERTY AND ADULTHOOD

Hormones, substances produced by the endocrine glands, play an enormous role in prenatal gonadal-sexual differentiation, as we saw earlier. This occurs again at puberty. Puberty is not a single event but a process through which secondary sexual characteristics appear along with the ability to reproduce sexually. There is increased production of sex hormones, under the control of three glands: the **pituitary gland,** located at the base of the brain, the **hypothalamus** in the brain, and the gonads. **Adrenal glands** also secrete higher levels of androgens. Growth hormone (GH), produced by the pituitary gland increases. Both sexes experience significant growth spurts, increased pubic and other body hair, oil-producing related acne, voice changes, and growth of genital tissues. But there is substantial individual variability in the timing and extent of the changes.

**Puberty** accentuates key biological differences in male and female bodies and in their reproductive cycles, with female menstruation and male ejaculation. But society often focuses on difference rather than parallels. Or it ignores how much variability there is within each sex.

When you consider human diversity, many sex-related traits are relatively minor. Take hairiness. Human populations vary enormously in their amount of body hair. Females in some populations are hairier than males in others. Height, another sex-related trait, shows greater variability across populations than among males and females of any single population. Average heights in human groups range from barely five feet to six feet and over, for both males and females.

TERMS

**pituitary gland** An endocrine gland at the base of the brain that produces hormones and regulates the release of hormones—including sex hormones—by other glands.

**hypothalamus** A region of the brain above the pituitary gland whose hormones control the secretions of the pituitary; also involved in the control of many bodily functions, including hunger, thirst, temperature regulation, and sexual functions.

**adrenal glands** Endocrine glands, located over the kidneys, that produce sex hormones.

**puberty** The period of biological maturation when individuals develop secondary sexual characteristics and become capable of sexual reproduction.

**menstrual cycle** The monthly ovarian cycle, regulated by hormones; in the absence of pregnancy, menstruation occurs.

**menarche** The first menstrual period, which is typically experienced during adolescence.

**menses** The portion of the menstrual cycle characterized by menstrual flow (bleeding).

**follicle** A saclike structure within the ovary, in which an egg (ovum) matures.

**endometrium** The lining of the uterus.

Although puberty is a biological process, virtually all cultures and religions attach significance to it.

**Puberty in Females** The first signs of puberty usually appear between the ages of 8 and 12. Physical changes include breast development, often followed by a rounding of the hips and buttocks. As breasts develop, hair appears in the pubic region and later in the underarms. A general increase in growth rate often follows between ages 9 and 15. Estrogen eventually stops this growth spurt, sooner in girls than in boys, producing typical average adult height differences.

Other body changes include increased blood supply to the clitoris, thickening of the vaginal walls, and doubling of the size of the uterus. The pelvic bone structure grows and widens, creating a space large enough to allow an infant's birth. For females, estrogen surges come from the ovaries, while the adrenal glands are the major producer of androgens, although some comes from the ovaries. Again, there is tremendous variability, influenced by a combination of genetic, social-cultural and environmental factors.

**The Menstrual Cycle** A major landmark of puberty for is the onset of the **menstrual cycle,** the monthly ovarian cycle that leads to menstruation (loss of blood and tissue lining the uterus) in the absence of pregnancy. The timing of **menarche** (the first *menstrual period*) varies with several factors, including race/ethnicity, genetics, and nutritional status. The typical range for the onset of menstruation is wide; some girls experience menarche as young as 9 or 10, and others when they are 16 or 17 years old. The current average age of menarche in the United States is around 12 years of age, although it has been dropping. Early menarche has been shown to correlate with higher than average weight, which may explain the current trend in the United States. Girls should check with a health care provider if their menstrual cycle does not begin during their mid-teens.

The day of the onset of bleeding is considered to be day 1 of the menstrual cycle. For the purposes of our discussion, a cycle of 28 days will be used as a model; however, normal cycles vary in length from 21 to 35 days. The menstrual cycle consists of the following four phases (Figure 6.3):

1. ***Menses.*** During **menses,** characterized by the menstrual flow (bleeding from the uterus), blood levels of hormones from the ovaries and the pituitary gland are relatively low. This phase of the cycle usually lasts from day 1 to about day 5.
2. ***Follicular phase*** (also *proliferative* or *estrogenic phase).* The pituitary gland begins to produce follicle-stimulating hormone (FSH) and luteinizing hormone (LH). Under the influence of FSH, an egg-containing ovarian **follicle** begins to mature, producing increasingly higher amounts of estrogen. Stimulated by estrogen, the **endometrium** (the uterine lining) thickens with large numbers of blood vessels and uterine glands.
3. ***Ovulation.*** A surge of a potent estrogen called *estradiol* from the follicle causes the pituitary gland to release

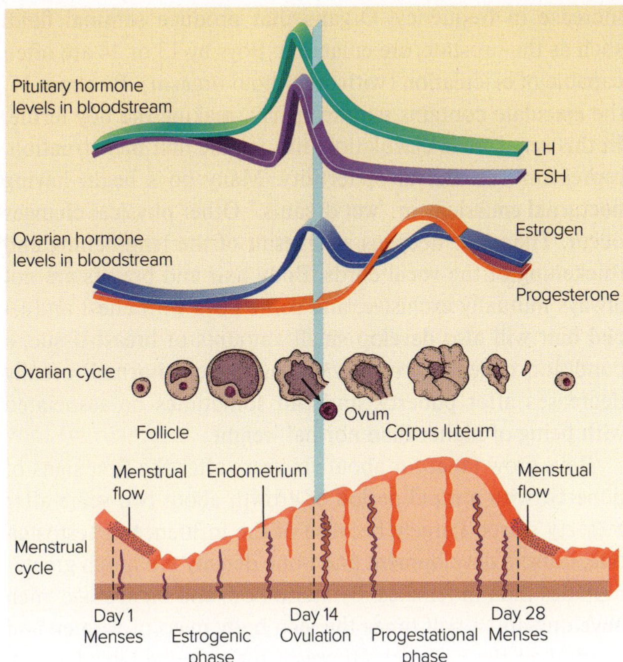


**FIGURE 6.3 The menstrual cycle.**

a large burst of LH and a smaller amount of FSH. The LH stimulates the developing follicle to release its ovum. This is known as **ovulation.** Ovulation theoretically occurs about 14 days prior to the onset of menstrual flow, with the window of greatest fertility occurring from a few days before ovulation to about one day after. This information has been used to attempt to predict the most fertile time during the menstrual cycle for fertility treatments and natural family planning methods. However, a recent study showed that even women with regular menstrual cycles often have unpredictable ovulation, and they can actually be fertile on any day of the month, including during menstruation. The "window of fertility" is especially unpredictable in teenagers and women who are approaching menopause.

4. ***Luteal phase.*** After ovulation, the follicle is transformed by LH into a glandular mass of cells called the *corpus luteum*, which manufactures progesterone and estrogen. If pregnancy occurs, the fertilized egg produces a hormone called human chorionic gonadotropin (hCG), which maintains the corpus luteum. hCG is the hormone detected by pregnancy tests.

If pregnancy does not occur, the corpus luteum degenerates, and estrogen and progesterone levels gradually fall and a new menstrual cycle begins.

**Menstrual Symptoms** Menstruation is a normal biological process, though physical or emotional symptoms associated with the menstrual cycle are common. **Dysmenorrhea,** discomfort associated with menstruation, can include any combination of the following symptoms: lower abdominal cramps, backache, vomiting, nausea, bloating, diarrhea, headache, and fatigue. Many of these symptoms can be attributed to uterine muscular contractions caused by chemicals called *prostaglandins*. Nonsteroidal anti-inflammatory drugs (NSAIDs) such as ibuprofen often relieve dysmenorrhea by blocking the effects of prostaglandins. Oral contraceptives are also effective in reducing dysmenorrheal symptoms in most women. Some people also obtain relief from rest, acupuncture, and other nonmedical treatments.

Another approach, suggested by sex researchers Masters and Johnson, is masturbation. Sex researcher Janet Hyde notes that this makes sense since part of menstrual discomfort comes from pelvic edema. While sexual arousal increases edema, orgasm dissipates it, thus relieving discomfort. It also helps reduce stress.

**Psychological Aspects** Cross-national studies reveal that women outside the United States may have different perceptions of the menstrual cycle. U.S. folk wisdom focuses on menstrual problems and mood fluctuations, especially negative emotions such as crankiness and depression. Lay terms, such as **PMS (premenstrual syndrome)** have emerged to describe physical and psychological premenstrual symptoms. But PMS is not a medical term. And research suggests there is no solid, scientific evidence for old folk beliefs. Methodologically sound studies find that mood swings are most strongly associated with stress, physical health, and social support rather than with the phase of the menstrual cycle.

This is not to say no women experience PMS. Some women do, and their symptoms can be severe. The American Psychiatric Association has a diagnosis called **premenstrual dysphoric disorder (PMDD).** This is a controversial category. Critics says it pathologizes women's experiences, is unsupported by scientific evidence, and reinforces old negative stereotypes about women's bodily functions. Cultural beliefs also shape how women perceive and experience menstruation. Research with college students found that women who had been falsely led to believe they were in the premenstrual phase reported more menstrual distress (e.g., water retention, pain) than those who were told they were around midcycle.

Researchers also investigated whether menstrual cycles affect performance, such as on cognitive tests, or of women athletes. Overall, there is no consistent evidence of cycle fluctuations in performance. Elite women athletes had higher testosterone levels than non-elite athletes, and feelings of

**TERMS**

**ovulation** The release of a mature egg (ovum) from an ovary.

**dysmenorrhea** Painful or problematic menstruation.

**PMS (premenstrual syndrome)** A nonmedical term that describes physical discomfort, psychological distress, and behavioral changes that some women experience before menstruation begins.

**premenstrual dysphoric disorder (PMDD)** A medical term for a severe form of PMS, where symptoms interfere with daily activities and relationships. A controversial category and applicable to only a small percentage of women.

> **Ask Yourself**
>
> **QUESTIONS FOR CRITICAL THINKING AND REFLECTION**
>
> Think about your own experience as you matured during puberty and adolescence. In what ways did these changes affect your life? How did they contribute to the person you are today?

competitiveness fluctuated with testosterone levels, highest during ovulation. But experience shapes our bodies and brains. So which is cause and which is effect, activities or hormone levels? Research on fluctuations in sex drive during the menstrual cycle also show contradictory results, some showing peaks around ovulation, others reporting peaks before or after ovulation.

Cultural expectations, the social environment, and prior learning affect how people experience their bodies. This does not mean that menstrual symptoms aren't real.

The following strategies provide relief for many women with premenstrual symptoms, and all of them can contribute to a healthy lifestyle at any time:

- ***Limit salt intake.*** Salt promotes water retention and bloating.
- ***Exercise.*** Women who exercise may experience fewer symptoms before and after menstrual periods.
- ***Don't use alcohol or tobacco.*** Alcohol and tobacco may aggravate certain symptoms of PMS and PMDD.
- ***Eat a nutritious diet.*** Choose a low-fat diet rich in complex carbohydrates from vegetables, fruits, and whole grains. Get enough calcium, and minimize your intake of sugar and caffeine.
- ***Relax and sleep.*** Stress reduction is always beneficial, and stressful events can trigger PMS symptoms. Try relaxation techniques during the premenstrual time and be sure to get sufficient sleep (7-8 hours per night).

If you suffer persistent premenstrual symptoms, keep a daily diary to track the types of symptoms, their severity, and their correlation with your menstrual cycle. Some people find help after being evaluated by a health care provider.

Avoid prescription medications, such as Prozac and Zoloft, which are expensive and may have negative side effects.

**Puberty in Males** Testicular growth usually begins at about age 10 or 11. The penis also begins to grow at this time, reaching adult size by about age 18. Pubic hair starts to develop as the genitals begin increasing in size, and underarm and facial hair gradually appear. Hair later develops on the chest, back, and abdomen. Facial hair often continues to get thicker and darker for several years after puberty. Erections increase in frequency. Organs that produce seminal fluid, such as the prostate, are enlarging. Boys by 13 or 14 are often capable of ejaculation (with or without orgasm). By about 15, the ejaculate contains mature sperm, making the boy fertile. In this sense male ejaculation, like female first menstruation, represents the arrival of fertility. Many boys begin having **nocturnal emissions** or "wet dreams." Other physical changes occur. The voice deepens as a result of the lengthening and thickening of the vocal cords. Body hair and breasts are not always mutually exclusive, and some boys with chest and facial hair will also develop small amounts of breast tissue, a condition called *gynecomastia.* This is very normal, usually decreases after puberty, and can sometimes be associated with being of higher than normal weight.

> **TERMS**
>
> **nocturnal emissions** Orgasm and ejaculation (wet dream) during sleep.
>
> **menopause** The cessation of menstruation, occurring gradually between the ages of 45 and 55.

Boys grow taller for about six years after the first signs of puberty, with a rapid period of growth about two years after puberty starts. Largely because of the influence of testosterone, muscle development and bone density are much greater in males than in females. By adulthood, and on average, men have one and a half times the lean body mass of women and nearly half the body fat. However, many individuals fall outside these averages.

**Cycles in Men** In the past, we assumed that only women have monthly biological and psychological cycles. Recent research has found weekly fluctuations in male testosterone levels, with weekend peaks. Men who wanted to have a child with their female partner displayed a 28-day cycle of testosterone levels. And men's testosterone levels increased the next morning after having sex with an unfamiliar partner.

## Aging and Human Sexuality

As humans age, sex hormone production declines, partially because gonads (ovaries, testes) become less responsive to gonad-stimulating hormones. Fewer germ cells (eggs, sperm) mature or are released, and for females there is eventual cessation. Growth hormone production declines, producing bone and muscle loss and an increased risk of *osteoporosis* (thin, porous bones). Blood flow may decrease to erectile tissue, affecting arousal and erection. Psychological and behavioral changes occur but are more complex and less well-studied.

**The Female *Climacteric*** Starting around age 40, for around 15 to 20 years, a woman's body transitions to a post-reproduction stage. Ovaries gradually stop releasing eggs and producing sex hormones, and there are changes in other body tissues and systems. **Menopause,** the cessation of menstruation, refers to one specific event in the process and typically occurs over a two-year period.

For some people, the drop in hormone production causes troublesome symptoms. The most common is the hot flash, a sensation of warmth rising to the face from the upper chest, with or without perspiration and chills. Other menopausal symptoms may include low libido (sexual desire), thinning hair, mood changes, and reduced bone density. As a result of decreased estrogen production during menopause, the vaginal walls thin and become less elastic, and lubrication diminishes. Sexual intercourse may become uncomfortable. However, using lubricants and hormonal creams can minimize these problems.

Like menstruation, menopause is a normal aging process rather than an illness requiring medication. Cross-cultural studies comparing Japanese with North American women dispel the idea that hot flashes and other menopausal reactions are universal, or even experienced as problems. A diet of fish and vegetables; an exercise regimen of cycling, walking, or farming; and cultural ideas about the meaning of bodily changes positively affected the Japanese experience of menopause among the women studied.

Within the United States, not all ethnic groups report the same level of symptoms nor treat them the same way. Apart from diet, smoking, and exercise, overall attitude, marital status, education, and other socioeconomic and cultural factors influence how women experience menopause. Menopause can be a positive event for women, freeing them from reproduction and pregnancy concerns. Some studies found women's sexual experiences improved after menopause.

Western medicine, however, promotes drugs for menopause. Doctors (encouraged by the pharmaceutical industry) once regularly prescribed hormone therapy (HT) during and after menopause. Post-menopausal American women took HT for decades until a large-scale 2002 research study called the Women's Health Initiative reported an increased risk of cardiovascular disease, dementia, and breast cancer, far outweighing a modest decrease in osteoporosis. As U.S. women stopped taking HT, there was a 7% decline in the U.S. breast cancer rate, the largest one-year drop in any cancer ever reported. It was even larger (12%) among women age 50 to 60, those most likely to have used HT. The FDA and NIH recommended HT be generally restricted to short-term relief in the lowest possible doses. Since then, new approaches, drugs, and alternative therapies have emerged, along with continued controversy. A major concern, according to Hyde (Hyde and Delamater, 2020: 252) are "bioidentical" compounded menopausal hormone therapy products "customized" for the patient. None are FDA approved or tested for safety or effectiveness. The Endocrine Society issued an official statement against their use. Yet they are an estimated 40% of menopausal hormone treatments used by U.S. women. Current approaches emphasize nondrug solutions, including CAM (complementary and alternative) treatments.

**Andropause** Testosterone production and male gonadal function decrease between the ages of 35 and 65, resulting in what is sometimes referred to as *male menopause* or *andropause.* Some prefer the term *aging male syndrome* because the process is much less obvious than female menopause. Symptoms vary widely, but they include loss of muscle mass, increased fat mass, decreased sex drive, erectile problems, depressed mood, irritability, difficulties with concentration, increased urination, loss of bone mineral density, and sleep difficulties. Many, though not all, of these conditions are related to declining levels of testosterone. Drug manufacturers have initiated advertising campaigns to persuade men to use prescription androgen/testosterone supplements. However, an FDA advisory panel advised against this except for men with medically diagnosed abnormal conditions, such as congenital hypogonadism.

Erection issues are normal with aging. Older men may need more direct physical stimulation and take longer to achieve an erection, and find it more difficult to maintain one. Orgasmic contractions may be less intense. These issues can often be handled through diet, exercise, behavioral modification, and patience. In some cases, prescription medications may be used to increase blood flow to the penis. On the positive side, the volume and force of ejaculation decrease, allowing some men to better control and prolong coitus and orgasm. Unlike females, males remain fertile (produce sperm) throughout their lives. However, the quantity and viability/quality of their sperm declines as they age. The pregnancy rate drops to 50% for heterosexual couples when a man is over age 35, regardless of the woman's age.

## Atypical Sexual Development

The two most common disorders of sex chromosomes are Klinefelter syndrome and Turner syndrome. In Klinefelter syndrome, the embyro carries two or more X chromosomes in addition to a Y chromosome. It occurs in about 1 in 500–1000 babies and causes infertility and atypical genitals. In Turner syndrome, which occurs in about 1 in 2500–4000 babies, the fetus has only a single complete X chromosome and is missing part or all of a second X chromosome, at least in some cells. This affects the ovaries, fertility, and bodily characteristics.

Other intersex conditions have different roots but may be more common. In congenital adrenal hyperplasia (CAH), the adrenal glands produce excess androgens, masculinizing the external genitals of an otherwise chromosomal XX female. The reverse case is androgen-insensitivity syndrome, where an XY fetus has tissues that are insensitive to testosterone, thus feminizing its external genitals. Other problems with key enzymes can also produce atypical sexual and reproductive structures. Some researchers estimate that at least 2% of all births in the United States have an intersex condition. Many, though not all, individuals will have other medical problems and will need medical help if they wish to have children.

The presence of individuals who do not neatly fit into male or female boxes raises many questions: Do we use chromosomes, external genitals, inner organs, or hormonal levels to determine if someone is a biological male or female? More important, why must we force people into one of two categories? Is it because we still feel that intersex persons will challenge and upset the traditional binary gender system?

Many adults have undergone surgeries as children so that others can assign them to a conventional sex and gender category. Some are calling for an end to early surgeries so that people with intersex conditions can choose what sex or gender is right for them, on their own time. In 2017, Germany began to legally recognize a third sex category, making it easier for parents and doctors to assign a sex to these children. Nepal, India, Pakistan, Bangladesh, Germany, New Zealand, and Australia, as well as some U.S. states, legally recognize a third option for people who do not identify as either male or female.

# SEXUAL AROUSAL AND RESPONSE

Sexual physiology consists of sexual arousal (excitement) and sexual response (how the body responds, once aroused). Research, particularly the pioneering work of William Masters and Virginia Johnson, has shown that human bodies, male and female, once sufficiently aroused, respond in biologically similar, measurable ways. Sexual arousal, however, is another matter. What is sexually stimulating, pleasurable, exciting, and with whom, is far more complex, variable, and shaped by one's experiences and society. There are some natural sources of arousal, parts of the body called **erogenous zones.** But humans find numerous creative ways to become sexually aroused. Essentially, arousal is in the mind, and even physical sensations must pass through and be processed, interpreted, given meaning, responded to or not, by the brain.

## Sexual Arousal

Sexual arousal requires some source of stimulation. Physical stimulation is the most direct form, but nonphysical sources, including thoughts, talking explicitly about sex, and vicarious experiences, are also important.

**Physical Stimulation** Touch is the most obvious and effective means of physical stimulation. Certain parts of the body have very dense nerve endings and are extremely responsive to stimulation. These include the genitals, particularly erectile tissues, such as the clitoris, penis, and labia. Other responsive areas are the perineum, nipples, breasts, inner thighs, buttocks, anal region, scrotum, and lips. Some people find other body parts stimulating, such as armpits, earlobes, hands, fingers, or the neck.

Even though culturally defined practices and individual preferences vary, most sexual encounters eventually involve some form of touching. For some people, including those with physical disabilities, encounters may also involve prosthetics or other objects. Of course, response to sexual touch, even in erogenous zones, is mediated by the brain. It is not just what is touched but how, for how long, and especially by whom.

QUICK STATS

**In the United States, up to 95% of men and 85% of women have masturbated.**

—Hyde and Delamater 2020

TERMS

**erogenous zones** Areas of the body that are particularly sensitive to sexual stimulation.

**vasocongestion** The accumulation of blood in tissues and organs by more blood flowing into an area than flowing out.

Smells are another source of sexual arousal. There is increasing evidence of human *pheromones* (biochemicals secreted outside the body) that can act as sexual attractants. Primary sources may be genital odors, especially vaginal secretions, and sweat, such as in armpits. Yet society and religion can shape one's response to potential sexual stimuli. This applies to other physical stimuli such as sounds or potential visual attractants, like genitals or breasts.

**Psychological Stimulation** Sexual arousal also has an important psychological component, regardless of the nature of the physical stimulation. Fantasies, memories, and mood can all generate sexual excitement. Erotic thoughts may be linked to an imagined person or situation or to a sexual experience from the past. Fantasies may involve activities a person may not wish to experience in reality, sometimes because they're dangerous, frightening, or forbidden.

Arousal is also powerfully influenced by emotions and attitudes about sex. How you feel about sex and the person or people you are with, and how they feel about you, matter tremendously in how sexually responsive you are likely to be. Even the most direct forms of physical stimulation carry emotional overtones. Kissing, caressing, and fondling express affection and caring. The emotional charge they give to a sexual interaction plays a significant role in sexual arousal—for some, as significant as the purely physical stimulation achieved by touching.

## The Sexual Response Cycle

*Sexual response cycle* describes the physiological processes that occur in humans once they are sexually aroused. Two physiological mechanisms explain most genital and bodily reactions during sexual arousal and orgasm (Figure 6.4): **vasocongestion** and muscular tension. Vasocongestion is the engorgement of tissues that results when more blood flows into an organ than is flowing out. Thus the penis and the clitoris become erect on the same principle that makes a garden hose become stiff when the water is turned on. Increased muscular tension culminates in rhythmic muscular contractions during orgasm.

There are several models of human sexual response, most of which are variations on the one described here. In this model, developed by William Masters and Virginia Johnson in 1966, four phases characterize the sexual response cycle:

1. ***The excitement phase.*** The clitoris, labia, and vaginal walls become engorged with blood. Tension increases in the vaginal muscles, and the vaginal walls become moist with lubricating fluid. The penis becomes erect as its tissues become engorged with blood. The testes expand and are pulled upward within the scrotum.
2. ***The plateau phase.*** This is an extension of the excitement phase during which reactions become more marked. The uterus rises, causing the inner one-third of the vaginal

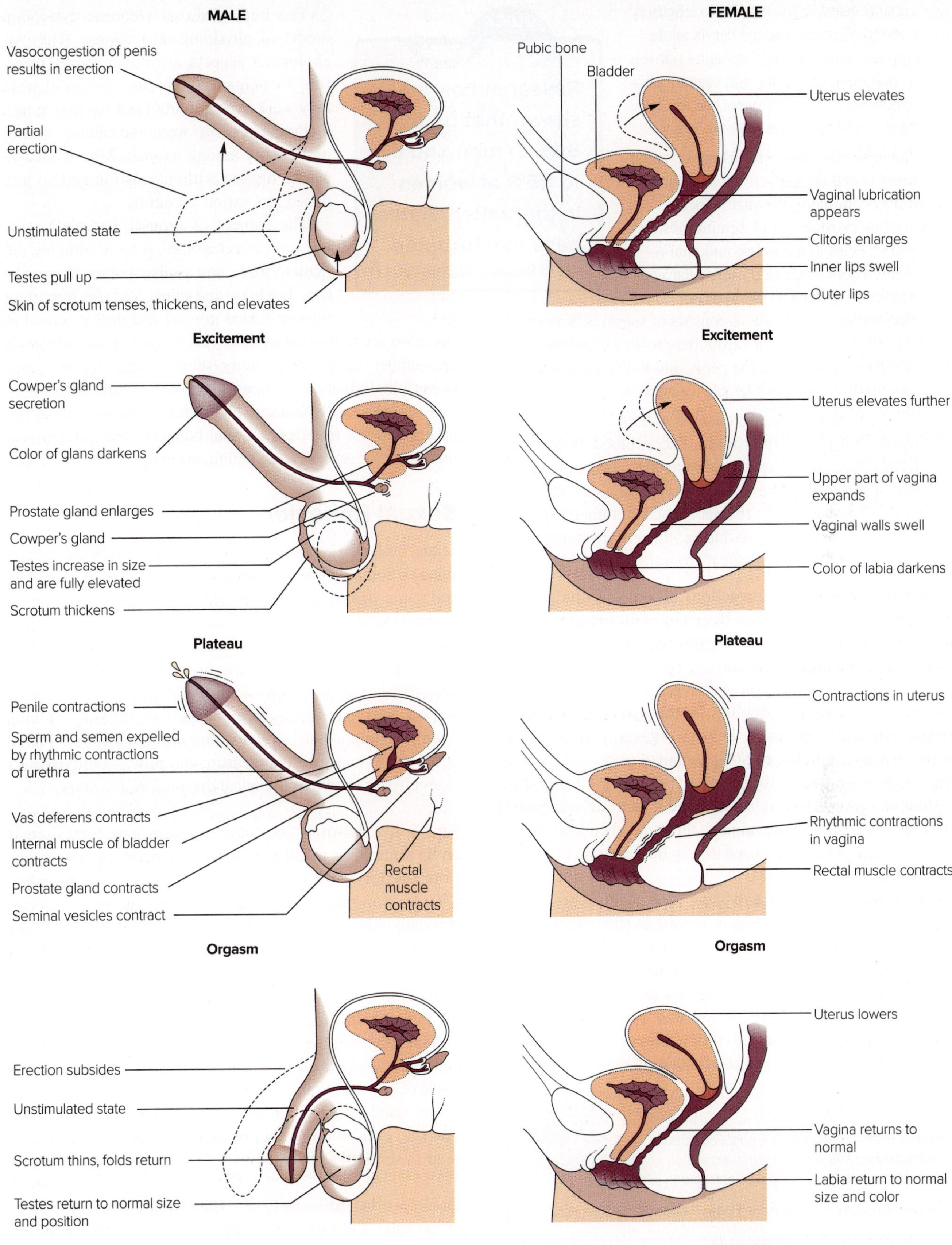


**FIGURE 6.4** **Stages of the sexual response cycle.**

canal (closest to the cervix) to lengthen and "tent" open near the cervix while the outer one-third of the vagina (closest to the opening) swells, and vaginal lubrication increases. The penis becomes harder, and the testes become larger.

3. ***The orgasmic phase.*** In this phase, sometimes called **orgasm,** rhythmic contractions occur along the vagina, penis, urethra, prostate gland, seminal vesicles, and muscles in the pelvic and anal regions. These involuntary muscular contractions can lead to two types of ejaculation: semen, which consists of sperm cells from the testes and secretions from the prostate gland and seminal vesicles, from the penis; and fluid from a woman's urethra, known as female ejaculation.
4. ***The resolution phase.*** All changes initiated during the excitement phase are reversed. Excess blood drains from tissues, the muscles in the region relax, and the genital structures return to their unstimulated states. Following ejaculation, the penis and scrotum are subject to a *refractory period* during which more stimulation will not lead to physiological arousal.

QUICK STATS

**Research has shown that up to 94% of men and up to 85% of women in the United States have masturbated.**

—Hyde and Delamater, 2020

More general physical reactions accompany the genital changes in these four phases. Beginning with the excitement phase, nipples become erect, breasts begin to swell, and the skin of the chest becomes flushed (this is more visible in people with lighter skin); these changes are more marked in women. The heart rate doubles by the plateau phase, and respiration becomes faster. During orgasm, breathing becomes irregular and the person may moan or cry out. A feeling of warmth leads to increased sweating during the resolution phase. Deep relaxation and a sense of well-being pervade the body and the mind as the brain chemicals dopamine and oxytocin are released during the response cycle.

**Gender and Sexual Response** All orgasms are physiologically the same, regardless of the site of stimulation (e.g., penile, clitoral, or vaginal). Clitoral stimulation is almost always involved in female orgasm, including during vaginal-penile intercourse. There are some sex differences. Females do not enter a refractory period and can have *multiple orgasms* within a short period of time. These are most likely to occur through mouth-genital stimulation or masturbation.

TERMS

**orgasm** The discharge of accumulated sexual tension with characteristic genital and bodily manifestations and a subjective sensation of intense pleasure; may occur simultaneously with ejaculation in males.

**erotic fantasy** Sexually arousing thoughts and daydreams.

**masturbation** Self-stimulation for the purpose of sexual arousal.

**cunnilingus** Oral stimulation of the vulva, clitoris, and vagina.

**fellatio** Oral stimulation of the penis.

The human sexual response cycle is a model of physiological response. The psychological aspects are much more subjective. Participants' own descriptions of what they were experiencing (and for how long), including orgasm, were enormously varied, particularly among women. Men tended to equate orgasm with ejaculation and so produced less varied accounts.

The subject of arousal, especially how emotions affect arousal, is more complex, difficult to study, and a subject of much speculation. The brain and spinal cord play important roles in sexual arousal and desire. Stored in the brain are individual experiences, shaped by one's biologic sex, gender, family, community, religion, and culture. These powerfully influence the how, when, why, if, and with whom we become sexually aroused. Nevertheless, learning about our bodies and the varieties of sexual behavior and techniques is important for sexual health and functioning.

## Sexual Behavior

Sexual desire varies among individuals and in different circumstances. Some people feel sexual but choose not to express it, and some people do not feel any sexual desire (asexuality). Health considerations and religious and moral beliefs may lead some people to celibacy, particularly until marriage or until an acceptable partner appears. Some people use the term abstinence to refer to the avoidance of coitus.

Not everyone emphasizes achieving orgasm. Talking openly is important. Direct communication about preferences can enhance sexual pleasure and protect both partners from physical and psychological discomfort and abuse.

**Self-Stimulation** Sex does not require a partner. There is **erotic fantasy,** or creating imaginary experiences that range from fleeting thoughts to elaborate scenarios. **Masturbation** is a common human sexual behavior. Masturbation involves manually stimulating the genitals, sometimes using devices like vibrators. Although commonly associated with adolescence, masturbation is practiced by many adults. It may be alone or may include a partner. Women find that stimulating their clitoris during coitus makes it easier to reach orgasm.

Masturbation gives a person control over the pace, time, and method of sexual release and pleasure. It can provide a sense of autonomy, and a way to avoid getting into unhealthy sexual relationships. Masturbation can be used to practice safe sex, explore one's own body, and understand what you want in sex with another person.

**Oral-Genital Stimulation** **Cunnilingus** (the stimulation of the vulva and vagina with the lips and tongue) and **fellatio** (the stimulation of the penis with the mouth) are common practices. Oral sex may be practiced either as part of foreplay or as a sex act culminating in orgasm. A recent study showed that more teens aged 15–19 had engaged in oral sex than had engaged in vaginal intercourse. The most common reasons given for postponing vaginal-penile intercourse were avoidance of pregnancy, the desire to remain technically a virgin, and the mistaken belief that STIs cannot be transmitted via oral sex. Some studies show that fellatio is more common among heterosexuals than cunnilingus, and many women report that male partners are reluctant to orally stimulate their genitals. Like all acts of sexual expression between two people, oral sex requires the cooperation and consent of both partners.

**Anal Intercourse** About one-third of women and men report having ever engaged in anal sex. Males who experience anal insertion by a penis, finger, or sex toy may find this induces orgasm or ejaculation. Because the anus is composed of delicate tissues that tear easily with friction, anal intercourse can be one of the riskiest of sexual behaviors for the transmission of HIV and other STIs. Practicing monogamy and using barrier devices such as condoms reduce the risk.

Those engaging in anal sex should use condoms and lubrication, be gentle, and cleanse before and after entry.

**Coitus (Sexual Intercourse)** The term *coitus* or *sexual intercourse* usually refers to heterosexual activity involving the vagina and penis. There are many sexual positions beyond the stereotypical "missionary" position with the man on top, and couples often rotate between them. The woman-on-top position has some advantages for clitoral stimulation and males delaying ejaculation. Side-to-side may be helpful during pregnancy, or when partners are tired or are obese. There is a huge literature, from the past and present, on coital techniques, positions, and practices. Coital pleasure depends on physical readiness: vaginal lubrication, penile erection, and other aspects of arousal. But it also depends on social and psychological factors, including being comfortable with and consenting to the behaviors involved.

## Sexual Disorders

The term **sexual disorder** (or *sexual dysfunction*) refers to disturbances in sexual desire, performance, or satisfaction. They are often classified into four types: desire, arousal, orgasmic, and sexual pain. Examples are an inability to get an erection or reach orgasm. Some sex researchers argue that conditions we now label medical disorders are not necessarily problems, permanent, nor require specialized drugs or medical therapy. Many physical conditions and drugs can interfere with sexual functioning. Psychological causes and relationship problems can be important. Moreover, sexual needs and satisfaction are highly individual. For these reasons, some say the term *sexual disorder* should only apply to a problem that causes a person mental distress.

**Desire and Arousal Disorders** In the first, sexual desire or interest in sexual activity is low. According to some studies, this is common in the United States, and higher among women than men. Sometimes it is a discrepancy between couples' desire for sex.

*Female sexual arousal disorder* refers to a lack of response to sexual stimulation, including lack of lubrication. It affects approximately 10% of women, according to some studies. This is often subjectively defined by the woman herself and increases with age. Lubricants are a partial solution.

**Erectile disorder (ED),** previously called *impotence* or *erectile dysfunction*, is the inability to achieve or maintain a penile erection sufficient for sexual intercourse. The condition is associated with aging (about 30% for men in their sixties), but ED can occur at any age. Recent studies suggest that rates of ED are increasing among men under age 40. It can produce severe psychological reactions, from embarrassment to depression. This is not surprising, given the strong symbolic association of erection with manhood and masculinity.

**Premature ejaculation** (PE), ejaculation before or just after vaginal insertion, is common among men, especially at younger ages. Surveys suggest it affects about 15% of men. As with ED, it can create psychological distress. The International Society for Sexual Medicine's definition includes not only length or lack of control over ejaculation but a third component, an individual's distress about the problem. Another, less common **orgasmic disorder** is delayed ejaculation, when a male is unable to have an orgasm or when it is quite delayed, despite a solid erection.

*Female orgasmic disorder (FOD)* is the inability to have an orgasm. It goes by many other names, including orgasmic dysfunction. In some estimates, 20% of women have difficulty reaching orgasm, although global numbers may be higher. Many women have orgasms in some situations but not others. Women are more likely to achieve orgasm from

### Ask Yourself

**QUESTIONS FOR CRITICAL THINKING AND REFLECTION**

What do you think about using medication to treat sexual dysfunction? What alternatives do you think should be considered before trying medication? Do you think the general public is appropriately educated about the side effects of such products? In your opinion, would the potential benefits of such products outweigh the risks? Who do you think is most qualified to determine if someone has a sexual dysfunction?

**TERMS**

**sexual disorder** A disturbance in sexual desire, performance, or satisfaction that causes distress.

**erectile disorder** The inability to achieve or maintain a penile erection sufficient for sexual activity.

**premature ejaculation** The inability to ejaculate when you wish to during sexual activity.

**orgasmic disorder** The inability to experience orgasm, despite engaging in the types of stimulation that would typically lead to one.

clitoral stimulation through self-stimulation, manual stimulation with a partner, oral sex, or the use of a vibrator than through penile–vaginal intercourse alone. Because many heterosexual couples do not engage in practices that might lead to female orgasm, and because women are sometimes discouraged from masturbating, many women believe they have an orgasmic disorder when simple behavior changes might solve the problem. Once again, disorder is a subjective definition.

Painful intercourse, or *dyspareunia*, refers to genital pain regularly experienced during sexual intercourse. It is more common in women but can occur in men. Possible causes include infection, lack of lubrication, endometriosis, past sexual trauma, fear of insertion, menopause, and scarring due to childbirth. *Vaginismus* is the spastic contractions of the outer third of the vagina that can make sexual intercourse difficult to impossible. This condition may include discomfort with inserting a tampon or a finger during a pelvic exam into the vaginal opening. This is not common in the general population, although it has significant consequences for heterosexual women in relationships.

**Causes of Sexual Disorder** Sexual disorders can be caused by physical, psychological, and interpersonal factors or a combination of all. A first step is to have a physical examination to explore possible medical causes. Erectile disorder is often associated with heart disease. Sexual health problems can be related to other *systemic disease*s like diabetes or poor immune function. Smoking, alcoholism, and excess weight can also lead to sexual problems. Sexual difficulties may be the first sign of serious health problems in the cardiovascular, nervous, or endocrine system since they affect sexual functioning. This is one reason people should think twice before buying treatments online. Being overweight is a risk factor for cardiovascular problems, and it can also affect hormonal balance. Extreme underproduction of testosterone or overproduction of prolactin can lead to ED in males.

Alcohol and many drugs can inhibit sexual response. Antidepressant drugs (especially SSRIs) may cause sexual dysfunction in up to 50% of people. Sometimes drugs are used to counteract the side effects of antidepressants. Other common medications that can inhibit sexual response include certain drugs that treat high blood pressure. If optimum sexual functioning is a concern, ask a health care provider for a medication that will not lead to sexual side effects.

Sexual disorders, especially ED and FOD, can also be caused by general ill health, fatigue, anxiety, and other sources of stress, including overwork, behavioral or lifestyle factors. Sexual inexperience or ignorance of sexual anatomy and functioning also contribute. But psychological, social, and cognitive factors play significant roles. Problems in a couple's relationship are a leading cause of sexual disorders. Anger, resentment, conflicts over power, difficulty with intimacy, distrust, and other relationship inequities can all feed into sexual response.

A group of sex therapists specializing in women have formulated what they call a New View of women's sexual problems. They are critical of the American Psychiatric Association's medicalized approach to sexual disorders and look to other causes. These include sociocultural, political, and economic factors such as inadequate sexuality education, unrealistic cultural norms about female bodies or sexuality, fatigue from family and work obligations, and partner issues relating to sexuality, power, and emotional or physical abuse. Only after exploring these sources do they turn to medical conditions and solutions.

**Treating Sexual Disorders** Approaches to treating sexual disorders vary with the type of problem and the cause. Most sexual disorders are treatable, often without drugs.

Pain disorders, like dyspareunia and vaginismus, are treated first by diagnosing and treating any underlying physical cause of the problem. Using generous amounts of lubricant during sexual activity is important. Sexual therapy for vaginismus involves gradual desensitization techniques. Dilators are inserted into the vagina in order to relax the vaginal muscles, stop the involuntary spasms, and help the vagina to gradually stretch.

Erectile disorder (ED) in males is often treated with drugs like Viagra (sildenafil citrate). These enhance the effects of nitric oxide, a chemical that relaxes smooth muscles in the penis. The relaxed muscles increase blood flow and allow a natural erection to occur in response to sexual stimulation.

Other medical treatments for erectile dysfunction are available, along with vacuum devices that pull blood into the penis, and in severe cases, penile implants. Hormone replacement therapy is an option for ED when testosterone levels are lower than the normal range, which is, however, quite variable. Exercise may also help improve erectile function, especially exercises that target the muscles of the pelvic floor.

Too often sexual difficulties are treated with drugs when nondrug strategies may be more appropriate. Psychosocial causes of dysfunction include troubled relationships, a lack of sexual skills, ineffective stimulation, religious-cultural prohibitions, anxiety, shame, prior experiences, and psychosexual trauma such as sexual abuse or rape. Some sexual problems are the result of rigid gender roles that lead men to believe they need to be the sexual aggressor, women to believe they should remain passive, and gender-nonconforming people to believe that they are sexually abnormal or deviant. None of these beliefs is based in biological or social fact. Many can be addressed through sex counseling. A therapist can promote open discussion between partners and suggest specific techniques.

Premature ejaculation is an example of a common sexual problem that responds well to nondrug therapy. On average, men typically ejaculate between 2 and 10 minutes after insertion and thrusting begin, but most men periodically ejaculate more quickly. Several nondrug techniques are helpful such as Kegel exercises, which strengthen and improve control of the pelvic muscles, and practicing masturbation to extend arousal.

Women who seek treatment for orgasmic dysfunction often have not learned what types of stimulation will excite them and bring them to orgasm. Sex therapists teach patients about their own anatomy and sexual responses and encourage them to experiment with masturbation, focusing on the clitoris, until they experience orgasm. Vibrators can be helpful during masturbation or intercourse. Previously taboo, they are now common and easy to obtain from retailers that specialize in sex-positive approaches. Once someone can masturbate to orgasm, they can transfer this learning to partner sexual encounters.

Drug companies have not given up on female sexual disorders. Testosterone replacement is currently used off-label to treat low desire. A prostaglandin cream that improves blood flow to the clitoris is being developed. In 2015, a drug called Addyi (flibanserin) was introduced as a treatment for hypoactive female sexual desire. Critics argue that low female sexual desire is more complicated than ED and that women might benefit more from education, behavioral changes, or therapy. Researchers who study sexual assault and coercion are concerned about young women using a drug that, when mixed with alcohol, can lead to unconsciousness, compromising their ability to refuse unwanted sex.

Given these issues, many sex researchers advocate using nondrug therapies first. They also suggest more critical reflection on what we've been taught is normal sexuality and whether that really fits our own needs, desires, and situations.

**Other Sexual Health Issues** Sexual health depends on doing regular genital self-examination, cleansing (but not douching) the genitals, and becoming comfortable with one's own body. Be alert to unusual discharges, odors, and sensations that might indicate a potential health problem. Don't let embarrassment about one's body or sexual activities keep you from self-examination or seeking out a health provider or counselor for advice.

Other common sexual health problems include inflammation of the vagina, prostate, and epididymis; endometriosis; and testicular torsion.

## GENDER AND SEXUALITY: BIOLOGIC SEX, GENDER ROLES, GENDER IDENTITY, SEXUAL ORIENTATION

The last 60 years has seen enormous challenges to old binary ways of thinking. Biologic sex and gender are now recognized as distinct. Gender is the set of socially created norms, expectations, behaviors, privileges, and character traits we attach to biologic sex. Gender roles and identities have to be learned. From at least birth on, humans are immersed in gendered worlds, learning, subtly or not, what it means to be male or female, through colors, names, body decoration, speech patterns, activities, and social encounters. Parents often choose gender-specific names, clothes, and toys for their children, and children may model their behavior after their same-gender parent. Family and friends create an environment that teaches children how to act gender appropriately. Teachers, television, books, social media, advertisements, and even strangers model gender roles. U.S. social, economic, and political institutions, and all aspects of popular culture, are at least partially organized around a binary system of gender. Not surprisingly, gender identity is a major part of who people are and how they live their lives, despite other identities. And heterosexuality forms an important part of traditional gender roles and gender identity.

But U.S. gender roles are not universal or inevitable. They vary cross-culturally, and they change over time and circumstances.

### Gender Nonconforming

More people are rejecting gender stereotypes and pursuing paths that fit their own interests, talents, preferences, sense of self. The concept of **androgyny** describes people who have a mixture of prototypical male and female traits. Androgynous adults are less gender stereotyped in their thinking; in how they look, dress, and act; in how they divide work in the home; in how they think about jobs and careers; and in how they express themselves sexually.

Some people use the term **gender nonconforming** or **nonbinary** to describe androgynous people. Androgynous people can have a strong sense of identity as a female or male, biologically, but reject their culture's gender stereotypes. For some people, questioning gender stereotypes and roles also means reassessing their sexual preferences, pursuing sexual partners to whom they are attracted (for whatever reasons), regardless of their biologic sex or gender identity.

### Transgender

Some people may reject the gender category associated with their biologic sex. The term *gender dysphoria* refers to psychological stress about a person's perceived gender identity and their gender assigned at birth. For example, a person assigned male because of a penis may feel more like a girl or a woman than a boy or a man. Or they may feel like neither and identify as nonbinary or gender nonconforming. Some intersex individuals or others with ambiguous genitals may have similar feelings. **Transgender** individuals often experience prejudice, even violence, which can have negative consequences on their physical and mental health. Some trans children may, from an early age, show intense and persistent distress about their assigned sex and associated gender and may view themselves as another sex or gender. They may be diagnosed with and treated for gender dysphoria.

**TERMS**

**androgyny** Possessing role and behavioral characteristics that are not from just one gender but from all genders.

**gender nonconforming** A term for people who question and may not identify with conventional gender categories.

**nonbinary** A gender identity that cannot be described in traditional categories and actively questions or refuses the male/female binary.

**transgender** A term describing an individual whose bodily sex category differs from their own gender identity.

Medical procedures are available for transgender people who wish to align their biologic sex with their perceived gender identity, called *gender-affirming treatment* or *sex reassignment*. This includes hormone therapy and genital surgery accompanied by psychotherapy. Hormonal treatments induce secondary sex characteristics such as breasts or facial hair, and surgery changes the appearance and function of the genitals or breasts. Not all transgender people desire surgical or hormonal treatment, but they may want to assume a gender identity different than their birth sex assignment. Trans individuals may have a variety of sexual preferences and orientations. Over 20 countries have legally recognized and awarded rights, to varying degrees, to transgender individuals. These may include formally identifying as neither male nor female.

QUICK
STATS
An estimated 2 million U.S. adults identify as transgender.
—Gallup, 2019

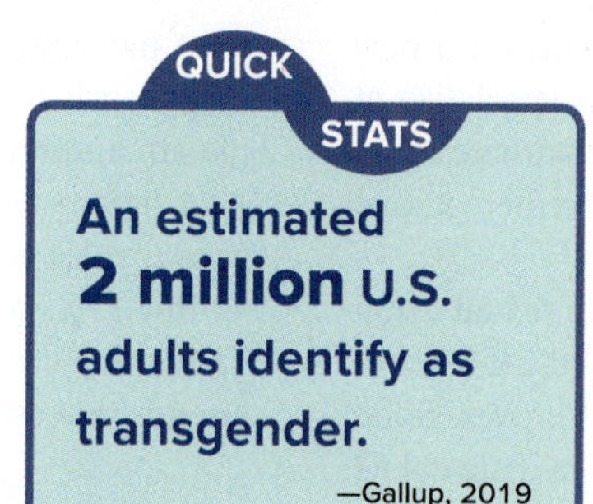

The language for nonbinary or gender-nonconforming people can be confusing. It is a reminder of how deeply embedded in language are traditional binary ideas of sex and gender, and of how many different ways there are to think about biologic sex, gender, and who we are as individuals. While some words may seem new, the people and behaviors they refer to have always been a part of humanity and recognized in some cultures.

## Sexual Orientation

Sexual orientation refers to which gender or genders we are attracted to emotionally and sexually. It exists along a continuum that ranges from exclusive heterosexuality through bisexuality to exclusive same-gender.

The labels and categories are in flux. Some in the gay community prefer the term *queer* or, for females, *lesbian*. Others reject old categories completely, using terms like **genderfluid** or *pansexual* to reflect a more shifting, expansive view of sexuality where attraction depends on the person and circumstances, regardless of sex or gender. These labels and categories are not universal. People in some societies may think of sex as a behavior, something you do, regardless of with whom, rather than as your sexual identity.

Sexual orientation involves feelings and self-concept, and someone may or may not express it through their behavior. Sexual orientation and behavior can change over time and with circumstances. Some married people with children enter into same-sex relationships later in life. And more younger people are willing to experiment with unconventional sexual partners. Many experts believe humans are born sexually fluid and potentially bisexual. However, In the United States, only approximately 3–5% of the population identify as bisexual.

While a majority of people are heterosexual, other sexual orientations are becoming more acceptable. Surveys in 2021 and 2022 show increases in the percentage of U.S. adults identifying as LGBT, now at least 6–8%, with the majority identifying as bisexual. This reflects growing acceptance of gender-nonconforming identities, especially among young people. LGBT communities exist around the world and provide support for "coming out" or acknowledging one's sexual orientation to oneself and others.

**TERMS**

**genderfluid** The term used to describe people who have a nonbinary gender identity or gender expression that may vary.

Cases of depression and attempted suicide, while higher for gender-nonconforming individuals than for heterosexuals, are mainly due to a lack of family and peer support, prejudice, and maltreatment. Children in gender-nonconforming families show adjustment and mental health patterns similar to those in heterosexual families. Gender-nonconforming people are as varied and diverse as heterosexuals. Some are in long-term, committed relationships, others are not. As of 2019, same-gender couples could marry in 30 countries, including the United States.

## The Origins of Sexual Orientation

Older theories of sexual orientation focused almost exclusively on same-sex attraction. More recent research includes explaining heterosexuality as well. Most experts agree they are far from fully understanding sexual orientation. Multiple factors interact in complex ways: genetic, hormonal, cultural, social, economic, historical, and psychological.

Some scientists continue looking for biological or genetic markers associated with same-gender sexual orientation, especially of males. But many researchers prefer sociological and psychological explanations: how much contact children have with different genders, their early experiences with heterosexuality or homosexuality, and family dynamics. Other research explores how gender nonstereotypic children are affected by others' labels, especially in homophobic societies with rigid gender stereotypes. In addition to producing anxiety, the labels get children questioning their own sexual identity, eventually labeling themselves as gay or trans.

Understanding sexual attraction and mate choices is extremely difficult, whether for heterosexuals or for gender-nonconforming people. Research shows most people prefer people who are like themselves socioeconomically, ethnically, in religion, culturally, in interests and activities, and regionally, even from the same neighborhood. But what about interracial, interreligious, even cross-national partnering? And why do most humans partner with people who are different when it comes to biologic sex, gender role, and gender identity? Scientists still have a long way to go in understanding human sexual preferences and orientation.

# SEXUALITY AND THE LIFE CYCLE

Our behavior is shaped by the interplay of our biological predispositions and our life experiences. Our life experiences are deeply influenced by the family, community, religion, society, and culture in which we have been raised.

## Childhood Sexual Behavior

The capacity for genital response is present at birth. Ultrasound studies suggest that penile erections can occur in utero, and both penile erections and vaginal lubrication are possible during infancy. Sexual behaviors emerge gradually; self-exploration and touching the genitals are common forms of play and have been observed among infants as young as six months. These behaviors often lead to more deliberate forms of masturbation, with or without orgasm.

Children are also likely to explore their playmates' genitals, often as part of games such as "playing house" or "playing doctor." By age 12, 40% of boys have engaged in sex play. The peak exploration age for girls is 9, by which time 14% have had such experiences.

## Adolescent Sexuality

At puberty, individuals may be biologically mature but not yet adults psychologically and socially. This can create confusion over what constitutes appropriate sexual behavior during adolescence. Most countries have laws about when someone is old enough to have sexual intercourse, sometimes referred to as the age of consent. In the United States, this age varies between 16 and 18, depending on the state.

Sexual fantasies and dreams increase in adolescence, often accompanying masturbation. Masturbation may be the most common sexual activity of teenagers. Family relationships and attitudes toward sex and teen perceptions of what is normal among peers strongly influence choices about sex. But popular culture plays an extraordinary role. Music videos and other highly sexualized commercial products target teenagers and present sexual scripts that are both unrealistic and harmful.

In the United States, sexual interaction often occurs in the context of dating or partying. It may involve sexual touching that produces arousal but not always orgasm. Teens may engage in oral or anal sex to avoid pregnancy and loss of virginity (especially for girls). But these behaviors have emotional and social consequences. They can lead to sexually transmitted infections unless safer sex practices are used. Same-gender attractions, with or without sexual encounters, are common in adolescence and are not necessarily related to adult sexual orientation.

**QUICK STATS**

**One of every five U.S. women will experience rape at some point in their lives, usually by someone they know.**

—CDC, 2018

## Adult Sexuality

Early adulthood is a time when people make important life choices—a time of increasing responsibility in terms of interpersonal relationships and family life. The average age at marriage in the United States is almost 30 for men and 28 for women. According to the Kinsey Institute, men are typically sexually active for 10 years before getting married, and women for 8 years. Today more people in their twenties believe that becoming sexually experienced rather than preserving virginity is an important prelude to selecting a mate. (See the box "Questions to Ask before Engaging in a Sexual Relationship.")

Popular culture projects the image that everyone is having sex. The reality is more complicated. Individual motivations for sex can change with age, from emphasizing physical release to a more emotional or social focus. Or the opposite occurs. Elderly people, despite stereotypes, often have active sex lives, adjusting their sexual behavior to reflect changes in their genitals, bodies, and motivations for having sex. Masturbation, alone or with another person, may become more common, along with forms of sex other than sexual intercourse. Age can release people from old expectations and inhibitions.

## Sexuality in Illness and Disability

Any disease or disability that affects mobility, well-being, self-esteem, or body image has the potential to affect sexual expression. People with chronic diseases or disabilities often have special needs regarding their sexual behavior. They may also confront the perception that they are asexual or have lost themselves as the sexual person they once knew. But more people are recognizing that disability is not a permanent obstacle to having and enjoying sexual experiences. Helpful resources, including educational videos, are now available.

## Force and Sexual Coercion

The use of force and coercion in sexual relationships is an enormous problem. **Sexual coercion** is not just about physical force. It includes all forms of coercion, verbal, emotional, economic, and social, through which one person gets another person to submit, unwillingly, to a sexual encounter. It can range from sexual harassment to forced sexual intercourse (penile, anal, oral). It usually involves unequal power relations, whether in a personal relationship or in the workplace or other institutional setting. Sexual coercion is not about desire. It's about *forcing* another person to submit. It's nonconsensual.

Historically, many societies, including the United States, did not grant the right to consent to or refuse sex to all individuals. Men had sexual rights over women, especially over women of comparably lower status. The legal concept of spousal rape is very recent in U.S. law and does not exist in all countries. Many Americans may not realize that one spouse has a right to refuse to have sex with the other. **Rape,** usually defined as nonconsensual oral, anal, or vaginal sex, is pervasive globally.

**TERMS**

**sexual coercion** The use of physical or psychological force or intimidation to make a person submit to sexual demands.

**rape** A criminal offense defined in most states as forcible sexual relations with a person against that person's will or when a person is incapable of providing consent to sexual activity.

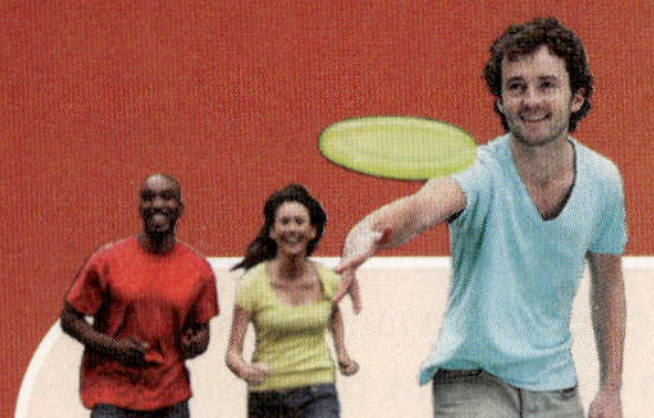

## WELLNESS ON CAMPUS
### Questions to Ask Before Engaging in a Sexual Relationship

#### Who Am I Sexually Attracted To?

- What are the characteristics that usually attract me to someone in a physical way?
- How comfortable am I with the people I find sexually attractive? What would I change if I could? Do I feel safe when I am with them?
- Are the people I am usually sexually attracted to the same types of people as those I consider having a long-term, stable relationship with? Why or why not?

#### What Sexual Behaviors Are Comfortable for Me Right Now?

- What has influenced my comfort level with these behaviors?
- What am I not entirely comfortable with, but would be willing to experiment with in order to please a partner? What level of trust would I need to establish with that partner in order to proceed? What would we need to talk about ahead of time?
- What exactly do I say in order to make my comfort level clear to my partner? What do I do if my partner tries to push me beyond my comfort level?

#### How Can I Express My Sexual Needs, Desires, and Concerns to a Potential Sexual Partner?

- When would be the best time to talk about these needs, desires, and concerns?
- How do I start the conversation?
- What will I do if my needs are not being met or my concerns are not taken seriously?

#### What Preparations Do I Need to Make in Order to Engage in the Safest Sex Possible?

- If I am engaging in heterosexual sexual activity, and I do not wish to reproduce, I need to obtain birth control. Have I consulted a health professional to figure out the best method of birth control for myself and my partner? Do I know how to employ this method correctly? Have we discussed what we plan to do if a pregnancy occurs?
- If I am engaging in any type of sexual activity with a partner, I need protection from sexually transmitted infections. Have I consulted a health professional to figure out the best method of STI protection for myself and my partner? Do I know how to employ this method correctly? Have I discussed with my partner their sexual history, including information about risky behavior and STIs? Do I understand the ways that sexual behaviors transmit these infections?
- What do I need from my partner in order to ensure that I feel emotionally safe before, during, and after our sexual behavior together?
- Do I engage in any behaviors that cause me to participate in sexual activity that I wouldn't otherwise be comfortable with, such as excessive drinking or drug use? What do I need to do in order to reduce or eliminate these behaviors?
- Do I make sure that the people I am being sexual with are actively consenting to the behaviors? Do I understand what constitutes sexual consent? Do I understand that I need to stop what I'm doing if the other person asks me to or is not communicating active and willing consent?
- Do I have trusted friends and adults with whom I can discuss my sexual concerns, questions, and relationships? If not, how can I go about finding those people so that I don't have to figure all of this out on my own or overly rely on a romantic partner?

Intimate partner sexual abuse occurs among people of all communities, socioeconomic levels, cultures, and religions. Child abuse figures are also startling high, with 25% of U.S. women and 8% of men reporting some form of sexual abuse prior to age 18. Although men can be victims, and women perpetrators, data show the vast majority of sexual abusers are male. Some research links this to deeply entrenched cultural attitudes about gender and sexuality, including male dominance, hostility toward women, and male entitlement to sex. These beliefs not only affect intimate relationships and families; they also affect society as a whole, perpetuating a toxic model of masculinity that permeates all aspects of society, from policing and college campuses to sports and politics.

Recent high-profile cases of abuse have been reported in Olympic gymnastics, higher education, Hollywood, law enforcement, the judicial system, and virtually all occupations. Nevertheless, most cases of sexual abuse and sexual coercion occur in private relationships and go unreported. Sexual health requires freedom from coercion, the right to consent or refuse to consent, without punishment–verbal, emotional, economic, or physical. The Rape, Abuse, and Incest National Network (RAINN) is an excellent resource for anyone wanting to learn more about how to resist and respond to sexually coercive situations and relationships.

#### Ask Yourself

**QUESTIONS FOR CRITICAL THINKING AND REFLECTION**

What do you consider to be appropriate sexual behavior? What behaviors do you think are inappropriate or wrong? What experiences have shaped your views of such behaviors? Have they changed in the past five years? What do you think they will be like five years from now?

## TAKE CHARGE
### Communicating about Sexuality

To talk with your partner about sexuality, follow the general suggestions for effective communication in Chapter 5. Getting started may be the most difficult part. Some people feel more comfortable if they begin by initiating a discussion about why people are so uncomfortable talking about sexuality. Talking about sexual histories—how partners first learned about sex or how family and cultural background influenced sexual values and attitudes—is another way to get started. Reading about sex can also be a good beginning: Partners can read an article or book and then discuss their reactions.

Be honest about what you feel and what you want from your partner. Cultural and personal obstacles to discussing sexual subjects can be difficult to overcome, but self-disclosure is important for successful relationships. Research indicates that when one person openly discusses attitudes and feelings, partners are more likely to do the same. If your partner seems hesitant to open up, try asking open-ended or either/or questions: "Where do you like to be touched?" or "Would you like to talk about this now or wait until later?"

If something is bothering you about your sexual relationship, choose a good time to initiate a discussion with your partner. Be specific and direct but also tactful.

If you are going to make a statement that your partner may interpret as criticism, try mixing it with something positive. If you want to say no to some sexual activity, say no unequivocally. Don't send mixed messages. If you are afraid of hurting your partner's feelings, offer an alternative if it's appropriate: "I am uncomfortable with that. How about . . .?"

If you're in love, you may think that the sexual aspects of a relationship will work out magically without discussion. However, partners who never talk about sex deny themselves the opportunity to increase their closeness and improve their relationship. Finally, it is never necessary to experience these thoughts, concerns, or feelings alone. Identify trusted friends and adults from whom you can seek advice and support.

## Responsible Sexual Behavior

Healthy sexuality is an important part of adult life. But there are potential consequences to most sexual behavior, including pregnancy, STIs, social embarrassment, and emotional changes in relationships. Every sexually active person should be aware of these consequences and accept responsibility for them. Consider the following with your partners:

**Open, Honest Communication** Each person needs to clearly indicate what sexual involvement means to them. Does it mean love, fun, a permanent commitment, or something else? The intentions of each person should be clear. (See the box "Communicating about Sexuality.")

**Agreed-On Sexual Activities** No one should pressure or coerce or force anyone to be sexual. Sexual behaviors should be consistent with the sexual values, preferences, and comfort level of all partners. Everyone has the right to refuse sexual activity at any time, including married couples, and including after sexual behavior has begun. Sexual activity should be explicitly and enthusiastically consented to by all people involved; the absence of a stated "no" does not indicate clear and enthusiastic consent to sexual activity. Some state legislatures and U.S. universities are considering adopting a "yes means yes" standard of consent for sexual activities.

**Sexual Privacy** Intimate relationships involving sexual activity are based on trust, and that trust can be violated if partners reveal private information about the relationship to others; this includes disseminating images that were shared privately. Sexual privacy also involves respecting other people—not engaging in activities in the presence of others that would make them uncomfortable. The question of how to handle bringing a partner back to a shared dorm room is a situation that many college students must address. Roommates should be respectful of one another and discuss the situation in advance to avoid embarrassing encounters.

**Safe Sex** Sexual partners should be aware of and practice safe sex to guard against STIs and unwanted pregnancies. Partners should be honest about their health and any medical conditions and work out a plan for protection.

**Contraception Use** If pregnancy is not desired, contraception should be used during penile-vaginal intercourse. Both partners need to take responsibility for protecting against unwanted pregnancy (See Chapter 7.)

**Sober Sex** The use of alcohol or drugs in sexual situations increases the risk of unplanned, unprotected sexual activity, especially for young adults, many of whom binge-drink during social events. Binge drinking also increases the risk of sexual assault. RAINN estimates that 11.2% of college students experience rape or sexual assault through physical force, violence, or incapacitation; college-aged women are almost five times as likely as men to be forced into an unwanted sexual experience. Unfortunately, a cycle then ensues for some of these women: those with a history of sexual assault are more likely to drink heavily. Approximately 30% of underage college women engage in such heavy episodic drinking, and women under age 21 also bear the highest risk for sexual assault in college. Alcohol and drugs impair judgment and should not be used in association with sexual activity. Be

> **Ask Yourself**
>
> **QUESTIONS FOR CRITICAL THINKING AND REFLECTION**
>
> If you are sexually active or plan to become active soon, how open have you been in communicating with your partner? Are you aware of your partner's feelings about sex and about their comfort level with certain activities? Do you and your partner share the same views on contraception, STI prevention, and ethical issues about sex?

honest with yourself; if you need to drink in order to engage in sexual activities, it may be a good idea to rethink your social life and relationships. This can be facilitated by talking with a trusted friend or a professional counselor. Someone who is intoxicated cannot legally consent to sex.

Aside from the dangers of mixing alcohol and sex, alcohol typically impairs sexual performance. Although alcohol may lower sexual inhibition, too much makes it difficult to achieve or keep an erection, decreases vaginal lubrication, and makes orgasm more difficult. Chronic overuse of alcohol reduces testosterone, ultimately causing erectile dysfunction, infertility, and body changes such as enlarged breasts in men. Women who overuse alcohol may experience menstrual abnormalities and decreased sexual function.

> **TERMS**
>
> **fertilization** The initiation of biological reproduction; the union of the nucleus of an egg cell with the nucleus of a sperm cell.
>
> **fertilized egg** The egg after penetration by a sperm; a *zygote*.

## CONCEPTION

The process of conception begins with the union of the nucleus of an egg cell (ovum) and the nucleus of a sperm cell—a process called **fertilization** (see Figure 6.5). Every month during a woman's fertile years, her body prepares itself for conception and pregnancy. In one of her ovaries, an egg matures and is released from its follicle. The egg, about the size of a fine grain of sand, travels through an oviduct, or fallopian tube, to the uterus in three to four days. The endometrium, which is the lining of the uterus, has already thickened for the implantation of a **fertilized egg,** that is, a *zygote*. If the egg is not fertilized, it lasts about 24 hours and then disintegrates. The woman's body then sheds the uterine lining during menstruation.

### Fertilization

Sperm cells are produced in the testes and ejaculated from the penis into the vagina during sexual intercourse (except in cases of artificial insemination or assisted reproduction; see the section "Treating Infertility"). Sperm cells are much smaller than eggs. The typical ejaculate contains millions of sperm, but only a few complete the journey through the uterus and up the fallopian tube to the egg. Many sperm cells do not survive the vagina's acidic environment.

Once through the cervix and into the uterus, many sperm cells are diverted to the wrong oviduct or get stuck along the way. Of those that reach the egg, only one will penetrate its hard outer layer. As sperm approach the egg, they release enzymes that soften this outer layer. Enzymes from hundreds of sperm must be released in order for the egg's outer layer to soften enough to allow a single sperm cell to penetrate. It then fuses with the nucleus

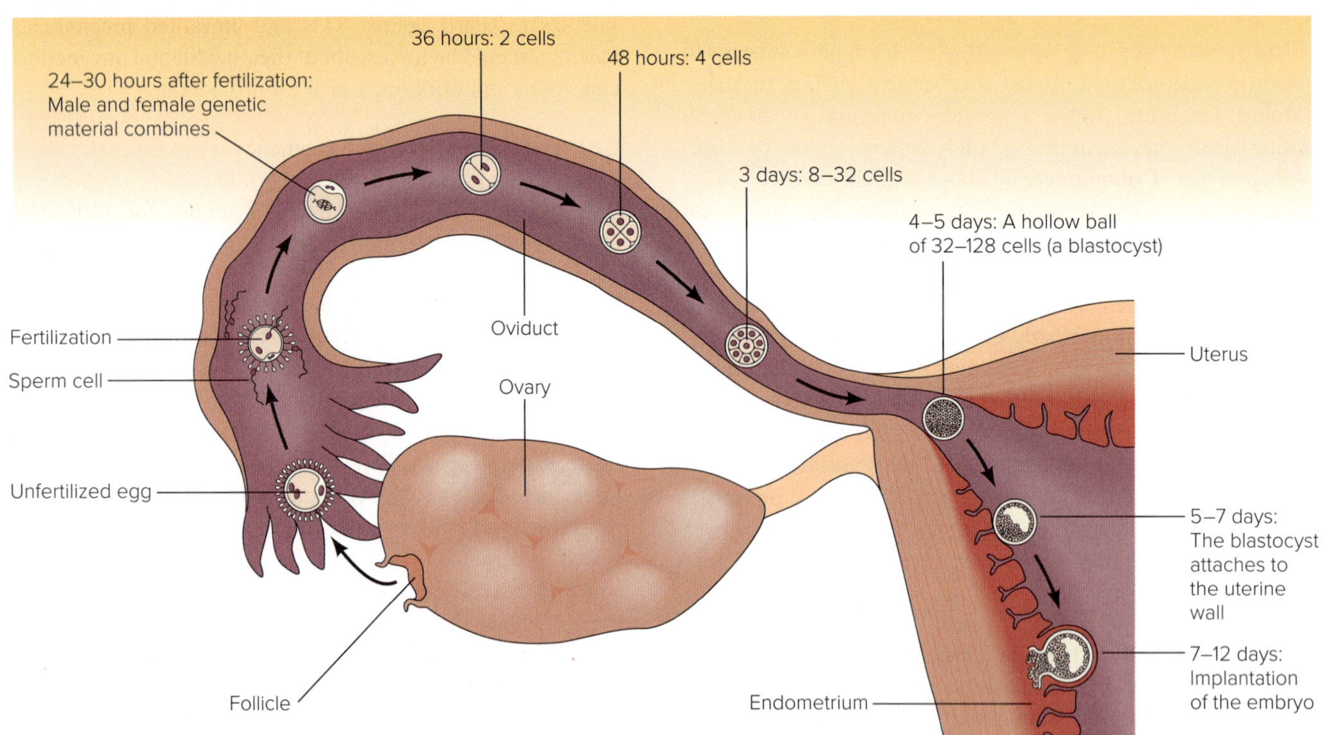


**FIGURE 6.5 Fertilization and early development of the embryo.**

## Ask Yourself

**QUESTIONS FOR CRITICAL THINKING AND REFLECTION**

If you don't have children now, do you plan to have them someday? Which skills and qualities make a good parent? Given what you know about yourself today, do you think you would be a good parent? What skills or qualities do you think you would need to develop?

of the egg, and fertilization occurs. The sperm's tail, its means of locomotion, is left behind on the egg's outer membrane, while the sperm's head is inside the egg. This event triggers a chemical change that makes the egg impenetrable to other sperm.

The ovum carries the hereditary characteristics of the mother and her family; sperm cells carry the hereditary characteristics of the father and his family. Each egg or sperm cell contains 23 chromosomes, each of which contains **genes,** which are packages of biochemical instructions for the developing baby. Genes provide the blueprint for a unique human based on the functional and health characteristics of their ancestors.

### Twins

In the usual course of events, one egg and one sperm unite to produce one fertilized egg and one baby. But if the ovaries release two eggs during ovulation and both eggs are fertilized, twins develop. These twins will be no more alike than siblings from different pregnancies because each will have come from a different fertilized egg. Twins who develop this way are referred to as **fraternal (dizygotic) twins;** they may be the same sex or different sexes. About 70% of twins are fraternal.

Twins can also develop from the early division of a single fertilized egg into two cells that develop separately. Because these babies share all genetic material, they will be **identical (monozygotic) twins.**

The most serious complication of multiple births is preterm delivery (delivery before the fetuses are adequately mature). The higher the number of fetuses a woman carries, the earlier in gestation she will deliver. This leads to higher rates of complications due to prematurity.

## INFERTILITY

More than 12% of the U.S. population (about 2 million couples) will seek infertility services due to difficulty conceiving. **Infertility** is defined as the inability to conceive after trying for a year or more. Infertility affects about 9% of American women of reproductive age (15–49 years) in the United States. Although the focus is often on women, one-fourth of the factors contributing to infertility are male, and in one-third (35%) of infertile couples, both partners have problems. Therefore, it is important that both partners be evaluated.

### Female Infertility

One-third of cases of female infertility usually result from one of two key causes—tubal blockage (14%) or failure to ovulate (21%). An additional one-third of cases of female infertility are due to anatomical abnormalities, benign growths in the uterus, thyroid disease, and other uncommon conditions; the remaining 28% of cases are unexplained.

Blocked oviducts are most commonly the result of *pelvic inflammatory disease* (*PID*), a serious complication of several STIs. Most cases of PID are associated with untreated cases of chlamydia or gonorrhea, both of which can occur without symptoms. Tubal blockages can also be caused by prior surgery or by *endometriosis,* a condition in which endometrial (uterine) tissue grows outside the uterus. Tubal blockage increases the risk of infertility and ectopic pregnancy, where the embryo develops outside the uterus.

Deterioration of organs through the wear and tear of aging also affects fertility. Beginning at around age 30, a woman's fertility naturally begins to wane. Age is probably the main factor in ovulation failure. Exposure to toxic chemicals, cigarette smoke, or radiation also appears to reduce fertility, as do genetic factors identifiable in your family history.

### Male Infertility

Male infertility accounts for about one-quarter of infertile couples. The leading causes of male infertility can be divided into four main categories: hypothalamic pituitary disease (1–2%), testicular disease (30–40%), disorders of sperm transport or posttesticular disorders (10–20%), and unexplained (40–50%). Some acquired disorders of the testes can lead to infertility, such as damage from drug use (including marijuana), smoking, infection, or environmental toxins.

### Treating Infertility

The cause of infertility can be determined for about 72–85% of infertile couples. Most cases of infertility are treated with conventional medical therapies. Surgery can repair oviducts, remove endometriosis, and correct anatomical problems in men and women. Fertility drugs can help women ovulate but may cause multiple births. If these conventional treatments don't work, couples can turn to **assisted reproductive technology (ART)** techniques, as described in the following sections. According to CDC data published in 2020, about 2% of births in the United States are the result of ART treatments.

Most infertility treatments are expensive and emotionally draining, with a live birth occurring in about a third of cases.

**TERMS**

**gene** The basic unit of heredity; a section of a chromosome containing biochemical instructions for making a particular protein.

**fraternal (dizygotic) twins** Twins who develop from separate fertilized eggs and thus are not genetically identical.

**identical (monozygotic) twins** Twins who develop from the division of a single zygote and thus are genetically identical.

**infertility** The inability to conceive after trying for a year or more.

**assisted reproductive technology (ART)** Advanced medical techniques used to treat infertility.

Some infertile couples choose not to try to have children, whereas others turn to adoption. Couples will need to balance the risks of age-related infertility with the competing demands of careers and academics.

**Intrauterine Insemination** Male infertility can sometimes be overcome by collecting and concentrating the man's sperm and introducing the semen by syringe into a woman's vagina or uterus, a procedure known as **artificial (intrauterine) insemination.** To increase the probability of success, the woman is often given fertility drugs to induce ovulation prior to the insemination procedure. The sperm can be provided by the woman's partner or a donor. Donor sperm are also used by single women and lesbian couples who want to conceive using artificial insemination. The success rate is about 5–20%. The wide range is due to age-related influences.

**IVF** A surgical technique used to overcome infertility, **in vitro fertilization (IVF)** involves surgically removing mature eggs from a woman's ovary and pairing the harvested eggs with sperm outside the woman's body (*in vitro*), in a laboratory dish. If eggs are successfully fertilized, one or more of the resulting embryos are inserted into the woman's uterus. The remaining embryos can then be frozen for future use.

There are disadvantages to IVF. Success rates determined by live birth rates vary from about 4% to 40% depending on the woman's age. It often costs more than $15,000 per procedure and may require five or more attempts to produce one live birth. IVF also increases the chance of twins or triplets, which in turn increases the risk of premature birth and maternal complications, including pregnancy-related hypertension and diabetes.

**Gestational Carrier** A *gestational carrier* is a fertile woman who agrees to carry a fetus for an infertile couple. The gestational carrier agrees to be artificially inseminated by the father's sperm or to undergo IVF with the couple's embryo, to carry the baby to term, and to give it to the couple at birth. In return, the couple pays her for her services and medical costs. It is estimated that 3% of all ART in the United States is performed through gestational carriers.

**Ask Yourself**

**QUESTIONS FOR CRITICAL THINKING AND REFLECTION**

Who gets to determine how and when a couple gets pregnant and has children? Can we stipulate reproductive behavior for other people?

**TERMS**

**artificial (intrauterine) insemination** The introduction of sperm into the vagina by artificial means.

**in vitro fertilization (IVF)** Combining eggs and sperm outside the body and inserting one or more fertilized eggs into the uterus.

**trimester** One of three 3-month periods of pregnancy.

# PREGNANCY

Pregnancy is usually discussed in terms of **trimesters**—three periods of about three months (or 13 weeks) each. During the first trimester, the mother experiences a few physical changes and some fairly common symptoms. During the second trimester, often the most peaceful time of pregnancy, the mother gains weight, looks noticeably pregnant, and may experience a general sense of well-being if she is happy about having a child. The third trimester is the hardest because the mother must breathe, digest, excrete, and circulate blood for herself and the growing fetus.

## Physical Changes with Pregnancy

Hormonal changes begin as soon as an egg is fertilized, and for the next nine months the body nourishes the fetus and adjusts to its growth (Figure 6.6).

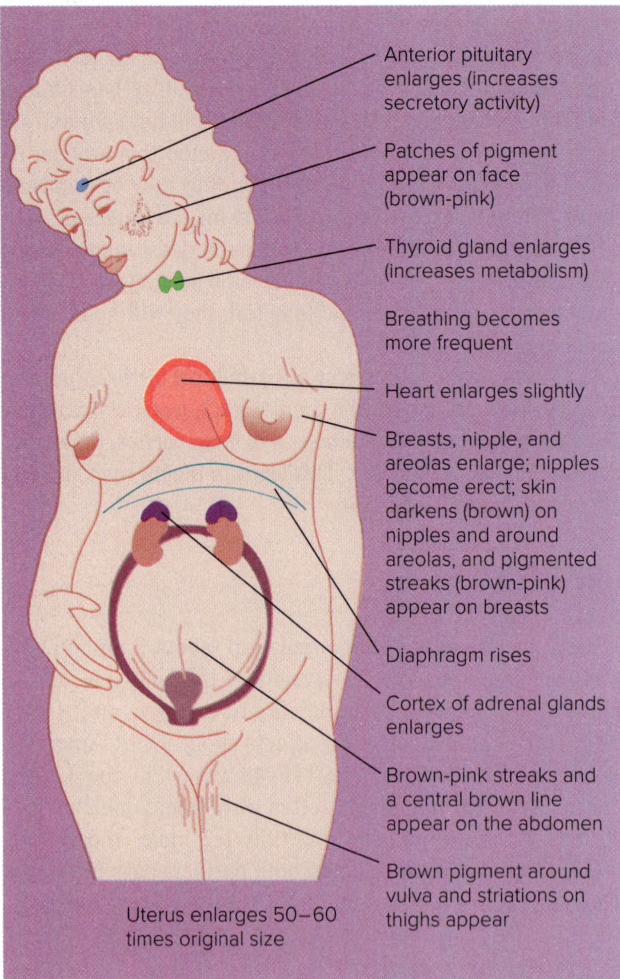


**FIGURE 6.6 Physiological changes during pregnancy.**

## CRITICAL CONSUMER
### Home Pregnancy Tests

Women have access to a variety of over-the-counter home pregnancy tests today, but generally speaking, these tests all work in the same way to determine whether a woman is pregnant. Pregnancy tests are designed to detect the presence of the hormone **human chorionic gonadotropin (hCG),** a hormone produced by the implanted fertilized egg, which is discussed in this chapter. Because the placenta releases hCG, the hormone can be detected in a woman's urine or blood when she is pregnant.

Although home pregnancy tests have become extremely accurate since their introduction in 1975, not all tests behave equally. A sensitive test will give a "positive" result with very low levels of hCG and can identify pregnancies earlier. A less sensitive test may not give an accurate result until hCG levels are much higher. Most kits will reliably detect 97% of pregnancies one week after a missed period.

Two types of home pregnancy tests are available—those that require the test strip to be dipped into urine, and those that require the user to urinate directly onto the test strip.

A clinical blood test is more accurate but not necessarily more sensitive than a home pregnancy test. A quantitative blood test, usually called a *beta hCG test,* measures the exact number of units of hCG in the blood. This type of test can detect even the most minimal level. Labs vary in what is considered a positive pregnancy test. Common cutoffs for positive are 5, 10, and 25 units. A level under 5 is considered negative.

Women need to use home pregnancy test kits with a clear understanding of their limitations. If you're comfortable waiting, a sensitive test taken a week after your period is due will almost certainly give you accurate results. If you elect to take the test as early as the day after you've missed your period, remember that a negative result cannot be relied upon. A positive result may mean either a viable pregnancy or a pregnancy destined to end shortly after it began. With either of those results, you should plan to test again a week later, just to be sure.

**Early Signs and Symptoms** Early recognition of pregnancy is important, especially for women with medical conditions. The following symptoms are not absolute indications of pregnancy, but they are reasons to visit a gynecologist, and maybe take a home pregnancy test (see the box "Home Pregnancy Tests"):

- ***A missed menstrual period.*** When a fertilized egg implants in the uterine wall, the endometrium is retained to nourish the embryo. A missed period within several weeks of having intercourse may indicate pregnancy.
- ***Light bleeding.*** Following implantation of the fertilized egg into the endometrial lining, a light bleed occurs in about 14% of pregnancies. Because this happens about when a period is expected, about two weeks after ovulation, the bleeding is sometimes mistaken for menstrual flow. It usually lasts only a few days.
- ***Nausea.*** Between 50% and 90% of pregnant women feel increased nausea, probably in reaction to surging levels of progesterone and other pregnancy hormones. Although this nausea is often called *morning sickness,* some will have symptoms all day long. It frequently begins during the 6th week and disappears by the 12th week. In some cases it continues throughout the pregnancy.
- ***Breast tenderness.*** Some women experience breast tenderness, swelling, and tingling, usually described as different from the tenderness experienced before menstruation.
- ***Increased urination.*** Increased frequency of urination can occur soon after the missed period.
- ***Sleepiness, fatigue, and emotional upset.*** These symptoms result from hormonal changes. Fatigue can be surprisingly overwhelming in the first trimester but usually improves significantly around the third month of pregnancy.

The first reliable physical signs of pregnancy can be distinguished about four weeks after a missed menstrual period. Increased uterine growth and blood flow contribute to softening of the uterus just above the cervix, called *Hegar's sign,* and a bluish discoloration to the cervix and labia minora, termed *Chadwick's sign.*

Four weeks after a woman misses her menstrual period, she is considered to be about eight weeks pregnant because pregnancy is calculated from the time of her last menstrual period rather than from the time of fertilization. The uterine lining buildup in the two weeks before fertilization is part of the gestation cycle, and the timing of ovulation and fertilization is often difficult to determine. Although a woman should see her physician to determine her due date, due dates can be approximated by subtracting three months from the date of the last menstrual period and then adding seven days. For example, a woman whose last menstrual period began on September 20 would have a due date of about June 27.

**Changes during Early Pregnancy** The most obvious changes occur in the reproductive organs. During the first three months, the uterus enlarges to about three times its nonpregnant size, but it still cannot be felt in the abdomen. By the fourth month, it is large enough to make the abdomen

**TERMS**

**human chorionic gonadotropin (hCG)** A hormone produced by a fertilized egg that encourages the body to support and maintain the pregnancy; it can be detected in the urine or blood of the mother shortly after conception.

| Table 6.1 Recommended Weight Gain during Pregnancy | |
|---|---|
| STATUS (BMI)* | WEIGHT GAIN (POUNDS) |
| Underweight (<18.5) | 28–40 |
| Normal (18.5–24.9) | 25–35 |
| Overweight (25–29.9) | 15–25 |
| Obese (>30) | 11–20 |

*BMI, or body mass index, allows comparison of body weight across different heights. (See Chapter 15 to calculate BMI.)

protrude. By the seventh or eighth month, the uterus pushes up under the rib cage, which makes breathing slightly more difficult. The breasts enlarge and are sensitive; by week 8, they may tingle or throb. The pigmented area around the nipple, called the *areola,* and the nipple itself darken and broaden. For some women, hyperpigmentation may show in the face or the midline of the abdomen.

Early in pregnancy, the muscles and ligaments attached to bones begin to soften and stretch. The joints between the pelvic bones loosen and spread, making it easier to have a baby but harder to walk. The circulatory system becomes more efficient to accommodate higher blood volume, and the heart pumps more rapidly. By the end of the second trimester, blood flows have already increased by 29%. By term, many women experience a blood volume expansion of 50% or greater. Much of the increased blood flow goes to the uterus and placenta (the organ that exchanges nutrients and waste between mother and **fetus**).

The average weight gain during a healthy pregnancy is 31.3 pounds, although actual weight change varies with the individual. Table 6.1 shows the weight gains recommended by the Institute of Medicine based on a woman's prepregnancy weight. About half the weight gain is directly related to the baby (to the placenta, for example); the rest accumulates over the woman's body as fluid and fat.

**Changes during the Later Stages of Pregnancy** By the end of the sixth month, the increased needs of the fetus place a burden on the mother's lungs, heart, and kidneys. Her back may ache from the pressure of the baby's weight and from having to throw her shoulders back to keep her balance while standing. Her body retains more water, perhaps up to three extra quarts of fluid. Her hands, legs, ankles, or feet may swell, and she may be bothered by leg cramps, heartburn, or constipation. Despite discomfort, both her digestion and her metabolism are working at top efficiency.

Near term, the uterus prepares for childbirth with a series of preliminary contractions, called **Braxton Hicks contractions.** Unlike true labor contractions, Braxton Hicks contractions are irregular with short duration; they are also often painless. To the mother, a contraction may initially feel only as though her abdomen is hard to the touch.

In the ninth month, increased joint laxity coupled by a softening cervix allows the baby to settle deeper into the pelvis. This process, called **lightening,** produces a visible change in the mother's abdominal profile. Pelvic pressure increases, and pressure on the diaphragm lightens. Breathing becomes easier; urination becomes more frequent. Sometimes, after a first pregnancy, lightening does not occur until labor begins.

TERMS

**fetus** The unfinished, developing product of human conception from its ninth week in the uterus to its birth.

**Braxton Hicks contractions** A pattern of late-pregnancy uterine contractions that are irregular in timing, short in duration, and painless and do not result in labor.

**lightening** A process in which the uterus sinks down because the baby's head settles into the pelvic area.

**blastocyst** The stage of embryonic development, days 4–7, before the cell cluster becomes the embryo and placenta.

### Emotional Responses to Pregnancy

Rapid changes in hormone levels can cause a pregnant person to experience unpredictable emotions. During the first trimester, a pregnant woman may fear that she will miscarry or that the child will not be normal. During the second trimester, a pregnant person can feel early fetal movements, and worries about miscarriages usually begin to diminish.

The third trimester is the time of greatest physical stress during the pregnancy. A woman may find that her physical abilities are limited by her size. Because some women feel physically awkward and sexually unattractive, they may experience periods of depression. But many also feel a great deal of happy excitement and anticipation.

## FETAL DEVELOPMENT

Now that we've seen what happens to the mother's body during pregnancy, let's consider the development of the fetus (Figure 6.7).

### The First Trimester

About 30 hours after an egg is first fertilized, the cell divides, and this process of cell division repeats many times. In these early stages, these cells can become any type of cell needed by the growing embryo. We call this ability to transform into multiple types of tissues *pluripotency.* While every cell contains a complete set of genetic instructions (chromosomes), cells that are destined to become liver tissue, for example, use a different part of the genetic instructions from cells that are destined to become eye tissue. This process is called *differentiation.*

On about the fourth day after fertilization, the cluster of rapidly developing cells arrives in the uterus as a **blastocyst,** a mostly hollow sphere of between 32 and 128 cells. The blastocyst attaches to the uterine wall on the sixth or seventh day,

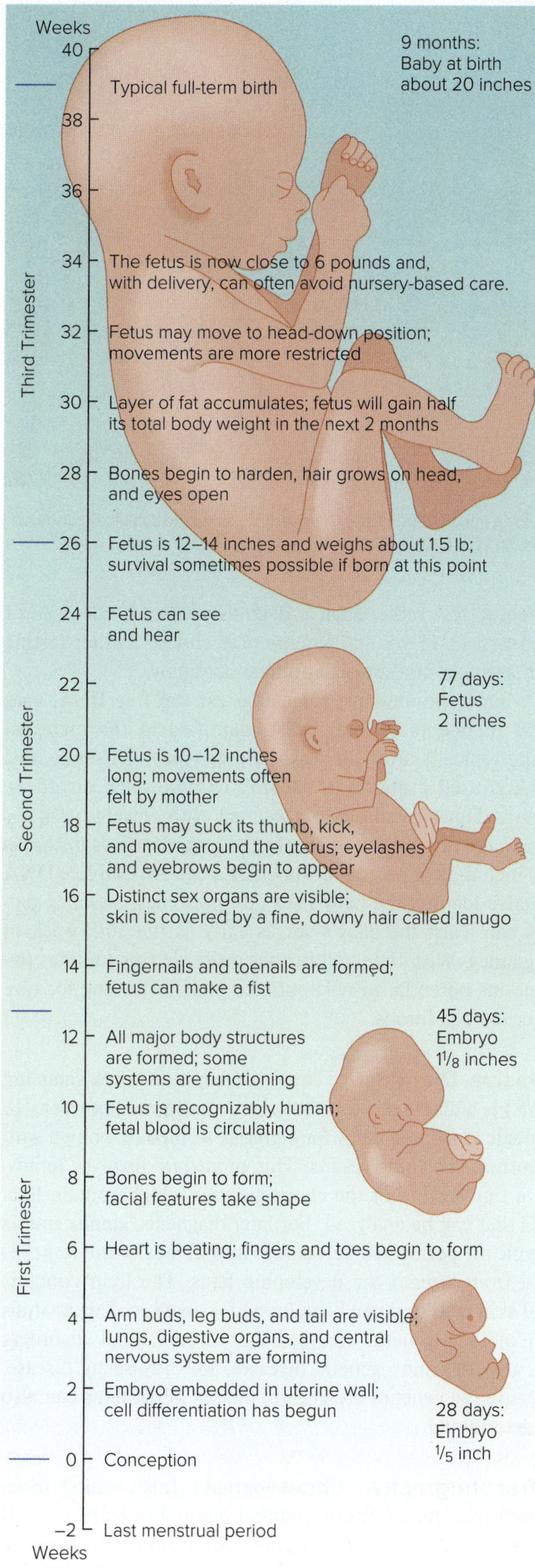


**FIGURE 6.7** **A chronology of milestones in prenatal development.**

allowing for implantation into the nourishing uterine lining. The blastocyst becomes an **embryo** by about the end of the second week after fertilization. The inner cells of the blastocyst separate into three layers. The innermost layer becomes the digestive and respiratory systems; the middle layer becomes muscle, bone, blood, kidneys, and sex glands; and the outer layer becomes the skin, hair, and nervous tissue.

The outermost shell of cells becomes the supporting structures of the pregnancy: the **placenta, umbilical cord,** and **amniotic sac.** A network of blood vessels called *chorionic villi* eventually forms the placenta. The human placenta allows a two-way exchange of nutrients and waste materials between the mother and fetus. The placenta brings oxygen and nutrients to the fetus and transports waste products out. The placenta does not provide a perfect barrier between fetal circulation and maternal circulation, however. Some genetic information is exchanged, and certain substances, such as alcohol as well as most vitamins, nutrients, sugar, and oxygen, pass freely from maternal circulation through the placenta to the fetus.

The period between weeks 2 and 9 is a time of rapid differentiation and change. All major body structures are formed during this time, including the heart, brain, liver, lungs, and sex organs. Eyes, nose, ears, arms, and legs also appear. Some organs begin to function, as well; the heart begins to beat, and the liver starts producing blood cells. Because body structures are forming, the developing organism is vulnerable to damage from environmental influences such as drugs and infections.

By the end of the second month, the fetal brain sends out impulses that coordinate the functioning of its other organs. The embryo is now a fetus, and further changes will be in the size and refinement of working body parts. In the third month, the fetus becomes active. By the end of the first trimester, at 13 weeks, the fetus is about an inch long and weighs less than one ounce.

## The Second Trimester

To grow during the second trimester, to about 14 inches and 1.5 pounds, the fetus requires large amounts of food, oxygen, and water, which come from the mother through the placenta. All body systems are operating, and the fetal heartbeat can be heard with a stethoscope. By the fourth or fifth month, the mother can detect early fetal movements that may feel like "flutters." A fetus born at 24–26 weeks has a better than

**TERMS**

**embryo** The stage of development between blastocyst and fetus; about weeks 2–8.

**placenta** The organ through which the fetus receives nourishment and empties waste via the mother's circulatory system; after birth, the placenta is expelled from the uterus.

**umbilical cord** The cord connecting the placenta and fetus, through which nutrients pass.

**amniotic sac** A membranous pouch enclosing and protecting the fetus; also holds amniotic fluid.

50% chance of survival. The age at which survival is possible depends on the development of lung tissue, which completes a critical step in weeks 24–26 of pregnancy. Prior to 23 weeks, survival without significant impairment is rare, occurring in 3–15% of cases.

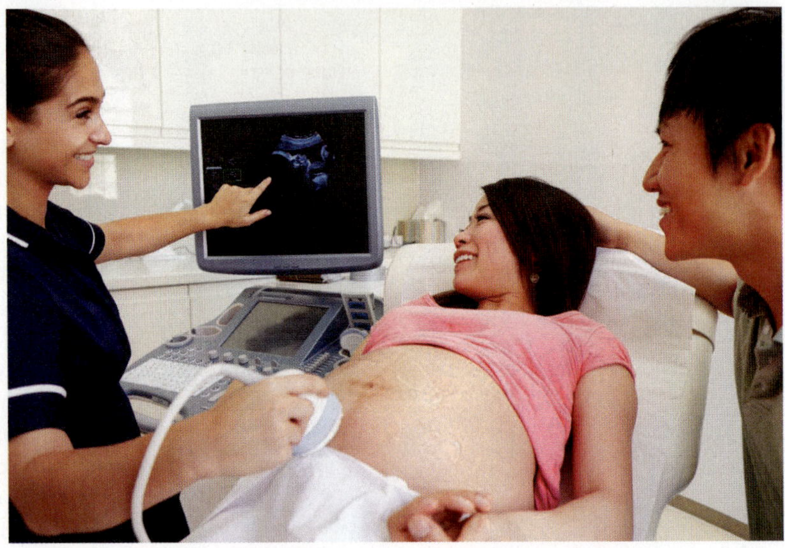

Ultrasonography provides information about the position, size, and physical condition of a fetus in the uterus. Monkey Business Images/Shutterstock

## The Third Trimester

The fetus gains most of its birth weight during the last three months of the pregnancy. Some of the weight is brown fat under the skin that insulates the fetus and supplies food. *Brown fat* is a special fat rich with blood supply that is found in hibernating mammals and newborns and is associated with protection against hypothermia. This is an important consideration because babies are often too small to generate much of their own heat and are too weak to move away from cold areas. The fetus also takes in other nutrients; about 85% of the calcium and iron the mother consumes goes into the fetal bloodstream.

The fetus also needs the immunity supplied by antibodies in the mother's blood during the final three months. The antibodies protect the fetus against many of the diseases to which the mother has acquired immunity.

## Diagnosing Fetal Abnormalities

About 2–4% of babies are born with a major birth defect. Information about the health and sex of a fetus can be obtained prior to birth through prenatal testing.

**Noninvasive Screening Tests** Maternal blood testing can be used to help identify fetuses with neural tube defects, Down syndrome, and other anomalies. Traditionally, blood is taken from the mother at 16–19 weeks of pregnancy and analyzed for four hormone levels—human chorionic gonadotropin (hCG), unconjugated estriol, alpha-fetoprotein (AFP), and inhibin-A. These four hormone levels, the **quadruple marker screen (QMS),** can be compared to appropriate standards, and the results are used to estimate the probability that the fetus has particular anomalies. This type of test is a screening test rather than a diagnostic test; in the case of abnormal QMS results, parents may choose further testing such as an amniocentesis or ultrasonography.

A newer noninvasive screening test, **cell-free DNA,** uses small fragments of fetal DNA identified in the maternal serum typically after 10 weeks of pregnancy. Currently, this DNA is used primarily to identify chromosomal disorders, such as Down syndrome, in women with elevated risk for *aneuploidy* (an abnormal number of chromosomes in the fetus) including in pregnant women over age 35. Cell-free DNA can also identify the baby's sex chromosomes, meaning parents can learn the baby's sex as early as the 10th week of pregnancy. With time and further research, this tool has tremendous potential to revolutionize prenatal testing for rare inherited conditions.

**Invasive Diagnostic Tests** **Chorionic villus sampling (CVS)** is a diagnostic test that can be performed in weeks 10 through 12 of pregnancy for high-risk women or women with abnormal screening results. This procedure involves removing a tiny section of the chorionic villi, which contain fetal cells that can be analyzed. For later diagnosis, **amniocentesis** is typically performed between 16 and 22 weeks and removes fluid from around the developing fetus. The fluid contains fetal skin cells that can be cultured for analysis. This analysis can include genetic analyses for chromosomal disorders but also for some genetic diseases, like Tay-Sachs disease. Because the genetics are known, the sex of the fetus can also be determined.

**Ultrasonography** **Ultrasonography** (also called *ultrasound*) uses high-frequency sound waves to create a visual image of the fetus in the uterus. Ultrasound can show the fetus's position, size, and gestational age, and it can identify the presence of certain anatomical problems. Ultrasound can also be used to determine the sex of the fetus.

**TERMS**

**quadruple marker screen (QMS)** A measurement of four hormones, used to assess the risk of fetal abnormalities.

**cell-free DNA** Fetal genetic material in the maternal blood supply, used to assess the risk of fetal genetic conditions, especially for fetuses already identified as having elevated risk.

**chorionic villus sampling (CVS)** Surgical removal of a tiny section of placental villi to be analyzed for genetic defects.

**amniocentesis** A process in which amniotic fluid is removed and analyzed to detect possible birth defects.

**ultrasonography** The use of high-frequency sound waves to view the fetus in the uterus; also known as *ultrasound*.

# THE IMPORTANCE OF PRENATAL CARE

Adequate prenatal care—as described in the following sections—is essential to the health of both mother and baby. All physicians recommend that women start getting regular prenatal checkups as soon as they become pregnant. Typically this means one checkup per month during the first eight months and then one checkup per week during the final month. Seventy-eight percent of pregnant women begin receiving adequate prenatal care by the fourth month of pregnancy; about 6% wait until the last trimester or receive no prenatal care at all.

## Regular Checkups

In the woman's first visit to her obstetrician, she will be asked for a detailed medical history and receive a complete physical exam. Her obstetrician will note any hereditary conditions that may assume increased significance during pregnancy. The tendency to develop gestational diabetes (diabetes during pregnancy only), for example, can be inherited; appropriate treatment during pregnancy reduces the risk of serious harm.

She returns for regular checkups throughout the pregnancy, during which her blood pressure and weight gain are measured, her urine is analyzed, and the fetus's size and position are monitored. Regular prenatal visits give the mother a chance to discuss her concerns and be assured that everything is proceeding normally. Physicians, midwives, health educators, and teachers of childbirth classes can provide the mother with valuable information.

## Blood Tests

A blood sample is taken during the initial prenatal visit to determine blood type and detect possible anemia or Rh incompatibilities. The **Rh factor** is a blood protein. If an Rh-positive father and an Rh-negative mother conceive an Rh-positive baby, the baby's blood will be incompatible with the mother's blood.

This condition is completely preventable with a serum called *Rh-immune globulin,* which coats Rh-positive cells as they enter the mother's body and prevents her immune system from recognizing them and forming antibodies. Blood may also be tested for evidence of hepatitis B, syphilis, rubella immunity, thyroid problems, and HIV infection.

## Prenatal Nutrition

A nutritious diet throughout pregnancy is essential for both the mother and her unborn baby. Not only does the baby get all its nutrients from the mother, but it also competes with her for nutrients not sufficiently available to meet both their needs. When a woman's diet is low in iron or calcium, the fetus receives most of it, and the mother may become deficient in the mineral. To meet the increased nutritional demands of her body, a pregnant woman shouldn't just eat more; she should make sure that her diet is nutritionally adequate.

To maintain her own health and help the fetus grow, a pregnant woman typically needs to consume about 250–500 extra calories per day. Breastfeeding an infant requires even more energy—about 500 or more calories per day. To ensure that she's getting enough calories and nutrients, a pregnant woman should talk to her physician or a registered dietician and determine what dietary changes she should make.

Supplements can help boost the levels of nutrients available to mother and child, helping with fetal development while ensuring that the mother doesn't become nutrient-deficient. Pregnant and lactating women, however, should not take supplements without the advice of their physicians because some vitamins, such as vitamin A, can be harmful if taken in excess. Pregnant women also should not take herbal dietary supplements without consulting a physician.

Two vitamins—vitamin D and folate—are particularly important to pregnant women. Pregnant women who do not get enough vitamin D are more likely to deliver low-birth-weight babies. Chronic vitamin D deficiency has been linked to other health problems, including heart disease.

If a woman does not get the recommended daily amount of folate, both before and during pregnancy, her child has an increased risk of neural tube defects, including spina bifida. Anyone capable of becoming pregnant should get at least 400 micrograms (0.4 milligram) of folic acid (the synthetic form of folate) daily from fortified foods or supplements, and also from folate occurring naturally in other foods. Pregnant women should get 400–800 micrograms (0.4–0.8 milligram) every day.

Food safety is another special dietary concern for pregnant women because foodborne pathogens can be especially dangerous to them and their unborn children. Germs and parasites such as *Listeria monocytogenes* and *Toxoplasma gondii* are both particularly worrisome. To avoid them, pregnant women should avoid eating undercooked and ready-to-eat meats (such as hot dogs and pre-packaged deli meats) and should wash produce thoroughly before eating it. Pregnant women should also follow the FDA's recommendations for consumption of fish and seafood.

## Avoiding Drugs and Other Environmental Hazards

Everything the mother ingests may eventually reach the fetus in some proportion. In addition to the food the mother eats, the drugs she takes and the chemicals she is exposed to affect the fetus. Some drugs harm the fetus but not the mother because the fetus is in the process of developing and because the proper dose for the mother is a proportionately massive dose for the fetus.

During the first trimester, when the major body structures are forming rapidly, the fetus is extremely vulnerable to environmental factors such as viral infections, radiation, drugs,

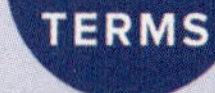


**Rh factor** A protein found in blood; Rh incompatibility between a mother and fetus can jeopardize the fetus's health.

and other **teratogens,** any of which can cause **congenital malformations,** or birth defects. As most organs are developing during the first trimester, exposures are of special concern during this critical window. The rubella (German measles) virus, for example, can cause congenital malformation of nerves supplying the eyes and ears in the first trimester, leading to blindness or deafness, but exposure to it later in the pregnancy does no damage. Another example, excess retinoic acid (vitamin A) exposure, can lead to spontaneous abortion and fetal malformations such as microcephaly and cardiac anomalies. Women who are taking medications known to cause birth defects must take care to avoid pregnancy.

QUICK STATS

**One to five percent of school-aged children in the United States have symptoms of fetal alcohol syndrome.**

—*Journal of American Medical Association*, 2018

**Alcohol** Alcohol is a potent teratogen. Although 1 in 10 pregnant women reports an alcohol exposure at some point, getting drunk just one time during pregnancy may be enough to cause damage in a fetus. A high level of alcohol consumption during pregnancy is associated with spontaneous miscarriage and stillbirth. Fetuses born to mothers who have consumed alcohol are at risk for **fetal alcohol syndrome (FAS).** A baby born with FAS is likely to be characterized by mental impairment, a small head and body size, unusual facial features, congenital heart defects, defective joints, impaired vision, and abnormal behavior patterns. Researchers doubt that any level of alcohol consumption is safe during pregnancy.

**Tobacco** Smoking is a preventable risk factor associated with miscarriage, low birth weight, preterm birth, infant death, and other pregnancy complications that may occur via direct damage to genetic material. Nicotine, the active ingredient in cigarette smoke, impairs oxygen delivery to the fetus and leads to faster fetal heart rates and reduced fetal breathing. Up to 34% of sudden infant death syndrome (SIDS) cases have been attributed to tobacco use.

**Caffeine** Caffeine, a powerful stimulant, puts both mother and fetus under stress by raising the level of the hormone epinephrine. Caffeine also reduces the blood supply to the uterus. A pregnant woman should limit her caffeine intake to no more than the equivalent of two cups of coffee per day.

**Drugs** Some prescription drugs, such as some blood pressure medications, can harm the fetus, so they should be used only under medical supervision. Antidepressant use in pregnancy can lead to withdrawal symptoms in newborns after delivery. Newborns may become fussy, with high-pitched, irritable cries, and develop difficulty feeding. Both prescription and over-the-counter drugs should be used only under a physician's direction. Large doses of vitamin A, for example, can cause birth defects.

Recreational drugs, such as cocaine, can increase the risk of miscarriage, stillbirth, growth abnormalities, major birth defects, and placental bleeding. Marijuana is associated with preterm birth and stillbirth. Methamphetamine use is associated with underweight babies.

TERMS

**teratogen** An agent or influence that causes physical defects in a developing fetus.

**congenital malformation** A physical defect existing at the time of birth, either inherited or caused during gestation.

**fetal alcohol syndrome (FAS)** A combination of birth defects caused by excessive alcohol consumption by the mother during pregnancy.

**Infections** Infections, including those that are sexually transmitted, are another serious problem for the fetus. The most common cause of life-threatening infections in newborns is group B streptococcus (GBS), a bacterium that can cause pneumonia, meningitis, and blood infections. As 25–30% of all pregnant women are carriers of GBS, screening at 36 weeks of pregnancy is recommended. A carrier or a woman who develops a fever during labor will be given intravenous antibiotics at the time of labor to reduce the risk of passing GBS to her baby.

Novel infections also pose the possibility of new risks. In 2020, the coronavirus pandemic raised new concerns about risks for pregnant people. A pregnant person with Covid-19 appears to bear a three times greater risk for needing intensive care or ventilation than a nonpregnant person. Those with severe disease are also at higher risk for complications in pregnancy, including preterm birth. Hand washing, mask wearing, and vaccination are the mainstays of prevention for coronavirus infection and are recommended by the CDC and women's health organizations in pregnancy.

Sexually transmitted infections, including syphilis, chlamydia, gonorrhea, and hepatitis B, are associated with increased risks during pregnancy and possible transmission to the infant at birth.

Nearly 90% of children diagnosed with human immunodeficiency virus (HIV) will have acquired it through pregnancy, birth, or breastfeeding.

## Prenatal Activity and Exercise

Physical activity during pregnancy contributes to mental and physical wellness (see the box "Physical Activity during Pregnancy"). Women can continue working at their jobs until late in their pregnancy, provided the work isn't so physically demanding that it jeopardizes their health. At the same time, pregnant women need more rest and sleep to maintain their own well-being and that of the fetus.

*Kegel exercises,* to strengthen the pelvic floor muscles, are recommended for pregnant women. These exercises are performed by alternately contracting and releasing the muscles used to stop the flow of urine. Each contraction should be held for about five seconds. Kegel exercises should be done several times a day for a total of about 50 repetitions daily.

## TAKE CHARGE
### Physical Activity during Pregnancy

Most pregnant people benefit from moderate-intensity physical activity. At least 2.5 hours of moderate aerobic activity per week is recommended during pregnancy and the postpartum period.

Maintaining a regular routine of physical activity throughout pregnancy can help a mother-to-be stay healthy and feel her best. Regular exercise can improve posture and decrease common pregnancy-related discomforts, such as backaches and fatigue. There is also evidence that physical activity may prevent gestational diabetes, relieve stress, and build stamina that can help during labor and delivery.

A person who was physically active before pregnancy should be able to continue her favorite activities in moderation, except for those that carry a risk of trauma, or unless there is a medical reason to reduce or stop exercise.

The American Congress of Obstetricians and Gynecologists (ACOG) offers advice regarding exercise during pregnancy. For example, downhill skiing or contact sports such as ice hockey, boxing, or soccer place pregnant people at risk for falls or abdominal trauma and should be avoided. Hot yoga and hot Pilates place the fetus at risk for overheating and are not recommended. In general, experts encourage low-impact aerobic activities such as walking or swimming over high-impact exercise. Physicians and pregnant women alike have concerns about exercise intensity. A good rule of thumb is never to exercise more than allows you to comfortably talk with a friend. If a pregnant person is out of breath while exercising, she should slow down! Experts also recommend proper hydration and dressing to avoid overheating.

A person who has never exercised regularly can safely start an exercise program during pregnancy after consulting with a health care provider. A routine of regular walking is considered safe. ACOG recommends that any pregnant person who exercises should stop if she experiences any of the following warning signs:

- Vaginal bleeding
- Increased shortness of breath
- Dizziness
- Headache
- Pain in the chest or calves
- Regular painful contractions
- Decreased fetal movement
- Leakage of amniotic fluid

For detailed information about physical activity, see Chapter 11.

SOURCES: American College of Obstetricians and Gynecologists. 2015. Committee Opinion No. 650: Physical activity and exercise during pregnancy and the postpartum period. *Obstetrics and Gynecology* 126(6): 1326–1327; U.S. Centers for Disease Control and Prevention. 2020. *Physical Activity Basics: Healthy Pregnant or Postpartum Women* (https://www.cdc.gov/physicalactivity/basics/pregnancy/index.htm).

## Preparing for Birth

Childbirth classes are almost a routine part of the prenatal experience for both mothers and fathers today. These classes typically teach details of the birth process as well as relaxation techniques to help deal with the discomfort of labor and delivery. Mothers learn and practice a variety of techniques so that they will be able to choose what works best for them during labor when the time comes. Their partners can help by supporting them emotionally and helping with her breathing and relaxing. They remain with the mother throughout labor and delivery, even when a cesarean section is performed.

# COMPLICATIONS OF PREGNANCY AND PREGNANCY LOSS

Complications can arise in pregnancy for myriad reasons: *maternal diseases and exposures* such as diabetes, hypertension, or tobacco use; *placental factors,* including abruption or placenta previa; or *fetal conditions* such as genetic conditions like Down syndrome or cystic fibrosis. Each complication benefits from early diagnosis, counseling, and, if possible, corrective action.

## Ectopic Pregnancy

In an **ectopic pregnancy,** the fertilized egg implants and begins to develop outside the uterus, usually in an oviduct. As the limited space of the oviduct cannot accommodate the rapid growth of a fertilized egg, ectopic pregnancies pose high risk of emergent bleeding through tubal rupture. Although ectopic pregnancies account for only 2% of all pregnancies, they contribute to 6% of all maternal deaths.

Ectopic pregnancies usually occur because of occlusion (blockage) of the fallopian tube, most often as a result of pelvic inflammatory disease, although smoking also increases a woman's risk for ectopic pregnancy. The embryo may spontaneously abort, or the embryo and placenta may continue to expand until they rupture the fallopian tube. Sharp pain on one side of the abdomen or in the lower back, usually in about the seventh or eighth week of pregnancy, may signal an ectopic pregnancy, and there may be irregular bleeding.

Ectopic pregnancy is considered an emergency and may require surgical removal of the embryo and the fallopian tube

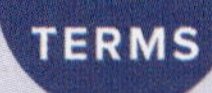


**ectopic pregnancy** A pregnancy in which the embryo develops outside the uterus, usually in an oviduct.

to save the mother's life. If diagnosed early, before the fallopian tube ruptures, ectopic pregnancy can often be treated successfully without surgery using the chemotherapy drug methotrexate.

## Spontaneous Abortion

A spontaneous abortion, or miscarriage, is the termination of pregnancy before the 20th week. Most miscarriages—about 60%—are due to chromosomal abnormalities in the fetus. Certain occupations that involve exposure to chemicals or radiation may increase the likelihood of a spontaneous abortion.

One miscarriage doesn't mean that later pregnancies will be unsuccessful. Seventy to ninety percent of women who miscarry eventually become pregnant again.

## Stillbirth

The terms *fetal death, fetal demise, stillbirth,* and *stillborn* all refer to the delivery of a fetus that shows no signs of life. Each year over 3 million stillbirths occur worldwide. In the United States, the stillbirth rate is a little more than 6 in 1000. Risk factors for stillbirth include smoking, maternal age greater than 40, multiple gestations, and chronic disease. Race is also a factor; Black women have twice as many stillbirths as non-Hispanic White, Hispanic, or Asian women. These biases are implicated in disparities in socioeconomic status and chronic disease.

## Preeclampsia

One in 25 pregnancies in the United States will be complicated by **preeclampsia,** a condition characterized by elevated blood pressure and the appearance of protein in the urine. Left untreated, preeclampsia will worsen over time, resulting in symptoms including headache, right upper-quadrant abdominal pain, vision changes, increased swelling, and weight gain. The most significant potential complications of preeclampsia are seizures, liver and kidney damage, bleeding, fetal growth restriction, and fetal death. Women with preeclampsia without severe features may be monitored closely outside of the hospital. More severe cases may require hospitalization for close medical management and early delivery.

**TERMS**

**preeclampsia** A condition of pregnancy characterized by high blood pressure and protein in the urine.

**placenta previa** A complication of pregnancy in which the placenta covers the cervical opening, preventing the mother from delivering the baby vaginally.

**placental abruption** A complication of pregnancy in which a normally implanted placenta separates prematurely from the uterine wall.

**gestational diabetes mellitus (GDM)** A form of diabetes that occurs during pregnancy.

## Placenta Previa

In **placenta previa,** the placenta either completely or partially covers the cervical opening, preventing the mother from delivering the baby vaginally. As a result, the baby must be delivered by cesarean section. This condition occurs in 1 in 250 live births. Risk factors include prior cesarean delivery, multiple pregnancies, intrauterine surgery, smoking, multiple gestations, and advanced maternal age.

## Placental Abruption

In **placental abruption,** a normally implanted placenta separates prematurely from the uterine wall. Patients experience abdominal pain, vaginal bleeding, and uterine tenderness. This causes 30% of all bleeding in the third trimester. The condition also increases the risk of fetal death. The risk factors for developing a placental abruption are maternal age, smoking, cocaine use, multiple gestation, trauma, preeclampsia, hypertension, and premature rupture of membranes.

## Gestational Diabetes

During gestation, about 7–18% of all pregnant women develop **gestational diabetes mellitus (GDM),** in which the body loses its ability to use insulin properly. In these women, diabetes occurs only during pregnancy. It is important to accurately diagnose and treat GDM because it can lead to preeclampsia, polyhydramnios (increased levels of amniotic fluid), large fetuses, birth trauma, operative deliveries, perinatal mortality, and neonatal metabolic complications. All women in pregnancy are therefore advised to test for GDM, which is a simple and straightforward procedure. GDM is usually treated by diet and exercise modification, and sometimes medication.

## Preterm Labor and Birth

When a pregnant woman goes into labor before the 37th week of gestation, she is said to experience *preterm labor.* Preterm labor is one of the most common reasons for hospitalizing pregnant women, but verifying true preterm labor from false labor can be difficult, and stopping it is even harder. About 30–50% of preterm labors resolve themselves, with the pregnancy continuing to full term. Preterm birth is the leading direct cause of newborn death, accounting for about one-third of all infant deaths. Preterm birth is also the main risk factor for newborn illness and death from other causes, particularly infection. Babies born prematurely appear to be at a higher risk of long-term health and developmental problems, including delayed development and learning problems.

Currently, the underlying causes for preterm labor remain poorly identified and require further research. Established risk factors for preterm birth include lack of prenatal care, smoking, drug use, stress, personal health history, infections or illness during pregnancy, obesity, exposure to environmental toxins, a previous preterm birth, and the carrying of multiple fetuses. However, only about half the women who give birth prematurely have any known risk factors.

> **Ask Yourself**
>
> **QUESTIONS FOR CRITICAL THINKING AND REFLECTION**
>
> Do you know anyone who has lost a child to miscarriage, stillbirth, or a birth defect? If so, how did they cope with their loss? What would you do to help someone in this situation?

### Labor Induction

If pregnancy continues well beyond the baby's due date, it may be necessary to induce labor artificially. This is one of the most common obstetrical procedures and is typically offered to pregnant women who have not delivered and are 7–14 days past their due dates.

### Low Birth Weight and Premature Birth

A **low-birth-weight (LBW)** baby is one that weighs less than 5.5 pounds at birth. LBW babies may be **premature** (born before the 37th week of pregnancy) or full-term. Babies who are born small even though they're full-term are referred to as *small-for-gestational-age* babies. Low birth weight affected 8.3% of babies born in the United States in 2019. About half of all cases are related to teenage pregnancy, cigarette smoking, poor nutrition, and poor maternal health. Other maternal factors include drug use, stress, depression, and anxiety. Adequate prenatal care is the best way to prevent LBW. Full-term LBW babies have fewer problems than premature infants.

### Infant Mortality and SIDS

The U.S. rate of **infant mortality,** the death of a child at less than 1 year of age, is near its lowest point ever—5.6 deaths for every 1000 live births as of 2019; however, that number remains far higher than rates in most of the developed world. Poverty and inadequate health care are key causes, with rates rising in poorer communities.

Forty-six percent of infant deaths are due to one of three leading factors: congenital abnormalities, prematurity/low birth weight, or **sudden infant death syndrome (SIDS).** SIDS is defined as a sudden and unexpected death of a child less than 1 year of age not explained by thorough investigation including autopsy. The CDC estimates that 33 babies die of SIDS for every 100,000 live births. Although statistics by race/ethnicity are difficult to compare across studies due to inconsistent data gathering, a 2020 CDC report shows that infant mortality rates are roughly twice as high for Black, Native Hawaiian, American Indian, and Alaska infants, compared to those of Hispanic, non-Hispanic white, and Asian infants.

Research suggests that abnormalities in the brain stem, the part of the brain that regulates breathing, heart rate, and other basic functions, underlie the risk for SIDS. Risk is increased greatly for infants with these innate differences if they are exposed to environmental risks such as tobacco smoke, alcohol, substance use, and, most important, sleeping stomach-side down. Because infants developmentally change how they sleep between 2 and 4 months of age, this is a time period of particular risk. Additionally, suffocation risk increases with the presence of many items common to cribs: fluffy pillows, mattresses, or plush toys. Therefore, current recommendations are to place babies to sleep back down, on a firm sleep surface, without soft bedding, plush toys, or additional clothing that might cause overheating. Several studies have found that the use of a pacifier significantly reduces the risk of SIDS.

## CHILDBIRTH

By the end of the ninth month of pregnancy, most women are tired of being pregnant; both parents are eager to start a new phase of their lives. Most couples find the actual process of birth to be an exciting and positive experience.

### Choices in Childbirth

Ninety-eight percent of babies in the United States in 2020 were delivered in hospitals. Less than 2% of births occur in freestanding birth centers where the environment may feel more comfortable while still remaining close to the medical resources of a hospital.

Health care providers will need to assess maternal and fetal health and make decisions together with prospective parents about appropriate care providers and delivery location.

### Labor and Delivery

The birth process occurs in three stages (Figure 6.8). **Labor** begins when hormonal changes in both the mother and the baby cause strong, rhythmic uterine **contractions.** These contractions exert pressure on the cervix and cause the lengthwise muscles of the uterus to pull on the circular muscles around the cervix, causing effacement (thinning) and dilation (opening) of the cervix. The contractions also pressure the baby to descend into the mother's pelvis, if it hasn't already. The entire process of labor and delivery usually takes between 2 and 36 hours, depending on the size of the baby, the baby's position in the uterus, the size of the

> **TERMS**
>
> **low birth weight (LBW)** Weighing less than 5.5 pounds at birth, often the result of prematurity.
>
> **premature** Born before the 37th week of pregnancy.
>
> **infant mortality** The death of a child at less than 1 year of age.
>
> **sudden infant death syndrome (SIDS)** The sudden death of an apparently healthy infant during sleep.
>
> **labor** A series of continuous, progressive uterine contractions that move the fetus through the birth canal and expel it with the placenta.
>
> **contraction** Shortening of the muscles in the uterine wall, which causes effacement and dilation of the cervix and assists in expelling the fetus.

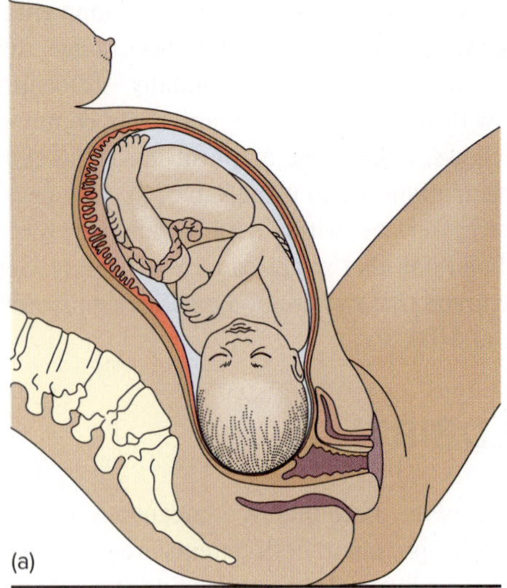


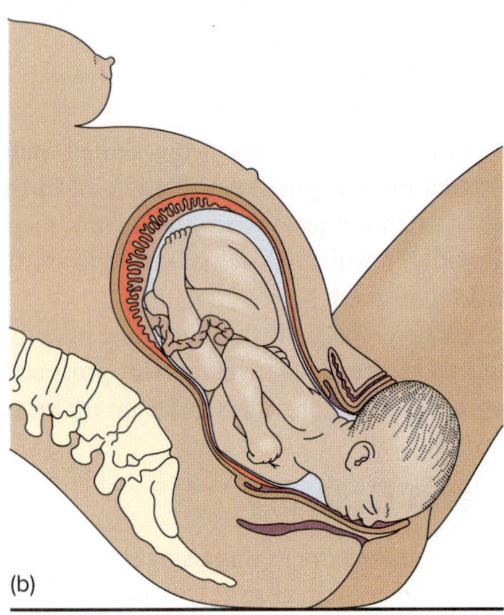


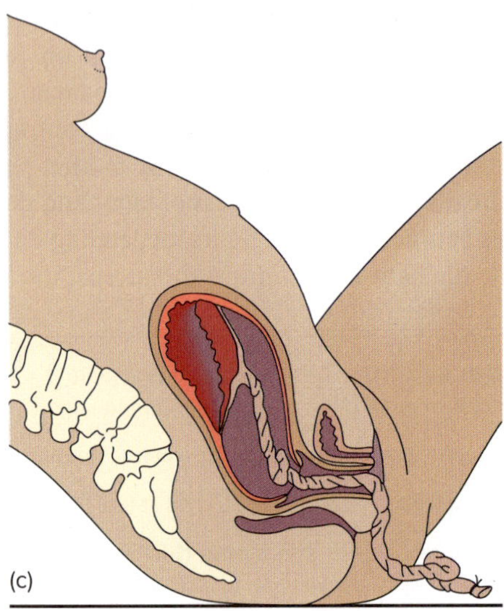


**FIGURE 6.8 Birth: labor and delivery.** (a) The first stage of labor contractions causes cervical effacement and dilation; (b) the second stage of labor: delivery of the baby; (c) the third stage of labor: expulsion of the placenta.

mother's pelvis, the strength of the uterine contractions, the number of prior deliveries, and other factors. The length of labor is generally shorter for subsequent births.

**The First Stage of Labor** The first stage of labor averages 13 hours for a first birth, although there is wide variation among women. It begins with cervical effacement and dilation and continues until the cervix is completely dilated. Contractions usually last about 30 seconds and occur every 15–20 minutes at first. They occur more often later. The prepared mother relaxes as much as possible during these contractions to allow labor to proceed without being blocked by tension. Early in the first stage, a small amount of bleeding may occur as a plug of slightly bloody mucus that blocked the opening of the cervix during pregnancy is expelled. In some women, the amniotic sac ruptures and the fluid rushes out; this is sometimes referred to as "breaking water."

The last part of the first stage of labor, called **active labor,** is characterized by strong and frequent contractions, much more intense than in the early stages of labor. Contractions may last 60–90 seconds and occur every 1–3 minutes. During active labor the cervix opens completely, to a diameter of about 10 centimeters. When the head of the fetus is flexed forward, to present its smallest diameter, the opening measures 9–10 centimeters. Therefore, a completely dilated cervix should permit the passage of the fetal head.

**The Second Stage of Labor** The second stage of labor is the "pushing phase." It begins with the cervix completely dilated to 10 cm and ends with the delivery of the baby. With uterine contractions and maternal pushing, the baby descends through the bones of the pelvis, past the cervix, and into the vagina, which it stretches open. Some women find this the most difficult part of labor; others find that the contractions and bearing down bring a sense of relief. The baby's head and body turn to fit through the narrowest parts of the passageway, and the soft bones of the baby's skull move together and overlap as it is squeezed through the pelvis. When the top of the head appears at the vaginal opening, the baby is said to be *crowning*.

As the head of the baby emerges, the physician or midwife will check to ensure that the umbilical cord is not around the neck. With a few more contractions, the baby's shoulders and body emerge. As the baby is squeezed through the pelvis, cervix, and vagina, amniotic fluid in the lungs is forced out by the pressure on the baby's chest. Once this pressure is released as the baby emerges from the vagina, the chest expands and the lungs fill with air for the first time. The baby will appear wet and often is covered with a cheesy substance called *vernix*. The baby's head may be oddly shaped at first, due to the molding of the soft plates of bone during birth, but it usually takes on a more rounded appearance within 24 hours.

**TERMS**

**active labor** The last part of the first stage of labor, during which the cervix becomes fully dilated; characterized by intense and frequent contractions.

**The Third Stage of Labor** In the third stage of labor, the uterus continues to contract until the placenta is expelled. This stage usually takes 5–30 minutes. The entire placenta must be expelled; if part remains in the uterus, it may cause bleeding and infection. Breastfeeding soon after delivery helps control uterine bleeding because it stimulates secretion of a hormone that makes the uterus contract.

The baby's physical condition is assessed with the **Apgar score,** a formalized system for assessing the baby's physical condition and whether medical assistance is needed. Heart rate, respiration, color, reflexes, and muscle tone are rated individually with a score of 0–2, and a total score between 0 and 10 is given at 1 and 5 minutes after birth. A score of 7–10 at 5 minutes is considered normal. Most newborns are also tested for 29 specific disorders, some of which are life-threatening. The American Academy of Pediatrics endorses these tests, but they are not routinely performed in every state.

**Pain Relief during Labor and Delivery** Women vary in how much pain they experience in childbirth. First babies are typically the most challenging to deliver because the birth canal has never stretched to this extent before. It is recommended that women and their partners learn about labor and what kinds of choices are available for pain relief. Childbirth preparation courses are a good place to start, and communicating with one's obstetrician or midwife is essential to assessing pain relief options. Pain can be modified by staying active in labor, laboring in water, and using breathing and relaxation techniques, including hypnosis.

Medical pain relief can come in the form of intravenous narcotics, which are short-acting and can be used only in early labor. If a baby is born under the influence of narcotics, it can appear floppy and without vigor. The most commonly used medical intervention for pain relief is the *epidural injection*. This procedure involves placing a thin plastic catheter between the vertebrae in the lower back. Medication that reduces the transmission of pain signals to the brain is given through this catheter. Regional anesthetic drugs are given in low concentration to minimize weakening of the leg muscles so that the mother can push effectively during the birth. The advantage of the epidural is that the medication is used in low amounts in the confined space of the spinal column, protecting the fetus from the effect of the medication. The mother is awake and is an active participant in the birth.

Local anesthesia is available for repair of any tear or **episiotomy** (a surgical incision of the perineum to allow easier delivery of the baby) if the mother has not used an epidural for the labor.

**Cesarean Delivery** In a **cesarean section,** the baby is removed through a surgical incision in the abdominal wall and uterus. Cesarean sections are necessary when a baby can't be delivered vaginally—for example, if the baby's head is bigger than the mother's pelvis or if the baby is not head down at the time of labor. If the mother has a serious health condition such as high blood pressure, a cesarean may be safer for her than labor and a vaginal delivery. Cesareans are more common among women who are overweight or have diabetes. Other reasons for cesarean delivery include abnormal or difficult labor, fetal distress, and the presence of a dangerous infection like herpes that can be passed to the baby during vaginal delivery.

Repeat cesarean deliveries are also very common. In 2019, 88.4% of American women who had had one child by cesarean had subsequent children delivered the same way. Although the risk of complications from a vaginal delivery after a previous cesarean delivery is low, there is a small (1%) risk of serious complications for the mother and baby if the previous uterine scar opens during labor (uterine rupture). For this reason, women and their physicians may choose to deliver by elective repeat cesarean.

Cesarean section is the most common hospital procedure performed in the United States. High rates have prompted health officials to examine ways to reduce cesarean sections, leading to a successful reduction over the past years. The safest mode of delivery for both mother and baby in an uncomplicated pregnancy is a vaginal delivery. Like any major surgery, cesarean section carries a longer recovery period and additional risks. Most cesarean deliveries are performed with regional anesthetic, which permits the mother to remain awake for the surgery with her partner present.

QUICK STATS

**32% of American babies born in 2019 were delivered by cesarean section.**

—Centers for Disease Control and Prevention, 2021

## The Postpartum Period

The **postpartum period,** a stage of about three months following childbirth, is a time of critical family adjustments.

### Ask Yourself

**QUESTIONS FOR CRITICAL THINKING AND REFLECTION**

If you are considering pregnancy, what are your views on labor and delivery options? If you have a child in the future, which facility, delivery, and pain management options do you think you would prefer? How might you support someone in labor? What steps do you think could be taken to help new parents at home? In the workplace?

TERMS

**Apgar score** A formalized system for assessing a newborn's need for medical assistance.

**episiotomy** An incision made in the perineum to widen the vaginal opening to facilitate birth and prevent uncontrolled tearing during delivery.

**cesarean section** A surgical incision through the abdominal wall and uterus, performed to deliver a fetus.

**postpartum period** The period of about three months after delivering a baby.

Parenthood begins literally overnight, and the transition can cause considerable stress.

**Breastfeeding** **Lactation,** the production of milk, begins about three days after childbirth. Prior to that time (sometimes as early as the second trimester), **colostrum** is secreted by the nipples. Colostrum contains antibodies that help protect the newborn from infectious diseases; it is also high in protein.

The American Academy of Pediatrics recommends breastfeeding exclusively for six months, then in combination with solid food until the baby is one year of age, and then for as long after that as a mother and baby desire. Currently only 25.6% of U.S. mothers breastfeed exclusively for six months. Human milk is perfectly suited to the baby's nutritional needs and digestive capabilities, and it supplies the baby with antibodies. Breastfeeding decreases the incidence of infant infection and diarrhea and appears to decrease diabetes and childhood obesity.

Breastfeeding is beneficial to the mother as well. It stimulates contractions that help the uterus return to normal more rapidly, contributes to postpregnancy weight loss, and may reduce the risk of breast and ovarian cancers. Nursing also provides a sense of closeness and emotional well-being for mother and child.

Some women find breastfeeding difficult: They may not have enough milk or the milk will not circulate properly. Sometimes babies refuse to nurse at the breast. Tenderness or infection of the nipples can also be a constraint. An advantage to bottlefeeding is that it is easier to tell how much milk an infant is taking in, and bottlefed infants tend to sleep longer. Bottlefeeding also allows the father or other caregiver to share in the nurturing process. Both breastfeeding and bottlefeeding can be part of loving, secure parent-child relationships.

**Postpartum Depression** The physical stress of labor, blood loss, fatigue, decreased sleep, fluctuating postpartum hormone levels, and anxieties of becoming a new parent all contribute to emotional instability postpartum. About 50–80% of new mothers experience "baby blues," characterized by episodes of sadness, weeping, anxiety, headache, sleep disturbances, and irritability. A mother may feel lonely and anxious about caring for her infant.

According to a 2018 CDC study, 13% of new mothers experience **postpartum depression.** Postpartum depression is characterized by a prolonged period of anxiety, guilt, fear, or self-blame; these feelings prevent the new mother from normal participation in everyday life or the normal care of her newborn. Those close to the affected woman may fear for the well-being of the mother or those in her care. Fortunately, postpartum depression can be prevented and treated effectively. Women with a history of depression or depression during pregnancy can benefit from early referral to an appropriate mental health care provider. Rest is a key component of recovery. The mother's support system should offer to take on important responsibilities to allow the mother to rest and recover, as well as encourage her to continue outside interests and share her concerns with a professional who can assess the need for medical therapy.

Some men also seem to get a form of postpartum depression, characterized by anxiety about their changing roles and feelings of inadequacy. Both mothers and fathers need time to adjust to their new roles as parents.

**Attachment** Another feature of the postpartum period is the development of attachment—the strong emotional tie that

**TERMS**

**lactation** The production of milk.

**colostrum** A yellowish fluid secreted by the mammary glands around the time of childbirth until milk comes in, about the third day.

**postpartum depression** An emotional low that may be experienced by the mother following childbirth.

## Ask Yourself

**QUESTIONS FOR CRITICAL THINKING AND REFLECTION**

What are some early signs or symptoms of depression? Consider ways you might start a conversation about depression or help a new mother find access to help. What kinds of things might you say or do?

## TIPS FOR TODAY AND THE FUTURE

A healthy sexual life is built on acceptance of yourself and good communication with your partners, as is recognizing that parenthood means making responsible choices and preparing for it long before pregnancy.

**RIGHT NOW YOU CAN:**

- Articulate to yourself your beliefs about sexual relationships. Consider whether you are acting in accordance with them. Your beliefs may be different from those of your partners, family, and caregivers.
- If you're in a sexual relationship, consider the information you and your partner have shared about sex. Are you comfortable that you know enough about each other to have a safe, healthy sexual relationship?
- Take some time to think about whether you really want to have children. Cut through the cultural, societal, family, and personal expectations that may stand in the way of making the decision you really want to make.

**IN THE FUTURE YOU CAN:**

- If you're in a sexual relationship, or if you plan to begin one, open (or reopen) a dialogue about sex. Make time to talk at length about the responsibilities and consequences of a sexual relationship.
- If you want to be a parent someday, start looking at the many sources of information about pregnancy, childbirth, and parenting. This is a good idea for anyone who plans to have a family.

grows between the baby and the adult who cares it. Parents can foster secure attachment relationships in the early weeks and months by responding sensitively to the baby's true needs. Parents who respond appropriately to the baby's signals of gazing, looking away, smiling, and crying establish feelings of trust in their child. They feed the baby when she's hungry, for example; respond when she cries; interact with her when she gazes, smiles, or babbles; and stop stimulating her when she frowns or looks away. A secure attachment relationship helps the child develop and function well socially, emotionally, and mentally.

## SUMMARY


- Human sexuality is a natural capacity, but how humans express their sexuality is profoundly shaped by culture and society.
- Language categories and labels are always changing in response to society's understanding of sex and gender. New terms for nonconforming identities and sexual orientations reflect the huge diversity that exists among human beings.
- Biologic sex is based on chromosomes and the genital structures that develop prenatally. Gender refers to the social roles and identities that are associated with one's biologic sex. Gender roles and identities are human creations and vary around the world and over time.
- At conception, all humans have the same undifferentiated sex organs: gonads, genitals, urogenital sinus, and ducts.
- In males, Wolffian ducts develop into the epididymis, vas deferens, and seminal vesicles connected through the urethra and penis. In females, Mullerian ducts become the uterus, fallopian tubes, and upper part of the vagina.
- Sexual activity involves stimulus and response. Sources of sexual stimulation are complex and can be physical and psychological.
- Physical, psychological, and social relationship problems can interfere with sexual functioning. Treatments for sexual disorders should consider all underlying sources and should not rely solely on medical approaches.
- Fertilization is a complex process culminating when a sperm penetrates the membrane of the egg released from the woman's ovary.
- Early signs and symptoms of pregnancy include a missed menstrual period; slight bleeding; nausea; breast tenderness; increased urination; fatigue and emotional upset; and a softening of the uterus just above the cervix.
- During pregnancy, the uterus enlarges until it pushes up into the rib cage; the breasts enlarge and may secrete colostrum; the muscles and ligaments soften and stretch; and the circulatory system, lungs, and kidneys become more efficient.
- The fetal anatomy is almost completely formed in the first trimester and is refined in the second; during the third trimester, the fetus grows and gains most of its weight, storing nutrients in fatty tissues.
- Important elements of prenatal care include good nutrition; avoidance of drugs, alcohol, tobacco, infections, and other harmful environmental agents or conditions; and regular physical activity.
- Pregnancy usually proceeds without major complications. Problems that can occur include ectopic pregnancy, spontaneous abortion, preeclampsia, low birth weight, and preterm birth.
- The first stage of labor begins with contractions that exert pressure on the cervix, causing effacement and dilation. The second stage begins with complete cervical dilation and ends when the baby is delivered. The third stage of labor is expulsion of the placenta.
- During the postpartum period, the mother's body begins to return to its prepregnancy state, and she may begin to breastfeed. Both mother and father must adjust to their new roles as parents as they develop a strong emotional bond with their baby.


## FOR MORE INFORMATION

*American Congress of Obstetricians and Gynecologists (ACOG).* Provides written materials relating to many aspects of preconception care, pregnancy, and childbirth.

http://www.acog.org

*American Psychological Association: Answers to Your Questions about Transgender People, Gender Identity, and Gender Expression.* Offers question-and-answer format sections on transgender and homosexuality.

http://www.apa.org/topics/sexuality/transgender.aspx

*Centers for Disease Control and Prevention, National Center on Birth Defects and Developmental Disabilities.* Provides information about a variety of topics related to birth defects, including fetal alcohol syndrome and the importance of folic acid.

http://www.cdc.gov/ncbddd

*Eunice Kennedy Shriver National Institute of Child Health and Human Development.* Provides information about reproductive and genetic problems; sponsors the "Safe to Sleep" campaign to fight SIDS.

http://www.nichd.nih.gov/sts

*The Guttmacher Institute.* A leading research and policy organization committed to advancing sexual and reproductive health and rights in the United States and globally. They provide a wealth of information and resources about sexual and reproductive health.

http://www.guttmacher.org

*Health Resources and Services Administration (HRSA): Maternal and Child Health.* Provides publications, videos, and other resources relating to maternal, infant, and family health.

http://www.mchb.hrsa.gov

*International Council on Infertility Information Dissemination.* Provides information about current research and treatments for infertility.

http://www.inciid.org

*The Kinsey Institute for Research in Sex, Gender, and Reproduction.* One of the oldest and most respected institutions doing research on sexuality.

http://www.kinseyinstitute.org

*Media Education Foundation.* Excellent series of videos analyzing gender and sexuality in mass media, popular culture, and advertising. Videos often include teaching guides.

http://www.mediaed.org/

*MedlinePlus* (National Library of Medicine). Excellent readable materials on human biology, including genes, chromosomes, typical and atypical.

https://medlineplus.gov/genetics/chromosome/y/

*National Women's Health Network.* A pioneering network for providing science, evidence-based information on women's health and reproductive issues and related products.

http://www.nwhn.org

*Rape, Abuse, and Incest National Network (RAINN).* This group provides information, counseling, and support for those concerned about sexual abuse, rape, and incest.

http://www.rainn.org

## SELECTED BIBLIOGRAPHY


Aguree, S., and A. D. Gernand. 2019. Plasma volume expansion across healthy pregnancy: A systematic review and meta-analysis of longitudinal studies. *BMC Pregnancy and Childbirth* 19(508).

American College of Obstetricians and Gynecologists. 2019. *ACOG Committee Opinion: Prepregnancy Counseling.* Washington, DC: American College of Obstetricians and Gynecologists.

Bauman, B., et al. 2020. Vital signs: Postpartum depressive symptoms and provider discussions about perinatal depression—United States, 2018. *Morbidity and Mortality Weekly Report* 69(19): 575–581.

Cantor, D., et. al. 2020. *Report on the AAU Campus Climate Survey on Sexual Assault and Sexual Misconduct.* Association of American Universities.

Centers for Disease Control and Prevention. 2018. *Let's Stop HIV Together* (https://www.cdc.gov/actagainstaids/campaigns/ottl/faq.html).

Centers for Disease Control and Prevention, American Society for Reproductive Medicine, Society for Assisted Reproductive Technology. 2018. *2016 Assisted Reproductive Technology National Summary Report.* Atlanta (GA): U.S. Department of Health and Human Services.

Centers for Disease Control and Prevention. 2022. *Breastfeeding Report Card United States, 2022* (http://www.cdc.gov/breastfeeding/data/reportcard.htm).

Child Care Aware of America. 2020. Picking up the pieces—Building a better child care system post COVID 19. (https://www.childcareaware.org/our-issues/research/the-us-and-the-high-price-of-child-care-2019/). Appendix 1 (https://usa.childcareaware.org/advocacy-publicpolicy/resources/research/costofcare/).

Cystic Fibrosis Foundation. 2021. *Patient Registry 2020 Annual Data Report.* Bethesda, MD.

Dietary Guidelines Advisory Committee. 2020. *Scientific Report of the 2020 Dietary Guidelines Advisory Committee: Advisory Report to the Secretary of Agriculture and the Secretary of Health and Human Services.* U.S. Department of Agriculture, Agricultural Research Service, Washington, DC.

Drake, P., A. K. Driscoll, and T. J. Mathew. 2018. Cigarette smoking during pregnancy: United States, 2016. *NCHS Data Brief, no 305.* Hyattsville, MD. National Center for Health Statistics.

Else-Quesi, N. M., and J. S. Hyde. 2018. *The Psychology of Women And Gender: Half the Human Experience+.* Los Angeles: SAGE.

Ely, D., and A. Driscoll. 2020. Infant mortality in the United States, 2018: Data from the Period Linked Birth/Infant Death File. *National Vital Statistics Reports* 69(7). Hyattsville, MD. National Center for Health Statistics.

Fine, C. 2017. *Testosterone Rex: Myths of Sex, Science, and Society.* New York: Norton.

Gregory, E., et al. 2021. Changes in home births by race and Hispanic origin and state of residence of mother: United States, 2018–2019 and 2019–2020. *National Vital Statistics Reports* 70(15). Hyattsville, MD. National Center for Health Statistics.

Herdt, G. and N. Polen-Petit. 2021. *Human Sexuality: Self, Society, and Culture,* 2nd ed. New York: McGraw Hill.

Human Rights Campaign Foundation. 2022. *We Are Here: Understanding the Size of the LGBTQ+ Community* (https://hrc-prod-requests.s3-us-west-2.amazonaws.com/We-Are-Here-120821.pdf).

Hyde, J. S., and J. Delamater. 2020. *Understanding Human Sexuality.* 14th ed. New York: McGraw Hill.

Johnson, J. L., et al. 2015. Trends in gestational weight gain: The pregnancy risk assessment monitoring system, 2000–2009. *American Journal of Obstetrics & Gynecology* 212(6): 806.e1–086.e8.

Jones, J. M. 2022. LGBT identification in U.S. ticks up to 7.1%. *Gallup* (https://news.gallup.com/poll/389792/lgbt-identification-ticks-up.aspx).

LaPonsie, M. 2021. How much does it cost to raise a child? *U.S. News & World Report* (https://money.usnews.com/money/personal-finance/articles/how-much-does-it-cost-to-raise-a-child).

Levey, T. 2018. Sexual Harassment Online. Shaming and Silencing Women in the Digital Age. Boulder, CO: Lynne Rienner.

Martin, J. A., et al. 2021. Births: Final data for 2019. *National Vital Statistics Reports* 70(2). Hyattsville, MD: National Center for Health Statistics.

Mattison, D. R., et al. (eds.). 2003. *Institute of Medicine (US) Roundtable on Environmental Health Sciences, Research, and Medicine.* Washington (DC): National Academies Press (US) (https://www.ncbi.nlm.nih.gov/books/NBK216221/).

May, P., et al. 2018. Prevalence of fetal alcohol spectrum disorders in 4 US communities. *Journal of American Medical Association* 319(5): 474–482.

Mukhopadhyay, C., and T. Blumenfield. 2020. Gender and sexuality. In *Perspectives: An Open Introduction to Cultural Anthropology*, 2nd ed. (https://perspectives.pressbooks.com/chapter/gender-and-sexuality/).

Nagoski, Emily. 2015. *Come As You Are.* New York: Simon & Schuster.

National Center for Health Statistics. 2021. *Infertility* (https://www.cdc.gov/nchs/nsfg/key_statistics/i-keystat.htm#infertilityservices)

Orenstein, P. 2020. *Boys and Sex: Young Men on Hookups, Love, Porn, Consent, and Navigating the New Masculinity.* New York: Harper.

Ottaviani, G. 2014. *Crib Death—Sudden Infant Death Syndrome (SIDS): Sudden Infant and Perinatal Unexplained Death: The Pathologist's Viewpoint.* Berlin: Springer International.

Perkins K. M., et al., NASS Group. 2016. Trends and outcomes of gestational surrogacy in the United States. *Fertility and Sterility* 106: 435–442.

Pruitt, S., et al. 2020. Racial and ethnic disparities in fetal deaths—United States, 2015–2017. *Morbidity and Mortality Weekly Report* 69(37): 1277–1282.

Rippon, G. 2019. *Gender and the Brain.* New York: Vintage Books edition 2020.

Rostosky, S. S., and E. D. B. Riggle. 2015. *Happy Together: Thriving as a Same-Sex Couple in Your Family, Workplace, and Community.* Washington DC: American Psychological Association.

Society for Maternal Fetal Medicine (SMFM). 2021. *COVID-19 and Pregnancy: What Maternal Fetal Medicine Subspecialists Need to Know.* Washington, DC: (https://smfm.org/covidclinical).

Sunderam, S., et al. 2020. Assisted reproductive technology surveillance—United States, 2017. *MMWR Surveillance Summaries* 69(9):1–20.

U.S. Department of Health and Human Services, Office on Women's Health. 2021. *Preconception Health.* Washington, DC (https://www.womenshealth.gov/pregnancy/you-get-pregnant/preconception-health/).

Wade, L. 2017. *American Hookup: The New Culture of Sex on Campus.* New York: Norton.

Xu, J., et al. 2021. Deaths: Final data for 2019. *National Vital Statistics Reports* 70(8). Hyattsville, MD: National Center for Health Statistics.


**Design Elements:** Assess Yourself icon: Aleksey Boldin/Alamy Stock Photo; Diversity Matters icon: Rawpixel Ltd/Getty Images; Wellness on Campus icon: Radius Images/Alamy Stock Photo; Take Charge icon: VisualCommunications/Getty Images; Critical Consumer icon: pagadesign/Getty Images.

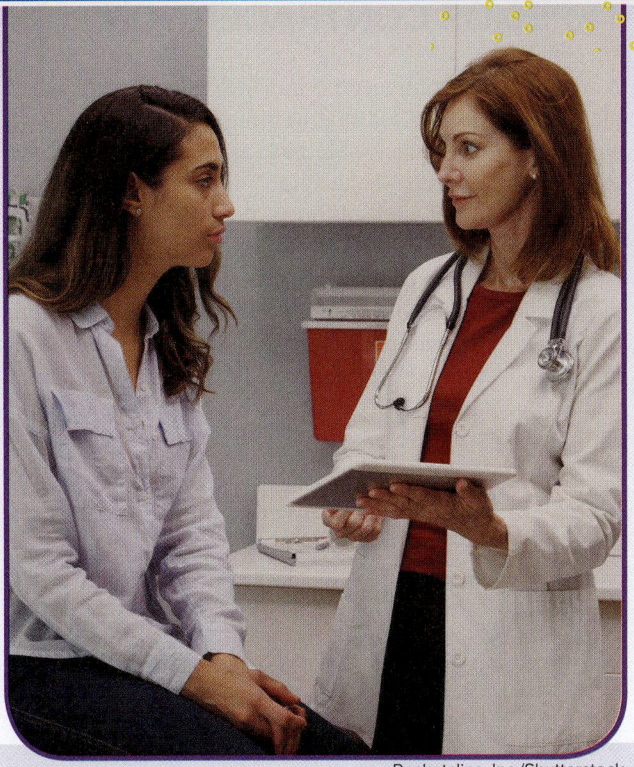
Rocketclips, Inc./Shutterstock

## CHAPTER OBJECTIVES

- Describe the types of long-acting and short-acting reversible contraceptives and how they work
- Explain approaches to emergency and permanent contraception
- Understand the pros and cons of different contraceptive methods
- Explain the role of abortion in people's reproductive lives
- Explain the methods of abortion and postabortion care
- Describe the legal restrictions placed on abortion in the United States

CHAPTER 7

# Contraception and Abortion

For thousands of years, people have used **birth control** to choose if and when they want to become pregnant and have a child. Records dating to the fourth century BCE describe foods, herbs, drugs, douches, and sponges used to prevent **conception,** the fusion of an ovum and a sperm that creates a fertilized egg, or *zygote*. Early attempts at **contraception** (the act of blocking conception through a device, substance, or method) followed the same principle as many contemporary birth control methods.

Today people can choose from many types of **contraceptives** to help prevent pregnancy and promote their overall sexual and reproductive health. All current methods of contraception are very effective in preventing pregnancy when used correctly. Of all unintended pregnancies, only 5% occur in women who use contraception consistently (Figure 7.1).[1]

Contraceptive methods not only prevent pregnancy associated morbidity and mortality, but they may also help prevent **sexually transmitted infections (STIs),** reduce the risk of certain cancers, and help manage menstruation-related problems and health conditions. Contraceptive information and services are fundamental not just to individual health, but also to community health and development. The World Health Organization works globally to ensure equitable access to evidence-based family planning information and services, recognizing that contraception helps meet multiple

[1]In this chapter, we use the word *women* to refer to people who have ovaries and uteri, and *men* to refer to individuals with sperm and testes. We recognize that these definitions do not align with how all individuals self-identify.

**TERMS**

**birth control** The practice of managing fertility and preventing unwanted pregnancies.

**conception** The fusion of ovum and sperm, resulting in a fertilized egg, or zygote.

**contraception** The prevention of conception through the use of a device, substance, or method.

**contraceptive** Any agent or method that can prevent conception.

**sexually transmitted infection (STI)** Any of several contagious infections contracted through intimate sexual contact.

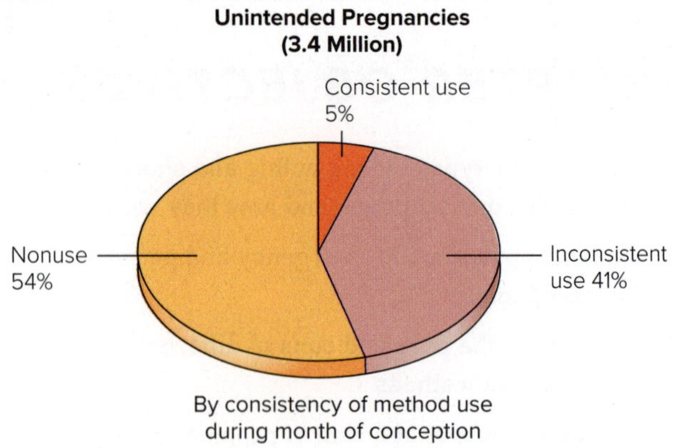

Unintended Pregnancies
(3.4 Million)

Consistent use
5%

Nonuse
54%

Inconsistent
use 41%

By consistency of method use
during month of conception

**FIGURE 7.1 The number of unintended pregnancies in relation to contraception use.**

SOURCES: Guttmacher Institute. 2018. Contraceptive use in the United States.

international development goals, including ensuring good health and well-being, and promoting gender equality. Contraception promotes gender equality by facilitating girls' educational attainment, women's engagement in the workforce, and women's ability to be economically self-sufficient.

# TYPES OF CONTRACEPTION

A wide range of contraceptive methods exists, enabling people to select the method that best meets their health needs and personal preferences. Methods are sometimes classified as "modern" versus "behavioral." Modern contraceptive methods consist of sterilization, **intrauterine devices (IUDs),** implants, injectables, pills, patches, rings, and **barrier methods.** Modern contraceptive methods are commonly discussed in terms of tiers of effectiveness in preventing pregnancy, but multiple considerations factor into which method best meets people's needs (Figure 7.2). Behavioral methods rely on knowledge about reproductive physiology and the menstrual cycle to determine when sex is least likely

> **TERMS**
>
> **intrauterine device method** A form of contraception that prevents the sperm from reaching the egg through chemical or hormonal changes.
>
> **barrier method** A contraceptive that acts as a physical barrier, blocking sperm from uniting with an egg.

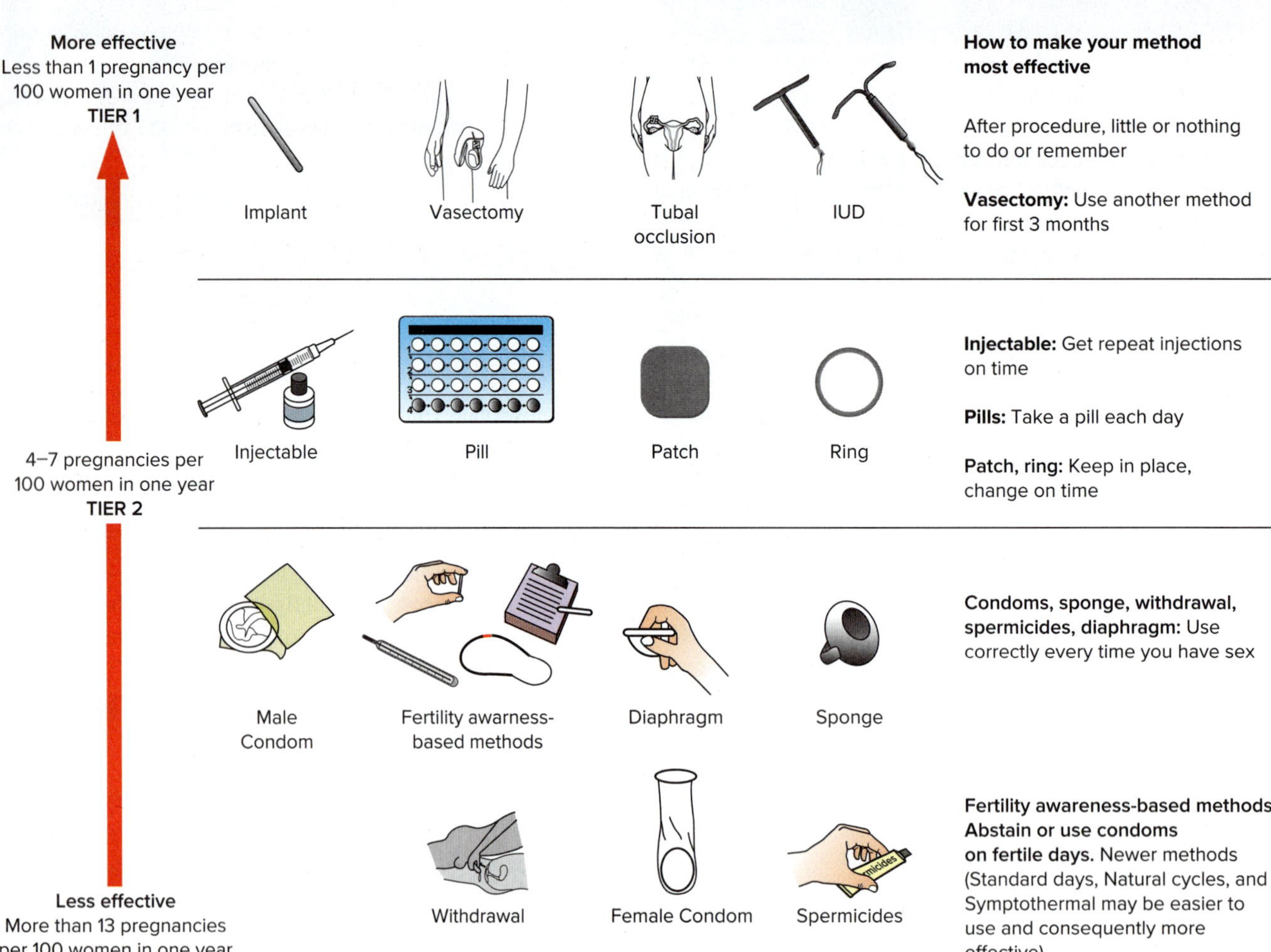


**FIGURE 7.2 Contraceptive effectiveness.**

SOURCE: Trussel, J. et al. 2018. Efficacy, safety, and personal considerations. In R. A. Hatcher, et al., eds. *Contraceptive Technology*, 21st ed. New York, NY: Ayer Company Publishers, Inc.

**Table 7.1 How Different Contraceptives Work**

| METHOD | MECHANISM |
|---|---|
| Surgery | Both female and male sterilization include a surgical procedure to remove or block part of the fallopian tubes or vas deferens. This permanently prevents the union of sperm and egg. |
| Intrauterine device (IUD) | IUDs prevent the sperm from reaching the egg through chemical or hormonal changes. The copper IUD induces a chemical reaction that is spermicidal. The hormonal IUD primarily works as a barrier method by making cervical mucus thicker and difficult for sperm to pass through. |
| Hormone | Hormonal methods are the largest category of methods and include the implant, injection, pill, patch, and ring. Hormonal methods primarily work by preventing ovulation, but they also alter cervical mucus to block sperm from entering the uterus. |
| Barrier | Barrier methods work by physically blocking the sperm from reaching the egg. Condoms are the most popular method based on this principle, but diaphragms and cervical caps are also in this category. |
| Behavioral | These methods rely on knowledge about male and female reproductive physiology and the menstrual cycle to prevent pregnancy. Periodic abstinence is used to avoid times in the cycle when fertility is highest. |

to result in a pregnancy. No one method of contraception is the best type for all people. In addition to discussing any medical conditions people may have with their health care provider, other factors influencing contraceptive choice include effectiveness, convenience, cost, reversibility, side effects and risks, and protection against STIs.

Table 7.1 explains how different contraception strategies prevent pregnancy and how their different mechanisms (ways in which they work) affect each method's effectiveness in pregnancy prevention. Contraceptive effectiveness is determined partly by the reliability of the method itself—that is, the failure rate if the method were always used exactly as directed (perfect use). Effectiveness is also determined by characteristics and behaviors of the person using the method. This includes the age-based **fertility** of the user, frequency of intercourse, and how consistently and correctly the method is used. This typical use **contraceptive failure rate** is based on studies that directly measure the percentage of unintended pregnancies in the first year of contraceptive use. For example, the 7% failure rate of oral contraceptives means 7 out of 100 typical users will become pregnant in the first year. This failure rate is likely to be lower for women who consistently take the pill and higher for those who often forget to take it; the *perfect use* failure rate of oral contraceptives is 0.3%.

Contraception is often divided into categories, or tiers, based on efficacy in preventing pregnancy. The most effective forms of contraception include sterilization, IUDs, and implants (Tier 1). With these methods, less than one pregnancy per 100 women occurs in a year. This contrasts with Tier 3 methods (barrier and behavioral methods of contraception), where 13 pregnancies per 100 women will typically occur over the course of a year. It is helpful to think about these rates in comparison with pregnancy. Among reproductive age individuals who are sexually active and not using contraception, 85 out of 100 women will become pregnant over the course of a year. It is important to note that only barrier methods provide some protection against STIs; all other contraceptive methods prevent pregnancy only. Figure 7.2 offers a graphic depiction of these tiers along with the typical use effectiveness ratings and tips on how to improve efficacy.

**Ask Yourself**

**QUESTIONS FOR CRITICAL THINKING AND REFLECTION**

Do you think the onus of contraception should fall equally on both partners? What can each partner do to enable the safest outcome? How could you begin a conversation about contraception while keeping you and your partner comfortable?

## WHICH CONTRACEPTIVE METHOD IS RIGHT FOR YOU?

The process of choosing and using a contraceptive method can be complex and what one seeks in a method may change over time, depending on one's health, relationship status, and personal preferences. Additionally, certain populations face unique challenges in accessing contraceptives (see the box "Barriers to Contraceptive Use"). Key considerations include those listed here.

1. ***The implications of an unplanned pregnancy and the efficacy of the method.*** For couples under age 30 who are having intercourse without contraception, 85% will become pregnant within a year.
2. ***Potential noncontraceptive benefits.*** Women with dysmenorrhea (painful menstruation), irregular periods, acne, endometriosis, severe premenstrual syndrome (PMS), and other medical problems may benefit from using a particular method of contraception.

**TERMS**

**fertility** The ability to reproduce.

**contraceptive failure rate** The percentage of women using a particular contraceptive method who experience an unintended pregnancy in the first year of use.

## DIVERSITY MATTERS
### Barriers to Contraceptive Use

Even in ideal circumstances, raising children is challenging. The ideal situation is that a person becomes pregnant only if and when they are ready to start a family. Why, then, when the stakes are so high, do so many unintended pregnancies occur? Well into the late 1960s, birth control was barely adequate, but now people have many choices for effective contraception. Why doesn't everyone who wishes to prevent pregnancy use contraception consistently?

A complex mix of factors relating to financial status, gender, age, culture, history, and policy can create barriers to effective contraception. For intrauterine devices, the cost for the medical exam, the IUD, the insertion of the IUD, and follow-up visits to a health care provider can range up to $1300, depending on health insurance. This cost may deter some candidates. In heterosexual couples, women tend to bear the brunt of the costs. When partners share in these burdens, it becomes easier to overcome them.

Another deterrent is family culture. A cofounder of the Women of Color Sexual Health Network, Bianca Laureano, writes about barriers young people may face when their parents or guardians do not believe in birth control. Laureano herself grew up in a Puerto Rican family who advised her that birth control kills Puerto Rican women.

Young people who are closely monitored by families that distrust birth control cannot wear a visible patch, nor use a method that requires visits to a physician, especially if a parent or guardian accompanies them. They must also continue having a menstrual cycle, so they cannot use Depo Provera, which, in some cases, causes menstrual bleeding to stop. In other cases, some young people do not want a contraceptive method that requires them to remember to take a pill each day (oral birth control pills) or to touch their genitals (for example, the NuvaRing).

Oral contraceptive pills are still the most widely used form of contraception. The people who use them most are younger, more educated, and more likely to be White (than Hispanic or Black). Long-acting reversible contraception (LARC) methods, such as implants and IUDs, are very effective, but have faced opposition. Historically, some doctors have discouraged younger people from using them. Now they have been shown to be safe, both in research and in the increased numbers of sexually active women aged 15–44 using IUDs successfully.

Still, people of color contend with an additional history of medical mistrust; some observers are concerned that campaigns targeting "at-risk" women focus too much on underrepresented racial and ethnic groups, the poor, and the young. In her book *Exposing Prejudice: Puerto Rican Experiences of Language, Race, and Class*, Bonnie Urciuoli gives a history of U.S. policies toward Puerto Rican immigrants, which included controlling their population through sterilization, enforced contraception, and migration. In *Killing the Black Body*, Dorothy Roberts describes the experiences of Black women throughout U.S. history—from being forced to bear children during slavery to having their fertility controlled by modern-day welfare policies. Thus, having less access to these methods is not the only reason women of color might not be using them.

In recent decades contraception use has increased and teen pregnancies have decreased. However, with government actions and public debates curtailing access to contraception and general reproductive rights, we still have a ways to go to equalize the burden of contraception and embrace its protective safeguards.

SOURCES: England, P., et al. 2016. Why do young, unmarried women who do not want to get pregnant contracept inconsistently? Mixed-method evidence for the role of efficacy. *Socius: Sociological Research for a Dynamic World* 2; Roberts, D. 1997. *Killing the Black Body: Race, Reproduction, and the Meaning of Liberty*. New York: Pantheon; Sweeney, M. M., and R. Kelly Raley. 2014. Race, ethnicity, and the changing context of childbearing in the United States. *Annual Review of Sociology* 40: 539–558; Urciuoli, B. 1996. *Exposing Prejudice: Puerto Rican Experiences of Language, Race, and Class*. Boulder, CO: Westview; Kaiser Family Foundation. 2019. *Oral Contraceptive Pills* (https://www.kff.org/womens-health-policy/fact-sheet/oral-contraceptive-pills/); Ome, M. 2020. The surprisingly fraught question of who pays for birth control. *The Atlantic*, 19 February.

3. ***Health risks.*** Pregnancy carries significant health risks that are generally much greater than the risks of contraception.
4. ***STI risk.*** Several activities besides vaginal intercourse (such as oral and anal sex) can put you at risk for an STI. Use condoms whenever any risk of STIs is present, even if already using another contraceptive method.
5. ***Convenience and comfort level.*** Many consider IUDs and implants to be the most convenient methods because they do not require any work on the part of the user once inside the body. Other methods may be convenient if incorporated into an existing routine.
6. ***Type of relationship.*** People who are not in an ongoing relationship may prefer to have a method to use at the time of intercourse, rather than every day. When the method depends on the cooperation of one's partner, communication and shared commitment are necessary, no matter how difficult.
7. ***Ease and cost of obtaining and maintaining each method.*** In the United States, methods should be covered at no or low cost to you. Remember that your student health clinic probably provides family planning services, and many communities have low-cost family planning clinics, such as Planned Parenthood.

8. ***Religious or philosophical beliefs.*** Talk with your health care provider about your concerns and beliefs to find a method that will meet your needs.

# PERMANENT CONTRACEPTION

**Sterilization** is permanent, and it is highly effective at preventing pregnancy. At present it is tied with the pill as the most commonly used contraceptive method in the United States, and it is by far the most common method used worldwide. It is especially popular among couples who have been married 10 or more years and have had all the children they intend to have. Regret after sterilization is relatively rare, and is most common in individuals under age 30 at time of sterilization. An important consideration is that, in nearly all cases, the procedure cannot be reversed.

## Male Sterilization: Vasectomy

The procedure for male sterilization, **vasectomy,** involves severing the vasa deferentia, two tiny ducts that transport sperm from the testes to the seminal vesicles. After surgery, the testes continue to produce sperm, but the sperm are absorbed into the body. Because the testes contribute only about 10% of the total seminal fluid, the actual quantity of ejaculate is reduced only slightly. Hormone production from the testes continues with very little change, and secondary sex characteristics are not altered.

Vasectomy is ordinarily performed in a physician's office and takes about 30 minutes. A local anesthetic is injected into the skin of the scrotum. Small incisions are made at the upper end of the scrotum where it joins the body, and the vas deferens on each side is exposed, severed, and tied off or sealed by electrocautery. Some doctors seal each of the vasa with a plastic clamp, which is the size of a grain of rice. The incisions are then closed with sutures, and a small dressing is applied. Pain and swelling are usually slight and can be relieved with ice compresses and a scrotal support. Bleeding and infection occasionally develop but can be treated easily. After the procedure, most men can return to work in two days. Men can have sex after vasectomy as soon as they feel no discomfort, usually after about a week.

**Advantages** Short office-based procedure with a low complication rate. Does not require ongoing medications or actions.

**Disadvantages** A follow-up visit, approximately three months after the procedure, is essential to confirm contraceptive effectiveness. A semen analysis is done at this time to confirm that no sperm are present. A backup method of contraception is needed until this time because sperm produced before the operation may still be present in the semen.

**Effectiveness** The overall failure rate for vasectomy is 0.15%. In a small number of cases, a severed vas rejoins itself.

## Female Sterilization

The most common method of female sterilization involves cutting or blocking the fallopian tubes, which prevents eggs from being fertilized by sperm. Ovulation and menstruation continue, but the unfertilized eggs are released into the abdominal cavity and absorbed. Hormone production by the ovaries and secondary sex characteristics are generally not affected.

**Tubal sterilization** (also called *tubal ligation*) can be performed during a hospital admission for childbirth, or at any point an individual requests it. Outside of pregnancy, the most commonly used method for tubal sterilization is **laparoscopy.** A laparoscope, a camera containing a small light, is inserted through a small abdominal incision, and the surgeon looks through it to locate the fallopian tubes. Instruments are passed either through the laparoscope or through a second small incision, and the tube is either completely removed or a large section of it is excised. Tubes can also be blocked by using a permanent clip or by electrocautery. General anesthesia is usually used. The operation takes about 30 minutes, and women can usually leave the hospital two to four hours after surgery. Tubal sterilization can also be performed shortly after a vaginal delivery through a small incision, or in the case of cesarean section, during the same surgery.

**Advantages** It is a permanent, female-controlled method. Research has shown that removing the tube, or even part of it for sterilization, significantly decreases a woman's risk of ovarian cancer.

**Disadvantages** Although tubal sterilization is riskier than vasectomy, with a rate of minor complications of about 6–11%, it is the more common procedure. Potential problems include bowel injury, wound infection, and bleeding. Serious complications are rare.

**TERMS**

**sterilization** Surgically altering the reproductive system to prevent pregnancy. Vasectomy is the procedure in males; tubal sterilization or hysterectomy is the procedure in females.

**vasectomy** The surgical severing of the ducts that carry sperm to the ejaculatory duct.

**tubal sterilization** Severing or blocking the oviducts to prevent eggs from reaching the uterus; also called tubal ligation.

**laparoscopy** Examining the internal organs by inserting a small camera through an abdominal incision.

## Ask Yourself

**QUESTIONS FOR CRITICAL THINKING AND REFLECTION**

What are your personal views on sterilization? Do you think it could be an option for you one day? Do you believe people should forgo considering sterilization until they have reached a certain point in their lives? When does sterilization become the best option?

**Effectiveness** The failure rate for tubal sterilization is about 0.5%. When pregnancies occur, an increased percentage of them are ectopic (occurring outside the uterus). Ectopic pregnancy is dangerous and can even cause maternal death, so any woman who suspects she might be pregnant after having tubal sterilization should seek medical help.

# LONG-ACTING REVERSIBLE CONTRACEPTION

**Long-acting reversible contraception (LARC)** consists of intrauterine devices (IUDs) and implants. These methods of contraception are very popular because of their convenience, high effectiveness, and in some cases, reduction in menstrual bleeding. Once placed, the user does not have to take a daily pill, interrupt foreplay for contraception, or obtain refills from the pharmacy. These methods have very high satisfaction rates, and they are suitable for nearly all individuals, including those who have never been pregnant.

## Intrauterine Devices (IUDs)

An **intrauterine device (IUD)** is a small object placed in the uterus as a contraceptive. Five different IUDs are now available in the United States. The Copper T-380A (also known as ParaGard®) provides protection for up to 12 years. Hormonal IUDs Mirena®, Liletta®, Kyleena®, and Skyla® release small amounts of progestin (a synthetic progesterone) and remain effective for three to seven years. Current evidence suggests that ParaGard works primarily by preventing fertilization. This IUD contains copper, which is thought to cause biochemical changes in the uterus that affect the movement of sperm and eggs. ParaGard may also interfere with the implantation of fertilized eggs in the uterine lining. The hormonal IUDs also work primarily by preventing fertilization. As a result of the slow release of very small amounts of progestin, the cervical mucus thickens and stops sperm. An IUD must be inserted and removed by a trained professional. It can be inserted at any time during the menstrual cycle, as long as the woman is not pregnant. The device is threaded into a sterile inserter that is introduced through the cervix, and the IUD is placed at the top of the uterus. IUDs have two threads attached that protrude from the cervix into the vagina. These threads are trimmed so that only 1 to 2 inches remain in the upper vagina (Figure 7.3), and they do not cause discomfort during vaginal intercourse for the woman or her sexual partner. A woman or a clinician can confirm the IUD is in place by touching the strings at the top of the vagina.

**TERMS**

**long-acting reversible contraception (LARC)** Intrauterine devices and implant methods of contraception, which last for several years, earn high satisfaction rates, and reduce rates of unintended pregnancy and abortion compared to other methods.

**intrauterine device (IUD)** A device inserted into the uterus as a contraceptive.

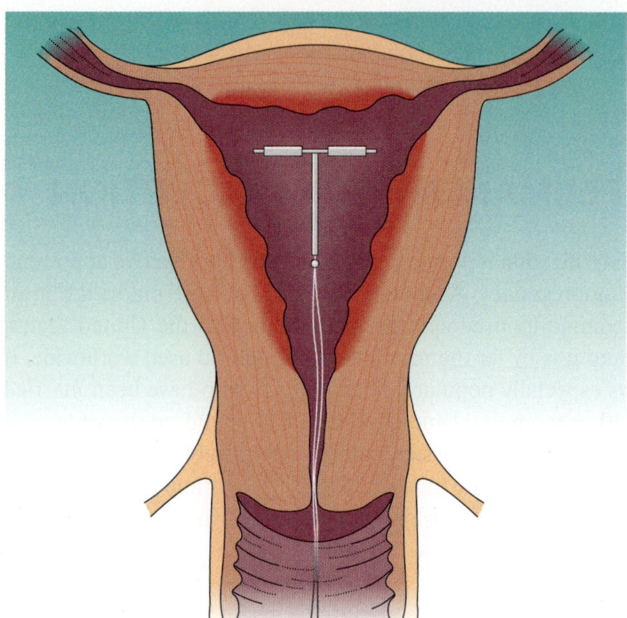

**FIGURE 7.3 An IUD (Copper T-380A, or ParaGard) properly positioned in the uterus.**

**Advantages** Intrauterine devices are highly effective and are simple and convenient to use, requiring no attention. They do not require the woman to anticipate or interrupt sexual activity. IUDs act mainly on the uterus and tend to be very safe, including for women with complex medical problems.

All hormonal IUDs reduce menstrual bleeding and cramping. The Mirena IUD has also been shown to prevent endometrial cancer (in the lining of the uterus) and even to reverse the endometrial changes that precede endometrial cancer. ParaGard has been shown to decrease the risk of endometrial cancer, but the reasons for this are less clear.

**Disadvantages** A trained provider is needed to place an IUD. Most IUD side effects are limited to the genital tract. Side effects differ between the types of IUD. Heavy menstrual flow and increased menstrual cramping sometimes occur with ParaGard, whereas hormonal IUDs cause a reduction in bleeding and cramping. Spontaneous expulsion of the IUD can happen, typically when the IUD is placed postpartum or if uterine fibroids are present. A very rare risk of IUD placement is perforation, where the IUD is placed through the wall of the uterus into the abdominal cavity. Surgery is needed to retrieve the IUD. An ultrasound at the end of placement can confirm its location. Infection following IUD placement is rare. IUDs are not suitable for women with suspected pregnancy, large tumors of the uterus, other anatomical abnormalities, or bleeding that has not been evaluated; hormonal IUDs are not to be used in women with certain hormonally responsive cancers.

**QUICK STATS**

**Contraception designed for women (e.g., female sterilization, IUDs, and pills) accounts for most contraceptive use worldwide.**

—United Nations, 2019

**Effectiveness** The typical first-year failure rate of IUDs is 0.8% for ParaGard, 0.5% for Skyla, and 0.2% for Mirena, Liletta, and Kyleena. Effectiveness can be increased by using a backup method for the first week of IUD use and by periodically making sure that the device is in place. If pregnancy occurs, the IUD may need to be removed to safeguard the woman's health and to maintain the pregnancy; removal depends on the location of the IUD with respect to the pregnancy. If an IUD must be left in place during pregnancy, there is an increased risk of complications.

## Contraceptive Implants

Contraceptive implants are placed under the skin of the upper arm and deliver a small but steady dose of progestin over a period of years. Implants are common globally, with brands such as Jadelle, Sino-implant, and Nexplanon in wide use.

In the United States, Nexplanon is in use. Nexplanon is a single implant and is considered to be one of the most effective forms of contraception (Figure 7.4). It is approved for use for three years by the Food and Drug Administration, and large studies support its effectiveness in preventing pregnancy for four years. Implants have several contraceptive effects. They cause hormonal shifts that inhibit ovulation and thin the uterine lining. The hormone also thickens the cervical mucus, inhibiting the movement of sperm.

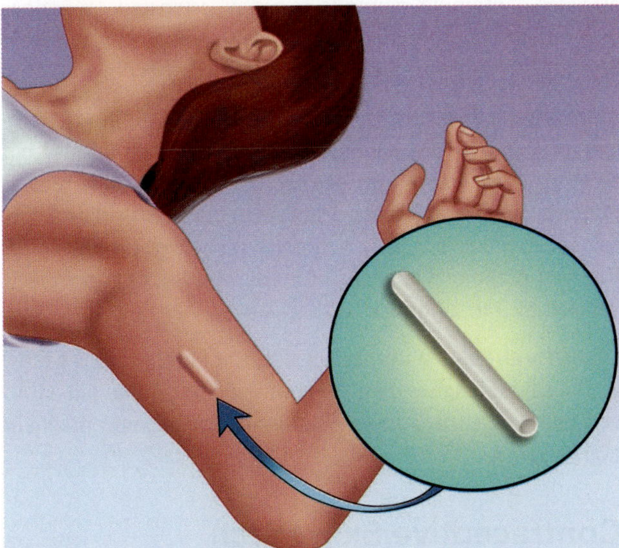

**FIGURE 7.4 Placement of contraceptive implant.** The Implanon/Nexplanon implant device has to be placed and removed by a trained medical professional.

**Advantages** Implants are highly effective and are simple and convenient to use, requiring no attention. They do not require the woman to anticipate or interrupt sexual activity. Implants contain progestin only, so they are very safe, including for women with complex medical problems or contraindications to estrogen (e.g., high blood pressure). The contraceptive effects of the implant are quickly reversed on removal. Like the hormonal IUDs, implants make menstrual bleeding irregular and light and reduce cramps for most users.

**Disadvantages** A trained provider is needed to place and remove the implant. Although the implants are barely visible, their presence may bother some women. Common side effects of contraceptive implants are menstrual irregularities, including longer menstrual periods, spotting between periods, or having no bleeding at all. Less common side effects include headaches, weight gain, breast tenderness, nausea, acne, and mood swings.

**Effectiveness** The overall failure rate for Nexplanon® is estimated at about 0.05%. Along with the IUDs and sterilization, implants are one of the most effective forms of contraception.

# SHORT-ACTING REVERSIBLE CONTRACEPTION

A variety of hormonal and barrier methods fall into the group of short-acting reversible contraceptives. For these methods, the user must take action on a daily, weekly, or monthly basis, or at the time of intercourse. Such short-acting methods include, among others, oral contraceptives, skin patches, and vaginal rings. A pelvic exam and/or pap test is not needed to begin contraception. Individuals with high blood pressure are usually not eligible to use an estrogen-containing method.

It is safe and effective to start methods like the pill, patch, ring, and injection at any point in a woman's cycle when it is reasonably certain she is not pregnant (i.e., hasn't had sex since her last period; is within seven days of her period starting or of having had an abortion; has been correctly and consistently using contraception; or is within four weeks of giving birth). If it has been five days or longer, she should either not have vaginal intercourse or should use a condom or other backup method.

## Oral Contraceptives: The Pill

**Oral contraceptives (OCs),** also known as *birth control pills* or "the pill," fall into two general categories: the combined hormonal pill containing progestin and estrogen, and progestin-only pills. Progestin's role is to prevent pregnancy, whereas estrogen, when added, promotes the effect of progestin in pregnancy prevention and makes bleeding more regular.

**The Combined Hormonal Pill** The most common type of OC is the *combination pill,* which contains varying amounts of estrogen and progestin. Traditionally, each one-month packet contains a three-week supply of "active" pills that combine varying types and amounts of estrogen and progestin, as well as a one-week supply of "placebo" pills that do not contain hormones. During the placebo week, vaginal bleeding occurs that is typically lighter than the women's period when not on the pill. There is no health benefit or reason to have a period while on contraception. Hormone-containing pills can be taken daily (referred to as "continuous use") to avoid periods, and newer formulations reflect this by having fewer placebo weeks or no placebo pills.

QUICK STATS

**Of women aged 15–49, 14% use the pill, 10% use an IUD or contraceptive implant, and 18% use female sterilization.**

—National Center for Health Statistics, 2020

**ADVANTAGES** The pill is relatively simple to use and does not hinder sexual spontaneity. Most women also appreciate the predictable regularity of periods, as well as the reduction in cramps and blood loss. Women who have significant problems associated with menstruation may benefit from menstrual suppression with continuous use (skipping placebo pills included in the pill pack). The pills are reversible, and fertility returns shortly after stopping.

Medical advantages include a decreased incidence of benign breast disease, acne, iron-deficiency anemia, colon and rectal cancer, endometrial cancer, and ovarian cancer. OC use can help reduce symptoms for women with dysmenorrhea (painful periods), endometriosis, and polycystic ovary syndrome.

**DISADVANTAGES** Consistency is key for the pill to be effective, but taking the pill daily is challenging. Studies show that over one year, more than half of pill users have a break in use, typically due to forgetting to take the pill or delayed refills.

Among women who experience problems with OCs, the most common issue is bleeding during mid cycle (called *breakthrough bleeding*), which is usually slight and tends to disappear after a few cycles. Morning nausea and swollen breasts may appear during the first few months of OC use, although these side effects are uncommon with the low-dose pills in current widespread use.

Birth control pills are not recommended for women with a history of blood clots (or a close family member with unexplained blood clots at an early age), heart disease or stroke, migraines with changes in vision, any form of cancer or liver tumor, or impaired liver function. Women with certain other health conditions or behaviors, including migraines without changes in vision, high blood pressure, cigarette smoking, and sickle-cell disease, require close monitoring when taking the pill.

**EFFECTIVENESS** If taken as directed, the failure rate is as low as 0.3%. However, the typical user has a 7% failure rate. The effectiveness of the pill can be affected by gastrointestinal illness (vomiting or diarrhea), and it also can interact with other medications such as certain antibiotics, antiseizure medications, and the herb St. John's wort.

**Progestin-Only Pills** The progestin-only pill is sometimes called the minipill because it contains only the one hormone. These work primarily as a barrier: they thicken the cervical mucus so that sperm cannot pass through. They also reduce the chance of ovulation. A new progestin-only pill, Slynd®, was released in 2021. This progestin-only pill has the advantage of a longer missed-pill window of 24 hours. With older types of progestin-only pills, the effectiveness could decrease if you forgot to take it for even a few hours.

**ADVANTAGES** Progestin-only pills are safe for nearly everyone to use, including people who have contraindications to estrogen-containing methods (e.g., hypertension, migraines with aura). They are safe to use immediately postpartum, and they add to the contraceptive effect of breastfeeding.

**DISADVANTAGES** As with all progestin-only methods, irregular bleeding is normal. Typically periods are lighter, but spotting is common, and periods may not follow a regular pattern. Consistency is important with both types of oral contraceptive pills, but it is critical with progestin-only pills. Risks of pregnancy increase if taking a progestin-only pill is delayed by 3 to 24 hours.

**EFFECTIVENESS** With perfect use, the failure rate is as low as 1%, slightly higher than the combined hormonal pill. However, in typical use, about 7% of women become pregnant every year.

TERMS

**oral contraceptive (OC)** Hormone compounds (made of estrogen and progestins) in pill form that prevent conception by preventing ovulation; also called the birth control pill or "the pill."

## Contraceptive Skin Patch

The contraceptive skin patch is a thin, one-inch-square patch that slowly releases both an estrogen and a progestin into the bloodstream. The patch works in the same way that the pill does, but the medication is delivered differently. The patch can be worn on the upper outer arm, abdomen, buttocks, or upper torso (excluding the breasts); it is designed to stick to skin even during bathing or swimming. Each patch is worn continuously for one week and is replaced on the same day of the week for three consecutive weeks. The fourth week is patch-free, allowing a woman to have her menstrual period. If the patch falls off partially, or completely, for more than a day, a new patch should be started and a backup method of contraception used for seven days.

**Advantages** Because the patch provides the same combination of hormones as a combined birth control pill, the advantages are the same. Compliance seems to be higher with the patch than with OCs, probably because the patch requires weekly instead of daily action.

**Disadvantages** Minor side effects are similar to those of OCs, although breast discomfort may be more common in patch users. Some women also experience skin irritation around the patch. More serious complications are thought to be similar to those of OCs, including an increased risk of side effects among women who smoke. However, because the contraceptive patch exposes users to higher doses of estrogen than most OCs, patch use may further increase the risk of blood clots. The patch is not used as commonly to avoid periods for this reason.

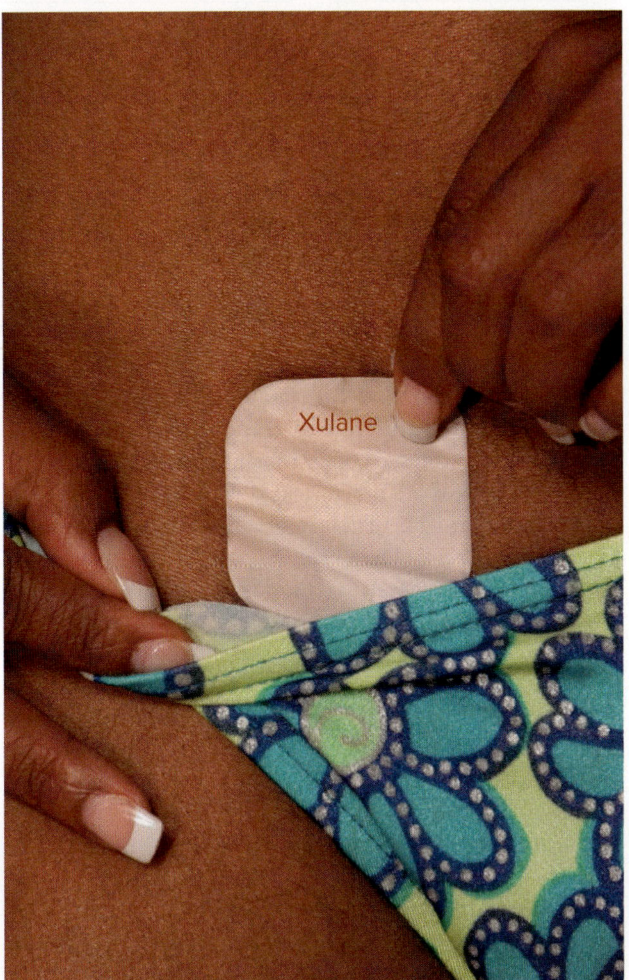

The contraceptive skin patch can be worn on several different parts of a woman's body; it remains on during bathing or swimming. Bob Pardue/Medical Lifestyle/Alamy Stock Photo

**Effectiveness** With perfect use, the patch's failure rate is very low (0.3%) in the first year of use. The typical failure rate is approximately 7%, similar to that of the oral contraceptive pill. Failure rates have been shown to be higher in women with obesity.

## Vaginal Contraceptive Ring

Currently two types of vaginal rings are used for contraception. These include the NuvaRing and Annovera. Both rings are soft, flexible, and contain a combination of estrogen and progestin to prevent pregnancy. The ring slowly releases hormones and maintains blood hormone levels comparable to those found with OC use. The ring prevents pregnancy in the same way as OCs. The NuvaRing ring is inserted vaginally and left in place for three weeks. During the fourth week, when the ring is removed, the next menstrual cycle occurs. A new ring is then inserted seven days later. Backup contraception must be used if the ring has been removed for more than three hours. Annovera is a newer ring that can be used for a year.

**Advantages** The ring offers one month of protection with no daily or weekly action required. It does not require a fitting by a clinician, and exact placement in the vagina is not as critical as it is for a diaphragm. Because the ring provides the same combination of hormones as a combined birth control pill, the advantages are similar. The medical benefits of the ring include, but are not limited to, lighter, less painful menses; decreased risk of uterine and ovarian cancer; decreased anemia; and the ability to control your cycle.

**Disadvantages** Side effects are roughly comparable to those seen with OC use, except for a lower incidence of nausea and vomiting. Other side effects may include vaginal discharge, vaginitis, and vaginal irritation. Medical risks also are similar to those found with OC use.

**Effectiveness** As with the pill and patch, the perfect use failure rate is around 0.3%. The ring's typical use failure rate is similar to the pill's at 7%.

## Injectable Contraceptives

Hormonal contraceptive injections were first developed in the 1960s, and their use is common worldwide. In the United States, only Depo-Provera is available. These injectables contain a larger dose of progestin, which is injected into the muscle of the arm or buttocks. The Depo-Provera injection prevents ovulation for about 12 weeks. A different dose and formulation of these medications have recently been developed to allow subcutaneous injection. This offers an advantage because people can be easily trained to give subcutaneous injections to themselves, a practice that increased in popularity during the COVID pandemic.

**Advantages** Injectable contraceptives are highly effective and require little action on the part of the user. Some users value injectables for the high degree of privacy they afford; the injections leave no trace, and no ongoing medications or supplies need to be stored at home. Depo-Provera is a progestin-only method and is safe to use for many women.

**Disadvantages** The most common side effects of Depo-Provera are changes in menstrual bleeding. Bleeding becomes light and irregular, and after one year of using Depo-Provera many women have no menstrual bleeding at all. Depo-Provera is the only contraceptive method that has been linked with weight gain. Return to fertility is slower after Depo-Provera than with other methods. It can take up to 12 months for cycles to normalize and fertility to return.

**Effectiveness** The perfect use failure rate is 0.2% for Depo-Provera. With typical use, the failure rate increases to 4% in the first year of use.

## Male (External) Condoms

The **male condom** is a thin sheath designed to cover the penis during sexual intercourse. Most brands available in the United States are made of latex, although condoms made of polyurethane and polyisoprene are also available. Condoms prevent sperm from entering the vagina and provide protection against most STIs. Condoms are the most widely used barrier method and the third most popular of all contraceptive methods used in the United States, after the pill and female sterilization. Many couples combine various contraceptives, using condoms for STI protection and another contraceptive method for greater protection against pregnancy.

The man or his partner must put the condom on the penis before it is inserted because the small amounts of fluid that may be secreted unnoticed prior to **ejaculation** often contain sperm capable of causing pregnancy. The rolled-up condom is placed over the head of the erect penis and unrolled down to the base of the penis, leaving a half-inch space (without air) at the tip to collect semen (Figure 7.5). Some brands of condoms have a reservoir tip designed for this purpose. Uncircumcised men must first pull back the foreskin of the penis. Partners must be careful not to damage the condom with fingernails, rings, or other rough objects.

> **TERMS**
>
> **male condom** A thin sheath that covers the penis during sexual intercourse; used for contraception and to prevent STI transmission.
>
> **ejaculation** An abrupt discharge of semen from the penis during sexual stimulation.
>
> **spermicide** A chemical agent that kills sperm.

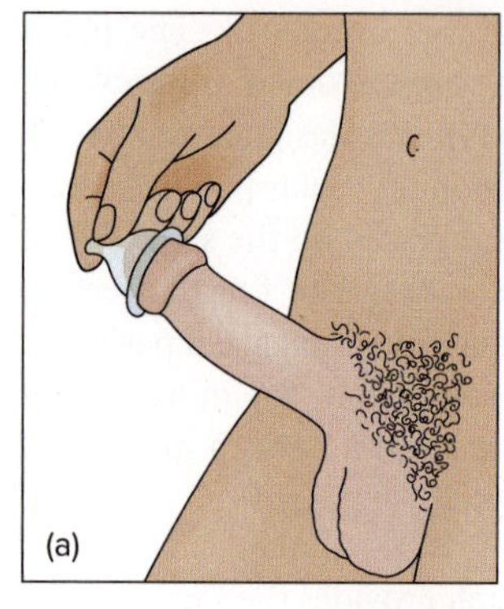


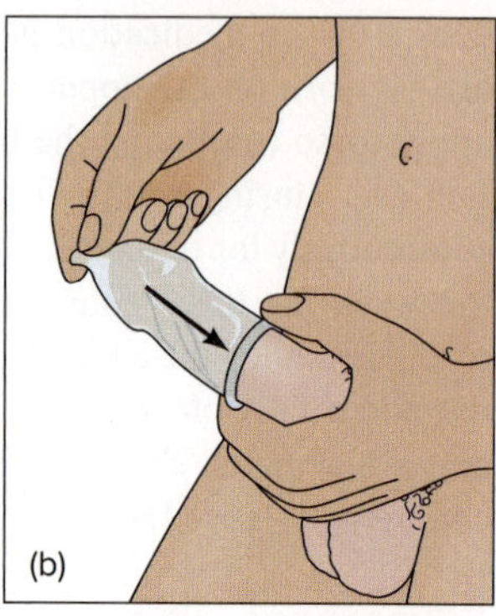


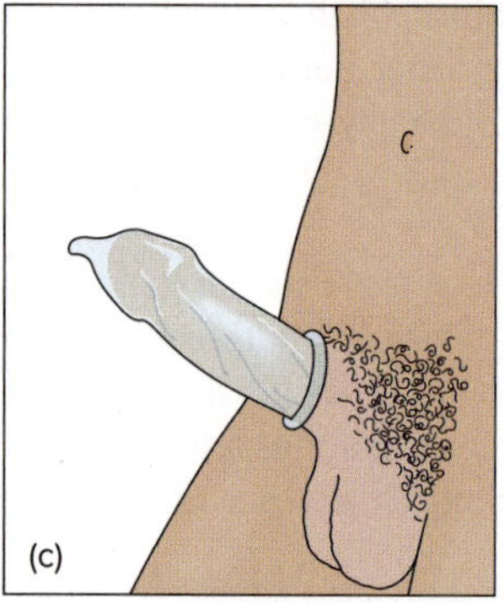


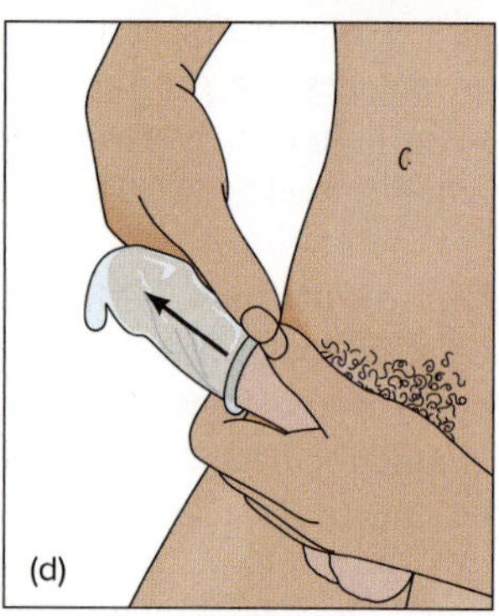


**FIGURE 7.5 Use of the male condom.** (a) Place the rolled-up condom over the head of the erect penis. Hold the top half-inch of the condom (with air squeezed out) to leave room for semen. (b) While holding the tip, unroll the condom onto the penis. Gently smooth out any air bubbles. (c) Unroll the condom down to the base of the penis. (d) To avoid spilling semen after ejaculation, hold the condom around the base of the penis as the penis is withdrawn. Remove the condom away from your partner, taking care not to spill any semen.

Many condoms are prelubricated with water-based or silicone-based lubricants. These lubricants make the condom more comfortable and less likely to break. Many people find that using extra, non-oil-based lubricant can be helpful. Prelubricated condoms are also available that contain the **spermicide** nonoxynol-9, the same agent found in many of the contraceptive creams that women use. However, spermicidal condoms are no more effective than condoms without spermicide. They cost more and have a shorter shelf-life than most other condoms. Further, condoms with nonoxynol-9 have been associated with urinary tract infections in women and, if they cause tissue irritation, an increased risk of HIV transmission.

Water-based lubricants can be used as needed. Any products that contain mineral or vegetable oil, including baby oil, many lotions, regular petroleum jelly, cooking oils (corn oil, shortening, butter, and so on), and some vaginal lubricants and antifungal or anti-itch creams should not be used with latex condoms. Such products can cause latex to start disintegrating within 60 seconds, thus greatly increasing the chance of condom breakage. (Polyurethane is not affected by oil-based products.)

**ADVANTAGES** Condoms are easy to purchase and are available without prescription or medical supervision. In addition to being free of medical side effects (other than occasional allergic reactions), latex condoms help protect against STIs. Condoms may also protect women from human papillomavirus (HPV), which causes cervical cancer. Condoms made of polyurethane are appropriate for people who are allergic to latex. However, they are more likely to slip or break than latex condoms and therefore may give less protection against STIs and pregnancy. Polyisoprene condoms, marketed under the brand name SKYN, are safe for most people with latex allergies, stretchier, and less expensive than polyurethane condoms. Condoms made of lambskin are also available but permit the passage of HIV and other disease-causing organisms and are less effective for pregnancy prevention. Except for abstinence or intercourse within a monogamous relationship with an uninfected partner, the correct and consistent use of latex male condoms offers the most reliable available protection against the transmission of HIV.

**QUICK STATS**

**More than 99% of women aged 15–44 who have ever had sexual intercourse have used at least one contraceptive method.**

—National Center for Health Statistics, 2018

**DISADVANTAGES** Condoms require both partners' participation and require correct use with every act of intercourse for maximum effectiveness. The two most common complaints about condoms are that they diminish sensation and interfere with spontaneity. Although some people find these drawbacks serious, others consider them only minor distractions. Many couples learn to creatively integrate condom use into their sexual practices. Indeed, condom use can be a way to improve communication and share responsibility in a relationship.

**EFFECTIVENESS** During the first year of typical condom use among 100 users, approximately 13 pregnancies will occur. And even with perfect use, the first-year failure rate is about 2%. If a condom breaks or is removed carelessly, a woman can reduce the risk of pregnancy by immediately using an emergency contraceptive (discussed later in the chapter).

## Female (Internal) Condoms

The female or internal condom is a clear, stretchy, disposable pouch with two rings that can be inserted into a vagina or anus. It can be inserted up to eight hours before intercourse. The one-size-fits-all condom, called the FC2, consists of a soft, loose-fitting, nonlatex rubber sheath with two flexible rings. The ring at the closed end is inserted into the vagina and placed at the cervix much like a diaphragm. The ring at the open end remains outside the vagina.

The manufacturer strongly recommends practicing inserting the female condom several times before actually using it for intercourse. Most women find that it is easy to use after practice. The FC2 comes prelubricated with a silicone lubricant, but extra lubricant or a spermicide can be used if desired. As with male condoms, users need to take care not to tear the condom during insertion or removal. Following intercourse, the woman should remove the condom before standing up. By twisting and squeezing the outer ring, she can prevent the spilling of semen. A new condom should be used for each act of sexual intercourse. A female condom should not be used with a male condom because tearing is more likely to occur.

**Advantages** Internal condoms can be inserted up to eight hours before sexual activity and are thus less disruptive than male condoms. Because the outer part of the condom covers the area around the vaginal opening as well as the base of the penis during intercourse, it offers potentially better protection against genital warts or herpes. The synthetic rubber pouch can be used by people who are allergic to latex. Because the material is thin and pliable, there is little loss of sensation. The FC2 is generously lubricated, and the material conducts heat well, increasing comfort and natural feel during intercourse. When used correctly, the internal condom should theoretically provide protection against HIV transmission and STIs comparable to that of the latex male condom. However, in research involving typical users, the internal condom was slightly less effective in preventing pregnancy and STIs. Effectiveness improves with careful practice and instruction.

**Disadvantages** While this is a method controlled by the receptive partner, it requires both partners' full cooperation. The outer ring of the internal condom, which hangs visibly outside the vagina, may be bothersome to some couples. During coitus, both partners must take care that the penis is inserted into the pouch, not outside it, and that the device does not slip inside the vagina. Internal condoms, like male condoms, are made for one-time use. A single internal condom costs about three to four times as much as a single male condom. Internal condoms are harder to find than male condoms. Some pharmacies do not currently carry them. You can buy the FC2 at Planned Parenthood and online.

**Effectiveness** The typical first-year failure rate of the female condom is 21%. For couples who follow instructions carefully and consistently, the failure rate is considerably lower, about 5%.

## Diaphragm with Spermicide

The **diaphragm** is rarely used in the United States, with only 0.3% of contraceptive users relying on it. The diaphragm is a dome-shaped cup of silicone with a flexible rim. When correctly used with spermicidal cream or jelly, the diaphragm covers the cervix, blocking sperm from the uterus. There are two diaphragms available in the United States: the Milex, which comes in two styles and multiple sizes, and the single-size Caya. Diaphragms are available in the United States only by prescription. Because of individual anatomical differences among women, the round Milex diaphragm must be carefully fitted by a trained clinician to ensure both comfort and effectiveness. The fit should be checked with each routine annual medical examination, as well as after childbirth, abortion, abdominal or pelvic surgery, or a weight change of more than 10 pounds. Caya comes in only one size and does not require fitting; it is oval in shape and designed to fit most women. Caya is contoured for easier use and includes grip "dimples" on the sides to help with insertion and a small dome to aid in removal of the device.

Spermicidal jelly or cream should be applied to the diaphragm before inserting it and checking its placement (Figure 7.6). If more than six hours elapse between the time of insertion and the time of intercourse, additional spermicide must be applied. The diaphragm must be left in place for at least six hours after the last act of coitus to give the spermicide enough time to kill all the sperm. With repeated intercourse, a condom should be used for additional protection.

To remove the diaphragm, the woman hooks the front rim (Milex) or small removal dome (Caya®) down from the pubic bone with one finger and pulls it out. After each use, a diaphragm should be washed with mild soap and water, rinsed, patted dry, and examined for holes or cracks. A diaphragm should be stored in its case.

**Advantages** A diaphragm can be inserted up to six hours before intercourse. Its use can be limited to times of sexual activity only, and it allows for immediate and total reversibility. The diaphragm is free of medical side effects (other than rare allergic reactions) and increased risk of urinary tract infection.

**Disadvantages** Diaphragms must always be used with a spermicide, so a woman must keep both of these supplies with her whenever she anticipates sexual activity. Diaphragms require extra attention because they must be cleaned and stored with care to preserve their effectiveness. Some women cannot wear a diaphragm because of their vaginal or uterine anatomy. In other women, diaphragm use can cause bladder infections and may need to be discontinued if repeated infections occur.

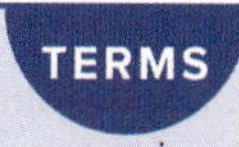


**diaphragm** A contraceptive device consisting of a flexible, dome-shaped cup that covers the cervix and prevents sperm from entering the uterus.

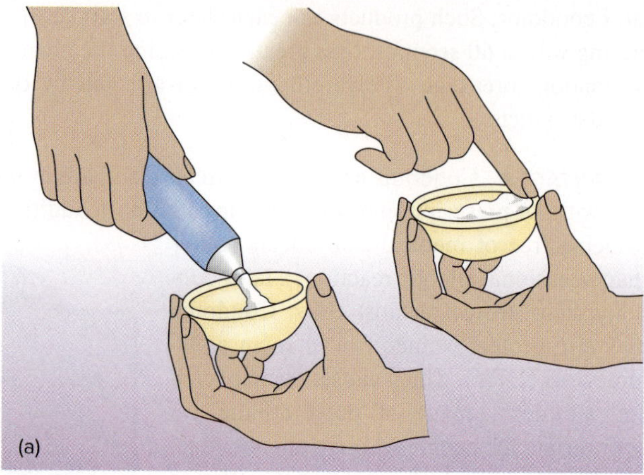


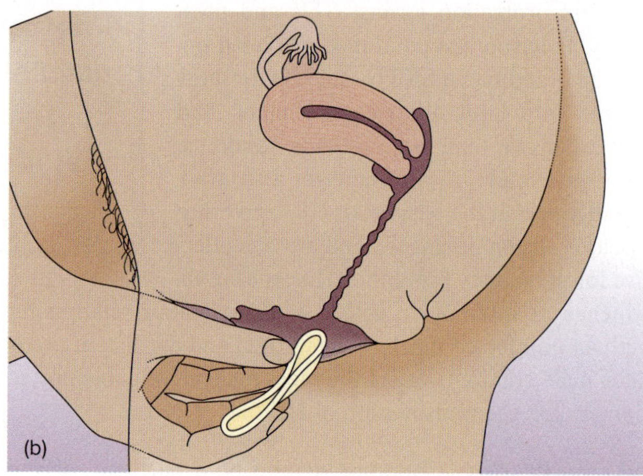


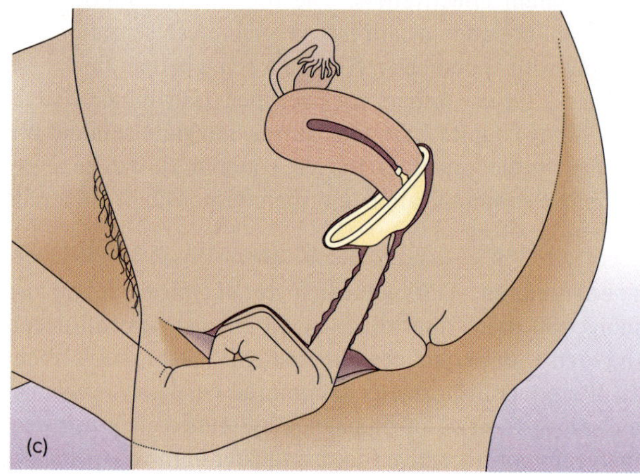


FIGURE 7.6 **Use of the diaphragm.** Wash your hands with soap and water before inserting the diaphragm. It can be inserted while squatting, lying down, or standing with one foot raised. (a) Place about a tablespoon of spermicidal jelly or cream in the concave side of the diaphragm, and spread it around the inside of the diaphragm and around the rim. (b) Squeeze the diaphragm into a long, narrow shape between the thumb and forefinger. Insert it into the vagina, and push it up along the back wall of the vagina as far as it will go. For the Caya, use the grip nubs to fold and grasp the device during insertion. (c) Check its position to make sure the cervix is completely covered and that the front rim of the diaphragm is tucked behind the pubic bone.

**Effectiveness** The typical failure rate is 17% during the first year of use. The main causes of failure are incorrect insertion, inconsistent use, and inaccurate fitting. If a diaphragm slips during intercourse, a woman should use emergency contraception.

## Cervical Cap

The **cervical cap,** another barrier device, is a small, flexible cup that fits snugly over the cervix and is held in place by suction. This cap is a clear silicone cup with a brim around the dome to hold spermicide and trap sperm, and a removal strap over the dome. It comes in three sizes and must be fitted by a trained clinician. It is used like a diaphragm, with a small amount of spermicide placed in the cup and on the brim before insertion. The cervical cap is reusable but must be replaced annually.

**Advantages** Advantages of the cervical cap are similar to those associated with diaphragm use. It is an alternative for women who cannot use a diaphragm because of anatomical reasons or recurrent urinary tract infections. The cap fits tightly, so it does not require backup condom use with repeated intercourse. It may be left in place for up to 48 hours.

**Disadvantages** Along with most of the disadvantages associated with the diaphragm, difficulty with insertion and removal is more common for cervical cap users.

**Effectiveness** Studies indicate that the average failure rate for the cervical cap is 16% for women who have never had a child and 32% for women who have had a child.

## Contraceptive Sponge

The **contraceptive sponge** is a round, absorbent device that fits snugly over the cervix. The sponge is made of polyurethane and is presaturated with the same spermicide used in contraceptive creams and foams. The spermicide is activated when moistened with a small amount of water just before insertion. The sponge, which can be used only once, acts as a barrier and a spermicide and absorbs seminal fluid.

**Advantages** The sponge offers advantages similar to those of the diaphragm and cervical cap. In addition, sponges can be obtained without a prescription or professional fitting, and they may be safely left in place for 24 hours without the addition of spermicide for repeated intercourse. Most women and men find the sponge to be comfortable and unobtrusive during sex.

**Disadvantages** Reported disadvantages include difficulty with removal and an unpleasant odor if the sponge is left in place for more than 18 hours. Allergic reactions, such as irritation of the vagina, are more common with the sponge than with other spermicide products, probably because the overall dose of spermicide contained in each sponge is significantly higher than that used with other methods. If irritation of the vaginal lining occurs, the risk of yeast infections and STIs (including HIV) may increase. The sponge is a single-use device and must be thrown away after each use. Additionally, the sponge cannot be used during menstruation.

**Effectiveness** The typical effectiveness of the sponge is the same as that of the diaphragm (14% failure rate during the first year of use) for women who have never experienced childbirth. For women who have had a child, however, the failure rate rises to 27%.

## Vaginal Spermicides and Gels

Spermicidal compounds developed for use with a diaphragm have been adapted for use without a diaphragm by combining them with a bulky base. Foams, creams, and jellies must be placed deep in the vagina near the cervical entrance and must be inserted no more than 60 minutes before intercourse. After an hour, their effectiveness is reduced drastically, and a new dose must be inserted. Another application is also required before each repeated act of coitus.

The spermicidal suppository is small and easily inserted like a tampon. The vaginal contraceptive film (VCF) is a paper-thin two-inch square of film that contains spermicide. It is folded over one or two fingers and placed high in the vagina, as close to the cervix as possible.

While not technically a spermicide, a newer product, Phexxi is a gel that is used in a similar way. It is inserted vaginally with a pre-filled applicator. Phexxi makes the vagina more acidic in the presence of sperm, making it harder for sperm to move, decreasing the chance of fertilization. It may be used with condoms and all other barrier methods.

**Advantages** The use of vaginal spermicides and gels is relatively simple and can be limited to times of sexual activity. They are readily available in most drugstores and do not require a prescription or a pelvic examination. An exception is Phexxi, which is available only by prescription. Spermicides allow complete and immediate reversibility, and the only medical side effects are occasional allergic reactions.

**Disadvantages** When used alone, vaginal spermicides must be inserted shortly before intercourse, so their use may be seen as a disruption. Some women find the slight increase in vaginal fluids after spermicide use unpleasant. Also, spermicides can alter the balance of bacteria in the vagina.

**TERMS**

**cervical cap** A small, flexible cup that fits over the cervix; used with spermicide.

**contraceptive sponge** A contraceptive device about two inches in diameter that fits over the cervix and acts as a barrier and spermicide and absorbs seminal fluid.

## Ask Yourself

**QUESTIONS FOR CRITICAL THINKING AND REFLECTION**

If you are sexually active, do you use any of the reversible methods described in the preceding sections? Based on the information given here, do you believe you are using your contraceptive perfectly, or in a way that increases your risk of an unintended pregnancy?

Because this may increase the occurrence of yeast infections and urinary tract infections, women who are especially prone to these infections may want to avoid spermicides. Also, this contraception method does not protect against STIs such as gonorrhea, chlamydia, or HIV. Overuse of spermicides can irritate vaginal tissues; if this occurs, the risk of HIV transmission may increase.

**Effectiveness** Vaginal spermicides on their own are not very effective. The typical failure rate is about 21% during the first year of use. Spermicide is generally recommended only in combination with other barrier methods or as a backup to other contraceptives. Emergency contraceptives provide a better backup than spermicides, however.

# BEHAVIORAL METHODS OF CONTRACEPTION

People may choose to use behavioral methods because of individual preferences, cultural prohibitions, religious convictions, or lack of access to contraceptive methods dispensed or administered by health care workers or pharmacies. These methods require active participation and cooperation from both partners.

## Abstinence

The decision not to engage in sexual intercourse for a chosen period of time, or **abstinence,** has been practiced throughout history for a variety of reasons. Until relatively recently, many people abstained because they had no other contraceptive measures. Concern about possible contraceptive side effects, STIs, and unwanted pregnancy may be factors. For others, the most important reason for choosing abstinence is a moral one, based on cultural or religious beliefs or strongly held personal values.

**TERMS**

**abstinence** Avoidance of sexual intercourse; can be a method of contraception.

**withdrawal** A method of contraception in which the man withdraws his penis from the vagina prior to ejaculation; also called coitus interruptus.

## Withdrawal

In **withdrawal,** or *coitus interruptus,* the male removes his penis from the vagina just before he ejaculates. Withdrawal has a high failure rate because the male has to overcome a powerful biological urge. Further, because preejaculatory fluid may contain viable sperm, pregnancy can occur even if the man withdraws prior to ejaculation. Sexual pleasure is often affected because the man must remain in control and the sexual experience of both partners is interrupted. The failure rate for typical use is about 22% in the first year. Withdrawal does not protect against STIs.

## Fertility Awareness–Based Methods

Sexual partners abstain from intercourse during the woman's fertile phase of their menstrual cycle. First day of a period is considered day 1 and on average, a woman will release one egg from her ovaries midway through the cycle (this is called ovulation). The egg exists for about 24 hours unless it is fertilized. Sperm can exist in the female genital tract for up to five days. Thus, the fertile phase is five days leading to ovulation and 24 hours after. Those wanting to prevent pregnancy should avoid vaginal-penile sex during those six "at-risk for pregnancy" days. While seemingly straightforward, in practice it is often difficult to determine correctly when a woman is in her fertile phase, making this approach about 75% effective with typical use.

It is only appropriate for women with regular menstrual cycles and for couples who agree to abstain from sex or use a barrier method during the at-risk days or when learning about the woman's cycle. The most common types of methods are described here:

1. *Calendar or rhythm method:* Track cycles on a calendar for at least six months before beginning. The first day of abstinence is calculated by subtracting 18 from the number of days in the shortest cycle. The last day is calculated by subtracting 11 from the number of days in the longest cycle.
2. *Temperature method*: Some women's basal (resting) body temperature (BBT) drops slightly just before ovulation and rises slightly after ovulation. Typically, fertile days begin on day 5 and end three days after the BBT increases. Dedicated thermometers can track these minor fluctuations.
3. *Mucus or Billings method:* Some women can detect a change in the texture of their cervical mucus and find that, at the time of ovulation, it is more likely to form an elastic thread when stretched between thumb and finger. After ovulation, these secretions become cloudy and sticky and decrease in quantity.
4. *Symptothermal technique:* Determining ovulation and predicting the fertile phase using at least two of the preceding methods is more effective than any of the methods alone.

## WELLNESS ON CAMPUS
## Contraception Use and Pregnancy Among College Students

College is a time of increased sexual activity for many young adults. Those who were sexually active in high school may engage with more sexual partners or in riskier behaviors once they enter college; those who abstained from intercourse during high school may begin to explore their sexuality once they enter this new environment.

This greater and newfound sexual activity among young women, especially, is often discussed in popular media and in scientific literature in connection with an increased risk for STIs, mental health issues, and other problems. To combat this negative focus surrounding women, research institutions such as the American Psychological Association and the Centers for Disease Control and Prevention encourage a new emphasis on women's comfort and happiness surrounding their sexual activities. Sexual exploration in a variety of relationship contexts (e.g., experiencing more than one relationship) is also increasingly seen as an important part of women's development of a safe, fulfilling sexual self and well-being. Studies have shown that young adults who avoid sexual activity may be deprived of opportunities for positive sexual experiences.

With more sexual partners and exploration, it becomes important for all partners to discuss safety and risks. Young adults tend to prefer romantic relationships to hookups, even during college. But if a committed romantic partner is not available, then casual sex may be perceived as acceptable in the short term. Over 50% of undergraduates reported engaging in sexual activity with an uncommitted partner.

Concerns about STIs and pregnancy are on the minds of many students. Male condoms were the most commonly used contraceptive, with about 65% of men using this method; women who used a contraceptive at last intercourse reported using the pill 51% of the time, IUDs 16%, and implants 9%. Of note, the withdrawal method was used by 30% of respondents; this method does not protect against STIs and has a high failure rate in preventing pregnancy.

Although the male condom is effective at preventing the transmission of a wide variety of STIs and the oral contraceptive pill is a highly effective form of contraception when used as directed, they must be used together to provide simultaneous protection against both pregnancy and STIs. This is particularly important for couples who are not in a long-term, mutually monogamous relationship. However, surveys show that college students use a male condom plus another form of contraception only about 45% of the time.

Around 1% of college women report having become pregnant in the previous year, many unintentionally. A disproportionate number of these pregnancies occur in students attending community colleges; recent data indicate that 10% of female dropouts at community colleges were due to unplanned births—as were 7% of all community college dropouts.

The consequences of pregnancy among college students can be significant. For example, studies have demonstrated that 60% of women who became pregnant while attending community college subsequently dropped out. Those who continue their education face added expenses and stress. Given the importance of education in achieving long-term career and financial goals, the implementation of effective contraception during the college years can have a significant impact on the lives of young women. Unfortunately, only 42% of students report that their college provided any information about pregnancy prevention.

SOURCES: Kaestle, C. E., and L. M. Evans. 2018. Implications of no recent sexual activity, casual sex, or exclusive sex for college women's sexual well-being depend on sexual attitudes. *Journal of American College Health* 66(1): 32–40; Hamilton, K. M., et al. 2019. Nonmedical use of prescription drugs during sexual activity as a predictor of condom use among a sample of college students. *Journal of American College Health* 67(5): 459–468; American College Health Association. 2019. American College Health Association-National College Health Assessment II: Reference Group Data Report. Spring 2019. Silver Spring, MD: American College Health Association (https://www.acha.org/documents/ncha/ncha-ii_spring_2019_us_reference_group_data_report.pdf).

## CONTRACEPTION AFTER PREGNANCY

Women can initiate contraception shortly after giving birth to provide enough time before having another child or to avoid future pregnancy; timing depends on her preferences, her health, and the method desired. In addition to the modern and behavioral methods of contraception discussed, women who are breastfeeding may use the *lactational amenorrhea method*, which is intentionally relying on breastfeeding as the way to prevent pregnancy. A person can use this method as long as she has not resumed her period, she is exclusively breastfeeding, and the baby is less than six months old. This method is not realistic for many, as 20–50% of women start menstruating within the first six months, and many postpartum women do not breastfeed for six months. Women can use lactational amenorrhea along with most other methods of contraception.

## EMERGENCY CONTRACEPTION

**Emergency contraception (EC)** refers to postcoital methods—those used after unprotected sexual intercourse but before the establishment of a pregnancy. An emergency contraceptive may be appropriate if a regularly used method has failed

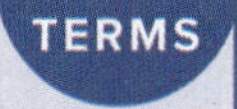


**emergency contraception (EC)** A birth control method used after unprotected sexual intercourse.

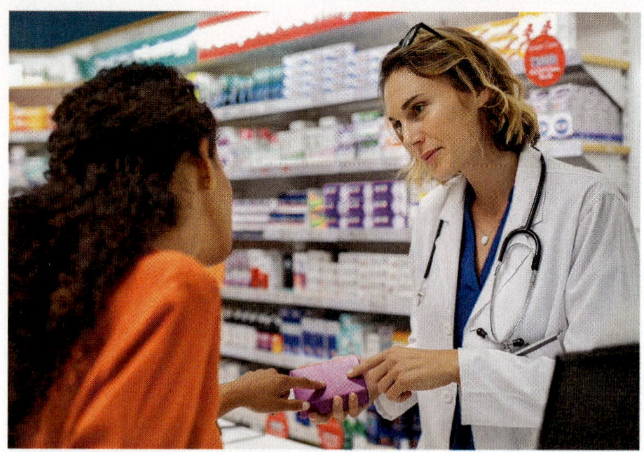

Rido/Shutterstock

(for example, if a condom breaks or pills were missed) or if a couple engaged in unprotected sex. There are pills and intrauterine devices (IUDs) that can be used for EC up to five days following intercourse. They do not interrupt an existing pregnancy and therefore, do not cause an abortion. EC pills are more commonly used than IUDs, though IUDs are more effective in preventing pregnancy.

There are two types of oral medications (pills), one containing a progestin, levonorgestrel (Plan B One-Step, Next Choice One Dose), and the other containing ulipristal (Ella®). Both types of medications delay ovulation and thereby lower the chances of sperm fertilizing an egg. Plan B One Step is available without a prescription at most pharmacies, health centers, and even vending machines at college campuses. Next Choice One Dose is available for persons 17 and older without a prescription.

To buy most emergency contraceptives, you need to ask at the pharmacy counter. It is recommended that you call ahead to make sure your pharmacy has EC on hand. They are most effective if taken as soon as possible, ideally within 72 hours, but they can be taken up to 120 hours (five days) after intercourse. Ulipristal EC maintains the same efficacy for 120 hours and is available only by prescription. Possible side effects of EC pills include nausea, stomach pain, headache, dizziness, and breast tenderness. People on birth control pills should wait five days after taking ulipristal (Ella) before resuming this method as it can interfere with Ella working. Some clinicians advise women to keep a package of emergency contraceptives on hand in case their regular contraception method fails or they have unprotected intercourse. Research has found that ready access to emergency contraception increases the rate of use and decreases the time to use. It does not result in more unprotected sex or STIs.

The most effective form of EC is the Paragard IUD when inserted within 120 hours (five days) of unprotected sex. A recent study suggests that the Mirena IUD might also be an effective EC method, but more research is needed before the Mirena IUD is implemented for this indication. How IUDs work in preventing pregnancy as ECs is not well understood, but it is clear that these do not disrupt an implanted embryo. The main benefits of selecting an IUD instead of an EC pill are that it is more likely to prevent pregnancy and it provides long-term contraception. However, an IUD may be more difficult to obtain, especially within five days, and its use includes the discomforts of the device's insertion.

> **Ask Yourself**
>
> **QUESTIONS FOR CRITICAL THINKING AND REFLECTION**
>
> Do you feel your sexual education up to this point in your life has been helpful? Do you feel it has prepared you to have a healthy, safe, and responsible sexual life?

## ABORTION

Even when using contraception, it is important to consider what one would do if they or their sexual partner becomes pregnant. Some may have an abortion (meaning ending the pregnancy), while others may continue the pregnancy and become parents or pursue adoption. The circumstances of one's life influence the decision, and someone may have an abortion at one point in their life and have a child at another. Abortion is common: nearly one in four American women (24%) have an abortion during their lifetime, and more than half (60%) of people who have an abortion already have children. It is also safe when done under the care of a trained medical professional.

We should also think about abortion independent of contraception. Some people become pregnant as a result of nonconsensual sex, or they did not know that they could get pregnant. In addition, some people want to have a child and intended to be pregnant but find out that continuing their pregnancy may seriously compromise their health or the health of their developing baby. In all these circumstances, the person may consider ending the pregnancy.

Having both the right and the access to abortion as well as having social institutions that support pregnancy and child rearing fully enable people to make decisions about their bodies and possible parenthood. Despite the importance of abortion to individuals and society, many people live in places where abortion services are not available due to laws, policies, and practices that make it difficult for medical institutions to offer them. Some 41% of women worldwide live under restrictive laws, and this is becoming more common in the United States. Places with the greatest abortion restrictions also have the highest abortion-related morbidity and mortality. In such settings, people still seek abortions but do so clandestinely in unsafe conditions, risking death or long-term problems such as injury to their reproductive organs and other physical, emotional, and social consequences. Unsafe abortion, defined as a procedure for terminating a pregnancy either by persons lacking the necessary skills or in an environment lacking minimal health standards, is a leading but preventable cause of pregnancy-related death and complications. Therefore, the World Health

While techniques to end pregnancy have changed over time, the practice of abortion goes back thousands of years. In the United States, until the 19th century, abortion was largely a private affair without any government or professional oversight.

The first anti-abortion campaign was launched in the mid-19th century, and doctors were at the forefront of this movement. They intended to raise the standard of abortion care, mandating that abortions be performed only by doctors in a hospital for women with health conditions that were life-threatening. For instance, it became illegal for a family who could not afford another child to ask a midwife to perform an abortion at home. Instead, the pregnant woman would need to be admitted to the hospital by a doctor and demonstrate that she needed an abortion to save her life. Unfortunately, the techniques used by physicians in hospitals to terminate pregnancies were not necessarily safer than techniques used by non-doctors in the community and were cost-prohibitive for many. Consequently, thousands of women who sought to end their pregnancies had no choice but to seek illegal abortions.

By the mid-20th century, the medical profession started to recognize the harms of criminalizing abortion. Also during this time, women's status improved as they entered the labor force and demanded a say over reproductive decisions and access to safe abortion. Abortion was legalized in the United States in 1973 with the landmark Supreme Court decision in *Roe v. Wade,* determining that abortion is a fundamental right under the due process clause of the 14th Amendment as a right of privacy. The decision to have an abortion was up to the woman and her doctor within certain constraints, such as how far along the woman was in her pregnancy.

Subsequently, legalization of abortion allowed significant improvements in its safety and technique. In terms of safety, the evolution of abortion care in the United States is overall a great success and has influenced abortion care worldwide; however, it is not without challenges. Isolating abortion services to abortion clinics has perpetuated the stigma for women seeking abortions and medical professionals who provide this care, implying that abortion is somehow different from other reproductive services. Some clinicians abstain from performing abortions for personal reasons, but a majority are not able to provide this procedure even if they want to because institutional rules or logistics make it extremely difficult or impossible to do so. Furthermore, it has made abortion clinics vulnerable to attacks by extremist individuals and groups that oppose abortion. Since the early 1990s there has been an increase in violence against abortion providers and abortion clinics, including vandalism, bombing, arson, and shootings, some of which have been fatal.

Using the legislative and legal systems to restrict abortion has become an important strategy in state and national politics by groups opposed to abortion and has shifted the conversation away from the area of health and reproductive justice. Over the last 50 years, some federal and many state laws have tested the limits of *Roe v. Wade* by making it more difficult for a woman to obtain an abortion. The biggest challenge presented has been the Supreme Court case, *Dobbs v. Jackson Women's Health Organization*. In June 2022, the Supreme Court gave states the right to ban abortion under any circumstance and at any point in a pregnancy. This ruling is expected to markedly restrict abortion access in 22 states, with 13 states having "trigger laws" in place to ban abortion immediately upon the overturn of *Roe v. Wade*.

Figure 7.7 depicts abortion rates since legalization. The number of abortions rose after legalization, reaching a peak in the early 1980s and then declining steadily. The drop has occurred across the nation and not just in states with the most significant restrictions. Other factors are likely contributing, such as declining pregnancy and birth rates from increased access and use of contraception.

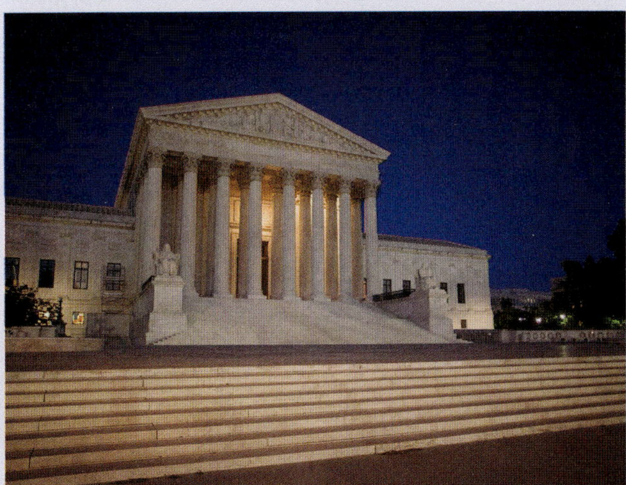

Mark Andersen/Rubberball/Getty Images

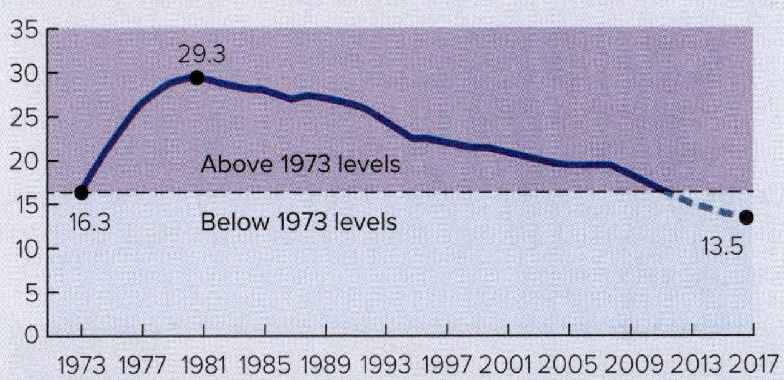


**FIGURE 7.7 The U.S. abortion rate reached a historic low in 2017.**

SOURCE: Guttmacher Institute. September 2019. Induced abortion in the United States (https://www.guttmacher.org/fact-sheet/induced-abortion-united-states).

Organization recognizes that access to safe, timely, affordable, and respectful abortion care is a critical public health and human rights issue.

## UNDERSTANDING ABORTION

The word **abortion** generally refers to a pregnancy ending. A **spontaneous abortion,** also called a miscarriage, is a pregnancy that ends on its own; it may be an emotionally trying event for some women and their families, and it is often experienced as a loss.

About 15% of pregnant women experience spontaneous abortions, which occur most frequently during the first trimester. Generally, chromosomal abnormalities lead to an abnormal pregnancy that is incompatible with life and that the body ultimately detects and ends. **Induced abortion,** or pregnancy termination, is a pregnancy that is intentionally ended. The rest of this chapter focuses on induced abortion.

The decision to have an abortion may be complex or straightforward, depending on the circumstances of one's life at that time, and is usually in the context of an unintended pregnancy. This is the reason for 95% of abortions in the United States. An **unintended pregnancy** includes pregnancies that are (1) *mistimed,* meaning that a woman or couple wanted to conceive but at a later date or (2) *unwanted,* meaning that a woman or couple did not want to conceive at all. Mistimed pregnancies account for 60% of unintended pregnancies. More than half of women with unintended pregnancies continue their pregnancies and give birth. The remainder of women with unintended pregnancies have either an induced abortion or a miscarriage in relatively equal proportions.

### Personal and Social Indicators

Several personal and social indicators are commonly given as reasons for terminating a pregnancy. These reasons include lack of financial resources; interference with the woman's work, educational aspirations, or ability to care for their children; reluctance to become a single parent; or problems in a relationship. Younger women who become pregnant often report that they are unprepared for the transition to motherhood, whereas older women regularly cite that a pregnancy would interfere with their responsibility to their existing children.

**TERMS**

**abortion** A pregnancy ending.

**spontaneous abortion** Also known as miscarriage or pregnancy loss; a pregnancy that ends on its own.

**induced abortion** An ongoing pregnancy that is ended deliberately; synonymous with pregnancy termination.

**unintended pregnancy** A mistimed (wrongly timed) or unwanted (not desired at all) pregnancy.

**viable** Able to survive outside the uterus.

Women who have abortions represent various ages, religions, races, and levels of education. Poverty has been identified as a key factor leading to an abortion. In 2014, 75% of American women undergoing an abortion were poor or low income by federal standards.

### Fetal and Maternal Indicators

Individuals may ultimately decide to end a pregnancy if they learn from genetic testing or ultrasound that the fetus has a significant abnormality. In addition, due to risks to their own health, pregnant women with serious medical conditions sometimes need to end their pregnancies. These conditions might include severe high blood pressure, a lung disease called pulmonary hypertension, severe kidney disease, advanced diabetes, and severe cardiac disease. Some conditions that already exist can worsen in pregnancy and permanently compromise a woman's health after pregnancy. If she knows that her health is at risk, ending the pregnancy before the fetus becomes **viable** (able to survive outside the uterus) may prevent a life-threatening problem.

### Personal Considerations for the Pregnant Woman

For a woman with an unintended or abnormal pregnancy, the decision about how to proceed is not political, especially as she tries to weigh the many short- and long-term ramifications for all those who are directly concerned. If she continues the pregnancy, how will her life change by having a child? Can she become a mother to this child? If she has other children, how will another child affect them? How does she feel about adoption? What are her long-term feelings likely to be? If she ends the pregnancy, does she feel like it contradicts her own moral or religious beliefs, and if so, can these be reconciled? What are her partner's feelings about having this child? Does she have the social and emotional resources to raise the child on her own? If she is young, what will be the effects on her own development? Will she be able to continue with her educational and personal goals? What about the ongoing financial responsibilities?

### Personal Considerations for the Partner

Partners are often involved in the decision-making process, and they may experience a range of emotions similar to those felt by pregnant women. Men and nonpregnant partners may also accompany pregnant women during the abortion process. Accompaniment may reflect an effort to share responsibility for the pregnancy as well as to provide emotional and practical support by providing transportation or helping to pay for the abortion. Supporting each other through the abortion process may strengthen their relationship. In some instances, partners disagree with the pregnant woman's decision, and they may try to control the outcome of the pregnancy or may be abusive. Many abortion facilities are sensitive to creating a safe space for pregnant women in such situations.

## Considering Adoption

Before abortions were legal, women with unintended pregnancies had the legal options of becoming a parent or pursuing adoption. Before 1979, about 9% of babies born to never-married women were relinquished for adoption, and in the mid-1990s to early 2000s, the number dropped to 1%. This decline may be due to a variety of factors, including an easing of the social stigma of single parenthood. Many children who are adopted are adopted by a relative or foster parent. Adoptions in which the child is not related to an adoptive parent(s) are more common among those with higher levels of income and educational attainment. The decision to go through an unintended pregnancy and then give the baby to another family may be emotionally difficult. Adoption is permanent: The adoptive parents will raise the child and have legal authority for their welfare. Many people can help a pregnant woman to consider her options, including her partner, friends, family members, a professional counselor, a family planning clinic, or family services, social services, or adoption agencies. A person who places the child for adoption should also consider the reaction and rights of the biological father. A woman can choose to have an abortion without the consent or knowledge of the father, but once the baby is born, the father has certain rights. These rights vary by state, but at a minimum, most states require that the biological father be notified of the adoption. Working with an adoption agency can help a person navigate the laws in each particular state.

# METHODS OF ABORTION

Abortion is an extremely safe medical procedure. To put it into perspective, it is safer than childbirth. The technique used to end the pregnancy depends on how far along a woman is in her pregnancy. Ultrasound (a device that shows an image of the developing fetus) is the most accurate way to determine this. If an ultrasound is not available, the date of the woman's last period and/or a gynecologic exam provide an estimate.

## First-Trimester Abortion

Most abortions (90%) in the United States take place in the first trimester. Women who are up to 2.5 months pregnant can choose between taking pills or having a procedure to end the pregnancy. Women who are 2.5 to 3.5 months pregnant undergo a procedure.

**Medication abortion** entails taking two medications, mifepristone and misoprostol. People who have a medication abortion take mifepristone in a doctor's office and then go home. They take the second medication, misoprostol, on their own. This second medication causes period-like cramps and causes the pregnancy tissue to pass out of the body, usually within four hours, but it can be up to 48 hours. The amount of bleeding is similar to that of a heavy period or miscarriage. Women return to see their provider one to two weeks later and have an ultrasound or a serum pregnancy test to confirm they are no longer pregnant. With the rise of telehealth and challenges in accessing abortion care, some people consult with a clinician virtually to determine their eligibility for a medication abortion. Then they receive the medications in the mail or at a designated clinic. The person has a follow-up virtual visit to confirm that the medications worked. Medication abortion successfully ends pregnancies 95–97% of the time. If the woman continues to be pregnant, she may repeat the medications or undergo an aspiration procedure.

**Aspiration abortion** is another way to end a pregnancy in the first trimester. It is also known as "suction abortion," or dilation and curettage (D&C). This is a procedure performed in a medical facility (usually in an outpatient clinic and rarely in a hospital) by a trained clinician. The woman is usually awake, and the procedure is done through the vagina exclusively (no cut on the abdomen). The clinician dilates the cervix (opening to the uterus) and inserts a slender tube into the uterus, which is attached to a vacuum device, and removes the pregnancy. The procedure may cause strong cramps and usually takes fewer than 10 minutes. Women undergoing the procedure receive a powerful oral or intravenous pain medication in addition to a numbing medication administered vaginally. The cramping subsides once the procedure is over. Women return home the same day, typically within 30 minutes to an hour after the pain medication has worn off. Aspiration abortions are successful 98% of the time.

**Medication vs. Aspiration Abortion in the First Trimester** Some women may have the option of selecting either medication or aspiration abortion to end a first-trimester pregnancy. A number of women feel that medication abortion allows them to take more control of the process and gives them more privacy than an aspiration abortion. It is also a noninvasive alternative to aspiration abortion because no instruments are introduced into the uterus. Most women who select a medication abortion are satisfied with this method.

A downside of medication abortion is that it takes longer to complete, typically at least 24 hours from the time the first pill is taken to the time the pregnancy passes, whereas an aspiration abortion takes about 10 minutes for the entire procedure. Side effects of one of the medications, misoprostol, include nausea, vomiting, diarrhea, fever, and abdominal pain for some women. Women undergoing a medication abortion are typically given additional medications to help with these symptoms. Vaginal bleeding is often more prolonged and in a few cases heavier than with aspiration abortion. The financial cost to the patient is generally about the same.

**TERMS**

**medical abortion** A method of ending an early first-trimester pregnancy by taking two sets of pills: mifepristone and misoprostol.

**aspiration abortion (D&C)** A vaginal procedure to end a first-trimester pregnancy that involves aspiration of the uterus; also known as suction abortion, suction curettage, or dilation and curettage.

## Second-Trimester Abortion

About 10% of abortions take place in the second trimester (between three and six months of pregnancy). Women who have an abortion at this stage in pregnancy may do so for a variety of reasons: They recognized they were pregnant later in the pregnancy; they had a difficult time finding a facility to have an abortion; they felt conflicted about ending the pregnancy and needed more time to decide; they discovered that the fetus had problems; or they became sick themselves, making it difficult or dangerous to continue the pregnancy. The approach to ending a second-trimester pregnancy depends on where the woman goes for care and how far along she is.

Some medical facilities offer termination of pregnancy by inducing labor with medications, a process called **induction abortion.** Other facilities may offer a surgical procedure called **dilation and evacuation (D&E),** the most common method of second-trimester pregnancy termination in the United States. While similar to a first-trimester procedural abortion, a D&E may take longer, and women typically receive stronger pain medications. Dilation and evacuation is typically done as outpatient surgery, but a woman may need to be seen the day before to take medications or to begin the process of dilating the cervix. Under moderate or deep sedation (woman asleep), the fetus is surgically removed from the uterus through the vagina, and suction is used to remove any remaining tissue; women can usually go home the same day. Soreness and cramping may occur for a day or two after the procedure, and some bleeding may last for one to two weeks. Second-trimester pregnancy termination is also very safe (Table 7.2).

**Table 7.2** Risks of Contraception, Pregnancy, and Abortion

| CONTRACEPTION | RISK OF DEATH |
|---|---|
| Oral contraceptives | |
| Nonsmoker | |
| Ages 15–34 | 1 in 1,667,000 |
| Ages 35–44 | 1 in 33,300 |
| Smoker | |
| Ages 15–34 | 1 in 57,800 |
| Ages 35–44 | 1 in 5,200 |
| IUDs | 1 in 10,000,000 |
| Barrier methods, spermicides | None |
| Fertility awareness-based methods | None |
| Tubal ligation | 1 in 66,700 |
| **PREGNANCY** | |
| Pregnancy | 1 in 6,900 |
| **ABORTION** | |
| Spontaneous abortion | 1 in 142,900 |
| Medical abortion | 1 in 200,000 |
| Surgical abortion | 1 in 142,900 |

SOURCE: Hatcher, R. A., et al. *Contraceptive Technology,* 20th revised ed. 2011, Ardent Media.

# POSTABORTION CONSIDERATIONS

The recovery after an abortion is rapid, usually lasting a few days, and most women do not need to significantly modify their everyday activities as part of recovery. Abortion does not cause infertility, jeopardize a woman's ability to have children in the future, compromise her reproductive organs, or increase her chances of cancer. The incidence of immediate problems following an abortion (infection, bleeding, trauma to the cervix or uterus, and incomplete abortion requiring another procedure) is rare. The potential for problems is reduced significantly by a woman's good health, early timing of the abortion, use of the suction method compared to an older technique using sharp curettage, performance by a well-trained clinician, and the availability and use of prompt follow-up care.

There has been concern that women who have an abortion face long-term mental health consequences and that they might be better off by having the child instead. Researchers have studied this possibility rigorously, most recently in the Turnaway Study. They compared women who successfully had an abortion to women who were "turned away" because their pregnancies were too far along for the medical facilities where they sought care (medical facilities and state laws determine limits for performing procedures, and the limits vary widely from one facility or region to another). Women who got an abortion and those who were turned away were similarly far along in their pregnancies. The study found that a person's feelings toward an unintended pregnancy and feelings toward having an abortion are mixed–many women felt regret about an unwanted pregnancy and also felt that the decision to have an abortion was the right decision for them.

Most women who were denied an abortion gave birth and adjusted to motherhood, happy to have that child. Nine percent of the women pursued adoption. Rates of mental health problems did not appear higher in women who had an abortion compared to women who gave birth or vice versa. This shows that abortion does not typically lead to mental health problems. The most profound measurable effect observed in the group of women who were denied an abortion and went on raise that child was economic. They had four times greater odds of ending up below the federal poverty level and three times greater odds of being unemployed compared to women who had abortions, despite having similar socioeconomic status before the pregnancy. As many women predict when making a decision to have an abortion, having a child significantly strains their resources.

**TERMS**

**induction abortion** A method to end a second-trimester pregnancy by administering medications to induce labor and delivery of a fetus.

**dilation and evacuation (D&E)** A vaginal surgical procedure to end a second-trimester pregnancy that involves surgical removal of the pregnancy from the uterus.

> ## Ask Yourself
> **QUESTIONS FOR CRITICAL THINKING AND REFLECTION**
> Suppose one of your friends has an unplanned pregnancy and does not know what to do. How would you begin discussing how she feels and what options are available to her? What kind of support would you be willing to offer?

## THE POLITIZATION OF ABORTION

Abortion is simultaneously one of the most common procedures in the United States (with a quarter of women having one by age 45) and the most polarized. Opinions about abortion have remained generally consistent over time. Although nearly half of Americans feel that abortion is morally wrong, an overwhelming majority supports legal availability of abortion services in some circumstances (see Figure 7.8).

While most Americans believe abortion should be legal, a well-organized anti-abortion minority has had much influence over state legislatures and courts aiming to take away this right. Over the years, their efforts have been largely successful in restricting people's access to abortion and more recently, as of the 2022 U.S. Supreme Court decision, making most abortions illegal again.

To understand how the country came to this crossroads, we must explore the legal protections that the 1973 landmark case of *Roe v. Wade* provided. *Roe v. Wade* legalized abortion in every state and created a uniform framework for all states to follow. The justices divided pregnancy into three parts, or *trimesters,* giving a woman less choice about abortion as her pregnancy advances toward full term. According to *Roe v. Wade,* in the first trimester, the abortion decision must be left to the judgment of the pregnant woman and her doctor. During the second trimester, similar rights remain up to the point when the fetus becomes viable. Today most clinicians define this point as 23–24 weeks of gestation. When the fetus is considered viable, a state may regulate and even bar all abortions except those considered necessary to preserve the pregnant person's life or health.

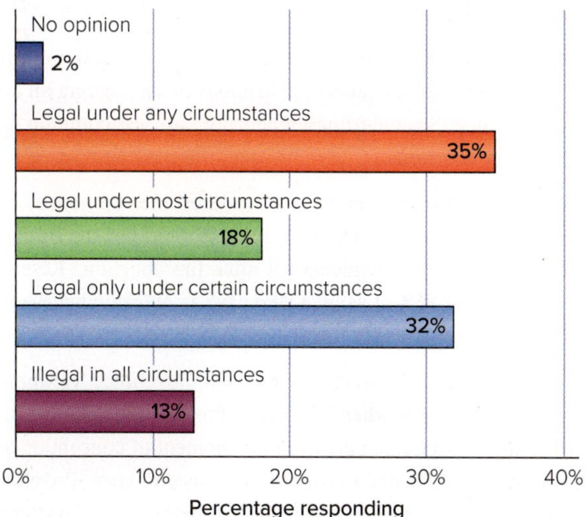


**FIGURE 7.8 Public opinion about abortion.**

SOURCE: "Abortion," In Depth: Topics A to Z. Gallup Inc. 2019.  http://www.gallup.com/poll/1576/abortion.aspx.

Three years after *Roe v. Wade,* Congress passed the Hyde Amendment, which prohibits the use of federal funds (such as Medicaid) to pay for an abortion unless the pregnancy arises from incest or rape or if the woman's life is endangered. In practice, this amendment affects women who rely on Medicaid to pay for medical services. They must pay out of pocket for abortion-related care, and if they are unable to pay or they take too long to raise funds, they may be compelled to continue their pregnancies.

In 1992, the U.S. Supreme Court case *Planned Parenthood of Southeastern Pennsylvania v. Casey* affirmed the right to abortion before viability but gave states the power to regulate abortion as long as no "undue burden" is imposed on women seeking these services. The "undue burden" test is ambiguous and more difficult to apply, creating many ways to make it more challenging for a person to have an abortion even if they maintain this right. Examples include mandatory waiting periods, parental consent for minors, and state-mandated counseling. These have generally not been considered to be an undue burden (and therefore not unconstitutional), whereas spousal consent has been deemed unconstitutional.

Since the composition of the Supreme Court became more conservative during the Trump presidency, some states have passed laws to ban abortions in the first trimester or early in the second trimester, directly challenging *Roe v. Wade*. Examples include prohibiting all abortions as early as at conception or after a fetal heartbeat can be detected by ultrasound, which happens before many women know they are pregnant (around six weeks). *Dobbs v. Jackson Women's Health Organization* bans all abortions after 15 weeks of gestation except in cases of medical emergencies and severe fetal anomalies. After the Supreme Court sided with Mississippi, laws banning or restricting abortion before viability were poised to go into effect in 21 states.

Unlike Mississippi, some states (mostly in the West and Northeast) passed laws in support of abortion rights and access. Some examples include protecting access to abortion clinics, allowing clinicians other than physicians to perform abortions, and requiring public and private health insurance to cover abortion services. For example, California has all of these laws supportive of abortion, and in 2019 the state enacted a law requiring public universities to provide medical abortion services in their health centers. It was the first state in the country to pass such a law.

> ## Ask Yourself
> **QUESTIONS FOR CRITICAL THINKING AND REFLECTION**
> How may restrictive abortion laws increase the number of women who have second-trimester abortions? Do these laws affect poor women differently than they do more affluent women? What about the variation among states in abortion laws and number of providers?

## TIPS FOR TODAY AND THE FUTURE

You may never have to face an unplanned pregnancy, but you should know what choices you would have, as well as where you stand on the issue of abortion.

**RIGHT NOW YOU CAN:**

- If you're sexually active, consider whether you are confident that you're doing everything possible to prevent an unwanted pregnancy.
- If you're sexually active, discuss your contraceptive method with your partner. Make sure you are using the method that works best for you.
- Examine your feelings about the possibility of becoming a parent, especially if it were to happen unintentionally.
- Consider your views on the morality of abortion, and under which circumstances it would be acceptable to you.

**IN THE FUTURE YOU CAN:**

- Talk to your physician about contraception and get their advice on choosing the best method for you.
- Occasionally discuss your contraceptive method with your partner to make sure it continues to meet your needs. A change in health status or lifestyle may make a different form of contraception preferable in the future.
- Talk to your partner about the possibility of pregnancy. How would you proceed? Do you share similar views and feelings, or do they differ? How would you resolve conflicts about this issue?
- Make sure you are using your contraceptive method correctly and consistently. Become familiar with emergency contraception in case your method fails.

## SUMMARY

- Barrier methods of contraception physically prevent sperm from reaching the egg; hormonal methods are designed to prevent ovulation, fertilization, and/or implantation; and surgical methods permanently block the movement of sperm or eggs to the site of conception.
- The choice of contraceptive method depends on effectiveness, convenience, cost, reversibility, side effects, risk factors, protection against STIs, and noncontraceptive benefits. Measures of effectiveness include failure rate and continuation rate.
- Hormonal methods may include a combination of estrogen and progestin, or a progestin alone. Hormones may be delivered via pills, patch, vaginal ring, IUD, implants, or injections.
- Hormonal methods prevent ovulation, inhibit the movement of sperm, and affect the uterine lining so that implantation is prevented.
- IUDs and implants can provide very effective long-term (3–12 years) contraception and are especially useful for women who want contraception for at least six months.
- Male condoms are simple to use, are immediately reversible, and provide STI protection; female condoms can be inserted hours before intercourse.
- The diaphragm, cervical cap, and contraceptive sponge cover the cervix and block sperm from entering; all need to be used with or contain spermicide.
- Vaginal spermicides come in the form of foams, creams, jellies, suppositories, and film. There's also a gel available by prescription that is used similarly.
- Behavioral methods of contraception include abstinence, withdrawal, and fertility awareness.
- Combining methods can increase contraceptive effectiveness and help protect against STIs. The most common combination is a hormonal method, such as the birth control pill, combined with condoms.
- The most commonly used emergency contraceptive, Plan B One-Step, is available without a prescription.
- Vasectomy sterilization involves severing the vas deferens. Female sterilization involves severing or blocking the oviducts so that the egg cannot reach the uterus.
- Issues to be considered in choosing a contraceptive include the individual health risks of each method, the implications of an unplanned pregnancy, STI risk, convenience and comfort level, type of relationship, the cost and ease of obtaining and maintaining each method, and religious or philosophical beliefs.
- From the first anti-abortion campaigns of the mid-19th century, through the landmark *Roe v. Wade* Supreme Court decision of 1973, which legalized abortion in the United States, and then its overturning in the 2022 case *Dobbs v. Jackson Women's Health Organization,* abortion is a health issue that has also become politicized.
- In medical terms there are two distinct types of abortion: *spontaneous abortion* and *induced abortion*. A spontaneous abortion is a pregnancy that ends on its own and is referred to as *miscarriage* or *pregnancy loss.* Induced abortion is an ongoing pregnancy that is ended deliberately.
- Most induced abortions take place in the first trimester of pregnancy. Methods include taking medications or undergoing an aspiration procedure. Second-trimester abortions are less common than first-trimester abortions.
- Women's and men's emotional responses after an abortion include relief, happiness, regret, guilt, sadness, or anger; the strongest feelings usually occur immediately after the abortion. Research suggests that over 95% of women who have an abortion believe that it was the right decision for them.
- The controversy between pro-life and pro-choice viewpoints focuses on the issue of when life begins. Pro-life groups believe that a fertilized egg is a human life from the moment of conception and that a woman is obligated to carry a pregnancy to term. Pro-choice groups distinguish between stages of fetal development and argue that the fetus does not have an equal status to the pregnant woman and that the woman should make the final decision regarding her pregnancy. Most Americans are not completely pro-life or pro-choice but fall somewhere on the spectrum.

• Overall, public opinion in the United States supports legal abortion in at least some circumstances and opposes overturning *Roe v. Wade.*

## FOR MORE INFORMATION

*Bedsider.Org.* Provides information on all methods of contraception. Describes how to use a method, typical side effects, cost, and how to get the method.

https://bedsider.org/

*Child Welfare Information Gateway.* A clearinghouse of information about many aspects of child rearing, including adoption.

http://www.childwelfare.gov

*Emergency Contraception website.* Provides extensive information and hotline about emergency contraception; sponsored by the Office of Population Research at Princeton University.

http://ec.princeton.edu and 888-NOT-2-LATE

*Guttmacher Institute.* Provides reproductive health research, policy analysis, and public education.

http://www.guttmacher.org

*It's Your Sex Life.* Provides information about sexuality, relationships, contraceptives, and STDs; geared toward teenagers and young adults. Provided by the Kaiser Family Foundation and MTV.

http://www.itsyoursexlife.com

*Kaiser Family Foundation: Women's Health Policy: Contraception.* Provides information and reports focused on how policies affect reproductive health care and access to contraceptives.

http://kff.org/other/womens-health-policy-contraception/

*Managing Contraception.* Provides brief descriptions and tips for using many forms of contraception. Features a detailed survey to help with contraceptive choices.

http://www.managingcontraception.com

*MedlinePlus: Abortion.* Managed by the U.S. National Library of Medicine and the National Institutes of Health, this site provides a list of informational resources about various aspects of abortion.

http://www.nlm.nih.gov/medlineplus/abortion.html

*National Abortion and Reproductive Rights Action League.* Provides information about the politics of the pro-choice movement. Also provides information about the abortion laws and politics in each state.

http://www.prochoiceamerica.org

*National Abortion Federation.* Provides information and resources on medical and political issues relating to abortion; managed by health care providers.

http://www.prochoice.org

*National Adoption Center.* A national agency focused on finding adoptive homes for children with special needs or who are currently in foster care.

http://www.adopt.org

*National Right to Life Committee.* Provides information about pregnancy continuation and the politics of the pro-life movement.

http://www.nrlc.org

*Plan B One-Step.* Contains a card you can print and hand to the pharmacist as an easy way to request EC.

http://www.planbonestep.com

*Planned Parenthood Federation of America.* Provides information on family planning, contraception, and abortion and offers counseling services.

http://www.plannedparenthood.org

*World Health Organization.* Provides information about contraception and abortion from a global perspective.

*https://www.who.int/health-topics/contraception*

*https://www.who.int/health-topics/abortion*

## SELECTED BIBLIOGRAPHY


Advancing New Standards in Reproductive Health. Turnaway Study. (http://www.ansirh.org/research/turnaway.php).

Altshuler, A. L., and P. D. Blumenthal. 2020. Behavioral methods of contraception. In: Shoupe, D. (eds.) *The Handbook of Contraception*, 3rd ed. Current Clinical Practice series. New York: Humana Press. https://doi.org/10.1007/978-3-030-46391-5_12

Altshuler, A. L., et al. 2016. Male partners' involvement in abortion care: A mixed methods systematic review. *Perspectives on Sexual and Reproductive Health* 48(4): 209–219.

Altshuler, A. L., et al. 2017. A good abortion experience: A qualitative exploration of women's needs and preferences in clinical care. *Social Science & Medicine* 191:109–116.

American Cancer Society. 2018. *Can Ovarian Cancer Be Prevented?* (https://www.cancer.org/cancer/ovarian-cancer/causes-risks-prevention/prevention.html).

American Cancer Society. 2020. *Risk Factors for Cervical Cancer* (https://www.cancer.org/cancer/cervical-cancer/causes-risks-prevention/risk-factors.html).

American College Health Association. 2019. *American College Health Association-National College Health Assessment II: Reference Group Data Report.* Spring 2019. Silver Spring, MD: American College Health Association (https://www.acha.org/documents/ncha/NCHA-II_SPRING_2019_US_REFERENCE_GROUP_DATA_REPORT.pdf).

American College of Obstetricians and Gynecologists. 2015. *Frequently Asked Questions: Induced Abortion* (http://www.acog.org/Patients/FAQs/Induced-Abortion).

Anawalt, B. D. 2007. Update on the development of male hormonal contraceptives. *Current Opinion in Investigational Drugs* 8(4): 318–323.

Bearak, J., et al. 2018. Global, regional, and subregional trends in unintended pregnancy and its outcomes from 1990 to 2014: Estimates from a Bayesian hierarchical model. *The Lancet Global Health* (6)4: PE380–E389.

Centers for Disease Control and Prevention. 2019. *About Teen Pregnancy* (https://www.cdc.gov/teenpregnancy/about/index.htm).

Cha, A. E. 2018. Nine organizations sue Trump administration for ending grants to teen pregnancy programs. *The Washington Post,* February 15 (https://www.washingtonpost.com/news/to-your-health/wp/2018/02/15/planned-parenthood-sues-trump-administration-for-ending-grants-to-teen-pregnancy-programs/).

Charles, V., et al. 2008. Abortion and long-term mental health outcomes: A systematic review of the evidence. *Contraception* 78(6): 436–450.

Cornell Law School Legal Information Institute. Dobbs v. Jackson Women's Health Organization. (https://www.law.cornell.edu/supct/cert/19-1392).

Cremer, M., and R. Masch. 2010. Emergency contraception: Past, present and future. *Minerva Ginecologica* 62(4): 361–371.

Critical Trials Arena. 2019. Phase I trial of male birth control pill reveals positive results (https://www.clinicaltrialsarena.com/news/trial-11-beta-mntdc/).

Curtin S. C., J. C. Abma, and K. Kost. 2015. 2010 pregnancy rates among U.S. women (http://www.cdc.gov/nchs/data/hestat/pregnancy/2010_pregnancy_rates.htm).

Dehlendorf, C., et al. 2011. Race, ethnicity and differences in contraception among low-income women. *Perspectives on Sexual and Reproductive Health* 43(3): 181–187.

Donovan, M. 2017. In real life: Federal restrictions on abortion coverage and the women they impact. *Guttmacher Policy Review* 20: 1–7.

Fine, P., et al. 2010. Ulipristal acetate taken 48–120 hours after intercourse for emergency contraception. *Obstetrics and Gynecology* 115: 257–263.

Finer, L. B., and M. R. Zolna. 2016. Declines in unintended pregnancy in the United States, 2008–2011. *New England Journal of Medicine* 374(9): 843–852.

Foster, D. G., et. al. 2018. Socioeconomic outcomes of women who receive and women who are denied wanted abortions. *American Journal of Public Health*. DOI:10.2105/AJPH.2017.304247

Guttmacher Institute. 2018. Global, regional, and subregional trends in unintended pregnancy and its outcomes from 1990 to 2014: Estimates from a Bayesian hierarchical model (https://www.guttmacher.org/article/2018/03/unintended-pregnancy-and-its-outcomes-global-regional-and-subregional-trends-1990).

Guttmacher Institute. 2018. Unintended pregnancy rates declined globally 1990–2014 (https://www.guttmacher.org/news-release/2018/unintended-pregnancy-rates-declined-globally-1990–2014).

Guttmacher Institute. 2019. Fact Sheet: Unintended Pregnancy in the United States (https://www.guttmacher.org/fact-sheet/unintended-pregnancy-united-states).

Guttmacher Institute. 2019. Fact Sheet: Induced Abortion in the United States (https://www.guttmacher.org/fact-sheet/induced-abortion-united-states).

Guttmacher Institute. 2022. State policy updates. Major developments in sexual & reproductive health (https://www.guttmacher.org/state-policy/explore/state-funding-%ADabortion-under-medicaid).

Guttmacher Insistute. 2022. *Abortion Policy in the Absence of Roe* (https://www.guttmacher.org/state-policy/explore/abortion-policy-absence-roe).

Harris, L. H. 2012. Recognizing conscience in abortion provision. *New England Journal of Medicine* 367(11): 981–983.

Jatlaoui, T. C., et al. 2018. Abortion surveillance United States, 2015. *MMWR Surveillance Summaries* 67(13): 1–45.

Jerman, J., R. K. Jones, and T. Onda. 2016. *Characteristics of U.S. Abortion Patients in 2014 and Changes Since 2008.* New York: Guttmacher Institute (https://www.guttmacher.org/sites/default/files/report_pdf/characteristics-us-abortion-patients-2014.pdf).

Joffe, C. 1995. *Doctors of Conscience. The Struggle to Provide Abortion Before and After* Roe v. Wade. Boston, MA: Beacon.

Jones, R. K., and J. Jerman. 2017a. Characteristics and circumstances of U.S. women who obtain very early and second-trimester abortions. *PLoS ONE* 12(1): e0169969.

Jones, R. K., et al. 2019. *Abortion Incidence and Service Availability in the United States, 2017.* New York: Guttmacher Institute (https://www.guttmacher.org/report/abortion-incidence-service-availability-us-2017).

Kossler, K., et al. 2011. Perceived racial, socioeconomic and gender discrimination and its impact on contraceptive choice. *Contraception* 84(3): 273–279.

Kulier, R., et al. 2011. Medical methods for first trimester abortion. *Cochrane Database Systematic Review* 11: CD002885.

Livingston, G., and D. Thomas. 2019. Why is the teen birth rate falling? *Fact Tank: News in the Numbers* (https://www.pewresearch.org/fact-tank/2019/08/02/why-is-the-teen-birth-rate-falling/).

Lyus, R., et al. 2011. Use of the Mirena LNG-IUS and ParaGard CuT380A intrauterine devices in nulliparous women. *Contraception* 81(5): 367–371.

Macmillan, C. 2019. What birth control is best for me? (https://www.yalemedicine.org/stories/best-birth-control-options/).

Mansour, D., et al. 2011. Fertility after discontinuation of contraception: A comprehensive review of the literature. *Contraception* 84(5): 465–477.

McNicholas, C. et al. 2015. Use of the etonogestrel implant and levonorgestrel intrauterine device beyond the U.S. Food and Drug Administration-approved duration. *Obstetrics & Gynecology* 125(3): 599–604.

Meyer, J. L., et al. 2011. Advance provision of emergency contraception among adolescent and young adult women: A systematic review of the literature. *Journal of Pediatric and Adolescent Gynecology* 24(1): 2–9.

Mohamad, A. M., et al. 2011. Combined contraceptive ring versus combined oral contraceptive. *International Journal of Gynecology and Obstetrics* 114(2): 145–148.

National Alliance of State Pharmacy Associations. 2019. Pharmacist prescribing: Hormonal contraceptives (https://naspa.us/resource/contraceptives/).

National Cancer Institute. 2018. Oral Contraceptives and Cancer Risk (https://www.cancer.gov/about-cancer/causes-prevention/risk/hormones/oral-contraceptives-fact-sheet).

National Center for Health Statistics. 2018. *National Survey of Family Growth: Contraception* (http://www.cdc.gov/nchs/nsfg/index.htm).

Planned Parenthood. 2020. *Title X: The Nation's Program for Affordable Birth Control and Reproductive Health Care* (https://www.plannedparenthoodaction.org/issues/health-care-equity/title-x).

Ramasamy, R., and P. N. Schlegel. 2011. Vasectomy and vasectomy reversal: An update. *Indian Journal of Urology* 27(1): 92–97 (http://www.ncbi.nlm.nih.gov/pmc/articles/PMC3114592/).

Raymond, E. G., and D. A. Grimes. 2012. The comparative safety of legal induced abortion and childbirth in the United States. *Obstetrics and Gynecology* 119(2.1): 215–219.

Riddle, J. 1999. *Eve's Herbs: A History of Contraception and Abortion in the West.* Cambridge, MA: Harvard University Press.

Rocca, C., et al. 2015. Decision rightness and emotional responses to abortion in the United States: A longitudinal study. *PLoS ONE* 10(7): e0128832.

Ross, L., and R. Solinger. 2017. *Reproductive Justice: A New Vision for the 21st Century.* Oakland: University of California Press.

Sedgh, G., et al. 2015. Adolescent pregnancy, birth, and abortion rates across countries: Levels and recent trends. *Journal of Adolescent Health.* 56(2): 223–230.

Sedgh, G., J. et al. 2016. Abortion incidence between 1990 and 2014: Global, regional, and subregional levels and trends. *Lancet* 388(10041): 258–267.

Sedgh, G., S. Singh, and R. Hussain. 2014. Intended and unintended pregnancies worldwide in 2012 and recent trends. *Studies in Family Planning* 45(3): 301–314.

Smith, T. W., and J. Son. 2013. *Final Report. Trends in Public Attitudes toward Abortion.* NORC, University of Chicago (http://www.norc.org/PDFs/GSS_abortion2013_final.pdf).

Stoll, B. J., et al. 2015. Trends in care practices, morbidity, and mortality of extremely preterm neonates, 1993–2012. *Journal of the American Medical Association* 314(10): 1039–1051.

Turok, D. K., et al. 2021. Levonorgestrel vs. copper intrauterine devices for emergency contraception. *New England Journal of Medicine* 384: 335.

United Nations, Department of Economic and Social Affairs, Population Division. 2019. *Contraceptive Use by Method 2019: Data Booklet* (ST/ESA/SER.A/435). (https://www.un.org/en/development/desa/population/publications/pdf/family/ContraceptiveUseByMethodDataBooklet2019.pdf).

U.S. Department of Health and Human Services. 2019. *Approval of Emergency Contraception* (https://www.womenshealth.gov/30-achievements/19).

Van der Wijden, C., and C. Manion. 2015. Lactational amenorrhoea method for family planning. *Cochrane Database of Systematic Reviews,* October 12(10): CD001329.

Van Vliet, H. A., et al. 2011. Triphasic versus monophasic oral contraceptives for contraception. *Cochrane Database of Systematic Reviews,* November 9(11): CD003553

Westwood R. 2022. Jackson Women's Health Org. is fully booked, with abortions facing a ban in 9 days. *National Public Radio,* June 25 (https://www.npr.org/2022/06/25/1107628722/jackson-womens-health-org-is-fully-booked-with-abortions-facing-a-ban-in-9-days).

Winner, B., et al. 2012. Effectiveness of long-acting reversible contraception. *New England Journal of Medicine* 366(21): 1998–2007.


**Design Elements:** Assess Yourself icon: Aleksey Boldin/Alamy Stock Photo; Diversity Matters icon: Rawpixel Ltd/Getty Images; Wellness on Campus icon: Radius Images/Alamy Stock Photo; Take Charge icon: VisualCommunications/Getty Images; Critical Consumer icon: pagadesign/Getty Images.

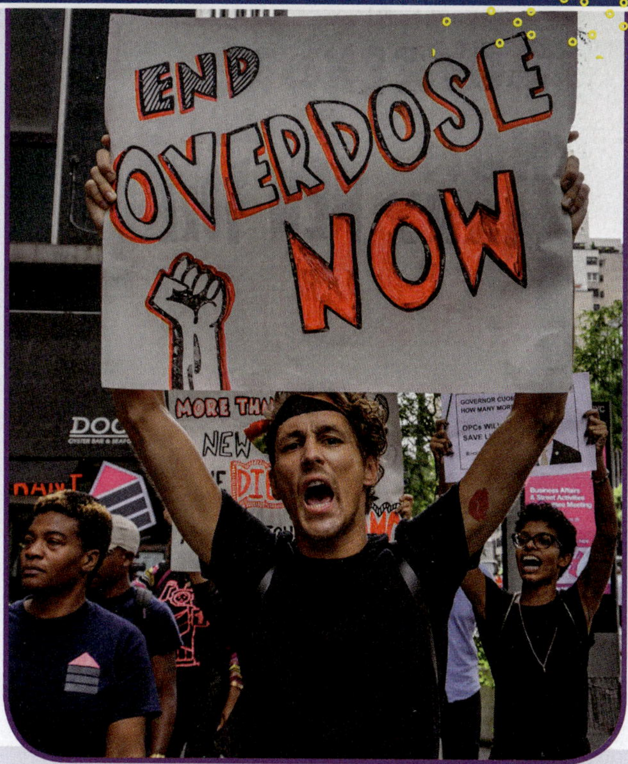

Erik McGregor/Pacific Press Media Production Corp./Alamy Stock Photo

## CHAPTER OBJECTIVES

- Define and discuss addiction
- Explain factors that contribute to drug use and misuse and addiction
- List risks associated with drug misuse
- Understand how drugs affect the body
- List and describe the effects of the six major groups of psychoactive drugs
- Outline ways to prevent drug-related problems

CHAPTER 8

# Drug Use and Addiction

The use of **drugs** for both medical and social purposes is widespread in the United States (Table 8.1). Many Americans believe that every problem has or should have a chemical solution. When feeling tired, many turn to caffeine or other stimulants; for insomnia, sleeping pills; for anxiety, prescription medication, alcohol, or other sedative drugs. Advertisements, social pressures, and the human desire for quick solutions to difficult problems all contribute to the prevailing wishful view that drugs can ease all pain. But benefits often come with the risk of harmful consequences, and drug use can—and in many cases does—pose serious or even life-threatening risks.

This chapter introduces the concepts of addiction and misuse, and then focuses on the major classes of misused drugs, their effects, their potential for addiction and impairment, and other issues related to their use. Alcohol and nicotine—two of the most widely used and most problematic psychoactive drugs—are discussed in Chapter 9.

## ADDICTION

Aside from death, the most serious drug-related risks are addiction and impairment of daily activities. The drugs most often associated with addiction and impairment are **psychoactive drugs**—those that alter a person's perception, mood, behavior, or consciousness. In the short term, psychoactive drugs can cause **intoxication,** a state in which, sometimes, unpredictable physical and emotional changes occur. People who are intoxicated may experience potentially serious

**TERMS**

**drug** Any chemical other than food intended to affect the structure or function of the body.

**psychoactive drug** A drug that can alter a person's consciousness or experience.

**intoxication** The state of being mentally affected by a chemical (literally, a state of being poisoned).

VITAL STATISTICS

**Table 8.1** Drug Misuse among Americans, 2020 (percent using in past month)

| | YOUNG ADULTS AGED 18–25 | YOUTHS AGED 12–17 | ALL AMERICANS AGED 12 AND OVER |
|---|---|---|---|
| ILLICIT DRUGS* | 4.8 | 1.2 | 3.4 |
| Marijuana and hashish | 3.0 | 5.9 | 11.8 |
| Cocaine | 1.3 | 0.0 | 0.7 |
| Heroin | 0.1 | 0.0 | 0.7 |
| Hallucinogens | 1.9 | 0.3 | 0.6 |
| Ecstasy | 0.6 | 0.1 | 0.2 |
| Inhalants | 0.5 | 0.4 | 0.3 |
| Methamphetamine | 0.2 | 0.0 | 0.6 |
| MISUSE OF PSYCHOTHERAPEUTICS | 2.3 | 0.7 | 1.9 |
| Pain relievers | 0.9 | 0.4 | 0.9 |
| Tranquilizers | 1.1 | 0.1 | 0.8 |
| Stimulants | 0.8 | 0.3 | 0.5 |

*Other than marijuana, which is permitted in many states.

SOURCE: Substance Abuse and Mental Health Services Administration. 2021. *Key substance use and mental health indicators in the United States: Results from the 2020 National Survey on Drug Use and Health* (HHS Publication No. PEP21-07-01-003, NSDUH Series H-56). Rockville, MD: Center for Behavioral Health Statistics and Quality.

changes in physical functioning. Their emotions and judgment may be affected in ways that lead to uncharacteristic and unsafe behavior. Recurrent drug use can have profound physical, emotional, and social effects.

## What Is Addiction?

Today scientists view **addiction** as a complex disease that involves disruption of the brain's systems related to reward, motivation, and memory. Dysfunction in these systems leads to biological, psychological, and social effects associated with pathologically pursuing pleasure or relief by substance use and other behaviors. Addiction is a chronic (ongoing, relapsing) condition that causes compulsive substance use despite harmful consequences to the addicted person and often to others.

Addiction is rooted in biological, psychological, social, environmental, and genetic factors. Chronic use of substances can lead to brain changes that cause intense cravings as well as distorted thinking, and problems with behaviors, interpersonal relationships, and emotional responses. Like other chronic conditions, addiction often involves cycles of relapse and remission. Without treatment, addiction is progressive and can result in disabling or deadly health consequences.

Although addiction is most often associated with drug use, many experts now extend the concept of addiction to other behaviors. One example is gambling disorder. Looking at the nature of addiction and a range of addictive behaviors can help us understand similar behaviors when they involve drugs. **Addictive behaviors** are any activities or uses of substances that are pursued compulsively for physical or psychological reward, despite unwanted physical, mental, or social consequences.

Although experts now agree that addiction is more fully defined by behavioral characteristics, they also agree that changes in the brain may underlie addiction. One such change is **tolerance,** in which the body adapts to a drug so that the initial dosage no longer produces the original emotional or psychological effects. To achieve the same **high,** the person using the drug requires larger and larger doses. The concept of addiction as a disease based in identifiable changes to the brain has led to many advances in the understanding and treatment of drug addiction.

The view that addiction is based in our brain chemistry does *not* imply that people are not responsible for their addictive behavior. All addictions involve an initial voluntary step. At the same time, nobody intends to one day develop a disorder. Vulnerabilities such as genetic risk, family history, or a stressful environment all contribute to the development of addiction.

TERMS

**addiction** A chronic disease that disrupts the brain's system of motivation and reward, characterized by a compulsive desire and increasing need for a substance or behavior, and by harm to the individual and/or society.

**addictive behavior** Compulsive behavior that is both rewarding and reinforcing and is often pursued to the marginalization or exclusion of other activities and responsibilities.

**tolerance** Lower sensitivity to a drug or substance so that a given dose no longer exerts the usual effect and larger doses are needed.

**high** The subjectively pleasing effects of a drug, usually felt quite soon after the drug is taken.

## Diagnosing Substance Misuse and Substance Use Disorder

It is important to note that you do not have to be addicted to a drug to suffer its serious consequences—in many cases you only have to misuse it once. **Substance misuse** is the use of a substance inconsistent with medical or legal guidelines. Misuse is a broad concept and can include the use of illegal drugs, prescription drugs in greater-than-prescribed amounts, another person's prescription drug, or even excessive use of a legal substance like alcohol. The situation in which a person takes prescribed painkillers to get high would be considered drug *misuse.*

The American Psychiatric Association (APA) provides criteria for diagnosing a **substance use disorder (SUD)** in the *Diagnostic and Statistical Manual of Mental Disorders (DSM-5),* which is the standard classification system used by mental health professionals. A person with problems associated with habitual drug use is classified as having an SUD based on symptoms ranging from mild to severe. The terms *SUD* (e.g., a person with an SUD) and *misuse* replace terms like *addict/addiction* and *abuse/abuser*, which have the potential to stigmatize people who misuse drugs; research has shown that stigmatization can keep people from seeking help. Some of these terms, however, are still commonly used in mental health literature.

Addiction is a psychological or physical dependence on a substance or behavior that produces undesirable, negative consequences. According to the APA, people with addiction are focused on a particular drug or behavior to the point that it takes over their lives; they use the substance or engage in the behavior compulsively despite knowing it will cause them problems.

The 11 *DSM-5* criteria for a substance use disorder are listed here, grouped in four categories. The severity of the disorder is determined by the number of criteria a person meets: 2–3 criteria indicate a mild disorder; 4–5 criteria point to a moderate disorder; 6 or more criteria are evidence of a severe disorder.

### Impaired Control

1. Taking the substance in larger amounts or over a longer period than was originally intended.
2. Expressing a persistent desire to cut down on or regulate substance use, but being unable to do so.
3. Spending a great deal of time getting the substance, using the substance, or recovering from its effects.
4. Craving or experiencing an intense desire or urge to use the substance.

### Social Problems

5. Failing to fulfill major obligations at work, school, or home.
6. Continuing to use the substance despite having persistent or recurrent social or interpersonal problems caused or worsened by the effects of its use.
7. Giving up or reducing important social, school, work, or recreational activities because of substance use.

### Risky Use

8. Using the substance in situations in which it is physically hazardous to do so.
9. Continuing to use the substance despite the knowledge of having persistent or recurrent physical or psychological problems caused or worsened by substance use.

### Drug Effects

10. Developing tolerance to the substance. When a person requires increased amounts of a substance to achieve the desired effect or notices a markedly diminished effect with continued use of the same amount, they have developed tolerance to the substance.
11. Experiencing withdrawal. In someone who has maintained prolonged, heavy use of a substance, a drop in its concentration within the body can result in unpleasant physical and cognitive **withdrawal** symptoms. Withdrawal symptoms vary for different drugs. For example, nausea, vomiting, and tremors are common withdrawal symptoms in people dependent on alcohol, opioids, or sedatives.

Physical dependence, in a narrow sense, can be a normal bodily response to the use of a substance. For example, regular coffee drinkers may experience caffeine withdrawal symptoms if they reduce their intake. Does this mean they have a substance use disorder? Not necessarily. The National Institute on Drug Abuse specifies that more criteria, such as compulsive use, are required to qualify for substance abuse and **dependence.** A person who regularly takes prescribed low-dose opioids for chronic pain can suffer withdrawals and therefore physical dependence without exhibiting signs of an addictive disorder.

**TERMS**

**substance misuse or abuse** The use of any substance in a manner inconsistent with legal or medical guidelines; may be associated with adverse social, psychological, or medical consequences; the use may be intermittent and with or without tolerance and physical dependence.

**substance use disorder** A cluster of symptoms involving cognitive, bodily, and social impairment related to the continued use of a substance; a single disorder measured on a continuum from mild to severe.

**withdrawal** Physical and psychological symptoms that follow the interrupted use of a drug that a person has become dependent on; symptoms may be mild or life threatening.

**dependence** Frequent or consistent use of a drug or behavior that makes it difficult for the person to get along without it; the result of physiological and/or psychological adaptation that occurs in response to the substance or behavior; typically associated with tolerance and withdrawal but can also be based solely on behavioral factors such as compulsive use.

## The Development of Substance Use Disorder

We all engage in activities that are potentially addictive. An addiction often starts when a person does something to bring pleasure or avoid pain. The activity may be drinking a beer, using the internet, playing the lottery, or shopping. If it works, the person is likely to repeat it. Reinforcement leads to an increasing dependence on the behavior. Tolerance—caused by physical changes to brain cells and reward pathways in the brain—develops, and the person needs more of the substance or behavior to feel the expected effect. Eventually the behavior becomes a central focus of the person's life, and other areas such as school performance or relationships deteriorate. The behavior no longer brings pleasure, but repeating it is necessary to avoid withdrawal.

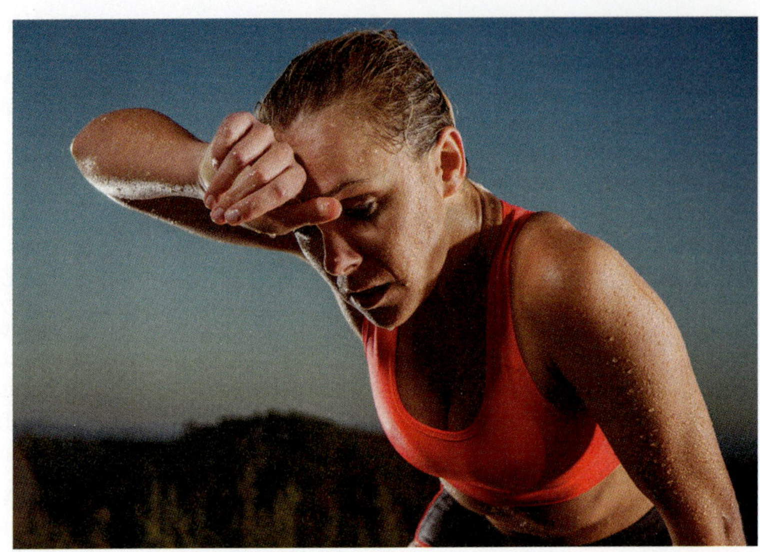

When taken to an extreme, even healthy activities such as exercise can become addictive. Erik Isakson/Blend Images LLC

Although many common behaviors are potentially addictive, most people who engage in them do not develop problems. This is because the development of an SUD includes factors such as personality, lifestyle, heredity, the social and physical environment, and the nature of the substance or behavior in question.

## Behavioral Addictions

For some people, behaviors unrelated to drugs can become addictive. Such behaviors can include eating, gambling, and playing video games. Any substance or activity that becomes the focus of a person's life at the expense of other needs and interests should be a sign there is a problem. Like substance addictions, behavioral or nondrug addiction symptoms also meet *DSM-5* criteria of craving, loss of control over the behavior, tolerance, withdrawal, and a repeating pattern of recovery and relapse. Behavioral addictions also promote changes in the brain similar to those changes associated with misuse of and addiction to alcohol, nicotine, or other drugs.

Gambling is the only disorder listed below included in the *DSM-5*; however, the *Manual* recommends that addiction to internet gaming should be further studied. The other behavioral addictions listed here have been variously classified as mood, obsessive-compulsive, and impulse control.

**Gambling Disorder** Gambling disorders, or pathological gambling, affects 0.5–1% of adult Americans. Some 75% of students report having gambled in the past year, and about 6% have a serious gambling problem that can result in psychological difficulties, unmanageable debt, and failing grades. The suicide rate of compulsive gamblers is 15 times higher than that of the general population.

Characteristic behaviors involved in a gambling disorder include preoccupation with gambling, unsuccessful efforts to quit, using gambling to escape problems, and lying to family members to conceal the extent of gambling. Also associated with the disorder are higher rates of crime, interpersonal violence, and child neglect.

**Gaming** Characteristic behaviors include preoccupation with video games, loss of interest in other activities, using gaming to relieve anxiety or guilt, and risking opportunities or relationships due to time spent gaming. The disorder is separate from gambling disorder and differs from general use of social media or the internet.

**Compulsive Exercising** When taken to a compulsive level, even healthy activity can turn into harmful addictions. For example, compulsive exercising is now recognized as a serious departure from normal behavior. Compulsive exercising is often accompanied by more severe psychiatric disorders such as anorexia nervosa and bulimia (see Chapter 12). Traits often associated with compulsive exercising include an excessive preoccupation and dissatisfaction with body image, use of laxatives or vomiting to lose weight, and development of other obsessive-compulsive symptoms.

**Work Addiction** People who are excessively preoccupied with work are often called *workaholics*. Work addiction, however, is based on a set of specific symptoms, including an intense work schedule, the inability to limit your own work schedule, the inability to relax when away from work, and failed attempts to reduce work intensity. Work addiction typically coincides with a well-known risk factor for cardiovascular disease—personality traits of competitiveness, ambition, drive, time urgency, restlessness, hyper-alertness, and hostility.

**Sex and Pornography Addiction** Behaviors associated with sex addiction include an extreme preoccupation with sex, a compulsion to have sex repeatedly in a brief period of time, a great deal of time and energy spent looking for partners, sex used as a means of relieving painful feelings, and a reduced control over sexual behaviors despite the experience of negative emotional, personal, and professional consequences.

Pornography addiction, often grouped under sex addiction, is characterized by excessive viewing of pornography, using it to avoid negative feelings, needing it to be increasingly more stimulating (tolerance), feeling distress when it is stopped (withdrawal), and continuing with it despite unwanted consequences. These behaviors may result in physical problems such as erectile dysfunction, psychological problems such as preoccupation with sexual thoughts, and social consequences such as losing interest in person-to-person sexual contact, difficulty becoming aroused, and emotional detachment.

**Compulsive Buying or Shopping** Someone with a shopping compulsion repeatedly gives in to the impulse to buy more than they need or can afford. They often buy luxury items rather than daily necessities, even though they are usually distressed by their behavior and its social, personal, and financial consequences. Some experts link compulsive shopping with neglect or abuse during childhood; it also seems to be associated with eating disorders, depression, and bipolar disorder.

**Internet Addiction** In the years since the internet became widely available, millions of Americans have become compulsive internet users—as many as one out of eight people fits this description; among college students, approximately one of seven. There is also a growing preoccupation with social media, mobile devices, and general screen time. Researchers are studying cell-phone behavior in the population as a whole as well as among its heaviest users—those under age 20.

QUICK STATS

**59.3 million Americans aged 12 and over used an illicit drug in the past year; this is over 20% of Americans.**

—Substance Abuse and Mental Health Services Administration, 2020

## WHY PEOPLE USE AND MISUSE DRUGS

Using drugs to alter consciousness is an ancient and universal pursuit. People have used alcohol for celebration and intoxication for thousands of years. But many drugs have addictive properties and change the chemistry of the brain; their use can open the door to the problems of misuse and dependence.

### Ask Yourself

**QUESTIONS FOR CRITICAL THINKING AND REFLECTION**

Have you ever repeatedly or compulsively engaged in a behavior that had negative consequences? What was the behavior, and why did you continue? Did you ever worry that you were losing control? Were you able to bring the behavior under control?

### The Allure of Drugs

The main factors in the initial use of drugs are availability and peer influence. Some people use drugs because they want to alter their mood—they want to feel a euphoric high, or they are in pursuit of a spiritual experience. Others use drugs as a way to escape boredom, anxiety, depression, feelings of worthlessness, or other distressing symptoms. They use drugs to cope with the difficulties they experience in life. Beginning in March 2020, pandemic-related stress, isolation, and job disruption likely elevated rates of drug misuse in the United States. The overdose death rate rose, exacerbated by more people using drugs alone and having less access to treatment. The sharpest rises in deaths happened among people ages 25–54, Black men, and American Indian/Alaska Native people.

### Risk Factors for Drug Misuse and Addiction

Can some people use psychoactive drugs without becoming addicted? The answer seems to lie in a combination of physical, psychological, and social factors. Research indicates that some people may be born with a brain chemistry or metabolism that makes them more vulnerable than others to addiction.

The causes and course of an addiction vary, but people with SUD share some characteristics. As mentioned, many use a substance or activity as a substitute for healthier coping strategies. People vary in their ability to manage their lives, and those who have trouble dealing with stress and painful emotions may be susceptible to addiction. For this reason, one-half of people with psychological disorders also have a substance use disorder.

Whether suffering from dual disorders or not, people with addictive disorders usually have a distinct preference for a particular addictive behavior. They also often have problems with impulse control and self-regulation and tend to be risk takers.

Drug misuse and addiction occur at all income and education levels, among all ethnic groups, and across all age groups (see the box "Drug Use among College Students"). Even if a person is not predisposed to addiction nor afforded many opportunities to experiment with drugs, casual or recreational use of them can lead to addiction. Some drugs are more likely than others to lead to addiction (Table 8.2).

**Factors Associated with Trying Drugs** Who are the young people most likely to try drugs? They share the following characteristics:

- ***Male.*** Males are more likely than females to use almost all types of illicit drugs. According to the National Institute on Drug Abuse, fewer women use marijuana. Women tend to use smaller amounts of heroin and for less time, and they are

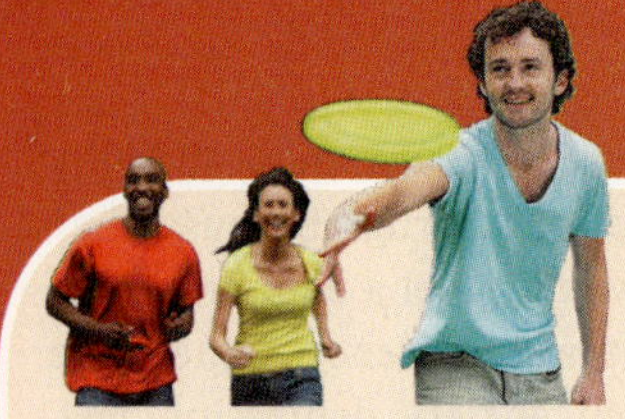

## WELLNESS ON CAMPUS
### Drug Use among College Students

Drug use in college has long been recognized as a significant health problem that affects many students. According to the most recent survey data from the National Survey on Drug Use and Health (NSDUH), almost 24% of young adults aged 18–25 reported using an illicit drug in the past 30 days, with marijuana the most commonly used drug (refer to Table 8.1). In recent years, rates of vaping marijuana tripled for high school seniors, but they leveled in 2020. Marijuana use was highest among people ages 19–30; 42% had used marijuana at least once in the past year.

Drug use on college campuses has been examined extensively, and many experts believe that no single factor can explain the widespread cause of this phenomenon. Family history, peer pressure, depression, anxiety, low self-esteem, and the dynamics of college life (for example, the drive to compete and a distorted perception of drug use among peers) have been suggested as potential explanations for college-age drug use.

Excessive alcohol use often accompanies illicit drug use, and the risk of combining drugs and alcohol increases with the number of drinks a young adult consumes during a single session. In March 2020, the National Survey of Substance Abuse Treatment Services reported on this issue. Of approximately one million people age 18 and older who were receiving substance use treatment, about one-third were using both alcohol and drugs.

The term *AOD* (alcohol and other drug) has been coined to refer to this type of substance use among college students. Further, AOD use and depression and/or anxiety are generally recognized as coexisting conditions that require a comprehensive approach to prevention and treatment. Despite the growing awareness among college counselors and other health professionals who work with college students, it is not entirely clear whether anxiety and depression precede the onset of alcohol and drug use or whether early precollege exposure to alcohol and drug use exacerbates more serious psychiatric disorders by the time a student enters college. A third line of research suggests that AOD use, depression, and anxiety share common causes such as genetic predisposition and family history.

However, one aspect of drug use among college students remains clear: AOD use has dramatic consequences for the educational, family, and community lives of students. Poor academic performance has been linked with AOD use. Further, driving while intoxicated remains one of the most dangerous outcomes associated with AOD use affecting families and communities.

Several AOD prevention programs are now under way at college campuses. Several federal laws have been enacted to address AOD use at schools. The 2016 Comprehensive Addiction and Recovery Act (CARA) was the first major federal addiction act in 40 years. It authorized over $181 million in spending to respond to the opioid epidemic through prevention and treatment programs, including some efforts focused on youths.

less likely than men to inject it. National overdose deaths from prescription drugs, cocaine, and heroin are consistently higher in males than in females. However, females are just as likely as males to develop a substance use disorder.

**Table 8.2** Psychoactive Drugs and Their Potential for Substance Use Disorder and Addiction

| | |
|---|---|
| Very high | Heroin |
| High | Nicotine, morphine |
| Moderate/high | Cocaine, pentobarbital |
| Moderate | Alcohol, ephedra, Rohypnol |
| Moderate/low | Caffeine, marijuana, MDMA (methylenedioxymethamphetamine), nitrous oxide |
| Low/very low | Ketamine, LSD (lysergic acid diethylamide), mescaline, psilocybin |

SOURCE: Adapted from Gable, R. S. 2006. "Acute toxicity of drugs versus regulatory status." Edited by J. M. Fish. *Drugs and Society: U.S. Public Policy,* 149–162. Lanham, MD: Rowman & Littlefield.

- ***Troubled childhood.*** Teens are more likely to try drugs if they have had behavioral issues in childhood, such as aggression, have suffered abuse, used tobacco at a young age, or suffer from certain mental or emotional problems.

- ***Thrill-seeker.*** Impulsivity and a sense of invincibility is a factor in drug experimentation.

- ***Dysfunctional family.*** A chaotic home life with poor supervision, constant tension or arguments, or parental abuse increases the risk of teen drug use. Having parents who misuse drugs or alcohol increases the risk for teen use.

- ***Trouble at school.*** Young people who are uninterested in school, or have problems at school, or have difficulty fitting in, are more likely to find a peer group that accepts drug use.

- ***Poor.*** Young people who live in disadvantaged areas are more likely to be around drugs at a young age.

- ***Adolescents engaged in risky sexual behavior.*** There is a relationship between drug use and risky sexual behavior, such as with adolescent girls who date boys two or more years older than themselves; they are more likely to use drugs.

**Factors Associated with Not Using Drugs** As a group, people who do not use drugs also share some characteristics. Not surprisingly, people who perceive drug use as risky and who disapprove of it are less likely to use drugs. Drug use is also less common among people who have positive self-esteem and self-concept and who are assertive, independent thinkers able to resist peer pressure. People with self-control, social competence, optimism, academic achievement, and religiosity (hold religious beliefs and attend religious services) are less likely to use drugs.

Home environments are also influential: Young people who communicate openly with and feel supported by their parents are also less likely to use drugs.

## RISKS ASSOCIATED WITH DRUG MISUSE

Tracking emergency department visits is one way to measure levels of drug misuse. Over 1.2 million visits were reported for 2017 (Table 8.3); the number of visits increased 44% from 2006 to 2014. The following are serious concerns:

- ***Intoxication.*** People who are intoxicated may act in uncharacteristic and unsafe ways because their physical and mental functioning are impaired. They are more likely to be injured from a variety of causes, to have unsafe sex, and to be involved in incidents of aggression and violence.

- ***Unexpected side effects.*** Psychoactive drugs have many physical and psychological effects that can range from nausea and constipation to paranoia, depression, and heart failure. Some drugs also carry the risk of fatal overdose.

- ***Unknown drug constituents.*** A drug may have been mixed with other drugs or substances to boost its effects. Illicit drugs can be contaminated or even poisonous.

**Table 8.3** Estimated Drug-Related Emergency Department (ED) Visits: 2017

| REASON FOR ED VISIT | NUMBER OF ED VISITS* |
|---|---|
| Alcohol | 1,284,000 |
| Opioid | 393,000 |
| Cannabis | 70,000 |
| Sedative | 43,000 |
| Hallucinogen | 15,000 |
| Inhalant | 3,000 |
| **All drug poisonings** | **2,171,056** |

*Includes people who were treated and released or who died; does not include people admitted to hospital.

SOURCE: Peterson, Cora, Mengyao Li , Likang Xu , Christina A Mikosz, and Feijun Luo. 2021. "Assessment of annual cost of substance use disorder in US hospitals." *JAMA Network Open* 4, no.3: e210242.

### Ask Yourself

**QUESTIONS FOR CRITICAL THINKING AND REFLECTION**

Have you ever tried a psychoactive drug for fun? What were your reasons for trying it? Whom were you with, and what were the circumstances? What was your experience? What would you tell someone who was thinking about trying a drug?

- ***Infection and injection drug use.*** Heroin is the most commonly injected drug, but people with an SUD can also inject cocaine, amphetamines, and other drugs. Many people who inject drugs share or reuse needles, syringes, and other injection supplies, which can become contaminated with the user's blood. Small amounts of blood can carry enough human immunodeficiency virus (HIV) and hepatitis C virus (HCV) to be infectious. According to the CDC, one in ten new diagnoses of HIV infection is due to injection drug use. Injection drug use also accounts for the majority of new HCV infections.

- ***Legal consequences.*** Many psychoactive drugs are illegal, so possessing them can result in large fines and imprisonment. According to the FBI, the highest arrest counts for all types of crimes were for drug use violations (estimated at 1.1 million out of 7.6 million total arrests in 2020).

## HOW DRUGS AFFECT THE BODY

Beyond a fairly predictable change in brain chemistry, the effects of a drug may vary depending on drug factors, user factors, and social factors.

### Changes in Brain Chemistry

The quicker a drug reaches the brain, the more likely the person becomes dependent on it. Once a psychoactive drug reaches the brain, it interferes with the way neurons (nerve cells that communicate with other cells) send, receive, and process signals sent by **neurotransmitters.** Drugs like cocaine and amphetamines increase the amount of dopamine, a neurotransmitter thought to play a key role in the process of reinforcement–the brain's way of telling itself, "I feel good; do the same thing again." This is a reward pathway. When a neuron releases a neurotransmitter, it travels across a gap, called a *synapse,* to signal another neuron.

Other drugs, like marijuana and heroin, mimic the brain's own chemical; these drugs don't activate neurons in the same way as a natural neurotransmitter, and they lead to abnormal messages being sent through the network.

The duration of a drug's effect depends on many factors and may range from 5 minutes (crack cocaine) to 12 or more hours (LSD). As drugs circulate through the body, they are

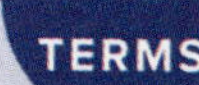
TERMS

**neurotransmitter** A brain chemical that transmits nerve impulses.

metabolized by the liver and eventually excreted by the kidneys in urine. Small amounts may also be eliminated in other ways, including in sweat, in breast milk, and via the lungs.

### Physical Factors

Certain physical characteristics help determine how a person will respond to a drug. Body mass is one variable: The effects of a certain dose of a drug on a 150-pound person will exceed its effect on a 200-pound person. Other variables include general health and genetic factors. For example, some people have an inherited ability to rapidly metabolize a cough suppressant called dextromethorphan, which also has psychoactive properties. These people must take a higher-than-normal dose to get a given cough suppressant effect.

If a person's biochemical state is already altered by another drug, this too can make a difference. Some drugs intensify the effects of other drugs, as is the case with alcohol and sedatives. Some drugs block the effects of other drugs, such as when a tranquilizer is used to relieve anxiety caused by cocaine. Interactions between drugs, including many prescription and over-the-counter (OTC) medications, can be unpredictable and dangerous.

One physical condition that requires special precautions is pregnancy. It can be risky for a woman to use any drugs at all during pregnancy, including alcohol and common OTC products like cough medicine.

### Psychological Factors

Sometimes a person's response to a drug is strongly influenced by expectations of how the drug will affect them. With large doses, the drug's chemical properties seem to have the strongest effect on the individual's response. But with small doses, psychological (and social) factors are often more important. If people believe that a given drug will affect them a certain way, they are more likely to experience those effects regardless of the drug's pharmacological properties. In one study, regular users of marijuana reported a moderate level of intoxication (high) after using a cigarette that smelled and tasted like marijuana but contained no THC, the active ingredient in marijuana. This is an example of the **placebo effect**—when a person receives an inert substance yet responds as if it were an active drug. In other studies, subjects who smoked low doses of real marijuana that they believed to be a placebo experienced no effects from the drug. Clearly the expectations had a greater effect than the drug itself.

**QUICK STATS**

**Overdoses claim more lives each year than firearms, suicide, homicide, or motor vehicle crashes: 100,000 in June 2020-May 2021.**

—Rand, 2022

**TERMS**

**placebo effect** A response to an inert or innocuous substance given in place of an active drug.

**opioid** Any of several natural or synthetic drugs that relieve pain and cause drowsiness and/or euphoria; examples are opium, morphine, and heroin; also called a *narcotic*.

**euphoria** An exaggerated feeling of well-being.

**Ask Yourself**

**QUESTIONS FOR CRITICAL THINKING AND REFLECTION**

Has an OTC medication (such as a decongestant) ever made you feel strange, drowsy, or even high? Did you expect to react to the medication that way? Do such reactions influence the way you use OTC drugs?

### Social Factors

The *setting* is the physical and social environment surrounding the drug use. If a person uses marijuana at home with trusted friends and pleasant music, the effects are likely to differ from the effects if the same dose is taken in an austere experimental laboratory with an impassive research technician. Similarly, a dose of alcohol that produces mild euphoria and stimulation at a noisy, active cocktail party might induce sleepiness and slight depression when taken at home while alone.

## GROUPS OF PSYCHOACTIVE DRUGS

The following sections and Figure 8.1 introduce six representative groups of psychoactive drugs: opioids, central nervous system (CNS) depressants, CNS stimulants, marijuana and other cannabis products, hallucinogens, and inhalants. Some of these drugs are classified according to how they affect the body. Others—the opioids and the cannabis products—are classified according to their chemical makeup.

### Opioids

**Opioids** are natural or synthetic (laboratory-made) drugs that relieve pain, cause drowsiness, and induce **euphoria.** Natural opioid-like hormones released by the brain, called endorphins, can inhibit pain and induce euphoria. Opium, morphine, heroin, methadone, codeine, hydrocodone, oxycodone, meperidine, and fentanyl are opioids. When taken at prescribed doses, opioids have beneficial medical uses, including pain relief and cough suppression. Opioids tend to reduce anxiety and produce lethargy, apathy, and an inability to concentrate.

Although the euphoria associated with opioids is an important factor in their misuse, many people experience a feeling of uneasiness when they first use these drugs. Even so, the misuse of opioids often results in addiction. Tolerance can

| Category | Representative drugs | Street names | Appearance | Methods of use | Short-term effects |
|---|---|---|---|---|---|
| Opioids | Heroin | Dope, H, junk, brown sugar, smack | White/dark brown powder; dark tar or coal-like substance | Injected, smoked, snorted | Relief of anxiety and pain; euphoria; lethargy, apathy, drowsiness, confusion, inability to concentrate; nausea, constipation, respiratory depression |
| | Opium | Big O, black stuff, hop | Dark brown or black chunks | Swallowed, smoked | |
| | Morphine | M, Miss Emma, monkey, white stuff | White crystals, liquid solution | Injected, swallowed, smoked | |
| | Oxycodone, codeine, hydrocodone | Oxy, O.C., killer, Captain Cody, schoolboy, vike | Tablets, powder made from crushing tablets | Swallowed, injected, snorted | |
| Central nervous system depressants | Barbiturates | Barbs, reds, red birds, yellows, yellow jackets | Colored capsules | Swallowed, injected | Reduced anxiety, mood changes, lowered inhibitions, impaired muscle coordination, reduced pulse rate, drowsiness, loss of consciousness, respiratory depression |
| | Benzodiazepines (e.g., Valium, Xanax, Rohypnol) | Candy, downers, tranks, roofies, forget-me pill | Tablets | Swallowed, injected | |
| | Methaqualone | Ludes, quad, quay | Tablets | Injected, swallowed | |
| | Gamma hydroxy butyrate (GHB) | G, Georgia home boy, grievous bodily harm | Clear liquid, white powder | Swallowed | |
| Central nervous system stimulants | Amphetamine, methamphet-amine | Bennies, speed, black beauties, uppers, chalk, crank, crystal, ice, meth | Tablets, capsules, white powder, clear crystals | Injected, swallowed, smoked, snorted | Increased and irregular heart rate, blood pressure, metabolism; increased mental alertness and energy; nervousness, insomnia, impulsive behavior; reduced appetite |
| | Cocaine, crack cocaine | Blow, C, candy, coke, flake, rock, toot, snow | White powder, beige pellets or rocks | Injected, smoked, snorted | |
| | Ritalin | JIF, MPH, R-ball, Skippy | Tablets | Injected, swallowed, snorted | |
| Marijuana and other cannabis products | Marijuana | Dope, grass, joints, Mary Jane, reefer, skunk, weed, pot | Dried leaves and stems | Smoked, swallowed | Euphoria, slowed thinking and reaction time, confusion, anxiety, impaired balance and coordination, increased heart rate |
| | Hashish | Hash, hemp, boom, gangster | Dark, resin-like compound formed into rocks or blocks | Smoked, swallowed | |
| Hallucinogens | LSD | Acid, boomers, blotter, yellow sunshines | Blotter paper, liquid, gelatin tabs, pills | Swallowed, absorbed through mouth tissues | Altered states of perception and feeling; nausea; increased heart rate, blood pressure; delirium; impaired motor function; numbness, weakness |
| | Mescaline (peyote) | Buttons, cactus, mesc | Brown buttons, liquid | Swallowed, smoked | |
| | Psilocybin | Shrooms, magic mushrooms | Dried mushrooms | Swallowed | |
| | Ketamine | K, special K, cat valium, vitamin K | Clear liquid, white or beige powder | Injected, snorted, smoked | |
| | PCP | Angel dust, hog, love boat, peace pill | White to brown powder, tablets | Injected, swallowed, smoked, snorted | |
| | MDMA (Ecstasy) | X, peace, clarity, Adam, Molly | Tablets | Swallowed | |
| Inhalants | Solvents, aerosols, nitrites, anesthetics | Laughing gas, poppers, snappers, whippets | Household products, sprays, glues, paint thinner, petroleum products | Inhaled through nose or mouth | Stimulation, loss of inhi-bition, slurred speech, loss of motor coordination, loss of consciousness |
| New psychoactive drugs | Synthetic opioids (e.g., carfentanil, fentanyl) | Apace, China Girl, Dance Fever, He-Man | Powder, tablets mimicking pharmaceutical opioid products | Lozenge, tablet, injected, smoked, snorted | Relaxation, euphoria, pain relief, confusion, drowsiness, dizziness |
| | Synthetic cathinones (e.g., mephedrone, "bath salts") | Bliss, Blue Silk, Flakka, Ivory Wave, Meow Meow, Vanilla Sky, White Lightning | Fine white, off-white, or slightly yellow-colored powder or crystals; can be tablets or capsules | Swallowed, smoked, vaporized, sniffed, snorted, and injected | Increased blood pressure, rapid heartbeat, panic attacks in some people |
| | Synthetic cannabinoids (e.g., K2, Spice) | Black Mamba, Bliss, Bombay Blue, Fake Weed, Genie, Spice, Zohai | Herbal material | Smoked, teas | Increased blood pressure and heartbeat, paranoia, panic attacks |

**FIGURE 8.1 Commonly misused drugs and their effects.**

SOURCES: Indiana Department of Health. 2021. *Signs and Symptoms of Drug Misuse* (https://www.in.gov/health/overdose-prevention/general-information/signs-and-symptoms-of-drug-misuse/).

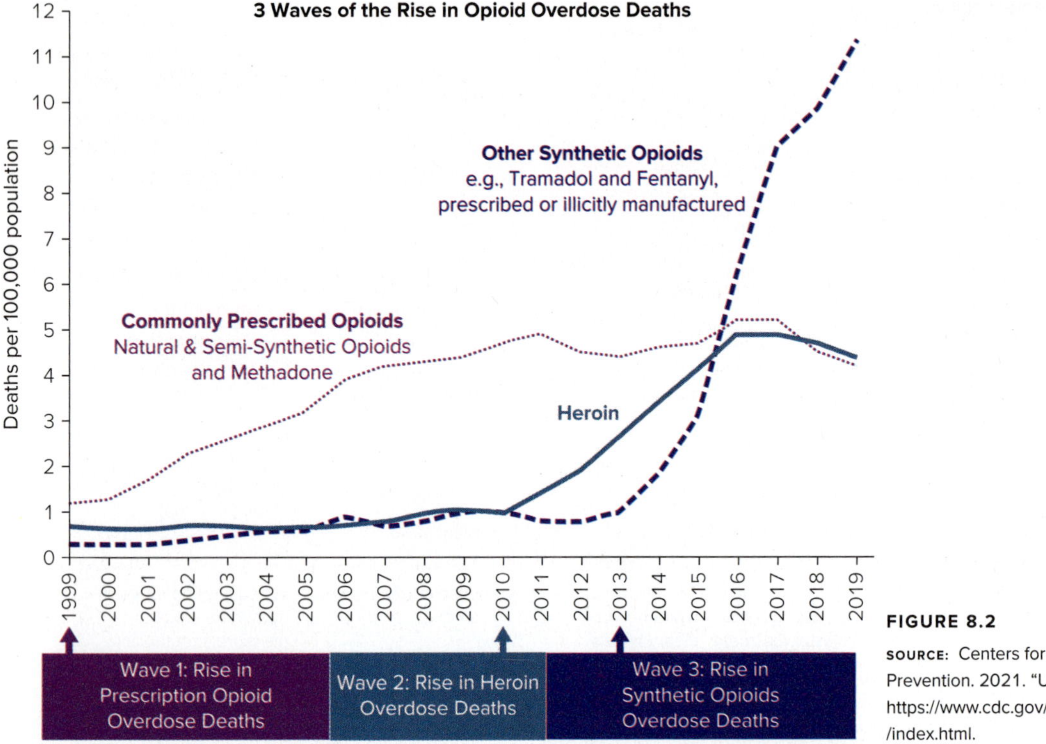


**FIGURE 8.2**

**SOURCE:** Centers for Disease Control and Prevention. 2021. "Understanding the Epidemic." https://www.cdc.gov/drugoverdose/epidemic/index.html.

develop rapidly and be pronounced. Withdrawal symptoms include cramps, chills, sweating, nausea, tremors, irritability, and feelings of panic.

The opioid epidemic in the United States claims the lives of around 130 people each day. According to the CDC, between 1999 and 2019 there were 500,000 deaths from opioid-related overdoses.

The opioid epidemic has emerged in three waves. The first wave began in the 1990s with prescription opioids like oxycodone, hydrocodone, and methadone. Health care providers began overprescribing opioid pain relievers as pharmaceutical companies reassured them that patients would not become addicted. This led to widespread misuse, and by 2011 there were around 16,000 overdose deaths on pills annually (Figure 8.2).

The second wave began in 2010 as those addicted shifted to heroin, a cheaper alternative to prescription pills. From 2010 to 2017, heroin deaths increased fivefold; in 2017, 15,000 people suffered fatal overdoses. The third wave surfaced with a rise in synthetic opioids like fentanyl and carfentanil, which are 50 times stronger than heroin. The third wave surfaced with a rise in synthetic opioids like fentanyl and carfentanil. Fifty times stronger than heroin, fentanyl and other synthetic opioids caused more than 36,000 overdose deaths in 2019. Between June 2020 and May 2021, there were more than 100,000 fatal overdoses; synthetic opioids (other than methadone) accounted for 64%.

When taken as prescribed in tablet form, these drugs treat moderate to severe chronic pain and do not typically lead to misuse. When taken in large doses or combined with other drugs, oxycodone and hydrocodone can cause fatal respiratory depression. Reports in the news recount people buying street-made pain medication and dying because the pills are contaminated with fentanyl.

In 2021, Congress established the Commission on Combating Synthetic Opioid Trafficking to understand why there has been an influx of synthetic opioids, and the source and destination of their trafficking.

**TERMS**

**depressant, sedative-hypnotic,** or **tranquilizer** A drug that decreases nervous or muscular activity, causing drowsiness or sleep.

**central nervous system (CNS)** The brain and spinal cord.

**sedation** The induction of a calm, relaxed, often sleepy state.

**barbiturates** CNS depressants used to treat seizures, headaches, and sometimes used in euthanasia.

**benzodiazepines** CNS depressants used for sleep and anxiety disorders.

## Central Nervous System Depressants

Central nervous system **depressants,** also known as **tranquilizers** or **sedative-hypnotics,** slow the **central nervous system (CNS).** They were mainly developed as antianxiety agents. The effects of these depressants can range from feeling relaxed with mild **sedation** to coma and death.

**Types** CNS depressants include alcohol as well as **barbiturates** (used for the treatment of seizures and migraines) and **benzodiazepines.** Other CNS depressants include methaqualone (Quaalude), ethchlorvynol (Placidyl), chloral hydrate, and gamma hydroxybutyrate (GHB). An additional class of sedative-hypnotics is called the "Z-drugs" and includes the sleeping pills known as Ambien (zolpidem), Lunesta (eszopiclone), and Sonata (zaleplon).

**Effects** CNS depressants reduce anxiety and cause mood changes, impaired muscular coordination, slurring of speech, and drowsiness or sleep. Mental functioning is also affected, but the degree varies from person to person and also depends on the kind of task the person is trying to do. Most people become drowsy with small doses, although a few become more active.

QUICK STATS

**Over 100 billion doses of oxycodone and hydrocodone were shipped nationwide in 2006–2014.**

—*The Washington Post*, 2020

**From Use to Misuse** The CNS depressants listed above are used for their calming properties in combination with **anesthetics** before operations and other medical or dental procedures. The use of Rohypnol and GHB (discussed in greater detail later in this chapter) is often associated with dance clubs and raves. The misuse of CNS depressants by a medical patient may begin with repeated use for insomnia and progress to dependence through increasingly larger doses at night, coupled with doses during stressful times of the day.

Most CNS depressants, including alcohol, can lead to addiction. Tolerance, sometimes for up to 15 times the usual dose, can develop with repeated use. CNS depressants can produce physical dependence even at ordinary prescribed doses. Withdrawal symptoms can be more severe than those accompanying opioid addiction and are similar to the DTs of alcoholism (see Chapter 9). They may begin as anxiety, shaking, and weakness but may turn into seizures and possibly cardiovascular collapse and death.

Too much depression of the central nervous system slows respiration and may stop it entirely. CNS depressants are particularly dangerous in combination with another depressant, such as alcohol, or with opioids, which are respiratory depressants.

**Club Drugs** Club drugs can lead to a substance use disorder and have many potential negative effects; they are particularly potent and unpredictable when mixed with alcohol.

**Rohypnol** (flunitrazepam) is a sedative that is 10 times more potent than Valium. Its effects, which are magnified by alcohol, include reduced blood pressure, dizziness, confusion, gastrointestinal disturbances, and loss of consciousness. People who use Rohypnol may develop physical and psychological dependence on the drug. Rohypnol has never been approved for medical use by the U.S. Food and Drug Administration (FDA); along with some other club drugs such as GHB, it is used as a "date rape drug." Because they can be added to beverages surreptitiously, these drugs may be unknowingly consumed by intended rape victims. In addition to depressant effects, some drugs also cause *anterograde amnesia*—the loss of memory of things occurring while under the influence of the drug. Rohypnol can be fatal if combined with alcohol.

**GHB** (gamma hydroxybutyrate) can be produced in clear liquid, white powder, tablet, and capsule form. GHB, used to treat narcolepsy, is a CNS depressant that, when taken in large doses or in combination with alcohol or other depressants, can cause sedation, loss of consciousness, respiratory arrest, and death. GHB may cause prolonged and potentially life-threatening withdrawal symptoms. GHB is often produced clandestinely, resulting in varying degrees of purity; it has been responsible for many poisonings and deaths.

## Central Nervous System Stimulants

Central nervous system **stimulants** speed up the activity of the nervous or muscular system. Under their influence, the heart rate accelerates, blood pressure rises, blood vessels constrict, the pupils and bronchial tubes dilate, and gastric and adrenal secretions increase. There is greater muscular tension and sometimes an increase in motor activity. Small doses usually make people feel more awake and alert, and less fatigued and bored. The most common CNS stimulants are cocaine, amphetamines, nicotine (see Chapter 9), ephedrine, and caffeine.

**Cocaine** Usually derived from the leaves of coca shrubs that grow high in the Andes in South America, cocaine is a potent CNS stimulant. Cocaine is usually snorted and absorbed through the nasal mucosa or injected intravenously, with fast, intense effects. Processing cocaine with baking soda and water yields the ready-to-smoke form of cocaine known as crack. Crack is typically used as small beads or pellets smokable in glass pipes.

**EFFECTS** The effects of cocaine are usually intense but short-lived. The euphoria lasts from 5 to 20 minutes and ends abruptly with irritability, anxiety, or slight depression. When cocaine is absorbed by either smoking or inhalation, it reaches the brain in about 10 seconds, and the effects are particularly intense. This is part of the appeal of smoking crack. The effects from IV injections occur almost as quickly—in about 20 seconds. Since the mucous membranes in the nose briefly slow absorption, the onset of effects from snorting takes 2–3 minutes. People with severe cocaine use disorder may inject cocaine intravenously every 10–20 minutes to maintain the effects.

TERMS

**anesthetic** A drug that produces a loss of sensation with or without a loss of consciousness.

**Rohypnol** (flunitrazepam) A sedative that is 10 times more potent than Valium; used as a "date rape drug."

**GHB** (gamma hydroxybutyrate) A central nervous system depressant that can be produced in clear liquid, white powder, tablet, and capsule form.

**stimulant** A drug that increases nervous or muscular activity.

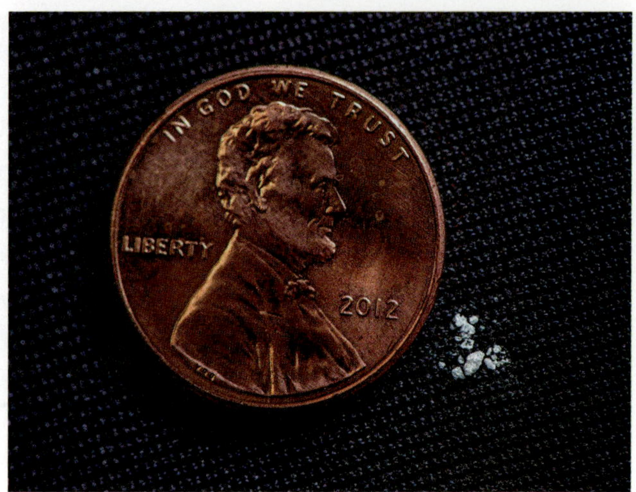


A potentially lethal dose of fentanyl. National Defense University

The larger the cocaine dose and the more rapidly it is absorbed into the bloodstream, the greater the immediate–and sometimes lethal–effects. Sudden death from cocaine is often the result of excessive CNS stimulation that causes convulsions and respiratory collapse, irregular heartbeat, extremely high blood pressure, blood clots, and possibly heart attack or stroke. Although rare, fatalities can occur in healthy young people; people aged 18–59 who use cocaine are seven times more likely than nonusers to have a heart attack. Chronic cocaine use produces inflammation of the nasal mucosa, which can lead to persistent bleeding and ulceration of the septum between the nostrils. The use of cocaine may also cause paranoia and aggressiveness. When stopping steady cocaine use, individuals experience a sudden "crash" characterized by depression, agitation, and fatigue, followed by a period of withdrawal.

**COCAINE USE DURING PREGNANCY** A woman who uses cocaine during pregnancy is at higher risk for miscarriage, premature labor, and stillbirth. Her infant may be at increased risk for defects of the genitourinary tract, cardiovascular system, central nervous system, and extremities. Infants whose mothers use cocaine may also be born intoxicated, and effects continue into childhood. They are typically irritable and jittery and do not eat or sleep normally. Cocaine also passes into breast milk and can intoxicate a breastfeeding infant.

### Amphetamines

Amphetamines (uppers) are a group of synthetic chemicals that are potent CNS stimulants. Some common drugs in this family are amphetamine (Benzedrine), dextroamphetamine (Dexedrine), and methamphetamine (Methedrine). Crystal methamphetamine (also called ice) is a smokable, high-potency form of methamphetamine, or "meth."

**EFFECTS** Small doses of amphetamines usually make people feel more alert. Amphetamines generally increase motor activity but do not measurably alter a normal, rested person's ability to perform tasks calling for challenging motor skills or complex thinking. When amphetamines improve performance, it is primarily by counteracting fatigue and boredom. In small doses, amphetamines increase heart rate and blood pressure and change sleep patterns.

Amphetamines are sometimes misused to curb appetite, but after a few weeks tolerance develops, and higher doses are necessary. When people stop taking the drug, their appetite usually returns, and they gain back the weight they lost unless they have made permanent changes in eating behavior.

**MISUSE AND ADDICTION** Much amphetamine misuse begins as an attempt to cope with a temporary situation. A student cramming for an exam or an exhausted long-haul truck driver can go a little longer by taking amphetamines, but the results can be disastrous. The likelihood of making bad judgments increases significantly. The stimulating effects may also wear off suddenly, and the person may precipitously feel exhausted or fall asleep ("crash").

Performance may deteriorate when students use drugs to study and then take tests in their normal, nondrug state. People taking antihistamines may also experience this problem. Repeated use of amphetamines can lead to severe disturbances in behavior, including a temporary state of paranoid **psychosis,** with delusions of persecution and episodes of unprovoked violence.

Methamphetamine is more addictive than other forms of amphetamine. It also is more dangerous because it is more toxic and its effects last longer. In the short term, meth can cause rapid breathing, increased body temperature, insomnia, tremors, anxiety, and convulsions. Meth use has been linked to high-risk sexual behavior and increased rates of sexually transmitted infections, including HIV infection. In the long term, the effects of meth can include weight loss, severe acne, hallucinations, paranoia, violence, and psychosis. Meth use may cause extensive tooth decay and tooth loss, a condition referred to as "meth mouth," but this may be due to poor hygiene associated with chronic meth use and severe drug dependence in general. Meth takes a toll on the heart; it can cause heart attack and stroke. People on methamphetamine have signs of brain damage similar to those seen in Parkinson's disease patients. These symptoms can persist even after drug use ceases, causing impaired memory and motor coordination problems. Withdrawal from meth causes symptoms that may include muscle aches and tremors, profound fatigue, deep depression, despair, and apathy. Addiction to methamphetamine is associated with pronounced psychological cravings and obsessive drug-seeking behavior.

Women who use amphetamines during pregnancy risk premature birth, stillbirth, low birth weight, and early infant death. Babies born to amphetamine-using mothers have a higher incidence of cleft palate, cleft lip, and deformed limbs. They may also experience symptoms of withdrawal.

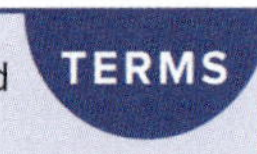


**psychosis** A severe mental disorder characterized by a distortion of reality; symptoms might include delusions or hallucinations.

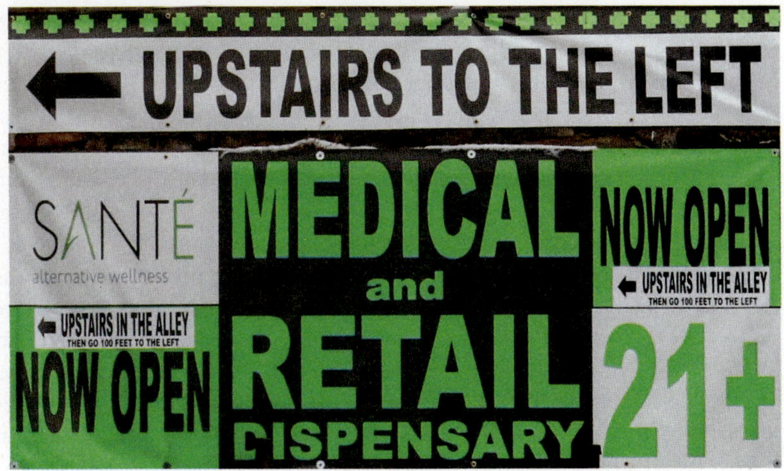


Some states permit the sale of both medical and recreational marijuana. The regulations typically differ for the two types of sales: In Colorado, for example, medical marijuana is taxed at a lower rate and is less expensive than recreational marijuana. KaraGrubis/iStock Editorial/Getty Images

**Stimulant ADHD Medications** Prescription stimulants such as Ritalin, Adderall, or Concerta in low dosages have a calming effect on people with attention-deficit/hyperactivity disorder (ADHD), allowing greater attention and focus. Studies have found that prescription stimulants do not enhance learning or thinking ability when taken by people who do not have ADHD. Taken in higher dosages, or by people who do not have ADHD, prescription stimulants can increase dopamine in a rapid and amplified manner (similar to methamphetamine), thereby disrupting normal communication between brain cells.

**Caffeine** Caffeine is a very popular psychoactive drug and also one of the most ancient. It is found in coffee, tea, cocoa, soft drinks, headache remedies, energy drinks, and OTC preparations. In ordinary doses, caffeine produces greater alertness and a sense of well-being. It also decreases feelings of fatigue or boredom, so using caffeine may enable a person to keep at physically tiring or repetitive tasks longer. Such use is usually followed, however, by a sudden crash. Caffeine does not noticeably influence a person's ability to perform complex mental tasks unless fatigue, boredom, or other factors have already affected normal performance.

Caffeine mildly stimulates the heart and respiratory system, increases muscular tremor, and enhances gastric secretion. Higher doses may cause nervousness, anxiety, irritability, headache, disturbed sleep, and gastric irritation or peptic ulcers. In people with high blood pressure, caffeine can cause blood pressure to rise even further above normal; in people with type 2 diabetes, caffeine may cause glucose and insulin levels to rise after meals.

Drinks containing caffeine are rarely harmful for most people, but some tolerance develops, and withdrawal symptoms of irritability, headaches, and even mild depression occur. People can usually avoid problems by simply decreasing their daily intake of caffeine. The average daily intake is about 280 mg.

## Marijuana and Other Cannabis Products

With close to 50 million users in 2020, marijuana is the most widely used federally illegal drug in the United States. At the time of this writing, 37 states and the District of Columbia (DC) have legalized medical marijuana, and 18 states and DC allow for recreational usage. Since the new laws took effect, general marijuana use among twelfth graders has remained steady, although the number of students vaping it has risen. More use has been reported among eighth and tenth graders, as well as college students. THC (tetrahydrocannabinol) is the main active ingredient in marijuana. The buds from the flowering tops may contain 10–20% THC or more. Hashish, a potent preparation made from the thick resin that exudes from the marijuana leaves, may contain up to 15% THC or more.

**Short-Term Effects and Uses** At low doses, marijuana typically gives an experience of euphoria, a heightening of subjective sensory experiences, a slowing down of the perception of passing time, and a relaxed attitude. These pleasant effects are the reason this drug is so widely used. With moderate doses, marijuana's effects become stronger, and the person can also expect to have impaired memory function, disturbed thought patterns, lapses of attention, and feelings of **depersonalization,** in which the mind seems to be separated from the body. There is growing evidence that adolescent initiation of cannabis use is associated with the development of psychiatric disorders such as depression, anxiety, and psychosis.

Very high doses produce feelings of depersonalization, marked sensory distortion, and changes in body image (such as a feeling that the body is very light). Inexperienced individuals sometimes think these sensations mean they are going crazy and become anxious or even panicky. Consuming food or candy infused with marijuana can increase the risk of an unexpected reaction. Edibles take longer to digest and produce a high; people often overconsume edibles in a mistaken attempt to speed up the process.

Physiologically, marijuana increases heart rate and dilates certain blood vessels in the eyes, which creates the characteristic bloodshot eyes. The user may also feel less inclined toward physical exertion and may feel particularly hungry or thirsty. Because THC affects parts of the brain that control balance, coordination, and reaction time, marijuana use impairs driving performance. The combination of alcohol

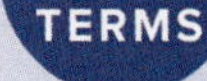


**depersonalization** A state in which a person loses their sense of reality or perceives their body as unreal.

and marijuana is even more dangerous: Even a low dose of marijuana, when combined with alcohol, significantly impairs driving performance and increases crash risk.

The U.S. Supreme Court has held that state laws permitting medical marijuana use cannot supersede federal law. Thus, anyone using marijuana can still be prosecuted under federal drug laws.

Research shows benefits for using cannabis to treat muscle spasms in multiple sclerosis and cancer-related pain that is not otherwise relieved by opioid medications.

**Long-Term Effects** The most probable long-term effect of smoking marijuana is respiratory damage, including impaired lung function and chronic bronchial irritation. Although no evidence links marijuana use to lung cancer, it may cause changes in lung tissue that promote cancer growth. People who use marijuana may be at increased risk for emphysema and cancer of the head and neck, and among people with chronic conditions like cancer and AIDS, marijuana use is associated with increased risk of fatal lung infections. (These are key reasons why the National Academy of Medicine has recommended the development of alternative methods of delivering the potentially beneficial compounds in marijuana.) People using it heavily may experience learning problems, as well as subtle impairments of attention and memory that may or may not be reversible following long-term abstinence. Long-term use may also affect sperm productivity and quality.

Studies show that marijuana use during pregnancy may affect the fetus's neural development. Children exposed to cannabis in-utero showed cognitive deficits, suggesting that maternal use of marijuana has interfered with the proper development of the brain. Babies born to mothers who used marijuana during pregnancy also had increased startles and tremors as well as difficulty adjusting to light. Their sleep patterns were altered, and they showed increased irritability. Moreover, THC rapidly enters breast milk and may impair an infant's early motor development. As children developed into adolescents, memory, impulsivity, and attention problems emerged.

## Hallucinogens

As shown in Figure 8.1, **hallucinogens** are a group of drugs whose primary pharmacological effect is to alter perceptions, feelings, and thoughts.

> **TERMS**
>
> **hallucinogen** Any of several drugs that alter perception, feelings, or thoughts; examples are LSD, mescaline, and PCP.
>
> **synesthesia** A condition in which a stimulus evokes not only the sensation appropriate to it but also another sensation of a different character, such as when a color evokes a specific smell.
>
> **altered states of consciousness** Profound changes in mood, thinking, and perception.
>
> **flashback** A perceptual distortion or bizarre thought that recurs after the chemical effects of a drug have worn off.

**LSD** LSD (lysergic acid diethylamide) is one of the most powerful psychoactive drugs. Tiny doses will produce noticeable effects in most people, such as an altered sense of time, visual disturbances, an improved sense of hearing, mood changes, and distortions in perception. Dilation of the pupils and slight dizziness, weakness, and nausea may also occur. With larger doses, people may experience a phenomenon known as **synesthesia:** feelings of depersonalization and other alterations in the perceived relationship between the self and external reality.

The immediate effects of low doses of hallucinogens are determined largely by expectations and setting. Reports of many effects vary because they involve subjective and unusual dimensions of awareness—the **altered states of consciousness** for which these drugs are famous. For this reason, hallucinogens have acquired a certain aura not associated with other drugs. People have taken LSD in search of a religious or mystical experience or in the hope of exploring new worlds. During the 1960s some psychiatrists gave LSD to their patients to help them talk about their feelings. In the past several years, the FDA has allowed clinical trials for psilocybin-assisted therapy for depression and approved esketamine (Spravato) for severe depression in patients who do not respond to other treatments.

A severe panic reaction, which can be terrifying, can result from taking any dose of LSD. Even after the drug's chemical effects have worn off, spontaneous **flashbacks** and other psychological disturbances can occur.

**MDMA** MDMA (methylenedioxymethamphetamine), and variants called Ecstasy (MDMA with a stimulant such as caffeine added) and Molly (a powder that often contains synthetic cathinone, or bath salts, discussed later), may be classified as a hallucinogen or a stimulant, having both hallucinogenic and amphetamine-like properties. Tolerance to MDMA develops quickly, leading people to take the drug more frequently, use higher doses, or combine MDMA with other drugs to enhance the drug's effects. High doses can cause anxiety, delusions, and paranoia. People using the drug may experience euphoria, increased energy, and a heightened sense of belonging. Using MDMA can produce dangerously high body temperature and potentially fatal dehydration with kidney failure; several cases have been reported of low total body salt concentrations (hyponatremia). Some experience confusion, depression, anxiety, paranoia, muscle tension, involuntary teeth clenching, blurred vision, nausea, and seizures. Even low doses can affect concentration, judgment, and driving ability.

**Other Hallucinogens** Most other hallucinogens have the same general effects as LSD, but there are some variations. For example, a DMT (dimethyltryptamine) or ketamine high does not last as long as an LSD high.

PCP (phencyclidine) reduces and distorts sensory input, especially proprioception—the sensation of body position and movement—and creates a state of sensory deprivation. The effects of ketamine are similar to those of PCP—confusion, agitation, aggression, lack of coordination, and distorted perceptions of sight and sound that produce feelings of dissociation from the environment and self—but they tend to be less predictable. Tolerance to either drug can develop rapidly.

Hallucinogenic effects can be obtained from certain mushrooms (*Psilocybe mexicana,* or "magic mushrooms"). Medical uses of psilocybin mushrooms and LSD were banned in the 1960s; however, research in recent years has renewed interest in potential uses of psilocybin to treat depression, post-traumatic stress disorder, anorexia, Alzheimer's disease, and addiction to alcohol, nicotine, and heroin. Johns Hopkins launched the Center for Psychedelic and Consciousness Research in 2019, the first research center of its kind in the United States.

## Inhalants

Inhaling certain chemicals can produce effects ranging from heightened pleasure to delirium and death. Inhalants fall into several major groups:

(1) volatile solvents, which are found in products such as paint thinner, glue, and gasoline

(2) aerosols, which are sprays that contain propellants and solvents

(3) nitrites, such as butyl nitrite and amyl nitrite

(4) anesthetics, which include nitrous oxide (laughing gas)

Inhalant use tends to be highest among younger adolescents and declines with age. Inhalant use is difficult to control because inhalants are easy to obtain. They are present in a variety of seemingly harmless products, from dessert-topping sprays to underarm deodorants, that are both inexpensive and legal. Using the drugs also requires no illegal or suspicious paraphernalia. People misusing inhalants get high by sniffing, snorting, "bagging" (inhaling fumes from a plastic bag), or "huffing" (placing an inhalant-soaked rag in the mouth).

Although different in makeup, nearly all inhalants produce effects similar to those of anesthetics, which slow down body functions. Low doses may cause feelings of slight stimulation; higher doses, feelings of less inhibition and less control. Sniffing high concentrations of the chemicals in solvents or aerosol sprays can cause loss of consciousness, heart failure, and death. High concentrations of any inhalant can also cause death from suffocation by displacing oxygen in the lungs and central nervous system. Deliberately inhaling from a bag or in a closed area greatly increases the chances of suffocation. Other possible effects of the excessive or long-term use of inhalants include damage to the nervous system, hearing loss, increased risk of cancer, and damage to the liver, kidneys, and bone marrow.

## Prescription Drug Misuse

The National Institute on Drug Abuse describes prescription drug misuse as the use of a medication without a prescription, in a way other than as prescribed, or to feel euphoria.

### Ask Yourself

**QUESTIONS FOR CRITICAL THINKING AND REFLECTION**

Do you know anyone who may be at risk for using inhalants? If so, would you try to intervene in some way? What would you tell a teenager to convince him or her to stop inhaling chemicals?

Over the past decade, misuse of prescription drugs has increased, and national surveys now show that prescription medications—such as those used to treat pain, ADHD, and anxiety—are being misused at a rate second only to marijuana, tobacco, and alcohol. In 2020, over 16,000 people died from drug overdoses involving prescription opioids.

## New Psychoactive Substances

In recent years, herbal or synthetic recreational drugs have become increasingly available. These drugs are part of a group called new psychoactive substances; they are intended to have pharmacological effects similar to those of illicit drugs while being chemically distinct from them and therefore either legal or impossible to detect in drug screening. The drugs fall into two main groups. One group is marketed as synthetic marijuana and sold as "herbal incense," or "herbal highs," with names such as Spice, K2, Genie, and Mr. Nice Guy. The other group is marketed as stimulants with properties like those of cocaine or amphetamine and sold as "bath salts" with names such as Zoom, Ivory Wave, and White Rush.

Spice and other synthetic mimics of THC are human-made chemicals that are either sprayed onto plant material for smoking or sold in liquid form for vaping devices. Their active ingredients are synthetic cannabinoids that act on brain cells to produce effects similar to those of THC, such as physical relaxation, but may also include psychotic effects like extreme anxiety, confusion, paranoia, and hallucinations. Misleadingly marketed as safe and natural, synthetic cannabinoids went through a period of initial popularity among teens and young adults. In 2011, 11.4% of high school seniors reported having used synthetic cannabinoids at least once during the year, but levels have since dropped.

The blends of ingredients vary widely, but these products typically contain more than a dozen different substances that give rise to a variety of drug combinations. Calls to poison control centers for exposure to synthetic cannabinoids typically involve symptoms like rapid heart rate, vomiting, violent behavior, and suicidal thoughts; these drugs can also raise blood pressure and cause liver damage and seizures. In 2018, hundreds of cases of severe bleeding and bruising in midwestern states were linked to synthetic cannabinoids contaminated with brodifacoum, a blood-thinning compound commonly used in rat poison.

"Bath salts," marketed as cocaine or methamphetamine substitutes, are widely available on the internet. They contain synthetic cathinones such as mephedrone, methylone, or methylenedioxypyrovalerone (MDPV). Similar in effect to MDMA (Ecstasy), these cathinones are synthetic but more powerful versions of the active ingredient found in the stimulant khat, a chewable leaf that is widely used in countries of the Middle East and Africa. The products are sold in small packets of salt-like crystals with warnings like "novelty only" and "not for human consumption." Bath salts, not to be confused with products like Epsom salts used for bathing, can be ingested by smoking, eating, injecting, or snorting. The effects of bath salts can be severe and include combative violent behavior, extreme agitation, confusion, hallucinations, hypertension, chest pain, and suicidal thoughts. Bath salts can be highly addictive; in 2018, researchers developed a vaccine that blunts the drug's effects on the brain, which could help people recovering from drug use who are experiencing a relapse.

# PREVENTING DRUG-RELATED PROBLEMS

New psychoactive drugs may present unexpected possibilities for therapy, social use, and misuse. Making honest and unbiased information about drugs available to everyone, however, may cut down on their misuse.

Although the use of some drugs, both legal and illegal, has declined dramatically since the 1970s, the use of others has increased. Efforts to address the problem include workplace drug testing, tougher law enforcement and prosecution, and treatment and education. Today, ingredients used to synthesize fentanyl and other synthetic opioids come frequently from suppliers in China; these chemicals are shipped to Mexico, where cartels produce the drugs and traffic them into the United States.

## Drugs, Society, and Families

The economic cost of drug misuse is staggering. Use and misuse of alcohol, nicotine, and illicit drugs and prescription drugs cost Americans more than $700 billion a year in increased health care costs, crime, and lost productivity. The cost of overdose fatalities is estimated at approximately $1 trillion a year. But the costs are more than just financial—they are also paid in human pain and suffering.

The criminal justice system is inundated with people accused of crimes related to drug possession, sale, or use. The FBI reports that roughly 1.55 million arrests were made for drug violations in 2019, and over 1 million for driving under the influence. In 2021, almost half of federal inmates (65,370) were in prison because of drug offenses. The Bureau of Justice Statistics reports that about half of all state and federal prisoners—roughly 850,000 men and women—meet diagnostic criteria for a substance use disorder. Many assaults and murders are committed when people try to acquire or protect drug territories, settle disputes about drugs, or steal from dealers. Violence and gun use are common in neighborhoods where drug trafficking is prevalent. People with SUDs commit more robberies and burglaries than criminals not on drugs. People under the influence of drugs, especially alcohol, are more likely to commit violent crimes like rape and murder than are people who do not use drugs.

**QUICK STATS**

**In 2020, 40 million people aged 12 or older had an SUD.**

—Substance Abuse and Mental Health Services Administration, 2021

To what extent is drug misuse also a health care issue for society? Due to the sensitive nature of drug use reporting, the use or death numbers and the demographics they represent are only estimates (see the box "The Trouble with Substance Use and the Surveys that Report It"). In the United States, alcohol and prescription and illicit drug use leads to hundreds of thousands of emergency department admissions and 188,000 deaths annually. People with SUDs who want to quit, especially among the urban poor, often have to wait months for acceptance into a residential care or other treatment program.

Children born to women who use drugs such as alcohol, tobacco, or cocaine may have long-term health problems. Drug misuse in families can become a vicious cycle. Children who observe adults using drugs may assume it is acceptable. Abuse, neglect, lack of opportunity, and unemployment become contributing factors to drug use, perpetuating the cycle.

## Legalizing Drugs

Pointing out that many social problems associated with drugs are related to prohibition (which failed for alcohol from 1920 to 1933) rather than to the effects of the drugs themselves, some people argue for drug legalization or decriminalization. Proposals range from making drugs such as marijuana and heroin available by prescription to allowing licensed dealers to sell some of these drugs to adults. Proponents argue that legalizing some currently illicit drugs—but putting controls on them similar to those used for alcohol, tobacco, and prescription drugs—could eliminate many problems. Some states have adopted policies that decriminalize possession of small amounts of marijuana—that is, possession for recreational use either is legal or is treated as a misdemeanor crime without significant penalty. Opponents of drug legalization argue that allowing easier access to drugs would expose many more people to possible addiction. Drugs would be cheaper and easier to obtain, and drug use would be more socially acceptable. Legalizing drugs could cause an increase in drug use among children and teenagers. Opponents point out that alcohol and tobacco—drugs that already are legal—are major causes of disease and death in our society.

## Treating Drug Addiction

In 2022, the Biden administration renewed its predecessor's declaration of a national public health emergency regarding the opioid epidemic, and a government commission has

# DIVERSITY MATTERS
## The Trouble with Substance Use Surveys

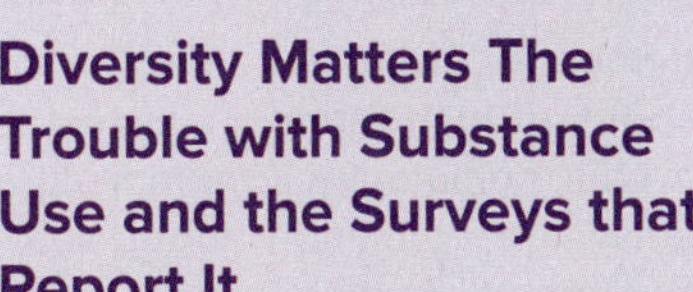

### Diversity Matters The Trouble with Substance Use and the Surveys that Report It

Surveys about sensitive topics such as drug use face challenges eliciting honest answers from participants, who may not want to disclose such personal information. Another challenge is getting a respondent pool that reflects the diversity of races, ethnicities, and genders in the general population. Even if a survey did get such a group of participants, our language often falls short in describing them. What if a survey wants to match its data collection with categories used 50 years ago? This comparison poses limits.

Such is the case with the U.S. Monitoring the Future (MTF) survey, a data collection of substance use for adolescents through adults. Nationally representative samples of eighth, tenth, and twelfth graders answer questions about their drug and alcohol use, as well as a variety of other subjects, ranging from attitudes toward religion, parental influence, and sex. The survey, funded by the National Institutes of Health and conducted by the University of Michigan, began in 1975. Partly because of its longitudinal scope, its race and gender categories are limited.

### Black, White, and Hispanic

For many years, Black high school seniors reported significantly lower rates of drug misuse compared to their White and Hispanic peers. In recent years, the gap has narrowed, due to increased rates of marijuana use among Black students and a leveling off of marijuana use among Whites. Black seniors reported higher use rates of crystal meth and a slightly higher rate of heroin use than Whites and Hispanics. But when marijuana is excluded from overall misuse rates, Black seniors show far lower rates than Whites and Hispanics.

Annual misuse rates for inhalants, methamphetamines, Oxycontin, Vicodin, and sedatives were similar among all groups. Hispanic twelfth graders reported the highest past-year misuse of synthetic marijuana, OTC cold medicine, and Ritalin. White seniors reported the highest nonmedical use of amphetamines, MDMA (Molly, ecstasy), and tranquilizers, and prescription and Adderall misuse. Hispanic and White seniors had higher rates of hallucinogen and cocaine use than Black seniors.

### Other Surveys, Other Challenges

Other studies such as the 2021 National College Health Assessment III demonstrates that trans/gender nonbinary students have higher rates of drug use compared to cis men and women. But their prevalence rates cover use only in the past three months or in a lifetime. The 2019 National Survey on Drug Use and Health offers rates on lesbian, gay, and bisexual (LGB) people, although it does not compare them to rates of non-LGB. The survey shows that American Indian and Alaska Natives (AIAN) have higher rates of substance use, although how much higher depends on the substance. Generally White, Black, and AIAN students have similar rates that also are higher than those of students who are Asian or Native Hawaiian and other Pacific Islander; participants identifying as multiple races have the highest rates.


Johnston, L. D., et al. 2020. *Demographic subgroup trends among adolescents in the use of various licit and illicit drugs, 1975–2019* (Monitoring the Future Occasional Paper No. 94). Ann Arbor, MI: Institute for Social Research, The University of Michigan; American College Health Association. 2021. *American College Health Association-National College Health Assessment III: Reference Group Executive Summary Spring 2021*. Silver Spring, MD: American College Health Association; Substance Abuse and Mental Health Services Administration. 2020. *2019 National Survey on Drug Use and Health: Lesbian, Gay, & Bisexual (LGB) Adults* (https://www.samhsa.gov/data/sites/default/files/reports/rpt31104/2019NSDUH-LGB/LGB%202019%20NSDUH.pdf).


been working on solutions. All insurance sold on health insurance exchanges or provided by Medicaid to certain newly eligible adults must include services for treatment of substance use disorders such as alcohol or drug addiction.

The 2016 United Nations General Assembly Special Session on Drugs put out recommendations, including the following: Eliminate stigma and discrimination toward people with substance use disorders; implement evidence-based prevention programs and treatment for addiction; engage scientific data and experts in policymaking, public health, education, law enforcement, and health care; support drug-related research; and ensure that scheduled medications are available for therapeutic use.

Treatment for addiction should assess for other mental disorders as well as infectious disease. Addiction is a mental disorder that often co-occurs with other mental illnesses, and drug-related behaviors put people at risk for diseases like HIV/AIDS, hepatitis B and C, and tuberculosis. Medically assisted detoxification is the first, not the only stage of treatment. Behavioral therapies and counseling, often combined with appropriate medications, are crucial components of effective treatment.

**Medication-Assisted Treatment** Medications are increasingly being used in addiction treatment to reduce the craving for the misused drug or to block its effects. Perhaps the best-known medication for drug use is methadone, a synthetic drug used as a substitute for heroin. Methadone prevents withdrawal reactions and reduces the craving for heroin. Its use enables heroin-addicted people to function normally in social and vocational activities, although they remain dependent on methadone. The drug buprenorphine, a partial opioid agonist, in combination with naloxone, approved for treatment of opioid addiction, reduces cravings and relapse

## TAKE CHARGE
### If Someone You Know Has a Drug Problem . . .

Changes in behavior and mood in someone you know may signal a growing dependence on drugs. Signs that a person's life is beginning to focus on drugs include the following:

- Sudden withdrawal or emotional distance
- Rebellious or unusually irritable behavior
- A loss of interest in usual activities or hobbies
- A decline in school performance
- A sudden change in the chosen group of friends
- Changes in sleeping or eating habits
- Frequent borrowing of money or stealing
- Secretive behavior about personal possessions, such as a backpack or the contents of a drawer
- Deterioration of physical appearance

If you believe a family member or friend has a drug problem, locate information about drug treatment resources available on campus or in your community. Communicate your concern, provide them with information about treatment options, and offer your support during treatment. If the person continues to deny having a problem, talk with an experienced counselor about setting up an intervention—a formal, structured confrontation designed to end denial by having family, friends, and other caring people present their concerns to the person using drugs. Participants in an intervention would indicate the ways in which the individual is hurting others as well as themself. If your friend or family member agrees to treatment, encourage them to attend a support group such as Narcotics Anonymous or Alcoholics Anonymous.

And finally, examine your relationship with the person with an SUD for signs of codependency. If necessary, get help for yourself; friends and family can often benefit from counseling.

but also leaves one dependent on buprenorphine. An opioid blocker called naltrexone in both oral and injection forms has also shown efficacy for the treatment of both opioid and alcohol use disorders. There is now a growing movement to intervene in emergency departments (EDs) with a brief course of either buprenorphine or naltrexone with coordination of outpatient addiction and primary care.

Medication therapy can appear efficacious and efficient and is therefore popular among patients and health care providers. However, the relapse rate remains high. Combining drug therapy with psychological and social services improves success rates, underscoring the importance of psychological factors in drug dependence.

**Treatment Centers** Treatment centers offer a variety of short-term and long-term services, including hospitalization, detoxification, counseling, and other mental health services. The therapeutic community is a specific type of residential program run in a completely drug-free environment. Administered by people recovering from an SUD, these centers use confrontation, strict discipline, and unrelenting peer pressure to attempt to resocialize the addicted individual with a different set of values. Halfway houses, which are transitional settings between a 24-hour-a-day program and independent living, are an important phase of treatment for some people.

**Groups and Peer Counseling** Groups such as Alcoholics Anonymous (AA) and Narcotics Anonymous (NA) have helped many people. People receiving treatment in drug substitution programs or substance use treatment centers are often urged or required to join a mutual-help group as part of their recovery. Many of these groups follow a 12-step program. Group members' first step is to acknowledge that they have a problem over which they have no control. Peer support is a critical ingredient of these programs, and members usually meet at least once a week. As part of a 12-step program, each member is paired with a sponsor to call on for advice and guidance in working through the 12 steps and getting support if the temptation to relapse becomes overwhelming. With such support, thousands of substance-dependent people have been able to recover, remain abstinent, and reclaim their lives. Chapters of AA and NA meet on some college campuses; community-based chapters are listed in the phone book, in local newspapers, and online. Other organizations provide an alternative to the 12 steps such as LifeRing Secular Recovery, Rational Recovery, SMART Recovery, Women for Sobriety, and Refuge Recovery.

Many colleges also have peer counseling programs, in which students are trained to help other students who have drug problems. A peer counselor's role may be as limited as referring a student to a professional with expertise in substance dependence for an evaluation or as involved as helping arrange a leave of absence from school for participation in a drug treatment program. Most peer counseling programs are founded on principles of strict confidentiality. Peer counselors may also be able to help students who are concerned about a classmate or loved one with an apparent drug problem (see the box "If Someone You Know Has a Drug Problem . . ."). Information about peer counseling programs is usually available from the student health center.

**Harm Reduction Strategies** Because many attempts at treatment are at first unsuccessful, some experts advocate the use of harm reduction strategies. The goal of harm reduction is to minimize the negative effects of drug use and misuse. A common example is the use of designated drivers to reduce alcohol-related motor vehicle crashes. Drug substitution programs such as methadone maintenance are another well-known form of harm reduction; although participants remain drug dependent, the negative consequences of their drug use are reduced. Additional examples of harm reduction strategies include the following:

- Syringe exchange programs, designed to reduce transmission of HIV and hepatitis C
- Safe injection facilities or sites where people using heroin can go to inject it under medical supervision
- Provision of easy-to-use forms of naloxone, a drug that rapidly reverses opioid overdose, to family members and caregivers of people using heroin. There are two FDA-approved formulations of naloxone: injectable and prepackaged nasal spray
- Free testing of street drugs for purity and potency to help people with SUDs avoid unintentional toxicity or overdose

**How Family and Friends Cope** Many treatment programs also offer counseling for those who are close to people with SUDs. Drug misuse takes a toll on friends and family members, and counseling can help people work through painful feelings of guilt and powerlessness. Codependency, in which a person close to someone with an SUD is controlled by their behavior, sometimes develops. The family member or friend may come to believe that love, approval, and emotional and physical security are contingent on their taking care of the person who is addicted. The family wants to help and may assume that their good intentions will persuade their loved one to stop using.

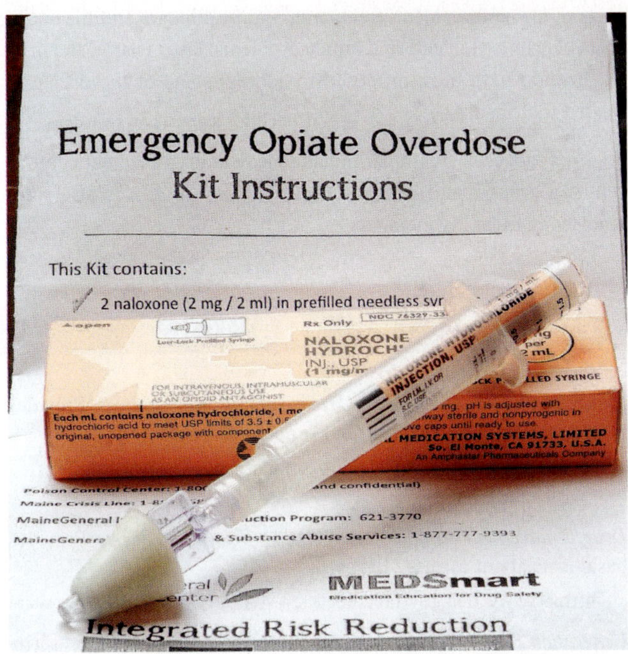

A naloxone kit is an example of a harm reduction strategy for people at risk of an opioid overdose. Portland Press Herald/Joe Phelan/Getty Images

Here are some less healthy behaviors:

- Giving someone countless chances to stop using drugs
- Making excuses or lying for someone to their friends, teachers, or employer
- Joining someone in drug use and blaming others for your behavior
- Lending money to someone to continue drug use
- Staying up late waiting for or going out searching for someone who uses drugs
- Feeling embarrassed or angry about the actions of someone who uses drugs
- Ignoring the drug use because the person got defensive when you brought it up
- Avoiding confronting a friend or relative who was obviously intoxicated or high on a drug

Many treatment programs involve the whole family. Support groups such as Al-Anon can help family members learn to recognize that they can't control or cure or enable or disable the problem. Rather, in an environment of social support, loved ones can find personalized paths of recovery and "detach with love."

## Preventing Drug Misuse

Obviously the best solution to drug misuse is prevention. Government attempts at controlling the drug problem have historically focused on stopping the production, importation, and distribution of illegal drugs. A national drug policy announced in 2010, however, redirects federal funding and efforts into stopping the demand for drugs. Developing persuasive antidrug educational programs may offer the best hope for solving the drug problem in the future. Indirect approaches to prevention involve building young people's self-esteem, improving their academic skills, and increasing their recreational opportunities. Direct approaches involve providing information about the adverse effects of drugs and teaching tactics that help students resist peer pressure to use drugs in various situations. Developing strategies for resisting peer pressure is one of the more effective techniques.

Prevention efforts need to focus on the different motivations individuals have for using and misusing specific drugs at different ages. For example, grade-school children seem receptive to programs that involve their parents or well-known adults such as professional athletes. Adolescents in

### Ask Yourself

**QUESTIONS FOR CRITICAL THINKING AND REFLECTION**

Do you have a substance use problem or a behavioral addiction? If so, how has it affected you? How has it affected others? Have you taken any steps to help yourself? Have friends or family offered help?

## TIPS FOR TODAY AND THE FUTURE

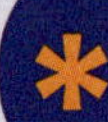

**RIGHT NOW YOU CAN:**

- Assess your own relationship with any substances you consume or behaviors in which you frequently engage.
- Consider whether you or someone you know might benefit from drug counseling. Find out what types of services are available on campus or in your area.

**IN THE FUTURE YOU CAN:**

- Think about the drug-related attitudes of people you know. For example, talk to two older adults and two fellow students about their attitudes toward legalizing marijuana. What might account for any differences in their opinions?
- Analyze media portrayals of drug use. As you watch television shows and movies, note the way they depict drug use among people of different ages and backgrounds. How realistic are the portrayals, in your view? Think about the influence they have on you and your peers.

junior or senior high school are often more responsive to peer counselors. Many young adults tend to be influenced by efforts that focus on health education. For all ages, it is important to provide nondrug alternatives–such as recreational facilities, counseling, greater opportunities for leisure activities, and places to socialize–that speak to the individual's or group's specific reasons for using drugs. Reminding young people that most people, no matter what age, are *not* users of illegal drugs, do *not* smoke cigarettes, and do *not* get drunk frequently is a critical part of preventing substance misuse.

## SUMMARY

- Some common behaviors are potentially addictive, including gambling, shopping, sexual activity, internet use, eating, exercising, and working.
- Addictions often persist despite adverse social, psychological, or medical consequences.
- Addiction involves taking a drug or engaging in a behavior compulsively, neglecting constructive activities because of it, and continuing to use or engage in it despite the adverse effects. Tolerance and withdrawal symptoms are often present.
- The development of addiction includes factors like genetics, heredity, age, gender, personality, lifestyle, social and physical environment, and the nature of the substance or behavior. People may use a substance or behavior as a means of alleviating stress or painful emotions.
- Drug misuse is use of a drug that is not consistent with medical or legal guidelines.
- Criteria for a substance use disorder are grouped in four categories: impaired control, social problems, risky use, and drug effects.
- Reasons for using drugs include the lure of the illicit, curiosity, rebellion, peer pressure, and the desire to alter mood or alleviate boredom, anxiety, depression, or other psychiatric symptoms.
- Risks associated with drug misuse include intoxication, unexpected side effects, ingestion of unknown drug constituents, injection-related infections and complications, and legal consequences.
- Psychoactive drugs affect the mind and body by altering brain chemistry. The effect of a drug depends on its properties and on how it's used (drug factors), the physical and psychological characteristics of the person using (personal factors), and the physical and social environment surrounding the drug use (social factors).
- Opioids relieve pain, cause drowsiness, and induce euphoria; they reduce anxiety and produce lethargy, apathy, and an inability to concentrate.
- CNS depressants slow down the overall activity of the central nervous system; they reduce anxiety and cause mood changes, impaired muscular coordination, slurring of speech, and drowsiness or sleep.
- CNS stimulants speed up the activity of the central nervous system, causing acceleration of the heart rate, a rise in blood pressure, dilation of the pupils and bronchial tubes, and an increase in gastric and adrenal secretions.
- Marijuana usually causes euphoria and a relaxed attitude at low doses; very high doses produce feelings of depersonalization and sensory distortion. Use during pregnancy may impair fetal growth.
- Hallucinogens alter perception, feelings, and thoughts and may cause an altered sense of time, visual disturbances, and mood changes.
- Inhalants are present in a variety of everyday products; they can cause delirium. Their use can lead to loss of consciousness, heart failure, suffocation, and death.
- Economic and social costs of drug misuse include the financial costs of law enforcement, treatment, and health care and the social costs of crime, violence, and family problems. Drug testing and drug legalization have been proposed to address some of the problems related to drug use.
- Approaches to treatment include medication, treatment centers, self-help groups, and peer counseling; many programs also offer counseling to family members.

## FOR MORE INFORMATION

*American Society of Addiction Medicine: Patient Resources.* Provides information about treatment and support groups.

https://www.asam.org/Quality-Science/resource-links/patient-resources

*Drug Enforcement Administration (DEA): Drug Facts Sheets.* Provides basic facts about misused drugs.

https://www.dea.gov/factsheets

*Generation Rx.* Works to educate people about the risks of prescription medication misuse.

https://www.generationrx.org/

## BEHAVIOR CHANGE STRATEGY
### Changing Your Drug Habits

This behavior change strategy focuses on one of the most commonly used drugs—caffeine. If you are concerned about your use of a different drug or another type of addictive behavior, you can devise your own plan based on this one and on the steps outlined in Chapter 1.

Like many Americans, you may find yourself relying on coffee (or tea, chocolate, or cola) to get through a busy schedule. When you are studying for exams, for example, the forced physical inactivity and the need to concentrate even when fatigued may lead you to over use caffeine. But caffeine doesn't help unless you are already sleepy. And it does not relieve any underlying condition (you are just more tired when it wears off). How can you change this pattern?

#### Self-Monitor

Keep a log of how much caffeine you eat or drink. Be sure to include all forms, such as chocolate and OTC medications, as well as colas, tea, and coffee. Use Table 4.1 in Chapter 4 to convert the amounts you drink into an estimate expressed in milligrams of caffeine.

#### Self-Assess

At the end of the week, add up your daily totals and divide by 7 to get your daily average in milligrams. At more than 250 mg per day, you may be experiencing some adverse symptoms. If you are experiencing at least five of the following symptoms, you may want to cut down:

- Restlessness
- Nervousness
- Excitement
- Insomnia
- Flushed face
- Excessive sweating
- Gastrointestinal problems
- Muscle twitching
- Rambling thoughts and speech
- Irregular heartbeat
- Periods of inexhaustibility
- Excessive pacing or movement

#### Set Limits

Can you restrict your caffeine intake to a daily total, and stick to this contract? If so, set a cutoff point, such as the amount of caffeine in one cup of coffee. If you cannot stick to your limit, you may want to cut out caffeine altogether: Abstinence can be easier than moderation for some people. If you experience caffeine withdrawal symptoms (headache, fatigue), you may want to cut your intake more gradually.

#### Find Other Ways to Keep Up Your Energy

Get enough sleep or exercise more, rather than drowning the problem in coffee or tea. Remember that exercise raises your metabolic rate for hours afterward—a handy fact to exploit when you need to feel more awake and want to avoid an irritable caffeine jag. And if you've been compounding your fatigue by not eating properly, try filling up on complex carbohydrates such as whole-grain bread or crackers instead of candy bars.

*Go Ask Alice.* A health question-and-answer resource produced by Columbia University; see "Alcohol & Other Drugs" in the Health Topics section.

http://goaskalice.columbia.edu

*Higher Education Center for Alcohol and Drug Misuse Prevention and Recovery.* Based at The Ohio State University, it promotes information and solutions to drug and alcohol use on college campuses.

http://hecaod.osu.edu/

*National Center on Addiction and Substance Abuse.* Provides information on addiction, including prevention and treatment.

http://www.centeronaddiction.org

*National Council on Problem Gambling.* Provides information and help for people with gambling problems and their families.

http://www.ncpgambling.org

*National Drug Information, Treatment, and Referral Hotlines (SAMHSA: see below)*

800-662-HELP

800-729-6686 (Spanish)

800-487-4889 (TDD for hearing impaired)

*National Institute on Drug Abuse (NIDA).* Develops and supports research on drug addiction prevention; provides background information on misused drugs.

http://www.drugabuse.gov

*Net Addiction: FAQs.* Provides background information on internet addiction disorder.

http://netaddiction.com

*Partnership for Drug-Free Kids: Drug Guide.* A comprehensive source of information on specific drugs.

http://www.drugfree.org/drug-guide

*Substance Abuse and Mental Health Services Administration (SAMHSA).* Provides statistics, information, and other resources related to substance misuse prevention and treatment.

http://www.samhsa.gov

The following additional organizations/websites provide support services:

*Cocaine Anonymous (CA)*

https://ca.org

*Gamblers Anonymous (GA)*
http://www.gamblersanonymous.org/ga/

*Marijuana Anonymous (MA)*
http://www.marijuana-anonymous.org

*Narcotics Anonymous (NA)*
http://www.na.org

*Overeaters Anonymous (OA)*
https://oa.org

*Refuge Recovery*
http://www.refugerecovery.org

*Sex Addicts Anonymous (SAA)*
https://saa-recovery.org

*SMART® Recovery*
http://www.smartrecovery.org

## SELECTED BIBLIOGRAPHY


American College Health Association. 2021. *American College Health Association-National College Health Assessment III: Reference Group Executive Summary Spring 2021.* Silver Spring, MD: American College Health Association (https://www.acha.org/NCHA/ACHA-NCHA_Data/Publications_and_Reports/NCHA/Data/Reports_ACHA-NCHAIII.aspx).

American Psychiatric Association. 2013. *Diagnostic and Statistical Manual of Mental Disorders,* 5th ed. Washington, DC: American Psychiatric Publishing.

American Psychiatric Association. 2016. Can you be addicted to the internet? *APA Blog* (https://www.psychiatry.org/news-room/apa-blogs/apa-blog/2016/07/can-you-be-addicted-to-the-internet).

American Psychiatric Association. 2022. *Addictions* (https://www.apa.org/topics/substance-use-abuse-addiction).

Centers for Disease Control and Prevention. 2019. *Annual Surveillance Report of Drug-Related Risks and Outcomes—United States, 2019.* Centers for Disease Control and Prevention, U.S. Department of Health and Human Services (https://www.cdc.gov/drugoverdose/pdf/pubs/2019-cdc-drug-surveillance-report.pdf).

Centers for Disease Control and Prevention. 2019. Syringe Services Programs (SSPs) Fact Sheet (https://www.cdc.gov/ssp/syringe-services-programs-factsheet.html).

Centers for Disease Control and Prevention. 2021. *Opioid Data Analysis and Resources* (https://www.cdc.gov/opioids/data/analysis-resources.html).

Consumer Reports National Research Center. 2017. Consumer Reports Examines: Do Americans take too many prescription medications? (https://www.consumerreports.org/media-room/press-releases/2017/08/consumer_reports_examines_do_americans_take_too_many_prescription_medications/).

Cox, C., M. Rae, and B. Sawyer. 2018. A look at how the opioid crisis has affected people with employer coverage. *Peterson-Kaiser Health System Tracker* (https://www.healthsystemtracker.org/brief/a-look-at-how-the-opioid-crisis-has-affected-people-with-employer-coverage/#item-start).

Drug Enforcement Administration, U.S. Department of Justice. 2017. *Drugs of Abuse: A DEA Resource Guide, 2017 Edition* (https://www.dea.gov/sites/default/files/drug_of_abuse.pdf).

European Monitoring Centre for Drugs and Drug Addiction. 2020. New psychoactive substances: global markets, glocal threats and the COVID-19 pandemic. An update from the EU Early Warning System (December). Publications Office of the European Union, Luxembourg.

Federal Bureau of Investigation. 2020. Arrests for drug abuse violations. *2019 Crime in the United States* (https://ucr.fbi.gov/crime-in-the-u.s/2019/crime-in-the-u.s.-2019/topic-pages/persons-arrested).

Federal Bureau of Investigation. 2021. *Federal Offenders in Prison-March 2021* (https://www.ussc.gov/research/quick-facts/federal-offenders-prison).

Law, T. 2022. Why overdose deaths skyrocketed after opioid prescriptions dropped. *Time,* September 19. (https://time.com/6214811/overdose-deaths-opioid-prescriptions/).

Lewis, T. 2020. Johns Hopkins scientists give psychedelics the serious treatment. *Scientific American* (January 16) (https://www.scientificamerican.com/article/johns-hopkins-scientists-give-psychedelics-the-serious-treatment/).

Miech, R. A., et al. 2021. *Monitoring the Future National Survey Results on Drug Use, 1975–2020: Volume I, Secondary school Students.* Ann Arbor: Institute for Social Research, The University of Michigan (http://monitoringthefuture.org/pubs.html#monographs).

National Academies of Sciences, Engineering, and Medicine. 2017. *The Health Effects of Cannabis and Cannabinoids: The Current State of Evidence and Recommendations for Research.* Washington, DC: The National Academies Press.

National Council on Problem Gambling. 2016. *What Is Problem Gambling?* (http://www.ncpgambling.org/help-treatment/faq/).

National Institute on Drug Abuse. n.d. College-Age & Young Adults (https://nida.nih.gov/drug-topics/college-age-young-adults).

National Institute on Drug Abuse. 2018. *Heroin Research Report* (https://nida.nih.gov/publications/research-reports/heroin/overview).

National Institute on Drug Abuse. 2018. *The Science of Drug Abuse and Addiction: The Basics* (https://archives.drugabuse.gov/publications/media-guide/science-drug-use-addiction-basics).

National Institute on Drug Abuse. 2020. *Sex and Gender Differences in Substance Use* (https://nida.nih.gov/publications/research-reports/substance-use-in-women/sex-gender-differences-in-substance-use).

National Institute on Drug Abuse. 2020. *Synthetic Cannabinoids (K2/Spice)* (https://nida.nih.gov/publications/drugfacts/synthetic-cannabinoids-k2spice).

National Institute on Drug Abuse. 2020. *What Is the Scope of Prescription Drug Misuse in the United States?* (https://nida.nih.gov/publications/research-reports/misuse-prescription-drugs/what-scope-prescription-drug-misuse).

National Institute on Drug Abuse. 2021. *Opioid Overdose Crisis* (https://nida.nih.gov/drug-topics/opioids/opioid-overdose-crisis).

O'Donnell J., et al. 2021. Trends in and characteristics of drug overdose deaths involving illicitly manufactured fentanyls—United States, 2019–2020. *Morbidity and Mortality Weekly Report* 70: 1740–1746. DOI: http://dx.doi.org/10.15585/mmwr.mm7050e3.

Office of National Drug Control Policy. 2016. *National Drug Control Strategy* (https://obamawhitehouse.archives.gov/ondcp/policy-and-research/ndcs).

Quest Diagnostics. 2019. *Workforce Drug Testing Positivity Climbs to Highest Rate Since 2004, According to New Quest Diagnostics Analysis* (https://newsroom.questdiagnostics.com/2019-04-11-Workforce-Drug-Testing-Positivity-Climbs-to-Highest-Rate-Since-2004-According-to-New-Quest-Diagnostics-Analysis).

The Recovery Village. 2021. *Pornography Facts and Statistics* (https://www.therecoveryvillage.com/process-addiction/porn-addiction/related/pornography-statistics/#gref).

Rich, S., S. Higham, and S. Horwitz. 2020. More than 100 billion pain pills saturated the nation over nine years. *The Washington Post,* 14 January (https://www.washingtonpost.com/investigations/more-than-100-billion-pain-pills-saturated-the-nation-over-nine-years/2020/01/14/fde320ba-db13-11e9-a688-303693fb4b0b_story.html).

Statista. 2022. Number of arrests for all offenses in the United States from 1990 to 2020 (https://www.statista.com/statistics/191261/number-of-arrests-for-all-offenses-in-the-us-since-1990/).

Substance Abuse and Mental Health Services Administration. 2021. *Key Substance Use and Mental Health Indicators in the United States: Results from the 2020 National Survey on Drug Use and Health* (HHS Publication No. PEP21-07-01-003, NSDUH Series H-56). Rockville, MD: Center for Behavioral Health Statistics and Quality, Substance Abuse and Mental Health Services Administration (https://www.samhsa.gov/data/).

Substance Abuse and Mental Health Services Administration. 2021. *National Survey of Substance Abuse Treatment Services (N-SSATS): 2020, Data on Substance Abuse Treatment Facilities* (https://www.samhsa.gov/data/sites/default/files/reports/rpt35969/2020%20NSSATS%20State%20Profiles_FINAL.pdf).

Swan, S. C., et al. 2017. Just a dare or unaware? Outcomes and motives of drugging ("drink spiking") among students at three college campuses. *Psychology of Violence* 7(2): 253–264 (https://doi.org/10.1037/vio0000060).

United States Commission on Combating Synthetic Opioid Trafficking. 2022. Final report (https://www.rand.org/content/dam/rand/pubs/external_publications/EP60000/EP68838/RAND_EP68838.pdf).

United States Sentencing Commission. 2021. *Federal Offenders in Prison* (https://ucr.fbi.gov/crime-in-the-u.s/2019/crime-in-the-u.s.-2019/topic-pages/persons-arrested).

United States Sentencing Commission. 2022. *Sourcebook* (www.ussc.gov/research/quickfacts/federal-offenders-prison).

U.S. Department of Labor, Bureau of Labor Statistics. 2022. Unintentional overdoses accounted for 388 workplace deaths in 2020. *Economics Daily* (https://www.bls.gov/opub/ted/2022/unintentional-overdoses-accounted-for-388-workplace-deaths-in-2020.htm).

U.S. Department of Justice, Federal Bureau of Investigation. 2019. *Crime in the United States: Persons Arrested* (https://ucr.fbi.gov/crime-in-the-u.s/2019/crime-in-the-u.s.-2019/topic-pages/persons-arrested).

Zielinski, M., et al. 2019. Codependency and prefrontal cortex functioning: preliminary examination of substance use disorder impacted family members. *The American Journal on Addictions* 28: 367–375.

**Design Elements:** Assess Yourself icon: Aleksey Boldin/Alamy Stock Photo; Diversity Matters icon: Rawpixel Ltd/Getty Images; Wellness on Campus icon: Radius Images/Alamy Stock Photo; Take Charge icon: VisualCommunications/Getty Images; Critical Consumer icon: pagadesign/Getty Images.

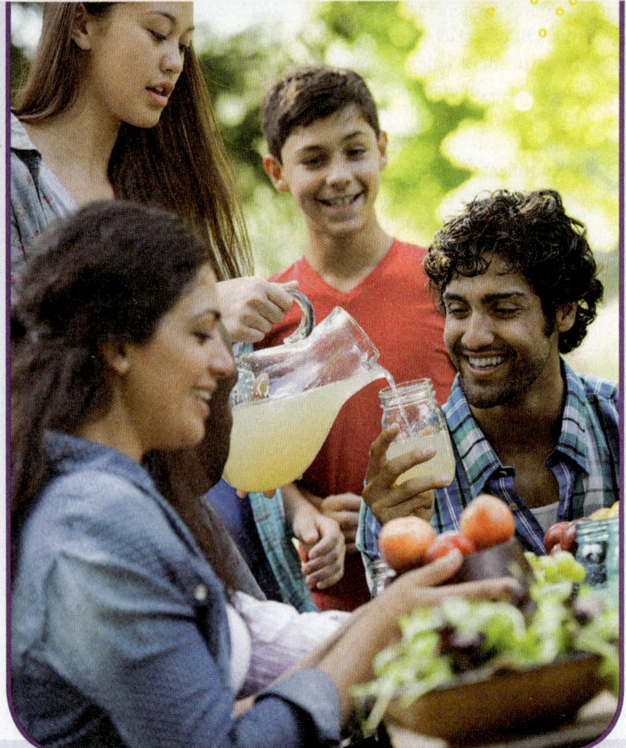
Mint Images Limited/Alamy

## CHAPTER OBJECTIVES

- Understand how alcoholic beverages work in your body
- Describe the immediate and long-term health effects of drinking alcohol
- Understand what constitutes excessive use of alcohol
- Evaluate the role of alcohol in your life, and list strategies for using it responsibly

CHAPTER 9

# Alcohol and Nicotine

Despite numerous prohibitions against it throughout history, alcohol has remained the most popular psychoactive drug in the Western world. Alcohol plays contradictory roles in human behavior. Used in moderation, alcohol can enhance social occasions by loosening inhibitions and creating pleasant feelings of relaxation. But alcohol can also be harmful. Like other drugs, alcohol produces physiological effects that can impair functioning in the short term and cause devastating damage in the long term.

Cigarette smoking is still the leading cause of preventable disease, disability, and death in the United States. Despite a significant drop in numbers of smokers since the 1960s, a sizeable 57 million adults in the United States still use nicotine products. And now the increasing availability and use of products such as electronic cigarettes have become an insidious inducement for young people. For many people, nicotine and alcohol become addictive, leading to a lifetime of recovery or to debilitation and death.

> **TERMS**
> **alcohol** The intoxicating ingredient in fermented or distilled beverages; a colorless, pungent liquid.

## ALCOHOL AND THE BODY

You have probably noticed that alcohol affects people in different ways. One person may seem to become intoxicated after just a drink or two, while another appears to tolerate a great deal of alcohol without apparent effect. These differences make alcohol's effects on the body seem mysterious and account for many misconceptions about alcohol use.

### Common Alcoholic Beverages

Technically speaking, there are many kinds of **alcohols,** which are organic compounds. In this book, however, the term *alcohol* refers only to ethyl alcohol (or ethanol). Several kinds of alcohol chemically resemble ethyl alcohol, such as

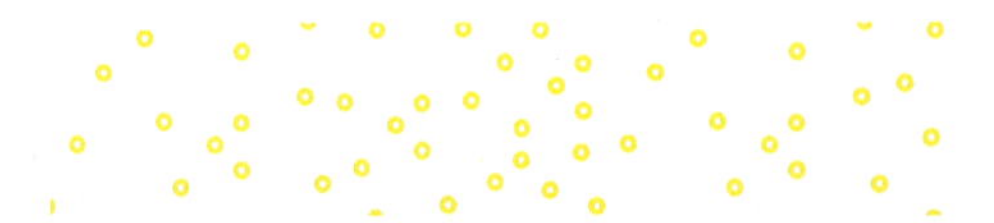

methanol (wood alcohol) and isopropyl alcohol (rubbing alcohol), but these are highly toxic; if consumed, they can cause serious illness, blindness, and death.

There are several basic types of alcoholic beverages. Ethanol is the psychoactive ingredient in each of them:

- Beer is a mild intoxicant brewed from a mixture of grains. By volume, beer usually contains 3–6% alcohol.

- Ales and malt liquors, which also have grain bases and are similar to beer in their processing, typically contain 6–8% alcohol by volume.

- Wines are made by fermenting the juices of grapes or other fruits. During *fermentation*, sugars from the fruit react with yeast to create ethanol and other by-products. In table wines, the concentration of alcohol is about 9–14%. A more potent type of wine, *fortified wine*, is called this because extra alcohol is added during its production. Fortified wines—such as sherry, port, and Madeira—contain about 20% alcohol.

- Hard liquor—such as gin, whiskey, rum, tequila, vodka, and liqueur—is made by *distilling* brewed or fermented grains or other plant products. Hard liquors usually contain 35–50% alcohol but can be much stronger.

The concentration of alcohol in a beverage is indicated by its **proof value,** which amounts to two times the percentage concentration. For example, if a beverage is 100 proof, it contains 50% alcohol by volume. Two ounces of 100-proof whiskey contain 1 ounce of pure alcohol. The proof value of hard liquor can usually be found on the bottle's label.

**"Standard Drinks" versus Actual Servings** When discussing alcohol consumption, the term **one drink** (or *a standard drink*) refers to the amount of a beverage that typically contains about 0.6 ounces or 14 grams of alcohol. A typical serving of most alcoholic beverages is larger (sometimes significantly larger) than a single standard drink. This is particularly true of mixed drinks, which often include more than one type of hard liquor.

**Caloric Content** Alcohol provides 7 calories per gram, and the alcohol in one drink (14–17 grams) supplies about 100–120 calories. Most alcoholic beverages also contain some carbohydrate; for example, one beer provides about 150 total calories. The "light" in light beer refers to calories; a light beer typically has close to the same alcohol content as a regular beer and about 100 calories. A 5-ounce glass of red wine has 100 calories; white wine has 96. A 3-ounce margarita supplies 157 calories, a 6-ounce cosmopolitan has 143 calories, and a 6-ounce rum and Coke contains about 180 calories.

## Absorption

The rate at which your body absorbs alcohol will affect how quickly you feel drunk or how quickly your behavior is impaired. In fact, the speed at which your blood alcohol concentration rises has been linked to the degree of impairment, more than the concentration itself. Several factors determine the rate of absorption: how fast you drink, how fast your stomach empties its contents, and how much and what type of food and other drugs are in your system. Food in the stomach slows the rate of absorption.

The kind of alcohol (volume, concentration, and nature) also affects absorption. For example, the carbonation in a beverage like champagne increases the rate of alcohol absorption, as do artificial sweeteners (commonly used in drink mixers). You may be surprised to know that drinking highly concentrated alcoholic beverages such as hard liquor slows absorption. Biological sex, race, and ethnicity also affect the rate of absorption.

How does alcohol get into the bloodstream? When a person drinks alcohol, a small amount is absorbed by the oral mucosa (the lining of the mouth). About 20% is absorbed in the stomach, and about 75% is absorbed through the upper part of the small intestine. Any remaining alcohol enters the bloodstream farther along the gastrointestinal (GI) tract. Once in the bloodstream, alcohol produces sensations of intoxication.

## Metabolism and Excretion

Once alcohol has been absorbed, it is metabolized, meaning that the body transforms it into usable substances and waste. The usable parts are transformed into energy and fat reserves in the following way.

The circulatory system quickly transports alcohol throughout the body. Because alcohol easily moves through most biological membranes, it is rapidly distributed throughout most body tissues. Although a small amount of alcohol is metabolized in the stomach, most is metabolized in the liver. There, several enzymes convert the alcohol to acetaldehyde, then to acetate. Individuals vary slightly in the enzymes they have, and thus they may react differently to alcohol. (See the box "Metabolizing Alcohol: Our Bodies Work Differently.")

About 2–10% of ingested alcohol is not metabolized in the liver or other tissues but is excreted unchanged by the lungs, kidneys, and sweat glands. Excreted alcohol causes the telltale smell on a drinker's breath and is the basis of breath and urine analyses for alcohol levels.

When alcohol enters the human brain, it affects neurotransmitters—the chemicals that carry messages between brain cells. These changes are temporary, creating many of the immediate effects of drinking alcohol. With chronic heavy use, however, alcohol's disruptive effects can become permanent, resulting in loss of brain function and changes in

**TERMS**

**proof value** Two times the percentage of alcohol, by volume, in an alcoholic beverage; a "100-proof" beverage is 50% alcohol by volume.

**one drink** The amount of a beverage that typically contains about 0.6 ounces of alcohol; also called a *standard drink*.

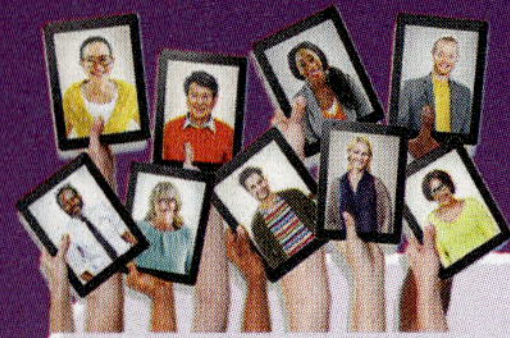

## DIVERSITY MATTERS
### Metabolizing Alcohol: Our Bodies Work Differently

Do you and your friends react differently to alcohol? If so, your reactions may be affected by genetic differences in alcohol metabolism. **Metabolism** refers to the chemical transformation of alcohol and other substances in your body into energy and waste. Alcohol is metabolized mainly in the liver, where an enzyme, alcohol dehydrogenase, converts the alcohol into a toxic substance called acetaldehyde. Acetaldehyde causes many of alcohol's noxious effects. Ideally it is quickly broken down to a less active by-product, acetate, by another enzyme, acetaldehyde dehydrogenase (ALDH). Acetate can then separate into water and carbon dioxide and easily be eliminated. But people vary in the length of time it takes to break down the toxins in alcohol and in how efficiently they can process them. Some differences in metabolism are associated with ethnicity and biological sex.

Some people, primarily those of Asian descent, inherit ineffective or inactive variations of that latter enzyme, acetaldehyde dehydrogenase. Others, including some people of African and Jewish descent, have forms of alcohol dehydrogenase that metabolize alcohol to acetaldehyde very quickly. Either way, toxic acetaldehyde builds up when these people drink alcohol. They experience a reaction called *flushing syndrome*. Their skin feels hot, their heart and respiration rates increase, and they may get a headache, vomit, or break out in hives. The severity of their reactions is affected by the inherited form of their alcohol-metabolizing enzymes. These adverse reactions to drinking makes some people so uncomfortable that they are unlikely to develop alcohol use disorder.

The body's response to acetaldehyde is the basis for treating alcohol misuse with the drug disulfiram (Antabuse), which inhibits the action of acetaldehyde dehydrogenase. When a person taking disulfiram ingests alcohol, acetaldehyde levels increase rapidly, and they develop an intense flushing reaction along with weakness, nausea, vomiting, and other disagreeable symptoms.

How people behave in relation to alcohol is influenced in complex ways by a wide range of factors, including liver size, body mass, and social and cultural influences. But individual choices and behavior are also strongly influenced by specific genetic characteristics.

brain structure. Alcohol interferes with the production of new brain cells (neurogenesis) in unborn children, young children, adolescents, and young adults, whose brains continue to develop until about age 21. Alcohol may also negatively affect neurogenesis in mature adults.

## Alcohol Intake and Blood Alcohol Concentration

**Blood alcohol concentration (BAC)** is the ratio of alcohol in a person's blood by weight, expressed as the percentage of alcohol measured in a deciliter of blood. BAC is affected by the amount of alcohol consumed in a given amount of time and by these individual factors:

- ***Body weight.*** In most cases, a smaller person develops a higher BAC than a larger person after drinking the same amount of alcohol (Figure 9.1). A smaller person has less overall body tissue into which alcohol can be distributed.

> **TERMS**
>
> **metabolism** The chemical transformation of food and other substances in the body into energy and wastes, first through breaking apart the components and then using them in other forms.
>
> **blood alcohol concentration (BAC)** The amount of alcohol in the blood expressed as the percentage of alcohol in a deciliter of blood; used as a measure of intoxication.

- ***Percentage of body fat.*** A person with a higher percentage of body fat will usually develop a higher BAC than a more muscular person of the same weight when they drink the same amount. Alcohol does not concentrate as much in fatty tissue as in muscle and most other tissues, in part because fat has fewer blood vessels.

- ***Sex.*** Women metabolize less alcohol in the stomach than men do because the stomach enzyme that breaks down alcohol before it enters the bloodstream is four times more active in men than in women. Hormonal fluctuations may also affect the rate of alcohol metabolism, making a woman more susceptible to high BACs at certain times during her menstrual cycle.

BAC also depends on the balance between the rate of alcohol absorption and the rate of alcohol metabolism. A man who weighs 150 pounds and has normal liver function metabolizes about 0.3 ounces of alcohol per hour, the equivalent of about half a 12-ounce bottle of beer or half a 5-ounce glass of wine.

The rate of alcohol metabolism varies among people and is determined largely by genetic factors and drinking behavior. Chronic drinking activates enzymes that metabolize alcohol in the liver, so people who drink frequently metabolize alcohol at a more rapid rate than nondrinkers. Other than that, nothing will sober you up faster than the time it takes for your sweat, urine, breath, and the enzyme alcohol dehydrogenase to eliminate the alcohol from your body. Although the rate of alcohol absorption can be slowed by factors like food,

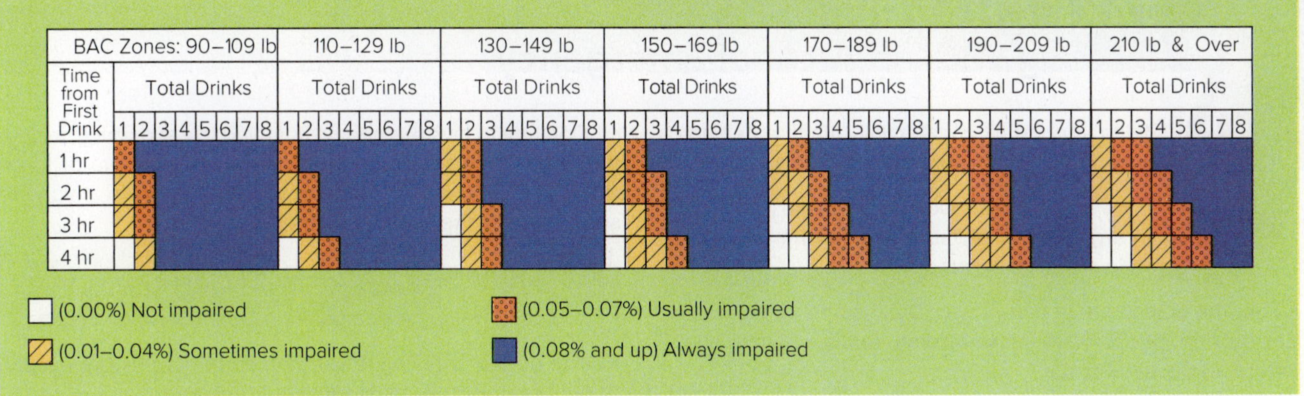


**FIGURE 9.1 Approximate blood alcohol concentration (BAC) and body weight.** This chart illustrates the BAC an average person of a given weight would reach after drinking the specified number of drinks in the time shown. The federal legal limit for BAC for drivers is 0.08%; for drivers under 21 years of age, many states have zero-tolerance laws that set BAC limits of 0.01% or 0.02%.

the metabolic rate *cannot* be influenced by exercise, breathing deeply, eating, drinking coffee, or taking other drugs. Whether a person is asleep or awake, the rate of alcohol metabolism is the same.

If a person absorbs slightly less alcohol each hour than can be metabolized in an hour, their BAC remains low. People can drink large amounts of alcohol this way over a long period of time without becoming noticeably intoxicated; however, they still run the risk of long-term health problems (described later in the chapter). If people drink more alcohol than they can metabolize (for example, two drinks within 30 minutes), the BAC will increase steadily, and they will become more and more intoxicated (see Figure 9.2).

**QUICK STATS**

**In the United States, the number of deaths related to alcohol spiked at 99,000 in 2020.**

—National Institutes of Health, 2022

## ALCOHOL'S IMMEDIATE AND LONG-TERM EFFECTS

The effects of alcohol consumption on health depend on the person, the circumstances, and the amount of alcohol consumed.

### Immediate Effects

The amount of alcohol in the blood is a primary factor determining the effects of alcohol. At low concentrations, alcohol tends to make people feel relaxed and jovial, but at higher concentrations, people are more likely to feel angry, sedated, or sleepy. In general, alcohol slows reactions, impairs coordination and judgment,

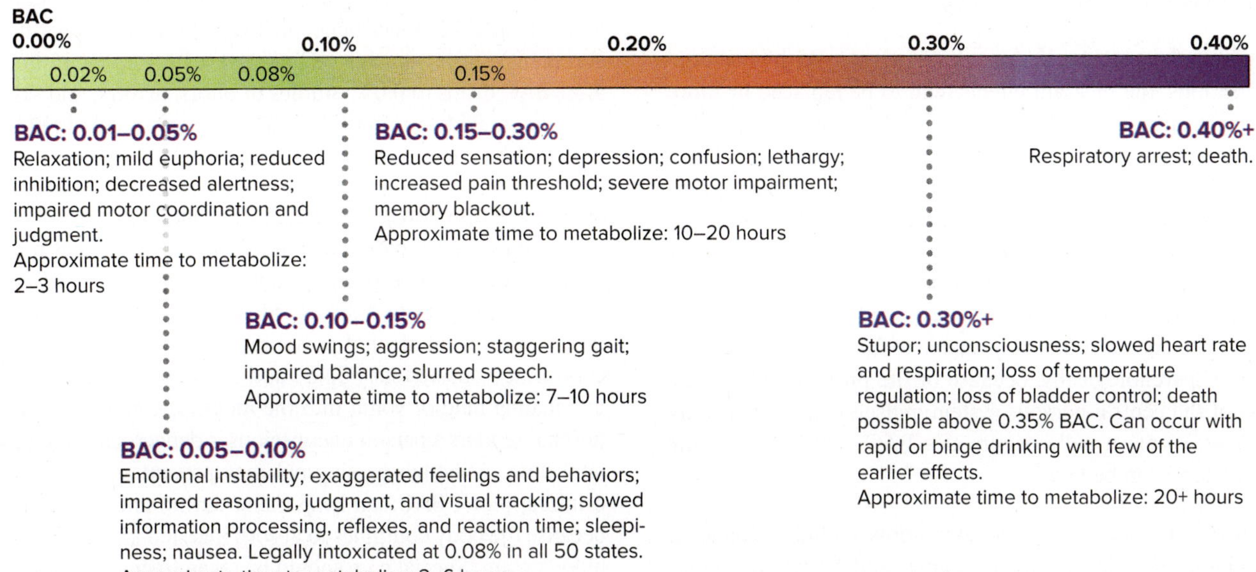


**FIGURE 9.2 Effects of blood alcohol concentration (BAC) at each stage of intoxication.**

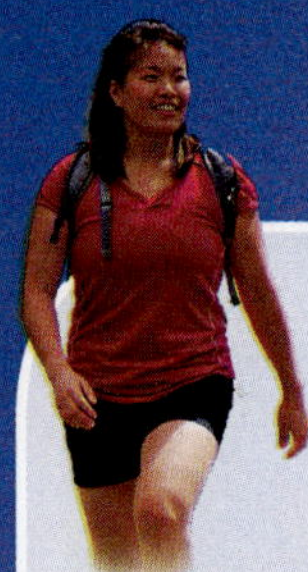

## TAKE CHARGE
### Dealing with an Alcohol Emergency

Being very drunk is potentially life-threatening. Helping a drunken friend could save a life.

- Be firm but calm. Don't engage the person in an argument or discuss her drinking behavior while she is intoxicated.
- Get the person out of harm's way. Don't let her drive, wander outside, or drink any more alcohol. Reduce stimuli and create a safe, quiet place.
- If possible without distressing the person, try to find out what and how much she drank, and when as well as what other drugs or medications she took, how much, and when.
- If the person is unconscious, don't assume she is just "sleeping it off." Place her on her side with her knees up. This position helps prevent choking if she vomits.
- Monitor airway, breathing, and circulation (check pulse).
- Stay with the person. You need to be ready to help if she vomits or stops breathing.
- Don't try to give the person anything to eat or drink, including coffee or other drugs. Don't give cold showers or try to make her walk around. None of these things help anyone to sober up, and they can be dangerous.

Call 911 immediately in any of the following instances:

- You can't wake the person even by shouting or shaking.
- The person is taking fewer than eight breaths per minute, or her breathing seems shallow or irregular.
- You think the person took other drugs with alcohol.
- The person has had an injury, especially a blow to the head.
- The person drank a large amount of alcohol in a short period of time and then became unconscious. Death caused by alcohol poisoning most often occurs when the blood alcohol level rises very quickly due to rapid ingestion of alcohol.

If you aren't sure what to do, call 911. You may save a life.

and eventually, sedates to inactivity. The senses become less acute.

**Low Concentrations of Alcohol** The effects of alcohol can first be felt at a BAC of 0.02–0.05%. These effects may include lightheadedness, relaxation, and a release of inhibitions. Most drinkers experience mild euphoria and become more sociable. When people drink in social settings, alcohol often seems to act as a stimulant, enhancing friendliness or confidence. This apparent stimulation occurs because alcohol depresses inhibitory centers in the brain.

**Higher Concentrations of Alcohol** At higher concentrations, the pleasant effects tend to be replaced by more negative ones: interference with motor coordination, verbal performance, and intellectual functions. Someone with a high blood alcohol concentration may have trouble regulating their emotions and may experience irritability or sadness.

When the BAC reaches 0.1%, most sensory and motor functioning is reduced, and many people become sleepy. Vision, smell, taste, and hearing become less acute. At 0.2%, most drinkers are completely unable to function, either physically or psychologically, because of the pronounced depression of the central nervous system, muscles, and other body systems. Coma usually occurs at a BAC of 0.35%, and any higher level can be fatal.

**Alcohol Hangover** The symptoms include headache, shakiness, nausea, diarrhea, fatigue, and impaired mental functioning. A hangover is probably caused by a combination of the toxic products of alcohol breakdown, dehydration, and hormonal effects. During a hangover, heart rate and blood pressure increase, making some individuals more vulnerable to heart attacks. Electroencephalography (brain wave measurement) shows slowing of brain waves for up to 16 hours after BAC drops to 0.0%. Studies of pilots, drivers, and skiers all indicate that coordination and cognition are impaired in a person with a hangover, increasing the risk of injury.

### Ask Yourself ?

**QUESTIONS FOR CRITICAL THINKING AND REFLECTION**

Have you ever had a hangover or watched someone else suffer through one? Did the experience affect your attitude about drinking? In what way?

**Alcohol Poisoning** Drinking large amounts of alcohol in a short time can rapidly raise the BAC into the lethal range. Alcohol, either alone or in combination with other drugs, is responsible for more toxic overdose deaths than any other drug. Death from alcohol poisoning may be caused either by central nervous system (CNS) and respiratory depression or by inhaling fluid or vomit into the lungs. The amount of alcohol that renders a person unconscious is dangerously close to a fatal dose. Although passing out may prevent someone from drinking more, BAC can keep rising during unconsciousness because the body continues to absorb ingested alcohol into the bloodstream. Special care should be taken to ensure the safety of anyone who has been drinking heavily, especially if they pass out (see the box "Dealing with an Alcohol Emergency").

**Using Alcohol with Other Drugs** Alcohol-drug combinations are a leading cause of drug-related deaths. Using alcohol while taking a medication that depresses the CNS increases the effects of both drugs, potentially leading to coma, respiratory depression, and death. Such drugs include barbiturates, Valium-like drugs, narcotics such as codeine, and over-the-counter antihistamines such as Benadryl. For people who consume three or more drinks per day, use of over-the-counter pain relievers like aspirin, ibuprofen, or acetaminophen increases the risk of stomach bleeding and liver damage. Some antacids, antibiotics, and diabetes medications can also interact dangerously with alcohol.

Many illegal drugs are especially dangerous when combined with alcohol. Life-threatening overdoses occur at much lower doses when heroin and other narcotics are combined with alcohol. When cocaine and alcohol are used together, they form a toxic substance in the liver called cocaethylene, which can produce effects that neither drug alone does. A trend among young drinkers involves mixing alcoholic beverages with caffeinated ones, especially highly caffeinated energy drinks (see the box "Alcoholic Energy Drinks").

**QUICK STATS**

**Despite a 13% decrease in travel in 2020 as compared to 2019, fatal alcohol-related crashes rose 9%.**

—National Highway Traffic Safety Administration, 2021

**Alcohol-Related Injuries and Violence** The combination of impaired judgment, weakened sensory perception, reduced inhibitions, impaired motor coordination, and increased aggressiveness and hostility that characterizes alcohol intoxication can be dangerous and deadly. Through homicide, suicide, automobile crashes, and other traumatic incidents, alcohol use is linked to about 99,000 deaths each year in the United States. Acute alcohol use is associated with an increased risk of suicide attempt. Among successful suicides, alcohol use is common as well; an analysis of studies involving over 420,000 participants reveals that alcohol use disorder is an important risk factor of suicide. Alcohol use more than triples the risk of fatal injuries during leisure activities such as swimming and boating. About 50% of fatal drownings, 40% of fatal burn injuries, and 65% percent of fatal falls happen to people who have been drinking.

**Alcohol and Aggression** Many arrests happen for drug- and alcohol-related offenses (domestic violence, driving under the influence of alcohol, public drunkenness, and property and drug offenses). Alcohol use is associated with 40% of all murders, assaults, and rapes. Alcohol impairment can also make people vulnerable to violent crimes and is frequently found in the bloodstream of victims as well as perpetrators. Some people may become violent under alcohol's influence.

The effects of alcohol can present an increased risk for people predisposed to aggressive or impulsive behavior. In many cases, people with alcohol use disorder may have an underlying psychiatric condition.

Alcohol misuse can contribute to problems with people outside and inside the home. Marital discord and domestic violence often exist in the presence of excessive alcohol consumption. Heavy drinking by parents is associated with abuse of their children, typically emotional or psychological abuse.

**Alcohol and Sexual Decision Making** Alcohol seriously impairs a person's ability to make safe decisions about sex. A recent survey of college students revealed that frequent binge drinkers were five times more likely to engage in unplanned sexual activity and five-and-a-half times more likely to have unprotected sex than non-binge drinkers. **Binge drinking** is a pattern of rapid, periodic drinking that brings a person's blood alcohol concentration up to 0.08% or higher, typically with five or more drinks for men, or four drinks for women, typically within about two hours. The difference between *bingeing* and *heavy drinking* is that heavy drinking involves bingeing on five or more days in the past month, according to the Substance Abuse and Mental Health Services Administration (SAMHSA).

Heavy drinkers are also more likely to have multiple sex partners and to engage in other forms of high-risk sexual behavior. Rates of sexually transmitted infections (including HIV) and unwanted pregnancy are higher among people who drink heavily than among people who drink moderately or not at all.

## Drinking and Driving

Drunk driving remains a serious problem in the United States, and it has increased since the start of the Covid-19 pandemic. In 2019, 10,142 Americans were killed in accidents involving alcohol-impaired drivers—close to one-third of all traffic fatalities for the year. Men are more likely than women to be driving drunk in fatal crashes. The National Highway Transportation Safety Administration reports that in 2019, for every fatal crash with an alcohol-impaired female driver, there were four with a male driver. Of all drivers involved in fatal crashes, those aged 21–24 had the highest percentage of BACs of 0.08% or higher.

People who drink are unable to drive safely because their judgment is impaired, their reaction time is slower, and their coordination is reduced. Some driving skills are affected at BACs of 0.02% and lower. At a BAC of 0.05%, visual perception, reaction time, and certain steering tasks are impaired. Any amount of alcohol impairs your ability to drive safely, and fatigue augments the effects of alcohol.

Can we predict which behaviors or traits factor into young adults' driving under the influence (DUI) of alcohol?

**TERMS**

**binge drinking** Periodically drinking alcohol to the point of severe intoxication: about four drinks (for women) and five drinks (for men) consumed within a period of about two hours.

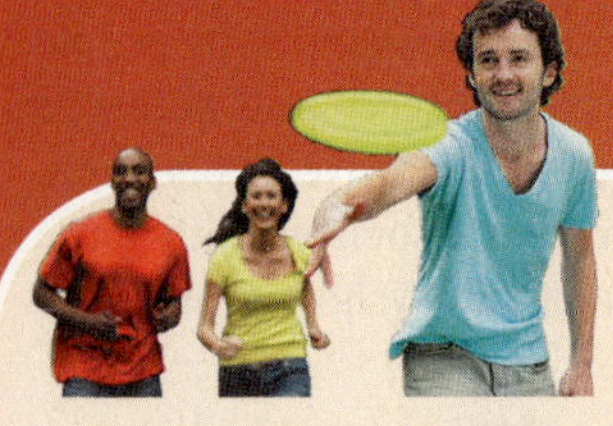

## WELLNESS ON CAMPUS
### Alcoholic Energy Drinks

A popular trend is to mix alcohol with energy drinks or other caffeinated beverages. In 2020, about one-fifth of college and noncollege groups consumed these mixed drinks—among others, espresso martinis, rum and coke, vodka Red Bull®, and Jägerbombs. This practice is dangerous for many reasons.

For one, combining energy drinks with alcohol increases alcohol absorption, but caffeine does not speed alcohol metabolism. This means that people who consume more caffeine–alcohol drinks reach higher BAC levels, consume more drinks, and spend more time drinking than those who consume alcohol by itself. There is also a greater correlation with alcohol dependence when people consume caffeine with alcohol than when they consume alcohol alone.

Another striking problem with these mixed drinks is that consumers *perceive* themselves to be more alert than they actually are. They expect the caffeine (sometimes five times greater than in a cup of coffee) to counteract the sedative effects of the alcohol, leading some drinkers to take risks they might not take with alcohol alone, such as driving a car. Along with impaired decision making, there is an increased risk for injury and aggression.

The myth that caffeine–alcohol drinks keep the drinker alert played a big role in a 2018 study about expectations. Some participants were led to believe that caffeine would offset negative effects of the alcohol. These participants showed more impairment in completing tasks than did the participants who did not expect the caffeine to help them remain sharp.

Some gender differences, however, emerged in a 2019 study on a predominantly female student sample: Up to a 0.13% blood alcohol level, the women overestimated the amount of alcohol in their blood as they drank more caffeine. In other words, caffeine did not increase their alertness, but instead their feelings of intoxication. Whatever the disparity between perception and actual levels of intoxication, making decisions after consuming any alcoholic beverages is often dangerous.

A growing body of evidence highlights the risks associated with energy drinks. These include risk-seeking behavior, such as substance abuse and aggression, mental health problems such as anxiety and stress, and physical problems such as increased blood pressure, obesity, kidney damage, fatigue, and stomachaches. According to SAMHSA, 1 in 10 emergency department visits of patients aged 12 and over in 2011 was related to highly caffeinated drinks. Nearly half the emergencies resulted from mixing the beverages with alcohol or other drugs.

In 2010, the FDA reported that premixed, commercial, caffeinated alcoholic beverages (CABs) are a public health concern and that adding caffeine to malt alcoholic beverages amounts to using an "unsafe food additive" that violates the Federal Food, Drug, and Cosmetic Act. Effectively, the FDA banned the sale of premixed drinks. Still, a general lack of regulation of energy drinks has led to vigorous marketing campaigns by CAB manufacturers, making unsubstantiated claims about the performance-enhancing properties of their product. It is important that each of us personally investigates what we are consuming.

SOURCES: Al-Shaar, L., et al. 2017. Health effects and public health concerns of energy drink consumption in the United States: A mini-review. *Frontiers in Public Health* 5 (https://doi.org/10.3389/fpubh.2017.00225); Marczinski, C. A., et al. 2018. Alcohol-induced impairment of balance is antagonized by energy drinks. *Alcoholism: Clinical and Experimental Research* 42(1): 144–152; Norberg, M. M., et al. 2019. Why are caffeinated alcoholic beverages especially risky? *Addictive Behaviors* 98 10.1016/j.addbeh.2019.106062; Schulenberg, J., et al. 2021. *Monitoring the Future National Survey Results on Drug Use, 1975-2020: Volume II, College Students and Adults Ages 19-60*. Ann Arbor: Institute for Social Research, The University of Michigan (http://www.monitoringthefuture.org/pubs.html); Substance Abuse and Mental Health Services Administration. 2014. *The DAWN Report: 1 in 10 Energy Drink-Related Emergency Department Visits Results in Hospitalization*. Rockville, MD: Substance Abuse and Mental Health Services Administration (http://www.samhsa.gov/data/sites/default/files /spot124-energy-drinks-2014.pdf).

Impulsivity—the tendency to act without thinking—is a predictor of DUI. However, the specific facets of impulsivity that predict DUI and how they vary with gender differences remain unclear. Men appear to exhibit higher sensation seeking and alcohol use than women. Women exhibit greater perception of risk and greater perseverance (staying focused on long, complex tasks). Men report more DUIs and have more of them, but the gender gap in both the prevalence of DUI arrests and fatalities is narrowing. Prevention strategies should be tailored to both biological sexes and all gender identities, and further studies are needed to characterize risk behaviors in women.

The *dose-response function* is the relationship between the amount of alcohol or drug consumed and the type and intensity of the resulting effect. Higher doses of alcohol are associated with a much greater probability of automobile crashes (Figure 9.3). A person driving with a BAC of 0.14% is over 40 times more likely to be involved in a crash than someone with no alcohol in their blood.

In addition to increasing the risk of injury and death, driving while intoxicated can have serious legal consequences. Drunk driving is against the law. The legal limit for BAC is 0.08% in the United States, but alcohol impairs the user even

**Ask Yourself**

**QUESTIONS FOR CRITICAL THINKING AND REFLECTION**

Have you ever witnessed or been involved in an alcohol emergency? Did you think the situation was urgent at the time? What were the circumstances surrounding the event? How did the people involved deal with it?

Blood alcohol concentration (%)
0.00
0.04
0.08
0.12
0.16
0.20
45
40
35
30
25
20
15
10
5
0
Relative probability of an automobile crash
0
1
2
3
4
5
6
Estimated number of drinks

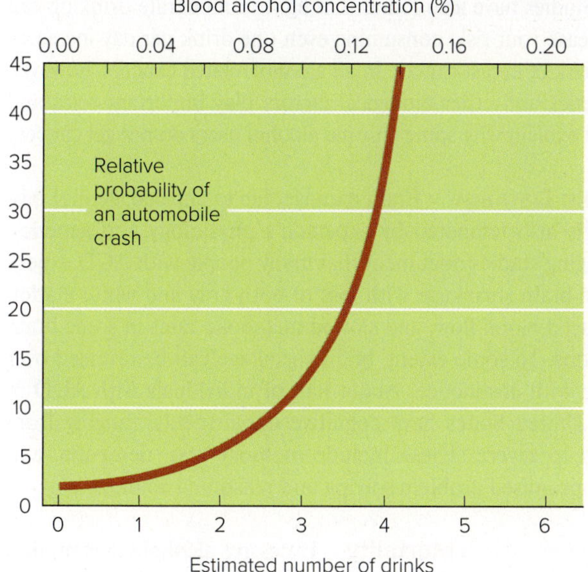

**FIGURE 9.3 The dose-response relationship between BAC and automobile crashes.**

at much lower BACs. Stiff penalties for drunk driving include fines, loss of license, confiscation of vehicle, and jail time. Under current zero-tolerance laws in many states, drivers under age 21 who have consumed *any* alcohol may have their licenses suspended. If you are out of your home and drinking, find alternative transportation, or appoint a *designated driver* who doesn't drink and can provide safe transportation home.

It's more difficult to protect yourself against someone else who drinks and drives. Learn to be alert to the erratic driving that signals an impaired driver. Warning signs include wide, abrupt, and illegal turns; straddling the lane marker; driving against traffic; driving on the shoulder; weaving, swerving, or nearly striking objects or other vehicles; following too closely; erratic speed; driving with headlights off at night; and driving with windows down in very cold weather. If you see any of these signs in another driver, avoid that vehicle by pulling off the road or turning at the nearest intersection. Report the driver to the police.

## Long-Term Effects of Chronic Misuse

Because alcohol is distributed throughout most of the body, it affects many organs and tissues (Figure 9.4).

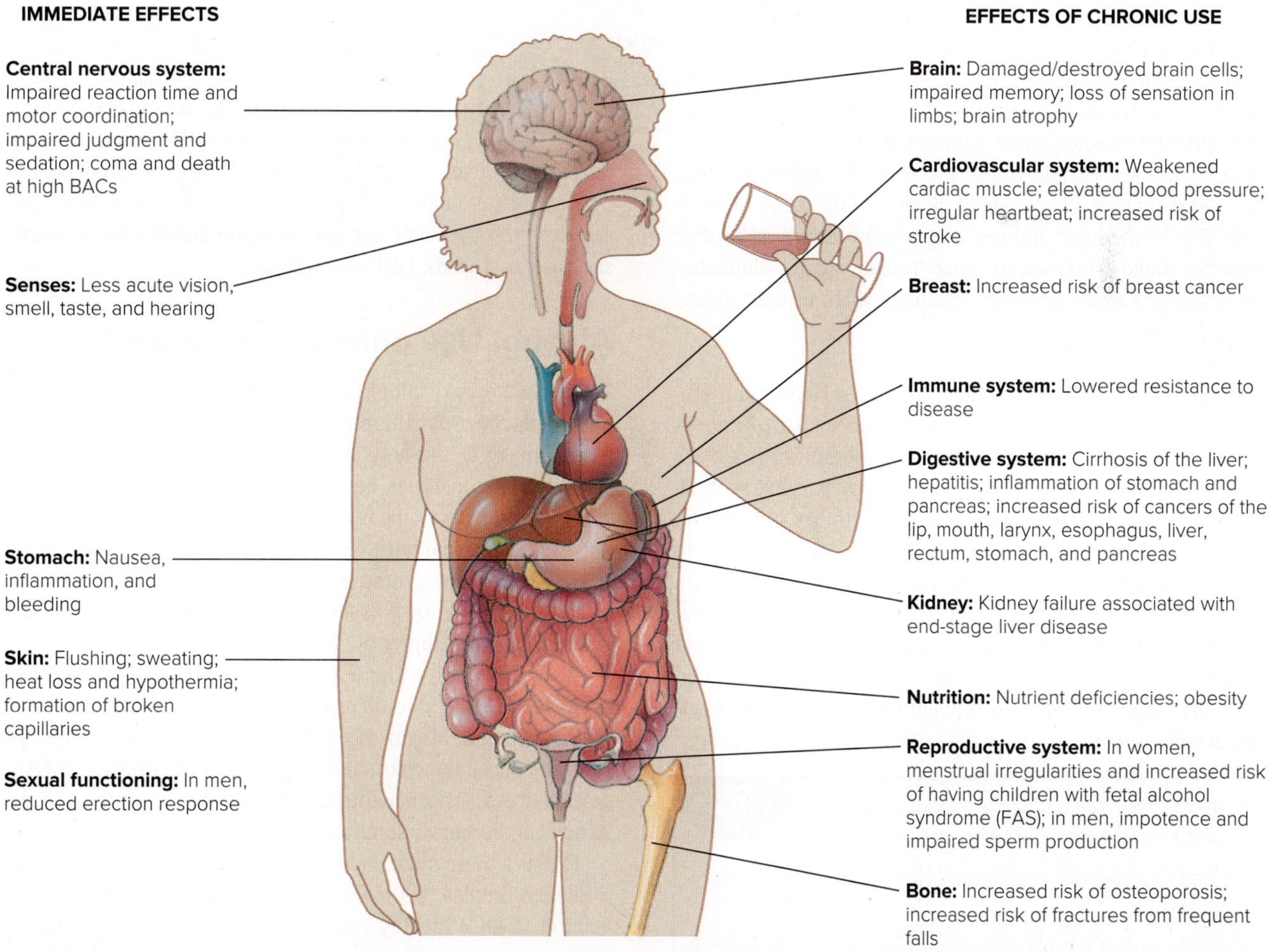

IMMEDIATE EFFECTS
Central nervous system: Impaired reaction time and motor coordination; impaired judgment and sedation; coma and death at high BACs
Senses: Less acute vision, smell, taste, and hearing
Stomach: Nausea, inflammation, and bleeding
Skin: Flushing; sweating; heat loss and hypothermia; formation of broken capillaries
Sexual functioning: In men, reduced erection response
EFFECTS OF CHRONIC USE
Brain: Damaged/destroyed brain cells; impaired memory; loss of sensation in limbs; brain atrophy
Cardiovascular system: Weakened cardiac muscle; elevated blood pressure; irregular heartbeat; increased risk of stroke
Breast: Increased risk of breast cancer
Immune system: Lowered resistance to disease
Digestive system: Cirrhosis of the liver; hepatitis; inflammation of stomach and pancreas; increased risk of cancers of the lip, mouth, larynx, esophagus, liver, rectum, stomach, and pancreas
Kidney: Kidney failure associated with end-stage liver disease
Nutrition: Nutrient deficiencies; obesity
Reproductive system: In women, menstrual irregularities and increased risk of having children with fetal alcohol syndrome (FAS); in men, impotence and impaired sperm production
Bone: Increased risk of osteoporosis; increased risk of fractures from frequent falls

**FIGURE 9.4 The immediate and long-term effects of alcohol misuse.**

**The Digestive System** Even in the short term, alcohol can alter the functioning of the liver, which is essential for digesting and absorbing fat. Within just a few days of heavy alcohol consumption, fat begins to accumulate in liver cells, resulting in the development of "fatty liver." If drinking continues, inflammation of the liver can occur, resulting in alcohol-associated hepatitis, a frequent cause of hospitalization and death among people with alcohol use disorder (AUD). Both fatty liver and alcohol-associated hepatitis are potentially reversible if the person stops drinking. With continued alcohol use, however, liver cells are replaced by fibrous scar tissue, a condition known as **cirrhosis.** As cirrhosis develops, a drinker may gradually lose their capacity to tolerate alcohol because fewer and fewer healthy cells remain in the liver to metabolize it.

Alcohol can inflame the pancreas, causing nausea, vomiting, abnormal digestion, and severe pain. Acute alcohol-associated pancreatitis generally occurs in binge drinkers. Unlike cirrhosis, which usually occurs after years of heavy alcohol use, pancreatitis can occur after one or two severe binge-drinking episodes. Acute pancreatitis is sometimes fatal; in survivors it can become a chronic condition.

**The Cardiovascular System** The effects of alcohol on the cardiovascular system depend on the amount of alcohol consumed. Higher doses of alcohol harm the cardiovascular system. In some people, more than two drinks a day will elevate blood pressure, making stroke and heart attack more likely. Some people with AUD show a weakening of the heart muscle, a condition known as **cardiac myopathy.** Binge drinking can cause "holiday heart," characterized by serious abnormal heart rhythms, which usually appear within 24 hours of a binge episode.

**Cancer** In 2000, the U.S. Department of Health and Human Services added alcoholic beverages to its list of known human carcinogens. Chronic alcohol consumption is a clear risk factor for cancers of the mouth, throat, larynx, esophagus, and breast (cancers also associated with use of tobacco, with which alcohol frequently acts as a cocarcinogen). Five or six daily drinks, especially combined with smoking, increases the risk of these cancers by a factor of 50 or more. Heavy drinking also puts users at risk for colorectal cancer and the most common form of liver cancer; and continued heavy drinking in people with hepatitis accelerates progression of this cancer.

Studies have also found that light to moderate drinking can increase your risk: consuming even one drink per day increases the risk of breast cancer. In all alcohol-related cancers, however, genetics and other biological factors play important roles and help explain why some chronic alcohol users do not get cancer.

**Brain Damage** Brain damage due to chronic alcohol misuse is also tempered by a person's physiology and genetics. Imaging studies document that many people with AUD experience brain shrinkage with loss of both gray and white matter, reduced blood flow, and slowed metabolic rates in some brain regions. To some extent, brain shrinkage can be reversed over time with abstinence. About half of individuals with AUD in the United States have cognitive impairments, ranging from mild to severe. These include memory loss, dementia, and compromised problem-solving and reasoning abilities.

**QUICK STATS**

**About 11% of pregnant women drink alcohol, and 3% engage in binge drinking.**

—Centers for Disease Control and Prevention, 2020

**Mortality** Excessive alcohol consumption is a factor in several leading causes of death for Americans. Average life expectancy is about 15 years less among people with alcohol use disorder than among people who do not have the disorder. Early in the coronavirus (Covid-19) pandemic, the World Health Organization put out the statement that alcohol consumption is associated with a range of diseases and mental health disorders that can compromise the body's immune system. Therefore, people should minimize their alcohol consumption at any time, and particularly during the Covid-19 pandemic. About half the deaths caused by alcohol are due to chronic conditions such as cirrhosis and cancer; the other half are due to acute conditions or events such as car crashes, falls, and suicide.

## Alcohol Use during Pregnancy

During pregnancy, alcohol and its metabolic product acetaldehyde easily cross the placenta, harming the developing fetus. Damage to the fetus depends on the amount of alcohol the mother consumes and the stage of fetal development. Early in pregnancy, heavy drinking can cause spontaneous abortion or miscarriage. Alcohol in early pregnancy, during critical fetal development periods, can also cause a collection of birth defects known as *fetal alcohol syndrome (FAS)*, which is discussed in Chapter 6.

Because rapid brain development continues throughout pregnancy, the fetal brain stays vulnerable to alcohol use until birth. Although effects of drinking later in pregnancy do not typically cause the characteristic physical deformities of FAS, getting drunk just once during the final three months of pregnancy can damage a fetal brain.

FAS is a permanent, incurable condition that causes lifelong disability. Studies by the Centers for Disease Control and Prevention (CDC) identify the number of FAS cases as ranging from two to nine infants for every 10,000 live births in the United States. About three times as many babies are born with **alcohol-related neurodevelopmental disorder (ARND).** Children with

**TERMS**

**cirrhosis** A disease in which the liver is severely damaged by alcohol, other toxins, or infection.

**cardiac myopathy** Weakening of the heart muscle through disease.

**alcohol-related neurodevelopmental disorder (ARND)** Cognitive and behavioral problems seen in people whose mothers drank alcohol during pregnancy.

ARND appear physically normal but often have significant learning and behavioral disorders. As adults, they are more likely to develop substance use disorders and to have criminal records. ARND must be treated as early as possible to avoid long-term physiological as well as social consequences. Treatments include medical care, medication, behavior and education therapy, parent training, and other approaches such as biofeedback, yoga, and art therapy. The whole range of FAS and ARND is commonly called *fetal alcohol spectrum disorder (FASD).*

No one is sure exactly how much alcohol causes FASD. Like other untoward effects of alcohol, genetics and individual differences in metabolism, along with environmental factors such as diet, are thought to affect vulnerability. The American Academy of Pediatrics stresses that no amount of alcohol at any point during pregnancy is considered safe.

Women who are trying to conceive, or who are sexually active without using effective contraception, should abstain from alcohol to avoid inadvertently harming their fetus in the first few days or weeks of pregnancy, before they know they're expecting. And because any alcohol consumed by a nursing mother quickly enters her milk, many physicians advise nursing mothers to abstain from drinking alcohol.

### Possible Health Benefits of Alcohol?

Earlier studies observed moderate drinkers over time and noted they had healthier hearts; but these observations show a correlation, not a causation. Light to moderate drinkers—those who have up to 14 drinks a week—tend to practice other, healthy behaviors such as smoking less and exercising more, and they tended to weigh less. Their lifestyle caused their healthier hearts, not their alcohol intake. The best practices for your heart health include no alcohol. But the risk of heart disease increases starting with an average of seven drinks a week; the risk increases rapidly as more drinks are consumed.

## EXCESSIVE USE OF ALCOHOL

Excessive use of alcohol affects more than just the drinker. Friends, family members, coworkers, strangers that drinkers encounter on the road, and society as a whole pay the physical, emotional, and financial costs of the misuse of alcohol. As discussed in Chapter 8, the *DSM-5* has refocused general understanding of **alcohol misuse.** It diagnoses behavior based on a continuum of mild, moderate, and severe symptoms. In this case, behaviors are symptoms. Meeting two of the following criteria indicates an **alcohol use disorder;** two to three symptoms indicates a mild disorder, four to five a moderate disorder, and six or more a severe disorder.

To determine a person's place on the disorder spectrum, ask these questions:

1. Do you often consume alcohol in large amounts over a long period?
2. Do you find that your efforts to control your alcohol use are unsuccessful?
3. Do you spend excessive time using alcohol or recovering from its effects?
4. Do you have a strong desire or craving to use alcohol?
5. Does your persistent alcohol use cause a failure to fulfill obligations at work, school, or home?
6. Do you continue using alcohol despite recurrent social or interpersonal problems caused by its effects?
7. Have you reduced important social or recreational activities because of your alcohol use?
8. Do you persist in using alcohol in situations that are physically risky?
9. Do you continue using alcohol despite knowing that it can cause or worsen a recurrent physical or psychological problem?
10. Do you have a need for increased amounts of alcohol to achieve a desired effect (increased tolerance)?
11. Do you experience symptoms of withdrawal, such as greater amounts of any of the following: sweating, increased pulse rate, hand tremor, insomnia, nausea, and anxiety?

### Alcohol Use Disorder: From Mild to Severe

**Alcohol misuse** is recurrent alcohol use that has negative consequences, such as drinking in dangerous situations (before driving, for instance) or drinking patterns that result in academic, professional, interpersonal, or legal difficulties. If a person drinks only once a month, but then drives while intoxicated, their alcohol use would be considered problematic. Nearly half of college student treatment admissions are for primary alcohol misuse.

Severe alcohol use disorder involves more extensive problems with alcohol use, usually involving physical tolerance and withdrawal.

How can you tell if you or someone you know has serious problems with alcohol? Look for the following warning signs:

- Drinking alone or secretively
- Using alcohol deliberately and repeatedly to perform or get through difficult situations
- Using alcohol as a way to "self-medicate" in order to dull strong emotions or negative feelings
- Feeling uncomfortable on certain occasions when alcohol is not available

**TERMS**

**alcohol misuse** Drinking in a manner, situation, amount, or frequency that could cause harm to the person who is engaging in drinking or to those around them.

**alcohol use disorder** A brain disorder characterized by the use of alcohol or impairment in functioning due to alcohol use in spite of negative health and interpersonal consequences for the person using it; characterized by tolerance to alcohol and withdrawal symptoms.

- Escalating alcohol consumption beyond an already established drinking pattern
- Consuming alcohol heavily in risky situations, such as before driving
- Getting drunk regularly or more frequently than in the past
- Drinking in the morning

## Binge Drinking

In 2020, almost one-third of Americans aged 18–25 reported that they engaged in binge drinking in the past month; almost 9% reported that they engaged in heavy drinking in the past month. Surprisingly, most binge drinkers are not alcohol dependent—that is, they do not have severe alcohol use disorder. If their judgment were not impaired, many would decide not to binge. Among Americans under age 21, most drinking occurs in the form of bingeing, and over 90% of the alcohol they drink is consumed while binge drinking. Over half the alcohol consumed by all adults in the United States is downed during binge drinking.

The price of binge drinking is significant to society as a whole. Binge drinking caused more than half the 90,000 deaths and three-fourths the estimated economic cost of excessive drinking—$249 billion—in 2010 (the latest available data). In addition to the economic impact, students also often mention that they experience negative consequences when they binge-drink (see the box "Peer Pressure and College Binge Drinking"). Frequent binge drinkers are three to seven times more likely than non-binge drinkers to engage in unplanned or unprotected sex, drive after drinking, get hurt or injured, fall behind in schoolwork, or argue with friends.

## Severe Alcohol Use Disorder

As mentioned earlier, AUD is usually characterized by tolerance to alcohol and withdrawal symptoms. Everyone who drinks—even if not suffering from an alcohol use disorder—develops tolerance after repeated alcohol use, whereas withdrawal symptoms suggest a severe disorder.

**Patterns and Prevalence** AUD occurs among people of all racial and ethnic groups and at all socioeconomic levels. The stereotype of the homeless, impoverished alcoholic accounts for less than 5% of all alcohol-dependent people and usually represents later stages of the disorder. Patterns of alcohol misuse vary, including these four common variations:

1. Regular daily intake of large amounts
2. Regular heavy drinking limited to weekends
3. Long periods of sobriety interspersed with binges of daily heavy drinking lasting for weeks or months
4. Heavy drinking limited to periods of stress

Once established, AUD often exhibits a pattern of exacerbations and remissions. The person may stop drinking and abstain from alcohol for days or months after a frightening problem develops. After a period of abstinence, the individual often attempts controlled drinking, which almost inevitably leads to an escalation in drinking and more problems. AUD is not hopeless, however. Many people achieve improvements in health, functioning, life circumstances, and well-being, if not permanent abstinence from alcohol.

**Health Effects** Tolerance and withdrawal can have a serious impact on health. As described in Chapter 8, *tolerance* means that a drinker needs more alcohol to achieve intoxication or the desired effect, that the effects of continued use of the same amount of alcohol are diminished, or that the drinker can function adequately at doses or a BAC that would produce significant impairment in a casual user. Heavy users of alcohol may need to consume about 50% more than they originally needed in order to experience the same degree of intoxication.

When people with severe alcohol use disorder stop drinking or sharply decrease their intake, they experience *withdrawal.* Symptoms include trembling hands (shakes or jitters), a rapid pulse and accelerated breathing rate, insomnia, nightmares, anxiety, and GI upset. More severe withdrawal symptoms include seizures (sometimes called "rum fits"), confusion, and **hallucinations** such as seeing visions or hearing voices. Still less common is **delirium tremens (the DTs)**, a medical emergency characterized by severe disorientation, confusion, epileptic-like seizures, and vivid hallucinations, often of vermin and small animals. The mortality rate from the DTs can be as high as 15%, especially in very debilitated people with preexisting medical illnesses.

People with AUD face all the physical health risks associated with intoxication and chronic drinking described earlier in the chapter. Some damage is compounded by nutritional deficiencies that often accompany AUD. A mental problem associated with alcohol use is profound memory gaps (commonly known as blackouts).

**Social and Psychological Effects** Alcohol misuse causes more serious social and psychological problems than all other forms of drug use combined. For every person with AUD, another three or four people are directly affected. More than half of all adults have a family history of AUD or problem drinking, and more than 7 million children live in a household where at least one parent is dependent on or has misused alcohol.

People suffering from an alcohol use disorder frequently have mental disorders. The prevalence of psychiatric conditions, including mood and thought disorders, is higher in people with AUD than in the general population. People with anxiety or panic attacks may try to use alcohol to lessen their anxiety, even though alcohol often intensifies these disorders. Alcohol use disorder often co-occurs with other substance use as well.

TERMS

**hallucination** A false perception that does not correspond to external reality, such as seeing visions or hearing voices that are not there.

**delirium tremens (the DTs)** A state of confusion brought on by the reduction of alcohol intake in an alcohol-dependent person; other symptoms are sweating, trembling, anxiety, hallucinations, and seizures.

## WELLNESS ON CAMPUS
## Peer Pressure and College Binge Drinking

College drinking is pervasive. Approximately 56% of college students drink alcohol and, of those, 24% report having binged on alcohol; the rate of binge drinking for college students was typically higher than similarly aged people not in college until 2020. Still, from 1980 through 2020, college students' prevalence of binge drinking declined 20 percentage points. In 2020, it declined to a new all-time low for the preceding four decades. It is possible that this significant decline was due in part to the pandemic, when students spent less time with friends.

Every year, more than 1800 college students aged 18–24 die from alcohol-related injuries. Another 600,000 sustain unintentional alcohol-related injuries; 700,000 are assaulted by other students who have been drinking; and close to 100,000 are victims of alcohol-related date rape or sexual assault.

These statistics have shocked many students, administrators, and parents into demanding changes in college attitudes and policies regarding alcohol.

### Peer Pressure

The pressure to think and act along certain peer-prescribed guidelines plays a major role in drinking motivations. Late adolescence and early adulthood are times of life in which we are particularly susceptible to frequent alcohol misuse, risky behavior, and peer pressure. A study of young adult men examined direct versus indirect peer pressure. The researchers found that indirect pressure, as in the ideas contributing to our beliefs about alcohol, had more influence than direct pressure, such as offers or dares to drink at parties. The most common motivations of the young adult men were to get high and to forget their worries, rather than to fit in socially or make their social gatherings more fun. Thus, the authors of the study recommend targeting motives over peer pressure as a way to change behaviors.

A vehicle for peer-pressuring young people in particular is the display of drinking and smoking on social media. A study of high school social media users emphasizes that exposure—at any time of day, in any setting, alone or with others—to a friend's risky displays contributed to their drinking and smoking. Parents and teachers could consider teaching adolescents about the effects of posting online about risky behaviors.

### Ten Ways to Decline a Drink

1. No thanks.
2. My religious beliefs or health condition prohibit me from drinking.
3. I have offered to be the designated driver.
4. I am an athlete or musician who cannot compromise my general performance.
5. I must do something tomorrow (e.g., work, an exam, a family function), and I won't be able to do it if I drink tonight.
6. I'm dancing (or DJing).
7. I already have a drink (whether alcoholic or not can be hard to tell).
8. I'm cutting calories.
9. I don't like the taste of alcohol.
10. The last time I drank I became violent.

### What Schools Are Doing

Some schools have attempted to shift classes to Fridays and even Saturdays after they found that binge drinking increases when students don't have Friday classes. Increasingly, incoming students are required to take a three-hour online class about alcohol. And some campuses apply stricter punishment for underage drinking and public drunkenness, with the likelihood of suspension for repeat offenders.

Many colleges ban ads for alcoholic drinks in college newspapers and during broadcasts of college athletic events. Flyers, posters, and other promotions for cheap drinks, such as two-for-one specials, happy hours, all you can drink, and ladies' night, are banned on many campuses. In these college communities, bars and restaurants that cater to students are discouraged from offering patrons cheap alcohol.

SOURCES: Huang, G. C., et al. 2014. Peer influences: The impact of online and offline friendship networks on adolescent smoking and alcohol use. *Journal of Adolescent Health* 54(5): 508–514; Schulenberg, J., et al. 2021. *Monitoring the Future national survey results on drug use, 1975–2020: Volume II, college students and adults ages 19–60.* Ann Arbor: Institute for Social Research, The University of Michigan; National Institute on Drug Abuse. 2015. *6 Tactful Tips for Resisting Peer Pressure to Use Drugs and Alcohol* (https://teens.drugabuse.gov/blog/post/6-tactful-tips-resisting-peer-pressure-to-use-drugs-and-alcohol); Studer, J., et al. 2014. Peer pressure and alcohol use in young men: A mediation analysis of drinking motives. *International Journal of Drug Policy* 25(4): 700–708.

**Causes of AUD** The precise causes of severe alcohol use disorder are unknown, but many factors are probably involved. Studies of twins and adopted children clearly demonstrate the importance of genetics. If one of a pair of fraternal twins has severe alcohol use disorder, the other has about twice the normal risk of developing the disorder. For the identical twin of a person with AUD, the risk of developing the disorder is about four times that of the general population. These risks persist even when the twins have little contact with each other or their biological parents. Similarly, adoption studies show an increased risk among children of parents with AUD, even if they were adopted at birth into nondrinking families. AUD in adoptive parents, by contrast, doesn't make their adopted children more or less likely to develop AUD. Some studies suggest that as much as 50–60% of a person's risk for AUD is determined by genetic factors.

Not all children of people with AUD develop the disorder, however, and it is clear that other factors are involved. A person's risk of developing AUD may be increased by having certain personality disorders, having grown up in a violent or

## CRITICAL CONSUMER
### Alcohol Advertising

Alcohol manufacturers spend $7 billion every year on advertising and promotions. They claim that the purpose is to persuade adults who already drink to choose a certain brand. But in reality, ads appeal far more broadly and subconsciously: They cleverly engage young people and children by clearly linking alcohol and good times.

Alcohol ads are common during sporting events and other shows popular with teenagers. Studies show that the more television adolescents watch, the more likely they are to take up drinking in their teens. New alcoholic drinks geared to the tastes of young people are heavily promoted. "Hard lemonade" and other drinks ("alcopops") have been described by teens as a way to get drunk without experiencing a bitter taste. Almost half of 14- to 18-year-olds report having tried them.

Alcohol manufacturers also reach out to young people at activities like concerts and sporting events. Product logos are heavily marketed through sales of T-shirts, hats, and other items. Many colleges allow alcohol manufacturers to advertise at campus events in exchange for sponsorship.

Many ads give the impression that drinking alcohol is a normal part of everyday life and good times. This message seems to work, as many young people believe that heavy drinking at parties is normal and fun. The use of famous musicians, athletes, or actors in commercials increases the appeal of alcohol by associating it with fame, wealth, sex, and popularity.

What ads don't show is the darker side of drinking. You never see hangovers, car crashes, slipping grades, or violence. Although some ads include a brief message such as "drink responsibly," the impact of such cautions is small compared to that of the image of happy, attractive young people having fun while drinking.

The next time you see an advertisement for alcohol, look critically and be aware of its effect on you.

SOURCE: Zenith. 2021. Alcohol adspend to beat market with 5.3% growth in 2021 as hospitality opens up (https://www.zenithmedia.com/alcohol-adspend-to-beat-market-with-5-3-growth-in-2021-as-hospitality-opens-up/).

otherwise troubled household, and imitating the alcohol misuse of peers and other role models. People who begin drinking excessively in their teens are especially prone to binge drinking and AUD later in life. Common psychological features of individuals who misuse alcohol are denial ("I don't have a problem") and rationalization ("I drink because I need to socialize with my clients"). Certain social factors have also been linked with AUD, including urbanization, disappearance of the extended family, a general loosening of kinship ties, increased mobility, and changing values. Advertising plays a part, too (see the box "Alcohol Advertising").

**Treatment** Some people with AUD recover without professional help. How often this occurs is unknown, but it is estimated that as many as one-third stop drinking on their own or reduce their drinking enough to eliminate problems.

Most people with AUD require a treatment program of some kind. Many different kinds of programs exist. No single treatment works for everyone, so a person may have to try different programs before finding the right one.

One of the oldest and best-known recovery programs is Alcoholics Anonymous (AA). In many communities, AA consists of self-help groups that meet several times each week and follow a 12-step program. Important steps for people in these programs include recognizing that they are "powerless over alcohol" and must seek help from a "higher power" to regain control of their lives. By verbalizing these steps, the person directly addresses the denial that is often prominent in AUD and other substance use disorders. Many AA members have a sponsor of their choosing who is available by phone for individual support and crisis intervention.

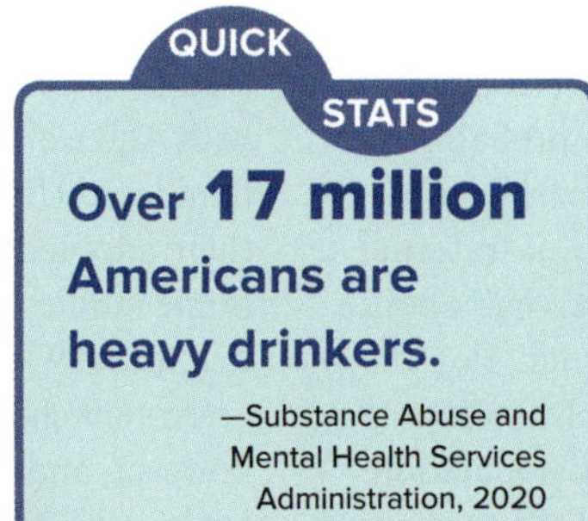


Other recovery approaches are available. Some, like Rational Recovery and Women for Sobriety, deliberately avoid any emphasis on higher spiritual powers. A more controversial approach to problem drinking is offered by the group Moderation Management, which encourages people to choose their own goals, which might include moderating their drinking rather than abstaining.

Al-Anon and Alateen are companion programs to AA for families and friends. In Al-Anon, family members and friends explore how they can cope with the stress of a loved one who drinks and focus on their own well-being.

Employee assistance programs and school-based programs represent another approach to AUD treatment. Inpatient hospital rehabilitation is useful for some people, especially if they have serious medical or mental health conditions or life stressors that are overwhelming.

There are also several pharmacotherapy treatments for AUD. All of these work best in combination with nonmedication programs:

- ***Disulfiram*** (Antabuse) inhibits the metabolic breakdown of acetaldehyde and causes patients to flush and feel ill when they drink, theoretically inhibiting impulse drinking. However, disulfiram is potentially dangerous if the user continues to drink.

- ***Naltrexone*** (ReVia, Depade) binds to a brain pleasure center that reduces the craving for alcohol and decreases its pleasant, reinforcing effects. When taken correctly, naltrexone usually does not make the user feel ill.

• ***Injectable naltrexone*** (Vivitrol) acts the same as oral naltrexone, but it is a single monthly shot administered by a health professional. Compliance with a monthly regimen may be better for some patients.

• ***Acamprosate*** (Campral) helps people maintain abstinence after they have stopped drinking. It is unclear how acamprosate works, but it appears to act on brain pathways related to alcohol craving.

A variety of other drugs to treat AUD are undergoing clinical trials—alone, in combination, or in combination with counseling therapies.

Alcohol treatment programs are successful in achieving an extended period of sobriety for about half of those who participate. Success rates of conventional treatment programs are about the same for men and women and for people from different racial and ethnic groups. Women and racial, ethnic, sexual, and gender minorities, as well as people with low socioeconomic status, often face major economic and social barriers to receiving treatment.

## Sex and Race Differences

People who misuse alcohol come from all socioeconomic levels and cultural groups, but notable differences appear in drinking patterns between men and women and among different racial and ethnic groups (Table 9.1).

VITAL STATISTICS

**Table 9.1** Alcohol Use and Binge Alcohol Use by Sex and Race/Ethnicity in 2020, Aged 21 and Over

| | PAST MONTH PREVALENCE (PERCENTAGE OF TOTAL POPULATION) | |
|---|---|---|
| | ALCOHOL USE | BINGE ALCOHOL USE |
| **Gender and Sex** | | |
| Male | 58.8 | 27.6 |
| Female | 52.1 | 21.2 |
| **Race and Ethnicity** | | |
| Not Hispanic or Latino | 56.5 | 23.7 |
| White | 59.6 | 24.5 |
| Black or African American | 50.6 | 23.5 |
| American Indian and Alaska Native | 35.3* | 22.7* |
| Native Hawaiian/Pacific Islander | 48.7* | 27.7* |
| Asian American | 39.3 | 13.9 |
| Two or more races | 49.2 | 24.0 |
| Hispanic or Latino | 49.4 | 27.4 |
| **Total Population** | **55.3** | **24.3** |

*(2019) [2020 was "low precision"]

SOURCE: Center for Behavioral Health Statistics and Quality. 2021. 2020 National Survey on Drug Use and Health: Detailed Tables. SAMHSA, Rockville, MD.

**Men** Men are more likely than women to drink alcohol, to misuse alcohol, and to develop alcohol use disorder. Men account for the majority of alcohol-related deaths and injuries in the United States. Among Euro-American men, excessive drinking often begins in the teens or twenties and progresses gradually through the thirties until the man exhibits clear signs of AUD by the time he is in his late thirties or early forties. Other men may remain controlled drinkers until later in life, sometimes developing AUD in association with retirement, the loss of friends and loved ones, boredom, illness, or psychological disorders.

**Women** Women tend to develop AUD at later ages and with fewer years of heavy drinking. It is not unusual for women in their forties or fifties to have clear AUD symptoms after years of controlled drinking.

Rates of alcohol misuse and dependence among women have increased in the past decade. Women with AUD develop cirrhosis and other medical complications more often and after a shorter period of heavy drinking than men, and have higher death rates—including deaths from cirrhosis—than men. Some alcohol-related health issues are unique to women, including increased risk of breast cancer and menstrual disorders, and complications during pregnancy. Women are more vulnerable to the anticlotting effects of alcohol, which can raise the risk of bleeding strokes. Women are less likely to seek early treatment for drinking problems, possibly because of the social stigma.

**Native Americans** American Indians/Alaska Natives have some of the highest rates of AUD; they are disproportionately affected by alcohol problems. A history of forced displacement from Indigenous lands, generations of massacre, and cultural genocide represent unique environmental stressors. Several studies have shown high levels of childhood trauma in some Indigenous communities. It is important for clinicians to take into account these particular traumas when working with members of Indigenous communities to create treatment plans.

**Black Americans** Black Americans use less alcohol than the average for American adults, but they face disproportionately high levels of alcohol-related birth defects, cirrhosis, cancer, hypertension, and other medical problems. In addition, Blacks are more likely than members of other racial or ethnic groups to be victims of alcohol-related homicides, criminal assaults, and injuries. African American women are more likely

### Ask Yourself

**QUESTIONS FOR CRITICAL THINKING AND REFLECTION**

Do you know anyone with a serious alcohol problem? From what you have read in this chapter, would you say that this person misuses alcohol or is dependent on it? What effects, if any, has this person's problem had on your life? Have you thought about getting support or help?

to abstain from alcohol use than White women, but among Black women who drink there is a higher percentage of heavy drinkers.

Treatments should address environmental and socioeconomic factors (e.g., poverty, unemployment, and limited education) that play a role in AUD. Programs designed to serve the Black community specifically can provide relevant care.

QUICK
STATS
50% of American adults report not drinking alcohol in the past month.
—SAMHSA
2020 National Survey on Drug Use and Health

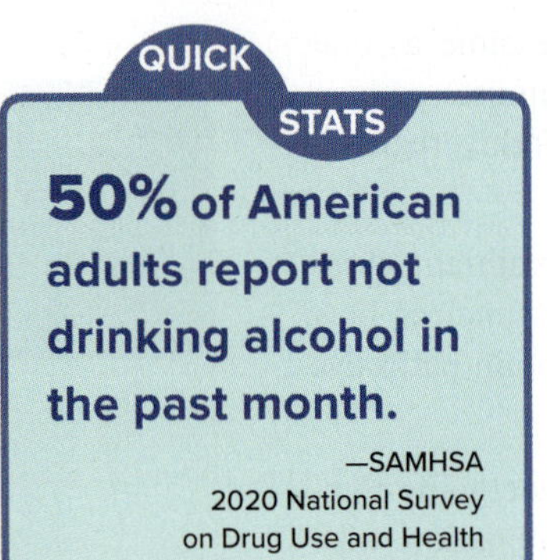

**Hispanic Americans** Drinking patterns among Latinos vary significantly, depending on their specific cultural background and level of acculturation and acculturative stress. Drunk driving and cirrhosis are the most common causes of alcohol-related death and injury among Latino men. Hispanic American women are more likely to abstain from alcohol than Native American, Euro, or African American women. Some may do better if treatment efforts integrate spirituality and traditional values, so care providers should have a good understanding of these specific cultural considerations. Familial country of origin also plays a large role. For example, rates of drinking among Puerto Rican Americans is higher than among Cuban Americans, so it's important to understand these cultural differences to provide effective treatment.

QUICK STATS

**One in nine high schoolers uses e-cigarettes.**

—Centers for Disease Control and Prevention, 2022

**Asian Americans** As a group, Asian Americans have lower-than-average rates of alcohol misuse. However, acculturation may greatly influence heavier alcohol use. Within this population, men consume much more alcohol than do women (60% versus 39%). For many Asian Americans, though, the genetically based physiological aversion to alcohol remains a deterrent to misuse. Ethnic agencies, health care professionals, and ministers seem to be the most effective sources of treatment for members of this group, when needed. Additionally, Asian Americans with AUD are largely an understudied and underserved population.

### Supporting Someone with an Alcohol Problem

Even when problems are acknowledged, there may be reluctance to get help—it takes hard work. You can't cure a friend's drinking problem, but you can support their efforts to seek appropriate help. Your best role might be to help obtain information about the available resources on campus. Consider asking if your friend would like to make an appointment at the student health center and whether they would like you to go with them to the appointment. Most student health centers will be able to recommend local options for self-help groups and formal treatment; the counseling center is another excellent source for help. Your friend can also check the phone book and the internet for local chapters of AA and other groups (see For More Information at the end of the chapter).

TERMS

**tobacco** The leaves of cultivated tobacco plants prepared for smoking, chewing, or use as snuff.

**psychoactive drug** A chemical substance that affects brain function and changes perception, mood, or consciousness.

**nicotine** A toxic, addictive substance found in tobacco and responsible for many of the effects of tobacco.

## WHO USES TOBACCO?

Rates of tobacco use vary based on gender, age, race and ethnicity, and education level (Figure 9.5). According to the CDC National Health Interview Survey, 13% of Americans aged 18 and over were cigarette smokers in 2020. About 25% of men and 14% of women reported that they currently used any tobacco product. Adults with a twelfth-grade education or less were much more likely to smoke cigarettes than were those who finished high school or college. Other groups with higher-than-average smoking rates include those who live below the poverty level, those without health insurance (or insured through Medicaid), those who have a physical disability or psychological disorder, those living in the Midwest or South, and LGBTQ people.

The number of people in the United States who smoke cigarettes (every day or some days) has been decreasing overall, however, with about a 66% decline since 1965. In fact, cigarette smoking is at an all-time low. The largest decrease has been in young adults (aged 18–24), although electronic cigarettes remain extremely popular among this age group.

College students, who make up 40% of young adults, often fit the "very light smoker" category, and most of those very light smokers use at least one type of alternative tobacco product. Advertisements may claim these products have lower health risks, but many pose considerable danger. These products also do not help very light smokers reduce their tobacco use.

## WHY PEOPLE USE TOBACCO

People start smoking for a variety of reasons; they usually become long-term smokers after becoming addicted to nicotine.

### Nicotine Addiction

The primary reason why people continue to use **tobacco** is that they have become addicted to a powerful **psychoactive drug: nicotine.** Although the tobacco industry long maintained that nicotine had not been proved to be addictive, scientific evidence overwhelmingly shows that it is highly addictive.

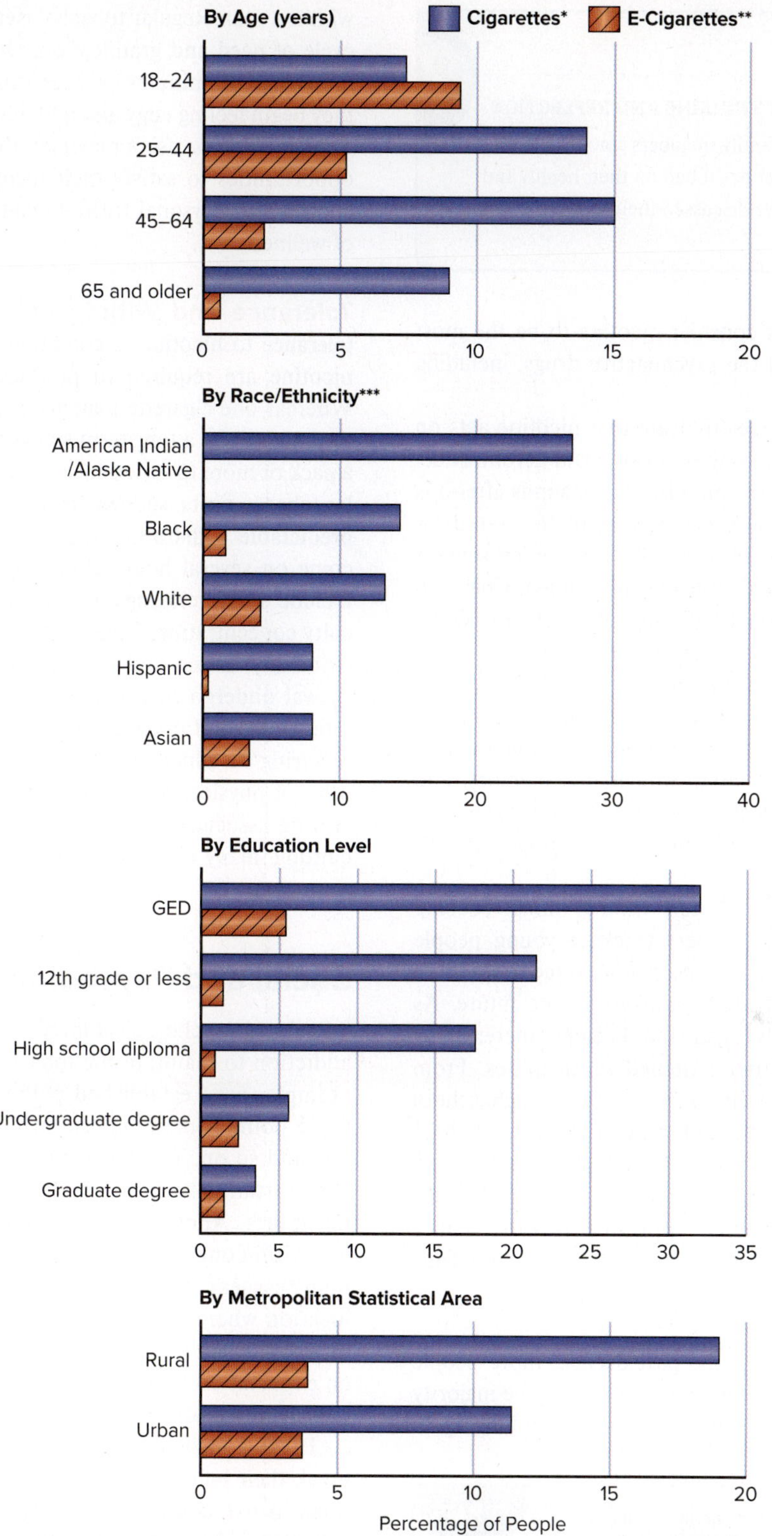


**FIGURE 9.5 Who is smoking and who is vaping?** Among U.S. adults in 2020, almost 19% were currently using any tobacco product. However, smoking and vaping rates vary significantly by age, race/ethnicity, education level, and where one lives.

*Current cigarette smoking = smoking ≥ 100 cigarettes during lifetime and now "every day" or "some days."

**Missing e-cigarette bars indicate no data available; current e-cigarette use = using e-cigs at least once ever and now using "every day" or "some days."

***Unless noted, all racial/ethnic groups are non-Hispanic; Hispanics can be of any race.

**SOURCE:** Cornelius, M. E., et al. 2022. Tobacco Product Use Among Adults—United States, 2020. *Morbidity and Mortality Weekly Report* 71: 397–405.

## Ask Yourself

**QUESTIONS FOR CRITICAL THINKING AND REFLECTION**

Do any of your friends or family members smoke cigarettes or use e-cigarettes? What effect has it had on their health and relationships? Have you ever discussed their tobacco use with them? Why or why not?

In fact, many researchers consider nicotine to be the most physically addictive of all the psychoactive drugs, including cocaine and heroin.

Some neurological studies indicate that nicotine acts on the brain in much the same way as cocaine and heroin. Nicotine reaches the brain via the bloodstream seconds after it is inhaled or absorbed through membranes of the mouth or nose. It triggers the release of powerful chemical messengers in the brain, including epinephrine, norepinephrine, and dopamine. But unlike street drugs, most of which are used to achieve a high, nicotine's primary attraction seems to lie in its ability to modulate everyday emotions.

At low doses, nicotine acts as a stimulant, increasing heart rate and blood pressure. In adults, nicotine can enhance alertness, concentration, information processing, memory, and learning. The opposite effect, however, occurs in teens who smoke; they show impairment in memory and other cognitive functions.

As more young people began vaping, more become addicted to nicotine. Researchers tracking young people since 2014 found that e-cigarette users were three times more likely to become daily cigarette smokers in the future. As participants in the study aged and became increasingly dependent on nicotine, they switched to cigarettes. From 2017 to 2018, rates climbed to over 20% of high school students and almost 5% of middle school students. A 2021 CDC investigation shows that 11% of high schoolers and almost 3% of middle schoolers reported vaping in the past month. Sleek advertisements, appealing flavors, and a perception of safety still loom large, and more campaigns against them are fighting back.

**Loss of Control** Within the past decade, more people are trying to quit and having more success. Still, the majority of smokers (94%) who attempt to quit start smoking again within a year. Regular tobacco users live according to a rigid cycle of need and gratification. On average, they can go no more than 40 minutes between doses of nicotine; otherwise, they begin feeling edgy and irritable and have trouble concentrating. Tobacco users may plan their daily schedule around opportunities to satisfy their nicotine cravings; this loss of control and personal freedom can affect all the dimensions of wellness.

**Tolerance and Withdrawal** Tobacco users build up **tolerance** to nicotine—a condition in which higher doses of nicotine are required to produce the same initial effect. Whereas one cigarette may make a beginning smoker nauseated and dizzy, a long-term smoker may have to chain-smoke a pack or more to experience the same effects. For most regular tobacco users, sudden abstinence from nicotine produces predictable **withdrawal** symptoms. These symptoms, which come on several hours after the last dose of nicotine, can include severe cravings, insomnia, confusion, tremors, difficulty concentrating, fatigue, muscle pains, headache, nausea, irritability, anger, and depression. Users experiencing withdrawal undergo measurable changes in brain waves, heart rate, and blood pressure, and they perform poorly on tasks requiring sustained attention. Although most of these symptoms of physical dependence pass in two or three days, the craving associated with addiction persists. Even years after quitting, many ex-smokers report intermittent, intense urges to smoke.

**TERMS**

**tolerance** A need for increasingly more of a substance to achieve the desired effect or a diminished effect with continued use of the same amount of the substance.

**withdrawal** Symptoms such as irritability, anxiety, and insomnia that can be relieved by taking more of an addictive substance.

**secondary reinforcers** Stimuli that are not necessarily pleasurable in themselves but that are associated with other stimuli that are pleasurable.

## Social and Psychological Factors

Social and psychological forces combine with physiological addiction to maintain the tobacco habit. Many people, for example, have established patterns of smoking or vaping while doing something else—while talking, working, drinking, and so on. The spit tobacco pattern is also associated with certain situations—studying, drinking coffee, or playing sports. Another social factor could be a norm that is less within one's control. For example, people experiencing homelessness may have to wait in line at a housing support location where others are smoking and offering them cigarettes. A certain position within the family could include an expectation that you take the first smoke, according to your family traditions.

These associations can make it more difficult for users to break their habits because the activities they associate with tobacco use continue to trigger urges. Such activities are called **secondary reinforcers;** they act together with physiological addiction to keep the user dependent on nicotine.

## Genetic Factors

Genetics play an important role in some aspects of tobacco use. Specific genes may affect how nicotine is metabolized in the body, increasing or decreasing one's risk for addiction. Inherited factors may be more important than social and environmental factors in smoking initiation and in the development of nicotine dependence.

### Why Start in the First Place?

In late 2019, the federal minimum age to purchase any tobacco product, including e-cigarettes, was raised from 18 to 21. Despite this, nearly 90% of all adult smokers report that they started smoking before age 18. The average age for starting smokers and smokeless tobacco users is around 15; for e-cigarettes, it is 17. The earlier people begin smoking, the more likely they are to become heavy smokers–and to die of tobacco-related disease.

Young people start using tobacco for a variety of reasons. Many young, White, male athletes, for example, begin using spit tobacco to emulate professional athletes. Young women commonly take up smoking because they think it will help them lose weight or stay thin. Most often, however, young people start using tobacco simply because their peers are already doing it; smoking or vaping gives them a way to fit in with a group.

**Rationalizing the Dangers** Making the decision to smoke requires minimizing or denying both the health risks and the tremendous costs–disability, emotional trauma, family stress, and financial expense involved in tobacco-related diseases such as cancer and emphysema. A sense of invincibility, characteristic of many young people, also contributes to the decision to use tobacco. They may persuade themselves they are too intelligent, too lucky, or too healthy to be vulnerable to tobacco's dangers. Many teenagers believe they can stop smoking when they want to. In fact, adolescents are more vulnerable to nicotine than are older tobacco users. Compared with older smokers, adolescents become heavy smokers and develop dependence after fewer cigarettes. Nicotine addiction can start within a few days of smoking and after just a few cigarettes. Over half of teenagers who try cigarettes progress to daily use, and about half of those who ever smoke daily progress to nicotine dependence. One National Institute on Drug Abuse (NIDA) survey revealed that about 75% of smoking teens state they wish they had never started.

**Emulating Smoking in the Media** Television ads for cigarettes have been banned for 50 years; however, just a few years ago, e-cigarette company JUUL began advertising on social media sites. Then they launched a $10 million TV ad campaign. By September 2019, in light of the epidemic of lung illnesses and multiple deaths attributable to vaping, many media corporations responded. CBS, Viacom, WarnerMedia, and others promised to ban e-cigarette advertising on their channels.

Tobacco imagery is widespread. A study conducted by Truth Initiative on people ages 15–24 found that, in 2020, 60% of favorite television shows, 38% of the top films released, and 23% of music videos for the top Billboard songs showed smoking or vaping. Studies find a direct causal relationship between media portrayals of smoking and smoking initiation. In general, the fictional portrayal of smoking or vaping in films and television does not reflect actual U.S. patterns of tobacco use. The prevalence of smoking among lead characters is three to four times that among comparable Americans.

## HEALTH HAZARDS

Tobacco adversely affects nearly every part of the body, including the brain, stomach, mouth, and reproductive organs.

### Tobacco Smoke: A Toxic Mix

Tobacco smoke contains thousands of chemical substances, several hundred of which are known to be harmful to humans, including acetone (found in nail polish remover), ammonia, hexamine (lighter fluid), and toluene (industrial solvent). Smoke from a typical unfiltered cigarette contains about 5 billion particles per cubic millimeter–50,000 times as many as are found in an equal volume of smoggy urban air. These particles, when condensed, form a brown, sticky mass called **cigarette tar.**

**Carcinogens and Poisons** When burned, cigarettes create more than 7000 chemicals. At least 69 of them are linked to cancer. Some, such as benzo(a)pyrene and urethane, are **carcinogens**–that is, they directly cause cancer. Other chemicals, such as formaldehyde, are **cocarcinogens;** they do not themselves cause cancer but combine with other chemicals to stimulate the growth of certain cancers, at least in laboratory animals. Other substances in tobacco cause health problems because they damage the lining of the respiratory tract or decrease the lungs' ability to fight off infection.

Tobacco also contains acutely poisonous substances, including arsenic, hydrogen cyanide, and nicotine. Cigarette smoke contains carbon monoxide, the deadly gas in automobile exhaust, in concentrations 400 times greater than is considered safe in industrial workplaces. Carbon monoxide displaces oxygen in red blood cells, depleting the body's supply of oxygen needed for extra work. Not surprisingly, smokers often complain of breathlessness when they exert themselves.

**Additives** Tobacco manufacturers use additives to manipulate the taste and effect of cigarettes and other tobacco products. Additives account for roughly 10%, by weight, of a cigarette, and include flavoring agents, humectants (compounds that keep tobacco from drying out), and chemicals

TERMS

**cigarette tar** A brown, sticky mass created when the chemical particles in tobacco smoke condense.

**carcinogen** Any substance that causes cancer.

**cocarcinogen** A substance that works with a carcinogen to cause cancer.

## Ask Yourself

**QUESTIONS FOR CRITICAL THINKING AND REFLECTION**

What has influenced your decision to try, continue, or quit smoking or vaping or using some other form of tobacco? Have you ever felt that images or messages in the media were encouraging you to use tobacco? How do you react to such messages?

that enhance nicotine's addicting properties. Some additives and their uses are described below:

- ***Sugars (such as licorice, cocoa, honey).*** These additives mask the bitter taste of tobacco, allowing for deeper inhalation. Burning sugar produces acetaldehyde, which is an addictive carcinogen.
- ***Other flavorings.*** Theobromine and glycyrrhizin are flavorings that also act as bronchodilators, opening the lungs' airways and making it easier for nicotine to get into the bloodstream.
- ***Ammonia.*** The main purpose of this additive is to boost nicotine delivery. Ammonia reduces the acidity of tobacco smoke and releases nicotine so it is more readily absorbed into the blood.
- ***Potassium citrate, aluminum, and clay.*** These additives make **sidestream smoke** (the uninhaled smoke from a burning cigarette) less obvious and objectionable. They are added to cigarette wrappers to convert particulate ash into an invisible gas with less irritating odor. These are intended to reduce social pressures from nonsmokers.

**QUICK STATS**

**More than 203 billion cigarettes were sold in the United States in 2020, the first time annual cigarette sales have increased in 20 years.**

—Federal Trade Commission, 2021

**"Reduced Harm" Cigarettes** There is no such thing as a safe cigarette, and smoking behavior is a more important factor in tar and nicotine intake than the type of cigarette smoked. Studies have found that people who smoke "light" cigarettes inhale up to eight times as much tar and nicotine as printed on the label. Studies also show that smokers of light cigarettes are less likely to quit than smokers of regular cigarettes. Use of light and low-tar cigarettes does not reduce the risk of smoking-related illnesses.

**Menthol Cigarettes** Menthol is a bronchodilator, which makes it easier for nicotine to enter the bloodstream. About 70% of African American smokers smoke these cigarettes, as compared to 30% of Euro-American smokers. Studies have found that African Americans absorb more nicotine than other groups and metabolize it more slowly; they also have lower rates of successful quitting. The anesthetizing effect of menthol, which may allow smokers to inhale more deeply and hold smoke in their lungs for a longer period, may be partly responsible for these differences.

## The Immediate Effects of Smoking

The beginning smoker often has symptoms of mild nicotine poisoning, including dizziness; rapid pulse; cold, clammy skin; nausea; and vomiting and diarrhea.

The effects of nicotine on smokers vary, largely depending on the size of the nicotine dose and how much tolerance the smoker has built up through previous smoking. Nicotine can either excite or tranquilize the nervous system, depending on dosage, and it has many other immediate effects (Figure 9.6). It stimulates the part of the brain called the **cerebral cortex.** It also stimulates the adrenal glands to release adrenaline, which accelerates heart rate, elevates blood pressure, and restricts blood flow to the heart. Nicotine inhibits the formation of urine and constricts blood vessels, especially in the skin. Higher blood pressure, faster heart rate, and constricted blood vessels require the heart to pump more blood.

## The Long-Term Effects of Smoking

Smoking is linked to many deadly and disabling diseases. Research indicates that the total amount of tobacco smoke inhaled is a key factor contributing to disease. People who begin smoking at early ages run a greater risk of disease than nonsmokers.

**Cardiovascular Disease** Cardiovascular disease is the most widespread cause of death for cigarette smokers, not lung cancer. **Coronary heart disease (CHD),** a form of cardiovascular disease, often results when the arteries that supply the heart muscle with blood develop **atherosclerosis.** In atherosclerosis, fatty deposits called **plaques** form on the inner walls of arteries, causing them to narrow and stiffen.

**TERMS**

**sidestream smoke** The uninhaled smoke from a burning cigarette.

**cerebral cortex** The outer region of the brain, which controls complex behavior and mental activity.

**coronary heart disease (CHD)** Cardiovascular disease caused by hardening of the arteries that supply oxygen to the heart muscle; also called *coronary artery disease.*

**atherosclerosis** Cardiovascular disease caused by the deposit of fatty substances (called *plaque*) in the walls of the arteries.

**plaque** A deposit on the inner wall of blood vessels; blood can coagulate around plaque and form a clot.

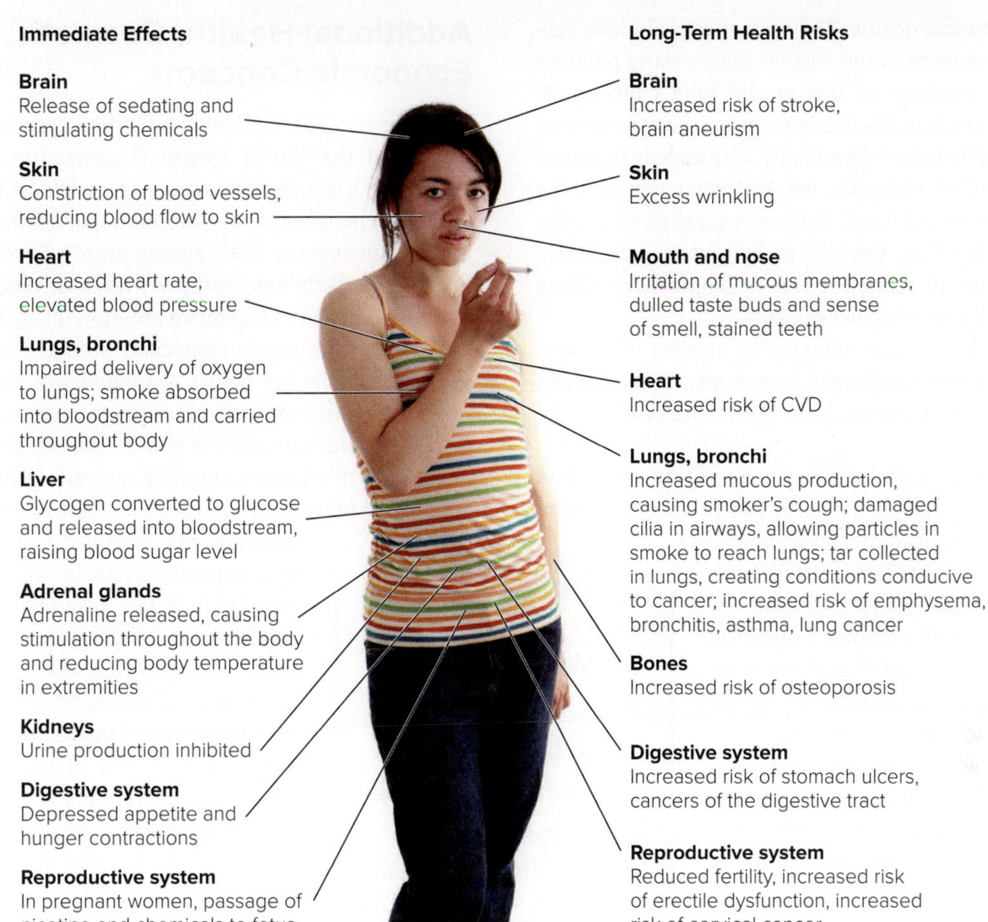


**FIGURE 9.6** **Tobacco use: Immediate effects and long-term health risks.**
Tim Large - Youth Social Issues/Alamy Stock Photo

Smoking and exposure to environmental tobacco smoke (ETS) accelerate the rate of plaque accumulation in the coronary arteries—50% for smokers, 25% for ex-smokers, and 20% for people regularly exposed to ETS. The crushing chest pain of **angina pectoris,** a primary symptom of CHD, results when the heart muscle, or *myocardium,* does not get enough oxygen. Sometimes a plaque forms at a narrow point in a main coronary artery. If the plaque completely blocks the flow of blood to a portion of the heart, that portion may die. This type of heart attack is called a **myocardial infarction.** CHD can also interfere with the heart's electrical activity, resulting in disturbances of the normal heartbeat rhythm.

Smokers have a death rate from CHD that is 70% higher than that of nonsmokers. New research shows that electronic cigarette smoking also significantly increases the risk of heart attack and CHD.

The risks of CHD decrease rapidly when a person stops smoking. This is particularly true for younger smokers, whose coronary arteries have not yet been damaged extensively.

QUICK STATS

Each year over **half a million** people die from smoking or environmental tobacco smoke. **16 million** live with serious illness due to smoking.

—Centers for Disease Control and Prevention, 2021

Cigarette smoking has been linked to other cardiovascular diseases, including the following:

- ***Stroke.*** A sudden interference with the circulation of blood in a part of the brain, resulting in the destruction of brain cells.
- ***Aortic aneurysm.*** A bulge in the aorta caused by a weakening in its walls.
- ***Pulmonary heart disease.*** A disorder of the right side of the heart, caused by changes in the blood vessels of the lungs.

## Lung Cancer and Other Cancers

About 30% of all cancer deaths are caused by smoking. Cigarette smoking is the primary cause of lung cancer and is responsible

TERMS

**angina pectoris** Chest pain due to coronary heart disease.

**myocardial infarction** A heart attack caused by the complete blockage of a main coronary artery.

for 87% of lung cancer deaths. The dramatic rise in lung cancer rates among women in the past 40 years clearly parallels the increase in smoking in this group; lung cancer now exceeds breast cancer as the leading cause of cancer deaths among women. The risk of developing lung cancer increases with the number of cigarettes smoked each day and the number of years of smoking. Evidence suggests that after 1 year without smoking, the risk of lung cancer decreases substantially. After 10 years, the risk of lung cancer among ex-smokers is half that of active smokers.

Research has also linked smoking to cancers of the trachea, mouth, pharynx, esophagus, larynx, pancreas, bladder, kidney, breast, cervix, stomach, liver, colon, and skin.

**Chronic Obstructive Pulmonary Disease** The stresses smoking places on the lungs can permanently damage lung function and lead to *chronic obstructive pulmonary disease* (*COPD*). COPD is a disorder that consists of several diseases, including emphysema and chronic bronchitis. It is caused by the overtaxing of smokers' lungs, which need to work harder to respond to the constant exposure to chemicals and irritants. COPD was the sixth leading cause of death in the United States in 2020.

QUICK STATS

**Smoking costs the United States $225 billion in direct medical care each year.**

—Centers for Disease Control and Prevention, 2021

In the U.S., cigarette smokers are up to 18 times more likely than nonsmokers to die from emphysema and chronic bronchitis. In a study of 605 people with COPD, 62% used tobacco.

**EMPHYSEMA** Smoking is the primary cause of **emphysema,** a disabling condition in which the air sacs in the walls of the lungs lose their elasticity and are gradually destroyed. The lungs' ability to take in oxygen and expel carbon dioxide is impaired. A person with emphysema is often breathless, gasps for air, and has the feeling of drowning. The heart must pump harder and may become enlarged. People with emphysema often die from a damaged heart. There is no known way to reverse this disease. In its advanced stage, emphysema leaves the victim bedridden and severely disabled.

**CHRONIC BRONCHITIS** Persistent, recurrent inflammation of the bronchial tubes characterizes **chronic bronchitis.** When the cell lining of the bronchial tubes is irritated, it secretes excess mucus. Bronchial congestion is followed by a chronic cough, which makes breathing more and more difficult. If smokers have chronic bronchitis, they face a greater risk of lung cancer, no matter how old they are or how many cigarettes they smoke.

TERMS

**emphysema** A disease characterized by a loss of lung tissue elasticity and destruction of the air sacs, impairing the lungs' ability to take in oxygen and expel carbon dioxide.

**chronic bronchitis** Recurrent, persistent inflammation of the bronchial tubes.

## Additional Health, Cosmetic, and Economic Concerns

Nicotine use has a number of other negative effects. The CDC and the World Health Organization conclude that smoking is a risk factor for more severe illness from Covid-19. Studies of people ages 13–24 found that a Covid-19 diagnosis was five times more likely among those who vaped and seven times more likely among those who both vaped and smoked cigarettes. People who smoke are more likely to develop and die from peptic ulcers (especially stomach ulcers) because smoking impairs the body's healing ability. Smoking also increases the risk of gastroesophageal reflux, which causes heartburn and can raise the risk of esophageal cancer.

Long-term cigarette smoking appears to hasten the thinning of the brain's cortex, which could lead to cognitive deterioration. Smoking affects blood flow and is an independent risk factor for erectile dysfunction. It is also linked to reduced fertility. Smokers are at increased risk for tooth decay and gum diseases, with symptoms appearing by the mid-twenties, and smoking dulls the senses of taste and smell. Over time it increases the risk of hearing loss and of macular degeneration and cataracts (serious eye conditions that can result in blindness).

Smokers have higher rates of motor vehicle crashes, fire-related injuries, and back

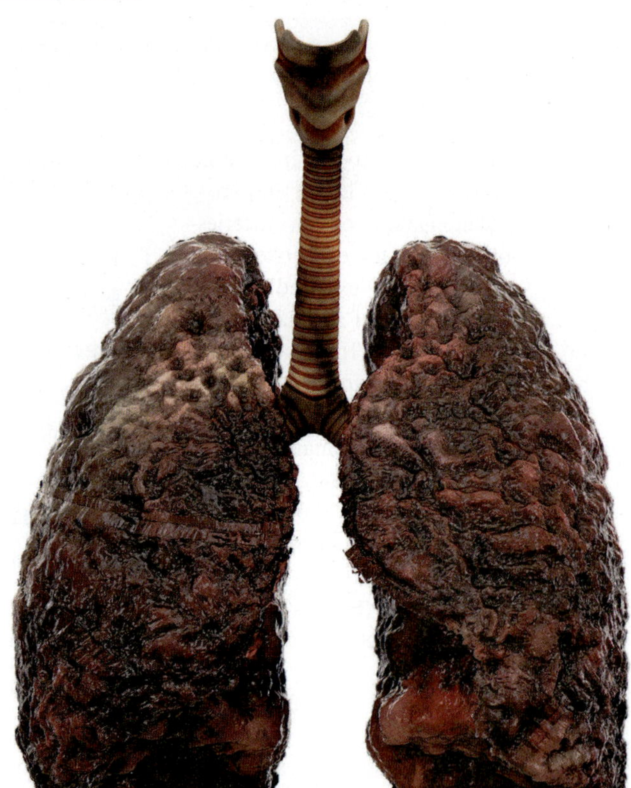

Tar deposits and other impurities eventually turn smokers' lungs black. Pavel Chagochkin/Shutterstock

pain. Smoking can cause premature skin wrinkling, premature baldness, stained teeth, discolored fingers, and a persistent tobacco odor in clothes and hair. In 2021, the average per-pack price of cigarettes was $6.28 so a pack-a-day habit can exceed $3600 per year. In addition, smoking contributes to osteoporosis, increases the risk of complications from diabetes, and accelerates the course of multiple sclerosis.

**Cumulative Effects** The cumulative effects of tobacco use fall into two general categories. The first is reduced life expectancy. A person who takes up smoking before age 15 and continues to smoke is only half as likely to live to age 75 as someone who never smokes.

The second category involves quality of life. Smokers become disabled at younger ages than nonsmokers and have more years of illness.

**Gender Differences in Health Hazards** Although overall risks of tobacco-related illness are similar for women and men, sex appears to make a difference in some diseases. Women, for example, are more at risk for smoking-related blood clots and strokes, and the risk is even greater for women using oral contraceptives. Among men and women with the same smoking history, the odds for developing three major types of cancer, including lung cancer, are 1.2–1.7 times higher in women.

Although the risks are elevated for everyone, men who smoke carry a greater risk of dying from bronchitis and emphysema and from cancer of the trachea, lung, and bronchus. They also increase their risk of erectile dysfunction and infertility due to reduced sperm density and motility. Women who smoke have higher rates of osteoporosis (a bone-thinning disease that can lead to fractures), thyroid-related diseases, and depression.

Women who smoke also have risks associated with reproduction and the reproductive organs. Smoking is associated with greater menstrual bleeding, greater duration of painful menstrual cramps, and more variability in menstrual cycle length. Smokers have a more difficult time becoming pregnant, and they reach menopause on average a year or two earlier than nonsmokers. In addition, smoking is a risk factor for cervical cancer.

## Risks Associated with Other Forms of Tobacco Use

Many smokers have switched from cigarettes to other forms of tobacco, such as spit tobacco, cigars, pipes, hookahs, and e-cigarettes. These alternatives, however, can be just as harmful.

**Smokeless (Spit) Tobacco** Smokeless tobacco, which is not burned, comes in several forms. Chewing tobacco is cured (aged) and sold in pouches. Often flavored, it is chewed or held between the cheek and gums to release the nicotine. Snuff, usually sold in small tins, is cured tobacco that has been finely cut or processed into a powder. Dry, powdered snuff is inhaled through the nose; powdered snuff also comes in lozenges or strips that are sucked on. Smokeless tobacco increases saliva production, and the resulting tobacco juice is usually spat out. Another product, called snus, is moist snuff contained in a pouch (like a teabag) and does not require spitting.

The nicotine in spit tobacco—along with flavorings and additives—is absorbed through the gums and lining of the mouth. Holding an average-size dip in the mouth for 30 minutes delivers about the same amount of nicotine as two or three cigarettes. Because of its nicotine content, spit tobacco is highly addictive. Some users keep it in their mouths even while sleeping.

Smokeless tobacco is not a safe alternative to cigarettes. Gums and lips become dried and irritated and may bleed. White or red patches may appear inside the mouth; this condition, known as *leukoplakia,* can lead to oral cancer. About 25% of regular smokeless tobacco users have *gingivitis* (inflammation), tooth loss, and recession of the gums and bone loss around the teeth, especially where the tobacco is typically placed. The senses of taste and smell are usually dulled.

One of the most serious effects of smokeless tobacco is an increased risk of oral cancer—cancers of the lip, tongue, cheek, throat, gums, roof and floor of the mouth, and larynx. Smokeless tobacco contains at least 28 chemicals known to cause cancer, and long-term snuff use may increase the risk of oral cancer by as much as 50 times. Surgery to treat oral cancer is often disfiguring and may involve removing parts of the face, tongue, cheek, or lip.

**Cigars and Pipes** About 3.5% of all U.S. adults smoke cigars; nearly 89% of cigar smokers are men. In government surveys, 2% of American high school students reported having smoked at least one cigar in the previous month.

Because cigar and pipe smoke is more alkaline than cigarette smoke, users of cigars and pipes do not need to inhale in order to ingest nicotine; instead they absorb nicotine through the gums and lining of the mouth. Cigars contain more tobacco than cigarettes and so contain more nicotine and produce more tar when smoked. Large cigars may contain as much tobacco as a whole pack of cigarettes and may take one or two hours to smoke.

The health risks of cigars depend on the number of cigars smoked and whether the smoker inhales. Because most cigar and pipe users do not inhale, they have a lower risk of cancer and cardiovascular and respiratory diseases than cigarette smokers. However, their risks are substantially higher than those of nonsmokers. For example, compared to nonsmokers, people who smoke one or two cigars per day without inhaling have six times the risk of cancer of the larynx. The risks are much higher for cigar smokers who inhale. Smoking a cigar immediately impairs the ability of blood vessels to dilate, reducing the amount of oxygen delivered to tissues, including the heart muscle, especially during stress. Pipe and cigar smoking are also risk factors for pancreatic cancer, which is almost always fatal.

The recent rise in cigar use among teens also raises concerns because nicotine addiction almost always develops in the teen or young adult years. More research is needed to determine if cigar use by teens will develop into nicotine addiction.

**Hookah** When puffing flavored tobacco through a water pipe—a **hookah**—the smoker inhales through a hose, drawing air over a piece of burning charcoal, heating the tobacco, and producing smoke that travels through the body of the pipe, an urn filled with water, and the hose.

Many people assume that hookahs provide a safer way of using tobacco. One study showed that over a quarter of college students believed hookahs did not contain tobacco, and over a third believed that hookahs did not contain nicotine. However, research has found hookah smoke contains many harmful chemicals, including 10 times more carbon monoxide than the smoke from a single cigarette. Depending on which toxic compound is measured, a single hookah session is the equivalent of smoking between 1 and 50 cigarettes.

**E-Cigarettes** Electronic cigarettes are battery-powered devices that look like traditional cigarettes, pens, or even USB flash drives. They use a changeable cartridge containing a liquid form of nicotine, flavorings, and other chemicals. When the user "smokes" or "vapes" an e-cig by sucking the filtered end, the battery heats the chemicals to create an inhalable vapor.

In addition to nicotine, carcinogens, and other toxic chemicals, e-cigarettes also produce nanoparticles, which have been linked to inflammation leading to asthma, stroke, and heart disease. One study found that vaping may make antibiotic-resistant bacteria even harder to kill. Another recent study linked e-cigarette flavorants to an irreversible respiratory disease called bronchiolitis obliterans, or "popcorn lung," in which the airways become inflamed and scarred, resulting in a permanent cough and shortness of breath. A recent study found that even nicotine-free e-cigarette solutions contain chemicals that damage lung cells.

In 2019, 2300 people across 49 states were sickened and 47 died from e-cigarette-associated lung injury. In response to the outbreak of vaping-related lung disease, the CDC recommends that people not use vaping products containing THC, nor purchase any type of vaping products, including those containing nicotine, from informal sources like friends, family, or at in-person or online dealers. They should also not add any substances to e-cigarette products that are not intended by the manufacturer.

No evidence submitted to the FDA supports the claim that e-cigarettes can be used as a smoking cessation product like nicotine gums and patches.

> **TERMS**
>
> **hookah** A pipe used for smoking specially flavored tobacco (e.g., apple, mint, cherry); sometimes called a water pipe or *shisha*.
>
> **environmental tobacco smoke (ETS)** Smoke that enters the atmosphere from the burning end of a cigarette, cigar, or pipe, as well as smoke that is exhaled by smokers; also called *secondhand smoke*.
>
> **mainstream smoke** Smoke that is inhaled by a smoker and then exhaled into the atmosphere.

> **Ask Yourself**
>
> **QUESTIONS FOR CRITICAL THINKING AND REFLECTION**
>
> Do you know anyone who has suffered from an illness related to tobacco use? If so, what problems did that person face? What was the outcome? Did the experience have any effect on your views about using tobacco?

## THE EFFECTS OF SMOKING ON THE NONSMOKER

Tens of thousands of nonsmokers die each year because of exposure to secondhand smoke, and the latest research points to similar devastating effects from thirdhand smoke. The medical and societal costs of tobacco use are enormous.

### Environmental Tobacco Smoke

The U.S. Environmental Protection Agency (EPA) has designated **environmental tobacco smoke (ETS)**—more commonly called *secondhand smoke* and *thirdhand smoke*—a Class A carcinogen. The National Toxicology Program classifies ETS as a "known human carcinogen." These designations put ETS in the same category as notorious cancer-causing agents like asbestos. The Surgeon General has concluded that for some people there is no safe level of exposure to ETS; even brief exposure can cause serious harm.

Environmental tobacco smoke consists of mainstream smoke and sidestream smoke. Smoke exhaled by smokers is referred to as **mainstream smoke.** Sidestream smoke enters the atmosphere from the burning end of a cigarette, cigar, or pipe. Nearly 85% of the smoke in a room where someone is smoking comes from sidestream smoke. Sidestream smoke is not filtered through either a cigarette filter or a smoker's lungs. It has twice as much tar and nicotine, three times as much benzo(a)pyrene, almost three times as much carbon monoxide, and three times as much ammonia as mainstream smoke.

In rooms where people are smoking, levels of carbon monoxide can exceed those permitted by federal air quality standards for outside air. In a typical home with the windows closed, it takes about six hours for 95% of the airborne cigarette smoke particles to clear. The carcinogens in the secondhand smoke from a single cigar exceed those of three cigarettes, and cigar smoke contains up to 30 times more carbon monoxide. E-cigarettes produce secondhand aerosol. While it contains fewer toxins than cigarette smoke, the Surgeon General has concluded that e-cigarette aerosol is not harmless; it may expose bystanders to nicotine, heavy metals, ultrafine particulates, volatile organic compounds, and other toxins.

**Thirdhand Smoke** A further complicating factor is *thirdhand smoke*, the toxic residues and chemicals that linger on indoor surfaces, curtains, and furniture, and in dust. Although it may seem like only a stale smell, thirdhand smoke contains the chemicals of secondhand smoke from tobacco: gases and particulate matter, including carcinogens and heavy metals such as arsenic, lead, and cyanide. Highly toxic particulates like nicotine can cling to walls and ceilings; gases can be absorbed into dust, fabrics, and upholstery. These toxic mixes can then recombine to form harmful compounds that remain at high levels long after smoking has stopped.

The transition from secondhand to thirdhand smoke is gradual, so the distinct chronic effects of each are not yet clear. The predicted health damage caused by thirdhand smoke ranges from 5% to 60% of total harm, much of which may currently be attributed to secondhand smoke. We do know that nicotine in thirdhand smoke forms carcinogens that are then inhaled, absorbed, or ingested, increasing the risk of respiratory illnesses and other tobacco-related health problems. Young children who crawl and put objects in their mouths are more likely to come in contact with contaminated surfaces and are therefore the most vulnerable to thirdhand smoke's harmful effects. Homes of former smokers remained polluted with thirdhand smoke for months after residents quit smoking. Nicotine could be measured in the bodies of nonsmokers who moved into homes that had been smoked in, cleaned, and left empty several months.

**ETS Effects** Nonsmokers subjected to ETS frequently develop coughs, headaches, nasal discomfort, and eye irritation. Other symptoms range from breathlessness to sinus problems. People with allergies tend to suffer the most. ETS causes an estimated 7300 lung cancer deaths and 34,000 deaths from heart disease each year in people who do not smoke. Exposure to ETS is also associated with a 20% increase in the progression of atherosclerosis and raises the risk of developing heart disease and stroke by up to 30%. ETS aggravates asthma and increases the risk for breast and cervical cancers.

Scientists have been able to measure changes that contribute to lung tissue damage and potential tumor promotion in the bloodstreams of healthy young people who spend just three hours in a smoke-filled room. After just 30 minutes of exposure to ETS, the function in the coronary arteries of healthy nonsmokers is reduced to the same level as that of smokers.

**Infants, Children, and ETS** Infants and children are perhaps the group most vulnerable to the harmful effects of ETS. Recent studies have shown that infants exposed to smoke from more than 21 cigarettes a day are more than *23 times* more likely to die of sudden infant death syndrome (SIDS) than are babies not exposed to ETS. The National Cancer Institute recently estimated that ETS causes up to 18,600 cases of low birth weight each year. Children under age 5 whose primary caregiver smokes 10 or more cigarettes per day have measurable blood levels of nicotine and tobacco carcinogens. Chemicals in tobacco smoke also show up in breast milk, and breastfeeding may pass more chemicals to the infant of a smoking mother than the infant receives through direct exposure to ETS.

ETS triggers bronchitis, pneumonia, and other respiratory infections in infants and toddlers up to age 18 months, resulting in as many as 15,000 hospitalizations each year. Higher levels of nicotine are found in the lungs of infants who die of SIDS than of other causes.

Older children suffer, too. ETS is a risk factor for asthma and aggravates symptoms in children who already have asthma. ETS is also linked to reduced lung function and fluid buildup in the middle ear, a contributing factor in middle-ear infections, a leading reason for childhood surgery. Children and teens exposed to ETS score lower on tests of reading and reasoning. Later in life, people exposed to ETS as children are at increased risk for lung cancer, emphysema, and chronic bronchitis.

## Smoking and Pregnancy

Smoking almost doubles a pregnant woman's chance of having a miscarriage, and it significantly increases her risk of ectopic pregnancy. Maternal smoking causes approximately 1000 infant deaths in the United States each year, primarily due to premature delivery and smoking-related problems with the placenta. Maternal smoking is a major factor in low birth weight, which puts newborns at high risk for infections and other serious problems. If a nonsmoking mother is regularly exposed to ETS, her infant is also at greater risk for low birth weight.

Babies born to mothers who smoke more than two packs a day perform poorly on developmental tests in the first hours after birth, compared to babies of nonsmoking mothers. Later in life, obesity, hyperactivity, short attention span, and lower scores on spelling and reading tests all occur more frequently in children whose mothers smoked during pregnancy than in those born to nonsmoking mothers. Prenatal tobacco exposure has also been associated with behavioral problems in children, including immaturity, emotional instability, physical aggression, and hyperactivity. Other research shows that teenagers whose mothers smoked during pregnancy have lower scores on tests of general intelligence and poorer performance on tasks requiring auditory memory than do children who were not exposed to cigarette smoke before birth.

### Ask Yourself

**QUESTIONS FOR CRITICAL THINKING AND REFLECTION**

What antismoking ordinances are in effect in your community? Does your school prohibit smoking on campus? Do you think these rules have been effective in reducing smoking or exposure to ETS? Do you support such regulations? Why or why not?

## WHAT CAN BE DONE TO COMBAT SMOKING?

There are many ways to act against this public health threat.

### Action at Many Levels

Since the 1980s, local government agencies—such as city councils, school boards, and county boards of commissioners—have been passing ordinances designed to discourage smoking in public places. Thousands of local ordinances across the nation now restrict or ban smoking in restaurants, stores, workplaces, and even public outdoor areas. In 2021, nearly 82% of Americans lived in municipalities that restrict or ban smoking in public buildings, workplaces, restaurants, and bars. Hundreds of colleges and universities now have totally smoke-free campuses or prohibit smoking in residential buildings. As local nonsmoking laws proliferate, evidence mounts that environmental restrictions are effective in encouraging smokers to quit.

State legislatures have passed many tough new anti-tobacco and anti-vaping laws. As of 2021, comprehensive smoke-free air laws were in effect in 28 states, the District of Columbia, Puerto Rico, and the U.S. Virgin Islands. Smoke-free legislation has contributed to a decline in heart disease morbidity and respiratory symptoms; a decrease in acute coronary events; and a decrease in rates of hospital admissions or deaths for cardiac events, other heart diseases, cerebrovascular accidents, and respiratory disease.

Additionally, studies have shown that smoking and vaping bans help increase tobacco cessation and reduce tobacco use among adults and youth.

**QUICK STATS**

**If smoking among U.S. youth continues at the current rate, 5.6 million of today's Americans younger than 18 will die early from a smoking-related illness.**

—Centers for Disease Control and Prevention, 2019

### FDA Regulation of Tobacco

In 2009, Congress first gave the FDA broad regulatory powers over the production, marketing, and sale of cigarettes. In 2016, this authority was extended to all tobacco products, including e-cigarettes, cigars, and hookah and pipe tobacco, banning their sale to minors and requiring identification for purchase.

WARNING
CIGARETTES CAUSE LUNG CANCER
Every cigarette you smoke increases your chance of getting lung cancer.
Health Canada

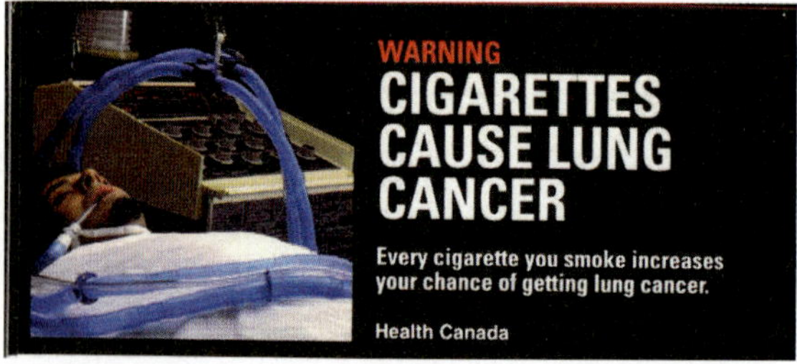

Canada's graphic cigarette labels have greatly helped reduce smoking rates. Staff/Getty Images News/Getty Images

**Ask Yourself**

**QUESTIONS FOR CRITICAL THINKING AND REFLECTION**

What are your views on the government's role in regulating tobacco products? Is current regulation enough, or should the government go further in controlling the production and marketing of these products? What events or experiences have shaped your views on this issue?

In 2017, the FDA proposed a new regulatory effort to decrease the level of nicotine in tobacco products. Still in the works, this plan would establish a maximum nicotine level to reduce youth use, addiction, and death. The FDA has enforced tougher rules on the marketing and sales of tobacco and vaping products, required additional standards and disclosures about the ingredients and by-products of smoking products, and raised the minimum age for purchase to 21.

### Individual Action

Nonsmokers have the right not only to breathe clean air but also to take action to help solve one of society's most serious public health threats. Here are just some of the many ways in which individuals can help support tobacco prevention and stop-smoking efforts: When a smoker violates a no-smoking designation, complain. If your favorite restaurant or shop doesn't have a nonsmoking policy, ask the manager to adopt one. If you see children buying tobacco, report this illegal activity to the facility manager or the police. Learn more about addiction and tobacco cessation so that you can better support the tobacco users you know. Vote for candidates who support anti-tobacco measures; contact local, state, and national representatives to express your views.

## HOW A TOBACCO USER CAN QUIT

Giving up tobacco is a long-term, intricate process. Research shows that tobacco users move through predictable stages—from being uninterested in stopping, to thinking about change, to making a serious effort to stop, to finally maintaining abstinence. But most attempt to quit several times before they finally succeed. Relapse is a normal part of the process.

### Benefits of Quitting

People who quit smoking find that food tastes better. Their sense of smell is sharper. Circulation improves, heart rate and blood pressure drop, and lung function and heart efficiency increase. Ex-smokers can breathe more easily, their coughing stops, and their capacity for exercise improves. Many

**Table 9.2** Benefits of Quitting Smoking

|  |  |
|---|---|
| **Within 20 minutes of your last cigarette:** | • Blood pressure drops to normal<br>• Pulse rate drops to normal<br>• Temperature of hands and feet increases to normal<br>• You stop polluting the air |
| **8 hours:** | • Carbon monoxide level in blood drops to normal<br>• Oxygen level in blood increases to normal |
| **24 hours:** | • Chance of heart attack decreases |
| **48 hours:** | • Nerve endings start regrowing<br>• Ability to smell and taste is enhanced |
| **2–3 months:** | • Circulation improves<br>• Walking becomes easier<br>• Lung function increases up to 30% |
| **1–9 months:** | • Coughing, sinus congestion, fatigue, and shortness of breath all decrease |
| **1 year:** | • Heart disease death rate is half that of a smoker |
| **5 years:** | • Stroke risk drops nearly to the risk for nonsmokers |
| **10 years:** | • Lung cancer death rate drops to 50% of that of continuing smokers<br>• Incidence of other cancers (mouth, throat, larynx, esophagus, bladder, kidney, and pancreas) decreases<br>• Risk of ulcer decreases |
| **15 years:** | • Risk of lung cancer is about 25% of that of continuing smokers<br>• Risks of heart disease and death are close to those of nonsmokers |

SOURCES: American Cancer Society. 2020. Benefits of Quitting Smoking Over Time (https://www.cancer.org/healthy/stay-away-fromtobacco/benefits-of-quitting-smoking-over-time.html); U.S. National Library of Medicine. 2022. Benefits of Quitting Tobacco (https://www.nlm.nih.gov /medlineplus/ency/article/007532.htm).

ex-smokers report feeling more energetic and alert. They experience fewer headaches. Even their complexions may improve.

Giving up tobacco provides immediate health benefits to people of all ages (Table 9.2). The younger people are when they stop smoking, the more pronounced the health improvements. And these improvements gradually but invariably increase as the period of nonsmoking lengthens. It's never too late to quit, though. According to a Surgeon General's report, people who quit smoking, regardless of age, live longer than people who continue to smoke.

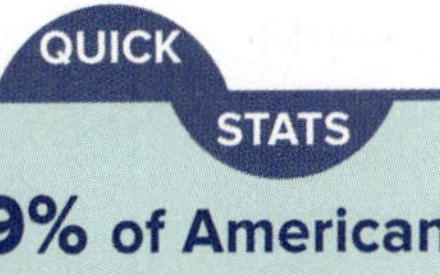


**69% of American college students report that they have never used tobacco or nicotine products.**

—American College Health Association, 2022

## Options for Quitting

More than two-thirds of adult tobacco users want to quit, and the majority will make an attempt this year. What are their options? No single method works for everyone, but each works for some people some of the time.

**Behavior Change** Choosing to quit requires developing a strategy for success (see the box "Strategies to Quit Smoking"). Some people quit cold turkey, whereas others taper off slowly. Over-the-counter and prescription products help many people. Support from others and regular exercise are behavioral factors that have been shown to increase the chances that a smoker will stop smoking permanently. Support can come from friends and family and/or formal group programs sponsored by organizations such as the American Cancer Society and the American Lung Association, or by a college health center or community hospital. Programs that combine group support with nicotine replacement therapy have rates of continued abstention as high as 35% after one year.

Most smokers in the process of quitting experience both physical and psychological effects of nicotine withdrawal, and exercise can help with both. For many smokers, tobacco use is associated with certain times and places–following a meal, for example. Resolving to walk after dinner instead of lighting up provides a distraction from cravings and eliminates the cues that trigger a desire to smoke. In addition, many people worry about weight gain associated with quitting. Although most ex-smokers do gain a few pounds, at least temporarily, incorporating exercise into a new tobacco-free routine lays the foundation for healthy weight management. The health risks of adding a few pounds are minimal compared to the risks of continued smoking.

The U.S. Department of Health and Human Services has a national toll-free number, 1-800-QUITNOW (1-800-784-8669), to serve as a single access point for smokers seeking information and assistance in quitting. Callers are routed to their state's smoking cessation quitline or, in states that have not established quitlines, to one maintained by the National Cancer Institute.

As with any significant change in health-related behavior, giving up tobacco requires planning, sustained effort, and support. It is an ongoing process, not a one-time event. The "Kicking the Tobacco Habit" box at the end of the chapter describes the steps that successful quitters follow.

**Smoking Cessation Products** Each year millions of Americans visit their doctors in the hope of finding a drug that can help them stop smoking. Although pharmacological options are limited, the few available drugs have proved successful.

**CHANTIX (VARENICLINE)** The newest smoking cessation drug, marketed under the name Chantix, works in two ways: It reduces

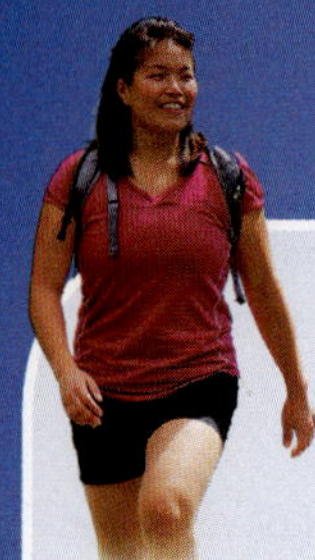

## TAKE CHARGE
## Strategies to Quit Smoking

The U.S. Public Health Service suggests a "5 Rs" strategy to enhance motivation to quit. If you are a smoker or are trying to help one, think about these areas of concern and see if they help develop a desire and readiness to make a real attempt at quitting.

- ***Relevance.*** Think about the personal relevance of quitting tobacco use. What would be the effects on your family and friends? How would your daily life improve? What is the most important way that quitting would change your life?
- ***Risks.*** Immediate risks include shortness of breath, infertility, and impotence, and long-term risks include cancer, heart disease, and respiratory problems. Remember, smoking is harmful both to you and to anyone you expose to your smoke.
- ***Rewards.*** The list of the rewards of quitting is almost endless, including improving immediate and long-term health, saving money, and feeling better about yourself. You can also stop worrying about quitting and set a good example for others.
- ***Roadblocks.*** What are the potential obstacles to quitting? Are you worried about withdrawal symptoms, weight gain, or lack of support? How can you overcome these barriers?
- ***Repetition.*** Revisit your reasons for quitting and strengthen your resolve until you are ready to prepare a plan. Most people make several attempts to quit before they succeed. Relapsing does not mean that you will never succeed.

nicotine cravings, easing the withdrawal process, and it blocks the pleasant effects of nicotine. The drug acts on neurotransmitter receptors in the brain.

Unlike most smoking cessation products currently on the market, Chantix is not a nicotine replacement. For this reason, smokers may be advised to continue smoking for the first few days of treatment to avoid withdrawal and to allow the drug to build up in their bodies. The approved course of treatment is 12 weeks, but the duration and recommended dosage depend on several factors, including the smoker's general health and the length and severity of their nicotine addiction.

Side effects reported with Chantix include nausea, headaches, vomiting, sleep disruptions, and changes in taste perception. People with kidney problems or who take certain medications should not take Chantix, and it is not recommended for women who are pregnant or nursing. Further, the FDA has been investigating reports of the drug causing adverse reactions, such as behavioral changes, agitation, depression, suicidal thoughts, and attempted suicide. Anyone taking Chantix should immediately notify their doctor of any sudden change in mood or behavior.

**ZYBAN (BUPROPION)** Bupropion is an antidepressant (prescribed under the name Wellbutrin) as well as a smoking cessation aid (prescribed under the name Zyban). As a smoking cessation aid, bupropion eases the symptoms of nicotine withdrawal and reduces the urge to smoke. Like Chantix, it acts on neurotransmitter receptors in the brain.

Bupropion users have reported an array of side effects, but they are rare. Side effects may be reduced by changing the dosage, taking the medicine at a different time of day, or taking it with or without food. Bupropion is not recommended for people with specific physical conditions or who take certain drugs. Zyban and Wellbutrin should not be taken together.

**NICOTINE REPLACEMENT PRODUCTS** The most widely used smoking cessation products replace the nicotine that the user would normally get from tobacco. The user continues to get nicotine, so withdrawal symptoms and cravings are reduced. Although still harmful, nicotine replacement products provide a cleaner form of nicotine without the thousands of

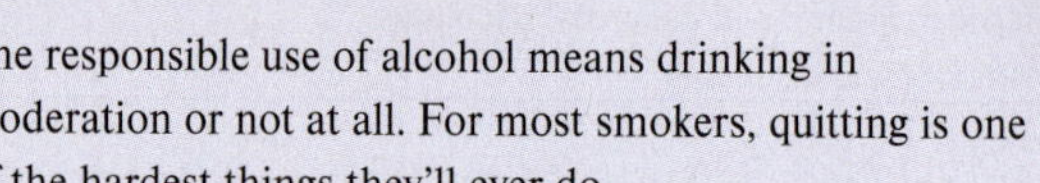

### TIPS FOR TODAY AND THE FUTURE

The responsible use of alcohol means drinking in moderation or not at all. For most smokers, quitting is one of the hardest things they'll ever do.

**RIGHT NOW YOU CAN:**

- Consider whether there is a history of alcohol abuse or dependence in your family.
- Think about your current drinking habits. For example, count the number of parties you attended in the past month and how many drinks you had at each one.
- If you smoke or vape, throw away the pack or device.
- If you use tobacco, go outside for a short walk or a stretch to limber up. Breathe deeply. Tell a friend you've just decided to quit.

**IN THE FUTURE YOU CAN:**

- Think about the next party you plan to attend. Decide how much you will drink at the party, and how you will get home afterward.
- Watch your friends' behavior at events where drinking is involved. Do any of them show signs of a drinking problem? If so, consider what you can do to help.
- Resolve to quit smoking or vaping. Research your options for quitting, and choose the one you think will work best for you.
- Recruit a friend or family member to help you quit smoking. Arrange to talk to this person whenever you feel the urge to smoke.

# BEHAVIOR CHANGE STRATEGY
## Kicking the Tobacco Habit

Congratulations! You've decided to quit smoking. You likely already know that your first day without cigarettes may be difficult. Here are six steps you can take to handle your "quit day" and be confident about being able to stay quit.

### 1. Make a Quit Plan

Having a quit plan helps you stay focused, confident, and motivated to quit. No single approach to quitting works for everyone. If you don't know what quit method might be right for you, visit the Explore Quit Methods website (http://smokefree.gov/explore-quit-methods) to learn more. As part of your plan, identify your reasons for quitting: for example, to be healthier, save money, smell better, relieve the worrying of your loved ones.

### 2. Set a Quit Date

Choose a date within the next two weeks. This will give you enough time to prepare:

- Start to get rid of smoking reminders—e.g., wash your clothes, clean your car, get rid of matches and ashtrays.
- Identify your smoking triggers. Triggers are the people, places, things, and situations that set off your urge to smoke. Some are emotional, such as feeling stressed or down; others are habitual, such as talking on the phone or drinking alcohol; still others are social, such as going to a bar or a party. Being aware of your triggers will help you avoid them or think of strategies for defusing them.
- Consider how you will fight the inevitable cravings—for example, think of ways to keep your hands and mouth busy; find new ways to relieve stress or improve your mood.

### 3. Stay Busy on Your Quit Day

Being busy will help you keep your mind off smoking and distract you from cravings. Try some of these activities:

- Go out for walks. Notice details about your neighborhood.
- Chew gum or hard candy.
- Keep your hands busy with a pen or toothpick.
- Drink lots of water.
- Relax with deep breathing.
- Go to a movie.
- Spend time with nonsmoking friends and family.
- Go to dinner at your favorite smoke-free restaurant.

### 4. Avoid Smoking Triggers

On your quit day, try to avoid all your triggers.

- Throw away all your cigarettes, lighters, and ash trays if you haven't already.
- Avoid caffeine, which can make you feel jittery. Try drinking water instead.
- Spend time with nonsmokers.
- Go to places where smoking isn't allowed.
- Get plenty of rest and eat healthy foods. Being tired can trigger you to smoke.
- Change your routine to avoid the things you associate with smoking.

### 5. Stay Positive

Quitting smoking is difficult. It happens one minute . . . one hour . . . one day at a time. Try not to think of quitting as forever. Pay attention to *today,* and the time will add up. Your quit day might not be perfect; what matters is that you don't smoke—not even one puff. Reward yourself for being smoke-free for 24 hours. You deserve it.

### 6. Ask for Help

You don't need to rely on willpower alone to be smoke-free. Tell your family and friends when your quit day is. Ask them for support on quit day and in the first few days and weeks after. Let them know exactly how they can support you. Don't assume they'll know. Be honest about your needs. If using nicotine replacement therapy is part of your plan, be sure to start using it first thing in the morning. Finally, Smokefree.gov has many tools to help you, including a text message program, apps to help you track cravings and monitor your progress, online chats with a cessation counselor, and a Facebook page.

SOURCES: Smokefree.gov. n.d. Build My Smoking Quit Plan (http://smokefree.gov/build-your-quit-plan); Smokefree.gov. n.d. *My Quit Day* (https://smokefree.gov/quit-smoking/pick-your-path/my-quit-day).

poisons and tars produced by burning tobacco. Less of the product is used over time as the need for nicotine decreases.

Nicotine replacement products come in several forms, including patches, gum, lozenges, nasal sprays, and inhalers. They are available in a variety of strengths and can be worked into many different smoking cessation strategies. Most are available without a prescription.

The nicotine patch is popular because it can be applied and forgotten until it needs to be removed or changed, usually every 16 or 24 hours. Placed on the upper arm or torso, it releases a steady stream of nicotine, which is absorbed through the skin. The main side effects are skin irritation and redness. Nicotine gum and nicotine lozenges have the advantage of allowing the smoker to use them whenever he or she craves nicotine. Side effects of nicotine gum include mouth sores and headaches; nicotine lozenges can cause nausea and heartburn. Nicotine nasal sprays and inhalers are available only by prescription.

Although all these products have proved to be effective in helping users stop smoking, experts recommend them only as one part of a complete smoking cessation program. Such a program should include regular professional counseling and physician monitoring.

## SUMMARY

- Although alcohol has long been a part of human celebrations, it is a psychoactive drug capable of causing dependence and AUD.
- After being absorbed into the bloodstream, alcohol is transported throughout the body. The liver metabolizes alcohol as blood circulates through it.
- If people drink more alcohol each hour than the body can metabolize, blood alcohol concentration (BAC) increases. The rate of alcohol metabolism depends on a variety of individual factors.
- At higher doses, alcohol interferes with motor and mental functioning; at very high doses, alcohol poisoning, coma, and death can occur. Effects may be increased if alcohol is combined with other drugs.
- Chronic alcohol use has negative effects on the digestive and cardiovascular systems and increases cancer risk and overall mortality.
- Alcohol misuse involves drinking in dangerous situations or drinking to a degree that causes academic, professional, interpersonal, or legal difficulties.
- AUD is characterized by more extensive problems with alcohol, usually involving tolerance and withdrawal.
- Physical consequences of alcohol misuse include the direct effects of tolerance and withdrawal, as well as all the problems associated with chronic drinking. Psychological problems associated with alcohol misuse include memory loss and additional mental disorders such as depression.
- AUD treatment includes mutual support groups like AA, job- and school-based programs, inpatient hospital programs, and pharmacological treatments.
- Supporting someone who misuses alcohol means not enabling them and finding support for yourself (i.e., Al-Anon and other family and friend groups) and potentially helping the person find useful information about available resources, e.g., treatment programs and support groups.
- Smoking is the largest preventable cause of premature disease and death in the United States. Nevertheless, millions of Americans use tobacco.
- Regular tobacco use causes physical dependence on nicotine, characterized by loss of control, tolerance, and withdrawal. Habits can become associated with tobacco use and trigger the urge for a cigarette.
- Tobacco and vape smoke is made up of thousands of chemicals, including some that are carcinogenic or toxic or that damage the respiratory system.
- Nicotine acts on the nervous system as a stimulant or a depressant. It can cause blood pressure and heart rate to increase, straining the heart.
- Cardiovascular disease is the most widespread cause of death for cigarette smokers. Cigarette smoking is the primary cause of lung cancer and is linked to many other cancers and respiratory diseases.
- Cigarette smoking is linked to ulcers, impotence, reproductive health problems, dental diseases, and other conditions. Tobacco use leads to lower life expectancy and to a diminished quality of life.
- The use of smokeless tobacco leads to nicotine addiction and is linked to a variety of cancers of the head and neck.
- Environmental tobacco smoke (ETS) contains high concentrations of toxic chemicals and can cause headaches, eye and nasal irritation, and sinus problems. Long-term exposure to ETS causes cancer and heart disease. Both secondhand and thirdhand smoke contribute to these devastating effects.
- Individuals and groups have many options for acting against tobacco use. Nonsmokers can use social pressure and legislative channels to assert their rights to breathe clean air.
- Giving up smoking is a difficult and long-term process. Many smokers benefit from stop-smoking programs, over-the-counter and prescription medications, and support groups.

## FOR MORE INFORMATION

*Al-Anon Family Group Headquarters.* Provides information and referrals to local Al-Anon and Alateen groups. The website includes a self-quiz to determine if you are affected by someone's drinking.

http://www.al-anon.alateen.org

*Action on Smoking and Health (ASH).* Provides statistics, news briefs, and other information.

http://ash.org

*Alcoholics Anonymous (AA) World Services.* Provides general information about AA, literature about alcoholism, and information about AA meetings and related 12-step organizations.

http://www.aa.org

*AlcoholScreening.Org.* Provides information about alcohol and health, referrals for treatment and support groups, and a drinking self-assessment.

http://www.alcoholscreening.org

*American Cancer Society (ACS).* Provides information about the dangers of tobacco, as well as tools for prevention and cessation for both smokers and users of smokeless tobacco; sponsors the annual Great American Smokeout.

http://www.cancer.org

*American Lung Association.* Provides information about lung diseases, tobacco control, and environmental health.

http://www.lung.org

*CDC's Tobacco Information and Prevention Source (TIPS).* Provides research results, educational materials, and tips on how to quit smoking; website includes special sections for kids and teens.

http://www.cdc.gov/tobacco

*Center for Responsive Politics (CRP).* A nonprofit, nonpartisan research group based in Washington, DC, that tracks the effects of money and lobbying on elections and public policy, including spending and lobbying by the tobacco industry.

http://www.opensecrets.org

*College Drinking: Changing the Culture.* Created by the National Institute on Alcohol Abuse and Alcoholism (NIAAA), this site gives comprehensive research-based information on issues related to alcohol abuse and binge drinking among college students.

http://www.collegedrinkingprevention.gov

*National Association for Children of Addiction (NACoA).* Provides information and support for children of alcoholics.

http://www.nacoa.org

*National Council on Alcoholism and Drug Dependence (NCADD).* Provides information and counseling referrals. Website URLs depend on your state and local chapter.

800-NCA-CALL (24-hour Hope Line)

*National Institute on Alcohol Abuse and Alcoholism (NIAAA).* Provides booklets and other publications on a variety of alcohol-related topics, including fetal alcohol syndrome, alcoholism treatment, and alcohol use and minorities.

http://www.niaaa.nih.gov

*National Institute on Alcohol Abuse and Alcoholism's Director's Blog.* NIAAA Director Dr. George F. Koob shares information about alcohol and stress, including Covid-19 information, and the neurobiology of alcohol and drug addiction.

https://www.niaaa.nih.gov/directors-blog-alcohol-poses-different-challenges-during-covid-19-pandemic

*Nicotine Anonymous.* A 12-step program for tobacco users.

http://www.nicotine-anonymous.org

*Smokefree.gov.* Provides step-by-step strategies for quitting as well as expert support via telephone or instant messaging.

http://www.smokefree.gov

*Substance Abuse and Mental Health Services Administration.* Provides statistics and information about alcohol abuse, including resources for people who want to help friends and family members overcome alcohol abuse problems.

http://www.samhsa.gov

*World No Tobacco Day (WNTD).* Provides information about the annual worldwide event to encourage people to quit smoking; includes general information about tobacco use and testimonials of ex-smokers.

https://www.who.int/tobacco/wntd/en/

See also the listings for Chapters 9, 15, and 16.

## SELECTED BIBLIOGRAPHY

Addiction Center. 2021. *Alcohol-Related Crime* (https://www.addictioncenter.com/alcohol/alcohol-related-crime/).

American Cancer Society. 2021. *Cancer Facts and Figures, 2021.* Atlanta, GA: American Cancer Society.

American College Health Association. 2019. *American College Health Association-National College Health Assessment IIc: Reference Group Executive Summary Spring 2019.* Hanover, MD: American College Health Association.

American College Health Association. 2021. *American College Health Association-National College Health Assessment III: Reference Group Executive Summary Spring 2021.* Hanover, MD: American College Health Association (https://www.acha.org/documents/ncha/NCHA-III_SPRING-2021_REFERENCE_GROUP_EXECUTIVE_SUMMARY_updated.pdf).

American Heart Association. 2022. Is drinking alcohol part of a healthy lifestyle? *American Heart Association News* (https://www.heart.org/en/healthy-living/healthy-eating/eat-smart/nutrition-basics/alcohol-and-heart-health).

American Lung Association. 2020. *Smokefree Air Laws* (http://www.lung.org/policy-advocacy/tobacco/smokefree-environments/smokefree-air-laws.html).

American Lung Association. 2020. *What's in a Cigarette?* (https://www.lung.org/stop-smoking/smoking-facts/whats-in-a-cigarette.html)

American Nonsmokers' Rights Foundation. 2021. *Overview List–Number of Smokefree and Other Tobacco-Related Laws* (http://no-smoke.org/wp-content/uploads/pdf/mediaordlist.pdf).

American Psychiatric Association. 2013. *Diagnostic and Statistical Manual of Mental Disorders,* 5th ed. *(DSM-5).* Washington, DC: American Psychiatric Publishing.

Armstrong, D., and Bloomberg. 2019. Slashing cigarette nicotine levels no longer on FDA's agenda. *Fortune* (https://fortune.com/2019/11/20/fda-nicotine-plan-cigarettes-no-longer-on-agenda/).

Berning, F., et al. 2020. Drug and alcohol prevalence in seriously and fatally injured road users before and during the COVID-19 public health emergency. *National Highway Traffic Safety Administration* (https://rosap.ntl.bts.gov/view/dot/50941).

Biddinger, K. J., et al. 2022. Association of habitual alcohol intake with risk of cardiovascular disease. *JAMA Network Open* 5(3): e223849.

Booker, B. 2019. TV broadcasters to stop taking e-cigarette ads. National Public Radio (https://www.npr.org/sections/health-shots/2019/09/19/762410165/tv-broadcasters-to-stop-taking-e-cigarette-ads).

Campaign for Tobacco-Free Kids. 2021. *State Cigarette Excise Tax Rates and Rankings.* Washington, DC: Campaign for Tobacco-Free Kids.

Campaign for Tobacco-Free Kids. 2021. *Tobacco Company Political Action Committee (PAC) Contributions to Federal Candidates* (https://www.tobaccofreekids.org/what_we_do/federal_issues/campaign_contributions).

Cao, Y., et al. 2015. Light to moderate intake of alcohol, drinking patterns, and risk of cancer: Results from two prospective US cohort studies. *British Medical Journal* 351: h4238.

Castilo-Carniglia, A., et al. 2019. Psychiatric comorbidities in alcohol use disorder. *Lancet Psychiatry* 6(12): 1068–1080.

Centers for Disease Control and Prevention. 2020. *Outbreak of Lung Injury Associated with the Use of E-Cigarette, or Vaping, Products* (https://www.cdc.gov/tobacco/basic_information/e-cigarettes/severe-lung-disease.html).

Centers for Disease Control and Prevention. 2020. *Smoking & Tobacco Use: Tobacco-Related Mortality* (https://www.cdc.gov/tobacco/data_statistics/fact_sheets/health_effects/tobacco_related_mortality/index.htm#cigs).

Centers for Disease Control and Prevention. 2021. Deaths from Excessive Alcohol Use in the United States. (https://www.cdc.gov/alcohol/features/excessive-alcohol-deaths.html.

Centers for Disease Control and Prevention. 2021. *Economic Trends in Tobacco* (https://www.cdc.gov/tobacco/data_statistics/fact_sheets/economics/econ_facts/index.htm).

Centers for Disease Control and Prevention. 2021. *Smoking & Tobacco Use: Secondhand Smoke* (https://www.cdc.gov/tobacco/basic_information/secondhand_smoke/index.htm).

Centers for Disease Control and Prevention. 2021. *State Tobacco Activities Tracking and Evaluation (STATE) System* (http://www.cdc.gov/STATESystem).

Centers for Disease Control and Prevention. 2022. *Binge Drinking* (https://www.cdc.gov/alcohol/fact-sheets/binge-drinking.htm).

Centers for Disease Control and Prevention. 2022. *Fetal Alcohol Spectrum Disorders (FASD)* (https://www.cdc.gov/ncbddd/fasd/data.html#ref).

Centers for Disease Control and Prevention. 2022. *Lesbian, Gay, Bisexual, and Transgender Persons and Tobacco Use* (https://www.cdc.gov/tobacco/disparities/lgbt/index.htm).

Centers for Disease Control and Prevention. 2022. *Smoking & Tobacco Use: Fast Facts and Fact Sheets* (https://www.cdc.gov/tobacco/data_statistics/fact_sheets/index.htm?s_cid=osh-stu-home-spotlight-001).

Centers for Disease Control and Prevention. n.d. *Electronic Cigarettes: What's the Bottom Line?* (https://www.cdc.gov/tobacco/basic_information/e-cigarettes/pdfs/Electronic-Cigarettes-Infographic-p.pdf

Center for Responsive Politics. 2021. *Tobacco: Industry Profile: Tobacco* (https://www.opensecrets.org/lobby/indusclient.php?id=A02).

Center for Responsive Politics. 2021. *Tobacco: Opensecrets* (https://www.opensecrets.org/industries/lobbying.php?cycle=2018&ind=A02).

College Drinking Prevention. n.d. *A Snapshot of Annual High-Risk College Drinking Consequences* (http://www.collegedrinkingprevention.gov/StatsSummaries/snapshot.aspx).

Cornelius, M. E., et al. 2022. Tobacco product use among adults–United States, 2020. *Morbidity and Mortality Weekly Report* 71: 397–405.

Cunningham, J. K., T. A. Solomon, and M. L. Muramoto. 2016. Alcohol use among Native Americans compared to whites: Examining the veracity of the 'Native American elevated alcohol consumption' belief. *Drug and Alcohol Dependence* 160: 65–75.

Daniel, C., et al. 2021. Electronic cigarettes: Their role in the lives of college students. *Journal of Pharmacy Practice* (https://doi.org/10.1177/08971900211026841).

Daube, M. 2015. Alcohol's evaporating health benefits. *British Medical Journal* 350: h407.

Division of Reproductive Health, National Center for Chronic Disease Prevention and Health Promotion. 2020. *Tobacco Use and Pregnancy* (https://www.cdc.gov/reproductivehealth/maternalinfanthealth/substance-abuse/substance-abuse-during-pregnancy.htm?CDC_AA_refVal=https%3A%2F%2Fwww.cdc.gov%2Freproductivehealth%2Fmaternalinfanthealth%2Ftobaccousepregnancy%2Findex.htm).

Drake, P., A. K. Driscoll, and T. J. Mathews. 2018. Cigarette smoking during pregnancy: United States, 2016. *NCHS Data Brief* 305. Hyattsville, MD: National Center for Health Statistics (https://www.cdc.gov/nchs/products/databriefs/db305.htm).

Ducharme, J. 2019. As the number of vaping-related deaths climbs, these states have implemented e-cigarette bans. *Time* (https://time.com/5685936/state-vaping-bans/).

Enoch, M.-A., and B. J. Albaugh. 2017. Genetic and environmental risk factors for alcohol use disorders in American Indians and Alaskan Natives. *The American Journal on Addictions* 26(5): 461–468.

Federal Trade Commission. 2019. *Federal Trade Commission Cigarette Report for 2017.* Washington, DC: Federal Trade Commission.

Federal Trade Commission. 2021. FTC report finds annual cigarette sales increased for the first time in 20 years (https://www.ftc.gov/news-events/press-releases/2021/10/ftc-report-finds-annual-cigarette-sales-increased-first-time-20).

Food and Drug Administration. 2019. *How FDA Is Regulating E-Cigarettes* (https://www.fda.gov/news-events/fda-voices/how-fda-regulating-e-cigarettes).

Gentzke, A. S., et al. 2022. Tobacco product use and associated factors among middle and high school students–National Youth Tobacco Survey, United States, 2021. *Morbidity and Mortality Weekly Report* 71(5): 1–30.

Gonçalves, A., et al. 2015. Relationship between alcohol consumption and cardiac structure and function in the elderly: The Atherosclerosis Risk in Communities Study. *Circulation: Cardiovascular Imaging* 8(6): e002846.

Hagström, H., et al. 2018. Alcohol consumption in late adolescence is associated with an increased risk of severe liver disease later in life. *Journal of Hepatology* 68(3): 505–510.

Kane, J. C., et al. 2016. Differences in alcohol use patterns between adolescent Asian American ethnic groups: Representative estimates from the National Survey on Drug Use and Health 2002–2013. *Addictive Behaviors* 64: 154–158.

Kaplan, R. M. 2020. Cancer deaths, smoking, and Rodney Dangerfield. *Health Affairs* (https://www.healthaffairs.org/do/10.1377/hblog20200417.775123/full/).

Kwok, A., A. L. Aimee, and G. Paton. 2019. Effect of alcohol consumption on food energy intake: A systematic review and meta-analysis. *British Journal of Nutrition* 121(5): 481–495.

Leone, R. M., et al. 2022. A laboratory study of the effects of men's acute alcohol intoxication, perceptions of women's intoxication, and masculine gender role stress on the perpetration of sexual aggression. *Alcoholism: Clinical & Experimental Research* 46: 166–176.

Lipari, R. N., and B. Jean-Francois. 2016. *A Day in the Life of College Students Aged 18 to 22: Substance Use Facts.* Rockville, MD: Center for Behavioral Health Statistics and Quality, Substance Abuse and Mental Health Services Administration.

LoConte, N. K., et al. 2017. Alcohol and cancer: A statement of the American Society of Clinical Oncology. *Journal of Clinical Oncology* 36(1): 83–93.

Luczak, S. E., et al. 2017. A review of the prevalence and co-occurrence of addictions in US ethnic/racial groups: Implications for genetic research. *The American Journal on Addictions* 26(5): 424–436.

Mascarenhas, L. 2021, Aug. 26. FDA blocks sale of 55,000 flavored e-cigarette products. *CNN Health* (www.cnn.com/2021/08/26/health/fda-blocks-ecig-products/index.html).

Matt, G., et al. 2017. When smokers quit: Exposure to nicotine and carcinogens persists from thirdhand smoke pollution. *Tobacco Control* 26(5): 548–556.

Moeller, F., Dougherty, D. n.d. *Antisocial Personality Disorder, Alcohol, and Aggression.* National Institute on Alcohol Abuse and Alcoholism (https://pubs.niaaa.nih.gov/publications/arh25-1/5-11.htm).

Mulia, N., et al. 2022. Effects of Medicaid expansion on alcohol and opioid treatment admissions in U.S. racial/ethnic groups. *Drug and Alcohol Dependence* 231: 109242.

Naimi, T. S. 2019. A fresh approach to the development of national alcohol guidelines. *Addiction* 114(4): 601–602.

National Center for Statistics and Analysis. 2021. Summary of motor vehicle crashes: 2019 data. *Traffic Safety Facts.* Report No. DOT HS 813 209. National Highway Traffic Safety Administration.

National Highway Traffic Safety Administration. 2021. 2020 fatality data show increased traffic fatalities during pandemic (https://www.nhtsa.gov/press-releases/2020-fatality-data-show-increased-traffic-fatalities-during-pandemic).

National Institutes of Health. n.d. *Rethinking Drinking* (https://www.rethinkingdrinking.niaaa.nih.gov/How-much-is-too-much/Whats-the-harm/What-Are-The-Consequences.aspx).

National Institute on Alcohol Abuse and Alcoholism. 2021. *Alcohol Facts and Statistics* (https://www.niaaa.nih.gov/publications/brochures-and-fact-sheets/alcohol-facts-and-statistics).

National Institute on Drug Abuse. 2018. *Cigarette Smoking Increases the Likelihood of Drug Use Relapse* (https://www.drugabuse.gov/news-events/nida-notes/2018/05/cigarette-smoking-increases-likelihood-drug-use-relapse).

Navasa, J. F.,et al. 2019. Sex differences in the association between impulsivity and driving under the influence of alcohol in young adults: The specific role of sensation seeking. *Accident Analysis & Prevention* 124: 174–179.

NIH/National Institute on Deafness and Other Communication Disorders. 2019. Genetic Vulnerability to Menthol Cigarette Use: Unexpected Sensory Variant Exclusive to African-Americans (https://www.nidcd.nih.gov/news/2019/researchers-find-genetic-vulnerability-menthol-cigarette-use).

Park-Lee E., et al. 2021. *Notes from the field:* E-cigarette use among middle and high school students–National Youth Tobacco Survey, United States. *Morbidity and Mortality Weekly Report* 70: 1387–1389.

Pierce, P. P., et al. 2021. Use of e-cigarettes and other tobacco products and progression to daily cigarette smoking. *Pediatrics* 147(2): e2020025122.

Porter, B., et al. 2020. Alcohol misuse and separation from military service: A dyadic perspective. *Addictive Behaviors* 110 (https://doi.org/10.1016/j.addbeh.2020.106512).

Rosenberry, Z. R., W. B. Pickworth, and B. Koszowski. 2018. Large cigars: Smoking topography and toxicant exposure. *Nicotine & Tobacco Research* 20(2): 183–191.

Schaeffer, K. 2019. Before recent outbreak, vaping was on the rise in U.S., especially among young people. *Pew Research Center* (https://www.pewresearch.org/fact-tank/2019/09/26/vaping-survey-data-roundup/).

Schulenberg, J. E., et al. 2021. *Monitoring the Future National Survey Results on Drug Use, 1975–2020: Volume II, College Students and Adults Ages 19-60.* Ann Arbor: Institute for Social Research, The University of Michigan (http://www.monitoringthefuture.org/pubs/monographs/mtf-vol2_2020.pdf).

Schulenberg, J. E., et al. 2019. *Monitoring the Future National Survey Results on Drug Use, 1975–2018; Volume II, College Students and Adults Ages 19–60.* Ann Arbor: Institute for Social Research, The University of Michigan.

Substance Abuse and Mental Health Services Administration. 2015. *Behavioral Health Trends in the United States: Results from the 2014 National Survey on Drug Use and Health* (HHS Publication No. SMA 15-4927, NSDUH Series H-41). Rockville, MD: Substance Abuse and Mental Health Services Administration.

Substance Abuse and Mental Health Services Administration. 2021. *Key substance use and mental health indicators in the United States: Results from the 2020 National Survey on Drug Use and Health* (HHS Publication No. PEP21-07-01-003, NSDUH Series H-56). Rockville, MD: Center for Behavioral Health Statistics and Quality.

Substance Abuse and Mental Health Services Administration Center for Behavioral Health Statistics and Quality. 2021. *Results from the 2020 National Survey on Drug Use and Health* (https://www.samhsa.gov/data/sites/default/files/reports/rpt35325/NSDUHFFRPDFWHTMLFiles2020/2020NSDUHFFR1PDFW102121.pdf).

Treat, T. A., et al. 2021. Selection and socialization accounts of the relation between fraternity membership and sexual aggression. *Psychology of Addictive Behaviors 35*(3): 337–350.

Tucker, J., Chandler, S., Witkiewitz K. 2020. Epidemiology of recovery from alcohol use disorder. *Alcohol Research* 40(3). National Institute on Alcohol Abuse and Alcoholism (https://arcr.niaaa.nih.gov/recovery-aud/epidemiology-recovery-alcohol-use-disorder#:~:text=Measures%20of%20functioning%20and%20well,low%2Drisk%20drinking%20without%20symptoms).

U.S. Department of Health and Human Services. 2020. *Smoking Cessation: A Report of the Surgeon General.* Atlanta, GA: HHS, Centers for Disease Control and Prevention, National Center for Chronic Disease Prevention and Health Promotion, Office on Smoking and Health.

U.S. Food and Drug Administration Center for Tobacco Products. 2020. *Vaporizers, E-Cigarettes, and other Electronic Nicotine Delivery Systems (ENDS).* (https://www.fda.gov/tobacco-products/products-ingredients-components/vaporizers-e-cigarettes-and-other-electronic-nicotine-delivery-systems-ends).

Vaeth, P. A. C., M. Wang-Schweig, and R. Caetano. 2017. Drinking, alcohol use disorder, and treatment access and utilization among U.S. racial/ethnic groups. *Alcoholism: Clinical and Experimental Research* 41(1): 61–69.

White, A. 2020. Gender differences in the epidemiology of alcohol use and related harms in the United States. *Alcohol Research* 40(2). National Institute on Alcohol Abuse and Alcoholism (https://arcr.niaaa.nih.gov/women-and-alcohol/gender-differences-epidemiology-alcohol-use-and-related-harms-united-states#article-toc10).

White, A. M., et al. 2022. Alcohol-related deaths during the COVID-19 pandemic. *JAMA* DOI: 10.1001/jama.2022.4308.

World Health Organization. 2020. Alcohol does not protect against COVID-19; access should be restricted during lockdown (http://www.euro.who.int/en/health-topics/disease-prevention/alcohol-use/news/news/2020/04/alcohol-does-not-protect-against-covid-19-access-should-be-restricted-during-lockdown).

Zhao, J., et al. 2017. Alcohol consumption and mortality from coronary heart disease: An updated meta-analysis of cohort studies. *Journal of Studies on Alcohol and Drugs* 78: 375–386.

**Design Elements:** Assess Yourself icon: Aleksey Boldin/Alamy Stock Photo; Diversity Matters icon: Rawpixel Ltd/Getty Images; Wellness on Campus icon: Radius Images/Alamy Stock Photo; Take Charge icon: VisualCommunications/Getty Images; Critical Consumer icon: pagadesign/Getty Images.

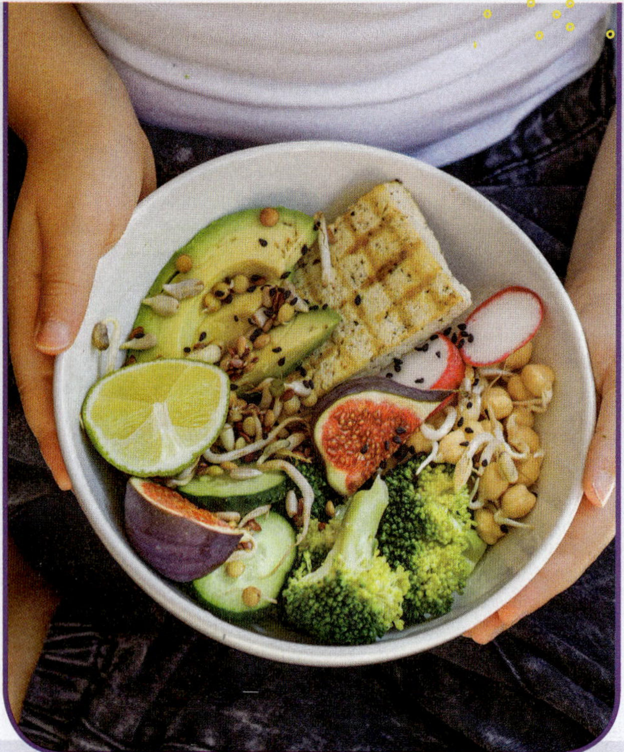

Nina Firsova/Alamy Stock Photo

## CHAPTER OBJECTIVES

- List the components of a healthy diet
- Explain how to make informed choices about foods
- Put together a personal nutrition plan

CHAPTER 10

# Nutrition Basics

This chapter examines the role of personal dietary choices and the basic principles of **nutrition.** It introduces the six classes of essential nutrients and explains their roles in health and disease. It also provides guidelines for designing a healthy diet plan. The chapter emphasizes the importance of making a personal commitment to eating right, engaging in physical activity, and staying educated about the role of our government in nutrition and public health policies to keep our food supply safe.

**TERMS**

**nutrition** The science of food and dietary supplements, and how the body uses them in health and disease.

**essential nutrients** Dietary components the body must get from foods or supplements because it cannot manufacture them to meet its needs.

**macronutrient** An important nutrient required by the body in relatively large amounts.

**micronutrient** An important nutrient required by the body in minute amounts.

**digestion** The process of breaking down foods into compounds the gastrointestinal tract can absorb and the body can use.

## COMPONENTS OF A HEALTHY DIET

If you're like most people, you think about your diet in terms of the foods you like to eat. More important for your health, though, are the nutrients contained in those foods. Your body requires proteins, fats, carbohydrates, vitamins, minerals, and water—about 45 **essential nutrients.** In this context, the word *essential* means that you must get these substances from food because your body is unable to manufacture them or make an adequate amount to meet your physiological needs. The body needs some essential nutrients in relatively large amounts; these **macronutrients** include protein, fat, carbohydrate, and water. **Micronutrients,** such as vitamins and minerals, are required in much smaller amounts.

Most nutrients become available to the body through the process of **digestion,** in which the foods we eat are broken down into compounds the gastrointestinal tract can absorb

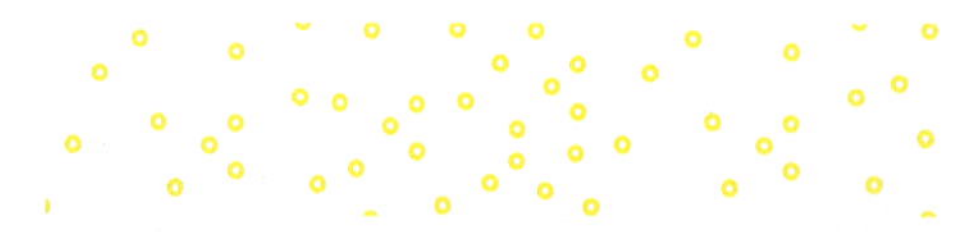

and that the body processes further and uses for normal body functions (Figure 10.1). An adequate diet must provide enough essential nutrients and energy to support and regulate various vital body functions.

The amount of energy in foods is expressed as **kilocalories (kcal)**. One kilocalorie represents the amount of heat required to raise the temperature of 1 liter of water by 1°C.

Although technically inaccurate, people usually refer to kilocalories as *calories*. This chapter uses the term *calorie* when discussing the energy unit, and food labels do as well. What's the difference between "energy" and "calorie?" **Energy** is the capacity to do work. Calories are used to measure energy. The energy in food is chemical energy, which the body converts to mechanical, electrical, or heat energy.

Of the six broad classes of essential nutrients, fat supplies the most energy per gram (9 calories) followed by protein and carbohydrate, which each supply 4 calories per gram.

QUICK STATS

**Worldwide, almost 768 million people (approximately 10% of the population) are undernourished.**

—Food and Agriculture Organization (FAO) of the United Nations, 2021

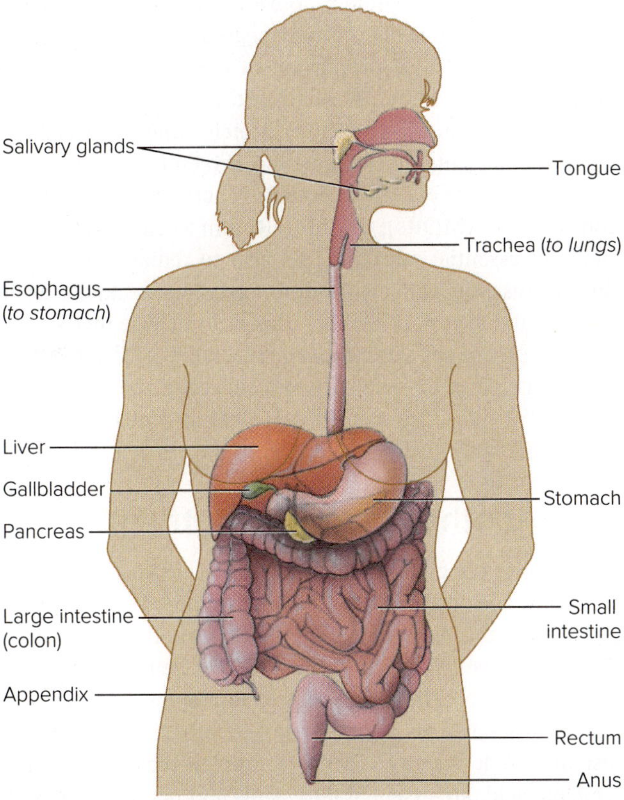

Salivary glands

Tongue

Trachea (*to lungs*)

Esophagus (*to stomach*)

Liver

Gallbladder

Stomach

Pancreas

Large intestine (colon)

Small intestine

Appendix

Rectum

Anus

**FIGURE 10.1 The digestive system.** Food is partially broken down by being chewed and mixed with saliva in the mouth. After traveling to the stomach via the esophagus, food is broken down further by stomach acids and other secretions. As food moves through the digestive tract, it is mixed by muscular contractions to facilitate further digestion and absorption. Most absorption of nutrients occurs via the lining of the small intestine. The large intestine reabsorbs excess water; the remaining solid wastes are collected in the rectum and excreted through the anus.

Alcohol, though not an essential component of our diet, also supplies energy, providing 7 calories per gram. (One gram equals about the weight of a small paperclip.) Certain calories consumed in excess of your energy needs may be converted into fat that is then stored in the body.

Just meeting energy needs is not enough. Our bodies also need an adequate amount of the essential nutrients to function properly. Many Americans consume sufficient or excess calories but not enough essential nutrients. Nearly all foods contain combinations of nutrients, although foods are sometimes classified according to their predominant nutrient; for example, pastas are considered carbohydrate foods even though they also contain other nutrients.

**Nutrient density** is an important concept related to food energy. Nutrient-dense foods such as brown rice, lean beef, and butternut squash are high in essential nutrients but relatively low in calories. Think of your daily calorie intake as a budget: You need to spend your calories wisely on nutrient-dense foods to obtain all essential nutrients while staying within your budget.

## Proteins—The Basis of Body Structure

**Proteins** form important parts of the body's main structural components: muscles and bones. They also form important parts of blood, enzymes, some hormones, and cell membranes.

### Amino Acids

The building blocks of proteins are called **amino acids.** Twenty common amino acids are found in food proteins. Nine of these amino acids are essential (sometimes called indispensable). As long as foods supply certain nutrients, the body can produce the other 11 amino acids.

### Complete and Incomplete Proteins

Individual protein sources are considered *complete* if they supply all the essential amino acids in adequate amounts and *incomplete* if they do not. Meat, fish, poultry, eggs, milk, cheese, and soy provide complete proteins. Incomplete proteins, which come from other plant sources such as nuts and legumes (dried

TERMS

**kilocalorie (kcal)** A measure of energy content in food; 1 kilocalorie represents the amount of heat needed to raise the temperature of 1 liter of water 1°C; commonly referred to as a *calorie*.

**energy** The capacity to do work, measured by calories. We get energy from certain nutrients in food.

**nutrient density** The ratio of a food's essential nutrients to its calories.

**protein** An essential nutrient that forms important parts of the body's main structures (muscles and bones) as well as blood, enzymes, hormones, and cell membranes; also provides energy.

**amino acid** One of the building blocks of proteins; 20 common amino acids are found in foods.

## Table 10.1 Goals for Protein, Fat, and Carbohydrate Intake

| | DAILY ADEQUATE INTAKE DISTRIBUTION (GRAMS)* | | ACCEPTABLE MACRONUTRIENT DISTRIBUTION RANGE (PERCENTAGE OF TOTAL DAILY CALORIES) |
|---|---|---|---|
| | MEN | WOMEN | |
| Protein** | 56 | 46 | 10–35 |
| Fat (total) | | | 20–35 |
| Linoleic acid | 17 | 12 | |
| Alpha-linolenic acid | 1.6 | 1.1 | |
| Carbohydrate | 130 | 130 | 45–65 |

*To meet daily energy needs, you must consume more than the minimally adequate amounts of the energy-providing nutrients listed here, which alone supply only 800–900 calories. Use the AMDRs to set overall daily goals.

**Protein-intake goals can be calculated more specifically by multiplying your body weight in pounds by 0.36.

**NOTE:** Individuals can allocate total daily energy intake among the three classes of macronutrients to suit individual preferences. To translate percentage goals into daily-intake goals expressed in calories and grams, multiply the appropriate percentages by your total daily energy intake and then divide the results by the corresponding calories per gram. For example, a fat limit of 35% applied to a 2200-calorie diet would be calculated as follows: 0.35 × 2200 = 770 calories of total fat; 770 ÷ 9 calories per gram = 86 grams of total fat.

**SOURCE:** Recommendations from Food and Nutrition Board, Institute of Medicine. 2005. *Dietary Reference Intakes for Energy, Carbohydrate, Fiber, Fat, Fatty Acids, Cholesterol, Protein, and Amino Acids.* Washington, DC: National Academies Press.

## Table 10.2 Protein Content of Common Food Items

| ITEM | PROTEIN (GRAMS)* |
|---|---|
| 3 ounces lean meat, poultry, or fish | 20–27 |
| ¼ block (3 ounces) tofu | 7 |
| 1 cup cooked beans (black, white, pinto) | 15–17 |
| 1 cup yogurt | 8–13 |
| 1 ounce cheese (cheddar, Swiss) | 6–8 |
| ½–1 cup cereals | 1–6 |
| 1 egg cooked | 6 |
| 1 cup ricotta cheese | 28 |
| 1 cup milk | 8 |
| 1 ounce nuts | 2–6 |

*For the specific protein content of a food, check the food label or the searchable USDA food composition database (https://fdc.nal.usda.gov/)

**SOURCE:** U.S. Department of Agriculture, Agricultural Research Service, Food Data Central (https://fdc.nal.usda.gov/).

beans, peas, and lentils), are good sources of most essential amino acids but are usually low in one or more.

Certain combinations of vegetable proteins create a complete protein. For example, legumes or grains (peanut butter or whole wheat bread) eaten separately lack certain essential amino acids; but eaten together, the combination makes up for the missing ones. Many traditional food pairings, such as beans and rice or corn and beans, have emerged as dietary staples because together they provide complementary proteins. About two-thirds of the protein in the typical American diet comes from animal sources (meat and dairy products); vegetarians should include a variety of vegetable protein sources in their diets to make sure they get enough of all the essential amino acids.

**Recommended Protein Intake** The Food and Nutrition Board of the National Academy of Medicine has established goals to help ensure adequate intake of protein as well as the other macronutrients (Table 10.1). For protein, adequate daily intake for adults is 0.8 gram per kilogram (0.36 gram per pound) of body weight. So, if you weigh 140 pounds, you should consume at least 50 grams of protein per day, and if you weigh 180 pounds, then 65 grams of protein per day represents adequate intake.

Most Americans meet or exceed the protein intake needed for adequate nutrition. If you consume substantially more protein than your body needs, the extra energy from protein is synthesized into fat for storage or burned for energy requirements, depending on your overall energy intake.

Consuming some protein above the amount needed for adequate nutrition is not harmful; suggested daily intake limits have been set as a proportion of overall calories rather than as specific amounts. The Food and Nutrition Board recommendations for how much protein (and other energy-supplying nutrients) to consume as a percentage of total daily energy intake are called Acceptable Macronutrient Distribution Ranges (AMDRs); the AMDRs aim to ensure adequate intake of essential nutrients and also to reduce the risk of chronic diseases. The AMDR for protein for adults aged 19 years and over is 10–35% of total daily calorie intake (see Table 10.2): For someone consuming a 2000-calorie diet, this percentage range corresponds to a suggested daily intake of between 50 and 175 grams per day. Healthy protein-rich food choices are described in detail later in the chapter.

## Fat—Another Essential Nutrient

At 9 calories per gram, fats, also known as *lipids,* are the most concentrated source of energy. The fats stored in your body represent usable energy, help insulate your body, and support and cushion your organs. Fats in the diet help your body to absorb fat-soluble vitamins, and they add important flavor and texture to foods. Fats are the major fuel for the body during rest and light activity. Two fats, linoleic acid and alpha-linolenic acid, are essential fatty acids and necessary components of the diet. They are used to make compounds that are key regulators of body functions such as the maintenance of blood pressure and the progress of a healthy pregnancy.

**Types and Sources of Fats** Called *triglycerides,* most fats in foods are fairly similar in basic composition, generally including a molecule of glycerol (an alcohol) with three fatty acid chains attached to it. Both animal fats and plant fats (oils) are made primarily of triglycerides.

**Table 10.3** Types of Fatty Acids

| TYPE OF FATTY ACID | FOUND IN* |
|---|---|
| Saturated | • Animal fats (especially fatty meats and poultry fat and skin)<br>• Butter, cheese, and other high-fat dairy products<br>• Palm and coconut oils |
| Monounsaturated | • Olive, canola, and safflower oils<br>• Avocados, olives<br>• Peanut butter (without added fat)<br>• Many nuts, including almonds, cashews, pecans, and pistachios |
| Polyunsaturated–omega-3† | • Fatty fish, including salmon, white albacore tuna, mackerel, anchovies, and sardines<br>• Compared to fish, lesser amounts are found in canola and soybean oils; tofu; walnuts; flaxseeds; and dark green leafy vegetables |
| Polyunsaturated–omega-6† | • Corn, soybean, and cottonseed oils (often used in margarine, mayonnaise, and salad dressings) |

*Food fats contain a combination of types of fatty acids in various proportions. For example, canola oil is composed mainly of monounsaturated fatty acids (62%) but also contains polyunsaturated (32%) and saturated (6%) fatty acids.

†The essential fatty acids are polyunsaturated: Linoleic acid is an omega-6 fatty acid and alpha-linolenic acid is an omega-3 fatty acid.

Within a triglyceride, differences in the fatty acid structure result in different types of fats. Depending on this structure, a fat may be saturated or unsaturated, monounsaturated or polyunsaturated. The essential fatty acids linoleic acid (omega-6) and alpha-linolenic acid (omega-3) are both polyunsaturated. Different types of fatty acids have different characteristics and therefore varied effects on health.

Food fats are usually composed of both saturated and unsaturated fatty acids. The dominant type of fatty acid determines the fat's characteristics. Food fats containing large amounts of saturated fatty acids or trans fatty acids are usually solid at room temperature; they are generally found naturally in animal products or in products containing hydrogenated oils. The leading sources of saturated fat in the American diet are red meats, whole milk, cheese, hot dogs, and lunch meats. Palm and coconut oils, also known as "tropical oils," although derived from plants, are also highly saturated and are solid or semisolid at room temperature. To find good sources of polyunsaturated fats, look for omega-3 fatty acids in fatty fish such as salmon, mackerel and sardines, and in walnuts, flaxseed, and canola or soybean oil. Look for the other main type of polyunsaturated fat, omega-6 fatty acids, in vegetable oils such as safflower, soybean, sunflower, walnut, and corn oils or items made from these. (See Table 10.3.)

### Hydrogenation and Trans Fats

When unsaturated vegetable oils undergo the chemical process known as **hydrogenation,** the result is a more solid fat from a liquid oil. The mixture contains both saturated and unsaturated fatty acids. Hydrogenation also changes some unsaturated fatty acids into **trans fatty acids**–known as artificial trans fats. Food manufacturers use hydrogenation to increase the stability of an oil so that it can be reused for deep frying, to improve the texture of certain foods (to make pie crusts flakier, for example), and to extend the shelf life of foods made with oil.

Trans fats added through hydrogenation (i.e., artificial trans fats) are associated with an increase in **low-density lipoprotein (LDL) cholesterol**, or "bad" cholesterol, and have been shown to increase the risk of cardiovascular disease, increase inflammation, damage the lining of the vascular system, and increase insulin resistance, which affects type 2 diabetes. Because of these health risks, the U.S. Food and Drug Administration (FDA) in 2015 banned the use of added trans fats. By 2021 the results of the ban dropped the level of artificial trans fat in our food supply to near zero, which is expected to reduce the incidence of coronary heart disease and prevent thousands of fatal heart attacks each year.

Small amounts of trans fats occur naturally in animal fat products such as beef, dairy, and lamb. A number of studies have found that natural trans fats have little or no effect on heart health.

### Recommended Fat Intake

Limits for total fat, saturated fat, and trans fat intake have been set by several government and research organizations at 20–35% of total daily calories. The recent Dietary Guidelines suggest that saturated fats be kept at <10% of total calories. It takes only 3–4 teaspoons (15–20 grams) of vegetable oil per day incorporated into your

**TERMS**

**hydrogenation** A chemical process by which hydrogen atoms are added to molecules of unsaturated fats, increasing the degree of saturation and turning liquid oils into solid fats. Hydrogenation produces a mixture of saturated fatty acids, and *cis* (standard) and *trans* forms of unsaturated fatty acids.

**trans fatty acid** A type of unsaturated fatty acid produced during the process of hydrogenation; trans fats have an atypical shape that affects their chemical activity. Trans fats are associated with an increase in LDL cholesterol and with endothelial dysfunction, attributes associated with risk of heart disease.

**cholesterol** A waxy substance in the blood and cells, needed for synthesis of cell membranes, vitamin D, and hormones.

**low-density lipoprotein (LDL) cholesterol** Blood fat that transports cholesterol to organs and tissues; excess amounts result in the accumulation of deposits in artery walls, causing hardening of the arteries and potentially cardiovascular disease.

diet to supply the essential fatty acids linoleic and linolenic, and most Americans consume sufficient amounts of the essential fats.

The latest federal guidelines place greater emphasis on choosing healthy unsaturated fats in place of saturated and trans fats. It is also important to avoid highly processed reduced-fat foods that substitute refined carbohydrates and added sugars for fats. Information about the types of fats present in a food can be found on the food label or, for unlabeled products, in nutrition guides and online. It is important to check ingredient labels for "partially hydrogenated oils:" As long as a product has no more than half a gram of trans fats, the label may claim zero.

## Carbohydrates—An Important Source of Energy

**Carbohydrates** are needed in the diet primarily to supply energy for body cells. Some cells, such as those in the brain, in (parts of) the nervous system, and in blood, prefer the carbohydrate glucose for fuel. During higher-intensity exercise, muscles also use energy from carbohydrates as their primary fuel source. Eating the equivalent of just three or four slices of bread supplies the body's daily minimum need for carbohydrates.

**Simple and Complex Carbohydrates** Carbohydrates are classified into two groups: simple and complex. *Simple carbohydrates* include single sugar molecules (monosaccharides) and double sugar molecules (disaccharides). The monosaccharides are glucose, fructose, and galactose. Glucose is the most common sugar and is used by both animals and plants for energy. Fructose is a very sweet sugar that is found in fruits, and galactose is the sugar in milk. The disaccharides are pairs of single sugars; they include sucrose or table sugar (fructose + glucose), maltose or malt sugar (glucose + glucose), and lactose or milk sugar (galactose + glucose). Simple carbohydrates add sweetness to foods; they are found naturally in fruits and milk and are added to soft drinks, fruit drinks, candy, sweet desserts, and a variety of other processed foods. As described below, diets high in added sugars are linked to obesity.

*Complex carbohydrates* include starches and most types of dietary fiber. Starches are found in a variety of plants, especially grains (wheat, rye, rice, oats, barley, and millet), legumes (dry beans, peas, and lentils), and tubers (potatoes and yams). Most other vegetables contain a mixture of complex and simple carbohydrates. Fiber, discussed in the next section, is found in grains, fruits, vegetables, legumes, and nuts.

TERMS

**carbohydrate** An essential nutrient, required for energy for cells; sugars, starches, and dietary fiber are all carbohydrates.

**glucose** A simple sugar that is the body's basic fuel.

**glycogen** A complex carbohydrate stored in the liver and muscles.

**whole grain** The entire edible portion of a grain (such as wheat, rice, or oats), consisting of the germ, endosperm, and bran; processing removes parts of the grain, often leaving just the endosperm.

During digestion, your body breaks down carbohydrates into single sugar molecules, such as **glucose,** for absorption. Once glucose is in the bloodstream, the pancreas releases the hormone insulin, which allows cells to take up glucose and use it for energy. The liver and muscles take up glucose to provide carbohydrate storage in the form of **glycogen.** Some people have problems controlling their blood glucose levels, a disorder called *diabetes mellitus* (Chapter 12).

**Refined versus Whole Grains** Complex carbohydrates from grains can be further divided into processed (refined) carbohydrates and whole grains (unrefined carbohydrates). Before they are processed, all grains are **whole grains,** consisting of an inner layer, the germ; a middle layer, the endosperm; and an outer layer, the bran. During processing, the germ and bran are often removed, leaving just the starchy endosperm. The refinement of whole grains transforms whole-wheat flour into white flour, brown rice into white rice, and so on.

Processed grains usually retain all the calories of their unrefined counterparts, but they tend to be much lower in fiber, vitamins, minerals, and other beneficial compounds–in other words, they are less nutrient dense. Processed grain products may be enriched or fortified with vitamins and minerals, but not all the nutrients lost in processing are replaced.

Whole grains tend to take longer to chew and digest than refined ones; they also enter the bloodstream more slowly. This slower digestive pace tends to make people feel full sooner and for a longer period. Also, a slower rise in blood glucose levels following the consumption of unrefined complex carbohydrates may help in the management of diabetes. Whole grains are also high in dietary fiber and so have all the benefits of fiber (discussed later).

Consumption of whole grains has been linked to a reduced risk of heart disease, diabetes, obesity, and cancer and plays an important role in gastrointestinal health and body weight management. For all these reasons, whole grains are recommended over those that have been processed. This does not mean that you should never eat processed carbohydrates such as white bread or white rice–simply that whole-wheat bread, brown rice, and other whole grains are healthier choices. See the box "Choosing More Whole-Grain Foods" for tips on increasing your intake of whole grains.

**Added Sugars** Food manufacturers or individuals sometimes add sugars to foods. The term *added sugars* refers to white sugar, brown sugar, high-fructose corn syrup, and other sweeteners added to processed foods. Naturally occurring sugars in fruit and milk are not considered added sugars. Foods high in added sugar tend to be higher in calories and lower in essential nutrients and fiber, thus providing "empty calories." High intake of added sugars from foods and sugar-sweetened beverages is associated with dental caries (cavities), excess body weight, and increased risk of type 2 diabetes, and it may also increase risk for hypertension, stroke, and heart disease.

Added sugars currently contribute about 250–300 calories in the typical daily American diet, representing about 13–17% of total energy intake. A limit of 10% is suggested by the U.S. Department of Agriculture (USDA) and the American Heart

## TAKE CHARGE
### Choosing More Whole-Grain Foods

Because whole-grain foods offer so many health benefits, federal dietary guidelines recommend six or more servings of grain products every day, with at least half of those servings from whole grains. Currently, however, Americans average less than one serving of whole grains per day.

#### What Are Whole Grains?

The first step in increasing your intake of whole grains is to correctly identify them. The following are whole grains:

| | |
|---|---|
| Whole wheat | Whole-grain corn |
| Whole rye | Popcorn |
| Whole oats | Brown rice |
| Oatmeal | Whole-grain barley |

More unusual choices include bulgur (cracked wheat), millet, kasha (roasted buckwheat kernels), quinoa, wheat and rye berries, amaranth, wild rice, graham flour, whole-grain kamut, whole-grain spelt, and whole-grain triticale.

Wheat flour, unbleached flour, enriched flour, and degerminated corn meal are not whole grains. Wheat germ and wheat bran are also not whole grains, but they are the constituents of wheat typically left out when wheat is processed and so are healthier choices than regular wheat flour, which typically contains just the grain's endosperm.

#### Checking Packages for Whole Grains

To find packaged foods—such as bread or pasta—that are rich in whole grains, read the list of ingredients and check for special health claims related to whole grains. The *first* item on the list of ingredients should be one of the whole grains in the preceding list. Product names and food color can be misleading. *When in doubt, always check the list of ingredients and make sure "whole" is the first word on the list.* The word "enriched" means that it is white flour to which some of the nutrients that were removed in the milling process have been added back.

The U.S. Food and Drug Administration (FDA) allows manufacturers to include special health claims for foods that contain 51% or more whole-grain ingredients. Such products may display a statement such as the following on their packaging:

"Rich in whole grain."
"Made with 100% whole grain."
"Diets rich in whole-grain foods may help reduce the risk of heart disease and certain cancers."

However, many whole-grain products do not carry such claims. This is one more reason to check the ingredient list to make sure you're buying a product made from one or more whole grains.

Association (AHA) recommends no more than 6% of calories per day, which is 100 calories or 6 teaspoons for women and 150 calories or 9 teaspoons for men. Major sources of added sugar in the U.S. diet are sugar-sweetened beverages, snacks, and sweets. Added sugars now appear on food labels as manufacturers have adopted the new Nutrition Facts food-labeling format.

The sugars in your diet should be those that occur naturally, coming mainly from whole fruits, which are excellent sources of vitamins and minerals, and from milk and other dairy products, which are high in protein and calcium. Dietary patterns low in added sugars are described in detail later in the chapter.

**Recommended Carbohydrate Intake** On average, Americans consume 200–300 grams of carbohydrate per day—well above the 130 grams needed to meet the body's minimum requirement for sufficient carbohydrate to run the brain. The AMDR for carbohydrates is 45–65% of total daily calories. That's about 225–325 grams of carbohydrate for someone who consumes 2000 calories per day. The focus should be on consuming a variety of foods rich in complex carbohydrates, especially whole grains.

Athletes can especially benefit from high-carbohydrate diets (60–70% of total daily calories), which can increase the amount of carbohydrates stored in their muscles and therefore provide more fuel for use during endurance events or long workouts. Carbohydrates consumed during prolonged athletic events (e.g., sports beverages and gels) provide fluid, electrolytes, and glucose to help fuel muscles and can extend the availability of glycogen stored in muscles. You should be aware, however, that overconsumption of carbohydrates often leads to underconsumption of other nutrients.

## Fiber—A Closer Look

**Dietary fiber** is the term given to nondigestible carbohydrates naturally present in plants such as whole grains, fruits, legumes, and vegetables. Instead of being digested, fiber helps move waste through the intestinal tract and provides bulk for feces in the large intestine, which in turn facilitates elimination. In the large intestine, bacteria break down some types of fiber into acids and gases, which explains why consuming too much fiber can lead to intestinal gas. Even though humans don't digest fiber, we need it for good health.

**Types of Fiber** There are two types of fiber: soluble and insoluble. Both types are important for health. **Soluble (viscous) fiber** such as that found in oat bran or legumes can delay stomach emptying, slow the movement of glucose into the blood after eating, and reduce absorption of cholesterol. Soluble fiber dissolves or swells in water (like oatmeal that

**TERMS**

**dietary fiber** Nondigestible carbohydrates and lignin that are intact in plants.

**soluble (viscous) fiber** Fiber that dissolves in water or is broken down by bacteria in the large intestine.

gets soft). In contrast, **insoluble fiber** does not dissolve in water, but it does soak up water. It increases fecal bulk and helps prevent constipation, hemorrhoids, and other digestive disorders. We can find insoluble fiber in all plants, and especially in wheat bran, or psyllium seed.

The Food and Nutrition Board gives three other descriptions of fiber. **Dietary fiber** refers to the nondigestible carbohydrates that are naturally present in plants such as grains, fruits, legumes, and vegetables. **Functional fiber** refers to nondigestible carbohydrates that have been either isolated from natural sources or synthesized in a laboratory and then added to a food product or dietary supplement. **Total fiber** refers to the sum of dietary and functional fiber in your diet.

A high-fiber diet can help reduce the risk of type 2 diabetes, heart disease, and cancer, as well as improve gastrointestinal health and aid in the management of metabolic syndrome and body weight. Many studies have linked high-fiber diets with a reduced risk of colon and rectal cancer. Other studies have suggested that it is the total dietary pattern–one rich in fruits, vegetables, and whole grains–that may be responsible for this reduction in risk (see Chapter 13). A high-fiber diet has also been linked to healthier gut bacteria, which may improve immunity and reduce the risk of obesity.

**Sources of Fiber** All plant foods contain some dietary fiber. Fruits, legumes, oats (especially oat bran), and barley all contain the viscous types of fiber that help lower blood glucose and cholesterol levels. Wheat (especially wheat bran), other grains and cereals, and vegetables are good sources of cellulose and other fibers that help prevent constipation. Psyllium, which is often added to cereals or used in fiber supplements and laxatives, improves intestinal health and also helps control glucose and cholesterol levels. The processing of packaged foods can remove fiber, so it is important to rely on fresh fruits and vegetables and foods made from whole grains as your main sources of fiber. Ideally, fiber should come from foods, not supplements.

**Recommended Fiber Intake** To reduce the risk of chronic disease and maintain intestinal health, the Food and Nutrition Board recommends a daily fiber intake of 38 grams for adult men and 25 grams for adult women. Americans generally consume about half this amount.

> **TERMS**
>
> **insoluble fiber** Fiber that does not dissolve in water and is not broken down by bacteria in the large intestine.
>
> **functional fiber** Nondigestible carbohydrates either isolated from natural sources or synthesized; these may be added to foods and dietary supplements.
>
> **total fiber** The total amount of dietary fiber and functional fiber in the diet.
>
> **vitamins** Carbon-containing substances needed in small amounts to help promote and regulate chemical reactions and processes in the body.
>
> **antioxidant** A substance that can reduce the breakdown of food or body constituents by free radicals; the actions of antioxidants include binding oxygen, donating electrons to free radicals, and repairing damage to molecules.

## Vitamins—Organic Micronutrients

**Vitamins** are organic (carbon-containing) substances required in small amounts to regulate various processes within living cells (Table 10.4). Humans need 13 vitamins; of these, 4 are fat-soluble (A, D, E, and K), and 9 are water-soluble (C, and the B vitamins thiamin, riboflavin, niacin, vitamin B-6, folate, vitamin B-12, biotin, and pantothenic acid). Solubility affects how a vitamin is absorbed, transported, and stored in the body. The water-soluble vitamins are absorbed directly into the bloodstream; fat soluble vitamins are usually carried in the blood and stored in the liver and fat tissues.

**Functions of Vitamins** Many vitamins help chemical reactions take place. They provide no energy to the body directly but help release the energy stored in carbohydrates, proteins, and fats. Other vitamins are critical in the production of red blood cells and the maintenance of the nervous, skeletal, and immune systems. Some vitamins act as **antioxidants,** which help preserve the health of cells.

**Sources of Vitamins** The human body does not manufacture most of the vitamins it requires and must obtain them from foods. Vitamins are abundant in fruits, vegetables, and grains. In addition, many processed foods, such as flour and breakfast cereals, contain added vitamins. There are a few vitamins made in the body: When exposed to sunlight, the skin makes vitamin D. Intestinal bacteria make vitamin K. Nonetheless, we still need additional vitamin D and vitamin K from foods. Table 10.4 lists good food sources of vitamins.

**Vitamin Deficiencies** If your diet lacks a particular vitamin, characteristic symptoms of deficiency can develop. For example, *scurvy* is a potentially fatal illness caused by a long-term lack of vitamin C. Children who do not get enough vitamin D can develop *rickets,* which can lead to disabling bone deformations. Low intake of folate during the early weeks of pregnancy increases a woman's risk of giving birth to a baby with a neural tube defect (a congenital malformation of the central nervous system). Vitamin A deficiency may cause blindness, and anemia can develop in people whose diet lacks vitamin B-12, folate, or B-6. Plant foods are not a source of B-12. Vegetarians and especially vegans must rely on fortified cereals or supplements for B-12.

**Vitamin Excesses** Extra vitamins in the diet can also be harmful, especially when taken as supplements for an extended period of time. Megadoses of fat-soluble vitamins

> **Ask Yourself** ?
>
> **QUESTIONS FOR CRITICAL THINKING AND REFLECTION**
>
> Experts say that two of the most important factors in a healthy diet are eating the "right" kinds of carbohydrates and eating the "right" kinds of fats. Based on what you've read so far in this chapter, which are the "right" carbohydrates and fats? How would you say your own diet stacks up when it comes to carbohydrates and fats?

## Table 10.4 Facts about Vitamins

| VITAMIN AND RECOMMENDED INTAKES* | IMPORTANT DIETARY SOURCES | MAJOR FUNCTIONS | SIGNS OF PROLONGED DEFICIENCY | TOXIC EFFECTS OF MEGADOSES |
|---|---|---|---|---|
| **Fat-soluble** | | | | |
| Vitamin A<br>Men: 900 μg<br>Women: 700 μg | Liver, milk, butter, cheese, fortified margarine, carrots, spinach, orange and deep green vegetables and fruits | Immune function and maintenance of vision; skin; and linings of the nose, mouth, and digestive and urinary tracts | Night blindness, scaling skin, increased susceptibility to infection, loss of appetite, anemia, kidney stones | Liver damage, miscarriage, birth defects, headache, vomiting, diarrhea, vertigo, double vision, bone abnormalities |
| Vitamin D<br>Men: 15 μg<br>Women: 15 μg | Fortified milk and margarine, fish oils, butter, egg yolks; sunlight on skin also produces vitamin D | Development and maintenance of bones and teeth, promotion of calcium absorption | Rickets (bone deformities) in children; bone softening, loss, and fractures in adults | Kidney damage, calcium deposits in soft tissues, depression, death |
| Vitamin E<br>Men: 15 mg<br>Women: 15 mg | Vegetable oils, whole grains, nuts and seeds, green leafy vegetables, asparagus, peaches | Protection and maintenance of cellular membranes | Red blood cell breakage and anemia, weakness, neurological problems, muscle cramps | Relatively nontoxic, but may cause excess bleeding or formation of blood clots |
| Vitamin K<br>Men: 120 μg<br>Women: 90 μg | Green leafy vegetables; smaller amounts widespread in other foods | Production of factors essential for blood clotting and bone metabolism | Hemorrhaging | None reported |
| **Water-soluble** | | | | |
| Biotin<br>Men: 30 μg<br>Women: 30 μg | Cereals, yeast, egg yolks, soy flour, liver; widespread in foods | Synthesis of fats, glycogen, and amino acids | Rash, nausea, vomiting, weight loss, depression, fatigue, hair loss | None reported |
| Folate<br>Men: 400 μg<br>Women: 400 μg | Green leafy vegetables, yeast, oranges, whole grains, legumes, liver | Amino acid metabolism, synthesis of RNA and DNA, new cell synthesis | Anemia, weakness, fatigue, irritability, shortness of breath, swollen tongue | Masking of vitamin B-12 deficiency |
| Niacin<br>Men: 16 mg<br>Women: 14 mg | Eggs, poultry, fish, milk, whole grains, nuts, enriched breads and cereals, meats, legumes | Conversion of carbohydrates, fats, and proteins into usable forms of energy | Pellagra (symptoms include diarrhea, dermatitis, inflammation of mucous membranes, dementia) | Flushing of the skin, nausea, vomiting, diarrhea, liver dysfunction, glucose intolerance |
| Pantothenic acid<br>Men: 5 mg<br>Women: 5 mg | Animal foods, whole grains, broccoli, potatoes; widespread in foods | Metabolism of fats, carbohydrates, and proteins | Fatigue, numbness and tingling of hands and feet, gastrointestinal disturbances | None reported |
| Riboflavin<br>Men: 1.3 mg<br>Women: 1.1 mg | Dairy products, enriched breads and cereals, lean meats, poultry, fish, green vegetables | Energy metabolism; maintenance of skin, mucous membranes, and nervous system structures | Cracks at corners of mouth, sore throat, skin rash, hypersensitivity to light, purple tongue | None reported |
| Thiamin<br>Men: 1.2 mg<br>Women: 1.1 mg | Whole-grain and enriched breads and cereals, organ meats, lean pork, nuts, legumes | Conversion of carbohydrates into usable forms of energy, maintenance of appetite and nervous system function | Beriberi (symptoms include muscle wasting, mental confusion, anorexia, enlarged heart, nerve changes) | None reported |
| Vitamin B-6<br>Men: 1.3 mg<br>Women: 1.3 mg | Eggs, poultry, fish, whole grains, nuts, soybeans, liver, kidney, pork | Metabolism of amino acids and glycogen | Anemia, convulsions, cracks at corners of mouth, dermatitis, nausea, confusion | Neurological abnormalities and damage |
| Vitamin B-12<br>Men: 2.4 μg<br>Women: 2.4 μg | Meat, fish, poultry, fortified cereals | Synthesis of blood cells, other metabolic reactions | Anemia, fatigue, nervous system damage, sore tongue | None reported |
| Vitamin C<br>Men: 90 mg<br>Women: 75 mg | Peppers, broccoli, spinach, brussels sprouts, citrus fruits, strawberries, tomatoes, potatoes, cabbage, other fruits and vegetables | Maintenance and repair of connective tissue, bones, teeth, and cartilage; promotion of healing; absorption of iron | Scurvy, anemia, reduced resistance to infection, loosened teeth, joint pain, poor wound healing, hair loss, poor iron absorption | Urinary stones in some people, acid stomach from ingesting supplements in pill form, nausea, diarrhea, headache, fatigue |

*Recommended intakes for adults aged 19–30; to calculate your personal Dietary Reference Intakes (DRIs) based on age, sex, and other factors, visit the Interactive DRI website (https://www.nal.usda.gov/fnic/dri-calculator/).

SOURCES: *Dietary Reference Intakes for Thiamin, Riboflavin, Niacin, Vitamin B6, Folate, Vitamin B12, Pantothenic Acid, Biotin and Choline* (1998); *Dietary Reference Intakes for Vitamin C, Vitamin E, Selenium, and Carotenoids* (2000); *Dietary Reference Intakes for Vitamin A, Vitamin K, Arsenic, Boron, Chromium, Copper, Iodine, Iron, Manganese, Molybdenum, Nickel, Silicon, Vanadium, and Zinc* (2001); and *Dietary Reference Intakes for Calcium and Vitamin D* (2011); Ross, A. C., et al., eds. 2014. *Modern Nutrition in Health and Disease,* 11th ed. Baltimore, MD: Lippincott Williams & Wilkins.

**Table 10.5** Facts about Selected Minerals

| MINERAL AND RECOMMENDED INTAKES* | IMPORTANT DIETARY SOURCES | MAJOR FUNCTIONS | SIGNS OF PROLONGED DEFICIENCY | TOXIC EFFECTS OF MEGADOSES |
|---|---|---|---|---|
| Calcium<br>Men: 1000 mg<br>Women: 1000 mg | Milk and milk products, tofu, fortified orange juice and bread, green leafy vegetables, bones in fish | Formation of bones and teeth, control of nerve impulses, muscle contraction, blood clotting | Stunted growth in children, bone mineral loss in adults, urinary stones | Kidney stones, calcium deposits in soft tissues, inhibition of mineral absorption, constipation |
| Fluoride<br>Men: 4 mg<br>Women: 3 mg | Fluoridated water, tea, marine fish eaten with bones | Maintenance of tooth and bone structure | Higher frequency of tooth decay | Increased bone density, mottling of teeth, impaired kidney function |
| Iodine<br>Men: 150 µg<br>Women: 150 µg | Iodized salt, seafood, processed foods | Essential part of thyroid hormones, regulation of body metabolism | Goiter (enlarged thyroid), cretinism (birth defect) | Depression of thyroid activity, hyperthyroidism in susceptible people |
| Iron<br>Men: 8 mg<br>Women: 18 mg | Meat and poultry, fortified grain products, dark green vegetables, dried fruit | Component of hemoglobin, myoglobin, and enzymes | Iron-deficiency anemia, weakness, impaired immune function, gastrointestinal distress | Nausea, diarrhea, liver and kidney damage, joint pains, sterility, disruption of cardiac function, death |
| Magnesium<br>Men: 400 mg<br>Women: 310 mg | Widespread in foods and water (except soft water); especially found in grains, legumes, nuts, seeds, green vegetables, milk | Transmission of nerve impulses, energy transfer, activation of many enzymes | Neurological disturbances, cardiovascular problems, kidney disorders, nausea, growth failure in children | Nausea, vomiting, diarrhea, central nervous system depression, coma; death in people with impaired kidney function |
| Phosphorus<br>Men: 700 mg<br>Women: 700 mg | Present in nearly all foods, especially milk, cereal, peas, eggs, meat | Bone growth and maintenance, energy transfer in cells | Impaired growth, weakness, kidney disorders, cardiorespiratory and nervous system dysfunction | Drop in blood calcium levels, calcium deposits in soft tissues, bone loss |
| Potassium<br>Men: 3400 mg<br>Women: 2600 mg | Meats, milk, fruits, vegetables, grains, legumes | Nerve function, body water balance | Muscular weakness, nausea, drowsiness, paralysis, confusion, disruption of cardiac rhythm | Cardiac arrest |
| Selenium<br>Men: 55 µg<br>Women: 55 µg | Seafood, meat, eggs, whole grains | Defense against oxidative stress, regulation of thyroid hormone action | Muscle pain and weakness, heart disorders | Hair and nail loss, nausea and vomiting, weakness, irritability |
| Sodium<br>Men: 1500 mg<br>Women: 1500 mg | Salt, soy sauce, salted foods, tomato juice | Body water balance, acid-base balance, nerve function | Muscle weakness, loss of appetite, nausea, vomiting; deficiency is rarely seen | Edema (excess fluid buildup), hypertension in sensitive people |
| Zinc<br>Men: 11 mg<br>Women: 8 mg | Whole grains, meat, eggs, liver, seafood (especially oysters) | Synthesis of proteins, RNA, and DNA; wound healing; immune response; ability to taste | Growth failure, loss of appetite, impaired taste acuity, skin rash, impaired immune function, poor wound healing | Vomiting, impaired immune function, impaired copper absorption |

*Recommended intakes for adults aged 19–30; to calculate your personal DRIs based on age, sex, and other factors, visit the Interactive DRI website (https://www.nal.usda.gov/fnic/dri-calculator/).

SOURCES: Institute of Medicine. 1998. *Dietary Reference Intakes for Thiamin, Riboflavin, Niacin, Vitamin B6, Folate, Vitamin B12, Pantothenic Acid, Biotin and Choline.* National Academies Press; Institute of Medicine. 2000. *Dietary Reference Intakes for Vitamin C, Vitamin E, Selenium, and Carotenoids.* National Academies Press; Institute of Medicine. 2001. *Dietary Reference Intakes for Vitamin A, Vitamin K, Arsenic, Boron, Chromium, Copper, Iodine, Iron, Manganese, Molybdenum, Nickel, Silicon, Vanadium, and Zinc.* National Academies Press; and Institute of Medicine. 2011. Ross, A. C., et al., eds. *Dietary Reference Intakes for Calcium and Vitamin D.* National Academies Press; Ross, A. C., et al., eds. 2014. *Modern Nutrition in Health and Disease.* 11th ed. Baltimore, MD: Lippincott Williams & Wilkins. www.nap.edu. Dietary Reference Intakes for Sodium and Potassium (2019).

are particularly dangerous because the excess is stored in the body rather than excreted, increasing the risk of toxicity. Even when vitamins are not taken in excess, relying on supplements for an adequate intake of vitamins can be a problem because many health benefits from other, nonvitamin ingredients in foods are likely to be missed.

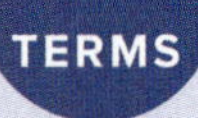


**minerals** Inorganic compounds needed in relatively small amounts for regulation, growth, and maintenance of body tissues and functions.

## Minerals—Inorganic Micronutrients

**Minerals** are inorganic (non-carbon-containing) elements you need in relatively small amounts to help regulate body functions, aid in the growth and maintenance of body tissues, and help release energy (Table 10.5). There are about

## TAKE CHARGE
## Eating for Healthy Bones

Osteoporosis is a condition in which the bones become dangerously thin and fragile over time. An estimated 10 million Americans over age 50 have osteoporosis, and another 44 million are at risk. Women account for about 80% of osteoporosis cases. Most of our adult bone mass is built by age 18 in girls and age 20 in boys. After bone density peaks between ages 25 and 35, bone mass is lost slowly over time and then at an increasing rate after menopause. To prevent osteoporosis, the best strategy is to build as much bone as possible during your youth and do everything you can to maintain it as you age. Up to 50% of bone loss is determined by controllable lifestyle factors such as resistance training and diet. Key nutrients for bone health include the following:

- **Calcium.** Getting enough calcium is important throughout life to build and maintain bone mass. Milk, yogurt, and calcium-fortified orange juice, bread, and cereals are all good sources.
- **Vitamin D.** Vitamin D is necessary for bones to absorb calcium. The National Academy of Medicine recommends a daily intake of 15 μg of vitamin D for most adults and 20 μg of vitamin D for men and women over the age of 70 years. Vitamin D can be obtained from foods and is manufactured by the skin when exposed to sunlight. Candidates for vitamin D supplements include people who don't eat many foods rich in vitamin D; those who don't expose their faces, arms, and hands to the sun (without sunscreen) for 5–15 minutes a few times each week; and people who live north of an imaginary line roughly between Boston and the Oregon–California border (where the sun is weaker).
- **Vitamin K.** Vitamin K promotes the synthesis of proteins that help keep bones strong. Broccoli and leafy green vegetables are rich in vitamin K.
- **Other nutrients.** Other nutrients that may play an important role in bone health include vitamin C, vitamin A, magnesium, potassium, phosphorus, fluoride, manganese, zinc, copper, and boron.

Several dietary substances may have a *negative* effect on bone health, especially if consumed in excess. These include alcohol, sodium, caffeine, and retinol (a form of vitamin A). Drinking lots of soda, which often replaces milk in the diet, has been shown to increase the risk of bone fractures in teenage girls.

The effect of protein intake on bone mass depends on other nutrients. Protein helps build bone as long as calcium and vitamin D intake are adequate. But if intake of calcium and vitamin D is low, high protein intake can lead to bone loss.

Weight-bearing aerobic exercise helps maintain bone mass throughout life, and strength training improves bone density, muscle mass, strength, and balance. Drinking alcohol only in moderation, refraining from smoking, and managing depression and stress are also important for maintaining strong bones. For people who develop osteoporosis, a variety of medications are available to treat the condition.

SOURCES: Movassagh, E. Z., and H. Vatanparast. 2017. Current evidence on the association of dietary patterns and bone health: A scoping review. *Advances in Nutrition* 8(1): 1–16; Institute of Medicine of the National Academies. 2011. *Dietary Reference Intakes for calcium and vitamin D;* Bone Health and Osteoporosis Foundation https://www.bonehealthandosteoporosis.org/

17 essential minerals. The major minerals, which the body needs in amounts exceeding 100 milligrams per day, include calcium, phosphorus, magnesium, sodium, potassium, and chloride. The essential trace minerals, which you need in minute amounts, include copper, fluoride, iodide, iron, selenium, and zinc.

Characteristic symptoms develop if an essential mineral is consumed in a quantity too large or too small for good health. For example, 90% of Americans consume too much sodium, which can raise blood pressure; as blood pressure increases, the risk for heart disease and stroke does as well. The minerals commonly lacking in the American diet are iron, calcium, potassium, and magnesium. Iron-deficiency **anemia** is a problem in some age groups, but particularly among menstruating women and among women who have had multiple pregnancies. Poor calcium and vitamin D intakes during childhood contribute to a risk of future **osteoporosis,** especially in women. The box "Eating for Healthy Bones" has tips for building and maintaining bone density; low fluoride intake contributes to dental caries; low iodine increases the risk of goiter.

## Water—Vital but Underappreciated

The human body is composed of about 50–60% water. Our need for other nutrients, in terms of weight, is much less than our need for water. We can live up to 50 days without food but only a few days without water.

Water is distributed among lean and other tissues and in blood and other body fluids. Water is used in the digestion and absorption of food and is the medium in which most chemical reactions take place within the body. Some water-based fluids, like blood, transport substances around the body, whereas other fluids serve as lubricants or cushions. Water also helps regulate body temperature.

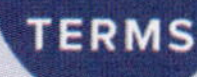


**anemia** A deficiency in the oxygen-carrying material, hemoglobin, in the red blood cells.

**osteoporosis** A condition in which the bones become thin and brittle over time and break easily; risk factors include age, sex, inactivity, and insufficient calcium intake.

Water is part of most foods, particularly liquids, fruits, and vegetables. The foods and beverages you consume provide 80–90% of your daily water intake; the remainder is generated through metabolism. You lose water each day in urine, feces, and sweat and through evaporation from your lungs.

Most people can maintain a healthy water balance by consuming beverages at meals and drinking fluids when thirsty. The Food and Nutrition Board has set levels of adequate water intake to maintain hydration. Under these guidelines, men need about 3.7 total liters of water daily, with 3.0 liters (about 13 cups) coming from beverages; women need 2.7 total liters, with 2.2 liters (about 9 cups) coming from beverages. All fluids, including those containing caffeine, can count toward your total daily fluid intake. If you exercise vigorously or live in a hot climate, you need to consume additional fluids to maintain a balance between water consumed and water lost. Severe dehydration causes weakness and can lead to death.

QUICK STATS

**Osteoporosis is more common in women; in people ages 65 and over with low bone mass, it occurs in about 25% of women and 5% of men.**

—Centers for Disease Control and Prevention, 2019

## Other Substances in Food

There are many other substances in food that are not essential nutrients but may influence health.

**Antioxidants** When the body uses oxygen or breaks down certain fats or proteins as a normal part of metabolism, it gives rise to substances called **free radicals.** Environmental factors such as cigarette smoke, exhaust fumes, radiation, excessive sunlight, high-fat diets, certain drugs, and stress can increase free radical production. A free radical is a chemically unstable molecule that reacts with fats, proteins, and DNA, damaging cell membranes and mutating genes. Free radicals have been implicated in aging, cancer, cardiovascular disease, and other degenerative diseases like arthritis.

Antioxidants found in foods can help protect the body from damage by free radicals in several ways. Some prevent or reduce the formation of free radicals; others remove free radicals from the body; still others repair some types of free radical damage after it occurs. Some antioxidants, such as vitamin C, vitamin E, and selenium, are also essential nutrients. Others—such as the carotenoids found in yellow, orange, and deep green vegetables—are not. Some of the top antioxidant-containing foods and beverages include berries, walnuts, artichokes, green tea, pecans, cloves, grape juice, dark chocolate, sour cherries, and red wine. Also high in antioxidants are brussels sprouts, kale, cauliflower, and pomegranates.

**Phytochemicals** Antioxidants fall into the broader category of **phytochemicals,** which are substances found in plant foods that may help prevent chronic disease. Researchers have identified and studied hundreds of compounds found in foods and how they affect our health, and many findings are promising. For example, certain substances found in soy foods may help lower cholesterol levels. Sulforaphane, a compound isolated from broccoli and other **cruciferous vegetables,** may render some carcinogenic compounds harmless. Allyl sulfides, a group of chemicals found in garlic and onions, appear to boost the activity of immune cells and lower total cholesterol concentrations. Carotenoids found in green vegetables may help preserve eyesight with age. Phytochemicals found in whole grains are associated with a reduced risk of cardiovascular disease, diabetes, and cancer. Currently, research on phytochemicals extends the role of nutrition to the prevention and treatment of many chronic diseases.

If you want to increase your intake of phytochemicals, eat a variety of fruits, vegetables, and unprocessed grains rather than relying on supplements. Like many vitamins and minerals, isolated phytochemicals may be harmful if taken in high doses. Another reason to get your phytochemicals from foods is that their health benefits could be the result of many chemical substances from whole foods working in combination. Eating more fruits and vegetables is a smart alternative to less healthy foods.

TERMS

**free radical** An electron-seeking compound that can react with fats, proteins, and DNA, damaging cell membranes and mutating genes in its search for electrons; produced through chemical reactions in the body and by exposure to environmental factors such as sunlight and tobacco smoke.

**phytochemical** A naturally occurring substance found in plant foods that may help prevent and treat chronic diseases like cancer and heart disease; *phyto* means "plant."

**cruciferous vegetables** Vegetables of the cabbage family, including cabbage, broccoli, brussels sprouts, kale, and cauliflower; the flower petals of these plants form the shape of a cross, hence the name.

**Dietary Reference Intakes (DRIs)** An umbrella term for four types of nutrient standards designed to prevent nutritional deficiencies and reduce the risk of chronic diseases. Adequate Intake (AI) and Recommended Dietary Allowance (RDA) are levels of intake considered adequate to prevent nutrient deficiencies and reduce the risk of chronic disease for most individuals in a population group; and Tolerable Upper Intake Level (UL) is the maximum daily intake that is unlikely to cause health problems.

# NUTRITIONAL GUIDELINES: PLANNING YOUR DIET

Scientific and government groups have created a variety of tools to help people design healthy diets. **Dietary Reference Intakes (DRIs)** are standards for nutrient intake designed to prevent nutritional deficiencies and reduce the risk of chronic diseases. ***Dietary Guidelines for Americans*** were established to promote health and reduce the risk of major chronic diseases through diet and physical activity. **MyPlate** provides a food guidance system to help people apply the *Dietary Guidelines for Americans* to their own diets

## Dietary Reference Intakes (DRIs)

The Food and Nutrition Board of the National Academy of Medicine establishes dietary standards, or recommended intake levels, for Americans of all ages. The current set of standards, the Dietary Reference Intakes (DRIs), was introduced in 1997. The DRIs are reviewed frequently and are updated as new nutrition-related information becomes available. The DRIs have a broad focus, being based on research that looks not just at the prevention of nutrient deficiencies but also at the role of nutrients in promoting health and preventing chronic diseases such as cancer, osteoporosis, and heart disease.

The DRIs include a set of four reference values used as standards for both recommended intakes and maximum safe intakes. The *Recommended Dietary Allowance (RDA)* is the amount that will cover about 97% of the healthy individuals in a given gender and life stage. If there is not enough information available to set an RDA, then an *Adequate Intake (AI)* is established. Regardless of whether an RDA or AI is used, it represents the best available estimate of intake for optimal health. The *Tolerable Upper Intake Level (UL)* is the maximum daily intake that is unlikely to cause health problems in a healthy person.

Because of lack of data, ULs have not been set for all nutrients. The absence of ULs does not mean that people can tolerate chronic intakes of these vitamins and minerals above recommended levels. Like all chemical agents, nutrients can produce adverse effects if intakes are excessive. There is no established benefit from consuming nutrients at levels above the RDA or AI.

The DRIs for many nutrients are found in Tables 10.1, 10.4, and 10.5. For a personalized DRI report for all nutrients, appropriate for your sex and life stage, visit the Interactive DRI website (https://www.nal.usda.gov/fnic/dri-calculator/).

Because the DRIs are too cumbersome to use as a basis for food labels, the FDA uses another set of dietary standards, the **Daily Values.** The Daily Values are based on several different sets of guidelines and include standards for fat, cholesterol, carbohydrate, dietary fiber, and selected vitamins and minerals. The Daily Values represent appropriate intake levels for a 2000-calorie diet. The Daily Value percentage on a food label shows how well that food contributes to your recommended daily intake, assuming you follow a 2000-calorie-per-day diet. Food labels are described in detail later in this chapter.

## Dietary Guidelines for Americans

To provide general guidance for choosing a healthy diet and reducing the risk of chronic diseases, the USDA and the U.S. Department of Health and Human Services issue the *Dietary Guidelines for Americans,* revising them every five years. The information in the *Dietary Guidelines* is used in developing federal food, nutrition, and health policies and programs and also serves as the basis for federal nutrition education materials.

The *Dietary Guidelines* are designed to help Americans make healthy and informed food choices. Over 70% of us are overweight or obese and yet at the same time undernourished in several key nutrients. The guidelines focus on the total diet and offer practical tips for how people can make *shifts* in their diet to integrate healthier choices. People do not eat individual nutrients or single foods but rather foods in combination, to form an overall **eating pattern** that has cumulative effects on health. The *2020–2025 Dietary Guidelines* point out the large discrepancy between the recommendations and the actual American diet, which includes too much added sugar, solid fat, refined grain, and sodium and not enough vegetables, fruits, high-fiber whole grains, low-fat milk and milk products, and seafood.

About 60% of all American adults have one or more preventable chronic diseases that are related to poor eating habits and inactivity; these include high blood pressure, type 2 diabetes, cardiovascular disease, and certain forms of cancer. The food and portion size choices you make at every meal can influence your risk for, or management of, many health conditions.

The *2020–2025 Dietary Guidelines* for the first time feature a whole life-span approach. Previously, the guidelines focused on children aged 2 and over. The new guidelines emphasize how diet during early life stages promotes health and prevents chronic disease throughout childhood and into adulthood. This means we take into account good nutrition for babies and children under 24 months, as well as for mothers who are pregnant and breastfeeding. Each of the guidelines is supported by an extensive review of scientific and medical evidence.

**General Recommendations** The *2020–2025 Dietary Guidelines* offer four primary recommendations:

1. **Follow a healthy dietary pattern at every life stage.** Nutrient needs vary over the life span and therefore require adjusting food and beverage choices throughout the life span to avoid disease risk.

2. **Customize and enjoy food and beverage choices to reflect personal preferences, cultural traditions, and budgetary considerations.** A healthy eating pattern is not a rigid prescription, but rather an adaptable framework.

**TERMS**

***Dietary Guidelines for Americans*** National nutritional recommendations issued jointly by the U.S. Department of Agriculture and the U.S. Department of Health and Human Services every five years; designed to promote health and reduce the risk of chronic diseases.

**MyPlate** The USDA food guidance system designed to help Americans make healthy food choices.

**Daily Values** A simplified version of the RDAs used on food labels; also included are values for nutrients with no RDA per se.

**eating pattern** The result of choices on multiple eating occasions over time, both at home and away from home.

3. **Focus on nutrient-dense foods and beverages and stay within calorie limits.** Meet your nutritional needs with recommended amounts of nutrient-dense foods and beverages across the food groups.
4. **Limit foods and beverages higher in added sugars, saturated fat, and sodium, and limit alcoholic beverages.** A healthy dietary pattern doesn't have much room for extra added sugars, saturated fat, or sodium, or for alcoholic beverages.

More than 38 million people in the United States, including 6 million children, live with food insecurity. The disproportionate lack of access to healthy and affordable foods that affects low-income, Black, and Hispanic households became even more apparent during the Covid-19 pandemic. Everyone has a role in supporting healthy eating in our homes and communities, and reaching out especially to those people who are isolated and marginalized.

QUICK STATS

**More than 70% of Americans consume too much added sugar and saturated fat; 89% have intakes that are too high for sodium.**

—U.S. Department of Health and Human Services and U.S. Department of Agriculture, 2018

The *Dietary Guidelines* acknowledge the challenges that make it difficult for Americans to reach their food and fitness goals. The *Guidelines* argue that all segments of our society, from families to food producers and restaurants to policymakers, have a responsibility in supporting healthy choices. Adopting an adaptable, healthy eating pattern and engaging in regular physical activity will go a long way toward improving health and reducing the risk of chronic disease in every life stage.

**Building Healthy Eating Patterns** The *Dietary Guidelines* highlight three healthy eating patterns:

- **Healthy U.S.-Style Pattern.** Based on the types and proportions of foods Americans typically consume, but in nutrient-dense forms and appropriate amounts.
- **Healthy Vegetarian Pattern.** Includes more legumes, processed soy products, nuts and seeds, and whole grains; it contains no meat, poultry, or seafood but is close to the Healthy U.S.-Style Pattern in amounts of all other food groups. Dairy and eggs are still included because the majority of vegetarians eat them; however, the plan can be vegan with plant-based substitutions.
- **Healthy Mediterranean-Style Pattern.** Reflecting a dietary pattern that includes more fruit and seafood and less dairy than the Healthy U.S.-Style Pattern. The Mediterranean diet has been associated with positive health outcomes such as lower rates of heart disease and lower total mortality.

All three patterns are based on amounts of food from different food groups (and subgroups) according to overall energy intake. They share an emphasis on whole fruits, vegetables, whole grains, beans, peas, and lentils, fat-free and low-fat milk and milk products, and healthy oils; they include less red meat and more seafood than the typical American diet.

A fundamental principle of all healthy dietary patterns is that people should eat nutrient-dense foods—foods with little or no solid fats, added sugars, and added refined starches—so that they can obtain all the needed nutrients without exceeding their daily energy requirements. In addition, people should strive to get their nutrients from foods rather than from dietary supplements, although supplements or fortification may be helpful for certain populations.

Following a healthy pattern allows you to meet all the DRIs for essential nutrients and stay within the AMDRs established by the Food and Nutrition Board for nutrients that supply energy. Table 10.6 compares the three patterns for a 2000-calorie diet. See the Nutrition Resources section at the end of the chapter for a more detailed breakdown of the recommendations for the three healthy dietary patterns.

Although the greatest emphasis of the *Dietary Guidelines* is on consuming an overall healthy eating pattern, specific recommendations have been set for dietary components of particular public health concern. The *Dietary Guidelines* recommend these actions for staying within calorie limits while sticking to a dietary pattern that has healthy amounts of vegetables, fruits, legumes, whole grains, nuts and seeds, with some vegetable oils, low-fat dairy, lean meat and poultry, and fatty fish (see Figure 10.2).

**FATS** Replace saturated fats with unsaturated fats, particularly polyunsaturated fat. Reducing saturated fats lowers the incidence of cardiovascular disease in adults and LDL cholesterol in all adults.

**BEVERAGES** Hydrate with water and drinks that don't have sugars added. Sugar-sweetened beverages, not including coffee and tea with added sugar, account for approximately one-third of all drinks that young children consume. They account for 50% of the beverages consumed by adolescents, and 60% of those consumed by adults. These beverages provide energy but contribute very little toward meeting nutrient and food group recommendations; rather, they increase overweight and obesity.

Alcohol has no confirmed health benefits: The current *Dietary Guidelines* specify at most one drink per day for women and two drinks per day for men on days when alcohol is consumed.

**SUGAR** Consume less than 10% of energy from added sugars. Added sugars account for about 13% of calories in the average American diet and are typically found in foods that provide little nutritional value. This high level of sugars is implicated in the development of obesity and diabetes. Nearly 70% of added sugars intake comes from five food categories: sweetened beverages, desserts and sweet snacks, coffee and tea (with their additions), candy and sugars, and breakfast cereals and bars.

About 85% of a person's calorie allowance each day is needed to meet food group recommendations, in a nutrient-dense form. The remaining calories can be used for added

**Table 10.6** USDA Healthy Food Patterns at the 2000-Calorie Level

| FOOD GROUP | HEALTHY U.S.-STYLE PATTERN | HEALTHY VEGETARIAN PATTERN | HEALTHY MEDITERRANEAN-STYLE PATTERN |
|---|---|---|---|
| **Vegetables** | **2½ c-eq/day** | **2½ c-eq/day** | **2½ c-eq/day** |
| Dark green | 1½ c-eq/wk | 1½ c-eq/wk | 1½ c-eq/wk |
| Red and orange | 5½ c-eq/wk | 5½ c-eq/wk | 5½ c-eq/wk |
| Beans, peas, and lentils | 1½ c-eq/wk | 3 c-eq/wk* | 1½ c-eq/wk |
| Starchy | 5 c-eq/wk | 5 c-eq/wk | 5 c-eq/wk |
| Other | 4 c-eq/wk | 4 c-eq/wk | 4 c-eq/wk |
| **Fruit** | **2 c-eq/day** | **2 c-eq/day** | **2½ c-eq/day** |
| **Grains** | **6 oz-eq/day** | **6½ oz-eq/day** | **6 oz-eq/day** |
| Whole grains | 3 oz-eq/day | 3½ oz-eq/day | 3 oz-eq/day |
| Refined grains | 3 oz-eq/day | 3 oz-eq/day | 3 oz-eq/day |
| **Dairy** | **3 c-eq/day** | **3 c-eq/day** | **2 c-eq/day** |
| **Protein Foods** | **5½ oz-eq/day** | **3½ oz-eq/day** | **6½ oz-eq/day** |
| Seafood | 8 oz-eq/wk | N/A | 15 oz-eq/wk |
| Meat, poultry, eggs | 26 oz-eq/wk | 3 oz-eq/wk (eggs) | 26 oz-eq/wk |
| Nuts, seeds, soy products | 5 oz-eq/wk | 15 oz-eq/wk | 5 oz-eq/wk |
| **Oils** | **27 g/day** | **27 g/day** | **27 g/day** |
| **Limit on calories for other uses (% of total calories)**** | 240 cal/day (12%) | 250 cal/day (13%) | 240 cal/day (12%) |

*For the Vegetarian Pattern, half of total beans, peas, and lentils intake counts as vegetables and half as protein foods.

**If all food choices to meet food group recommendations are in nutrient-dense forms, a small number of calories remain within the overall calorie limit of the pattern (i.e., limit on calories for other uses). Calories up to the specified limit can be used to consume added sugars, added refined starches, solid fats, or alcohol, or to eat more than the recommended amount of food in a food group.

NOTE: c-eq = cup-equivalent, the amount of a food or beverage product that is considered equal to 1 cup from the vegetables, fruits, or dairy food groups; oz-eq = ounce-equivalent, the amount of a food product that is considered equal to 1 ounce from the grain or protein food groups; N/A = not applicable.

SOURCE: U.S. Department of Agriculture and U.S. Department of Health and Human Services. *Dietary Guidelines for Americans, 2020–2025,* 9th ed. December 2020. Available at DietaryGuidelines.gov.

sugars; solid, more saturated, fats; more nutrient-dense foods; or for alcoholic beverages.

**Making Shifts to Align with Healthy Eating Patterns** Every food choice is an opportunity to move toward a healthy eating pattern. Making small positive dietary changes over time can cumulatively make a big difference and support your efforts at maintaining a healthy body weight, meeting nutrient needs, and reducing your risk for chronic disease. See the box "Positive Changes to Improve Your Diet."

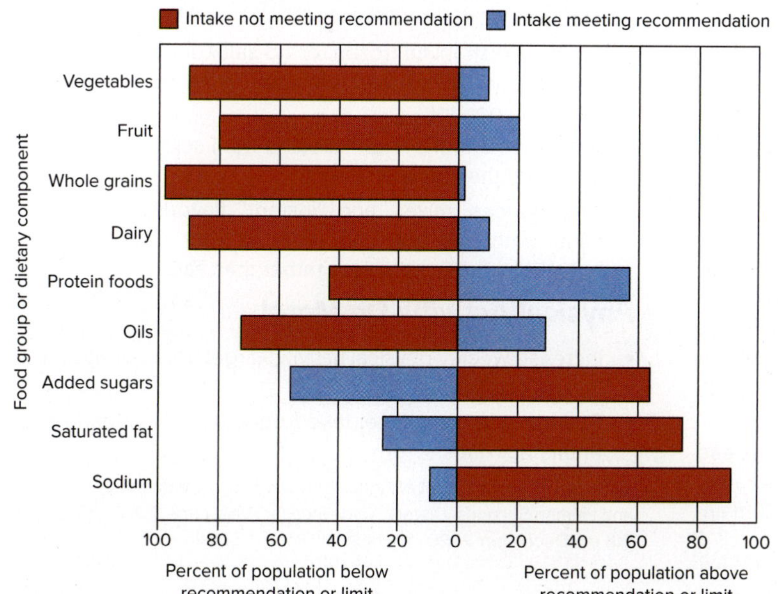


**FIGURE 10.2 Dietary intakes compared to recommendations.** The bars show the percentages of the U.S. population age 1 year and over who are below, at, or above each dietary goal or limit. The center (0) line is the goal or limit. For most people, meaning those represented by the orange sections of the bars, shifting toward the center line will improve eating patterns. For example, nearly 90% of people do not eat enough vegetables—they fall below the recommendation. Within the area of the graph demonstrating our consumption of foods we should limit—added sugars, saturated fat, and sodium— the data represent ages of U.S. Americans 19–30. The orange bars show that over 90% of people exceed the recommended limit for sodium intake.

SOURCE: U.S. Department of Agriculture. Analysis of what we eat in America, NHANES 2013–2016, ages 1 and older, 2 days dietary intake data, weighted. Recommended intake ranges: Healthy U.S.-Style Dietary Patterns (see *Dietary Guidelines for Americans,* 2020–2025 (www.dietaryguidelines.gov/sites/default/files/2020-12/Dietary_Guidelines_for_Americans_2020-2025.pdf).

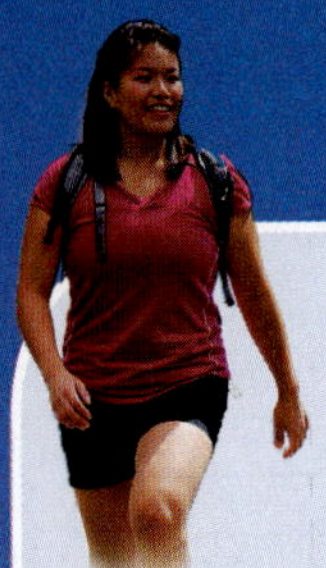

## TAKE CHARGE
## Positive Changes to Improve Your Diet

Remember to focus on nutrient-dense options for the majority of your food choices: Use your calorie budget wisely. The tips here focus on the types of changes and swaps needed for the majority of Americans to move toward the dietary pattern recommended in the *Dietary Guidelines*.

### Vegetables: Eat More

- Increase the vegetable content of mixed dishes while decreasing the amounts of other food components that you may overconsume—for example, cut the meat or cheese in half and double the vegetables in a soup, stew, or casserole.
- Always choose a green salad or a vegetable as a side dish.
- Incorporate vegetables into most meals and snacks.
- Replace foods high in calories, saturated fat, or sodium, such as some meats, poultry, cheeses, and snack foods, with vegetables.

### Fruits: Increase Fruit Intake, Especially Whole Fruits

- Choose more fruits as snacks, in salads, as side dishes, and as desserts in place of foods with added sugars such as cookies, pies, cakes, and ice cream.

### Grains: Swap Processed for Whole Grains

- Shift from refined to whole-grain versions of commonly eaten foods—from white to 100% whole-wheat breads, white to whole-grain pasta, and white to brown rice (see the section on whole grains earlier in the chapter for more information on using food labels to identify whole grains).
- Cut back on refined-grain desserts and sweet snacks that are high in added sugars, solid fats, or both. Choose smaller portions and eat them less often. For healthy swaps, try plain popcorn instead of buttered and bread instead of a croissant or biscuit, for example.

### Dairy: Increase Intake

- Drink fat-free or low-fat milk (or soy beverage) with meals, choose yogurt as a snack, or use yogurt as an ingredient in salad dressings, spreads, and other prepared dishes.
- Favor milk and yogurt for additional dairy servings; cheese has more sodium and saturated fat and less potassium, vitamin A, and vitamin D than milk and yogurt.

### Protein: Add Variety and Make More Plant-Based Choices

- Increase low-mercury seafood intake if yours is low: Try seafood as the protein choice in meals twice per week in place of meat, poultry, or eggs—for example, a tuna sandwich or a salmon steak.
- Use legumes or nuts and seeds in mixed dishes instead of some meat or poultry—for example, bean chili instead of a mixed-meat dish or almonds instead of ham on a main-dish salad.

### Oils: Choose Healthier Fats

- Use oils rather than solid fats in food preparation where possible—for example, vegetable oil in place of butter, stick margarine, shortening, lard, or coconut oils when cooking.
- Increase intake of foods that naturally contain oils, such as seafood and nuts, in place of some meat and poultry.
- Choose options for salad dressings and spreads made with oils instead of solid fats.

### Saturated Fats: Reduce to Less Than 10% of Calories per Day

- Substitute foods high in unsaturated fats for foods high in saturated fats; for example, use oils rather than solid fats for food preparation.
- Read food labels to identify the types of fats in prepared foods; compare and choose lower-fat forms of foods and beverages that contain solid fats (e.g., lower-fat milk instead of 2% or whole).
- Adjust proportions of ingredients in mixed dishes to increase vegetables, whole grains, lean meat, and lower-fat cheeses in place of some of the fatty meat or regular cheeses.
- Consume foods higher in solid fats less often and in smaller portions.

### Added Sugars: Reduce as Much as Possible

- Choose beverages with no added sugars, such as water, in place of sugar-sweetened beverages.
- Reduce portion sizes of sugar-sweetened beverages, and choose them less often.
- Limit servings and decrease portion sizes of grain-based and dairy desserts and sweet snacks.
- Choose unsweetened or no-sugar-added versions of canned fruit, fruit sauces, and yogurt.

### Sodium: Lower Intake

- Read food labels to compare sodium content, choosing products with less sodium.
- Choose fresh, plain frozen, or no-salt-added canned vegetables and fresh protein sources rather than processed meat and poultry.
- Eat at home more often; cooking from scratch allows you to control the sodium content.
- Limit sauces, mixes, and "instant" flavoring packs that come with rice and noodles; use your own flavorings based on herbs and spices rather than salt.

### Physical Activity: Do More!

- Increase weekly physical activity; target transportation and leisure activities.
- Reduce sedentary time; take frequent breaks during sedentary activities.

SOURCE: U.S. Department of Agriculture and U.S. Department of Health and Human Services. *Dietary Guidelines for Americans, 2020–2025*, 9th ed. December 2020. Available at DietaryGuidelines.gov.

People have many options for incorporating the recommendations of the *Dietary Guidelines* into healthy eating patterns that (1) meet nutrient needs; (2) stay within calorie limits; (3) accommodate cultural, ethnic, traditional, and personal preferences; and (4) take into account food cost and availability.

**Supporting Healthy Eating Patterns** Making healthy choices can be challenging, but ultimately each person makes decisions about what, where, when, and how much to eat. Individuals are more likely to shift their eating patterns toward the guidelines if we make a collaborative effort across all segments of society. By doing so, we create a culture in which healthy lifestyle choices at home, school, work, and everywhere else are easy, accessible, affordable, and normative.

## USDA's MyPlate

To help consumers put the *Dietary Guidelines for Americans* into practice, the USDA issues the food-guidance system called MyPlate. MyPlate provides a simple graphic showing how to use the five food groups to build a healthy plate at each meal (Figure 10.3). If you need to make changes in your dietary pattern, use MyPlate to build a healthy eating style by focusing on variety, amount of food consumed, and nutrition. Follow the recommendations in the *Dietary Guidelines* to limit saturated fat, added sugars, and sodium. Start with small changes; they will add up over time.

You can get a personalized MyPlan version of MyPlate recommendations by visiting MyPlate.gov. Using the daily food plan feature, you can determine the amount of each food group you need daily based on your calorie allowance. Your plan is personalized based on your age, gender, weight, height, and level of physical activity.

**Energy Intake and Portion Sizes** To build a healthy eating style, your food group goals should be based on an appropriate level of energy intake. Table 10.7 provides ranges for calorie intake for weight maintenance. Everyone is different, however, and the number of calories you need will vary depending on multiple factors. If your weight is stable, your current energy intake is in balance with calories expended; you can set a more personal calorie goal by carefully tracking your food intake for several days to determine your current calorie intake. Once you select a calorie level for your eating plan, monitor your body weight and adjust calorie intake and physical activity based on changes in weight over time. The *Dietary Guidelines* recommend that adults who are obese or overweight shift their eating and physical-activity behaviors to prevent additional weight gain and/or promote weight loss.

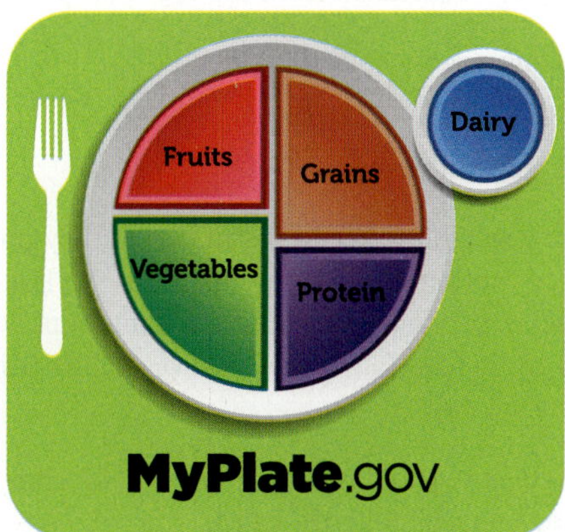


**FIGURE 10.3 MyPlate.** The USDA's MyPlate is designed as a simple graphic to help Americans apply the *Dietary Guidelines* to their own diets.

SOURCE: U.S Department of Agriculture, www.myplate.gov

**Table 10.7 USDA Estimated Daily Calorie Intake Levels to Maintain Energy Balance**

| AGE (YEARS) | SEDENTARY* | MODERATELY ACTIVE** | ACTIVE† |
|---|---|---|---|
| **FEMALE*** ** | | | |
| 16–18 | 1,800 | 2,000 | 2,400 |
| 19–25 | 2,000 | 2,200 | 2,400 |
| 26–30 | 1,800 | 2,000 | 2,400 |
| 31–50 | 1,800 | 2,000 | 2,200 |
| 51–60 | 1,600 | 1,800 | 2,200 |
| 61 & up | 1,600 | 1,800 | 2,000 |
| **MALE** | | | |
| 16–18 | 2,400 | 2,800 | 3,200 |
| 19–20 | 2,600 | 2,800 | 3,000 |
| 21–25 | 2,400 | 2,800 | 3,000 |
| 26–35 | 2,400 | 2,600 | 3,000 |
| 36–40 | 2,400 | 2,600 | 2,800 |
| 41–45 | 2,200 | 2,600 | 2,800 |
| 46–55 | 2,200 | 2,400 | 2,800 |
| 56–60 | 2,200 | 2,400 | 2,600 |
| 61–65 | 2,000 | 2,400 | 2,600 |
| 66–75 | 2,000 | 2,200 | 2,600 |
| 76 & up | 2,000 | 2,200 | 2,400 |

*A lifestyle that includes only the light physical activity associated with typical day-to-day life.

**A lifestyle that includes physical activity equivalent to walking about 1.5–3 miles per day at 3–4 miles per hour (30–60 minutes a day of moderate physical activity), in addition to the light physical activity associated with typical day-to-day life.

***Estimates for females do not include those who are pregnant or breastfeeding.

†Active means a lifestyle that includes physical activity equivalent to walking more than 3 miles per day at 3–4 miles per hour (60 or more minutes a day of moderate physical activity), in addition to the light physical activity associated with typical day-to-day life.

SOURCE: U.S. Department of Health and Human Services and U.S. Department of Agriculture. 2020. *Dietary Guidelines for Americans 2020–2025*. 9th ed. https://www.dietaryguidelines.gov/sites/default/files/2020-12/Dietary_Guidelines_for_Americans_2020-2025.pdf).

## TAKE CHARGE
### Judging Portion Sizes

Studies have shown that most people underestimate the size of their food portions, in many cases by as much as 50%. If you need to retrain your eye, try using measuring cups and spoons and an inexpensive kitchen scale when you eat at home. With a little practice, you'll learn the difference between 3 and 8 ounces of chicken or meat and what a half-cup of rice really looks like. For quick estimates, use the following equivalents:

- 1 teaspoon margarine = the tip of your thumb
- 1 ounce cheese = your thumb, four dice stacked together, or an ice cube
- 3 ounces chicken or meat = a deck of cards
- 1 cup pasta = a small fist or a tennis ball
- ½ cup rice or cooked vegetables = an ice cream scoop or one-third of a can of soda
- 2 tablespoons peanut butter = a Ping-Pong ball or a large marshmallow
- 1 medium potato = a computer mouse
- 2-ounce muffin or roll = a plum or a large egg
- 2-ounce bagel = a hockey puck or a yo-yo
- 1 medium fruit (apple or orange) = a baseball
- ¼ cup nuts = a golf ball
- small cookie or cracker = a poker chip

Most people underestimate not only the number of calories they consume but also the size of their portions. See the box "Judging Portion Sizes" for strategies to improve the accuracy of your estimates. MyPlate doesn't use number of portions as the basis of recommendations; instead, amounts are listed in terms of cup-equivalents and ounce-equivalents. These units of measurement allow for the alignment of servings of foods that differ—those that are concentrated versus those that are more airy or contain more water. For example, ½ cup of blueberries and ¼ cup of raisins both count as ½ cup-equivalent of fruit.

**QUICK STATS**

**Only about 12% of adults meet fruit recommendations and about 10% meet vegetable recommendations.**

Centers for Disease Control and Prevention 2022

**Fruits: Focus on Whole Fruits** People who eat more vegetables and fruits as part of an overall healthy diet are likely to have a reduced risk of some chronic diseases. Fruits are rich in carbohydrates, dietary fiber, some minerals, especially potassium, and many vitamins, especially vitamin C. A 2000-calorie diet should include 2 cups of fruit daily. Each of the following counts as 1 cup-equivalent from the fruit group:

- 1 cup fresh, canned, or frozen fruit
- 1 cup fruit juice (100% juice)
- 1 small whole fruit
- ½ cup dried fruit

Choose whole fruits often; they are higher in fiber and often lower in energy than fruit juices. Fruit *juices* typically contain more nutrients and less added sugar than fruit *drinks*. When buying canned fruits, choose those packed in 100% fruit juice or water rather than in syrup.

**Vegetables: Vary Your Veggies** Together, fruits and vegetables should make up half your plate. Vegetables contain carbohydrates, dietary fiber, vitamin A, vitamin C, folate, potassium, and other nutrients. They are naturally low in calories and fat and contain no cholesterol. A 2000-calorie diet should include 2½ cups of vegetables daily. Each of the following counts as 1 cup-equivalent from the vegetable group:

- 1 cup raw or cooked vegetables
- 2 cups raw leafy salad greens
- 1 cup vegetable juice

Because vegetables vary in the nutrients they provide, eat a variety to obtain maximum nutrition. MyPlate recommends weekly servings from the five subgroups within the vegetables group (see Table 10.6). Eat vegetables from several subgroups each day.

- Dark green vegetables (e.g., broccoli, bok choy, romaine lettuce, spinach, collards, kale)
- Red and orange vegetables (e.g., tomatoes, carrots, sweet potatoes, red peppers, winter squash)
- Beans and peas (e.g., split and black-eyed peas; lentils; soybeans; black, kidney, navy, pinto, and white beans)

- Starchy vegetables (e.g., corn, potatoes, green peas)
- Other vegetables (e.g., artichokes, asparagus, beets, cauliflower, green beans, head lettuce, onions, mushrooms, zucchini)

**Grains: Make Half Your Grains Whole Grains** Foods from this group are usually low in fat and rich in complex carbohydrates, dietary fiber (if grains are unrefined), and vitamins and minerals, including thiamin, riboflavin, iron, niacin, folic acid (if enriched or fortified), magnesium, selenium, and zinc. A 2000-calorie diet should include 6 ounce-equivalents each day, with half of those servings from whole grains. The following items count as 1 ounce-equivalent:

- 1 slice of bread
- 1 small (2½-inch diameter) muffin
- 1 cup ready-to-eat cereal flakes
- ½ cup cooked cereal, rice, grains, or pasta
- 1 6-inch tortilla

Choose foods that are typically made with little fat or sugar (bread, rice, pasta) over those that are high in fat and sugar (croissants, chips, cookies).

**Protein Foods: Vary Your Protein Routine** This group includes meat, poultry, seafood, beans, peas, and lentils, eggs, nuts and seeds, and soy products. These foods provide protein, niacin, iron, vitamin B-6, zinc, and thiamin. The animal foods in this group also provide vitamin B-12. A 2000-calorie diet should include 5½ ounce-equivalents daily. Each of the following counts as 1 ounce-equivalent:

- 1 ounce cooked lean meat, poultry, or fish
- ¼ cup cooked dried beans (legumes) or tofu
- 1 egg
- 1 tablespoon peanut butter
- ½ ounce nuts or seeds

Choose a variety of lean meats and skinless poultry, select a variety of protein foods, and watch serving sizes carefully. Choose plant proteins regularly, such as black beans, lentils, or tofu, every day, and include at least 8 ounces of cooked seafood per week. Vegetarian options in the protein foods group include beans, peas, and lentils, processed soy products, and nuts and seeds.

**Dairy: Move to Low-Fat and Fat-Free Dairy** This group includes milk and milk products, such as yogurt and cheeses that retain their calcium, as well as calcium-fortified soy milk. Foods from this group are high in protein, carbohydrate, calcium, potassium, zinc, magnesium, riboflavin, vitamin A, vitamin B12, and vitamin D (if fortified). Choosing lower-fat dairy will reduce energy intake and saturated fat intake. A 2000-calorie diet should include 3 cups of milk or the equivalent daily. Each of the following counts as 1 cup-equivalent:

- 1 cup milk
- 1 cup yogurt
- ½ cup ricotta cheese
- 1½ ounces natural cheese
- 2 ounces processed cheese

Cottage cheese is lower in calcium than most other cheeses; ½ cup is equivalent to ¼ cup milk. Ice cream is also lower in calcium and higher in sugar and fat than many other dairy products; one scoop counts as ⅓ cup milk.

QUICK STATS

**Top sources of calories in the U.S. diet are burgers, sandwiches, tacos, and burritos (15%); desserts and sweet snacks (8%); rice/pasta and grain dishes (6%); and sweetened beverages (6%).**

—U.S. Department of Health and Human Services and U.S. Department of Agriculture, 2020

**Oils** Included in this category are oils and fats that are liquid at room temperature; they come mostly from plant and fish sources. Also included are soft margarines, soft vegetable oil table spreads, mayonnaise, and some salad dressings that have no trans fats. Oils are major sources of vitamin E and unsaturated fatty acids, including essential fatty acids, but they are *not a food group.* A 2000-calorie diet should include 6 teaspoons (27 g) of oils per day. A 1-teaspoon serving is the equivalent of the following:

- 1 teaspoon vegetable oil or soft margarine
- 1 tablespoon mayonnaise-type salad dressing

Foods that are mostly oils include nuts, olives, avocados, and some fish. The following portions include about 1 teaspoon of oil: 8 large olives, ⅙ medium avocado, ½ tablespoon peanut butter, and ⅓ ounce roasted nuts. Food labels can help you identify the types and amounts of fat in various foods.

**Solid Fats and Added Sugars** If you choose nutrient-dense foods from all food groups, you will have a small proportion of your daily calorie budget left to "spend" on additional food choices. For those wanting to maintain weight, these calories may be used to increase the amount of nutrient-dense food from a food group, to consume foods that contain solid fats or added sugars, or to consume alcohol. People who are trying to lose weight and improve their health should limit solid fats and added sugars as much as possible. The average American consumes about 500 calories daily from solid fats and added sugars—far higher than the recommended limits.

**Physical Activity** Daily physical activity improves health, reduces the risk of chronic diseases, and helps people manage body weight. The MyPlate recommendation for

**Food Group Amounts for 2,000 Calories a Day for Ages 14+ Years**

| 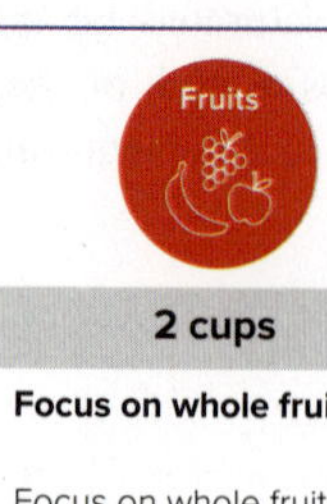 Fruits |  Vegetables | 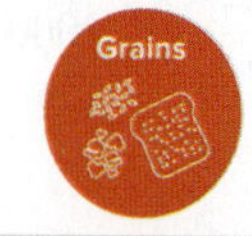 Grains | 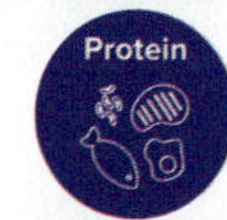 Protein |  Dairy |
|---|---|---|---|---|
| **2 cups** | **2½ cups** | **6 ounces** | **5½ ounces** | **3 cups** |
| **Focus on whole fruits** | **Vary your veggies** | **Make half your grains whole grains** | **Vary your protein routine** | **Move to low-fat or fat-free dairy milk or yogurt (or lactose-free dairy or fortified soy versions)** |
| Focus on whole fruits that are fresh, frozen, canned, or dried. | Choose a variety of colorful fresh, frozen, and canned vegetables—make sure to include dark green, red, and orange choices. | Find whole-grain foods by reading the Nutrition Facts label and ingredients list. | Mix up your protein foods to include seafood; beans, peas, and lentils; unsalted nuts and seeds; soy products; eggs; and lean meats and poultry. | Look for ways to include dairy or fortified soy alternatives at meals and snacks throughout the day. |

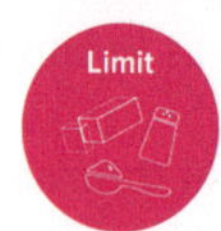


**Choose foods and beverages with less added sugars, saturated fat, and sodium.**
**Limit:**
- Added sugars to < **50 grams** a day.
- Saturated fat to < **22 grams** a day.
- Sodium to < **2,300 milligrams** a day.

**Be active your way:**
Children 6 to 17 years old should move **60 minutes** every day. Adults should be physically active at least **2½ hours** per week.

**FIGURE 10.4** **MyPlate food group amounts and recommendations for a 2000-calorie diet.**

SOURCE: MyPlate.gov. 2021. *MyPlate Daily Checklist for 2,000 Calories* (https://www.myplate.gov/myplate-plan/results/2000-calories-ages-14-plus).

adults is 2½ hours of moderate physical activity or 1¼ hours of vigorous aerobic physical activity per week, equivalent to the 150 minutes of moderate activity or 75 minutes of vigorous activity recommended in the *2018 Physical Activity Guidelines for Americans*, 2nd edition. In addition, muscle-strengthening activities that involve all major muscle groups should be done on two or more days a week. See Figure 10.4 for a summary of the MyPlate recommendations for a 2000-calorie diet.

## DASH Eating Plan

Other food-group plans have been proposed by a variety of experts and organizations, some to address the needs of special populations. One well-studied eating plan is called Dietary Approaches to Stop Hypertension (DASH). It was developed to help people control high blood pressure, and it is tailored with special attention to sodium, potassium, and other nutrients that affect blood pressure. Figure 4 in the Nutrition Resources section at the end of the chapter provides a more detailed look at the DASH Eating Plan.

## Choosing a Plant-Based Diet

People following a plant-based diet choose a diet with one basic difference from the diets described previously—they restrict or exclude foods of animal origin (meat, poultry, fish, eggs, and milk) and instead choose more plant-based foods. Commonly referred to as vegetarian, plant-based diets are lower in total fat, saturated fat, cholesterol, and animal protein and higher in complex carbohydrates, dietary fiber, magnesium, folate, vitamins C and E, carotenoids, and phytochemicals. **Vegetarians** generally have a lower body mass index than nonvegetarians and have diet patterns associated with lower mortality rates and lower rates of heart disease, obesity, hypertension, and type 2 diabetes. Many people adopt a vegetarian diet for health reasons, whereas others do so out of concern for the environment, for financial reasons, or for reasons related to ethics or religion. Since meat, dairy, and eggs are the only food sources for vitamin B-12 and for highly bioavailable iron, vegetarians must rely on fortified cereals and supplements.

> **TERMS**
> **vegetarian** Someone who follows a diet that restricts or eliminates foods of animal origin.

**Types of Plant-Based Diets** There are various vegetarian styles. The wider the variety of foods eaten, the easier it is to meet nutritional needs. *Vegans* eat only plant foods. *Lacto-vegetarians* eat plant foods and dairy products. *Lacto-ovo-vegetarians* eat plant foods, dairy products, and eggs. Others can be categorized as partial vegetarians, semivegetarians, or pesco-vegetarians. The latter–also called pescatarians or pescetarians–have diets that are mainly plant-based but also include fish and other seafood. Partial vegetarians generally eat plant foods, dairy products, eggs, and usually a small selection of poultry, fish, and other seafood. Many other people choose vegetarian meals frequently but are not strictly vegetarians. A quarter of Americans make dietary choices to limit their meat intake. Including some animal protein (such as dairy products and eggs) in a vegetarian diet makes planning easier, but it is not necessary.

**A Plant-Based Food Plan** Figure 2 in the Nutrition Resources section at the end of the chapter outlines the USDA's Healthy Vegetarian diet plan for a 2000-calorie diet.

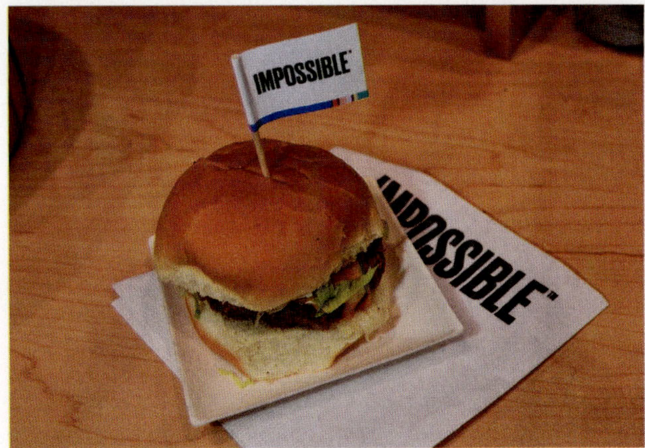


John D. Ivanko/Alamy Stock Photo

Adapting MyPlate for vegetarians requires only a few key modifications: For the meat and beans group, vegetarians can focus on the nonmeat choices of dry beans, nuts, seeds, eggs, and soy foods like tofu. Vegans and other vegetarians who do not consume any dairy products must find other rich sources of calcium. Fruits, vegetables, and whole grains are healthy choices for people following all types of vegetarian diets.

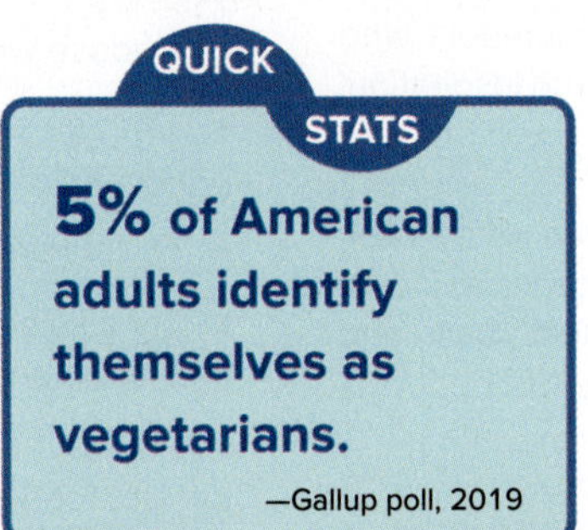


People following a more plant-based diet may choose to include meat alternatives—foods that approximate the taste and texture of meat but are made from vegetarian ingredients such as soy, gluten, or legumes. Many new plant-based products mimic beef patties, sausages, chicken strips, and similar animal foods. Recently developed products like the Impossible Burger and the Beyond Burger are promoted as especially meat-like and are even created to "bleed" like beef, but these are highly processed foods. As with any processed food, consider the overall nutritional profile of meat alternatives you select.

Unlike most animal proteins, most plant proteins do not contain all the necessary amino acids for good health. Thus, a healthy vegetarian diet must emphasize a wide variety of plant foods in order to include all the necessary amino acids. Choosing minimally processed and unrefined foods will maximize nutrient value and provide ample dietary fiber. Daily consumption of a variety of plant foods in amounts that meet total energy needs can provide all needed nutrients, except vitamin B-12 and possibly calcium, iron, zinc, and vitamin D.

## Dietary Challenges for Various Population Groups

The *Dietary Guidelines for Americans* and MyPlate can help nearly anyone create a healthy diet. However, some population groups face special dietary challenges.

**College Students** Convenient foods are not always the healthiest choices. Students who eat in buffet-style dining halls can easily overeat, and the foods offered are not necessarily high in nutrients or low in fat, sodium, and added sugars. The same is true of meals at fast-food restaurants. See the box "Eating Strategies for College Students" for tips on making healthy eating convenient and affordable.

**Pregnant and Breastfeeding Women** Good nutrition is essential to a healthy pregnancy. Before conception, nutrition counseling can help a woman establish a balanced eating plan and healthy body weight for pregnancy. During pregnancy and while breastfeeding, women have special nutritional needs and are often advised to take nutrient supplements (discussed in more detail later in this chapter and in Chapter 6).

**Older Adults** Nutrient needs do not change much as people age, but because older adults tend to become less active, they don't need as much energy intake to maintain body weight. At the same time, older adults absorb some nutrients less efficiently (e.g., vitamin B-12) because of age-related changes in the digestive tract. For these reasons, older adults should focus on eating nutrient-dense foods. Foods fortified with vitamin B-12 and/or B-12 supplements are recommended for people over age 50, and calcium and vitamin D supplements may be recommended for older adults to reduce bone loss and lower the risk of osteoporosis. Antioxidants from fruits and vegetables are important in older adults to reduce age-related changes in vision, immunity, and cognitive functioning. Because constipation is a common problem for older adults, eating high-fiber foods and drinking enough fluids are important goals.

**Athletes** Key dietary concerns for athletes are meeting their increased energy requirements and drinking enough fluids during practice and throughout the day to remain fully hydrated. Endurance athletes and athletes in heavy training may also benefit from increasing the amount of carbohydrates in the diet to 60–70% of total daily energy intake; this increase should take the form of complex, rather than simple, carbohydrates. Athletes who need to maintain a low body weight—such as skaters, gymnasts, and wrestlers—must avoid unhealthy eating patterns, which can lead to eating disorders. Eating for exercise is discussed in more detail in Chapter 11; see Chapter 12 for information about eating disorders.

**People with Special Health Concerns** People with diabetes benefit from a well-balanced diet that is low in simple sugars and high in complex carbohydrates. People with high blood pressure need to control their weight and limit their sodium consumption. If you have a health concern that requires a special diet, discuss your situation with a physician or registered dietitian nutritionist.

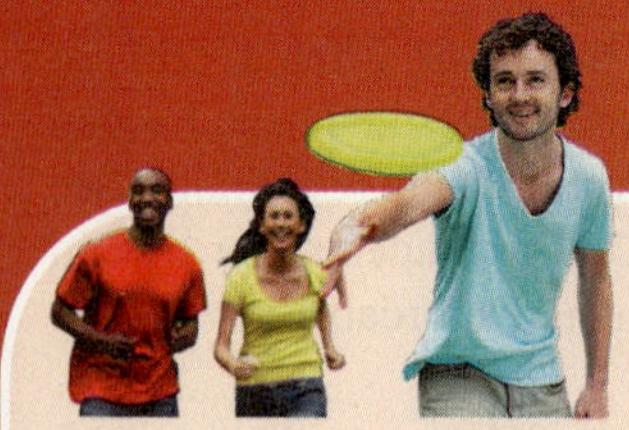

## WELLNESS ON CAMPUS

### Eating Strategies for College Students

#### All the Time

- Eat a colorful, varied, and plant-based diet. The more colorful your diet is, the more varied and rich in fruits and vegetables it will be. Fruits and vegetables are typically inexpensive, delicious, and nutrient-dense.
- Don't skip meals, especially breakfast. You'll have more energy in the morning and be less likely to grab an unhealthy snack later on. Skipping meals leads to poorer food choices throughout the day.
- Choose healthy snacks—fruits, vegetables, whole grains, and cereals.
- Drink lower-fat milk, water, mineral water, or 100% fruit juice more often than soft drinks or sweetened beverages.
- Pay attention to portion sizes. Enjoy your food, but eat less.
- Plan to eat meals with friends and family members who choose healthy foods and can provide support and inspiration.
- Combine physical activity with healthy eating.
- Choose plant-based (meatless) meals more often. Ask about vegetarian options when eating out or consider cooking your own meat-free burgers, tacos, or "meat" balls and spaghetti.

#### Eating in the Dining Hall

- Choose a meal plan that includes breakfast.
- Decide what you want to eat before you get in line, and stick to your choices.
- Build your meals around whole grains and vegetables. Ask for small servings of meat and high-fat main dishes.
- Choose leaner poultry, fish, or bean dishes without added sugar or high sodium rather than high-fat meats and fried entrees.
- Ask that gravies and sauces be served on the side; limit your intake.
- Choose broth-based or vegetable soups, not cream soups.
- At the salad bar, load up on leafy greens, beans, and fresh vegetables. Avoid mayonnaise-coated salads, bacon, croutons, and high-fat dressings. Put dressing on the side, and dip your fork into it rather than pouring it over the salad.
- Choose fruit for dessert rather than baked goods.
- Skip the soda machine and opt for water or low-fat dairy for your beverage choices.

#### Eating in Fast-Food Restaurants

- Most fast-food chains can provide a brochure with the nutritional content of their menu items. Ask for it, or check the restaurant's website for nutritional information. Order small single burgers with no cheese instead of double burgers with many toppings. If possible, get them broiled instead of fried.
- Ask for items to be prepared without mayonnaise, tartar sauce, sour cream, or other high-fat sauces. Ketchup, mustard, and fat-free mayonnaise or sour cream are better choices and are available at many fast-food restaurants.
- Choose whole-grain bread for burgers and sandwiches.
- Choose chicken items made from chicken breast, not processed chicken.
- Order vegetable pizzas without extra cheese.
- Try a salad or fruit as a side item. If you can't resist french fries or onion rings, get the smallest size.
- For food truck meals, use the same strategies suggested for fast-food restaurants: Choose lean proteins and ask for condiments on the side. If your favorite food truck doesn't have healthy options, ask that they be added to the menu.

#### Eating on the Run

- When you need to eat in a hurry, carry healthy foods in your backpack or a small insulated lunch sack (with a frozen gel pack to keep fresh food from spoiling). Also carry a refillable water bottle.
- Carry items that are small and convenient but nutritious, such as fresh fruits or vegetables, whole-wheat buns or muffins, snack-size cereal boxes, and water.
- When buying beverages from vending machines, choose water or 100% fruit juice. When buying snacks, choose whole-grain crackers, pretzels, nuts or seeds, baked chips, low-fat popcorn, or low-fat granola bars.

## A PERSONAL PLAN: MAKING INFORMED CHOICES ABOUT FOOD

Understanding the basics of good nutrition should get you started on creating a healthy diet that works for you. But eating for health involves other skills, as well. For example, it's helpful to be able to interpret the labels on food products and dietary supplement labels. Everyone who handles and prepares food should know how to avoid foodborne illnesses and environmental contaminants. In addition to understanding the nutritional content of foods, you can be an even smarter consumer if you know about other food contents, such as additives, and the various ways foods can be processed before going to market. The sections that follow address these issues.

## CRITICAL CONSUMER
## Using Food Labels

The Nutrition Facts panel on a food label is designed to help consumers make food choices based on the nutrients that are most important to good health. In addition to listing nutrient content by weight, the label puts the information in the context of a daily diet of 2000 calories, with the understanding that your calorie needs may be higher or lower depending on your age, gender, height, weight, and physical activity level.

Food labels contain uniform serving sizes. This means that if you look at different brands of salad dressing, for example, you can compare calories and fat content based on the serving amount. Food label serving sizes, however, may be larger or smaller than MyPlate serving-size equivalents.

The Nutrition Facts label had been in use without major changes since the 1990s. Based on research into how consumers use food labels as well as changes to the nutrients of most concern to Americans, the FDA announced changes to the look and content of the label in 2016 and the new food labels are now in effect. Some new features include:

- Adding added sugars, vitamin D, and potassium to all labels; Vitamins A and C will no longer be required because deficiencies in these vitamins are rare today
- Removing the listing for "Calories from Fat" because research shows the type of fat is more important than the amount
- Revising Daily Values for certain nutrients to reflect the latest recommendations
- Updating serving-size labeling for certain packages to be more realistic and to reflect amounts typically eaten at one time
- Refreshing the design to highlight calorie content and serving size and to make other parts of the label easier to read

You can explore the new Nutrition Facts Label at the following interactive site: https://www.accessdata.fda.gov/scripts/InteractiveNutritionFactsLabel/#intro

SOURCE: U.S. Food and Drug Administration. 2021. *Changes to the Nutrition Facts Label* (https://www.fda.gov/food/food-labeling-nutrition/changes-nutrition-facts-label)

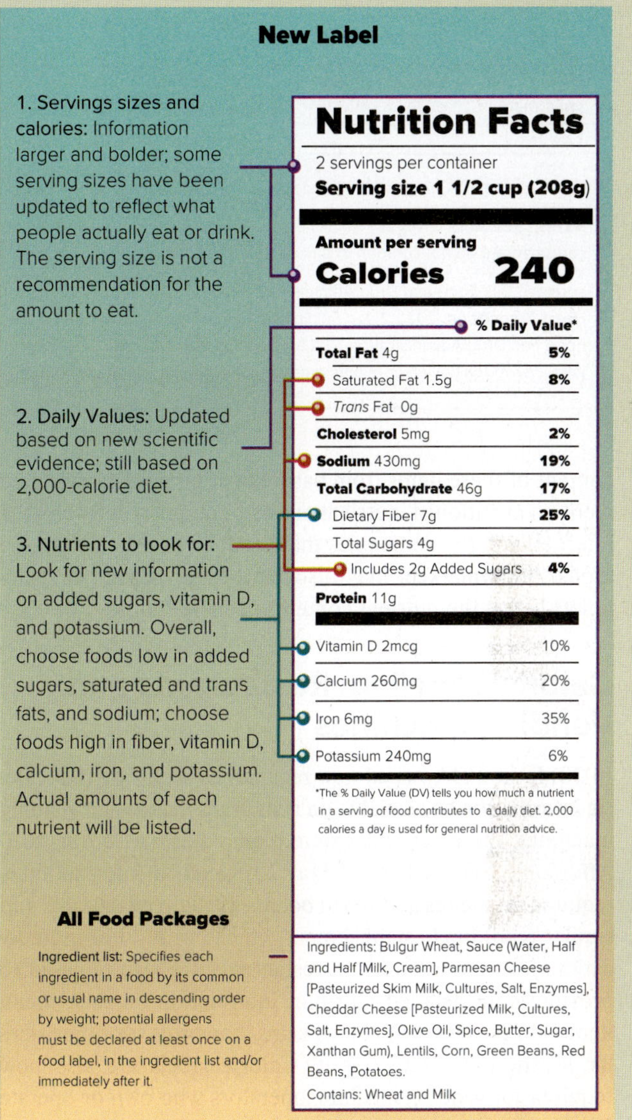


## Reading Food Labels

All processed foods regulated by either the FDA or the USDA include standardized nutrition information on their labels. Every food label shows serving sizes and the amounts of fat, saturated fat, trans fat, cholesterol, sodium, total carbohydrate, dietary fiber, total sugars, added sugars, and protein in each serving. To make informed choices about food, learn to read and *understand* food labels (see the box "Using Food Labels").

Food label regulations also require that foods meet strict definitions if their packaging includes terms such as *light, low-fat,* or *high-fiber* (Table 10.8). The FDA recently proposed an update to the nutrient content claim "healthy:" Products would need to contain a significant portion of food from at least one of the food groups or subgroups recommended by the Dietary Guidelines as part of healthy dietary patterns and remain below certain limits for saturated fats, sodium, and added sugars. For example, a cereal would need to contain ¾ ounces of whole grains and no more than 1 gram of saturated fat, 230 milligrams of sodium and 2.5 grams of added sugars.

Fresh meat, poultry, fish, fruits, and vegetables are not required to have food labels, and many of these products are not packaged. You can find information about the nutrient

**Table 10.8** Food Package Nutrient Claims

| TERM | DEFINITION |
|---|---|
| Healthy* | A significant portion from at least one of the food groups recommended by the Dietary Guidelines as part of healthy dietary patterns and below certain limits for saturated fats, sodium, and added sugars |
| Good source | 10–19% of the Daily Value for a particular nutrient per serving |
| High, rich in, or excellent source of | 20% or more of the Daily Value for a particular nutrient per serving |
| High fiber | 5 grams or more of fiber per serving |
| Low in | 5% or less of the Daily Value for a particular nutrient per serving |

*In 2022, the FDA proposed this redefinition of the "healthy" nutrient content claim.

NOTES: See more terms at the links below. The FDA has not yet defined nutrient claims relating to carbohydrates, so foods labeled low- or reduced-carbohydrate do not conform to any approved standard.

SOURCE: U.S. Food and Drug Administration. 2018. *FDA Nutrient Content Claims* (http://www.fda.gov/Food/LabelingNutrition/ucm2006880.htm); American Heart Association. 2022. *Food Packaging Claims* (https://www.heart.org/en/healthy-living/healthy-eating/eat-smart/nutrition-basics/food-packaging-claims); Food and Drug Administration. 2022. *FDA Proposes Updated Definition of 'Healthy' Claim on Food Packages to Help Improve Diet, Reduce Chronic Disease* (https://www.fda.gov/news-events/press-announcements/fda-proposes-updated-definition-healthy-claim-food-packages-help-improve-diet-reduce-chronic-disease).

content of these items from basic nutrition books, registered dietitian nutritionist, nutrient analysis computer software, the internet, and the companies that produce or distribute these foods. Supermarkets may also have large posters or pamphlets listing the nutrient contents of these foods.

## Calorie Labeling: Restaurants and Vending Machines

In 2014, the FDA issued new regulations requiring that calorie information be available on restaurant menus and vending machines; these new rules were required as part of the 2010 Affordable Care Act. As of May 2018, calorie information is required on menus and menu boards in chain restaurants and similar retail food establishments (those with 20 or more locations). In addition, chain restaurants are also required to provide more detailed nutrition information on their menu items—on posters, tray liners, signs, handouts, or other similar locations—so look for it! Calorie labels are also now required for vending machine operators who own or operate 20 or more machines.

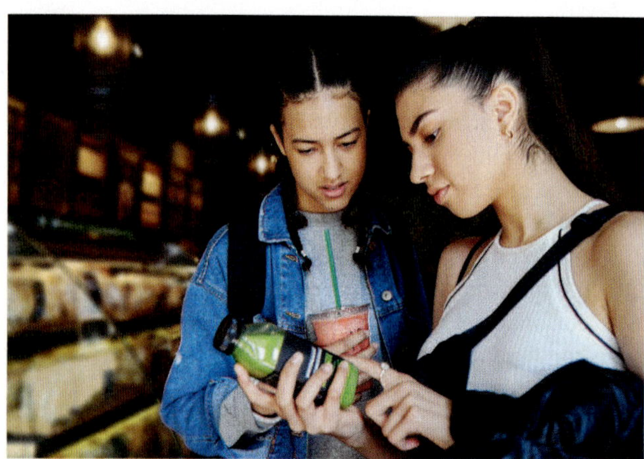

We Are/Getty Images

## Dietary Supplements

National food guidance encourages people to meet their nutritional needs with a nutritionally balanced diet of whole foods rather than with vitamin and mineral supplements. Although dietary supplements are sold over the counter, they are not necessarily proven effective or safe, especially when consumed over a long period of time. Some vitamins and minerals are dangerous when taken in excess. Large doses of particular nutrients can also cause health problems by affecting the absorption of certain vitamins or minerals or interacting with medications. For this reason, it is prudent to talk to your doctor, pharmacist, or a registered dietitian nutritionist before taking any high-dosage supplement.

**People Who Benefit from Supplements** In establishing the DRIs, the Food and Nutrition Board recommended supplements of particular nutrients for specific groups:

- Women who are capable of getting pregnant should get 400 μg per day of folic acid (the synthetic form of the vitamin folate) from fortified foods and supplements in addition to folate from a varied diet. This level of folate can reduce the risk of neural tube defects in a developing fetus. Enriched breads, flours, cornmeal, rice, noodles, and other grain products are fortified with folic acid. Folate is found naturally in leafy green vegetables, legumes, oranges, and strawberries.
- People over age 50 should eat foods fortified with vitamin B-12, take a B-12 supplement, or combine the two to meet the RDA of 2.4 μg daily. Up to 30% of people over age 50 may have trouble absorbing protein-bound B-12 in foods.
- Because of the oxidative stress caused by smoking, smokers should get 35 mg more vitamin C per day than the RDA set for their age and sex. Supplements aren't usually necessary, however, because this extra vitamin C can easily be found in foods. For example, one cup of sliced strawberries has about 100 mg of vitamin C.

Other people may benefit from supplementation based on their physical condition, the medicines they take, or their dietary habits.

Before deciding whether to take a vitamin or mineral supplement, consider whether you already eat a fortified breakfast cereal every day. Many breakfast cereals contain almost as many nutrients as a multivitamin pill. If you elect to take a supplement, choose one that contains 50–100% of the Daily Values for vitamins and minerals. Avoid supplements containing large doses at levels exceeding the tolerable upper intake level (UL).

**Reading Supplement Labels** Dietary supplements include vitamins, minerals, amino acids, herbs, phytochemicals enzymes, and other compounds. They are available as tablets, capsules, liquids, and powders. Although dietary supplements are often thought to be safe and sometimes labeled "natural," they can contain powerful bioactive chemicals that have the potential for harm.

In the United States, dietary supplements are not legally considered drugs and are not regulated the same way drugs are. Before a drug is approved by the FDA and put on the market, it must undergo clinical studies to determine safety, effectiveness, side effects and risks, possible interactions with other substances, and appropriate dosages. The FDA does not authorize or test dietary supplements, and supplement manufacturers are not required to demonstrate either safety or effectiveness prior to marketing. Although dosage guidelines exist for some of the compounds in dietary supplements, dosages for many are not well established, and purity can vary widely.

Dietary supplement manufacture is not closely regulated, and there is no guarantee that a product even contains a given ingredient, let alone in the appropriate amount. In addition, herbs can be contaminated or misidentified at any stage from harvest to packaging.

To provide consumers with more reliable and consistent information about supplements, the FDA requires supplements to have labels similar to those found on foods (see the box "Using Dietary Supplement Labels" for more information). Label statements and claims about supplements are also regulated.

QUICK
STATS
Each year, 1 in 6 Americans gets sick by consuming contaminated foods or beverages.
—Centers for Disease Control and Prevention, 2021

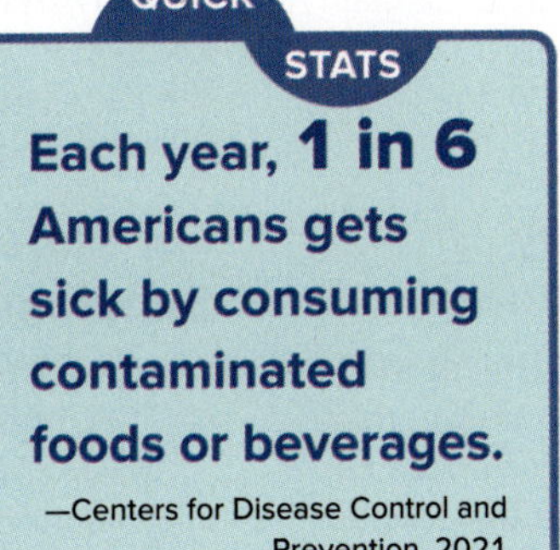

## Protecting Yourself against Foodborne Illness

The CDC estimates that approximately 48 million illnesses, 128,000 hospitalizations, and 3000 deaths occur each year in the United States due to foodborne illnesses. Symptoms include diarrhea, vomiting, fever, pain, headache, and weakness. Although the effects of foodborne illnesses are usually not serious, some groups, such as children, pregnant women, individuals with immune deficits, and older adults, are more at risk for severe complications such as rheumatic diseases, seizures, blood poisoning, hemolytic uremic syndrome, and death.

Thirty-one known **pathogens**—disease-causing microorganisms including bacteria, viruses, and parasites—cause many cases of foodborne illness every year. Food can be contaminated with pathogens through improper handling, and pathogens can grow if food is prepared or stored improperly. According to the CDC, 8 pathogens contribute to the vast majority of illnesses, hospitalizations, and deaths related to foodborne illnesses: *Salmonella* (most often found in eggs, on vegetables, and on poultry); *Norovirus* (most often found in salad ingredients and shellfish); *Campylobacter jejuni* (most often found in meat and poultry); *Toxoplasma* (most often found in meat); *Escherichia coli* (E. coli) O157:H7 (most often found in meat and water); *Listeria monocytogenes* (most often found in lunch meats, sausages, and hot dogs); *Clostridium perfringens* (most often found in meat and gravy); and *Staphylococcus aureus* (most often resulting from improper hand washing leading to food contamination). *Salmonella* is the leading cause of foodborne hospitalizations.

Other causes of foodborne illness include the bacteria *Vibrio vulnificus,* and *Yersinia enterocolytica;* the hepatitis A virus; the parasites *Trichinella spiralis* (found in pork and wild game), *Anisakis* (found in raw fish), *Giardia lamblia, Cyclospora cayetanensis,* and tapeworms; and certain molds. The known pathogens account for about 9 million illnesses annually. In addition to these, there are many other unspecified agents, such as biotoxins and metals, that account for about 37 million illnesses annually.

Food safety experts encourage people to follow four basic food safety principles: ***Clean*** hands, food contact surfaces, and vegetables and fruits. ***Separate*** raw, cooked, and ready-to-eat foods while shopping, storing, and preparing foods. ***Cook*** foods to a safe temperature. ***Chill*** (refrigerate) perishable foods promptly.

If you think you may be having a bout of foodborne illness, drink plenty of fluids to prevent dehydration and consult a physician. For more details on handling food safely, see the box "Safe Food Handling."

Although pathogens are usually destroyed during cooking, the U.S. government has taken steps to bring down levels of contamination by improving national surveillance and testing.

## Organic Foods

Some people who are concerned about pesticides and other environmental contaminants choose foods that are **organic.**

**TERMS**

**pathogen** A microorganism that causes disease.

**organic** A designation applied to foods grown and produced according to strict guidelines limiting the use of pesticides, nonorganic ingredients, hormones, antibiotics, irradiation, genetic engineering, and other practices.

# CRITICAL CONSUMER
## Using Dietary Supplement Labels

Since 1999, specific types of information have been required on the labels of dietary supplements. In addition to basic information about the product, labels include a "Supplement Facts" panel, modeled after the "Nutrition Facts" panel used on food labels (see the label illustrated in this box). Under the Dietary Supplement Health and Education Act (DSHEA) and food labeling laws, supplement labels can make three types of health-related claims:

- ***Nutrient content claims,*** such as "high in calcium," "excellent source of vitamin C," or "high potency." The claims "high in" and "excellent source of" mean the same as they do on food labels. A "high-potency" single-ingredient supplement must contain 100% of that nutrient's Daily Value; a "high-potency" multi-ingredient product must contain 100% or more of the Daily Value of at least two-thirds of the nutrients present for which Daily Values have been established.
- ***Health claims,*** if they have been authorized by the FDA or another authoritative scientific body. The association between adequate calcium intake and lower risk of osteoporosis is an example of an approved health claim. Since 2003, the FDA has also allowed so-called qualified health claims for situations in which there is emerging but as yet inconclusive evidence for a particular claim. These claims must include qualifying language such as "scientific evidence suggests but does not prove [the claim]."
- ***Structure–function claims,*** such as "antioxidants maintain cellular integrity" or "this product enhances energy levels." Because these claims are not reviewed by the FDA, they must carry a disclaimer (see the sample label).

### Tips for Choosing and Using Dietary Supplements

- Check with your physician before taking a supplement. Many are not meant for children, older adults, women who are pregnant or breastfeeding, people with chronic illnesses or upcoming surgery, or people taking prescription or over-the-counter medications. When you visit your doctor, bring a list of all dietary supplements you are taking. Do not take megadoses (more than double the DRI levels) without your doctor's approval.
- Choose brands made by nationally known food and drug manufacturers or house brands from large retail chains. Due to their size and visibility, such sources are likely to have high manufacturing standards.
- Look for the "USP" (United States Pharmacopeial Convention) verification mark on the label, indicating that the product meets minimum safety and purity standards developed under the USP Dietary Supplement Verification Program. The USP mark means that the product (1) contains the listed ingredients, (2) has the declared amount and strength of ingredients, (3) will dissolve effectively, (4) has been screened for harmful contaminants, and (5) has been manufactured using safe, sanitary, and well-controlled procedures. The National Nutritional Foods Association (NNFA) has a self-regulatory testing program for its members; other associations and laboratories, including ConsumerLab.com, also test and rate dietary supplements.

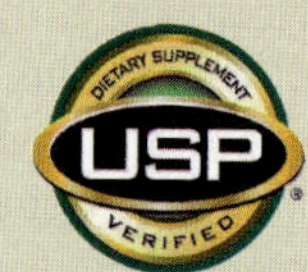


Courtesy The United States Pharmacopeial Convention. Registered trademark of The United States Pharmacopeial Convention.

- Follow the label's cautions, directions for use, and dosage.
- If you experience side effects, stop using the product and contact your physician. Report any serious reactions to the FDA's MedWatch monitoring program (800-FDA-1088 or online at http://www.fda.gov/Safety/MedWatch/default.htm).

### For More Information about Dietary Supplements

NIH Office of Dietary Supplements (http://ods.od.nih.gov)
FDA (http://www.fda.gov/food/dietarysupplements)
USDA (https://www.nal.usda.gov/legacy/fnic/general-information-and-resources-dietary-supplements)

Statement of identity and net quantity

Structure-function claim

Directions for use and storage

Warnings may appear on some labels

Disclaimer accompanying structure-function claim

***MOOD ENHANCER DIETARY SUPPLEMENT***

60 capsules

***Specially formulated to enhance your mood, maintain healthy energy levels, and help you deal with daily stresses.****

DIRECTIONS FOR USE: Take one capsule twice daily with a meal.

Keep out of reach of children. Store in a cool, dry place, tightly closed. Color variation is normal in this product.

WARNING: FOR ADULTS ONLY. Do not exceed the recommended dosage. Do not use if you are pregnant, lactating, or taking prescription antidepressant or anti-anxiety medication. Do not use with alcohol. Do not use if you have allergies to the ragweed family. Limit exposure to the sun as St. John's wort may cause increased sensitivity to light. Discontinue use in the event of a rash.

PHENYLKETONURICS: CONTAINS PHENYLALANINE.

*This statement has not been evaluated by the Food and Drug Administration. This product is not intended to diagnose, treat, cure, or prevent any disease.

**Supplement Facts**

Serving Size 1 capsule

| Amount per capsule | % Daily Value* |
|---|---|
| **Vitamin $B_6$** (as pyroxidine hydrochloride) 2.0 mg | 100% |
| **Folic acid** 200 mcg | 50% |
| **Vitamin $B_{12}$** (as cyanocobalamin) 6 mcg | 100% |
| **St. John's wort aerial parts extract** 300 mg (*Hypericum perforatum*) | † |
| **Kava root extract** 250 mg (*Piper methysticum*) | † |
| **Siberian ginseng root extract** 200 mg (*Eleutherococcus senticosus*) | † |
| **Phenylalanine** (as L-phenylalanine hydrochloride) 100 mg | † |

*Percent Daily Values are based on a 2000 calorie diet.
†Daily Value not established.

Other ingredients: Rice flour, gelatin, water.

Standardization levels: St. John's wort: 0.3% hypericin; kava: 30% kavalactones; Siberian ginseng: 1% eleutherosides.

*Made by JKS Herbal Supplements, P.O. Box 2000, San Francisco, CA 94444.*

Serving size

Source and amount of ingredients with established Daily Values

Name, source, and amount of ingredients without established Daily Values

Standardization levels may appear on some labels

Address to write to for more product information

## TAKE CHARGE
### Safe Food Handling

- Thoroughly wash your hands with warm, soapy water for 20 seconds before and after handling food, especially raw meat, fish, shellfish, poultry, or eggs.
- Don't buy food in containers that leak, bulge, or are severely dented. Refrigerated foods should be cold, and frozen foods should be solid when you buy them.
- Refrigerate perishable items as soon as possible after purchase. Use or freeze fresh meats within 3–5 days and fresh poultry, fish, and ground meat within 1–2 days.
- Store raw meat, poultry, fish, and shellfish in containers in the refrigerator so that the juices don't drip onto other foods. Keep these items away from other foods, surfaces, utensils, or serving dishes to prevent cross-contamination.
- Thaw frozen food in the refrigerator or in the microwave oven, not on the kitchen counter. Cook foods immediately after thawing.
- Make sure counters, cutting boards, dishes, utensils, and other equipment are cleaned thoroughly with hot, soapy water before and after use. Wash dishcloths frequently.
- If possible, use separate cutting boards for meat, poultry, and seafood and for foods that will be eaten raw. Replace cutting boards once they become worn or develop hard-to-clean grooves.
- Thoroughly rinse and scrub fruits and vegetables with a brush, if possible, or peel off the skin.
- Cook foods thoroughly, especially beef, poultry, fish, pork, wild game, and eggs; cooking kills most microorganisms. Use a food thermometer to ensure that foods are cooked to a safe temperature. Hamburgers should be cooked to at least 160°F. Turn or stir microwaved food to make sure it is heated evenly throughout. When eating out, order hamburger cooked well-done and make sure foods are served piping hot.
- Keep hot foods hot (140°F or above) and cold foods cold (40°F or below). Harmful bacteria can grow rapidly between these two temperatures. Refrigerate foods within two hours of purchase or preparation, and within one hour if the air temperature is above 90°F. Refrigerate foods at or below 40°F and freeze at or below 0°F. Use refrigerated leftovers within 3–4 days.
- Don't eat raw animal products, including raw eggs in homemade hollandaise sauce or eggnog. Use only pasteurized milk and juice, and look for pasteurized eggs, which are now available in some states.
- Cook eggs until they're firm, and fully cook foods containing eggs. Store eggs in the cooler parts of the refrigerator, not in the door, and use them within 3–5 weeks.
- Avoid raw sprouts. Even sprouts grown under clean conditions in the home can be risky because bacteria may be present in the seeds. Cook sprouts before eating them.
- Read the food label and package information, and follow safety instructions such as "Keep Refrigerated" and the "Safe Handling Instructions."
- According to the USDA, "When in doubt, throw it out." Even if a food looks and smells fine, it may not be safe. If you aren't sure that a food has been prepared, served, and stored safely, don't eat it.

Additional precautions are recommended for people at particularly high risk for foodborne illness—pregnant women, very young children, older people, and people with weakened immune systems or certain chronic illnesses. If you are a member of one of these groups, don't eat or drink any of the following products: unpasteurized juices; raw sprouts; unpasteurized (raw) milk and products made from unpasteurized milk; raw or undercooked meat, poultry, eggs, fish, or shellfish; and soft cheeses such as feta, Brie, Camembert, or blue-veined cheeses. To protect against *Listeria,* avoid ready-to-eat foods such as hot dogs, luncheon meats, and cold cuts unless they are reheated until they are steaming hot.

To be certified as organic by the USDA, foods must meet strict production, processing, handling, and labeling criteria. Organic crops must meet limits on pesticide residues. For meat, milk, eggs, and other animal products to be certified organic, animals must be given organic feed and access to the outdoors and may not be given antibiotics or growth hormones. The use of genetic engineering, ionizing radiation, and sewage sludge is prohibited. Products can be labeled "100% organic" if they contain all organic ingredients and "organic" if they contain at least 95% organic ingredients; all such products may carry the USDA organic seal. A product with at least 70% organic ingredients can be labeled "made with organic ingredients" but cannot use the USDA seal.

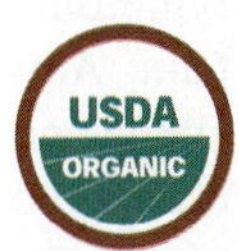


Some experts also recommend buying organic beef, poultry, eggs, dairy products, and baby food. Fruits and vegetables that carry little pesticide residue whether grown conventionally or organically include asparagus, avocados, bananas, broccoli, cauliflower, corn, kiwi, mangoes, onions, papaya, pineapples, and peas. All foods are subject to strict pesticide limits; the debate about the health effects of small amounts of residue is ongoing.

Organic farming is better for the environment. Benefits include sustainable farming practices, preservation of biodiversity, healthier soil, protection of water supplies, reduced use of fossil fuels, improved animal welfare, protection of ecosystems, and safer conditions for farmworkers. Buying organic food, buying locally grown foods, and participating in a community garden are ways to support food production that benefits and sustains the environment.

## Guidelines for Fish Consumption

Overall, fish and shellfish are healthy sources of protein, omega-3 fats, and other nutrients. Prudent choices can minimize the risk of any possible negative health effects. Consuming foods with mercury can cause brain damage in fetuses and young children. High mercury concentrations are most likely to be found in predator fish—large fish that eat smaller fish.

According to 2021 FDA and Environmental Protection Agency (EPA) guidelines, women who are or may become pregnant and nursing mothers should follow these guidelines to minimize their exposure to mercury:

- Do not eat shark, swordfish, king mackerel, marlin, orange roughy, bigeye tuna, or tilefish (from the Gulf of Mexico).
- Eat 2–3 servings (8–12 ounces) a week of a variety of fish and shellfish that are lower in mercury, such as shrimp, canned light tuna, salmon, pollock, and catfish. Limit consumption of albacore tuna to 1 serving (4 ounces) per week.
- Check advisories about the safety of recreationally caught fish from local lakes, rivers, and coastal areas; if no information is available, limit consumption to 4 ounces per week.

The same FDA/EPA guidelines apply to children, although they should consume smaller servings.

## Additives in Food

According to the FDA's "Substances Added to Food" inventory, over 3000 substances are intentionally added to foods to maintain or improve nutritional quality, maintain freshness, help in processing or preparation, or alter taste or appearance. The most widely used food additives are sugar, salt, and corn syrup; these three plus citric acid, baking soda, vegetable colors, mustard, and pepper account for 98% by weight of all food additives used in the United States.

Additives having potential health concerns include nitrates and nitrites, used in processed meats and associated with the synthesis of cancer-causing agents in the stomach; BHA (butylated hydroxyanisole) and BHT (butylated hydroxytoluene), used to maintain freshness and possibly associated with an increased risk of some cancers; and sulfites, used to keep vegetables from turning brown and associated with severe reactions in sensitive people.

TERMS

**genetically modified organism (GMO)**
A plant, animal, or microorganism in which genes have been added, rearranged, or replaced through genetic engineering.

## Functional Foods and Food Biotechnology

The American diet contains numerous functional foods. This phrase generally refers to foods containing components that may provide positive health benefits. Two of the earliest functional foods introduced in the United States were iodized salt and milk fortified with vitamins A and D. More recently, manufacturers began fortifying breads and grains with folic acid to reduce the incidence of neural tube defects. Some foods are made functional by the addition of an ingredient with proven health-promoting or disease-preventing components. To be considered functional, a food must be able to claim a health benefit beyond what you would normally get consuming the food in nonfortified form.

Food biotechnology techniques, such as crossbreeding, have been used by farmers for thousands of years to improve productivity and develop desirable qualities in animals and crops. Modern biotechnology tools, such as genetic engineering and cloning, allow for more precise, productive, and efficient development of crops and livestock.

Genetic engineering involves altering the characteristics of a plant, animal, or microorganism by adding, rearranging, or replacing genes in its DNA; the result is a **genetically modified organism (GMO).** New DNA may come from related species or from entirely different types of organisms. Many GM crops are already grown in the United States. For example, most soybean crops in the United States have been genetically modified to be resistant to some herbicides used to kill weeds, and most GM corn crops carry genes for herbicide resistance or pest resistance. Products made with GMOs include juice, soda, nuts, tuna, frozen pizza, spaghetti sauce, canola oil, chips, salad dressings, and soup.

The potential benefits of GM foods cited by supporters include improved yields overall and in difficult growing conditions, increased disease resistance, improved nutritional content, lower prices, and less pesticide use. Critics of biotechnology argue that unexpected harmful effects may occur: Gene manipulation could elevate levels of naturally occurring toxins or allergens, permanently change the gene pool, reduce biodiversity, and produce pesticide-resistant insects. The National Academies of Science, Engineering and Medicine (NASEM) published an extensive report analyzing research on GMOs, concluding that they were not a risk to human health. Research into many aspects of GMO agriculture is ongoing.

## Food Allergies and Food Intolerances

For some people, consuming a particular food causes symptoms such as itchiness, swollen lips, or abdominal pain. Adverse reactions like these may be due to a food allergy or a food intolerance, and symptoms may range from annoying to life-threatening.

## Ask Yourself

**QUESTIONS FOR CRITICAL THINKING AND REFLECTION**

What is the least healthy food you eat every day (either during meals or as a snack)? Identify at least one substitute that would be healthier and just as satisfying.

A true **food allergy** is a reaction of the body's immune system to a food or food ingredient, usually a protein. The immune system perceives the reaction-provoking substance, or allergen, as foreign and acts to destroy it. This immune reaction can occur within minutes of ingesting the food, resulting in symptoms that affect the skin (hives), gastrointestinal tract (cramps or diarrhea), respiratory tract (asthma), or mouth (swelling of the lips or tongue). The most severe response is a systemic reaction called *anaphylaxis,* which involves a potentially life-threatening drop in blood pressure and narrowing of airways blocking normal breathing. Repeated exposure to the allergen may result in more severe symptoms.

Food allergies are estimated to affect 4–8% of infants and children and 6.6–10% of adults in the United States. Although numerous food allergens have been identified, just eight foods account for more than 90% of the food allergies in the United States: cow's milk, eggs, peanuts, tree nuts (walnuts, cashews, and so on), soy, wheat, fish, and shellfish and, as of 2023, sesame is joining the list as the ninth allergen. Food labels are now required to state the presence of the nine most common allergens in plain language in the ingredient list.

Many people who believe they have food allergies may actually suffer from a much more common source of adverse food reactions—a **food intolerance.** In the case of a food intolerance, the problem usually lies with metabolism rather than with the immune system. Typically the body cannot adequately digest a food or food component, often because of some type of chemical deficiency; in other cases, the body reacts to a particular compound in a food. Lactose intolerance is a fairly common food intolerance.

A more serious condition may be intolerance of gluten, a protein component of some grains. In recent decades, the prevalence of celiac disease has risen in Western populations. Currently, up to 1% of Americans have a hereditary autoimmune disease that causes the body to attack the small intestine when gluten is ingested and can lead to other debilitating medical problems. An additional 18 million people, or about 6% of the population, is believed to have gluten sensitivity, a less severe problem with the protein in wheat, barley, and rye and other foods that gives elasticity to dough and stability to the shape of baked goods.

Food intolerance reactions often produce symptoms similar to those of food allergies, such as diarrhea or cramps, but reactions are typically localized and not life-threatening. Many people with food intolerances can consume small amounts of the food that affects them; exceptions are gluten and sulfite, which must be avoided by sensitive individuals. Through trial and error, most people with food intolerances can adjust their intake of the trigger food to an appropriate level.

**TERMS**

**food allergy** An adverse reaction to a food or food ingredient in which the immune system perceives a particular substance (allergen) as foreign and acts to destroy it.

**food intolerance** An adverse reaction to a food or food ingredient that doesn't involve the immune system; intolerances are often due to a problem with metabolism.

## TIPS FOR TODAY AND THE FUTURE

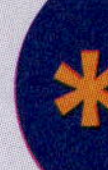

Opportunities to improve your diet present themselves every day, and small changes add up.

**RIGHT NOW YOU CAN:**

- Substitute a healthy snack for an unhealthy one.
- Drink a glass of water and put a reusable water bottle in your backpack for tomorrow.
- Plan to make healthy selections when you eat out, such as steamed vegetables instead of french fries, or fish instead of steak.

**IN THE FUTURE YOU CAN:**

- Visit the MyPlate website at MyPlate.gov and use the online tools to create a personalized nutrition plan and begin tracking your eating habits.
- Learn to cook healthier meals. Hundreds of free websites and low-cost cookbooks provide recipes for healthy dishes.

## SUMMARY

- To function at its best, the human body requires about 45 essential nutrients in certain relative proportions. People get these nutrients from foods; the body cannot synthesize most of them.
- Proteins, made up of amino acids, form muscles and bones and help make up blood, enzymes, hormones, and cell membranes. Foods from animal sources provide complete proteins; plants provide incomplete proteins and must be combined in order to attain the right balance of amino acids, especially if no or limited animal protein is in the diet. Protein intake should be 10–35% of total daily energy intake.
- Fats, a concentrated source of energy, also help to insulate the body and cushion the organs; 3–4 teaspoons of vegetable oil per day supplies the essential fats. Dietary fat intake should be 20–35% of total daily energy intake. In general, you can still eat high-fat foods, but avoid trans fats and limit the size of your portions and balance your intake with low-fat foods.

## BEHAVIOR CHANGE STRATEGY
# Improving Your Diet by Choosing Healthy Beverages

After reading this chapter and completing the dietary assessment, you can probably identify several ways to improve your diet. As an example here, we focus on choosing healthy beverages to increase intake of nutrients and decrease intake of empty calories from added sugars and fat. This model can be applied to any change you want to make to your diet.

### Gather Data and Establish a Baseline

Begin by tracking your beverage consumption in a journal. Write down the types and amounts of beverages you drink, including water. Also note where you were at the time and whether you got the beverage there or brought it with you. At the same time, investigate your options. Find out what other beverages you can easily find during your daily routine. This information will help you put together a successful plan for change.

### Analyze Your Data and Set Goals

Evaluate your beverage consumption by dividing your typical daily consumption between healthy and less healthy choices. Use the following guide as a basis, and add other beverages to the lists as needed:

| CHOOSE MORE OFTEN | SERVINGS DAILY | CHOOSE LESS OFTEN | SERVINGS DAILY |
|---|---|---|---|
| Water: plain, mineral, sparkling | | Regular soda | |
| Lower-fat milk | | Whole milk | |
| Fruit juice (100%) | | Fruit beverages made with little fruit juice | |
| Unsweetened or noncaloric sweetened herbal tea | | Sugar-sweetened beverages such as iced tea and sports drinks | |
| Others | | Others | |

How many beverages do you consume daily from each category? What would be a healthy and realistic goal for change? For example, if your beverage consumption is currently evenly divided between the "choose more often" and "choose less often" categories (four from each list), you might set a final goal for your behavior change program of increasing your healthy choices by two (to six from the "more often" list and two from the "less often" list).

### Develop a Plan for Change

Once you've set your goal, you need to develop strategies that will help you choose healthy beverages more often. Consider the following possibilities:

- Keep healthy beverages on hand. If you live in a dorm, rent a small refrigerator or keep water in a reusable bottle and other healthy choices in the dorm kitchen's refrigerator.
- Plan ahead, and carry a reusable bottle with water or 100% juice in your backpack every day.
- Check food labels on beverages for serving sizes, energy content, and nutrients; compare products to find the healthiest choices; and watch your serving sizes. Use this information to make your "choose more often" list longer and more specific.
- If you eat out frequently, examine all the beverages available at the places you typically eat your meals. You'll probably find that plain water or other healthy choices are available.

You may also need to make changes in your routine to decrease the likelihood that you'll make unhealthy choices. For example, your journal might reveal that you always buy a soda after class when you pass a particular vending machine. If this is the case, try another route that bypasses the machine. Guard against impulse buying by carrying water or a healthy snack with you every day.

To complete your plan, try some of the other behavior change strategies described in Chapter 1: Develop and sign a contract, set up a system of rewards, involve other people in your program, and develop strategies for challenging situations. Once your plan is complete, take action. Keep track of your progress by continuing to monitor and evaluate your beverage consumption.

- Carbohydrates supply energy to the brain and other parts of the nervous system as well as to red blood cells. The body needs about 130 grams of carbohydrates a day, but more is recommended. Carbohydrates should make up 45–65% of total daily energy intake.

- Fiber includes nondigestible carbohydrates provided mainly by plants. A high-fiber diet can help people manage diabetes and high cholesterol levels and improve intestinal health.

- The 13 vitamins needed in the diet are organic substances that regulate various processes within living cells and promote specific chemical reactions. Deficiencies or excesses can cause serious illnesses and even death.

- The approximately 17 minerals needed in the diet are inorganic substances that regulate body functions, aid in the growth and maintenance of body tissues, and help in the release of energy from foods.

- Water helps digest and absorb food, transport substances around the body, and regulate body temperature.

- Dietary Reference Intakes (DRIs) are standards for nutrient intake designed to prevent nutritional deficiencies and reduce the risk of chronic diseases.

- The *Dietary Guidelines for Americans* are designed to help people make healthy and informed food choices. Following the guidelines promotes health and reduces the risk of chronic disease.

- Choosing the right amount of foods from each food group in MyPlate every day ensures that you get enough necessary nutrients without overconsuming calories.

- A plant-based diet can meet human nutritional needs but must be planned carefully to prevent potential micronutrient deficiencies, especially of vitamin B-12 and readily bioavailable iron.

- Almost all foods have labels that show how much fat, cholesterol, protein, fiber, and sodium they contain. Serving sizes are standardized, and health claims are regulated carefully. Dietary supplements also have uniform labels that provide supplement facts.

- Food additives, environmental containments, and foodborne illnesses from *Salmonella*, *E. coli*, *Norovirus*, and other microorganisms can pose threats to health. Other dietary issues of concern to some people include genetic modification of foods and food allergies and intolerances.

## FOR MORE INFORMATION

*Academy of Nutrition and Dietetics (formerly the American Dietetic Association).* Provides a variety of nutrition-related educational materials.

http://www.eatright.org

*American Diabetes Association.* An organization with the aim of leading the fight against the deadly consequences of diabetes and fighting for those affected by diabetes.

http://www.diabetes.org

*The Dietary Guidelines.* The official site for the *Dietary Guidelines for Americans, 2020.*

https://www.dietaryguidelines.gov

*FDA Center for Food Safety and Applied Nutrition.* Offers information about topics such as food labeling, food additives, dietary supplements, and foodborne illness.

http://www.fda.gov/food

*Foodsafety.gov.* Provides access to government resources relating to food safety and nutrition.

http://www.foodsafety.gov

*Fruit and Veggies: More Matters.* A nonprofit organization designed to increase consumption of fruits and vegetables to five or more servings a day to improve the health of Americans.

https://fruitsandveggiesmorematters.com/

*Mayo Clinic: Nutrition Basics.* Medical, nutrition, and health information and tools for healthy living.

https://www.mayoclinic.org/healthy-lifestyle/nutrition-and-healthy-eating/basics/nutrition-basics/hlv-20049477

*MyPlate.* Provides personalized dietary plans and interactive food and activity tracking tools.

https://www.myplate.gov/

*National Academies' Food and Nutrition Board.* Provides information about the Dietary Reference Intakes and related guidelines.

http://www.nap.edu/read/11537/chapter/1

*Nutrition.gov.* A USDA-sponsored website that provides reliable information to help consumers make healthy eating choices.

http://www.nutrition.gov

*USDA Food and Nutrition Information Center.* Provides a variety of materials and extensive links such as the DRI calculator and FoodCentral with all the nutrient lists, and is a leader in online global nutrition information.

https://www.nal.usda.gov/legacy/fnic

## SELECTED BIBLIOGRAPHY

American Heart Association. 2017. *The Facts on Fat* (https://www.heart.org/en/healthy-living/healthy-eating/eat-smart/fats/the-facts-on-fats).

American Heart Association. 2021. *How Does Plant-Forward (Plant-Based) Eating Benefit Your Health?* (https://www.heart.org/en/healthy-living/healthy-eating/eat-smart/nutrition-basics/how-does-plant-forward-eating-benefit-your-health).

American Heart Association. 2021. *Saturated Fats* (https://www.heart.org/en/healthy-living/healthy-eating/eat-smart/fats/saturated-fats).

Billingsley, H. E., S. Carbone, and C. J. Lavie. 2018. Dietary fats and chronic noncommunicable diseases. *Nutrients* 10(10): 1385. DOI: 10.3390/nu10101385.

Bone Health and Osteoporosis Foundation. 2022. *Food and Your Bones—Osteoporosis Nutrition Guidelines* (https://www.nof.org/patients/treatment/nutrition/).

Centers for Disease Control and Prevention. 2018. *Burden of Foodborne Illness: Findings* (https://www.cdc.gov/foodborneburden/2011-foodborne-estimates.html).

Centers for Disease Control and Prevention. 2018. *Estimates of Foodborne Illness in the United States* (https://www.cdc.gov/foodborneburden/index.html).

Centers for Disease Control and Prevention. 2020. *Foodborne Germs and Illnesses* (http://www.cdc.gov/foodsafety/foodborne-germs.html).

Centers for Disease Control and Prevention. 2021. Sodium https://www.cdc.gov/heartdisease/sodium.htm

Centers for Disease Control and Prevention. 2022. Overweight & Obesity. *Adult Obesity Facts: Obesity Is a Common, Serious and Costly Disease* (https://www.cdc.gov/obesity/data/adult.html).

Centers for Disease Control and Prevention. 2022. Overweight & Obesity. *Childhood Obesity Facts: Prevalence of Childhood Obesity in the United States* (https://www.cdc.gov/obesity/data/childhood.html).

Coleman-Jensen, A., M. P. Rabbitt, C. A. Gregory, and A. Singh. 2021. *Household Food Security in the United States in 2020,* ERR-298, U.S. Department of Agriculture, Economic Research Service.

Council for Responsible Nutrition. *Dietary Supplements–Safe, Regulated and Beneficial* (https://www.crnusa.org/resources/dietary-supplements-safe-beneficial-and-regulated).

Dietary Guidelines Advisory Committee. 2020. *Scientific Report of the 2020 Dietary Guidelines Advisory Committee: Advisory Report to the Secretary of Agriculture and the Secretary of Health and Human Services.* U.S. Department of Agriculture, Agricultural Research Service, Washington, DC.

Environmental Protection Agency. 2021. EPA-FDA advice about eating fish and shellfish. (https://www.epa.gov/fish-tech/epa-fda-advice-about-eating-fish-and-shellfish).

FAO, IFAD, UNICEF, WFP, and WHO. 2021. *The State of Food Security and Nutrition in the World 2021.* Transforming food systems for food security, improved nutrition and affordable healthy diets for all. (https://www.fao.org/documents/card/en/c/cb4474en).

Grosse, Charlene C. S. J., et al. 2020. The role of a plant-based diet in the pathogenesis, etiology and management of the inflammatory bowel diseases. *Expert Review of Gastroenterology & Hepatology*. (DOI: 10.1080/17474124.2020.1733413).

Harvard Medical School. 2019. *The Truth about Fats: The Good, the Bad, and the In-Between* (https://www.health.harvard.edu/staying-healthy/the-truth-about-fats-bad-and-good).

The Hunger Project. 2022. *Know Your World: Facts about Hunger and Poverty* (http://www.thp.org/knowledge-center/know-your-world-facts-about-hunger-poverty/).

ISAAA. 2019. Brief 55-2019: Executive Summary. Biotech Crops Drive Socio-Economic Development and Sustainable Environment in the New Frontier. (https://www.isaaa.org/resources/publications/briefs/55/executivesummary/default.asp).

Islam, M. A., et al. 2019. Trans fatty acids and lipid profile: A serious risk factor to cardiovascular disease, cancer and diabetes. *Diabetes & Metabolic Syndrome* 13(2):1643–1647.

Micha, R., et al. 2017. Association between dietary factors and mortality from heart disease, stroke, and type 2 diabetes in the United States. *Journal of the American Medical Association* 317(9): 912–924.

National Academy of Sciences. 2016. *Genetically Engineered Crops: Experience and Prospects* (https://www.nationalacademies.org/news/2016/05/genetically-engineered-crops-experiences-and-prospects-new-report).

National Institutes of Health. 2022. *Bone Basics* (https://www.bones.nih.gov/health-info/bone/bone-basics).

U.S. Department of Agriculture, 2022. *Biotechnology.* (*https://www.usda.gov/topics/biotechnology).*

U.S. Department of Agriculture. 2022. *MyPlate* (https://www.myplate.gov/).

U.S. Department of Agriculture, Agricultural Research Service, *Food Data Central.* 2022. (https://fdc.nal.usda.gov/).

U.S. Department of Agriculture, Agriculture Research Service. 2022. *What We Eat in America.* (https://www.ars.usda.gov/northeast-area/beltsville-md-bhnrc/beltsville-human-nutrition-research-center/food-surveys-research-group/docs/wweianhanes-overview).

U.S. Department of Agriculture, Economic Research Service. 2020. *Biotechnology* (https://www.ers.usda.gov/topics/farm-practices-management/biotechnology).

U.S. Department of Agriculture and U.S. Department of Health and Human Services. 2020. *Dietary Guidelines for Americans, 2020–2025,* 9th ed. Available at DietaryGuidelines.gov.

U.S. Food and Drug Administration. 2018. *Substances Added to Food.* (https://www.fda.gov/food/food-additives-petitions/substances-added-food-formerly-eafus).

U.S. Food and Drug Administration. 2022. *Agricultural Biotechnology. Feed Your Mind* (https://www.fda.gov/food/consumers/agricultural-biotechnology)

U.S. Food and Drug Administration. 2019. *Calories on the Menu.* (https://www.fda.gov/food/nutrition-education-resources-materials/calories-menu).

World Health Organization. 2022. Joint child malnutrition estimates (https://www.who.int/gho/child-malnutrition/en/).

World Health Organization. 2020. Noncommunicable diseases: Childhood overweight and obesity (https://www.who.int/news-room/questions-and-answers/item/noncommunicable-diseases-childhood-overweight-and-obesity).

Wu, J. H. Y., R. Micha, and D. Mozaffarian. 2019. Dietary fats and cardiometabolic disease: Mechanisms and effects on risk factor and outcomes. *Nature Reviews Cardiology* 16(10):581-601. [https://doi.org/10.1038/s41569-019-0206-1]

Yang, W. S., et al. 2019. Association between plasma N-6 polyunsaturated fatty acid levels and the risk of cardiovascular disease in a community-based cohort study. *Scientific Reports* 9(1):19298. DOI: 10.1038/s41598-019-55686-7.

Zhang, P., et al. 2019. Dietary fats in relation to total and cause-specific mortality in a prospective cohort of 521120 individuals with 16 years of follow-up. *Circulation Research* 124(5):757–768. DOI: 10.1161/CIRCRESAHA.118.314038.

# Nutrition Resources

## Healthy U.S.-Style Food Patterns

| CALORIE LEVEL OF PATTERN | 1,000 | 1,200 | 1,400 | 1,600 | 1,800 | 2,000 | 2,200 | 2,400 | 2,600 | 2,800 | 3,000 | 3,200 |
|---|---|---|---|---|---|---|---|---|---|---|---|---|
| **FOOD GROUP OR SUBGROUP** | **Daily Amount of Food From Each Group** (Vegetable and protein foods subgroup amounts are per week.) | | | | | | | | | | | |
| **Vegetables (cup eq/day)** | **1** | **1 ½** | **1 ½** | **2** | **2 ½** | **2 ½** | **3** | **3** | **3 ½** | **3 ½** | **4** | **4** |
| | Vegetable Subgroups in Weekly Amounts | | | | | | | | | | | |
| Dark-Green Vegetables (cup eq/wk) | ½ | 1 | 1 | 1 ½ | 1 ½ | 1 ½ | 2 | 2 | 2 ½ | 2 ½ | 2 ½ | 2 ½ |
| Red and Orange Vegetables (cup eq/wk) | 2 ½ | 3 | 3 | 4 | 5 ½ | 5 ½ | 6 | 6 | 7 | 7 | 7½ | 7½ |
| Beans, Peas, Lentils (cup eq/wk) | ½ | ½ | ½ | 1 | 1½ | 1½ | 2 | 2 | 2 ½ | 2 ½ | 3 | 3 |
| Starchy Vegetables (cup eq/wk) | 2 | 3 ½ | 3 ½ | 4 | 5 | 5 | 6 | 6 | 7 | 7 | 8 | 8 |
| Other Vegetables (cup eq/wk) | 1 ½ | 2 ½ | 2 ½ | 3 ½ | 4 | 4 | 5 | 5 | 5 ½ | 5 ½ | 7 | 7 |
| **Fruits (cup eq/day)** | **1** | **1** | **1 ½** | **1 ½** | **1 ½** | **2** | **2** | **2** | **2** | **2 ½** | **2 ½** | **2 ½** |
| **Grains (ounce eq/day)** | **3** | **4** | **5** | **5** | **6** | **6** | **7** | **8** | **9** | **10** | **10** | **10** |
| Whole Grains (ounce eq/day) | 1 ½ | 2 | 2 ½ | 3 | 3 | 3 | 3 ½ | 4 | 4 ½ | 5 | 5 | 5 |
| Refined Grains (ounce eq/day) | 1 ½ | 2 | 2 ½ | 2 | 3 | 3 | 3 ½ | 4 | 4 ½ | 5 | 5 | 5 |
| **Dairy (cup eq/day)** | **2** | **2 ½** | **2 ½** | **3** | **3** | **3** | **3** | **3** | **3** | **3** | **3** | **3** |
| **Protein Foods (ounce eq/day)** | **2** | **3** | **4** | **5** | **5** | **5 ½** | **6** | **6 ½** | **6 ½** | **7** | **7** | **7** |
| | Protein Foods Subgroups in Weekly Amounts | | | | | | | | | | | |
| Meats, Poultry, Eggs (ounce eq/wk) | 10 | 14 | 19 | 23 | 23 | 26 | 28 | 31 | 31 | 33 | 33 | 33 |
| Seafood (ounce eq/wk) | 2-3 | 4 | 6 | 8 | 8 | 8 | 9 | 10 | 10 | 10 | 10 | 10 |
| Nuts, Seeds, Soy Products (ounce eq/wk) | 2 | 2 | 3 | 4 | 4 | 5 | 5 | 5 | 5 | 6 | 6 | 6 |
| **Oils (grams/day)** | **15** | **17** | **17** | **22** | **24** | **27** | **29** | **31** | **34** | **36** | **44** | **51** |
| **Limit on Calories for Other Uses (kcal/day)*** | **130** | **80** | **90** | **100** | **140** | **240** | **250** | **320** | **350** | **370** | **440** | **580** |
| Limit on Calories for Other Uses (%/day) | 13% | 7% | 6% | 6% | 8% | 12% | 11% | 13% | 13% | 13% | 15% | 18% |

Food group amounts shown in cup equivalents (c-eq) or ounce equivalents (oz-eq). Oils are shown in grams (g).
Quantity equivalents for each food group are:

- Grains, 1 ounce equivalent is: ½ cup cooked rice, pasta, or cooked cereal; 1 ounce dry pasta or rice; 1 slice bread; 1 cup ready-to-eat cereal flakes.
- Fruits and vegetables, 1 cup equivalent is: 1 cup raw or cooked fruit or vegetable, 1 cup fruit or vegetable juice, 2 cups leafy salad greens.
- Protein Foods, 1 ounce equivalent is: 1 ounce lean meat, poultry, or seafood; 1 egg; ¼ cup cooked beans or tofu; 1 Tbsp peanut butter; ½ ounce nuts/seeds.
- Dairy, 1 cup equivalent is: 1 cup milk or yogurt, 1½ ounces natural cheese such as cheddar cheese or 2 ounces of processed cheese.

*All foods are assumed to be in nutrient-dense forms, lean or low-fat, and prepared without added fats, sugars, refined starches, or salt. If all food choices to meet food group recommendations are in nutrient-dense forms, a small number of calories remain within the overall calorie limit of the pattern. Calories up to the specified limit can be used for added sugars, added refined starches, solid fats, alcohol, or to eat more than the recommended amount of food in a food group. The overall eating pattern also should not exceed the limits of less than 10% of calories from added sugars and less than 10% of calories from saturated fats. At most calorie levels, amounts that can be accommodated are less than these limits. For adults of legal drinking age who choose to drink alcohol, a limit of up to one drink per day for women and up to two drinks per day for men within limits on calories for other uses applies; and calories from protein, carbohydrate, and total fats should be within the Acceptable Macronutrient Distribution Ranges (AMDRs).

**FIGURE 1 Healthy U.S.-Style Food Patterns.**

**SOURCE:** U.S. Department of Agriculture and U.S. Department of Health and Human Services. 2020. *Dietary Guidelines for Americans 2020–2025*. 9th ed. (https://www.dietaryguidelines.gov).

# Nutrition Resources

## Healthy Vegetarian Patterns

| CALORIE LEVEL OF PATTERN | 1,000 | 1,200 | 1,400 | 1,600 | 1,800 | 2,000 | 2,200 | 2,400 | 2,600 | 2,800 | 3,000 | 3,200 |
|---|---|---|---|---|---|---|---|---|---|---|---|---|
| **FOOD GROUP OR SUBGROUP** | **Daily Amount[a] of Food From Each Group** (Vegetable and protein foods subgroup amounts are per week.) | | | | | | | | | | | |
| **Vegetables (cup eq/day)** | **1** | **1 ½** | **1 ½** | **2** | **2 ½** | **2 ½** | **3** | **3** | **3 ½** | **3 ½** | **4** | **4** |
| | Vegetable Subgroups in Weekly Amounts | | | | | | | | | | | |
| Dark-Green Vegetables (cup eq/wk) | ½ | 1 | 1 | 1 ½ | 1 ½ | 1 ½ | 2 | 2 | 2 ½ | 2 ½ | 2 ½ | 2 ½ |
| Red and Orange Vegetables (cup eq/wk) | 2 ½ | 3 | 3 | 4 | 5 ½ | 5½ | 6 | 6 | 7 | 7 | 7½ | 7½ |
| Beans, Peas, Lentils (cup eq/wk) | ½ | ½ | ½ | 1 | 1 ½ | 1 ½ | 2 | 2 | 2 ½ | 2 ½ | 3 | 3 |
| Starchy Vegetables (cup eq/wk) | 2 | 3 ½ | 3 ½ | 4 | 5 | 5 | 6 | 6 | 7 | 7 | 8 | 8 |
| Other Vegetables (cup eq/wk) | 1 ½ | 2 ½ | 2 ½ | 3 ½ | 4 | 4 | 5 | 5 | 5 ½ | 5 ½ | 7 | 7 |
| **Fruits (cup eq/day)** | **1** | **1** | **1 ½** | **1 ½** | **1 ½** | **2** | **2** | **2** | **2** | **2 ½** | **2 ½** | **2 ½** |
| **Grains (ounce eq/day)** | **3** | **4** | **5** | **5 ½** | **6 ½** | **6 ½** | **7 ½** | **8 ½** | **9 ½** | **10 ½** | **10 ½** | **10 ½** |
| Whole Grains (ounce eq/day) | 1 ½ | 2 | 2 ½ | 3 | 3 ½ | 3 ½ | 4 | 4 ½ | 5 | 5 ½ | 5 ½ | 5 ½ |
| Refined Grains (ounce eq/day) | 1 ½ | 2 | 2 ½ | 2 ½ | 3 | 3 | 3 ½ | 4 | 4 ½ | 5 | 5 | 5 |
| **Dairy (cup eq/day)** | **2** | **2 ½** | **2 ½** | **3** | **3** | **3** | **3** | **3** | **3** | **3** | **3** | **3** |
| **Protein Foods (ounce eq/day)** | **1** | **1 ½** | **2** | **2 ½** | **3** | **3 ½** | **3 ½** | **4** | **4 ½** | **5** | **5 ½** | **6** |
| | Protein Foods Subgroups in Weekly Amounts | | | | | | | | | | | |
| Eggs (ounce eq/wk) | 2 | 3 | 3 | 3 | 3 | 3 | 3 | 3 | 3 | 4 | 4 | 4 |
| Beans, Peas, Lentils (cup eq/wk)[b] | 1 | 2 | 4 | 4 | 6 | 6 | 6 | 8 | 9 | 10 | 11 | 12 |
| Soy Products (ounce eq/wk) | 2 | 3 | 4 | 6 | 6 | 8 | 8 | 9 | 10 | 11 | 12 | 13 |
| Nuts, Seeds (ounce eq/wk) | 2 | 2 | 3 | 5 | 6 | 7 | 7 | 8 | 9 | 10 | 12 | 13 |
| **Oils (grams/day)** | **15** | **17** | **17** | **22** | **24** | **27** | **29** | **31** | **34** | **36** | **44** | **51** |
| **Limit on Calories for Other Uses (kcal/day)[c]** | **170** | **140** | **160** | **150** | **150** | **250** | **290** | **350** | **350** | **350** | **390** | **500** |
| Limit on Calories for Other Uses (%/day) | 17% | 12% | 11% | 9% | 8% | 13% | 13% | 15% | 13% | 13% | 13% | 16% |

[a]Food group amounts shown in cup equivalents (c-eq) or ounce equivalents (oz-eq). Oils are shown in grams (g). Quantity equivalents for each food group are:

- Grains, 1 ounce equivalent is: ½ cup cooked rice, pasta, or cooked cereal; 1 ounce dry pasta or rice; 1 slice bread; 1 cup ready-to-eat cereal flakes.
- Fruits and vegetables, 1 cup equivalent is: 1 cup raw or cooked fruit or vegetable, 1 cup fruit or vegetable juice, 2 cups leafy salad greens.
- Protein Foods, 1 ounce equivalent is: 1 ounce lean meat, poultry, or seafood; 1 egg; ¼ cup cooked beans or tofu; 1 tbsp peanut butter; ½ ounce nuts/seeds.
- Dairy, 1 cup equivalent is: 1 cup milk or yogurt, 1½ ounces natural cheese (e.g. cheddar cheese) or 2 ounces of processed cheese.

[b]About half of total beans and peas are shown as vegetables, in cup eqs, and half as protein foods, in ounce eqs. Total beans and peas in cup eq is amount in vegetables plus the amount in protein foods/4:

| | 1600 | 1800 | 2000 | 2200 | 2400 | 2600 | 2800 | 3000 |
|---|---|---|---|---|---|---|---|---|
| Total beans/peas/lentils | 2 c-eq/wk | 3 c-eq/wk | 3 c-eq/wk | 3.5 c-eq/wk | 4 c-eq/wk | 5 c-eq/wk | 5 c-eq/wk | 6 c-eq/wk |

[c]All foods are assumed to be in nutrient-dense forms, lean or low-fat, and prepared without added fats, sugars, refined starches, or salt. If all food choices to meet food group recommendations are in nutrient-dense forms, a small number of calories remain within the overall calorie limit of the pattern. Calories up to the specified limit can be used for added sugars, added refined starches, solid fats, alcohol, or to eat more than the recommended amount of food in a food group. The overall eating pattern also should not exceed the limits of less than 10% of calories from added sugars and less than 10% of calories from saturated fats. At most calorie levels, amounts that can be accommodated are less than these limits. For adults of legal drinking age who choose to drink alcohol, a limit of up to one drink per day for women and up to two drinks per day for men within limits on calories for other uses applies; and calories from protein, carbohydrate, and total fats should be within the Acceptable Macronutrient Distribution Ranges (AMDRs).

**FIGURE 2 Healthy Vegetarian Food Patterns.**

SOURCE: U.S. Department of Agriculture and U.S. Department of Health and Human Services. 2020. *Dietary Guidelines for Americans, 2020–2025*. 9th ed. Available at DietaryGuidelines.gov.

# Nutrition Resources

## Healthy Mediterranean-Style Patterns

| CALORIE LEVEL OF PATTERN | 1,000 | 1,200 | 1,400 | 1,600 | 1,800 | 2,000 | 2,200 | 2,400 | 2,600 | 2,800 | 3,000 | 3,200 |
|---|---|---|---|---|---|---|---|---|---|---|---|---|
| **FOOD GROUP OR SUBGROUP** | **Daily Amount of Food From Each Group** (Vegetable and protein foods subgroup amounts are per week.) | | | | | | | | | | | |
| **Vegetables (cup eq/day)** | **1** | **1 ½** | **1 ½** | **2** | **2 ½** | **2 ½** | **3** | **3** | **3 ½** | **3 ½** | **4** | **4** |
| | Vegetable Subgroups in Weekly Amounts | | | | | | | | | | | |
| Dark-Green Vegetables (cup eq/wk) | ½ | 1 | 1 | 1 ½ | 1 ½ | 1 ½ | 2 | 2 | 2 ½ | 2 ½ | 2 ½ | 2 ½ |
| Red and Orange Vegetables (cup eq/wk) | 2 ½ | 3 | 3 | 4 | 5 ½ | 5 ½ | 6 | 6 | 7 | 7 | 7 ½ | 7 ½ |
| Beans, Peas, Lentils (cup eq/wk) | ½ | ½ | ½ | 1 | 1 ½ | 1 ½ | 2 | 2 | 2 ½ | 2 ½ | 3 | 3 |
| Starchy Vegetables (cup eq/wk) | 2 | 3 ½ | 3 ½ | 4 | 5 | 5 | 6 | 6 | 7 | 7 | 8 | 8 |
| Other Vegetables (cup eq/wk) | 1 ½ | 2 ½ | 2 ½ | 3 ½ | 4 | 4 | 5 | 5 | 5 ½ | 5 ½ | 7 | 7 |
| **Fruits (cup eq/day)** | **1** | **1** | **1 ½** | **2** | **2** | **2 ½** | **2 ½** | **2 ½** | **2 ½** | **3** | **3** | **3** |
| **Grains (ounce eq/day)** | **3** | **4** | **5** | **5** | **6** | **6** | **7** | **8** | **9** | **10** | **10** | **10** |
| Whole Grains (ounce eq/day) | 1 ½ | 2 | 2 ½ | 3 | 3 | 3 | 3 ½ | 4 | 4 ½ | 5 | 5 | 5 |
| Refined Grains (ounce eq/day) | 1 ½ | 2 | 2 ½ | 2 | 3 | 3 | 3 ½ | 4 | 4 ½ | 5 | 5 | 5 |
| **Dairy (cup eq/day)** | **2** | **2 ½** | **2 ½** | **2** | **2** | **2** | **2** | **2 ½** | **2 ½** | **2 ½** | **2 ½** | **2 ½** |
| **Protein Foods (ounce eq/day)** | **2** | **3** | **4** | **5 ½** | **6** | **6 ½** | **7** | **7 ½** | **7 ½** | **8** | **8** | **8** |
| | Protein Foods Subgroups in Weekly Amounts | | | | | | | | | | | |
| Meats, Poultry, Eggs (ounce eq/wk) | 10 | 14 | 19 | 23 | 23 | 26 | 28 | 31 | 31 | 33 | 33 | 33 |
| Seafood (ounce eq/wk) | 3 | 4 | 6 | 11 | 15 | 15 | 16 | 16 | 17 | 17 | 17 | 17 |
| Nuts, Seeds, Soy Products (ounce eq/wk) | 2 | 2 | 3 | 4 | 4 | 5 | 5 | 5 | 5 | 6 | 6 | 6 |
| **Oils (grams/day)** | **15** | **17** | **17** | **22** | **24** | **27** | **29** | **31** | **34** | **36** | **44** | **51** |
| **Limit on Calories for Other Uses (kcal/day)** | **130** | **80** | **90** | **120** | **140** | **240** | **250** | **280** | **300** | **330** | **400** | **540** |
| Limit on Calories for Other Uses (%/day) | 13% | 7% | 6% | 8% | 8% | 12% | 11% | 12% | 12% | 12% | 13% | 17% |

Food group amounts shown in cup equivalents (c-eq) or ounce equivalents (oz-eq). Oils are shown in grams (g).
Quantity equivalents for each food group are:

- Grains, 1 ounce equivalent is: ½ cup cooked rice, pasta, or cooked cereal; 1 ounce dry pasta or rice; 1 slice bread; 1 cup ready-to-eat cereal flakes.
- Fruits and vegetables, 1 cup equivalent is: 1 cup raw or cooked fruit or vegetable, 1 cup fruit or vegetable juice, 2 cups leafy salad greens.
- Protein Foods, 1 ounce equivalent is: 1 ounce lean meat, poultry, or seafood; 1 egg; ¼ cup cooked beans or tofu; 1 Tbsp peanut butter; ½ ounce nuts/seeds.
- Dairy, 1 cup equivalent is: 1 cup milk or yogurt, 1½ ounces natural cheese such as cheddar cheese or 2 ounces of processed cheese.

*All foods are assumed to be in nutrient-dense forms, lean or low-fat, and prepared without added fats, sugars, refined starches, or salt. If all food choices to meet food group recommendations are in nutrient-dense forms, a small number of calories remain within the overall calorie limit of the pattern. Calories up to the specified limit can be used for added sugars, added refined starches, solid fats, alcohol, or to eat more than the recommended amount of food in a food group. The overall eating pattern also should not exceed the limits of less than 10% of calories from added sugars and less than 10% of calories from saturated fats. At most calorie levels, amounts that can be accommodated are less than these limits. For adults of legal drinking age who choose to drink alcohol, a limit of up to one drink per day for women and up to two drinks per day for men within limits on calories for other uses applies; and calories from protein, carbohydrate, and total fats should be within the Acceptable Macronutrient Distribution Ranges (AMDRs).

**FIGURE 3 Healthy Mediterranean-Style Patterns.**

**SOURCE:** U.S. Department of Agriculture and U.S. Department of Health and Human Services. 2020. *Dietary Guidelines for Americans 2020–2025*. 9th ed. (https://www.dietaryguidelines.gov).

# Following the DASH Eating Plan

## FOR 1,800 TO 2,000 CALORIES PER DAY

### Grains

6–8 SERVINGS PER DAY

**Sources of fiber and magnesium**

**SERVING SIZE**

**1 slice** bread

**1 oz** dry cereal

**½ cup** cooked rice, pasta, or cereal

**EXAMPLES**

Oatmeal, grits, brown rice, unsalted pretzels and popcorn, whole grain cereal, whole wheat bread, rolls, pasta, English muffin, pita bread, bagel

### Vegetables

4–5 SERVINGS PER DAY

**Sources of potassium, magnesium, and fiber**

**SERVING SIZE**

**1 cup** raw leafy vegetable

**½ cup** cut-up raw or cooked vegetable

**½ cup** vegetable juice

**EXAMPLES**

Broccoli, carrots, collards, green beans, green peas, kale, lima beans, potatoes, spinach, squash, sweet potatoes, tomatoes

### Fruits

4–5 SERVINGS PER DAY

**Sources of potassium, magnesium, and fiber**

**SERVING SIZE**

**1 medium** fruit

**¼ cup** dried fruit (unsweetened)

**½ cup** fresh, frozen, or canned fruit, or fruit juice

**EXAMPLES**

Apples, apricots, bananas, dates, grapes, oranges, grapefruit, grapefruit juice, mangoes, melons, peaches, pineapples, raisins, strawberries, tangerines

### Dairy

2–3 SERVINGS PER DAY

**Sources of calcium and protein**

**SERVING SIZE**

**1 cup** milk

**1 cup** yogurt

**1½ oz** cheese

**EXAMPLES**

Fat-free (skim) or low-fat (1%) milk or buttermilk; fat-free, low-fat, or reduced-fat cheese; fat-free or low-fat regular or frozen yogurt; fortified soy beverage; lactose-free products

### Lean Meats, Fish, Poultry, and Eggs

6 SERVINGS OR LESS PER DAY

**Sources of protein and magnesium**

**SERVING SIZE**

**1 oz** cooked meats, fish, or poultry

**1** egg

**EXAMPLES**

Chicken or turkey without skin; salmon, tuna, trout; lean cuts of beef, pork, and lamb

### Fats and Oils

2–3 SERVINGS PER DAY

**Sources of energy and vitamin E**

**SERVING SIZE**

**1 tsp** soft margarine

**1 tsp** vegetable oil

**1 tbsp** mayonnaise

**2 tbsp** salad dressing

**EXAMPLES**

Soft margarine, vegetable oil (such as canola, corn, olive, or safflower), low-fat mayonnaise, light salad dressing

### Nuts, Seeds, and Legumes

4–5 SERVINGS PER WEEK

**Sources of energy, magnesium, protein, and fiber**

**SERVING SIZE**

**⅓ cup** or **1½ oz** nuts (unsalted)

**2 tbsp** peanut butter

**2 tbsp** or **½ oz** seeds

**½ cup** cooked legumes (dry beans and peas)

**EXAMPLES**

Almonds, hazelnuts, mixed nuts, peanuts, walnuts, sunflower seeds, peanut butter, kidney beans, lentils, split peas

### Sweets and Added Sugars

5 SERVINGS OR LESS PER WEEK

**Sweets should be low in fat**

**SERVING SIZE**

**1 tbsp** sugar

**1 tbsp** jelly or jam

**½ cup** sorbet, gelatin

**1 cup** lemonade

**EXAMPLES**

Fruit-flavored gelatin, fruit punch, hard candy, jelly, maple syrup, sorbet and ices, sugar

**FIGURE 4 The DASH Eating Plan.**

SOURCE: National Institutes of Health, National Heart, Lung, and Blood Institute. 2020. "Following the DASH Eating Plan for 1800-2000 Calories per day."

**Design Elements:** Assess Yourself icon: Aleksey Boldin/Alamy Stock Photo; Diversity Matters icon: Rawpixel Ltd/Getty Images; Wellness on Campus icon: Radius Images/Alamy Stock Photo; Take Charge icon: VisualCommunications/Getty Images; Critical Consumer icon: pagadesign/Getty Images.

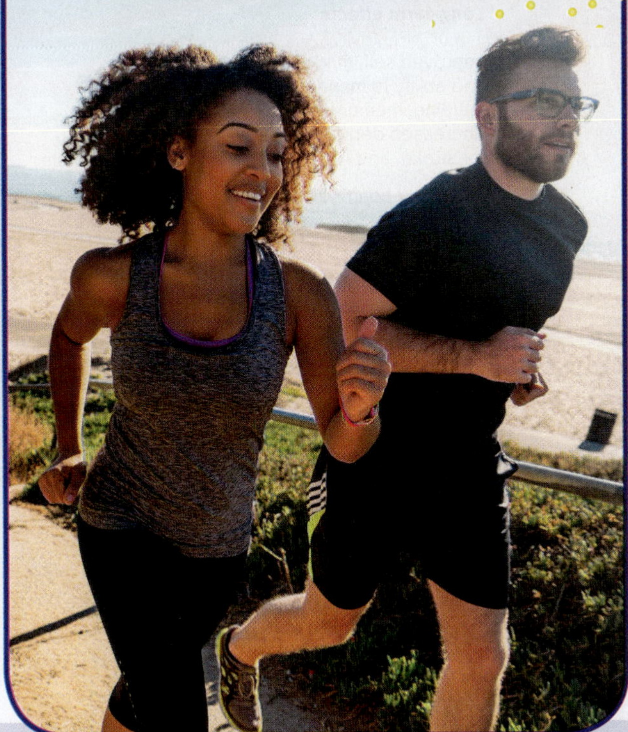

Kevin Kozicki/Getty Images

## CHAPTER OBJECTIVES

- **Describe the benefits of exercise**
- **Define physical fitness**
- **Explain the components of an active lifestyle**
- **Put together a personalized exercise program**
- **Explain strategies for staying on track with an exercise program**

CHAPTER 11

# Exercise for Health and Fitness

Your body is a beautiful moving machine. It readily adapts to practically any level of activity and exercise: The more you ask of your body, the stronger and more fit it becomes. The opposite is also true. Left unchallenged, bones lose their density, joints stiffen, muscles weaken, and the body's energy systems degenerate. To be truly healthy, human beings must be active.

This chapter gives you essential information to create a physical fitness program that will work for you.

## THE BENEFITS OF EXERCISE

The human body is adaptable. The greater the demands, the more it adjusts and the more fit it becomes. Over time, immediate, short-term adjustments translate into long-term changes and improvements (Figure 11.1).

According to a 2021 meta-analysis, physically active people have a reduced risk of dying prematurely from all causes, with the greatest benefits found for people with the highest levels of physical activity and fitness (Figure 11.2). Physical inactivity is a predictor of premature death and is as important a risk factor as smoking, high blood pressure, obesity, and diabetes.

### Improved Cardiorespiratory Functioning

During exercise, the cardiorespiratory system (heart, lungs, and circulation system) must work harder to meet the body's increased demand for oxygen. Regular cardiorespiratory endurance exercise improves the functioning of the heart and the ability of the cardiorespiratory system to carry oxygen to body tissues. Exercise directly affects the health of your arteries, keeping them from stiffening or clogging with a plaque and reducing the risk of cardiovascular disease. Exercise also improves sexual function and general vitality.

### More Efficient Metabolism and Improved Cell Health

Endurance exercise improves metabolism, which converts food to energy and builds tissue. This process involves oxygen, nutrients, hormones, and enzymes. A physically fit person's

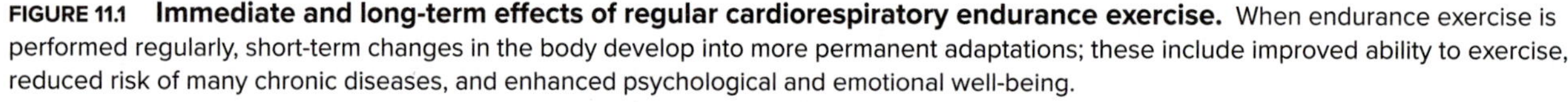


**FIGURE 11.1 Immediate and long-term effects of regular cardiorespiratory endurance exercise.** When endurance exercise is performed regularly, short-term changes in the body develop into more permanent adaptations; these include improved ability to exercise, reduced risk of many chronic diseases, and enhanced psychological and emotional well-being.

body can more efficiently use carbohydrates and fats and better regulate hormones. Exercise may also protect cells from damage from free radicals, which are destructive chemicals produced during metabolism (see Chapter 10), and from inflammation caused by obesity, high blood pressure or cholesterol, nicotine, and overeating. Training activates antioxidants that prevent free radical damage and maintain cell health. Regular physical activity and exercise prevent the deterioration of telomeres, which form the protective ends of chromosomes vital for cell health and repair.

## Improved Body Composition

Healthy body composition means that the body has a high proportion of fat-free mass and a relatively small proportion of fat. Too much body fat, particularly abdominal fat, is linked to various health problems, including heart disease, high blood pressure, cancer, and diabetes.

Exercise can improve body composition in several ways. Endurance exercise increases daily calorie expenditure. It can also slightly raise *metabolic rate,* the rate at which the body burns calories, for several hours after an exercise session. Strength training increases muscle mass, tipping the body composition ratio toward fat-free mass and away from fat. It can also help with losing fat because metabolic rate is directly proportional to fat-free mass: The more muscle mass, the higher the metabolic rate.

## Disease Prevention and Management

Regular physical activity and exercise lower your risk of many chronic, disabling diseases.

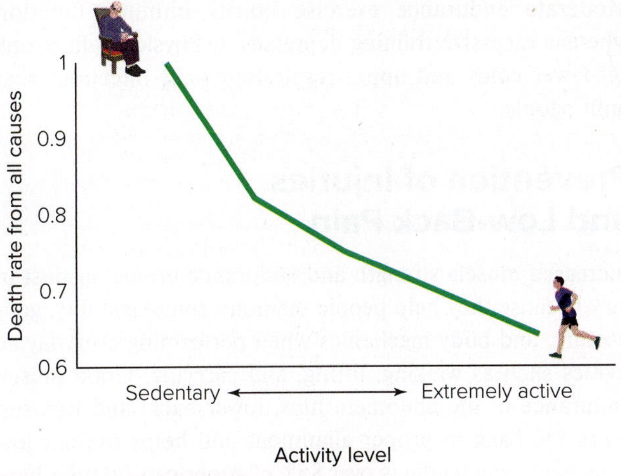


VITAL STATISTICS

**FIGURE 11.2 Exercise promotes longevity.** The risk of death each year from all causes decreases with increased amounts and intensities of weekly physical activity.

SOURCES: Adapted from a composite of 13 studies involving over 900,000 men and women. Tarp, J., et al. 2021. Fitness, fatness, and mortality in men and women from the UK Biobank: Prospective Cohort Study. *Journal of the American Heart Association* 10(6): e019605; Physical Activity Guidelines Advisory Committee. *Physical Activity Guidelines Advisory Committee Report, 2008*. Washington, DC: 2008. U.S. Department of Health and Human Services; Schnohr, P., et al. 2015. Dose of jogging and long-term mortality: The Copenhagen City Heart Study. *Journal of the American College of Cardiology* 65(5): 411–419.

**Cardiovascular Disease** A sedentary lifestyle is one of six major risk factors for cardiovascular disease (CVD), including heart attack and stroke. Sedentary people have CVD death rates significantly higher than those of fit individuals. Physical inactivity increases the risk of CVD by as much as 240%.

The benefits of physical activity begin at moderate levels of exercise and increase as the amount and intensity of activity rise. Exercise positively affects CVD risk factors, including cholesterol levels, insulin resistance, and blood pressure. Exercise also directly interferes with the disease process itself, lowering the risk of heart disease and stroke.

**BLOOD FAT LEVELS** Elevated concentrations of lipids (fats), such as high cholesterol and triglycerides or low-density lipoproteins, are linked to heart disease because they contribute to the formation of fatty deposits on the linings of arteries. When blood clots block a narrowed artery, a heart attack or stroke can occur.

Cholesterol is carried in the blood by lipoproteins, which are classified according to size and density. Cholesterol carried by low-density lipoproteins (LDLs) sticks to the walls of coronary arteries. High-density lipoproteins (HDLs) pick up excess cholesterol in the bloodstream and bring it back to the liver for excretion from the body. High LDL levels and low HDL levels increase the risk of cardiovascular disease. Cardiorespiratory endurance exercise and strength training promote healthy blood lipids by increasing HDL and decreasing LDL and triglycerides, reducing the risk of CVD.

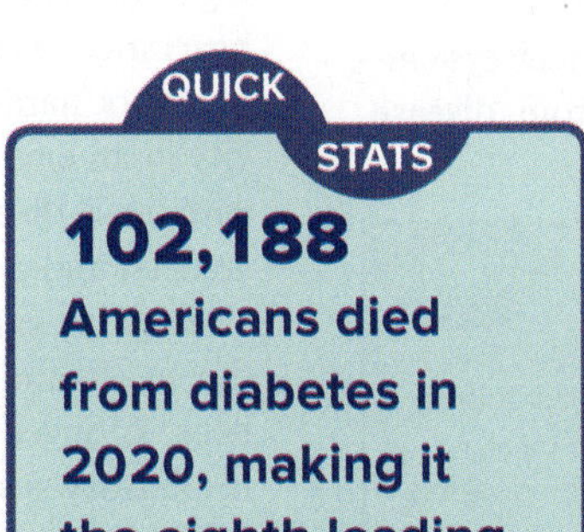


**CORONARY ARTERY DISEASE** Coronary artery disease (CAD) involves the blockage of one of the coronary arteries. These blood vessels supply the heart with oxygenated blood. An obstruction in a coronary artery can cause a heart attack. Exercise directly interferes with the disease process that causes coronary artery blockage. It also enhances the function of cells lining the arteries that help regulate blood flow.

**STROKE** The most common kind of stroke occurs when a blood vessel leading to the brain is blocked or leaks, often through the same disease process that leads to heart attacks. Regular exercise and higher fitness levels reduce the risk of stroke.

**Cancer** Studies have shown a relationship between increased physical activity and reduced cancer risk. Specifically, an analysis of 1.44 million study subjects concluded that higher levels of leisure-time physical activity were associated with lower risks for 13 of 26 types of cancer, including kidney, colon, head and neck, bladder, rectal, and liver cancer. Most of these associations applied whether the participants were overweight/obese or had a smoking history. Exercise may decrease the risk of colon cancer by speeding the movement of food through the gastrointestinal tract (quickly eliminating potential carcinogens), lowering blood-insulin levels, enhancing immune function, and reducing blood fats. Physical activity may be necessary during high school and college years to prevent breast cancer later in life.

**Osteoporosis** Exercise protects against osteoporosis, a disease that results in lost bone density and bone strength. Weight-bearing exercise, which includes almost everything except swimming, helps build bone during childhood and the teens and twenties. Older people with denser bones can better endure bone loss with aging. Strength training and impact exercises such as jumping rope help maintain bone and muscle health throughout life. With stronger bones and muscles and better balance, fit people are less likely to experience debilitating falls and bone fractures.

**Type 2 Diabetes** Diabetes increases the risk of heart disease, blindness, and neural disease. Exercise prevents type 2 diabetes, the most common form of the disease. Exercise burns excess sugar and makes cells more sensitive to insulin. When people have *insulin resistance*, they produce insulin but fail to use it effectively. Instead of the insulin enabling their cells to absorb and burn excess calories, insulin-resistant people store the extra calories as fat.

## Improved Psychological and Emotional Wellness

Physically active people enjoy many social, psychological, and emotional benefits, including:

- ***Reduced anxiety and depression.*** Exercise reduces anxiety symptoms, such as worry and self-doubt, and is associated with a lower risk for panic attacks, generalized anxiety disorder, and social anxiety disorder. Exercise also relieves feelings of sadness and hopelessness and can be as effective as psychotherapy in treating mild to moderate cases of depression.

- ***Improved sleep.*** Regular physical activity and exercise help people fall asleep more quickly—and enhance sleep quality.

- ***Reduced stress.*** Exercise reduces the overall response to all forms of stressors and helps people deal more effectively with stress.

- ***Enhanced self-esteem, self-confidence, and self-efficacy.*** Exercise can boost self-esteem and self-confidence by providing opportunities for people to succeed and excel. Exercise also improves body image. Sticking with an exercise program increases people's belief in their ability to be active, boosting self-efficacy.

- ***Enhanced creativity and intellectual functioning.*** In studies of people of all ages, physically active people score higher than sedentary people on creativity and mental function tests. Exercise improves alertness and memory in the short term. Over time, exercise helps maintain reaction time, short-term memory, and nonverbal reasoning skills and enhances brain metabolism.

- ***Improved work productivity.*** Studies show that workers' quality of work, time management abilities, and mental and interpersonal performance are better on days they exercise.

- ***Increased opportunities for social interaction.*** Exercise provides many chances for people to have positive interactions with other people.

## Improved Immune Function

Exercise can positively or negatively affect the immune system—the physiological processes that protect us from disease. Moderate endurance exercise boosts immune function, whereas excessive training depresses it. Physically fit people get fewer colds and upper respiratory tract infections than unfit people.

## Prevention of Injuries and Low-Back Pain

Increased muscle strength and endurance protect against injury because they help people maintain spinal stability, good posture, and body mechanics when performing everyday activities such as walking, lifting, and carrying. Good muscle endurance in the abdomen, hips, lower back, and legs supports the back in proper alignment and helps prevent low-back pain, which afflicts over 85% of Americans in their lives.

## Improved Wellness for Life

Although people differ in the maximum levels of fitness they can achieve through exercise, the wellness benefits of exercise are available to everyone. Exercising regularly may be the most important thing you can do now to improve the quality of your life.

# WHAT IS PHYSICAL FITNESS?

**Physical fitness** is a set of physical attributes that allow the body to respond or adapt to the demands and stress of physical effort—to perform moderate to vigorous physical activity levels without becoming overly tired.

Some components of fitness are related to specific activities or sports, whereas others relate to general health. **Health-related fitness** includes cardiorespiratory endurance, muscular strength and endurance, flexibility, and body composition. Health-related fitness helps you withstand physical challenges and protects you from diseases.

## Cardiorespiratory Endurance

People with good **cardiorespiratory endurance** can perform prolonged, large-muscle, dynamic exercises at moderate to high intensity. When cardiorespiratory fitness is low, the heart must work hard during normal daily activities and may not work hard enough to sustain high-intensity physical activity in an emergency. Poor cardiorespiratory fitness is linked with heart disease, diabetes, colon cancer, stroke, depression, anxiety, and premature death from all causes.

Regular **cardiorespiratory endurance training** conditions the heart and metabolism. Endurance training makes the heart stronger and improves the function of the entire cardiorespiratory system. As cardiorespiratory fitness improves, related physical processes also improve. The heart pumps more blood per heartbeat, resting heart rate and blood pressure decreases, blood volume increases, blood supply to tissues improves, the body can cool itself better, and metabolic health improves, which helps the body process fuels and regulate cell function.

**TERMS**

**physical fitness** The body's ability to respond or adapt to the demands and stress of physical effort.

**health-related fitness** Physical capabilities that contribute to health, including cardiorespiratory endurance, muscular strength, muscular endurance, flexibility, and body composition.

**cardiorespiratory endurance** The ability of the body to perform prolonged, large-muscle, dynamic exercise at moderate to high levels of intensity.

**cardiorespiratory endurance training** Exercise intended to improve cardiorespiratory endurance.

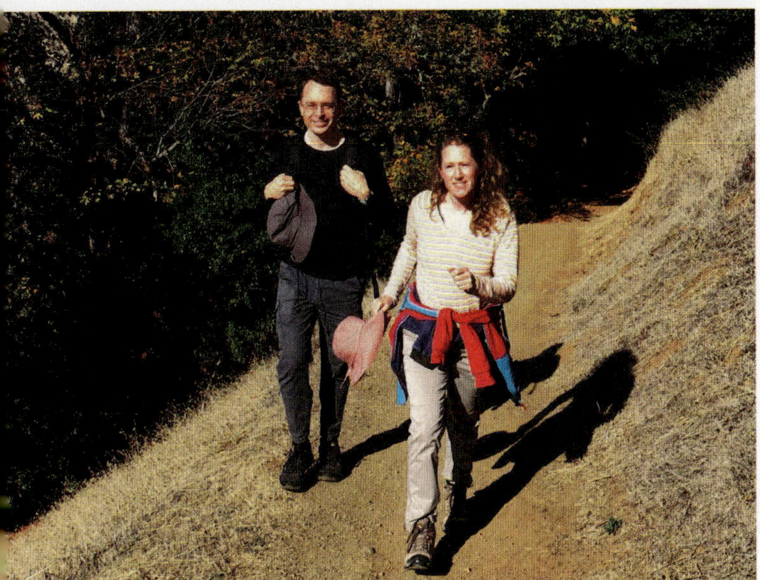

Cardiorespiratory endurance is a critical component of a fitness plan and, in this case, a mountaintop marriage proposal. Claire Insel

A healthy heart can better withstand the strains of daily life, the stress of occasional emergencies, and the wear and tear of time.

Endurance training also improves the function of the body's chemical systems, particularly in the muscles and liver, enhancing the body's ability to use energy from food and do more exercise with less effort. You can develop cardiorespiratory endurance through activities that involve continuous, rhythmic movements of large muscle groups, such as the legs. Such activities include walking, jogging, cycling, and group aerobics.

## Muscular Strength and Endurance

**Muscular strength** is the amount of force a muscle can produce with a single maximum effort. It depends on factors such as the size of muscle cells and the ability of nerves to activate muscle cells. Strong muscles are essential for everyday activities, such as climbing stairs, as well as for emergencies. Strong muscles help keep the skeleton in proper alignment, preventing back and leg pain and providing the support necessary for good posture. Recreational activities also require muscular strength: Strong people can hit a tennis ball harder, kick a soccer ball farther, and ride a bicycle uphill more quickly.

Muscle tissue is an essential element of overall body composition. Greater muscle mass makes possible a higher rate of metabolism and faster energy use, which help people to maintain healthy body weight.

Strength training helps maintain muscle mass, function, and balance in older people, greatly enhancing their quality of life and preventing injuries. Strength training promotes cardiovascular health, reduces the risk of osteoporosis (bone loss), and prevents premature death from all causes.

**Muscular endurance** is the ability to resist fatigue and sustain a level of muscle tension, to hold a muscle contraction for a long time, or to contract a muscle repeatedly.

Muscular endurance helps people cope with the physical demands of everyday life and enhances performance in sports and work. Stressing the muscles with a more significant load (weight) than they are accustomed to develops muscular endurance and muscular strength. How much power or endurance develops depends on the type and amount of stress applied.

## Flexibility

**Flexibility** is the ability of joints to move through their full range of motion. It depends on joint structure, the length and elasticity of connective tissue, and nervous system activity. Flexible, pain-free joints are important for good health and well-being. Inactivity causes the joints to become stiffer with age. Stiffness often causes older people to assume unnatural body postures that stress joints and muscles. Stretching exercises can help ensure a healthy range of motion for all major joints.

## Body Composition

**Body composition** refers to the proportion of fat and **fat-free mass** (muscle, bone, and water) in the body. Healthy body composition involves a high ratio of fat-free mass and an acceptably low level of body fat, adjusted for age and sex. The best way to lose fat is through a lifestyle that includes a sensible diet and exercise. The best way to add muscle mass is through resistance training such as weight training.

## Skill-Related Components of Fitness

In addition to the five health-related components of physical fitness, the ability to perform a particular sport or activity may depend on **skill-related fitness** components such as:

- ***Speed.*** The ability to perform a movement quickly.
- ***Power.*** The ability to exert force rapidly, based on strength and speed.
- ***Agility.*** The ability to change the body's position quickly and accurately.

**TERMS**

**muscular strength** The force a muscle can produce with a single maximum effort.

**muscular endurance** The ability of a muscle or group of muscles to remain contracted or to contract repeatedly for an extended period.

**flexibility** The joints' ability to move through their full range of motion.

**body composition** The proportion of fat and fat-free mass (muscle, bone, and water) in the body.

**fat-free mass** The nonfat components of the human body, consisting of skeletal muscle, bone, and water.

**skill-related fitness** Physical abilities that contribute to performance in a sport or activity, including speed, power, agility, balance, coordination, and reaction time.

- ***Balance.*** The ability to maintain equilibrium while either moving or stationary.
- ***Coordination.*** The ability to perform motor tasks accurately and smoothly using body movements and the senses.
- ***Reaction and movement time.*** The ability to respond quickly to a stimulus.

Skill-related fitness is sport specific and is best developed through practice. For example, playing basketball best develops the speed, coordination, and agility needed to play basketball, whereas swimming does not enhance basketball skills. Playing a sport can be fun, help build fitness, and contribute to other wellness areas.

## COMPONENTS OF AN ACTIVE LIFESTYLE

Despite the many benefits of an active lifestyle, levels of physical activity and exercise remain low for all populations of Americans.

**Physical activity** is any body movement carried out by the skeletal muscles that requires energy. Different types of physical activity can be arranged on a continuum based on the amount of energy they need. Quick, easy movements such as standing up or walking down a hallway require little energy or effort. More intense, sustained activities such as cycling five miles or running in a race require considerably more.

**Exercise** refers to a subset of repetitive activity planned and structured to improve or maintain physical fitness. A person must perform enough exercise to stress the body and cause long-term physiological changes to develop fitness.

Moderate-intensity physical activity is essential to health and confers wide-ranging health benefits, but more intense exercise is necessary to improve physical fitness. This important distinction between physical activity and exercise is critical in understanding the guidelines discussed in this chapter.

**QUICK STATS**

**Only 23.2% of high school students get at least 60 minutes of physical activity every day.**

—Centers for Disease Control and Prevention, 2020

### Increasing Physical Activity and Exercise

The current guidelines include the following critical recommendations for adults:

- For substantial health benefits, adults should do at least 150 minutes (2.5 hours) a week of moderate-intensity aerobic physical activity, or 75 minutes a week of vigorous-intensity aerobic physical activity, or an equivalent combination of moderate- and vigorous-intensity aerobic activity. As a rule of thumb for calculating a weekly total, 1 minute of vigorous-intensity activity is the equivalent of 2 minutes of moderate-intensity activity. Any amount of moderate- to vigorous-intensity activity contributes to these goals.

- For additional and more extensive health benefits, adults should increase their aerobic physical activity to 300 minutes (5 hours) a week of moderate-intensity activity, or 150 minutes a week of vigorous-intensity activity, or an equivalent combination of moderate- and vigorous-intensity activity. Adults can enjoy additional health benefits by engaging in physical activity beyond this amount.

  The Health and Retirement Study found that people who exercised vigorously had a lower death rate than those who exercised at moderate intensities or did no physical activity. After 16 years, the survival rate was 84% in those doing vigorous exercise, 78% in those doing moderate-intensity physical activity, and only 65% in those doing no physical activity.

- Adults should also do muscle-strengthening activities, such as moderate- or high-intensity weight training or body-weight exercise involving all major muscle groups on two or more days a week. These activities provide additional health benefits—for example, they prevent muscle loss and falls in older adults.

- Everyone should avoid inactivity. Spend less time in front of a screen because such inactivity decreases metabolic health, contributes to a sedentary lifestyle, and increases the risk of obesity.

- Physical activity benefits people of all ages and racial and ethnic groups, including people with disabilities. The benefits of exercise outweigh the dangers.

These levels of exercise promote health and wellness by lowering the risk of high blood pressure, stroke, heart disease, type 2 diabetes, colon cancer, and osteoporosis and by reducing feelings of mild to moderate depression and anxiety.

What's the difference between moderate- and vigorous-intensity physical activity? Moderate-intensity exercise is an activity that causes a noticeable increase in heart rate, such as brisk walking. Vigorous-intensity exercise is an activity that causes rapid breathing and a substantial increase in heart rate, such as jogging. Brisk walking, dancing, swimming, cycling, and yard work can all help you meet the physical activity recommendations. You can burn the same number of calories by doing a moderate-intensity exercise for a longer time or a higher-intensity activity for a shorter time.

The daily total of physical activity can be accumulated in multiple bouts of 10 or more minutes—for example, two 10-minute bike rides to and from class and a brisk 10-minute

**TERMS**

**physical activity** Any body movement carried out by the skeletal muscles requiring energy.

**exercise** Planned, structured, repetitive body movement intended to improve or maintain physical fitness.

## TAKE CHARGE
### Making Time for Physical Activity

"Too little time" is a common excuse for not being physically active. Learning to manage your time successfully is crucial to maintaining a wellness lifestyle. Begin by keeping a record of how you spend your time. List each type of activity and the total time you engaged in it—for example, sleeping, 7 hours; eating, 1.5 hours; studying, 3 hours; and so on. Prioritize your activities according to how important they are to you, from essential to somewhat important to not important.

Change your daily schedule by subtracting time from other activities to make time for physical activity. Look carefully at your leisure-time activities and your transportation methods—these are areas where it is easy to build in physical activity. For example, you may reduce the total time you spend playing computer games to be available for an after-dinner bike ride or a walk with a friend. You may watch 10 fewer minutes of television in the morning to change your 5-minute drive to class into a 15-minute walk.

Here are just a few ways to incorporate more physical activity into your daily routine:

- Take the stairs instead of the elevator or escalator.
- Walk to the mailbox, post office, store, bank, or library.
- Do at least one chore every day that requires physical activity: Wash the windows or your car, clean your room or house, mow the lawn, or rake the leaves.
- Take study or work breaks to avoid sitting for over 30 minutes at a time. Get up and walk around the library, your office, or your home or dorm; go up and down a flight of stairs.
- When you take public transportation, get off one stop early and walk to your destination.
- Take the dog for a walk every day.
- If weather or neighborhood safety rule out walking outside, look for alternative locations—an indoor track, an enclosed shopping mall, or even a long hallway.
- Seize every opportunity to get up and walk around. Move more and sit less.

### Ask Yourself

**QUESTIONS FOR CRITICAL THINKING AND REFLECTION**

When you think about exercise, do you think of only one or two of the five health-related fitness components, such as muscular strength or body composition? If so, where do you think your thoughts come from? What role do the media play in shaping your ideas about fitness?

walk to the store. In this lifestyle approach to physical activity, people can choose enjoyable activities and fit them into their daily routine. Everyday tasks at school, work, and home can be structured to contribute to the daily activity total (see the box "Making Time for Physical Activity").

## Reducing Sedentary Time

Regardless of whether we meet physical activity goals, too much sedentary time—sitting too much—is detrimental to health. Sedentary time is associated with an increased risk of disease and death independent of activity level. The risk of adverse outcomes from sedentary time was lower among people with higher levels of exercise.

How does excessive sedentary time affect health? Although not understood, sedentary time is associated with poor metabolic functioning, including unhealthy blood glucose levels, insulin, blood fats, and a large waist circumference. A study that looked at the impact of increased sedentary time in moderately active individuals found that sitting for over 30 or 60 minutes resulted in elevated glucose and insulin levels. Sedentary time also affects blood fats and inflammation. These factors can contribute to type 2 diabetes, metabolic syndrome, heart disease, and cancer.

What does this mean for an individual? Studies have found that average American adults spend more than half their waking day in sedentary activities, such as using a computer, studying, or watching television. Fortunately, the evidence so far suggests that frequent breaks from sedentary time—2 minutes every 20 or 30 minutes, for example—protect against some impacts of sedentary time. So, take frequent breaks when you are engaged in passive activities, whether at work or school or during leisure time. Try the strategies suggested in the box "Move More, Sit Less," and invent your own.

### Ask Yourself

**QUESTIONS FOR CRITICAL THINKING AND REFLECTION**

Does your current lifestyle include enough exercise—150 minutes of moderate-intensity activity a week—to support health and wellness? Do you go beyond this level to have enough vigorous activity and exercise to build physical fitness? What changes could you make in your lifestyle to start developing physical fitness?

## TAKE CHARGE
### Move More, Sit Less

Regular exercise provides substantial wellness benefits, but it does not cancel out all the adverse effects of too much sitting during the day. Advances in technology promote sedentary behavior: We can now work or study at a desk, watch TV or play video games in our leisure time, order takeout and delivery for meals, and shop and bank online. To avoid the adverse health effects of too little daily activity, try some of the following strategies:

- Stand up and walk when you are at work or making personal phone calls.
- Take the stairs whenever and wherever you can; walk up and down escalators instead of riding them.
- At work, walk to a coworker's desk rather than emailing or calling, take the long route to the restroom, and take a walk break whenever you take a coffee or snack break. Drink plenty of water so that you must take frequent restroom breaks.
- Set reminders to get up and move: Use commercial breaks while watching TV to remind yourself to move or stretch. Set the clock function on your computer or phone to remind you to get up at least every hour at work or while using a digital device. Moving every 20 or 30 minutes is even better.
- Engage in active chores and leisure activities.
- Track your sedentary time to get a baseline, and then continue monitoring to note any improvements. You can also use a step counter to track your general activity level and movement patterns.

## DESIGNING YOUR EXERCISE PROGRAM

The best exercise program has two primary characteristics: It promotes your health and is fun for you to do. Exercise can provide some of the most pleasurable moments of your day, once you make it a habit. A little thought and planning will help you achieve these goals.

Figure 11.3 shows a physical activity pyramid. The wide section at the bottom of the pyramid shows activities you should engage in more frequently throughout the day: walking, climbing stairs, doing yard work, and sweeping the floor. From there, work up to meeting the goal of 150 minutes of

Sedentary Activities
Watching television, surfing the internet, talking on the telephone
Limit your sedentary activities
Strength Training
2–3 nonconsecutive days per week (all major muscle groups)
Biceps curls, push-ups, abdominal curls, bench press, calf raises
Flexibility Training
At least 2–3 days per week, ideally 5–7 days per week (all major joints)
Calf stretch, side lunge, step stretch, hurdler stretch
Cardiorespiratory Endurance Exercise
3–5 days per week (20–60 minutes)
Walking, jogging, bicycling, swimming, aerobic dancing, in-line skating, cross-country skiing, dancing, basketball
Moderate-Intensity Physical Activity
150 minutes per week; for weight loss or prevention of weight regain 60–90 minutes per day
Walking to the store or bank, climbing stairs, working in your yard, walking your dog, cleaning your room

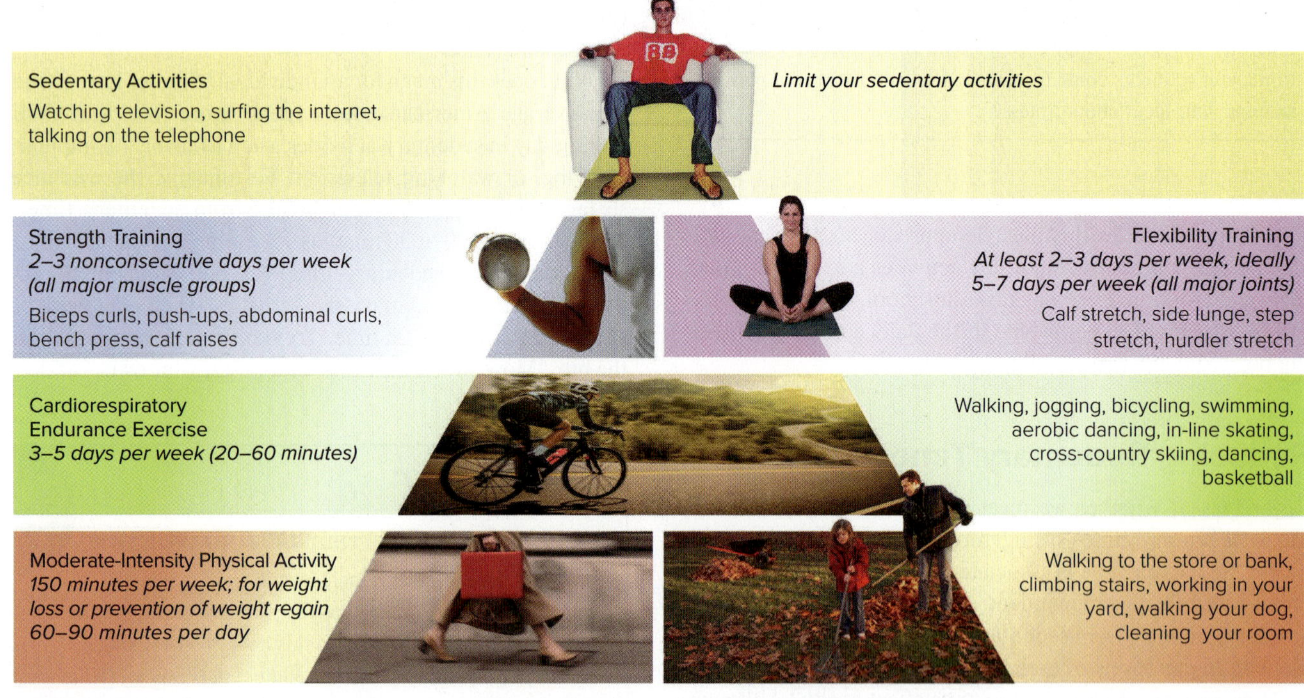

**FIGURE 11.3 Physical activity pyramid.** Make activities at the base of the pyramid part of your everyday life; limit your time in the sedentary activities listed at the top. George Doyle/Stockbyte/Getty Images; Ryan McVay/Photodisc/Getty Images; Seth Foley/McGraw Hill; Rattanasak Khuentana/Shutterstock; Doug Menuez/Forrester Images/Photodisc/Getty Images; UpperCut Images/Alamy Stock Photo

## TAKE CHARGE
### Interval Training: Pros and Cons

Few exercise techniques are more effective at improving fitness rapidly than *high-intensity interval training (HIIT)*—a series of very brief, high-intensity exercise sessions interspersed with short rest periods or low-intensity exercise. The four components of interval training are distance, repetition, intensity, and rest, defined as follows:

- ***Distance*** refers to either the distance or the time of the exercise interval.
- ***Repetition*** is the number of times the exercise is repeated.
- ***Intensity*** is the speed at which the exercise is performed.
- ***Rest*** is the time spent recovering between exercises.

Canadian researchers found that six high-intensity interval training sessions (HIIT) on a stationary bike increased muscle oxidative capacity by almost 50%, muscle glycogen by 20%, and cycle endurance capacity by 100%. The subjects made these remarkable improvements by exercising only 15 minutes in two weeks. Each workout consisted of 4–7 repetitions of high-intensity exercise (each repetition consisted of 30 seconds at near-maximum effort) on a stationary bike. Follow-up studies showed that practicing HIIT three times per week for six weeks improved endurance and aerobic capacity just as well as training five times per week for 60 minutes for six weeks. These studies (and more than 100 others) showed the value of high-intensity training for building aerobic capacity and endurance.

You can use interval training in your favorite aerobic exercises. The type of exercise you select is not essential if you exercise at a high intensity. HIIT training can even be used to help develop sports skills. For example, a runner might do 4–7 repetitions of 200-meter sprints at near-maximum effort. A tennis player might practice volleys against a wall as fast as possible for 4–8 repetitions lasting 30 seconds each. A swimmer might swim 4–8 repeats of 50 meters at 100% effort. It is essential to rest 3–5 minutes between repetitions, regardless of the type of exercise being performed.

If you add HIIT to your exercise program, do not practice interval training more than three days per week. Intervals are exhausting and quickly lead to injury. Let your body tell you how many days you can tolerate. If you become overly tired after interval training three days per week, cut back to two days. If you feel good, try increasing the intensity or number of intervals (but not the number of days per week) and see what happens. As with any exercise program, begin HIIT training slowly and progress conservatively. Although the Canadian studies showed that HIIT training produced substantial fitness improvements, it is best to integrate HIIT into a total exercise program.

High-intensity interval training appears to be safe and effective in the short term. Still, there are concerns about the long-term safety and effectiveness of this type of training, so consider the following issues:

- Maximal-intensity training could be dangerous for some people. A physician might be reluctant to give certain patients the green light for this type of exercise.
- Always warm up with several minutes of low-intensity exercise before practicing HIIT. Maximal-intensity exercise without a warm-up can cause cardiac arrhythmias (abnormal heart rhythms) even in healthy people.
- High-intensity interval training might trigger overuse injuries in unfit people. For this reason, it is essential to start gradually, especially for someone at a low level of fitness. Before starting HIIT, exercise at submaximal intensities for at least four to six weeks. Cut back on interval training or rest if you feel overly fatigued or develop extremely sore joints or muscles.

moderate-intensity exercise per week. Be active whenever you can. If weight management concerns you, begin by achieving the goal of 150 minutes per week and then gradually increase your activity level to 300 minutes per week while reducing caloric intake, especially from added sugars and other empty calories (see Chapter 10).

For even greater benefits, look to the next two levels of the pyramid, which illustrate parts of a formal exercise program. They take up less of your time than the activities on the lower two levels of the pyramid, but they will develop all the health-related components of physical fitness. New research shows that high-intensity interval training–repetitions of high-intensity exercise followed by rest–builds fitness rapidly in less time than traditional aerobic training (see the box "Interval Training: Pros and Cons"). The remaining sections of this chapter will show you how to develop a personalized exercise program. For a summary of the health and fitness benefits of different physical activity levels, see Figure 11.4.

## First Steps

Are you thinking about starting a formal exercise program? A little planning can help make it a success.

**Medical Clearance** Previously inactive men over 40 and women over 50 should get a medical examination before beginning an exercise program. Diabetes, asthma, heart disease, and extreme obesity are conditions that may call for a modified program. If you have an increased risk of heart disease

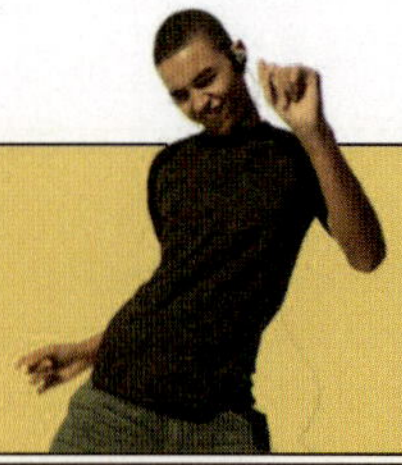

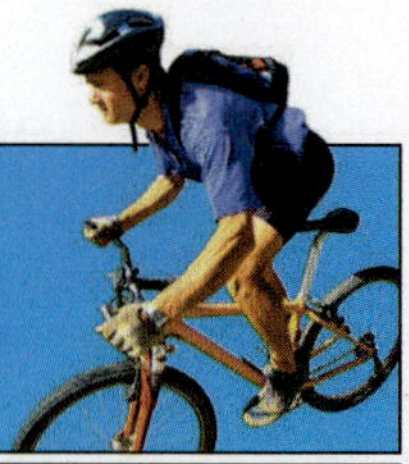

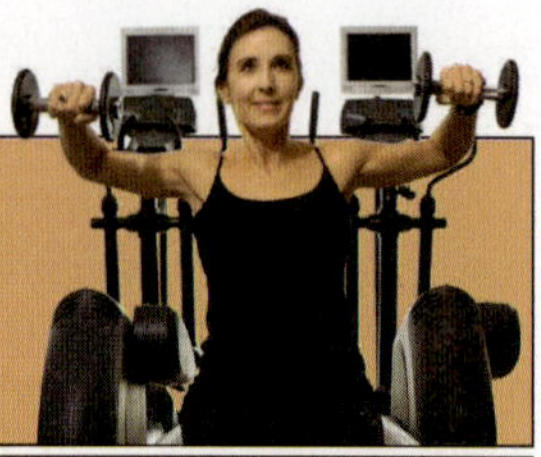

| | Lifestyle physical activity | Moderate exercise program | Vigorous exercise program |
|---|---|---|---|
| **Description** | Moderate physical activity (150 minutes per week; muscle-strengthening exercises 2 or more days per week) | Cardiorespiratory endurance exercise (20–60 minutes, 3–5 days per week); strength training (2–3 nonconsecutive days per week); and stretching exercises (2 or more days per week) | Cardiorespiratory endurance exercise (20–60 minutes, 3–5 days per week); interval training; strength training (3–4 nonconsecutive days per week); and stretching exercises (5–7 days per week) |
| **Sample activities or program** | *One of the following:*<br>• Walking to and from work, 15 minutes each way<br>• Cycling to and from class, 10 minutes each way<br>• Yard work for 30 minutes<br>• Dancing (fast) for 30 minutes<br>• Playing basketball for 20 minutes | • Jogging for 30 minutes, 3 days per week<br>• Weight training, 1 set of 8 exercises, 2 days per week<br>• Stretching exercises, 3 days per week | • Running for 45 minutes, 3 days per week<br>• Intervals: running 400 m at high effort, 4 sets, 2 days per week<br>• Weight training, 3 sets of 10 exercises, 3 days per week<br>• Stretching exercises, 6 days per week |
| **Health and fitness benefits** | Better blood cholesterol levels, reduced body fat, better control of blood pressure, improved metabolic health, and enhanced glucose metabolism; improved quality of life; reduced risk of some chronic diseases.<br><br>Greater amounts of activity can help prevent weight gain and promote weight loss. | All the benefits of lifestyle physical activity, plus improved physical fitness (increased cardiorespiratory endurance, muscular strength and endurance, and flexibility) and even greater improvements in health and quality of life and reductions in chronic disease risk. | All the benefits of lifestyle physical activity and a moderate exercise program, with greater increases in fitness and somewhat greater reductions in chronic disease risk.<br><br>Participating in a vigorous exercise program may increase risk of injury and overtraining. |

FIGURE 11.4 **Health and fitness benefits of different amounts of physical activity and exercise.** Rubberball Productions/Photodisc/Getty Images; Tyler Stableford/Brand X Pictures/Superstock; Thinkstock Images/Stockbyte/Getty Images

because of smoking, high blood pressure, or obesity, get a physical checkup, including an **electrocardiogram (ECG or EKG),** before beginning an exercise program.

**Basic Physical Training Principles** To put together an effective exercise program, you should first understand the basic principles of physical training.

TERMS

**electrocardiogram (ECG or EKG)** A recording of the changes in electrical activity of the heart.

**specificity** The training principle that the body adapts to the particular type and amount of stress placed on it.

**progressive overload** The training principle that placing increasing amounts of stress (in the form of exercise) on the body causes adaptations that improve fitness.

**SPECIFICITY** To develop a fitness component, you must perform exercises designed explicitly for that component. This is the principle of **specificity.** Weight training, for example, develops muscular strength but is less effective for developing flexibility or cardiorespiratory endurance. Specificity also applies to the skill-related fitness components and to the different parts of the body. A well-rounded exercise program includes exercises geared to each fitness element, other parts of the body, and specific activities or sports.

**PROGRESSIVE OVERLOAD** Your body adapts to the demands of exercise by improving its functioning. When the amount of exercise, or overload, is increased progressively, fitness improves. This training principle is called **progressive overload.** Low-intensity activity does not increase fitness; excessively intense exercise may cause injury. The appropriate amount depends on your current level of fitness, your genetic capacity to adapt to exercise, your fitness goals, and the fitness components being developed.

**Ask Yourself**

**QUESTIONS FOR CRITICAL THINKING AND REFLECTION**

Which benefits of exercise are most important and why? For example, is there a history of heart disease or diabetes in your family? Have you thought about how regular exercise could reduce your risks for specific conditions?

The overload needed to maintain or improve a particular fitness level is determined in four dimensions, represented by the acronym FITT, which stands for frequency, intensity, time, and type. Two more dimensions to consider when designing an exercise program are volume and progression.

**REST AND RECUPERATION** Fitness gains occur following exercise as the body adapts to training stress. Adequate rest is as essential to this process as training. Overtraining is an imbalance between training and recovery. It leads to injury, illness, and excessive fatigue.

**REVERSIBILITY** The body adjusts to lower physical activity levels just as it adjusts to higher levels. This is the principle of **reversibility.** When you stop exercising, you can lose up to 50% of fitness improvements within two months. Try to exercise consistently, and don't quit if you miss a few workouts.

**INDIVIDUAL DIFFERENCES** There are significant individual differences among people in their ability to improve fitness, achieve a desirable body composition, and perform and learn sports skills. Studies show that some people on a diet and exercise program improve fitness by 50%, whereas others on the same program improve by only 2-3%. It is more difficult for those whose bodies don't respond to exercise to change fitness or body fat levels. More than 800 genes are associated with endurance performance, and 100 of those determine individual differences in exercise capacity. However, regardless of heredity, physical training improves fitness. Elite athletes start with a genetic advantage. But everyone can improve fitness and reap the health benefits of exercise.

### Selecting Activities

If you have been inactive, begin by gradually increasing the amount of moderate-intensity exercise in your life (the bottom of the activity pyramid shown in Figure 11.3). Once your body adjusts to your new activity level, you can choose additional activities for your exercise program.

Be sure the activities you choose contribute to your overall wellness and make sense for you. Are you competitive? If so, try racquetball, basketball, or squash. Do you prefer to exercise alone? Then consider cross-country skiing, hiking, or road running. Have you been sedentary? A walking program may be an excellent place to start. If you think you may have trouble sticking with an exercise program, find a structured activity that you can do with a friend, a personal trainer, or a group.

## Cardiorespiratory Endurance Exercise

Exercises that condition your heart and lungs and improve your metabolism should play a central role in your fitness program.

### Frequency

The optimal workout schedule for endurance training is 3-5 days per week. Beginners should start with 3 days and work up to 5 days. Training more than 5 days a week often leads to injury for recreational athletes. Although you get health benefits from exercising vigorously only 1 or 2 days per week, you risk injury because your body never gets a chance to adapt fully to regular exercise training.

### Intensity

The most misunderstood aspect of conditioning, even among experienced athletes, is exercise intensity. Intensity is crucial in attaining significant training effects—that is, in increasing the body's cardiorespiratory capacity. A primary purpose of endurance training is to increase **maximal oxygen consumption** ($\dot{V}O_{2max}$). $\dot{V}O_{2max}$ represents the cells' maximum ability to use oxygen and is considered the best measure of cardiorespiratory capacity. Training intensity is crucial for improving $\dot{V}O_{2max}$.

One of the easiest ways to determine precisely how intensely you should work involves measuring your heart rate. It is not necessary or desirable to exercise at your maximum heart rate—the fastest heart rate possible before exhaustion sets in—to improve your cardiorespiratory capacity. Beneficial effects occur at lower heart rates with a much lower risk of injury. Your **target heart rate zone** is the range of rates within which you should exercise to obtain cardiorespiratory benefits. To determine the intensity at which you should exercise, see the box "Determine Your Target Heart Rate."

If you have been sedentary, start exercising at the lower end of your target heart rate range (65% of maximum heart rate) for at least 4-6 weeks. For people with a deficient initial level of fitness, a lower training intensity of 55-64% of maximum heart rate may be sufficient to achieve improvements in maximal oxygen consumption, especially at the start of an exercise program. Intensities of 70-85% of maximum heart rate are appropriate for people with an average fitness level.

**TERMS**

**reversibility** The training principle that fitness improvements are lost when demands on the body are lowered.

**maximal oxygen consumption ($\dot{V}O_{2max}$)** The body's maximum ability to transport and use oxygen.

**target heart rate zone** The range of heart rates that should be reached and maintained during cardiorespiratory endurance exercise to obtain benefits.

## TAKE CHARGE
## Determine Your Target Heart Rate

One of the best ways to monitor the intensity of cardiorespiratory endurance exercise is to measure your heart rate. It isn't necessary to exercise at your maximum heart rate to improve maximal oxygen consumption. Fitness adaptations occur at lower heart rates with a much lower risk of injury.

According to the American College of Sports Medicine, your target heart rate zone—rates you should exercise to experience cardiorespiratory benefits—is between 65% and 90% of your maximum heart rate. To calculate your target heart rate zone, follow these steps:

1. Estimate your maximum heart rate (MHR) by subtracting your age from 220, or have it measured precisely by undergoing an exercise stress test in a doctor's office, hospital, or sports medicine lab. (*Note:* The formula to estimate MHR carries an error of about ±10–15 beats per minute [bpm] and can be wildly inaccurate for some people, particularly older adults and young children.)
2. Multiply your MHR by 65% and 90% to calculate your target heart rate zone. Very unfit people should use 55% of MHR for their training threshold.

For example, a 19-year-old would calculate her target heart rate zone:

MHR = 220 − 19 = 201

65% training intensity = 0.65 × 201 = 131 bpm

90% training intensity = 0.90 × 201 = 181 bpm

To gain fitness benefits, the young woman in our example would have to exercise at an intensity that raises her heart rate to between 131 and 181 bpm.

An alternative method for calculating the target heart rate range uses heart rate reserve, the difference between the maximum and resting heart rates. With this method, the target heart rate equals resting heart rate plus between 50% (40% for very unfit people) and 85% of heart rate reserve. Although some people (particularly those with deficient fitness levels) will obtain more accurate results using this more complex method, both methods provide reasonable estimates of an appropriate target heart rate zone.

As your program progresses and your fitness improves, you will need to jog, cycle, or walk faster to reach your target heart rate zone. To monitor your heart rate during exercise, count your pulse while you're still moving or immediately after you stop exercising. Count beats for 15 seconds and multiply that number by 4 to see if your heart rate is in your target zone. Table 11.1 shows target heart rate ranges and 15-second counts based on the maximum heart rate formula.

Heart rate monitors are helpful if close heart rate tracking is important in your program. They can be integrated into workout information provided by smartphone apps.

When shopping for a heart rate monitor, do your homework. Quality, reliability, and warranties vary. Ask personal trainers for recommendations and look for product reviews in consumer magazines or online.

Another way scientists describe fitness is as the capacity to increase metabolism (energy usage level) above rest. One **MET** represents the body's resting metabolic rate—that is, the energy or calorie requirement of the body at rest. Exercise intensity is expressed in multiples of resting metabolic rate. Exercise intensities of less than 3-4 METs are considered low. Activities that increase metabolism by 6-8 METs are classified as moderate-intensity exercises and are suitable for most people beginning an exercise program. Vigorous exercise increases metabolic rate by over 10 METs. Table 11.2 lists the MET ratings for various activities.

**TERMS**

**MET** A measure of the metabolic cost of an exercise. One MET represents the body's resting metabolic rate—the energy or calorie requirement of the body at rest.

**Table 11.1** Target Heart Rate Range and 15-Second Counts

| AGE (YEARS) | TARGET HEART RATE RANGE (bpm)* | 15-SECOND COUNT (beats) |
|---|---|---|
| 20-24 | 127-180 | 32-45 |
| 25-29 | 124-176 | 31-44 |
| 30-34 | 121-171 | 30-43 |
| 35-39 | 118-167 | 30-42 |
| 40-44 | 114-162 | 29-41 |
| 45-49 | 111-158 | 28-40 |
| 50-54 | 108-153 | 27-38 |
| 55-59 | 105-149 | 26-37 |
| 60-64 | 101-144 | 25-36 |
| 65+ | 97-140 | 24-35 |

*Target heart rates lower than those shown here are appropriate for individuals with a very low initial level of fitness. Ranges are based on the following formula: target heart rate = 0.65 to 0.90 of maximum heart rate, assuming maximum heart rate = 220 − age.

**Table 11.2** Approximate MET and Caloric Costs of Selected Activities for a 154-Pound Person

| ACTIVITY | METS | CALORIC EXPENDITURE (kilocalories/min) |
|---|---|---|
| Rest | 1 | 1.2 |
| Light housework | 2-4 | 2.4-4.8 |
| Bowling | 2-4 | 2.5-5 |
| Walking | 2-7 | 2.5-8.5 |
| Archery | 3-4 | 3.7-5 |
| Dancing | 3-7 | 3.7-8.5 |
| Hiking | 3-7 | 3.7-8.5 |
| Horseback riding | 3-8 | 3.7-10 |
| Cycling | 3-8 | 3.7-10 |
| Basketball (recreational) | 3-9 | 3.7-11 |
| Swimming | 4-8 | 5-10 |
| Tennis | 4-9 | 5-11 |
| Fishing (fly, stream) | 5-6 | 6-7.5 |
| In-line skating | 5-8 | 6-10 |
| Skiing (downhill) | 5-8 | 6-10 |
| Rock climbing | 5-10 | 6-12 |
| Scuba diving | 5-10 | 6-12 |
| Skiing (cross-country) | 6-12 | 7.5-15 |
| Jogging | 8-12 | 10-15 |

NOTE: Intensity varies greatly with effort, skill, and motivation.

SOURCE: Adapted from American College of Sports Medicine. 2022. *ACSM's Guidelines for Exercise Testing and Prescription,* 11th ed. Philadelphia: Wolters Kluwer.

**Time (Duration)** A total of 20–60 minutes per workout is recommended for cardiorespiratory endurance training. Exercise can be done in a single session or several sessions lasting 10 or more minutes. The total duration of exercise depends on its intensity. To improve cardiorespiratory endurance during a moderate-intensity activity such as walking or slow swimming, exercise for 45–60 minutes. For high-intensity exercise performed at the top of your target heart rate zone, a duration of 20 minutes is sufficient. Start with less vigorous activities and gradually increase intensity.

**Type** The best exercises for developing cardiorespiratory endurance stress much of the body's muscle mass for a prolonged period. These include walking, jogging, running, swimming, bicycling, and group exercise. Many popular sports and recreational activities, such as racquetball, tennis, basketball, and soccer, are also good if the skill level and intensity of the game are sufficient to provide a vigorous workout.

**Volume of Activity** Exercise volume for cardiorespiratory endurance can be estimated using several measures. Each of the following is approximately equivalent: 150 minutes per week of moderate-intensity activity; 1000 calories per week in moderate-intensity exercise; 5400 to 7900 steps or more per day; and 500 to 1000 MET-min per week (exercise intensity in METs times minutes of exercise).

**Progression** The rate of progression depends on your goals, fitness, health, age, and adaptation to training. Most benefits occur at moderate training intensities for about 150 minutes per week for general health. Higher levels of fitness require more intense training programs. Increasing intensity is most important for improving fitness, while increasing time and frequency can promote a healthy body composition by increasing overall energy expenditure with moderate-intensity activity.

Fitness determines your capacity to improve. Untrained people can make rapid gains, whereas highly fit people slowly improve. Genetics also determines how fast you will improve. People vary in their response to similar training programs. Finally, health and age influence your adaptability and capacity for training progression.

**The Warm-Up and Cool-Down** Warm up before exercise and cool down afterward. Warming up enhances your performance and decreases your chances of injury. A warm-up session should include low-intensity movements like those in the activity that will follow. For example, hit forehands and backhands before a tennis game or jog slowly for 400 meters before progressing to an 8-minute mile. A warm-up might include low-intensity whole-body exercises such as walking lunges, jumping jacks, or arm circles. During the warm-up, don't do static stretching exercises because they can temporarily decrease muscle strength and power. Do static stretching at the end of your workout, when your body temperature is elevated and you are no longer concerned with muscle performance.

Cooling down after exercise is essential to restore the body's circulation to its normal resting condition. When you are at rest, a relatively small percentage of your total blood volume is directed to muscles, but during exercise, as much as 90% of the heart's output is directed to them. During recovery, continuing to exercise at a low level is important for a smooth transition to the resting state. Cooling down helps regulate the return of blood to your heart. After exercising, avoid taking a hot shower until you have cooled down.

## Exercises for Muscular Strength and Endurance

Any program designed to promote health should include exercises that develop muscular strength and endurance.

**Types of Strength-Training Exercises** Muscular strength and endurance can be developed in many ways, from weight training to calisthenics. Common exercises such as curl-ups, push-ups, pull-ups, and unweighted squats maintain the muscular strength of most people if they practice them several times a week. To condition and tone your whole body, choose exercises that work the major muscles of the shoulders, chest, back, arms, abdomen, and legs.

To increase muscular strength and endurance, you must do **resistance exercise**—exercises in which your muscles must exert force against significant resistance. Resistance can be provided by weights, exercise machines, your body weight, or even objects such as rocks.

**Isometric (static) exercises** involve applying force without movement, such as when you contract your abdominal muscles. This type of exercise is valuable for toning and strengthening muscles. Isometrics can be practiced anywhere and do not require any equipment. For maximum strength gains, hold an isometric contraction maximally for 6 seconds, and do 3–10 repetitions. Don't hold your breath: Doing so can restrict blood flow to your heart and brain. Within a few weeks, you will notice the effect of this exercise. Isometrics are particularly useful when recovering from an injury.

**Isotonic (dynamic) exercises** involve applying force with movement, as in weight training exercises such as the bench press. These exercises are the most popular for increasing muscle strength and are most valuable for developing strength that can be transferred to other forms of physical activity. They include exercises using barbells, dumbbells, kettlebells, weight machines, and body weight (as in push-ups or pull-ups).

**Core Training** The core muscles include those in the abdomen, pelvic floor, sides of the trunk, back, buttocks, hips, and pelvis. They stabilize the midsection when you sit, stand, reach, walk, jump, twist, squat, throw, or bend. During any dynamic movement, the core muscles and active muscles work together. Some shorten to cause movement, whereas others contract and hold to provide stability, lengthen to brake the movement, or send signals to the brain about the activities and positions of the muscles, joints, and bones. When specific core muscles are weak or tired, the nervous system steps in and uses other muscles. This substitution causes abnormal stress on the joints, decreases power, and increases the risk of injury.

For over 100 years, traditional core training included dynamic exercises such as sit-ups, back extensions, and twists. However, scientists have confirmed that spinal stability and stiffness are more critical for health and performance than core movement strength. Isometric core exercises like side bridges build core stiffness, strengthen core muscles, improve endurance, reduce low back pain, and boost sports performance. Greater core stiffness transfers strength and speed to the limbs, increases the load-bearing capacity of the spine, and protects the internal organs during sports movements.

The best exercises for low-back health are whole-body exercises that force the core muscles to stabilize the spine in many different directions. Exercises that focus on the core muscles include the lunge, side bridges, stir-the-pot, and bird dogs. These exercises are generally safe for beginning exercisers and, with physician approval, people with back pain.

**TERMS**

**resistance exercise** Exercise that forces muscles to contract against increased resistance; also called *strength training*.

**isometric (static) exercise** The application of force without movement.

**isotonic (dynamic) exercise** The application of force with movement.

**Sex Differences in Muscular Strength** Within a given genetic population, men are generally stronger than women because their bodies are typically larger overall. A more significant proportion of their total body mass is muscle. But when strength is expressed per unit of muscle tissue, men are only 1–2% stronger than women in the upper body and about equal to women in the lower body. Individual muscle cells are more prominent in men, but the functioning of the cells is the same in both sexes.

Three factors that help explain the strength disparities between men and women are testosterone levels, skeletal size, and nerve conduction velocity. Testosterone promotes the growth of muscle tissue in both males and females, but testosterone levels are about 6–10 times higher in men than in women, so men develop larger muscles. Also within a given genetic population, men are usually bigger than women, which gives them more leverage. Nerve conduction velocity in the brain and central nervous system is about 4% faster in men than in women, which slightly increases muscle activation speed.

Most women will not develop large muscles from strength training. Resistance exercise helps women reduce their overall body fat levels and reduce fat in the midsection. Losing muscle over time is a much greater health concern for women than small gains in muscle weight in response to strength training, mainly because any increases in muscle weight are typically more than balanced with loss of fat weight. Men and women lose muscle mass and power as they age, but because men start with more muscle when they are young and don't lose power as quickly as women, older women often have more significant impairment of muscle function than older men.

**Choosing Equipment** Many people prefer weight machines to free weights because they are safe, convenient, and easy to use. You set the resistance, sit down at the machine, and exercise. Free weights require more care, balance, and coordination to use, but they strengthen your body in ways that are more adaptable to real life.

**Choosing Exercises** A complete weight training program works all the major muscle groups: neck, upper back, shoulders, arms, chest, core, thighs, buttocks, and calves. Different exercises work different muscles, so it usually takes about 8–10 exercises to get a complete workout for general fitness. For example, you can do bench presses to develop the chest, shoulders, and upper arms; pull-ups to work the biceps and upper back; squats to build the legs and buttocks; toe raises to work the calves; and so on.

**Frequency** For general fitness, the American College of Sports Medicine (ACSM) recommends a strength workout frequency of at least two nonconsecutive days per week. This schedule allows your muscles one or more rest days between workouts to avoid soreness and injury. If you enjoy weight training and would like to train more often, try working different muscle groups on alternate days.

**Intensity and Time** The amount of weight (resistance) you lift in weight training exercises is equivalent to intensity in cardiorespiratory endurance training. The number of repetitions of each exercise is equal to time. To improve fitness, do enough repetitions of each exercise to fatigue your muscles temporarily. The number of repetitions needed to cause fatigue depends on the resistance: The heavier the weight, the fewer repetitions to reach fatigue. Heavy weights and few repetitions (1–5) build strength, whereas lighter weights and more repetitions (10–25) build endurance. For a general fitness program to build both strength and endurance, do 8–12 repetitions of each exercise. For people over 50 years of age, 10–15 repetitions of each exercise using a lighter weight is recommended.

The first few weight training sessions should be devoted to learning the exercises. To start, choose a weight you can move easily through 8–12 repetitions. Add weight when you can do over 12 repetitions. If adding weight means you can do only 7 or 8 repetitions before your muscles fatigue, stay with that weight until you can again complete 12 repetitions. If you can do only 4–6 repetitions after adding weight, or if you can't maintain good form, you've added too much and should take some off. As a general guideline, add approximately a half-pound of additional weight for every 10 pounds you are currently lifting.

For developing strength and endurance for general fitness, a single set (a group of repetitions) of each exercise is sufficient, provided you use enough weight to fatigue your muscles. Doing more than one set of each exercise may increase strength development further, and most serious weight trainers do at least three sets of each exercise. If you do more than one set of an exercise, rest long enough between sets (1–5 minutes) to allow your muscles to recover.

**Volume** For weight training, the volume of a specific exercise during a workout would be the weight lifted multiplied by the number of reps and sets. Choose a training volume that promotes progress and that you will do consistently. Change the components occasionally, increasing the weight on some days and the sets and reps on other days.

**Progression** Training intensity is the most critical factor promoting improvements in strength and power. You will progress rapidly when you begin training, but progress slows as you become more fit. Set fitness goals and progress systematically by adding weight or sets as you gain strength and power. After achieving your goal, maintain strength by training one to three times per week.

**A Caution about Supplements** No nutritional supplement or drug will change a weak person into a strong person. Those changes require regular training that stresses the body and causes physiological adaptations. Supplements or medications promising quick, significant gains in strength rarely work and are often dangerous, expensive, or illegal. Over-the-counter supplements are not regulated carefully, and their long-term effects have not been studied systematically. Performance-enhancing drugs such as **anabolic steroids** and growth hormone have potentially dangerous side effects.

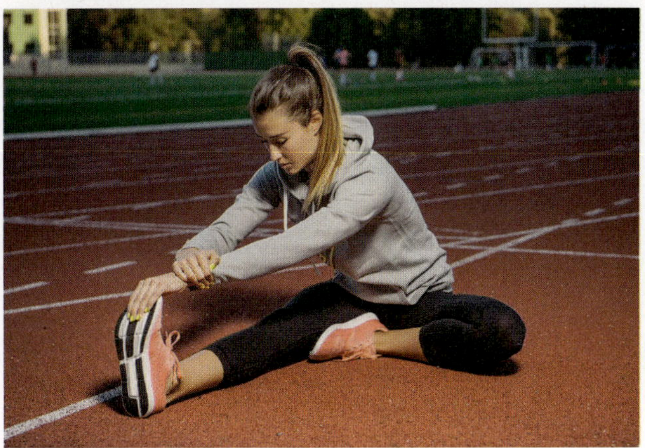

When performed regularly, stretching exercises help maintain or improve the range of motion in joints. Brian Caissie/fStop/Getty Images

## Flexibility Exercises

Flexibility, or stretching, exercises are essential for maintaining the normal range of motion in the body's major joints. Some activities, such as running, can decrease flexibility because they require only a partial range of motion. Like a good weight training program, a good stretching program includes exercises for all the body's major muscle groups and joints: neck, shoulders, back, hips, thighs, hamstrings, and calves. Flexibility training is essential for preventing low-back injuries and maintaining low-back health in tandem with core training.

**Proper Stretching Technique** Timing determines the best stretching technique: Do static stretching after a workout and dynamic or active stretching before a workout. *Static stretching* involves extending to a specific position and then holding it. *Dynamic stretching* is done by actively moving through the joints' ranges of motion. *Ballistic stretching* (known as "bouncing") is dangerous and counterproductive. The safest and most convenient technique for increasing flexibility may be active static stretching with a passive assist. For example, you might do a seated stretch of your calf muscles by contracting the muscles on the top of your shin and by grabbing your feet and pulling them toward you.

**Frequency** Do stretching exercises at least 2 or 3 days per week (but 5–7 days is optimal). If you stretch during your cool-down after cardiorespiratory endurance exercise or strength training, you may develop more flexibility because your muscles are warmer then and can be pushed farther.

**Intensity, Time, Volume, and Progression** Do stretching exercises statically. Stretch to the point of mild discomfort, hold the position for 10–30 seconds, rest for 30–60 seconds,

**TERMS**

**anabolic steroids** Synthetic male hormones used to increase muscle size and strength.

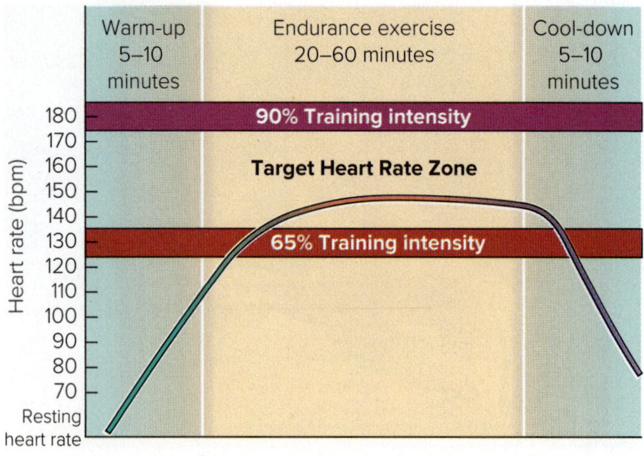


**Frequency:** 3–5 days per week

**Intensity:** 55/65–90% of maximum heart rate, 40/50–85% of heart rate reserve plus resting heart rate, or an RPE rating of about 4–8 (lower intensities—55–64% of maximum heart rate and 40–49% of heart rate reserve—apply to people who are quite unfit; for average individuals, intensities of 70–85% of maximum heart rate are appropriate)

**Time (duration):** 20–60 minutes (one session or multiple sessions lasting 10 or more minutes)

**Type of activity:** Cardiorespiratory endurance exercises, such as walking, jogging, biking, swimming, cross-country skiing, and rope skipping

FIGURE 11.5 **The FITT principle for a cardiorespiratory endurance program.** Longer-duration exercise at lower intensities can often be as beneficial for promoting health as shorter-duration, high-intensity exercise.

and then repeat, trying to stretch a bit farther. A total of 90 seconds of discontinuous flexibility exercise per joint is recommended. Older adults might benefit more from holding a stretch for 30–60 seconds.

Increase your intensity gradually. Improved flexibility takes many months to develop. There are significant individual differences in joint flexibility. Don't feel you have to compete with others during stretching workouts. Progressively build flexibility, striving for a normal but not excessive range of motion. Extremely flexible joints lose stability.

## Training in Specific Skills

The final component in your fitness program is learning the skills required for the sports or activities in which you participate. By taking the time and effort to acquire competence, you can achieve a sense of mastery and add a new physical skill to your repertoire.

The first step in learning a new skill is getting help. Sports like tennis, golf, and skiing require mastery of basic movements and techniques, so instruction from a qualified teacher or coach can save you hours of frustration and increase your enjoyment. Skill is also important in conditioning activities such as jogging, swimming, and cycling. Even if you learned a sport as a child, additional instruction now can help you refine your technique, get over stumbling blocks, and relearn skills that you may have misremembered.

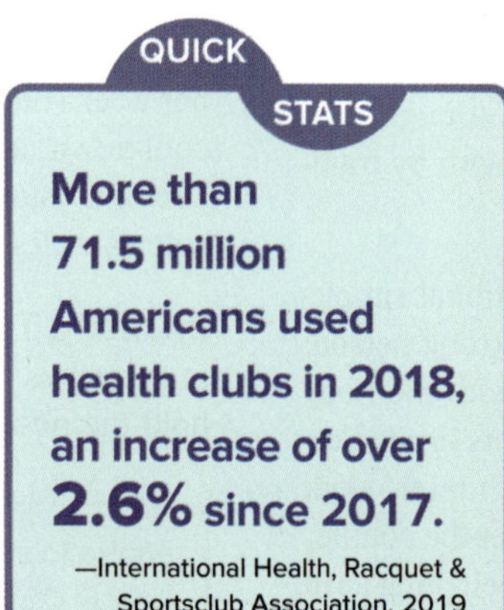


## Putting It All Together

Now that you know the essential components of a fitness program, you can put them all together in a program that works for you. See Figure 11.5 for a summary of the FITT principle for the health-related components of fitness.

# GETTING STARTED AND STAYING ON TRACK

Once a program fulfills your basic fitness needs and suits your tastes, adhering to a few fundamental principles will help you improve quickly, have fun, and minimize the risk of injury.

## Selecting Instructors, Equipment, and Facilities

Once you've chosen the activities for your program, you may need to look for the appropriate information, instruction, and equipment or find a suitable facility.

One of the best places to get help is an exercise class, where an expert instructor can teach you the basics of training and answer your questions. A qualified personal trainer can also start you on an exercise program or a new form of training. Ensure that your instructor or trainer has proper qualifications, such as a college degree in exercise physiology, kinesiology, or physical education and certification by the American College of Sports Medicine, National Strength and Conditioning Association, International Sports Science Association, or another professional organization.

Many apps and websites provide fitness programs, including ongoing support and feedback via email. Many of these sites charge fees, so review the sites, decide which ones seem most appropriate, and go through a free trial period before subscribing. Also, remember to consider the reliability of the information at fitness apps and websites, especially those that advertise or sell products.

Appropriate safety equipment is essential, such as pads and helmets for skateboarding. You can often find bargains through mail-order companies and discount or used equipment stores if you shop around.

Before you invest in a new piece of equipment, investigate it. Try it out at a local gym to ensure that you'll use it regularly. Footwear is an essential piece of equipment for almost any activity; see the "What to Wear" box for shopping strategies.

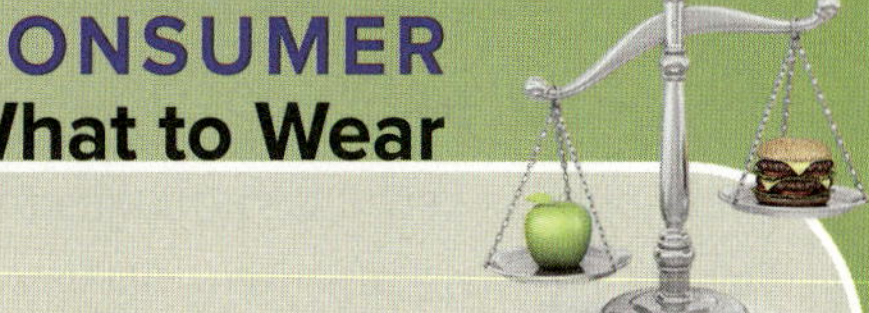

# CRITICAL CONSUMER
## What to Wear

### Clothing

Modern exercise clothing is attractive, comfortable, and functional. Shorts made of elastic material, such as spandex, hug the body, supplying support. If you prefer, you can wear running shorts and a T-shirt. The main requirement for workout clothes is that they let you move easily but are not so loose that they get caught in the exercise machines or on fences when running outside. Don't wear street clothes when exercising because they can interfere with movement, and sweat, oil, and dirt can ruin them. If you run or cycle on the street, wear bright-colored clothing so that motorists can see you, and cyclists should wear a helmet to prevent head injury in case of an accident.

### Specifics for Women and Men

- ***For women.*** Wear a good sports bra whenever you exercise. Breast support is important when running, playing volleyball, or weight training, The breasts can be injured if barbells press too firmly against them when you are weight-training or if they aren't properly supported when you run. A good sports bra should support the breasts in all directions, contain minimal elastic material, absorb moisture freely, and be easily laundered. Seams, hooks, and catches should not irritate the skin. You might buy a bra with an underwire for added support and a pocket in which to insert padding if you do exercises that could cause injury.
- ***For men.*** Wear a protective cup and jockstrap when participating in contact sports, such as football, baseball, cricket, hockey, wrestling, and karate. These protections can help guard against male infertility.

### Footwear

Footwear is perhaps the most important item of equipment for almost any activity. Shoes protect and support your feet and improve traction. When you jump or run, you place as much as six times more force on your feet than when you stand still. Shoes can help cushion against the stress this additional force places on your lower legs, preventing injuries. Some athletic shoes are also designed to help prevent ankle rollover, another common source of injury.

When choosing athletic shoes, first consider the activity you've chosen for your exercise program. Shoes appropriate for different activities have distinctive characteristics. Foot type is another important consideration. If your feet roll inward excessively, you may need additional stability features on the inner side of the shoe to counteract this movement. If your feet roll outward excessively, you may need highly flexible and cushioned shoes that promote foot motion. Most women will get a better fit if they choose shoes specially designed for women's feet rather than downsized versions of men's shoes.

### Barefoot Shoes or Minimalist Footwear

Two-thirds of runners experience an injury every year. Humans have evolved to run, so some scientists blame running shoes for the high injury rate. Most runners strike heel first when using heavily padded running shoes. Barefoot runners strike the

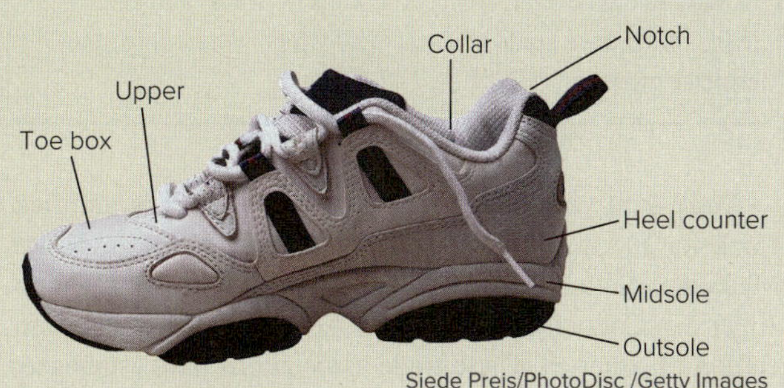

Siede Preis/PhotoDisc /Getty Images

ground with their forefoot (at least they're supposed to), which better uses the shock absorbing capacity of the skeleton. Some researchers speculated that using "minimalist" footwear allows people to run more naturally, which should cut down on the injury rate. Other research suggests that traditional running shoes provide a physiological advantage that makes running easier. We need more research to determine whether barefoot running is safe and viable or just the latest running fad.

### Successful Shopping

For successful shoe shopping, remember the following strategies:

- Shop late in the day or, ideally, following a workout. Your foot size increases during the day and after exercise.
- Wear socks like those you plan to wear during exercise.
- Try on both shoes and wear them around for 10 minutes or more. Try walking on an uncarpeted surface. Approximate the movements of your activity: walk, jog, run, jump, and so on.
- Check the fit and style carefully:
  - Is the toe box roomy enough? Your toes will spread out when your foot hits the ground or you push off. There should be at least one thumb's width of space from the longest toe to the end of the toe box.
  - Do the shoes have enough cushioning? Do your feet feel supported when you bounce up and down? Try bouncing on your toes and on your heels.
  - Do your heels fit snugly in the shoe? Do they stay put when you walk, or do they slide up?
  - Are the arches of your feet on top of the shoes' arch supports?
  - Do the shoes feel stable when you twist and turn on the balls of your feet? Try twisting from side to side while standing on one foot.
  - Do you feel any pressure points?
- If you exercise at dawn or dusk, choose shoes with reflective sections for added visibility and safety.
- Replace athletic shoes about every three months or 300–500 miles of jogging or walking.

**Ask Yourself**

**QUESTIONS FOR CRITICAL THINKING AND REFLECTION**

Think of a few physical activities and sports that you would like to do, but haven't. Given your current fitness and skill level, which ones could you reasonably incorporate into your exercise program?

Make sure your health club or fitness center is certified. Look for the displayed names American College of Sports Medicine, National Strength and Conditioning Association, American Council on Exercise, or Aerobics and Fitness Association of America. These trade associations have established standards to help protect consumer health, safety, and rights.

## Eating and Drinking for Exercise

When they begin a fitness program, most people need not change their eating habits. Many athletes and other physically active people succumb to buying aggressively advertised vitamins, minerals, and protein supplements, but usually a well-balanced diet contains all the energy and nutrients needed to sustain an exercise program (see Chapter 10).

A balanced diet is also the key to improving body composition when you exercise more. One promise of a fitness program is decreased body fat and increased muscle mass. As a general rule, fat increases if you consume more calories than you expend through metabolism and exercise. However, body fat control is determined by the amount and kind of calories you consume. Reduce your added sugars and trans fats intake, and be physically active.

An essential principle is to keep your body well hydrated by drinking enough fluids when exercising. Your body depends on water to sustain many chemical reactions and to maintain the correct body temperature. Sweating during exercise depletes the body's water supply and can lead to dehydration if fluids are not replaced. Severe dehydration can cause reduced blood volume, accelerated heart rate, elevated body temperature, muscle cramps, heatstroke, and other serious problems.

Drinking fluids before and during exercise is essential to prevent dehydration and enhance performance. Thirst receptors in the brain make you want to drink fluids, but during heavy or prolonged exercise or exercise in hot weather, thirst alone isn't a good indication of how much fluid you need to drink. Drink at least 16 ounces of fluid two to four hours before exercise and then drink enough during exercise to prevent significant fluid loss in sweat. Don't drink more than one quart per hour during exercise because consuming too much water is dangerous. After training, let thirst be your guide to your fluid needs. You can also check your weight before and after an exercise session; any weight loss is due to fluid loss that needs to be replaced.

Carry fluids when you exercise so that you can replace your fluids when they're depleted. Cool water is an excellent fluid replacement for exercise sessions lasting less than 60–90 minutes. For longer workouts, the ACSM recommends sports drinks that contain water and small amounts of electrolytes (sodium, potassium, and magnesium) and simple carbohydrates (sugar, usually in the form of sucrose or glucose). After your workout, replace any lost fluids. Nonfat or low-fat milk, for those who can tolerate dairy products, are excellent postexercise fluid replacement beverages because they promote long-term hydration. Milk is digested more slowly than water or sports beverages and contains electrolytes.

## Managing Your Fitness Program

How can you tell when you're in shape? When do you stop improving and start maintaining? How can you stay motivated? These questions are essential for your program to become an integral part of your life.

**Starting Slowly, Getting in Shape Gradually** As Table 11.3 shows, an exercise program can be divided into three stages. In the initial stage, the body adjusts to the new type and level of activity. In the improvement stage, fitness increases. In the maintenance stage, the targeted level of fitness is sustained over the long term.

When beginning a program, start slowly to give your body time to adapt to the stress of exercise. Choose activities carefully according to your fitness level.

**Table 11.3** Sample Progression for a Walking and Running Program

| STAGE/WEEK | FREQUENCY (days/week) | INTENSITY* (beats/minute) | TIME (duration in minutes) |
|---|---|---|---|
| Initial stage | | | |
| 1 | 3 | 120–130 | 15–20 |
| 2 | 3 | 120–130 | 20–25 |
| 3 | 4 | 130–145 | 20–25 |
| 4 | 4 | 130–145 | 25–30 |
| Improvement stage | | | |
| 5–7 | 3–4 | 145–160 | 25–30 |
| 8–10 | 3–4 | 145–160 | 30–35 |
| 11–13 | 3–4 | 150–165 | 30–35 |
| 14–16 | 4–5 | 150–165 | 30–35 |
| 17–20 | 4–5 | 160–180 | 35–40 |
| 21–24 | 4–5 | 160–180 | 35–40 |
| Maintenance stage | | | |
| 25+ | 3–5 | 160–180 | 20–60 |

*The target heart rates shown here are based on calculations for a healthy 20-year-old. The program progresses from an initial target heart rate of 50% to a maintenance range of 70–90% of maximum heart rate.

SOURCE: Adapted from American College of Sports Medicine. 2022. *ACSM's Guidelines for Exercise Testing and Prescription*, 11th ed. Philadelphia: Wolters Kluwer.

**Exercising Consistently** Consistency is the key to getting into shape without injury. Steady fitness improvement comes when you overload your body consistently. The best way to ensure consistency is to record the details of your workouts in a journal: how far you ran, how much weight you lifted, and so on. This record will help you evaluate your progress and plan workout sessions intelligently. Table 11.3 shows how the overload increases gradually over time in a sample walking-running program.

**Assessing Your Fitness** When are you in shape? It depends. One person may be out of shape running a mile in 5 minutes, but another may be in condition running a mile in 12 minutes. Your ultimate fitness level depends on your goals, program, and natural ability. The important thing is to set goals that make sense for you.

**Preventing and Managing Athletic Injuries** If an injury is not cared for properly, it can escalate into a chronic problem. If you learn how to deal with injuries, they won't derail your fitness program (Table 11.4). Some injuries require medical attention. See a physician right away if you suffer a head or eye injury, a possible ligament injury, a broken bone, or an internal disorder such as chest pain, fainting, or intolerance to heat. Also, seek medical attention for apparently minor injuries that do not get better within a reasonable time.

For minor cuts and scrapes, stop the bleeding and clean the wound with soap and water. Treat soft-tissue injuries (muscles and joints) with the R-I-C-E (REST - ICE - COMPRESSION - ELEVATION) principle.

After 36–48 hours, apply heat to relieve pain, relax muscles, and reduce stiffness if the swelling has disappeared. Immerse the affected area in warm water or use warm compresses, a hot water bottle, or a heating pad.

To prevent injuries, follow six basic guidelines:

1. Stay in condition: Haphazard exercise programs invite injury.
2. Warm up thoroughly before exercising.
3. Use proper body mechanics when lifting objects or executing sports skills.
4. Don't exercise when you're ill or overtrained (experiencing extreme fatigue due to overexercising).
5. Use the proper equipment.
6. Don't return to your regular exercise program until athletic injuries have healed.

**Table 11.4** Care of Common Exercise Injuries and Discomforts

| INJURY | SYMPTOMS | TREATMENT |
|---|---|---|
| Blister | Accumulation of fluid in one spot under the skin | Don't pop or drain it unless it interferes too much with your daily activities. If it does pop, clean the area with antiseptic and cover with a bandage. Do not remove the skin covering the blister. |
| Bruise (contusion) | Pain, swelling, and discoloration | R-I-C-E: rest, ice, compression, elevation. |
| Fracture and/or dislocation | Pain, swelling, tenderness, loss of function, and deformity | Seek medical attention, immobilize the affected area, and apply cold. |
| Joint sprain | Pain, tenderness, swelling, discoloration, and loss of function | R-I-C-E. Apply heat when swelling has disappeared. Stretch and strengthen affected area. |
| Muscle cramp | Painful, spasmodic muscle contractions | Gently stretch for 15–30 seconds at a time and/or massage the cramped area. Drink fluids and increase dietary salt intake if exercising in hot weather. |
| Muscle soreness or stiffness | Pain and tenderness in the affected muscle | Stretch the affected muscle gently; exercise at a low intensity; apply heat. Nonsteroidal anti-inflammatory drugs, such as ibuprofen, help some people. |
| Muscle strain | Pain, tenderness, swelling, and loss of strength in the affected muscle | R-I-C-E. Apply heat when swelling has disappeared. Stretch and strengthen the affected area. |
| Plantar fasciitis | Pain and tenderness in the connective tissue on the bottom of the foot | Apply ice, take nonsteroidal anti-inflammatory drugs, and stretch. Wear night splints when sleeping. |
| Shin splint | Pain and tenderness on the front of the lower leg; sometimes also pain in the calf muscle | Rest. Apply ice or heat to the affected area several times a day and before exercise; wrap with tape for support. Stretch and strengthen muscles in the lower legs. Purchase good-quality footwear and run on soft surfaces. |
| Side stitch | Pain on the side of the abdomen | Stretch the arm on the affected side as high as possible; if that doesn't help, try bending forward while tightening the abdominal muscles. |
| Tendinitis | Pain, swelling, and tenderness of the affected area | R-I-C-E. Apply heat when swelling has disappeared. Stretch and strengthen the affected area. |

SOURCE: Fahey, T. D., P. M. Insel, W. T. Roth and C. E. Insel. 2022. *Fit and Well: Core Concepts and Labs in Physical Fitness and Wellness,* 15th ed. New York: McGraw Hill. 

# BEHAVIOR CHANGE STRATEGY
## Planning a Personal Exercise Program

Although most people recognize the importance of incorporating exercise into their lives, many find it difficult to do. No single strategy will work for everyone, but the general steps outlined here should help you create an exercise program that fits your goals, preferences, and lifestyle. A carefully designed contract and program plan can help you convert your vague wishes into a detailed plan of action. And the strategies for program compliance outlined here and in Chapter 1 can help you enjoy and stick with your program for the rest of your life.

### Step 1: Set Goals

Setting specific goals to accomplish by exercising is an important first step in a successful fitness program because it establishes the direction you want to take. Your goals might be specifically related to health, such as lowering your blood pressure and risk of heart disease, or they might relate to other aspects of your life, such as improving your tennis game or the fit of your clothes. If you can decide why you're starting to exercise, it can help you keep going. Make sure your goals meet the SMART criteria described in Chapter 1.

Think carefully about your reasons for incorporating exercise into your life, and then fill in the Fitness Goals portion of the Personal Fitness Contract.

### Step 2: Select Activities

As discussed in the chapter, the success of your fitness program depends on the consistency of your involvement. Select activities that encourage your commitment: The right program will be its own incentive to continue, but poor activity choices provide obstacles and can turn exercise into a chore.

When choosing activities for your fitness program, consider the following:

- Is this activity fun? Will it hold my interest over time?
- Will this activity help me reach the goals I have set?
- Will my current fitness and skill level enable me to participate fully in this activity?
- Can I easily fit this activity into my daily schedule? Are there any special requirements (e.g., facilities, partners, equipment) that I must plan for?
- Can I afford any special costs required for equipment or facilities?
- If I have special exercise needs due to a particular health problem, does this activity conform to those exercise needs? Will it enhance my ability to cope with my specific health problem?

Using these guidelines listed, select several sports and activities. Fill in the Program Plan portion of the Personal Fitness Contract, including the fitness components your choices will develop and the frequency, intensity, and time standard you intend to meet for each activity. Does your program meet the criteria of a complete fitness program discussed in the chapter?

### Step 3: Make a Commitment

Complete your Personal Fitness Contract by signing it and having it witnessed by someone who can help make you accountable for your progress. By completing a contract, you make a firm commitment and will be more likely to follow through until you meet your goals.

### Step 4: Begin and Maintain Your Program

Start slowly and increase your intensity and duration gradually to allow your body time to adjust. Be realistic and patient—meeting your goals will take time. The important first step is to break your established pattern of inactivity. The following guidelines may help you start and stick with your program:

- ***Set aside regular periods for exercise.*** Choose times that fit in best with your schedule and stick to them. Allow an adequate amount of time for warm-up, cool-down, and a shower.
- ***Take advantage of any opportunity for exercise that presents itself.*** For example, walk to class or take stairs instead of an elevator.
- ***Do what you can to make your program fun and avoid boredom.*** Do stretching exercises or jumping jacks to music, or watch the evening news while riding your stationary bicycle.
- ***Exercise with a group that shares your goals and general level of competence.*** The social side of exercise is an important motivator for many people.
- ***Vary the program.*** Change your activities periodically. Alter your route or distance if biking or jogging. Change racquetball partners, or find a new volleyball court.
- ***Establish mini-goals or a point system, and work rewards into your program.*** Until you reach your main goals, a series of small rewards will help you stick with your program. Rewards should be things you enjoy that are easily obtainable.
- ***Focus on the positive.*** Concentrate on the improvements you get from your program, and how good you feel during and after exercise. Visualize what it will be like to reach your goals, and keep these images in your mind as an incentive to stick to your program.
- ***Revisit and revise.*** If your program turns out to be unrealistic, revise it. Expect to make many adjustments in your program along the way.
- ***Expect fluctuation and lapses.*** On some days your progress will be excellent, but on others you'll barely be able to drag yourself through your scheduled activities. Don't let

lapses discourage you or make you feel guilty. Instead make a renewed commitment to your exercise program.

- ***Plan ahead for difficult situations.*** Think about what circumstances might make it tough to keep up with your fitness routine, and develop strategies for sticking with your program. For example, devise a plan for your program during vacation, travel, bad weather, and so on.
- ***Renew your attitude.*** If you notice you're slacking off, try to list the negative thoughts and behaviors that are causing you to lose interest. Devise a strategy to reduce negative thoughts and behaviors. Make changes in your program plan and reward system to help renew your enthusiasm and commitment.

## Step 5: Record and Assess Your Progress

Keeping a record that notes the daily results of your program will help remind you of your ongoing commitment to your program and give you a sense of accomplishment. It can also help you identify problems. Create daily and weekly program logs that you can use to track your progress, or use one of the many available apps for exercise tracking. Record the activity frequency, intensity, time, and type. Post or check your log frequently to remind you of your activity schedule and to provide incentive for improvement.

SOURCE: Adapted from Kusinitz, I., and M. Fine. 1995. *Your Guide to Getting Fit*, 3rd ed. Mountain View, CA: Mayfield.

**Personal Fitness Contract**

I, ________________, am contracting with myself to follow an exercise program to work at the following goals. I will begin my program on ________________.

**Fitness Goals**

1. ________________
2. ________________
3. ________________
4. ________________
5. ________________
6. ________________

**Program Plan**

| Activities | Components (Check ✔) CRE | MS | ME | F | BC | Frequency (Check ✔) M | Tu | W | Th | F | Sa | Su | Intensity | Time |
|---|---|---|---|---|---|---|---|---|---|---|---|---|---|---|
| 1. | | | | | | | | | | | | | | |
| 2. | | | | | | | | | | | | | | |
| 3. | | | | | | | | | | | | | | |
| 4. | | | | | | | | | | | | | | |
| 5. | | | | | | | | | | | | | | |

Note: You should conduct activities for achieving CRE goals at your target heart rate.

I agree to maintain a record of my activity, assess my progress periodically, and, if necessary, revise my goals.

Signed ________________ Date ________________

Witness ________________

You can minimize the risk of injury by following safety guidelines, respecting signals from your body that something may be wrong, and treating injuries promptly. Use particular caution in heat or humidity (over 80°F and over 60% humidity): Exercise slowly, frequently rest in the shade, wear clothing that breathes, and drink plenty of fluids. Slow down or stop if you feel uncomfortable. During hot weather, exercise in the early morning or evening when temperatures are lowest.

**Staying with Your Program** Once you have attained your desired level of fitness, you can maintain it by exercising regularly at a consistent intensity, 3–5 days a week. If you exercise at the same intensity over a long period, your fitness will level out and can be maintained efficiently.

Adapt your program to changes in environment or schedule. Don't use wet weather or a new job as an excuse to give up your fitness program. If you walk in the summer, dress appropriately and walk in the winter. (Exercise is usually safe even in frigid temperatures if you dress warmly in layers and don't stay out too long.) If you can't go out because of darkness or an unsafe neighborhood, walk in a local shopping mall or on campus or join a gym.

What if you run out of steam? Although good health is an important *reason* to exercise, it's a poor *motivator*. You'll find specific suggestions for staying with your program in the Behavior Change Strategy box at the end of the chapter.

## TIPS FOR TODAY AND THE FUTURE

Physical activity and exercise offer benefits in nearly every area of wellness. Even a low to moderate level of activity provides valuable health benefits.

**RIGHT NOW YOU CAN:**

- Go outside and take a brisk 15-minute walk.
- Look at your calendar for the rest of the week and write in some physical activity—such as walking, running, or playing Frisbee—on as many days as you can. Schedule the training for a specific time and stick to it.
- Call friends and invite them to plan a regular exercise program with you.

**IN THE FUTURE YOU CAN:**

- Schedule a session with a qualified personal trainer who can evaluate your fitness level and help you set personalized fitness goals.
- Create seasonal workout programs for the summer, spring, fall, and winter. Develop programs varied but consistent with your overall fitness goals.

**TERMS**

**cross-training** Participating in two or more activities to develop a variety of fitness components.

**Cross-training** can add variety to your workouts. Cross-training emphasizes whole-body, high-intensity training using deadlifts, cleans, squats, presses, jerks, kettlebell exercises, snatches, plyometrics, sled pulls, and weight carrying. Cross-trainers learn to handle their body weight by practicing gymnastics, pull-ups, dips, kettlebell swings and snatches, rope climbing, push-ups, Olympic lifts, handstands, pirouettes, flips, and splits. They also do aerobics such as running, cycling, rope skipping, and rowing, but the emphasis is on speed and intensity. Cross-training programs attempt to develop well-rounded fitness by including exercises that build cardiovascular and respiratory endurance, stamina, strength, flexibility, power, speed, coordination, agility, balance, and accuracy.

## SUMMARY

- Exercise improves the functioning of the heart and the ability of the cardiorespiratory system to carry oxygen to the body's tissues. It also increases metabolic efficiency and improves body composition.
- Exercise lowers the risk of cardiovascular disease by improving blood fat levels, reducing high blood pressure, and interfering with the disease process that causes coronary artery blockage.
- Exercise reduces the risk of cancer, osteoporosis, and diabetes. It improves immune function and psychological health and helps prevent injuries and low-back pain.
- The five components of physical fitness most important to health are cardiorespiratory endurance, muscular strength, muscular endurance, flexibility, and body composition.
- Most people should accumulate at least 150 minutes of moderate-intensity or 75 minutes of vigorous-intensity exercise each week. Longer-duration or more vigorous activity produces additional health and fitness benefits.
- Cardiorespiratory endurance exercises stress a large portion of the body's muscle mass. Endurance exercise should be performed 3–5 days per week for 20–60 minutes per day. Intensity can be evaluated by measuring the heart rate.
- Warming up before exercising and cooling down afterward improve your performance and decrease your chances of injury.
- Exercises that develop muscular strength and endurance involve exerting force against a significant resistance. A strength-training program for general fitness typically involves one or more sets of 8–12 repetitions of 8–10 exercises performed on at least two nonconsecutive days per week.
- A good stretching program includes exercises for the body's major muscle groups and joints. Do active, static stretches at least 2–3 days per week. Hold each stretch for 10–30 seconds and do 2–4 repetitions for a total of 90 seconds per muscle group. Stretch when muscles are warm.
- Individuals should choose instructors, equipment, and facilities carefully to enhance enjoyment and prevent injuries.

- A well-balanced diet contains all the energy and nutrients needed to sustain a fitness program. When exercising, remember to drink enough fluids.

- Rest, ice, compression, and elevation (R-I-C-E) are treatments for minor muscle and joint injuries.

- People can maintain the desired fitness level by exercising 3–5 days a week consistently.

- Strategies for maintaining an exercise program over the long term include having meaningful goals, varying the program, and trying new activities.

## FOR MORE INFORMATION

*American College of Sports Medicine (ACSM).* The principal professional organization for sports medicine and exercise science. Provides brochures, publications, and audio- and videotapes.

http://www.acsm.org

*American Council on Exercise (ACE).* The website promotes exercise and fitness and features fact sheets on consumer topics, including choosing shoes, cross-training, and steroids.

http://www.acefitness.org

*Backfitpro.* This site provides excellent information on preventing back pain and promoting core fitness. Stuart McGill, a biomechanist and professor emeritus from the University of Waterloo in Canada, maintains the site.

http://www.backfitpro.com/

*CDC Physical Activity Information.* Provides information about the benefits of physical activity and suggestions for incorporating moderate physical activity into daily life.

http://www.cdc.gov/physicalactivity/

*Disabled Sports USA.* Provides sports and recreation services to people with physical or mobility disorders.

http://www.disabledsportsusa.org

*International Health, Racquet, & Sportsclub Association (IHRSA): Health Clubs.* Provides guidelines for choosing a health or fitness facility and links to clubs that belong to IHRSA.

http://www.ihrsa.org

*Dan John.* An excellent website for people serious about improving strength and fitness, written by a world-class athlete and coach in track and field and Highland games.

http://danjohn.net

*MedlinePlus: Exercise and Physical Fitness.* Provides links to news and reliable information about fitness and exercise from government agencies and professional associations.

https://medlineplus.gov/fitnessandexercise.html

*President's Council on Physical Fitness and Sports (PCPFS).* Provides information about PCPFS programs and publications, including fitness guides and fact sheets.

http://www.fitness.gov

http://www.presidentschallenge.org

*Robert Wood Johnson Foundation.* Promotes Americans' health and health care through research and distribution of information on healthy lifestyles; publishes an annual report on the status of the national obesity problem.

http://www.rwjf.org

*Shape America.* A professional organization dedicated to promoting quality health and physical education programs.

https://www.shapeamerica.org

*StrongFirst.* A school of strength, directed by kettlebell master Pavel Tsatsouline, teaches people how to reach high levels of strength and fitness without interfering with work, school, family, or sport. The program offers clinics and web-based information.

http://www.strongfirst.com

## SELECTED BIBLIOGRAPHY


American College of Sports Medicine. 2019. *ACSM's Complete Guide to Fitness & Health.* Champaign, IL: Human Kinetics.

American College of Sports Medicine. 2019. *ACSM's Health/Fitness Facility Standards and Guidelines,* 5th ed. Champaign, IL: Human Kinetics.

American College of Sports Medicine. 2022. *ACSM's Guidelines for Exercise Testing and Prescription,* 11th ed. Philadelphia: Wolters Kluwer.

Ballin, M., et al. 2020. Cardiovascular disease and all-cause mortality in male twins with discordant cardiorespiratory fitness: A nationwide cohort study. *American Journal of Epidemiology.* 189(10): 1114–1123.

Bangsbo, J., et al. 2019. Copenhagen consensus statement 2019: Physical activity and ageing. *British Journal of Sports Medicine.* 53: 856–858.

Bonet, J. B., et al. 2020. Inter-individual different responses to continuous and interval training in recreational middle-aged women runners. *Frontiers in Physiology* 11: 579835.

Brooks, G. A., et al. 2020. *Exercise Physiology: Human Bioenergetics and Its Applications,* 5th ed. New York: Amazon.

Burtscher, J., et al. 2019. The upper limit of cardiorespiratory fitness associated with longevity: An update. *AIMS Public Health* 6(3): 225–228.

Callahan M. J., et al. 2021. Can high-intensity interval training promote skeletal muscle anabolism? *Sports Medicine.* 51(3): 405–421.

Centers for Disease Control and Prevention. 2019. *2018 National Health Interview Survey.* National Center for Health Statistics (https://www.cdc.gov/nchs/nhis/releases/released201905.htm#7A).

Centers for Disease Control and Prevention. 2021. *Physical Activity Basics* (http://www.cdc.gov/physicalactivity/basics).

Da Silva, M. A. R., et al. 2020. The effects of concurrent training combining both resistance exercise and high-intensity interval training or moderate-intensity continuous training on metabolic syndrome. *Frontiers in Physiology* 11: 572.

Dietary Guidelines Advisory Committee. 2020. *Scientific Report of the 2020 Dietary Advisory Committee.* Washington, DC: U.S. Department of Agriculture, Agricultural Research Service.

Ekblom-Bak, E., et al. 2021. Cardiorespiratory fitness and lifestyle on severe COVID-19 risk in 279,455 adults: A case control study. *International Journal of Behavioral Nutrition and Physical Activity.* 18:135.

Fahey, T. D., and F. I. Katch. 2021. *Anabolic Steroids Demystified. Chico,* CA: Fortius Press.

Fahey, T. D., et al. 2022. *Fit & Well: Core Concepts and Labs in Physical Fitness and Wellness,* 15th ed. New York: McGraw Hill.

Gaesser, G., and S. Blair. 2019. The health risks of obesity have been exaggerated. *Medicine & Science in Sports & Exercise.* 51(1): 218–221.

Gibala, M. J. 2021. Physiological basis of interval training for performance enhancement. *Experimental Physiology.* 106(12): 2324–2327.

Hall, K. D. 2021. Energy compensation and metabolic adaptation: "The Biggest Loser" study reinterpreted. *Obesity* (Silver Spring) 30(1): 11–13.

International Health, Racquet & Sportsclub Association. 2019. Latest IHRSA Data: Over 6B Visits to 39,570 Gyms in 2018. (https://www.ihrsa.org/about/media-center/press-releases/latest-ihrsa-data-over-6b-visits-to-39-570-gyms-in-2018/)

Kerns J. C., et al. 2017. Increased physical activity associated with less weight regain six years after "the biggest loser" competition. *Obesity* (Silver Spring). 25(11): 1838-1843.

Kim, Y., et al. 2018. The combination of cardiorespiratory fitness and muscle strength, and mortality risk. *European Journal of Epidemiology* 33(10): 953-964.

King, A.C., K. E. Powell, and W. E. Kraus. 2019. The U.S. Physical Activities Guidelines Advisory Committee report–introduction. *Medicine & Science in Sports & Exercise* 51(6): 1203-1205.

Lavie, C. J., et al. 2019. Sedentary behavior, exercise, and cardiovascular health. *Circulation Research* 124(5): 799-815.

Loprinzi, P. D., E. Frith, and M. K. Edwards. 2018. Resistance exercise and episodic memory function: A systematic review. *Clinical Physiology Functional Imaging* DOI: 10.1111/cpf.12507.

Maughan, R. J., et al. 2016. A randomized trial to assess the potential of different beverages to affect hydration status: Development of a beverage hydration index. *American Journal of Clinical Nutrition* 103: 717-723.

McGill, S. M., et al. 2012. Kettlebell swing, snatch, and bottoms-up carry: Back and hip muscle activation, motion, and low back loads. *Journal of Strength & Conditioning Research* 26: 16-27.

McGill, S. M., et al. 2013. Low back loads while walking and carrying: Comparing the load carried in one hand or in both hands. *Ergonomics* 56(2): 293-302.

Moore, S. C., et al. 2016. Association of leisure-time physical activity with risk of 26 types of cancer in 1.44 million adults. *JAMA Internal Medicine*. DOI: 10.1001/jamainternmed.2016.1548.

Muntaner-Mas, A., et al. 2019. A systematic review of fitness apps and their potential clinical and sports utility for objective and remote assessment of cardiorespiratory fitness. *Sports Medicine* 49(4): 587-600.

O'Donovan, G., et al. 2017. Association of "weekend warrior" and other leisure-time physical activity patterns with risks for all-cause, cardiovascular disease, and cancer mortality. *JAMA Internal Medicine* 177(3): 335-342.

Pedersen, B. K. 2019. Which type of exercise keeps you young? *Current Opinion in Clinical Nutrition & Metabolic Care*. 22(2): 167-173.

Physical Activity Guidelines Advisory Committee. 2008. *Physical Activity Guidelines Advisory Committee Report, 2008*. Washington, DC: U.S. Department of Health and Human Services.

Poon, E. T., et al. 2021. Interval training versus moderate-intensity continuous training for cardiorespiratory fitness improvements in middle-aged and older adults: A systematic review and meta-analysis. *Journal of Sports Sciences*. 39(17): 1996-2005.

Ramakrishnan, R., et al. 2021. Objectively measured physical activity and all-cause mortality: A systematic review and meta-analysis, *Preventive Medicine* 143: 106356.

Rivera-Torres, S., et al. 2019. Adherence to exercise programs in older adults: Informative report. *Gerontology and Geriatric Medicine* 5:1-10.

Ross, R.E., et al. 2019. High-intensity aerobic exercise acutely increases brain-derived neurotrophic factor. *Medicine & Science in Sports & Exercise* 51(8): 1698-1709.

Sant'Ana, L. O., et al. 2020. Effects of cardiovascular interval training in healthy elderly subjects: A systematic review. *Frontiers of Physiology* 11: 739.

Shiroma, E. J., et al. 2017. Strength training and the risk of type 2 diabetes and cardiovascular disease. *Medicine & Science in Sports & Exercise* 49(1): 40-46.

Song, J., et al. 2017. Do inactive older adults who increase physical activity experience less disability: Evidence from the osteoarthritis initiative. *Journal of Clinical Rheumatology* 23(1): 26-32.

Tarp, J., et al. 2021. Fitness, fatness, and mortality in men and women from the UK Biobank: Prospective Cohort Study. *Journal of the American Heart Association*. 10(6): e019605.

Thompson, W. R. 2020. Worldwide survey of fitness: Trends for 2020. *ACSM's Health & Fitness Journal* 20(6): 8-17.

U.S. Department of Health and Human Services. 2020. *Healthy People 2020*. Washington, DC: U.S. Department of Health and Human Services (http://www.healthypeople.gov).

U.S. Department of Health and Human Services. 2018. *Physical Activity Guidelines for Americans*, 2nd ed. Washington, DC: U.S. Department of Health and Human Services.

Viana, R. B., et al. 2019. Is interval training the magic bullet for fat loss? A systematic review and meta-analysis comparing moderate-intensity continuous training with high-intensity interval training (HIIT). *British Journal of Sports Medicine* 53(10): 655-664.

Zaccardi, F., et al. 2019. Comparative relevance of physical fitness and adiposity on life expectancy: A UK Biobank observational study. *Mayo Clinics Proceedings* 94(6): 985-994.

**Design Elements:** Assess Yourself icon: Aleksey Boldin/Alamy Stock Photo; Diversity Matters icon: Rawpixel Ltd/Getty Images; Wellness on Campus icon: Radius Images/Alamy Stock Photo; Take Charge icon: VisualCommunications/Getty Images; Critical Consumer icon: pagadesign/Getty Images.

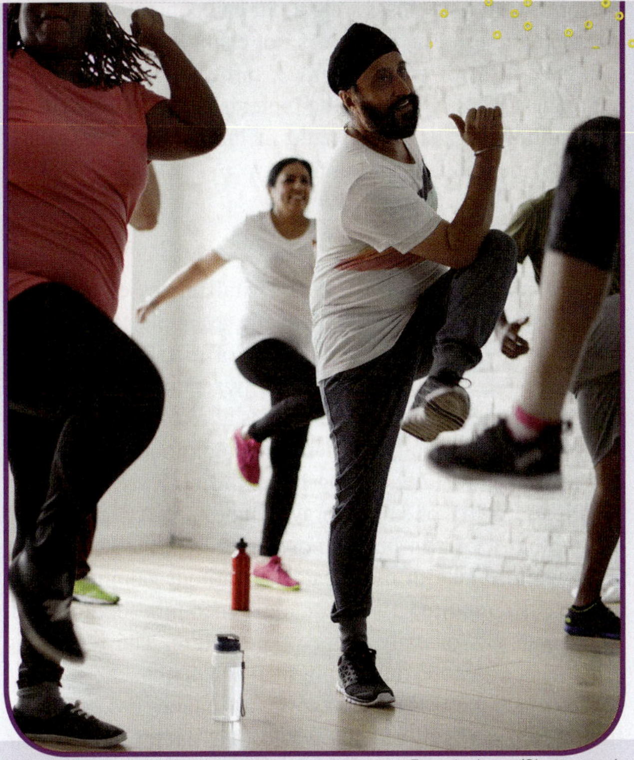
Rawpixel.com/Shutterstock

## CHAPTER OBJECTIVES

- Explain factors that influence weight and body composition
- Discuss methods for assessing body weight and body composition
- Explain the effects of too much or too little body fat on wellness
- Explain the relationship between body image and eating disorders and the associated health risks
- Describe lifestyle factors associated with successful weight management
- Name and describe approaches to overcoming weight challenges

CHAPTER 12

# Weight Management

Social pressure to achieve a given body shape or size can contribute to unhealthy thought patterns around weight. Although dietary and physical activity choices fall primarily within our control, many other genetic and environmental factors contribute to weight that we cannot change. Therefore, a first goal should be to value and appreciate our bodies no matter their size and shape, so that we are motivated to keep them as healthy as possible.

At the same time, achieving and maintaining a healthy body weight is a public health priority and a challenge for many Americans. According to standards developed by the National Institutes of Health (NIH), the prevalence of obesity among Americans is over 42% in adults (Figure 12.1). Of children ages 2-11 years, 13-20% have obesity, and among adolescents ages 12-19 years, about 21% have obesity.

## FACTORS THAT INFLUENCE WEIGHT

As individuals, we make many choices every day that affect weight management—what we eat, what physical activity we engage in, and how much sleep we get. But those individual choices and their impacts are influenced by many other forces, both inside and outside our bodies. Our weight, shape, and body composition depend on multiple genetic, metabolic, hormonal, psychological, cultural, and socioeconomic factors. Many of these influences are beyond our control, but we can make choices that significantly affect our health.

### Genetic Factors

Genes influence body size and shape, body fat distribution, and metabolic rate. Since the 1990s scientists have identified

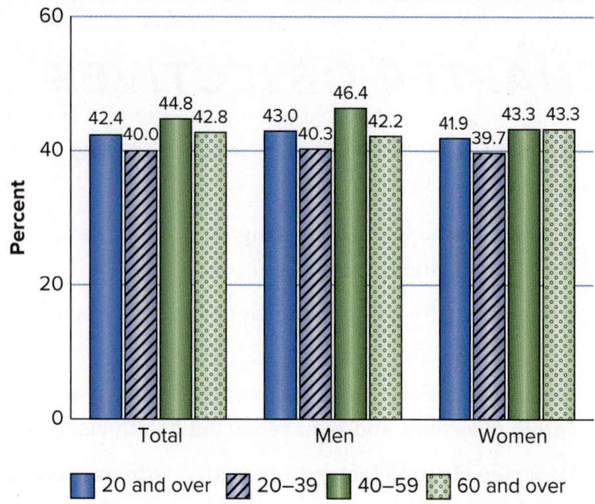


**FIGURE 12.1 Prevalence of obesity and severe obesity among adults: United States, 2017–2018.**

SOURCE: Hales, C. M., et al. 2020. Prevalence of obesity and severe obesity among adults: United States, 2017–2018. *NCHS Data Brief* 360. Hyattsville, MD: National Center for Health Statistics.

over 1100 independent genes and genetic markers that influence our weight, and they can place certain people at a higher risk of developing obesity. These genetic markers explain about 6% of the variation in weight and body mass index (BMI) among individuals.

The *set-point theory* suggests that our bodies are designed to maintain a healthy and generally stable weight within a narrow range, or at a "set point," despite the variability in energy intake and expenditure. This theory is based on the idea that the rate at which our body burns calories adjusts according to the amount of food that we eat. Can we change our set point? It appears that when we maintain changes in our activity level and in our diets over a long period of time, our set point does change. Therefore, the set-point theory does not imply that we cannot maintain weight loss, but it can help us understand why weight loss is often difficult.

## Fat Cells

The amount of fat (adipose tissue) the body stores is a function of the number and size of fat (adipose) cells, which is influenced by both genetic and lifestyle factors. Some people are born with an above-average number of fat cells and thus have the potential for storing more energy as body fat. Additionally, most people gain new fat cells during childhood and early adolescence. However, it is the size of fat cells that changes during periods of weight gain or weight loss. If a person with obesity loses weight, fat cell content is depleted, but the number of fat cells does not change. Fat tissue is not a passive form of energy storage; rather, fat cells send out chemical signals in order to be replenished. These signals affect multiple organs and systems, including those controlling appetite, metabolism, and immunity.

TERMS

**resting metabolic rate (RMR)** The energy required (in calories) to maintain vital body functions while the body is at rest, including respiration, heart rate, body temperature, and blood pressure.

**energy balance** A condition that occurs when energy intake equals energy expenditure; the key to achieving and maintaining a healthy body weight.

## Metabolism

Metabolism is the sum of all the vital processes by which food energy and nutrients are made available to and used by the body. The largest component of metabolism, **resting metabolic rate (RMR),** is the energy required to maintain vital body functions while the body is at rest, including respiration, heart rate, body temperature, and blood pressure. As shown in Figure 12.2, resting metabolism (RMR) accounts for about 65–70% of daily energy expenditure. A higher RMR means that a person burns more calories while at rest and can therefore take in more calories without gaining weight. The energy required to digest food accounts for up to an additional 10% of daily energy expenditure. The remaining 20–30% is expended during physical activity.

Together, these three categories of energy use represent the "energy out" side of what is known as **energy balance,** the relationship between the energy taken into the body through food and drink ("energy in") and the energy expended. Research suggests that it is more difficult to successfully maintain energy balance, and stable body weight, in our modern environment than it was in the past. Some people inherit a higher or lower RMR than others; RMR may vary by as much as 25% among same-weight individuals. The primary determinant of RMR is the amount of muscle a person has. Men, who tend to have a higher proportion of muscle mass than women, generally have a higher RMR. This is because muscle tissue is more metabolically active than fat, requiring more energy to support its activities.

A number of factors reduce metabolic rate, making weight management challenging. Low-calorie intake and weight loss reduce RMR. When energy intake declines and weight is lost, the body responds by trying to conserve energy, reducing both RMR and the energy required to perform physical tasks.

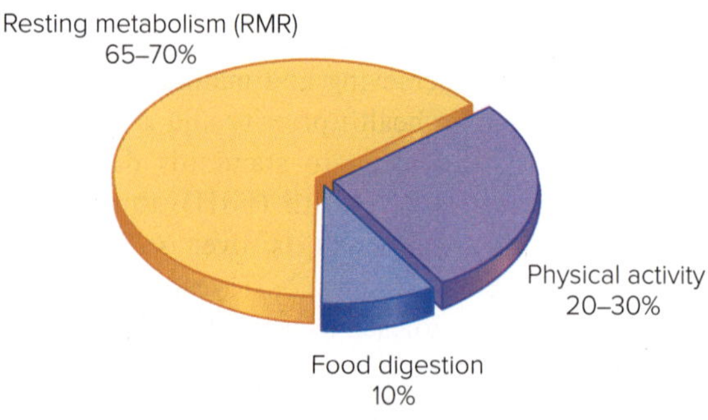


**FIGURE 12.2 Where does food energy go?** Energy in food you consume is expended through resting metabolism (maintaining vital body functions while at rest), physical activity, and digestion. Resting metabolism is the largest component of the "energy out" side of energy balance.

In essence, the body "defends" the original starting weight. Consider two people of the same size and activity level who both currently weigh 150 pounds, but one of whom used to weigh 170 pounds; the individual who lost weight will need to consume fewer calories to maintain the 150-pound weight than the person who had always been at that weight. This physiological response of the body points to the importance of preventing significant weight fluctuations in adulthood.

Exercise can have a modest positive effect on RMR: It temporarily raises RMR, and resistance training can increase muscle mass, which in turn boosts metabolism. In one study, a regular resistance training program increased RMR by an average of 5% in healthy adults. While relatively small, this degree of increase in RMR can still be helpful over the long term in maintaining a healthy weight. Resistance training may also protect against age-related declines in RMR.

## Hormones

Hormones play a role in the accumulation of body fat, especially for women. Hormonal changes at puberty, during pregnancy, and at menopause contribute to the amount and location of fat accumulation. For example, during puberty, hormones cause the development of secondary sex characteristics such as larger breasts, wider hips, and added fat under the skin. This addition of body fat at puberty is normal and healthy.

**QUICK STATS**

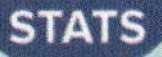

**Only 23% of U.S. adults meet the guidelines for both aerobic and muscle-strengthening activity.**

—Centers for Disease Control and Prevention, 2021

In addition to insulin, two other hormones thought to be linked to obesity are leptin and ghrelin. Secreted by the body's fat cells, leptin is carried to the brain, where it appears to let the brain know how big or small the body's fat stores are. With this information, the brain can regulate appetite and metabolic rate accordingly, decreasing appetite to prevent over-accumulation of fat. Leptin levels are higher in people who are obese, but obesity may cause the body to be less responsive to leptin's signals, a phenomenon known as leptin resistance. Low-calorie diets may reduce leptin and cause an increase in appetite.

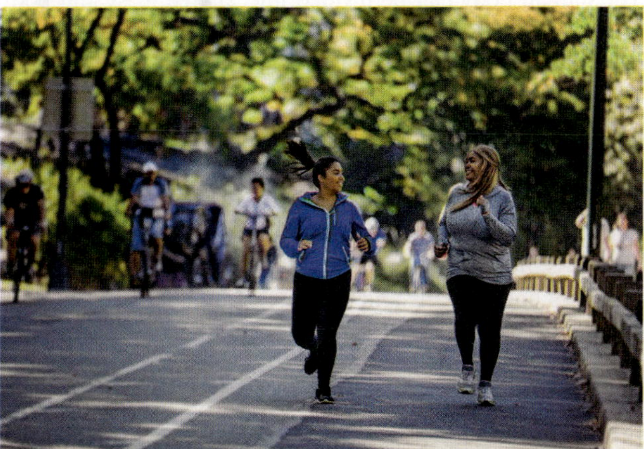

Regular physical activity is a key lifestyle strategy for weight loss and maintenance. LeoPatrizi/E+/Getty Images

The hormone ghrelin, released by the stomach, is responsible for increasing appetite. Ghrelin levels are high when a person is hungry. Once hunger is satisfied, ghrelin levels go down and typically stay low for approximately three hours after a meal. Adequate sleep and a diet high in whole grains and protein tend to promote lower ghrelin levels.

In recent years, research has focused on ways to recover sensitivity to leptin, based on the theory that leptin resistance is precipitated by problems with leptin transport across the blood-brain barrier.

## Gut Microbiota

The human intestine houses millions of bacteria that form the intestinal flora (gut flora). These bacteria help digest the foods you eat, and they produce some vitamins, such as vitamin K. Studies show that lean people differ from overweight people in the composition of their intestinal flora, suggesting that intestinal flora may be involved in the development of obesity. Diets high in processed foods have been linked to less diverse intestinal microbiota. Such diets have also been linked to a higher proportion of bacteria types associated with increased energy absorption and hormonal changes that increase appetite—both factors that can contribute to obesity.

## Sleep

Short sleep duration and sleep debt are associated with increased BMI and abdominal obesity, and researchers are still investigating how they might be linked. One possibility is that lack of sleep may affect hormone levels, appetite regulation, and metabolism. In a recent review article, studies showed that inadequate sleep was associated with inflammation, elevated levels of ghrelin, reduced levels of leptin, and impaired insulin sensitivity. Short sleep duration is also associated with increased snacking and overall energy intake. Another factor is that use of multimedia devices may contribute to sleep deprivation and increase both energy intake and sedentary time. Getting adequate sleep is critical for overall wellness.

### Ask Yourself

**QUESTIONS FOR CRITICAL THINKING AND REFLECTION**

Does anyone in your family struggle with their weight? If so, can you identify factors that may contribute to their weight challenges, such as heredity, eating patterns, or psychosocial factors? Has the person tried to address these challenges? How is the situation handled in your family? Do family members help the situation or make it worse?

## Food Marketing and Public Policy

The environment in which many Americans live and work can be "obesogenic"—meaning it encourages overconsumption of calories and discourages physical activity. This combination promotes weight gain rather than weight maintenance or loss. Food marketing and pricing, food production and distribution systems, and national agricultural policies all impact individual food choices.

The food industry promotes the sale of high-calorie processed foods at every turn. For example, vending machines offer mainly chocolate bars and unhealthy snacks, airlines offer complimentary soft drinks, and restaurants provide all-you-can-eat fried food buffets. Children are especially vulnerable to marketing that pushes ultra-processed foods high in sugar, salt, fat, and additives. Because they have a stronger preference for sweets than adults do, children are targeted from a young age and encouraged to make unhealthy choices.

Many experts observe that U.S. agricultural policy encourages farmers to produce corn and its by-product, high fructose corn syrup, at the expense of fruits and vegetables. As a result, over the past 30 years, the price of fruits and vegetables has risen much faster than the prices of other consumer goods, while the price of sugar, sweets, and carbonated drinks have declined. Issues of price and availability of healthy food can have a profound effect on food choices. Low-income neighborhoods often have only fast-food venues offering high-calorie, highly processed foods.

Public policies can also have a positive influence. For example, the Nutrition Facts label was updated to make it easier to understand the amount of calories and added sugars in a given food product. Food manufacturers were required to comply with the new label updates beginning January 1, 2020. Similarly, regulations requiring chain restaurants and vending machine operators to post calorie information should help consumers make more informed choices.

Rather than leaving all discussion to policymakers, public health experts are encouraging people to mobilize grassroots campaigns against the way food is currently distributed and marketed.

## Food Perceptions and Behaviors

Much of our behavior is acquired—that is, learned. Some cultural norms dictate eating meat-based protein with every meal; other norms prescribe almost no meat ever. Some of us learn that breakfast is the most important meal. Others wait to sit down only at noon or in the evening.

**TERMS**

**binge eating** A pattern of eating in which normal food consumption is interrupted by episodes of high consumption.

**essential fat** Fat incorporated in various tissues of the body; critical for normal body functioning.

**adipose tissue** Connective tissue in which fat is stored.

**subcutaneous fat** Fat located under the skin.

Food is an integral part of social gatherings and celebrations, and this can make eating patterns difficult to change. Eating can also provide a powerful distraction from difficult feelings—loneliness, anger, boredom, anxiety, shame, sadness, or inadequacy. It can be used to combat low moods, low energy levels, and low self-esteem. When eating becomes the primary means of regulating emotions, **binge eating** or other unhealthy eating patterns can develop.

As the world grows smaller through easier travel and wider internet distribution, an imposing set of norms and body ideals spreads to communities and individuals. Social pressures to get thin can seem omnipresent, but certain groups, such as upper-income women, may develop even more expectations to achieve this ideal. All the while, the food industry pushes highly processed foods, even into products sold for babies. Adding sugars and salt to baby and children's foods promotes a preference for these tastes early in life. If the prevalence of obesity goes down as family income level goes up, this disparity may reflect greater access to healthful, unprocessed foods, to more education about nutrition, and to more physical activity among upper-income women.

Biocultural perspectives—ideas that combine biological with social explanations—can intervene in arguments that people develop overweight because they have low incomes, are sedentary, or live in urban areas. As the chapter examines the health consequences of overweight and obesity, keep in mind how cultural politics get tangled up with claims coming from medical research. Discrimination comes in many forms.

# EVALUATING BODY WEIGHT AND BODY COMPOSITION

There are different methods for measuring and evaluating the health risks associated with body weight and body composition. First, let's look at the concept of body composition in more detail.

## Body Composition

The human body can be divided into fat-free mass and body fat. Fat-free mass is composed of all the body's nonfat tissues: bone, water, muscle, connective tissue, organ tissues, and teeth. Body composition measures how much of a person's total weight is composed of body fat and how much is fat-free mass.

A certain amount of body fat is necessary for the body to function. Fat is incorporated into the nerves, brain, heart, lungs, liver, mammary glands, and other body organs and tissues. It is the main source of stored energy in the body. It also cushions body organs and helps regulate body temperature. This minimum **essential fat** makes up about 3–5% of total body weight in men and about 8–12% in women. The percentage is higher in women due to such factors as fat deposits in the breasts and uterus.

Most of the fat in the body is stored in fat cells, or **adipose tissue,** located under the skin (**subcutaneous fat**) and around

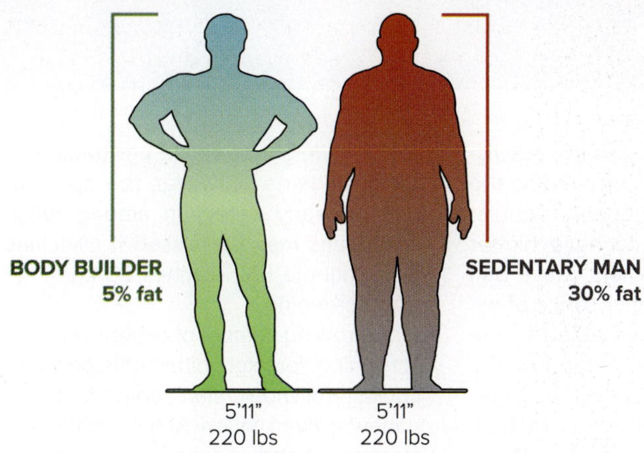


**FIGURE 12.3 Two people with the same height and weight but different percent body fat.**

major organs (**visceral fat** or *intra-abdominal fat*). People have a genetically determined number of fat cells, but these cells can increase or decrease in size depending on how much fat is being stored. The amount of stored fat depends on several factors, including age, sex, metabolism, diet, and activity level. Stored body fat comes from calories consumed in excess of calories expended in metabolism, physical activity, and exercise. These factors are discussed in detail in the next section.

When looking at body composition, one important consideration is the proportion of the body's total weight that is fat—the **percent body fat.** For example, two people of the same height and weight can differ widely in percent body fat (see Figure 12.3), and as a result, can have very different risk levels for chronic disease. Assessment methods based on body weight alone are less accurate than those based on body fat because they do not take body composition into account.

## Defining Healthy Weight, Overweight, and Obesity

Many people struggle with body dissatisfaction and are concerned about their weight, but weight alone has significant limitations as a marker of health. Body composition and lifestyle are much more important determinants of disease risk. Still, large-scale studies have determined weight ranges consistent with higher chronic disease risk on a population level.

**Overweight** is defined as total body weight above the recommended range for good health, whereas **obesity** is a more serious degree of overweight that carries multiple health risks, including a shorter life span. Both terms are used to identify weight ranges that are associated with increased likelihood of certain health problems (see Table 12.1).

**TERMS**

**visceral fat** Fat located around major organs; also called *intra-abdominal fat.*

**percent body fat** The percentage of total body weight that is composed of fat.

**overweight** Body weight above the recommended range for good health.

**obesity** Severe overweight, characterized by an excessive accumulation of body fat; may also be defined in terms of some measure of total body weight.

**VITAL STATISTICS**

**Table 12.1** Body Mass Index (BMI) Classification and Disease Risk

| | | | DISEASE RISK RELATIVE TO NORMAL WEIGHT AND WAIST CIRCUMFERENCE[a] | |
|---|---|---|---|---|
| CLASSIFICATION | BMI ($KG/M^2$) | OBESITY CLASS | MEN ≤ 40 IN. (102 CM) WOMEN ≤ 35 IN. (88 CM) | >40 IN. (102 CM) >35 IN. (88 CM) |
| Underweight[b] | <18.5 | | – | – |
| Normal[c] | 18.5–24.9 | | – | – |
| Overweight | 25.0–29.9 | | Increased | High |
| Obese | 30.0–34.9 | I | High | Very high |
| | 35.0–39.9 | II | Very high | Very high |
| Extreme obesity | ≥40.0 | III | Extremely high | Extremely high |

[a]Disease risk for type 2 diabetes, hypertension, and cardiovascular disease. The waist circumference cutoff points for increased risk are 40 inches (102 cm) for men and 35 inches (88 cm) for women.

[b]Research suggests that a low BMI can be healthy in some cases, as long as it is not the result of smoking, an eating disorder, or an underlying disease process. A BMI of 17.5 or less is sometimes used as a diagnostic criterion for the eating disorder anorexia nervosa.

[c]Increased waist circumference can also be a marker for increased risk, even in people of normal weight.

SOURCES: Adapted from National Heart, Lung, and Blood Institute. n.d. *Aim for a Healthy Weight: Classification of Overweight and Obesity by BMI, Waist Circumference, and Associated Disease Risks* (https://www.nhlbi.nih.gov/health/educational/lose_wt/BMI/bmi_dis.htm); U.S. Department of Health and Human Services, Centers for Disease Control and Prevention. 2021. *About BMI for Adults* (http://www.cdc.gov/healthyweight/assessing/bmi/adult_bmi/index.html#Athlete); National Heart, Lung, and Blood Institute. *Assessing Your Weight and Health Risk* (http://www.nhlbi.nih.gov/health/public/heart/obesity/lose_wt/risk.htm).

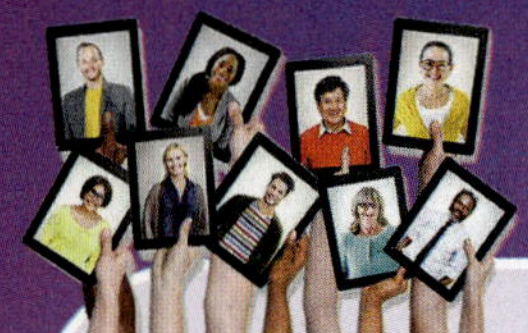

## DIVERSITY MATTERS
## Is BMI Biased?

Body mass index (BMI) is widely used to define weight status and assess health risk. However, the validity of this tool across races and ethnicities has recently been questioned. Developed in 1832 by Belgian mathematician Adolphe Quetelet, it was not originally intended as a health assessment metric, but as a parameter to define the size of an "average man." Thus the data for "Quetelet's Index" (which later became known as body mass index) came primarily from studies of white, European men. For this reason, BMI may be an inaccurate weight status indicator for people not of European descent.

A large study of over 40,000 adults in the United States found this to be the case: Traditional BMI standards classified nearly 50% as overweight and nearly 30% as obese. But based on markers such as blood pressure, triglycerides, cholesterol, and blood glucose, they classified as metabolically healthy. Conversely, over 30% of people classified as having "normal" weight status were not metabolically healthy.

Using the standard BMI categories, Black women are particularly likely to be misclassified as "overweight" or "obese." People of African descent tend to have more muscle mass and less visceral fat (abdominal fat surrounding the vital organs) than European populations. They also tend to have higher bone density. These factors cause BMI to be higher, even in the absence of excess body fat. This is reflected in the fact that 82% of Black women in the United States are classified as overweight or obese, compared to only 63% of white women. As a result, Black women may be subject to unfair stigmatization and pressure to lose weight, even when weight loss may be unnecessary from a health-risk standpoint. In fact, risk for chronic disease (i.e., cardiovascular disease and diabetes) statistically increases at a BMI of 33 kg/m$^2$ in Black women, compared to a BMI of 30 kg/m$^2$ in white women. Thus, the BMI threshold of 30 kg/m$^2$ to define obesity may be inappropriate for Black women.

For other populations, BMI may catch disease risk too late. Americans of Asian descent, for instance, are twice as likely as Euro-Americans to have an elevated risk for cardiometabolic disease when BMI is within the "normal" range. Health organizations have historically recommended screening for cardiovascular disease and diabetes in patients who are overweight or obese per traditional BMI standards. However, the opportunity for early detection among Asian Americans may be missed if clinicians wait until the BMI reaches 25 kg/m$^2$ to start screening.

A growing number of experts feel that screening for high blood glucose and cholesterol should start sooner for these patients, even when BMI is within the standard "healthy" range. The American Diabetes Association has responded by revising its diabetes screening guidelines for Asian Americans to recommend that screening begin at a BMI of 23 kg/m$^2$ instead of 25 kg/m$^2$. In summary, BMI is often the first marker that clinicians consider in evaluating health status. Data show that BMI is a relatively poor proxy for health, and it often misclassifies health risk in people who are not of European descent.

SOURCES: Dodgen, L., and E. Spence-Almaguer. 2017. Beyond Body Mass Index: Are weight-loss programs the best way to improve the health of African American women? *Preventing Chronic Disease* 14: 160573; Tomiyama, A., et al. 2016. Misclassification of cardiometabolic health when using body mass index categories in NHANES 2005–2012. *International Journal of Obesity* 40:883–886.

Several methods can be used to measure and evaluate body weight and percent body fat. They can help you establish reasonable goals and set a starting point for current and future decisions about weight loss and weight gain.

## Body Mass Index

**Body mass index (BMI)** is a measure of body weight that is often used to estimate weight status and classify the health risks of body weight. Although useful for examining aggregate data on a population level, particularly in populations of European descent, there are limitations when using BMI to evaluate weight and disease risk of an individual. (See the box "Is BMI Biased?")

> **TERMS**
>
> **body mass index (BMI)** A measure of relative body weight that takes height into account and is highly correlated with more direct measures of body fat; calculated by dividing total body weight (in kilograms) by the square of height (in meters).

### Calculating Your BMI

BMI is calculated by dividing your body weight (expressed in kilograms or pounds) by the square of your height (expressed in meters or inches). You can look up your BMI in the chart in Figure 12.4, or you can use the following formula to calculate it more precisely:

$$\text{BMI} = \frac{\text{weight in kg}}{(\text{height in meters})^2}$$

$$\textit{or} \quad \frac{\text{weight in pounds}}{(\text{height in inches})^2} \times 703 \text{ (conversion factor)}$$

Body weight status is categorized as underweight, healthy weight, overweight, or obese, compared with what is considered healthy for a given height. Under standards issued by the National Institutes of Health and adopted by the Dietary Guidelines for Americans, a BMI between 18.5 and 24.9 is considered healthy, a BMI of 25 or above is classified as overweight, and a BMI of 30 or above is classified as obese. A person with a BMI below 18.5 is classified as underweight. Because BMI only considers weight and height, and because

| | <18.5 Underweight | | 18.5–24.9 Normal | | | | | | 25–29.9 Overweight | | | | | 30–34.9 Obesity (Class I) | | | | | 35–39.9 Obesity (Class II) | | | | | ≥40 Extreme obesity |
|---|---|---|---|---|---|---|---|---|---|---|---|---|---|---|---|---|---|---|---|---|---|---|---|---|
| BMI | 17 | 18 | 19 | 20 | 21 | 22 | 23 | 24 | 25 | 26 | 27 | 28 | 29 | 30 | 31 | 32 | 33 | 34 | 35 | 36 | 37 | 38 | 39 | 40 |
| Height | Body Weight (pounds) | | | | | | | | | | | | | | | | | | | | | | | |
| 4' 10" | 81 | 86 | 91 | 96 | 101 | 105 | 110 | 115 | 120 | 124 | 129 | 134 | 139 | 144 | 148 | 153 | 158 | 163 | 168 | 172 | 177 | 182 | 187 | 192 |
| 4' 11" | 84 | 89 | 94 | 99 | 104 | 109 | 114 | 119 | 124 | 129 | 134 | 139 | 144 | 149 | 154 | 159 | 163 | 168 | 173 | 178 | 183 | 188 | 193 | 198 |
| 5' | 87 | 92 | 97 | 102 | 108 | 113 | 118 | 123 | 128 | 133 | 138 | 143 | 149 | 154 | 159 | 164 | 169 | 174 | 179 | 184 | 190 | 195 | 200 | 205 |
| 5' 1" | 90 | 95 | 101 | 106 | 111 | 117 | 122 | 127 | 132 | 138 | 143 | 148 | 154 | 159 | 164 | 169 | 175 | 180 | 185 | 191 | 196 | 201 | 207 | 212 |
| 5' 2" | 93 | 98 | 104 | 109 | 115 | 120 | 126 | 131 | 137 | 142 | 148 | 153 | 159 | 164 | 170 | 175 | 181 | 186 | 191 | 197 | 202 | 208 | 213 | 219 |
| 5' 3" | 96 | 102 | 107 | 113 | 119 | 124 | 130 | 136 | 141 | 147 | 153 | 158 | 164 | 169 | 175 | 181 | 186 | 192 | 198 | 203 | 209 | 215 | 220 | 226 |
| 5' 4" | 99 | 105 | 111 | 117 | 122 | 128 | 134 | 140 | 146 | 152 | 157 | 163 | 169 | 175 | 181 | 187 | 192 | 198 | 204 | 210 | 216 | 222 | 227 | 233 |
| 5' 5" | 102 | 108 | 114 | 120 | 126 | 132 | 138 | 144 | 150 | 156 | 162 | 168 | 174 | 180 | 186 | 192 | 198 | 204 | 210 | 216 | 222 | 229 | 235 | 241 |
| 5' 6" | 105 | 112 | 118 | 124 | 130 | 136 | 143 | 149 | 155 | 161 | 167 | 174 | 180 | 186 | 192 | 198 | 205 | 211 | 217 | 223 | 229 | 236 | 242 | 248 |
| 5' 7" | 109 | 115 | 121 | 128 | 134 | 141 | 147 | 153 | 160 | 166 | 173 | 179 | 185 | 192 | 198 | 204 | 211 | 217 | 224 | 230 | 236 | 243 | 249 | 256 |
| 5' 8" | 112 | 118 | 125 | 132 | 138 | 145 | 151 | 158 | 165 | 171 | 178 | 184 | 191 | 197 | 204 | 211 | 217 | 224 | 230 | 237 | 244 | 250 | 257 | 263 |
| 5' 9" | 115 | 122 | 129 | 136 | 142 | 149 | 156 | 163 | 169 | 176 | 183 | 190 | 197 | 203 | 210 | 217 | 224 | 230 | 237 | 244 | 251 | 258 | 264 | 271 |
| 5' 10" | 119 | 126 | 133 | 139 | 146 | 153 | 160 | 167 | 174 | 181 | 188 | 195 | 202 | 209 | 216 | 223 | 230 | 237 | 244 | 251 | 258 | 265 | 272 | 279 |
| 5' 11" | 122 | 129 | 136 | 143 | 151 | 158 | 165 | 172 | 179 | 187 | 194 | 201 | 208 | 215 | 222 | 230 | 237 | 244 | 251 | 258 | 265 | 273 | 280 | 287 |
| 6' | 125 | 133 | 140 | 148 | 155 | 162 | 170 | 177 | 184 | 192 | 199 | 207 | 214 | 221 | 229 | 236 | 243 | 251 | 258 | 266 | 273 | 280 | 288 | 295 |
| 6' 1" | 129 | 137 | 144 | 152 | 159 | 167 | 174 | 182 | 190 | 197 | 205 | 212 | 220 | 228 | 235 | 243 | 250 | 258 | 265 | 273 | 281 | 288 | 296 | 303 |
| 6' 2" | 132 | 140 | 148 | 156 | 164 | 171 | 179 | 187 | 195 | 203 | 210 | 218 | 226 | 234 | 242 | 249 | 257 | 265 | 273 | 281 | 288 | 296 | 304 | 312 |
| 6' 3" | 136 | 144 | 152 | 160 | 168 | 176 | 184 | 192 | 200 | 208 | 216 | 224 | 232 | 240 | 248 | 256 | 264 | 272 | 280 | 288 | 296 | 304 | 312 | 320 |
| 6' 4" | 140 | 148 | 156 | 164 | 173 | 181 | 189 | 197 | 206 | 214 | 222 | 230 | 238 | 247 | 255 | 263 | 271 | 280 | 288 | 296 | 304 | 312 | 321 | 329 |

**FIGURE 12.4 Body mass index (BMI).** To determine your BMI, find your height in the left column. Move across the appropriate row until you find the weight closest to your own. The number at the top of the column is the BMI at that height and weight.

SOURCES: U.S. Department of Health and Human Services and U.S. Department of Agriculture. 2020. *2020–2025 Dietary Guidelines for Americans*, 9th ed. (https://www.dietaryguidelines.gov/sites/default/files/2021-03/Dietary_Guidelines_for_Americans-2020–2025.pdf).

it is more useful for evaluating epidemiological trends in populations than the weight status of individuals, it is often combined with waist circumference and/or body composition to provide more accurate assessments of health status.

QUICK STATS

**In 1970, 15% of adult Americans were obese. Currently, over 40% are.**

—National Center for Health Statistics, 2021

## Estimating Body Composition

Methods for determining percent body fat provide an estimate of the amount of body fat (or adipose tissue) and the amount of fat-free mass (or lean tissue) you have (See Figure 12.5.)

A healthy body fat range for men is considered to be about 12–20%, and for women, about 20–30%. Men with more than 25% body fat are considered to have obesity, as are women with more than 33% body fat.

**Bioelectrical Impedance Analysis (BIA)** In this method, a person stands barefoot on a machine that resembles a scale, uses a handheld machine, or lies down with spot electrodes attached at various points on the body that are also connected to a bioelectrical machine. A very low level of electrical current is sent between electrodes through the body. Percent body fat is calculated from the measurements of resistance to the current. For the most accurate results, the person being tested must have followed guidelines for food and fluid intake, and restrictions on exercise. When protocols are followed precisely, BIA can estimate your body fat within a margin of error of about 3–4%.

**Skinfold Measurement** Skinfold measurement is a simple and practical way to assess body composition based on the amount of subcutaneous fat. A technician measures the thickness of skinfolds at several different sites on the body with a device, called a skinfold caliper, that painlessly "pinches" the skin and its underlying fat at specific sites on the body. The measurements are used in formulas that calculate body fat percentages. The accuracy of this method is highly dependent on the expertise of the practitioner.

**Scanning Procedures** High-tech scanning procedures are very accurate means of assessing body composition, but the costs are much higher compared to other methods. These procedures include computed tomography (CT), magnetic resonance imaging (MRI), dual-energy X-ray absorptiometry (DEXA), and dual-photon absorptiometry. Other procedures include near infrared reactance (Futrex 1100) and total body electrical conductivity (TOBEC). Considered to be very accurate, these techniques are generally offered only at medical or research facilities.

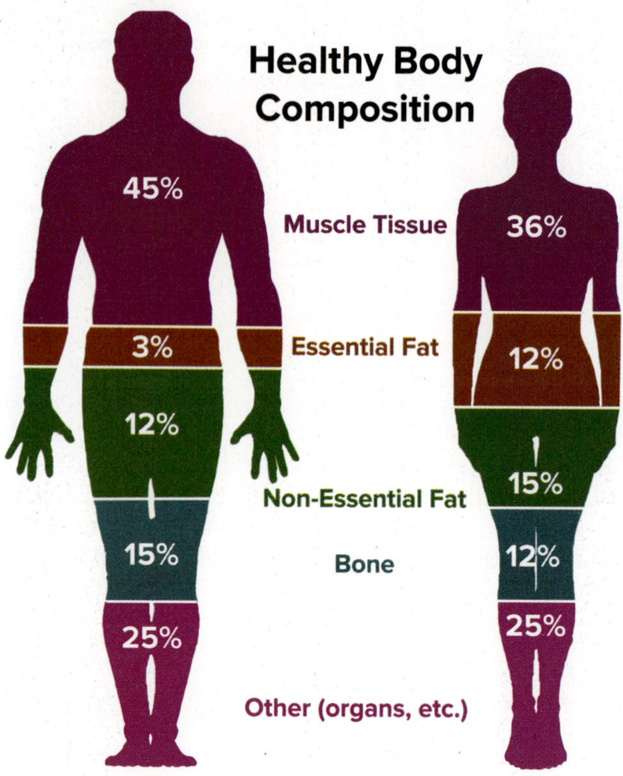


**FIGURE 12.5** **Healthy body composition.**

SOURCES: Diabetes Prevention Institute. "Body Composition."

## Body Fat Distribution

How is fat distributed throughout the body? The location of fat on your body has important implications for your health and affects your risk for various diseases.

Two of the simplest methods for measuring body fat distribution are waist circumference measurement and waist-to-hip ratio calculation. In the first method, waist circumference is measured using a tape measure placed around the abdomen at the top of the hip bone. A waist circumference of greater than 40 inches (102 cm) for men or greater than 35 in (88 cm) for women is associated with an increased risk for chronic disease for most adults. In the second method, both waist circumference and hip circumference are measured, and a mathematic formula (waist circumference divided by hip circumference) is used to find your waist-to-hip ratio (WHR). A WHR above 0.94 for young men and above 0.82 for young women is associated with an increased risk of heart disease and diabetes.

People who tend to store fat in the upper regions of their bodies, particularly in the abdominal area, are said to have an *android,* or apple-shaped, pattern of fat distribution store fat in the hips, buttocks, and thighs as subcutaneous fat are said to have a *gynoid,* or pear-shaped, pattern of fat distribution.

Abdominal obesity increases the risk of high blood pressure, diabetes, early-onset heart disease, stroke, certain types of cancer, and mortality. This risk is independent of a person's BMI.

The reason for the increased risk associated with abdominal obesity is that visceral fat is more easily mobilized and sent into the bloodstream, increasing disease-related blood fat levels. Visceral fat contains many biologically active substances such as inflammatory chemicals and growth factors, which can adhere to the lining of blood vessels, cause insulin resistance, and negatively affect cardiovascular health.

## What Is the Right Weight for You?

There are limits to the changes you can make to body weight and body shape, both of which are influenced by heredity. The changes that can and should be made are lifestyle changes, as described throughout this chapter.

To answer the question of what you should weigh, assess your health and body composition status and let your lifestyle be your guide. As described in Chapter 10, the *Dietary Guidelines for Americans 2020–2025* recommends that adults with overweight or obesity make healthful changes to their dietary habits and increase their physical activity to improve their health, prevent additional weight gain, or promote weight loss. Instead of focusing on a particular weight, focus on living a lifestyle that includes a healthy dietary pattern, getting plenty of exercise, thinking positively, and learning to cope with stress. Then let the pounds fall where they may. For some, their weight will be somewhat higher than societal standards—but right for them. By letting a healthy lifestyle determine your weight, you can avoid developing unhealthy patterns of eating and a negative body image. Later in the chapter, we'll take a closer look at lifestyle recommendations for healthy weight management.

# BODY FAT AND WELLNESS

The amount and distribution of fat in the body—both too much and too little—can have profound effects on health. Obesity doubles mortality rates and can reduce life expectancy by 10–20 years. Compared with those of healthy weight, people with obesity have an increased risk of death from all causes. Obesity is associated with a number of chronic conditions such as diabetes, CVD, many kinds of cancer, impaired immune function, gallbladder and kidney diseases, skin problems, erectile dysfunction, sleep and breathing disorders, back pain, arthritis, and other bone and joint disorders. Obesity is also associated with complications of pregnancy, menstrual irregularities, urine leakage (stress incontinence), increased surgical risk, and psychological disorders and problems (such as depression, low self-esteem, and body dissatisfaction). According to the World Health Organization, at least 2.8 million people die each year as a result of having overweight or obesity.

In addition, studies show a decrease in the quality of life (measured by such things as self-image, bullying, bodily pain, quality of food intake, physical activity, and screen time) in children and adolescents with overweight and obesity compared to those of normal weight. It is also important to realize that modest weight losses—5-10% of total body weight—can lead to significant health improvements.

There is debate over the health risks for people who have overweight but not obesity (those with a BMI of 25.0–29.9). Many researchers and clinicians argue that health risks depend far more on lifestyle than on weight, and that people who are overweight but metabolically healthy are not necessarily at increased risk of chronic disease.

## Diabetes

According to the American Diabetes Association, more than 37 million Americans have one of the two major types of **diabetes mellitus,** a disease that disrupts normal metabolism. An estimated 1.4 million Americans are diagnosed with diabetes every year, and an estimated 96 million people 18 and older are believed to have prediabetes.

People with obesity are more than three times as likely as people without obesity to develop type 2 diabetes, and the incidence of this disease among Americans has increased dramatically as the rate of obesity has climbed.

Diabetes involves a disruption in the process of metabolism. In normal metabolism, the pancreas secretes insulin, which stimulates cells to take up blood sugar (glucose) to produce energy (Figure 12.6). In diabetes, this process is disrupted, causing a buildup of glucose in the bloodstream. Diabetes is associated with kidney failure; nerve damage; circulation problems and amputations; retinal damage and blindness; and increased rates of heart attack, stroke, and hypertension. As of 2020, diabetes was the eighth leading cause of death in the United States.

**Types of Diabetes** About 1.6 million Americans have a form of diabetes known as type 1 diabetes. This is an autoimmune disease that usually begins in childhood or adolescence and is not related to obesity. In type 1 diabetes, the body's immune system, triggered by a viral infection or some other environmental factor, destroys the insulin-producing cells in the pancreas. Little or no insulin is produced, so daily doses of insulin are required. The remaining people with diabetes have type 2 diabetes, a disease that is strongly associated with excess body fat, particularly abdominal (visceral) fat. In type 2 diabetes, the pancreas doesn't produce enough insulin, or body cells are resistant to insulin (called *insulin resistance*), or both. About 25% of people with type 2 diabetes are unaware of their condition. About one-third of people with type 2 diabetes must take insulin; others may take medications that increase insulin production or stimulate the cells to take up glucose.

A third type of diabetes, called *gestational diabetes,* occurs in about 7% of women during pregnancy. The condition usually resolves after pregnancy, but about half of women who experience it eventually develop type 2 diabetes. *Prediabetes* is a condition in which blood sugar levels are higher than normal but not high enough for a diagnosis of diabetes. More than 80% of American adults with prediabetes don't even know they have it, and most will develop type 2 diabetes unless they adopt preventive lifestyle measures.

**Warning Signs and Risk Factors** In the early stages, diabetes has no symptoms; possible warning signs include: frequent urination, extreme hunger or thirst, unexplained weight loss, extreme fatigue, blurred vision, frequent infections, slow wound healing, tingling or numbness in the hands or feet, and generalized dry skin and itching with no rash.

The major risk factors for diabetes are age, obesity, physical inactivity, a family history of diabetes, and lifestyle. Race and ethnicity also play a role, with Native Americans, Alaska Natives, African Americans, and Hispanics having higher rates than Asian Americans and white Americans. Excess body fat reduces cell sensitivity to insulin, and insulin resistance is almost always a precursor of type 2 diabetes. More than 90% of people with type 2 diabetes have overweight or obesity.

Screening involves a blood test to check glucose levels after either a period of fasting or the administration of a set dose of glucose. A fasting glucose level of 126 mg/dl or higher indicates diabetes; a level of 100–125 mg/dl indicates prediabetes. If you are concerned about your risk for diabetes, talk with your physician about being tested.

It is estimated that 90% of cases of type 2 diabetes could be prevented if people adopted healthy lifestyle behaviors. For people with prediabetes, lifestyle measures are more effective than medication for delaying or preventing the development of diabetes. Regular exercise and a healthy diet are often sufficient to control type 2 diabetes. There is no cure for diabetes, but it can be successfully managed by keeping blood sugar levels within safe limits through diet, exercise, and, if necessary, medication.

## Heart Disease and Other Chronic Conditions

Obesity is one of the six major controllable risk factors for heart disease. Excess body fat is strongly associated with hypertension, unhealthy cholesterol and triglyceride levels, and impaired heart function. Many people with overweight and obesity—especially those who are sedentary and eat a poor diet—also suffer from a group of symptoms called *metabolic syndrome*. Symptoms include insulin resistance, high blood pressure, high blood glucose, unhealthy cholesterol levels, chronic inflammation, and abdominal fat. Metabolic syndrome increases the risk of heart disease, especially in men.

Obesity is also a risk factor for certain types of cancer.

**TERMS**

**diabetes mellitus** A disease that disrupts normal metabolism, interfering with cells' ability to take in glucose for energy production.

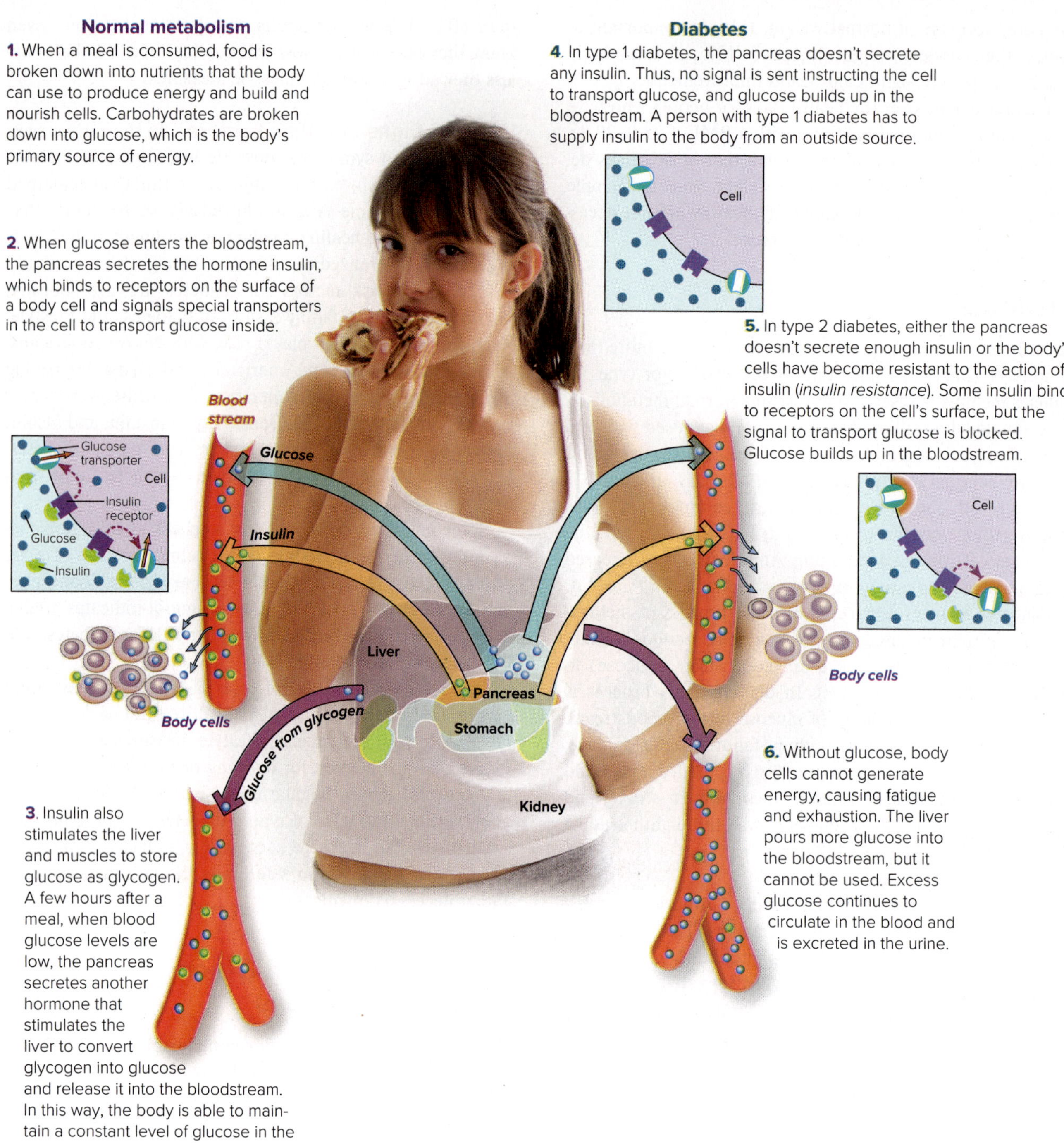


**FIGURE 12.6 Diabetes mellitus.** During digestion, carbohydrates are broken down in the small intestine into glucose, a simple sugar that enters the bloodstream. The presence of glucose signals the pancreas to release insulin, a hormone that helps cells take up glucose; once inside a cell, glucose can be converted to energy. In diabetes, this process is disrupted, resulting in a buildup of glucose in the bloodstream.
webphotographeer/iStock/Getty Images

## Problems Associated with Very Low Levels of Body Fat

Health experts have generally viewed very low levels of body fat—less than about 12% for women and 5% for men—as a threat to wellness. Extreme leanness has been linked with reproductive, circulatory, and immune system disorders. Extremely lean people may experience muscle wasting and fatigue. They are also more likely to suffer from dangerous eating disorders.

In physically active women and girls, particularly those involved in sports where weight and appearance are important (ballet, gymnastics, skating, and distance running, for example), a condition called the **female athlete triad** may develop. The triad consists of three interrelated disorders: abnormal eating patterns (and excessive exercising), followed by **amenorrhea** (absence of menstruation), followed by decreased bone density (premature osteoporosis). Prolonged amenorrhea can cause bone density to erode to a point that a woman in her twenties will have the bone density of a woman in her sixties or older. Left untreated, the triad can lead to decreased physical performance, increased incidence of bone fractures, disturbances of heart rhythm and metabolism, and even death.

## BODY IMAGE AND EATING DISORDERS

The collective picture of the body as seen through the mind's eye, **body image** consists of perceptions, images, thoughts, attitudes, and emotions. A negative body image is characterized by dissatisfaction with the body in general or some part of the body in particular. Most Americans, including those who are not overweight, are unhappy with their body weight or with some aspect of their appearance. People may be dissatisfied with their bodies for a variety of reasons, including sociocultural factors.

Losing weight does not necessarily improve body image. In fact, improvements in body image may occur in the absence of changes in weight or appearance. Developing a positive body image is an important aspect of psychological wellness and an important component of successful weight management. The Health at Every Size (HAES) movement reframes the paradigm from weight loss to disease prevention. Instead of focusing on our body shape and size, proponents of HAES encourage eating healthfully, enjoying physical activity, listening to body cues for hunger and satiety (rather than external cues like mealtimes), and fighting against fat stigma and for social justice. By not using weight changes as a marker for health, individuals may be more likely to continue in behaviors that have an independent benefit on health.

### Severe Body Image Problems

Poor body image can cause significant psychological distress. A person can become preoccupied with a perceived defect in appearance, thereby damaging self-esteem and interfering with relationships. Adolescents and adults who have a negative body image are more likely to diet restrictively, eat compulsively, or develop some other form of disordered eating.

When a person's dissatisfaction with his or her own body becomes extreme, the condition is called *body dysmorphic disorder* (*BDD*). Although many people are dissatisfied with some part of their body or their appearance, these concerns usually do not constantly occupy their thoughts. Individuals with BDD are constantly preoccupied and upset about body imperfections. They cannot seem to stop checking or obsessing about their appearance, often focusing on perceived flaws that are not obvious to others. Low self-esteem is common in people with body dysmorphia. Individuals with BDD may spend hours every day thinking about their flaws and looking at themselves in mirrors, so that their preoccupation can interrupt daily activities, such as work and socializing. Some people with BDD may seek repeated cosmetic surgeries. BDD affects about 2% of Americans, males and females in equal numbers. It usually begins before age 18 but can begin in adulthood, and it occurs in people with other mental health disorders such as major depression and anxiety.

Left untreated, BDD can lead to depression, social phobia, and thoughts of suicide. An individual with BDD needs to get professional evaluation and treatment. Medication and therapy can help people with BDD.

In some cases, body image may bear little resemblance to fact. People suffering from the eating disorder anorexia nervosa typically have a severely distorted body image—they believe themselves to be overweight even when they have become emaciated. Distorted body image is also a hallmark of *muscle dysmorphia,* a disorder experienced by some bodybuilders and other active people who see themselves as small and out of shape despite being very muscular. Those who suffer from muscle dysmorphia may let obsessive exercise—particularly muscle-building exercise—interfere with their work and relationships. They may also use steroids and other potentially dangerous muscle-building drugs.

### Eating Disorders

Problems with body weight and weight control are not limited to excessive body fat. A growing number of people, especially adolescent girls and young women, experience **eating disorders**—psychological disorders characterized by severe disturbances in body image, eating patterns, and eating-related behaviors. The main categories of eating disorders include anorexia nervosa, bulimia nervosa, binge-eating disorder, and other specified feeding or eating disorder (OSFED). During their lifetimes, one in seven males and one in five females will suffer from an eating disorder. Many more people have abnormal eating habits and attitudes about food that disrupt their lives, even though these habits do not meet the criteria for a clinically diagnosable eating disorder.

**TERMS**

**female athlete triad** A condition consisting of three interrelated disorders: abnormal eating patterns (and excessive exercising) followed by lack of menstrual periods (amenorrhea) and decreased bone density (premature osteoporosis).

**amenorrhea** The absence of menstruation.

**body image** The mental representation a person holds about their body at any given time, consisting of perceptions, images, thoughts, attitudes, and emotions about the body.

**eating disorder** A serious disturbance in eating patterns or eating-related behavior, characterized by a negative body image and concerns about body weight or body fat.

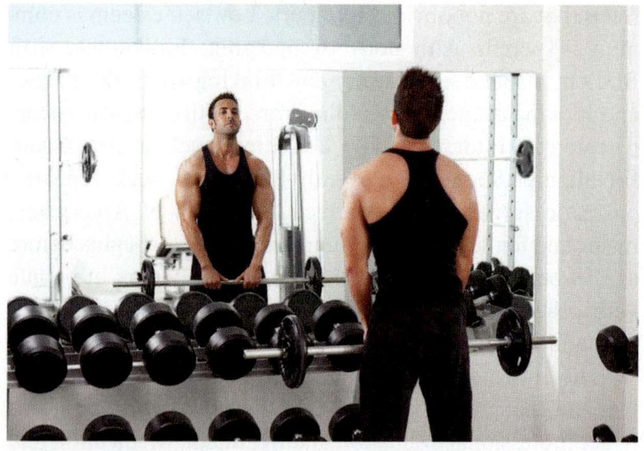

Exercise is a healthy practice, but people with muscle dysmorphia sometimes exercise compulsively, building their lives around their workouts. Compulsive exercise can lead to injuries and problems with work and relationships. Antonio Balaguer Soler/123RF

Many factors are involved in the development of an eating disorder. Heredity and how genes interact with the environment appear to play an important role in the development of eating disorders. Cultural messages, as well as family, friends, and peers, shape attitudes toward the self and others. Comparing yourself negatively with others can damage self-esteem and increase vulnerability. Young people who see themselves as lacking control over their lives are also at high risk for eating disorders. About 90% of eating disorders begin during adolescence.

Certain turning points in life, such as leaving home for college, can trigger an eating disorder. An eating disorder may become a means of coping: The abnormal eating behavior temporarily reduces anxiety and gives the person a sense of control. Restrictive dieting–whether for weight control, managing a medical condition, or other reasons–is another possible trigger for the development of eating disorders.

> **Ask Yourself**
>
> **QUESTIONS FOR CRITICAL THINKING AND REFLECTION**
>
> Describe your own body image in the fewest words possible. Do you think your self-image is in line with the way others see you? Make a list of 5 things you appreciate about your body, with a focus on what your body allows you to do and experience (opposed to what it looks like).

> **TERMS**
>
> **anorexia nervosa** An eating disorder characterized by a refusal to maintain body weight at a minimally healthy level and an intense fear of gaining weight or becoming fat; self-starvation.
>
> **purge** The use of vomiting, laxatives, excessive exercise, restrictive dieting, enemas, diuretics, or diet pills to compensate for food that has been eaten and that the person fears will produce weight gain.
>
> **bulimia nervosa** An eating disorder characterized by recurrent episodes of binge eating and purging—overeating and then using compensatory behaviors such as vomiting, laxatives, and excessive exercise to prevent weight gain.

### Anorexia Nervosa

A person with **anorexia nervosa** does not eat enough food to maintain a reasonable body weight. Up to 4% of women and 0.3% of men suffer from anorexia nervosa in their lifetimes. Anorexia typically develops during puberty and the late teenage years, with an average age of onset of about 19 years.

**CHARACTERISTICS OF ANOREXIA NERVOSA** People with anorexia nervosa have an intense fear of gaining weight or becoming fat. Their body image is so distorted that even when emaciated they think they are overweight. People with anorexia nervosa may engage in compulsive behaviors or rituals that help keep them from eating, though some may also binge and **purge.** A purge occurs when a person uses vomiting, laxatives, excessive exercise, restrictive dieting, enemas, diuretics, or diet pills to compensate for food that she or he has eaten and that the person fears will produce weight gain. Some people also use vigorous and prolonged exercise to reduce body weight as a way to purge. Although people with anorexia nervosa often express a great interest in food, and tend to enjoy preparing and serving food to others, their own diet becomes more and more restricted. People with anorexia nervosa often hide or hoard food without eating it.

People with anorexia are typically introverted, emotionally reserved, and socially insecure. They are often model children who rarely complain and are eager to please others and win their approval. Although school performance is typically above average, they are often critical of themselves and not satisfied with their accomplishments. For people with anorexia nervosa, their entire sense of self-esteem may be tied up in their evaluation of their body shape and weight.

**HEALTH RISKS OF ANOREXIA NERVOSA** Because of severe weight loss and extreme thinness, people with anorexia nervosa often become intolerant of cold and develop low blood pressure and heart rate. They develop dry skin that is often covered by fine body hair like that of a newborn. Their hands and feet may swell and take on a blue tinge. Females with this disease typically stop menstruating.

Anorexia nervosa has been linked to a variety of medical complications, including disorders of the cardiovascular, gastrointestinal, endocrine, and skeletal systems. When body fat is virtually gone and muscles are severely wasted, the body turns to its own organs in a desperate search for protein. Death can occur from heart failure caused by electrolyte imbalances. About 5–20% of people with anorexia nervosa eventually die of starvation, cardiac arrest, or other medical complications–the highest death rate for any psychiatric disorder. Other coinciding medical conditions (*comorbidities*) that people with anorexia nervosa commonly have are depression, obsessive-compulsive disorders, and anxiety disorders. About half the fatalities related to anorexia are suicides.

### Bulimia Nervosa

A person suffering from **bulimia nervosa** engages in recurrent episodes of binge eating followed by purging. Bulimia is often difficult to recognize because sufferers conceal their eating habits and usually maintain a normal weight, although they may experience weight fluctuations of 10–15 pounds. Although bulimia usually begins in adolescence or young adulthood, it has begun to emerge at increasingly younger (11–12 years) and older (40–60 years) ages; the average age of onset is about 20 years.

**CHARACTERISTICS OF BULIMIA NERVOSA** During a binge, a person with bulimia nervosa may rapidly consume thousands of calories. This is followed by an attempt to get rid of the food by purging, usually by vomiting or using laxatives or diuretics. During a binge, people with bulimia feel as though they have lost control and cannot stop or limit how much they eat. Some binge and purge only occasionally; others do so many times every day.

People with bulimia may appear to eat normally, but they are rarely comfortable around food. Binges usually occur in secret and can become nightmarish—uncontrollably raiding the kitchen for food, going from one grocery store to another to buy food, or stealing food. During the binge, food acts as an anesthetic, blocking out feelings. Afterward, people with bulimia feel physically drained and emotionally spent. They usually feel deeply ashamed and disgusted with both themselves and their behavior and terrified that they will gain weight from the binge.

Major life changes such as leaving for college, getting married, having a baby, or losing a job can trigger a binge-purge cycle. At such times, stress is high and the person may have no good outlet for emotional conflict or tension. As with anorexia nervosa, bulimia sufferers are often insecure and depend on others for approval and self-esteem. They may hide difficult emotions such as anger and disappointment from themselves and others. Binge eating and purging become a way of dealing with feelings.

**HEALTH RISKS OF BULIMIA NERVOSA** The binge-purge cycle of bulimia places a tremendous strain on the body and can have serious health effects. Contact with vomited stomach acids erodes tooth enamel. People with bulimia often develop tooth decay due to frequent vomiting as well as the tendency to binge on foods that are high in simple sugars. Repeated vomiting or the use of laxatives, in combination with deficient calorie intake, can damage the liver and kidneys and cause cardiac arrhythmia. Chronic hoarseness and esophageal tearing with bleeding may also result from vomiting. More rarely, binge eating can lead to rupture of the stomach. Although many women with bulimia maintain their weight within normal ranges, even a modest weight loss can cause menstrual problems. Bulimia is associated with increased depression, excessive preoccupation with food and body image, and sometimes cognitive dysfunction.

### Binge-Eating Disorder

**Binge-eating disorder** affects over 1% of American adults and is about twice as common in women as in men. It is characterized by uncontrollable eating, usually followed by feelings of guilt and shame about weight gain. Common eating patterns are eating more rapidly than normal, eating until uncomfortably full, eating when not hungry, and preferring to eat alone. Binge eaters may eat large amounts of food throughout the day, with no planned mealtimes. Many people with binge-eating disorder mistakenly see rigid dieting as the only solution to their problem. However, rigid dieting usually causes feelings of deprivation and a return to overeating.

Compulsive overeaters rarely eat because of hunger. Instead food is used as a means of coping with stress, conflict, and other difficult emotions or to provide solace and entertainment. People who do not have the resources to deal effectively with stress may be more vulnerable to binge-eating disorder. Inappropriate overeating often begins during childhood. In some families, eating may be used as an activity to fill otherwise empty time. Parents may reward children with food for good behavior or withhold food as a means of punishment, thereby creating distorted feelings about the experience of eating.

### Other Patterns of Disordered Eating

Eating habits and body image run along a continuum from healthy to severely disordered. Where an individual falls along that continuum can change depending on life stresses, illnesses, and many other factors. People who have feeding or eating disorders that can cause significant distress or impairment, but who do not meet the criteria for another feeding or eating disorder, may be classified as having **other specified feeding or eating disorders (OSFED),** according to the American Psychiatric Association's *Diagnostic and Statistical Manual of Mental Disorders*, 5th edition. OSFED is the most commonly diagnosed eating disorder in adults and adolescents. Examples include atypical anorexia nervosa, a condition in which the person exhibits all the classic behaviors of anorexia nervosa but weight is not below normal; bulimia nervosa with limited duration, a condition with less frequent bulimic episodes; purging disorder, a condition of forced purging without binge eating; and night eating syndrome, in which the individual engages in excessive nighttime food consumption. OSFED is present in approximately 30% of people who seek treatment for an eating disorder. OSFED is a serious mental illness, and affected people often have extremely disturbed eating habits, body image distortion, and intense fear of gaining weight.

Avoidant restrictive food intake disorder (ARFID) is a DSM-5 diagnosis that was previously referred to as selective eating disorder. ARFID is similar to anorexia nervosa—both conditions involve severe limitations of amount and types of foods consumed—but individuals with ARFID do not have the same fears about body weight and shape as those with anorexia nervosa.

**TERMS**

**binge-eating disorder** An eating disorder characterized by episodes of binge eating and a lack of control over eating behavior in general.

**other specified feeding or eating disorders (OSFED)** A feeding or eating disorder that causes significant distress or impairment but does not meet the criteria for another feeding or eating disorder.

Although not an official mental health diagnosis, the term *orthorexia* describes extreme obsession with healthy eating to the point that it is actually damaging to one's health and well-being. People with orthorexia are often compulsive about checking ingredient lists and nutritional labels and exhibit an inability to eat anything not on their narrow list of foods that they have deemed "pure" or "acceptable."

How do you know if you have disordered eating habits? When thoughts about food and weight dominate your life, you have a problem. If you're convinced that your worth as a person hinges on how you look and how much you weigh, it's time to get help. Other danger signs include frequent feelings of guilt after a meal or snack, any use of vomiting or laxatives after meals, or overexercising or severely restricting your food intake to compensate for what you've already eaten. If you suspect you have an eating problem, don't go it alone or delay getting help. Disordered eating habits can progress into a full-blown eating disorder. Check with your student health or counseling center.

**Treating Eating Disorders** The treatment of eating disorders must address both problematic eating behaviors and the misuse of food to manage stress and emotions. In many cases, anorexia nervosa treatment first involves averting a medical crisis by restoring adequate body weight; then the psychological aspects of the disorder can be addressed. The treatment of bulimia nervosa or binge-eating disorder involves first stabilizing the eating patterns, then identifying and changing the patterns of thinking that led to disordered eating, and then improving coping skills. Concurrent problems, such as depression, anxiety, and other mental disorders may be present and must also be addressed.

Treatment of eating disorders usually involves a combination of psychotherapy and medical management. The therapy may be done individually or in a group; sessions involving the entire family may be recommended. Medical professionals, including physicians, dentists, gynecologists, and registered dietitian nutritionists, can evaluate and manage the physical damage caused by the disorder. If a patient is severely depressed or emaciated, hospitalization may be necessary.

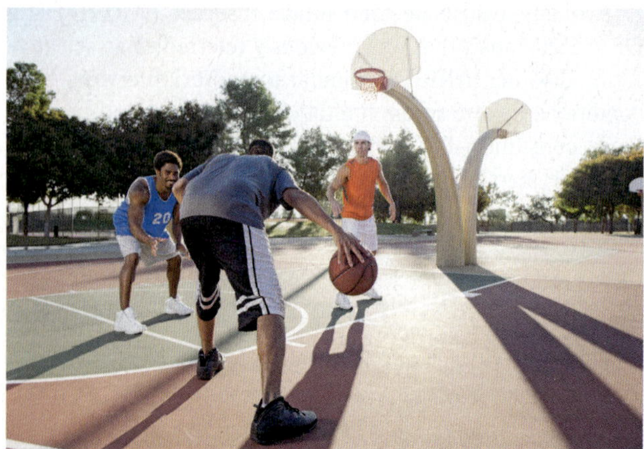


A balanced, realistic attitude toward weight management is part of overall wellness. Many healthy people do not fit society's image of ideal body size and shape. Dave and Les Jacobs/Blend Images LLC

**Ask Yourself**

**QUESTIONS FOR CRITICAL THINKING AND REFLECTION**

Do you know someone you suspect may suffer from an eating disorder? Have you ever experienced disordered eating patterns yourself? If so, can you identify the reasons for them?

## ADOPTING A HEALTHY LIFESTYLE FOR SUCCESSFUL WEIGHT MANAGEMENT AND DISEASE PREVENTION

Slow weight gain—just one or two pounds per year—can add up over time and contribute significantly to overweight and obesity, so weight management is important for everyone, not just for people who are currently overweight (see the box "The Freshman 15: Fact or Myth?").

A good time to develop a lifestyle for successful weight management is during your teens and early adulthood, when many behavior patterns form.

### Dietary Patterns and Eating Habits

In contrast to *dieting,* which may involve some form of food restriction, a *diet* or *dietary pattern* refers to your daily food choices over the long term. Everyone has a diet, but not everyone is dieting. You need to develop a way of eating that you enjoy and that enables you to maintain a healthy weight and body composition. Use the healthy dietary patterns recommended by the Dietary Guidelines for Americans, MyPlate, or the DASH Eating Plan as the basis for a healthy diet (see Chapter 10). For weight management, pay special attention to total calories, especially sugars, portion sizes, energy and nutrient density, and eating habits.

**Total Calories** MyPlate suggests approximate daily energy (calorie) needs based on age, sex, height, weight, and physical activity level. However, individual energy balance may be a more important consideration for weight management than total calories consumed. Also, because of individual variations in RMR and other factors, your energy needs may differ from those estimated by MyPlate.

If weight loss is your goal, increase your physical activity and include strength training to build muscle mass and

**Ask Yourself**

**QUESTIONS FOR CRITICAL THINKING AND REFLECTION**

How do you view your own body composition? Where do you think you've gotten your ideas about how your body should look and perform? In light of what you've read in this chapter, do the ideals and images promoted in our culture seem reasonable? Do they seem healthy?

## WELLNESS ON CAMPUS
### The Freshman 15: Fact or Myth?

According to popular belief, college students typically gain 15 pounds in their first year at school—the infamous "freshman 15." Is this the fate of all college students, or is it a myth that adds stress for body-conscious young adults?

In reality, the truth lies somewhere between these two scenarios. Many first-year college students gain weight, but usually not 15 pounds. More than 60% of college students gain an average of 7.5 pounds during their freshman year. First-year men tend to gain more weight than women.

The reasons most often responsible for the weight gain include stress and a changed environment and lifestyle—newfound food independence, different eating habits, and social comparisons that come with the influence of roommates and friends. Another part of the transition from high school to university life is a drop in physical activity. Leaving high school has been associated with a decline both in moderate-vigorous physical activity and in diet quality. The unhealthy snacks widely available to college students, especially during times of higher stress such as the end of the semester, may also contribute.

Even small weight increases can pose a health risk or contribute to lower self-esteem. Changes in body composition—specifically, increased body fat—can become a troublesome pattern for students. Although men gain more weight than women, their weight gain involves less fat and more lean mass than women's weight gain. Even if they don't have a spike in weight during their first year, college-educated individuals tend to experience a moderate but steady weight gain during and after college.

More important, whether the weight gain is 5 pounds, 15 pounds, or even more, freshman weight gain is avoidable! In addition to the healthy eating strategies for college students described in Chapter 10, follow these tips and guidelines for avoiding freshman weight gain:

- Listen to your hunger cues, eating when you are hungry (and not for emotional or social reasons) and stopping when you are satisfied.
- Before you snack, ask yourself if you are really hungry or if you are eating out of stress, boredom, or anxiety.
- Watch portion sizes, and avoid second and third servings; many people underestimate portion sizes by up to 25%.
- Make healthy choices in the dining hall—if you are not sure what to eat, you can find a registered dietitian nutritionist (RDN) in the campus health center who will advise you.
- Avoid getting "too hungry"; don't go longer than 3–4 hours without eating.
- Plan ahead so that you have healthy snacks handy.
- Don't skip breakfast, and avoid late-night eating.
- Try not to drink your calories—limit high-calorie smoothies, coffee drinks, and alcoholic beverages.

SOURCES: Vadeboncoeur, C., N. Townsend, and C. Foster. 2015. A meta-analysis of weight gain in first year university students: Is freshman 15 a myth? *BMC Obesity* 2: 22; Brawley, T. 2019. 8 ways to beat the 'freshman 15.' *Oregon Health & Science University* (https://news.ohsu.edu/2019/10/15/8-ways-to-beat-the-freshman-15). Hootman, K. C., K. A. Guertin, and P. A. Cassano. 2018. Stress and psychological constructs related to eating behavior are associated with anthropometry and body composition in young adults. *Appetite* 125: 287–294; Winpenny, E. M., et al. 2020. Changes in physical activity, diet, and body weight across the education and employment transitions of early adulthood: A systematic review and meta-analysis. *Obesity Reviews* 21(4): e12962.

aerobic-type exercises to burn calories (see Chapter 11). This physical activity should be combined with moderate calorie reduction targeting added sugars, refined carbohydrates and other processed foods, and solid fats. A focus on calorie sources can be just as important as total energy intake for successful weight loss.

Maintaining weight loss may be more difficult than losing the weight. To maintain weight loss, you will need to maintain some degree of the calorie restriction you used to lose the weight (recall that RMR drops in response to calorie restriction and weight loss). Therefore, you need to adopt a practical level of food intake that provides all the essential nutrients and that you can live with over the long term. Many people have found that *intuitive eating* provides an effective approach to long-term weight maintenance without the need for counting calories. Intuitive eating encourages trust in one's body and reconnection with the innate hunger and satiety cues we were born with. It aims to simplify eating and help people achieve freedom from incessant thoughts about food, weight, and calories.

**Portion Sizes** Overconsumption of total calories is often tied closely to portion sizes. Many Americans are unaware that the portions of packaged foods and of foods served at restaurants have increased in size, and most of us significantly underestimate the amount of food we eat. Bigger portion sizes correlate with higher calorie content, so being mindful of portion sizes can be helpful for maintaining a healthy body weight.

**Quality of Food Choices: Energy (Calorie) Density and Nutrient Density** Experts recommend that you pay attention to foods that are nutrient dense–that is, foods that are relatively low in calories but high in nutrients. As you increase your consumption of foods high in nutrient density, you will want to decrease foods in your diet that are high in *energy density.* Energy density refers to the number of calories per ounce or gram in a food. Ice cream, potato chips, croissants, crackers, cakes, and cookies are examples of foods high in energy density; in general, diets high in energy density are associated with higher rates of obesity. Foods that are low in energy density have more volume and bulk—that is, they are relatively heavy but have few calories, often due to high water and fiber content. For example, for the same 100 calories, you could eat 21 baby carrots or 4 pretzel twists; you are more likely to feel full after eating the serving of carrots because it weighs 10 times as much as the serving of pretzels (10 ounces versus 1 ounce).

Strategies for increasing the nutrient density of your diet while at the same time lowering its energy density include the following:

- Eat whole fruits with breakfast and for dessert.
- Add extra vegetables to sandwiches, casseroles, stir-fry dishes, pizza, pasta dishes, and fajitas.
- Start meals with a bowl of broth-based soup; include a green salad or fruit salad.
- Snack on fresh fruits and vegetables rather than crackers, chips, or other processed snack foods.
- Limit serving sizes of energy-dense foods such as butter, mayonnaise, cheese, fatty meats, croissants, and other sources of solid fats.
- Pay special attention to your beverage choices. Many sweetened drinks are low in nutrients and high in calories from added sugar; for example, a can of regular soda may have more than 35 grams of added sugar but no other nutrients, while the same amount of low-fat milk has no added sugars and is rich in many essential nutrients.
- Limit processed foods, especially those high in added sugars and refined carbohydrates; these are usually energy dense, nutrient poor, and high on the glycemic index, meaning they may increase rather than reduce your appetite.

Processed foods labeled "fat-free" or "reduced fat" may be high in calories and refined carbohydrates; such products may also contain sugar and fat substitutes.

**Eating Habits** Equally important to weight management are healthful eating patterns. Eating regular meals with whole, unprocessed foods that are nutrient dense can help to fuel healthy metabolism, maintain muscle mass, and prevent between-meal hunger that often leads to unhealthy snacking. Labeling some foods off-limits is generally not effective because it promotes feelings of deprivation, restriction, and punishment. A more sensible principle is, "everything in moderation." No foods need to be entirely off-limits, though some should be eaten judiciously.

Intermittent fasting can reduce overall calorie consumption. Keep in mind that it will also likely reduce RMR, since metabolism adjusts over time to match the amount of energy (calories) provided. One recent systematic review of 27 intermittent fasting trials found that weight loss ranging from 0.8% to 13.0% of baseline weight could be achieved with intermittent fasting. Another, 2022 study found that intermittent fasting did not result in more body weight or fat loss than just restricting calories. Additional research in the coming years can clarify the potential role of intermittent fasting as a weight management strategy. Besides weight loss, other proposed longer-term benefits of intermittent fasting include reduced blood pressure, lower inflammation, reduced cancer risk, slower aging, and diabetes prevention.

## Physical Activity and Exercise

Physical activity and exercise burn calories and keep the metabolism geared to using food for energy instead of storing it as fat. Exercise has a positive effect on metabolism. When people exercise, they increase the number of calories their bodies burn at rest (RMR). They also increase their muscle mass, which is associated with a higher metabolic rate. The exercise itself also burns calories, raising total energy expenditure. The higher the energy expenditure, the more the person can eat without gaining weight. In contrast, energy restriction alone will cause a loss in fat-free mass and a decrease in metabolic rate.

## Emotions and Coping Strategies

The way you think about yourself influences, and is influenced by, how you feel and how you act. In fact, research on people who struggle with their weight indicates that many of these individuals suffer from low self-esteem and the negative emotions that accompany it. Often people with low self-esteem mentally compare the actual self to an internally held picture of an "ideal self," an image based on perfectionistic goals and beliefs about how they and others should be. The more these two pictures differ, the larger the negative impact on self-esteem and the more likely the presence of negative emotions.

Besides the internal picture of ourselves, we all carry on an internal dialogue about events happening to us and around us. This *self-talk* can be self-deprecating or positively motivating, depending on our beliefs and attitudes (see Chapter 3). Having realistic beliefs and goals and practicing positive self-talk and problem solving support a healthy lifestyle.

Appropriate coping strategies help you deal with the stresses of life. They are also an important lifestyle factor in weight management. Many people use eating as a way to cope; others may cope by turning to drugs, alcohol, smoking, or gambling. Those who overeat might use food to alleviate loneliness or to serve as a pickup for fatigue, as an antidote to boredom, or as a distraction from problems. Some people even overeat to punish themselves for real or imagined transgressions.

Those who recognize that they are misusing food in such ways can analyze their eating habits with fresh eyes. They can consciously attempt to find new coping strategies and begin to use food appropriately—to fuel life's activities, to foster growth, and to bring pleasure, but *not* as a way to manage stress.

# APPROACHES TO OVERCOMING A WEIGHT PROBLEM

Each year, Americans spend more than $70 billion on various weight-loss plans and products. If you have overweight or obesity, you may already be creating a plan to lose weight and keep it off. You have many options. The "right" weight for you can evolve naturally. Combine modest cuts in energy intake with exercise, and avoid very-low-calorie diets.

According to the Centers for Disease Control and Prevention, reasonable weight loss for someone with obesity is 5–10% of body weight over six months. For example, for someone who weighs 200 pounds, a 5% weight loss would be 10 pounds. The person in this example may still be in the "overweight" or "obese" range, but this degree of weight loss can reduce the chronic disease risks related to obesity. Modest weight loss can also be easier to maintain. Even more modest weight loss, in the 3–5% range, and the lifestyle change used to achieve and maintain it, is likely to improve blood pressure, reduce cholesterol and glucose levels, and reduce the risk for diabetes.

To prevent the potentially dangerous consequences of rapid weight loss, don't try to lose weight more rapidly than 0.5–2.0 pounds per week. This rate of weight loss will initially require an energy (calorie) deficit of approximately 250–1000 calories per day. In general, a low-calorie diet provides 1200–1500 calories per day. Most low-calorie diets cause a rapid loss of body water at first. After this phase, weight loss declines, and dieters are often misled into believing that their efforts are not working. They give up, not realizing that the large initial fluid loss is not as significant as smaller fat losses that occur later in the diet.

QUICK
STATS
A 16-ounce whole-milk latte has 265 calories; beverages can have a significant impact on calorie intake.
—CDC, "Rethink Your Drink," 2022

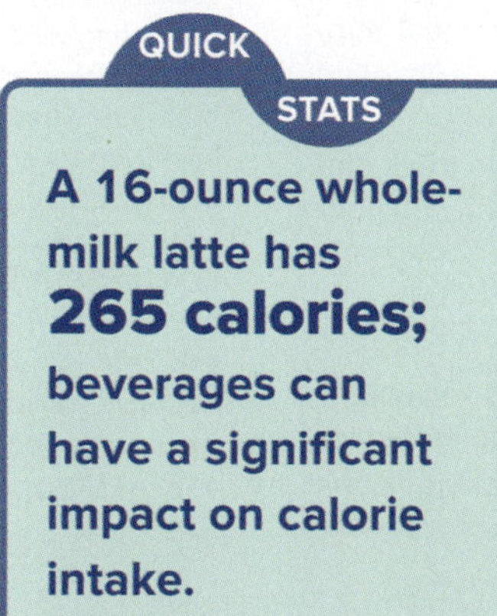

The National Institutes of Health has a planning tool that provides individual energy intake estimates for reaching a goal weight within a specific time period and to maintain it afterward (https://www.niddk.nih.gov/bwp). The tool can provide a starting point for planning, as well as a reality check on your goals.

Alternatively, you can set goals based on factors other than calories or pounds. You might instead monitor waist circumference or waist-to-hip ratio as a marker of health status related to body composition. Or aim for specific changes in dietary or activity patterns, such as fewer processed foods or more steps per day (see the Critical Consumer box "Apps and Wearables for Weight Management".).

Maintaining weight loss is usually a bigger challenge than losing weight. Without lasting lifestyle changes, most weight lost during a period of dieting is regained. Weight management is a lifelong project. When planning a weight-management program, include strategies that you can maintain over the long term, both for food choices and for physical activity. A registered dietitian nutritionist can create a personalized weight management plan and help set you up for long-term success. For more strategies, refer to the section "Adopting a Healthy Lifestyle for Weight Management and Disease Prevention."

> **Ask Yourself**
>
> **QUESTIONS FOR CRITICAL THINKING AND REFLECTION**
>
> Have you ever used food as an escape when you were stressed out or distraught? Were you aware of what you were doing at the time? How can you avoid using food as a coping mechanism in the future?

## Weight-Loss Plans and Products

Many people who try to lose weight by themselves fall prey to one or more of the hundreds of diet books, websites, social media programs, and over-the-counter supplements that promise jaw-dropping results with little to no basis in science. Although some plans and products have a sound premise, many make empty promises and do a better job of slimming your wallet than your waistline.

The list of top-selling diet books/plans has little in common with the dietary patterns most recommended by dietitians and other nutrition professionals for weight loss. If you decide to try a particular plan, look for one that advocates a balanced approach to diet that promotes overall wellness and that you can maintain over the long term.

Among the plans most recommended by dietitians are those described in Chapter 10: Mediterranean-style diets, the DASH dietary plan, and a flexible semivegetarian diet. These are backed by research and are considered sustainable and family-friendly. They do not require purchasing special foods or supplements.

Many of the current top-selling diet books/plans are based on a low-carbohydrate, high-protein or high-fat approach—sometimes referred to as ketogenic or "keto" plans. The original ketogenic diet was developed to treat epilepsy and includes about 90% of total calories from fat; it is typically prescribed by a health care provider and closely monitored.

While certain groups may benefit from ketogenic-style diets, it is not an approach generally recommended as the top choice for long-term weight management. Potential safety concerns are increased "bad" LDL cholesterol, lack of fiber and micronutrients, stress on the liver and kidneys, and changes to the microbiome. A study comparing diets for weight loss found that a low-carbohydrate diet ("paleo") was less effective for weight loss than the Mediterranean diet.

The number of dietary supplements and other weight-loss aids on the market has also increased over the past several decades. These products typically promise a quick and easy

## CRITICAL CONSUMER
### Apps and Wearables for Weight Management

A wide and ever-growing range of wearable trackers and weight-loss apps are available to consumers. You can find hundreds of smartphone apps to help you keep a nutrition journal and calculate your daily intake of calories and nutrients. You can also pair such apps with wearable trackers that can monitor your physical activity and calculate the calories you burn throughout the day. The apps may also synchronize data with a website that can display your results and progress in multiple formats; some also let you share your results across your social media networks or with a group of behavior change "buddies."

Do these digital tools help with weight loss and weight maintenance? Research findings have been mixed. As with any health habit, tracking alone is unlikely to create permanent behavior change. Apps and wearables for weight management may be most effective when you pair tracking with evidence-based behavior change techniques, such as reviewing goals, developing a specific action plan, planning for relapse prevention, and providing prompts, personalized feedback, rewards, and opportunities for motivational support. Pairing a digital tool with in-person or phone counseling from a health professional may further boost success.

If you decide to use a wearable and/or an app to track diet and exercise for your weight-management program, consider the following:

- Does the app track what you want to track and is it easy to use? Try it for a week or more: Did you stick with it?
- Does the app incorporate evidence-based behavior change strategies? What does it offer besides tracking? Look for apps with motivation components (e.g., feedback, rewards and challenges, and a system of points or levels).
- If you want to share your results with friends on social media, is that functionality supported? Can you join other app users in a supportive group?
- How was the app developed? Has it undergone scientific evaluation? Were behavior change medical experts involved in its development? If users claim the app has provided some level of effectiveness or success, what evidence is provided to back up the claim? Satisfaction or popularity ratings do not necessarily reflect effectiveness for supporting weight loss.

Even with the help of digital devices and programs, weight management is still primarily a matter of personal effort, perseverance, and a commitment to lifestyle changes that last for life.

SOURCES: Patel, M. L., L. N. Wakayama, and G. G. Bennett. 2021. Self-monitoring via digital health in weight loss interventions: A systematic review among adults with overweight and obesity. *Obesity* 29(3): 478–499; Abedtash, H. and R. J. Holden. 2017. Systematic review of the effectiveness of health-related behavioral interventions using portable activity sensing devices (PASDs). *Journal of the American Medical Informatics Association* (https://doi.org/10.1093/jamia/ocx006); Ross, K. M., and R. R. Wing. 2016 Impact of newer self-monitoring technology and brief phone-based intervention on weight loss: A randomized pilot study. *Obesity* 24(8): 1653–1659; Jakicic, J. M., et al. 2016. Effect of wearable technology combined with lifestyle intervention on long-term weight loss: The IDEA randomized clinical trial. *JAMA* 316(11): 1161–1171.

path to weight loss. Most of these products are marketed as dietary supplements and so are subject to fewer regulations than over-the-counter (OTC) medications. According to the Federal Trade Commission (FTC), more than half of advertisements for weight-loss products make representations that are likely to be false.

There is little information about effectiveness, proper dosage, drug interactions, and side effects of compounds marketed as dietary supplements.

## Weight-Loss Programs

Noncommercial programs such as Take Off Pounds Sensibly (TOPS) and Overeaters Anonymous (OA) mainly provide group support Commercial weight-loss programs typically provide group support, nutrition education, physical activity recommendations, and behavior modification advice. Some also make packaged foods available to assist in following dietary advice. Medically supervised clinical programs are usually located in a hospital or other medical setting and are designed to help those with severe obesity.

A responsible and safe weight-loss program should have the following features:

- Healthy eating plans that reduce calories but do not exclude specific foods or food groups
- Tips on ways to increase moderate-intensity physical activity
- Tips on healthy habits that also keep your cultural needs in mind, such as lower-fat versions of your favorite foods
- A goal of slow and steady weight loss
- A recommendation for medical evaluation and care if you have health problems, are taking medication, or are planning to follow a special formula diet that requires monitoring by a doctor
- A plan to keep the weight off after you have lost it
- Information on all fees and costs, including those of supplements and prepackaged foods, as well as data on risks and expected outcomes of participating in the program

You should also consider whether a program fits your lifestyle and whether you are truly ready to make a commitment to it. A strong commitment and a plan for maintenance are especially important because only 10–15% of program participants maintain their weight loss; the rest gain back all they had lost or more.

## Prescription Drugs and Surgery

Prescription weight-loss drugs are not for people who want to lose only a few pounds. The latest federal guidelines advise people to try lifestyle modification for at least six months before trying drug therapy. Prescription drugs are recommended only for people who have been unable to lose weight with nondrug options and who have a BMI over 30 (or over 27 if an additional risk factor such as diabetes or high blood pressure is present).

For a medicine to cause weight loss, it must (1) reduce energy consumption, (2) increase energy expenditure, and/or (3) interfere with energy absorption. The medications most often prescribed for weight loss are appetite suppressants that reduce feelings of hunger or increase feelings of fullness. Appetite suppressants usually work by increasing levels of catecholamine or serotonin, brain chemicals that affect mood and appetite. Although some medications are approved only for short-term use, most experts agree that medications must be safe to use over the long term in order to be effective for treatment of obesity.

Surgical intervention—known as bariatric surgery—may be necessary as a treatment of last resort. Bariatric surgery may be recommended for patients with a BMI greater than 40, or greater than 35 with obesity-related illnesses. The goal is to promote weight loss by reducing the amount of food the patient can eat. Bariatric surgery modifies the gastrointestinal tract. One method partitions the stomach with staples or a band, while another modifies the way the stomach drains (gastric bypass). Potential complications from surgery include nutritional deficiencies, fat intolerance, nausea, vomiting, and reflux. As many as 10–20% of patients may require follow-up surgery to address complications.

## Gaining Weight

A program for weight gain should be gradual and should include both exercise and dietary changes. People may want to gain weight if they've lost pounds during an illness, if they are older and have unintentionally lost weight, if they are below their healthy weight, or if they want to build strength and muscle. Like excess weight, underweight is also linked to certain health risks. Classified as a BMI of less than 18.5, about 2% of adults have underweight; many of these are people aged 18–24. Women are four times as likely as men to need to gain weight.

If you're classified as underweight, it's important to determine why, because the reasons may affect how you can proceed to gain weight. Busy schedules may not allow enough time for healthy diets and regular meals; worry and stress can interfere with appetite. Underweight may also result from certain medical conditions, like an overactive thyroid.

The foundation of a successful and healthy program for weight gain is a combination of strength training and in most cases a high-carbohydrate, high-protein diet that also contains healthy fats. Strength training will help you add weight as muscle rather than fat.

Energy balance is also important in a program for gaining weight. You need to consume more calories than your body needs in order to gain weight, but you need to choose those extra calories wisely. Fatty, sweet, high-calorie foods may seem like an obvious choice, but consuming empty calories from solid fats and added sugars can jeopardize your health and your weight-management program. Your body is more likely to convert excess dietary fat into fat tissue than into muscle mass.

A better strategy is to consume additional calories as protein, healthy fats, and complex carbohydrates from whole grains, fruits, and vegetables. To gain primarily muscle weight instead of fat, try these strategies for consuming extra calories:

- Don't skip any meals. If you fill up too fast, try eating five or six smaller meals.
- Add two or three snacks to your daily eating routine. Try trail mix, smoothies, and nut butters on crackers.
- Try a sports drink or supplement that has at least 60% of calories from carbohydrates, as well as significant amounts of protein, vitamins, and minerals. (But don't use supplements to replace meals because they don't contain all of the components of food.)

### TIPS FOR TODAY AND THE FUTURE

Many approaches work, but the best recipe for weight management is the one that will work for you. This means that the results for a particular plan will vary from person to person based on individual metabolism, overall health, starting weight, age, physical activity level, and how prepared you are to follow the plan.

**RIGHT NOW YOU CAN:**

- Assess your weight management needs. Do you need to gain weight, lose weight, or stay at your current weight?
- List five things you can do to add more physical activity (not just exercise) to your daily routine.
- Identify the foods you regularly eat that may be sabotaging your ability to manage your weight.

**IN THE FUTURE YOU CAN:**

- Make an honest assessment of your current body image. Is it accurate and fair, or is it unduly negative and unhealthy? If your body image presents a problem, consider getting professional advice on how to view yourself realistically.
- Keep track of your energy needs to determine whether your energy balance equation is correct. Use this information as part of your long-term weight management efforts.

- Eat quality proteins and fats to add calories: lean red meats, pork, chicken with the skin on (roasted or broiled, not deep fried), salmon and other oily fish, beans, whole milk, eggs, cheese, full-fat yogurt, soy/almond/coconut/rice milks, nut or seed butters, tofu, olives, avocado, and vegetable oil.
- Load up on carbohydrates: potatoes, brown rice, and whole-grain pasta, breads, and other whole grains.

Finally, remember your own genetics. Realize that you can change your body shape only so much through diet and exercise. Drastic changes may not be healthful or sustainable, or even possible. All bodies can, however, be healthy.

## SUMMARY

- Accepting that bodies come in all shapes and sizes, and that there is no universal, perfect body or diet is an important first step toward healthy living.
- Weight management involves more than a simple balance of energy in and energy out. It also includes genetic, metabolic, hormonal, psychological, cultural, and socioeconomic factors.
- Standards for assessing body weight and body composition include body mass index (BMI) and percent body fat.
- Body composition is the relative amounts of fat-free mass and fat in the body. *Overweight* and *obesity* refer to ranges for BMI and percent body fat that exceed what is typically associated with good health.
- Too much or too little body fat is linked to health problems; the distribution of body fat can also be a significant risk factor for many kinds of health problems.
- Dissatisfaction with body image and body weight can lead to physical problems and serious eating disorders, including anorexia nervosa, bulimia nervosa, binge-eating disorder, and other specified feeding or eating disorders (OSFED).
- Health at Every Size (HAES) is a movement that reframes the weight management paradigm from weight loss to disease prevention. It encourages eating healthfully, enjoying physical activity, listening to body cues for hunger and satiety, and fighting against fat stigma.
- Nutritional guidelines for weight management include consuming a moderate number of calories; limiting portion sizes, energy density, and the intake of simple sugars, refined carbohydrates, and solid fats; and redeveloping trust in your body's hunger and satiety signals to enable intuitive eating.
- Activity guidelines for weight management emphasize daily physical activity and regular sessions of cardiorespiratory endurance exercise and strength training.
- The sense of well-being that results from a well-balanced diet can reinforce commitment to a healthy lifestyle, improve self-esteem, and lead to realistic, as opposed to negative, self-talk. Those who are successfully managing their weight find strategies other than eating to cope with stress.
- People needing weight-management guidance can consult a registered dietitian nutritionist, read reliable science-based books, or join a weight-management program. In cases of extreme obesity, weight loss may require medical supervision.

## FOR MORE INFORMATION

*Academy of Nutrition and Dietetics (AND):* Find a Nutrition Expert. Find a qualified registered dietitian nutritionist or food and nutrition practitioner.

https://www.eatright.org/find-a-nutrition-expert

*American Diabetes Association.* Provides information, a free newsletter, and referrals to local support groups; the website includes an online diabetes risk assessment.

http://www.diabetes.org

*Calorie Control Council.* Includes a variety of interactive calculators, including an Exercise Calculator that estimates the calories burned from various forms of physical activity.

http://www.caloriecontrol.org

*Centers for Disease Control and Prevention: Obesity and Overweight.* The home page for accessing all the CDC's information about overweight and obesity, their health risks, statistics, and diet and exercise.

http://www.cdc.gov/obesity/index.html

*FDA Center for Food Safety and Applied Nutrition: Dietary Supplements.* Provides background facts and information on the current regulatory status of dietary supplements, including compounds marketed for weight loss.

http://www.fda.gov/Food/DietarySupplements/default.htm

*National Heart, Lung, and Blood Institute (NHLBI): Aim for a Healthy Weight.* Provides information and tips on diet and physical activity, as well as a BMI calculator.

http://www.nhlbi.nih.gov/health/educational/lose_wt/

*National Institute of Diabetes and Digestive and Kidney Diseases (NIDDK): Body Weight Planner.* Provides individual energy-intake estimates for reaching a goal weight within a specific time period and maintaining it afterward.

www.niddk.nih.gov/bwp

*National Institute of Diabetes and Digestive and Kidney Diseases (NIDDK): Weight Management.* Provides information and referrals for problems related to obesity, weight control, and nutritional disorders.

https://www.niddk.nih.gov/health-information/weight-management

***Resources for People Concerned about Eating Disorders:***

*Eating Disorder Referral and Information Center*

http://www.edreferral.com

*Eating Disorders Coalition for Research, Policy and Action*

http://www.eatingdisorderscoalition.org

*MedlinePlus: Eating Disorders*

http://www.nlm.nih.gov/medlineplus/eatingdisorders.html

*National Association of Anorexia Nervosa and Associated Disorders*

630-577-1330 (help line)

http://www.anad.org

*National Eating Disorders Association*

800-931-2237

http://www.nationaleatingdisorders.org

*National Institute of Mental Health: Eating Disorders*

http://www.nimh.nih.gov/health/topics/eating-disorders/index.shtml

See also the listings in Chapters 10 and 11.

## SELECTED BIBLIOGRAPHY

American Diabetes Association. 2022. *Statistics About Diabetes* (https://www.diabetes.org/about-us/statistics/about-diabetes).

American Psychiatric Association. 2013. *Diagnostic and Statistical Manual of Mental Disorders,* 5th ed. (https://doi-org.ezproxy.frederick.edu/10.1176/appi.books.9780890425596).

Barrack, W., et al. 2018. Disordered eating among a diverse sample of first-year college students. *Journal of the American College of Nutrition* 38(2): 141–148.

Beleigoli, A. M., et al. 2019. Web-based digital health interventions for weight loss and lifestyle habit changes in overweight and obese adults: Systematic review and meta-analysis. *Journal of Medical Internet Research* 21(1): e298. DOI: 10.2196/jmir.9609.

Bentley, J. 2017. *US Trends in Food Availability and Dietary Assessment of Loss-Adjusted Food Availability* 1970–2014. USDA. A report summary from the Economic Research Service (https://www.ers.usda.gov/webdocs/publications/82220/eib166%20summary.pdf?v=0).

Bratland-Sanda, S. 2019. Defining compulsive exercise in eating disorders: Acknowledging the exercise paradox and exercise obsessions. *Journal of Eating Disorders* 7(1): 8.

Bratland-Sanda, S., et al. 2019. Defining compulsive exercise in eating disorders: Acknowledging the exercise paradox and exercise obsessions. *Journal of Eating Disorders* 7: 8.

Buttitta, M., A. Rousseau, and A. Guerrien. 2017. A new understanding of quality of life in children and adolescents with obesity: Contribution of the self-determination theory. *Current Obesity Reports* 6(4):432–437.

Calugi, S., et al. 2020. The association between weight maintenance and session-by-session diet adherence, weight loss and weight-loss satisfaction. *Eating and Weight Disorders* 25(1): 127–133.

Centers for Disease Control and Prevention. 2020. *National Diabetes Statistics Report, 2020 Estimates of Diabetes and Its Burden in the United States.* (https://www.cdc.gov/diabetes/pdfs/data/statistics/national-diabetes-statistics-report.pdf).

Centers for Disease Control and Prevention. 2020. *Physical Activity Facts* (https://www.cdc.gov/healthyschools/physicalactivity/facts.htm).

Centers for Disease Control and Prevention. 2021. *Obesity and Overweight* (https://www.cdc.gov/nchs/fastats/obesity-overweight.htm).

Centers for Disease Control and Prevention. 2021. *Physical Activity. Recommendations and Guidelines* (https://www.cdc.gov/physicalactivity/resources/recommendations.html).

Centers for Disease Control and Prevention. 2021. *Prediabetes* (https://www.cdc.gov/diabetes/basics/prediabetes.html).

Centers for Disease Control and Prevention. 2022. *Leading Causes of Death* (https://www.cdc.gov/nchs/fastats/leading-causes-of-death.htm).

Centers for Disease Control and Prevention. 2022. *Overweight and Obesity* (https://www.cdc.gov/obesity/).

Christian, C., et al. 2020. Eating disorder core symptoms and symptom pathways across developmental stages: A network analysis. *Journal of Abnormal Psychology* 129(2):177–190.

Dues, K., et al. 2019. Adolescent body weight perception: Association with diet and physical activity behaviors. *Journal of School Nursing* 1–9. DOI: 10.1177/1059840518824386.

Dumas, A-A., and S. Desroches. 2019. Women's use of social media: What is the evidence about their impact on weight management and body image? *Current Obesity Reports* 8(1): 18–23.

Eatright. Academy of Nutrition and Dietetics. 2021. *Orthorexia* (https://www.eatright.org/health/diseases-and-conditions/eating-disorders/orthorexia-an-obsession-with-eating-pure).

Ebbing, C. B., et al. 2018, November 14. Effects of a low carbohydrate diet on energy expenditure during weight loss maintenance: Randomized trial. *BMJ* 363: k4583.

Food and Drug Administration. 2022. *What You Need to Know About Dietary Supplements* (https://www.fda.gov/Food/ResourcesForYou/Consumers/ucm109760.htm).

Freedhoff, Y., and K. D. Hall. 2016. Weight loss diet studies: We need help not hype. *Lancet* 388(10047): 849–851.

Fryar, C. D., et al. 2016. Prevalence of overweight, obesity, and extreme obesity among adults aged 20 and over: United States, 1960–1962 through 2013–2014. Centers for Disease Control and Prevention (https://www.cdc.gov/nchs/data/hestat/obesity_adult_13_14/obesity_adult_13_14.htm).

Galmiche, M., et al. 2019. Prevalence of eating disorders over the 2000–2018 period: A systematic literature review. *American Journal of Clinical Nutrition* 109(5): 1402–1413.

Gibson, A. A., and A. Sainsbury. 2017. Strategies to improve adherence to dietary weight loss interventions in research and real-world settings. *Behavioral Sciences (Basel).* 7(3). pii: E44.

Global BMI Mortality Collaboration. 2016. Body-mass index and all-cause mortality: Individual-participant-data meta-analysis of 239 prospective studies in four continents. *Lancet* 388(10046): 776–786.

Golden, N. H., M. Schneider, and C. Wood. Committee on Nutrition, Committee on Adolescence and Section on Obesity. 2016. Preventing obesity and eating disorders in adolescents. *Pediatrics* 138(3): e1–12.

Gray L. A., et al. 2018. Family lifestyle dynamics and childhood obesity: Evidence from the millennium cohort study. *BMC Public Health* 18: 500 (https://doi.org/10.1186/s12889-018-5398-5).

Hales, C. M., et al. 2018. Differences in obesity prevalence by demographic characteristics and urbanization level among adults in the United States, 2013–2016. *Journal of the American Medical Association* 319(23): 2419–2429.

Hales C. M., et al. 2020. *Prevalence of Obesity And Severe Obesity Among Adults: United States, 2017–2018.* NCHS Data Brief, No. 360. Hyattsville, MD: National Center for Health Statistics (https://www.cdc.gov/nchs/products/databriefs/db360.htm).

Hall, K. D., et al. 2016. Energy expenditure and body composition changes after an isocaloric ketogenic diet in overweight and obese men. *American Journal of Clinical Nutrition* 104(2): 324–333.

Harvard University T. H. Chan School of Public Health. 2022. *Toxic Food Environment: How Our Surroundings Influence What We Eat* (https://www.hsph.harvard.edu/obesity-prevention-source/obesity-causes/food-environment-and-obesity/).

Healthy People 2030. *Physical Activity,* Office of Disease Prevention and Health Promotion, Centers for Disease Control and Prevention (https://health.gov/healthypeople/objectives-and-data/browse-objectives/physical-activity).

Hills, R. D. et al. 2019. Gut Microbiome: Profound implications for diet and disease. *Nutrients Open Access* 11(7): 1613. (https://doi.org/10.3390/nu11071613).

Hyde, P. N., et al. 2019. Dietary carbohydrate restriction improves metabolic syndrome independent of weight loss. *JCI Insight* 4(12).

Izquierdo, A. G., et al. 2019. Leptin, obesity, and leptin resistance: Where are we 25 years later? *Nutrients* 11(11): 2704 (10.3390/nu11112704\).

Jane, M., et al. 2018. Social media for health promotion and weight management: A critical debate. *BMC Public Health* 18: 932.

Jin, Y., C. Ha, H. Hong, and H. Kang. 2017. The relationship between depressive symptoms and modifiable lifestyle risk factors in office workers. *Journal of Obesity & Metabolic Syndrome* 26(1): 52–60.

Johnson, S. S. 2019. The art of health promotion. Editor's desk: Masterful Microbes: The gut microbiome and food as medicine. *American Journal of Health Promotion* 35(5): 820–834.

Karazsia, B. T., S. K. Murnen, and T. L. Tylka. 2017. Is body dissatisfaction changing across time? A cross-temporal meta-analysis. *Psychological Bulletin* 143(3): 293–320.

Kennerly, A. M., and A. Kirk. 2018. Physical activity and sedentary behavior of adults with type 2 diabetes: a systematic review. *Practical Diabetes* 35(3): 86–89 (https://doi.org/10.1002/pdi.2169).

Krebs, G., L. Fernandez de la Cruz, and D. Mataix-Cols.2017. Recent advances in understanding and managing body dysmorphic disorder. *Evidence-Based Mental Health* 20(3):71–75.

LeBlanc, E. L., et al. 2018. *Behavioral and Pharmacotherapy Weight Loss Interventions to Prevent Obesity-Related Morbidity and Mortality in Adults: An Updated Systematic Review for the U.S. Preventive Services Task Force.* Rockville (MD): Agency for Healthcare Research and Quality (U.S.); 2018 Sep. Report No.: 18-05239-EF-1. U.S. Preventive Services Task Force Evidence Syntheses, formerly Systematic Evidence Reviews.

Liu, D., et al. 2022. Calorie restriction with or without time-restricted eating in weight loss. *The New England Journal of Medicine* 386: 1495–1504.

Loos, R., and G. Yeo 2022. The genetics of obesity: From discovery to biology. *Nature Reviews Genetics* 23(3): 120–133 (10.1038/s41576-021-00414-z).

Moehlecke, M. et al. 2016. Determinants of body weight regulation in humans. *Archives of Endocrinology and Metabolism* 60(2): 152–162.

Mozzafarian, D. 2016. Dietary and policy priorities for cardiovascular disease, diabetes, and obesity: A comprehensive review. *Circulation* 133(2): 187–225.

Nagata, J. M., K. T. Ganson, and S. B. Austin. 2020. Emerging trends in eating disorders among sexual and gender minorities. *Current Opinion in Psychiatry* 33(6): 562–567.

National Association of Anorexia Nervosa and Associated Disorders (ANAD). n.d. *Eating Disorders Statistics* (http://www.anad.org/education-and-awareness/about-eating-disorders/eating-disorders-statistics/).

National Center of Diabetes and Digestive and Kidney Diseases. 2021. *Overweight and Obesity Statistics.* (https://www.niddk.nih.gov/health-information/health-statistics/overweight-obesity#prevalence).

National Center for Health Statistics. 2019. *Health, United States, 2019:* Hyattsville, MD (https://www.cdc.gov/nchs/data/hus/hus19-508.pdf).

National Eating Disorders Association. n.d. *Other Specified Feeding or Eating Disorders* (https://www.nationaleatingdisorders.org/learn/by-eating-disorder/osfed).

National Eating Disorders Association. 2022. *Avoidant Restrictive Food Intake Disorder (ARFID)* (https://www.nationaleatingdisorders.org/learn/by-eating-disorder/arfid).

National Eating Disorders Association. 2022. *Statistics and Research on Eating Disorders* (https://www.nationaleatingdisorders.org/statistics-research-eating-disorders).

National Eating Disorders Association. 2022. *What Are Eating Disorders?* (https://www.nationaleatingdisorders.org/what-are-eating-disorders).

National Institute of Diabetes and Digestive and Kidney Diseases. 2017. *Choosing a Safe and Successful Weight-Loss Program* (https://www.niddk.nih.gov/health-information/weight-management/choosing-a-safe-successful-weight-loss-program#whatLook).

National Institutes of Health, National Institute of Diabetes and Digestive and Kidney Diseases. 2020. *Definition and Facts for Bariatric Surgery* (https://www.niddk.nih.gov/health-information/weight-management/bariatric-surgery/definition-facts).

National Institutes of Health. Office of Dietary Supplements. 2020. *Dietary Supplement: What You Need to Know* (https://ods.od.nih.gov/factsheets/WYNTK-Consumer/).

NCD Risk Factor Collaboration. 2016. Trends in adult body-mass index in 200 countries from 1975 to 2014: A pooled analysis of 1698 population-based measurement studies with 19.2 million participants. *Lancet* 387(10026): 1377–1396.

Nunez, C., et al. 2017. Obesity, physical activity and cancer risks: Results from the Cancer, Lifestyle and Evaluation of Risk Study (CLEAR). *Cancer Epidemiology* 47: 56–63

Ogilvie R. P., and S. R. Patel. 2017. The epidemiology of sleep and obesity. *Sleep Health* 3(5): 383–388.

Pearl, R. L., et al. 2020. Effects of a cognitive-behavioral intervention targeting weight stigma: A randomized controlled trial. *Journal of Consulting and Clinical Psychology*. DOI: 10.1037/ccp0000480.

Rinninella, E., et al. 2019. Food components and dietary habits: Keys for a healthy gut microbiota composition. *Nutrients* 11(10): 2393.

Ross, R., et al. 2020. Waist circumference as a vital sign in clinical practice: A consensus statement from the IAS and ICCR Working Group on Visceral Obesity. *Nature Reviews Endocrinology* 16: 177–189 (https://www.nature.com/articles/s41574-019-0310-7)

Rouhani, M. H., et al. 2016. Associations between dietary energy density and obesity: A systematic review and meta-analysis of observational studies. *Nutrition.* 32(10): 1037–1047.

Schiller, J. S., T. C. Clarke, and T. Norris. 2022. Early release of selected estimates based on data from the January–September 2021 National Health Interview Survey. National Center for Health Statistics (https://www.cdc.gov/nchs/nhis.htm).

Sheikh, V. K., and H. A. Raynor. 2016. Decreases in high-fat and/or high-added-sugar food group intake occur when a hypocaloric, low-fat diet is prescribed within a lifestyle intervention: a secondary cohort analysis. *Journal of the Academy of Nutrition and Dietetics* 116(10): 1599–1605.

Shrestha, N., et al. 2019. Effectiveness of interventions for reducing non-occupational sedentary behaviour in adults and older adults: A systematic review and meta-analysis. *British Journal of Sports Medicine* 53(19): 1206–1213.

Sicat, M. 2018. Defining obesity's interplay among environment, behavior and genetics. *Obesity Medicine Association* (https://obesitymedicine.org/obesity-and-genetics/).

Siegel, K. R., et al. 2016. Association of higher consumption of foods derived from subsidized commodities with adverse cardiometabolic risk among US adults. *JAMA Internal Medicine* 176(8): 1124–1132.

Slomski A. 2019. Low-carb diets help maintain weight loss. *Journal of the American Medical Association* 321(4): 355.

Smethers, A. D., and B. J. Rolls. 2018. Dietary management of obesity: Cornerstones of healthy eating patterns. *Medical Clinics of North America* 102(1): 107–124.

Thaler, L., and H. Steiger. 2017. Eating disorders and epigenetics. *Advances in Experimental Medicine and Biology* 978: 93–103.

The Global Health Observatory. 2022. Body Mass Index (BMI). *World Health Organization* (https://www.who.int/data/gho/data/themes/topics/topic-details/GHO/body-mass-index).

Tronieri, J. S., et al. 2019. Early weight loss in behavioral treatment predicts later rate of weight loss and response to pharmacotherapy. *Annals of Behavioral Medicine* 53(3): 290–295.

Udo, T., and C. M. Grilo. 2018. Prevalence and correlates of DSM-5 eating disorders in nationally representative sample of United States adults. *Biological Psychiatry* 84(5): 345–354.

USDA Nutrition.gov. n.d. *Online Tools* (https://www.nutrition.gov/topics/basic-nutrition/online-tools).

USDA Economic Research Service. 2016. *Recent Evidence on the Effects of Food Store Access on Food Choice and Diet Quality* (https://www.ers.usda.gov/amber-waves/2016/may/recent-evidence-on-the-effects-of-food-store-access-on-food-choice-and-diet-quality/).

U.S. Department of Health and Human Services. 2018. *Physical Activity Guidelines for Americans,* 2nd ed. Washington, DC: U.S. Department of Health and Human Services (https://health.gov/sites/default/files/2019-09/Physical_Activity_Guidelines_2nd_edition.pdf).

U.S. Department of Health and Human Services. 2020. *Healthy People 2030: Nutrition and Weight Status Workgroup* (https://health.gov/healthypeople/about/workgroups/nutrition-and-weight-status-workgroup).

U.S. Department of Health and Human Services and U.S. Department of Agriculture. 2020. *2020–2025 Dietary Guidelines for Americans,* 9th ed. (https://www.dietaryguidelines.gov/sites/default/files/2021-03/Dietary_Guidelines_for_Americans-2020-2025.pdf).

van Eeden A. E., D. van Hoeken, and H. W. Hoek. 2021. Incidence, prevalence and mortality of anorexia nervosa and bulimia nervosa. *Current Opinion in Psychiatry* 34(6): 515–524.

Vaughan, K. L., and J. A. Mattison. 2018. Watch the clock, not the scale. *Cell Metabolism* 27(6): 1159–1160.

Ward, Z. J., et al. 2019. Estimation of eating disorders prevalence by age and associations with mortality in a simulated nationally representative US cohort. *JAMA Network Open* 2(10): e1912925.

World Health Organization. 2021. *Obesity* (https://www.who.int/features/factfiles/obesity/en/).

Yoon, C., et al. 2020. Disordered eating behaviors and 15-year trajectories in body mass index: Findings from Project Eating and Activity in Teens and Young Adults (EAT). *Journal of Adolescent Health* 66(2): 181–188.

Zuraikat, F. M., et al. 2018. Comparing the portion size effect in women with and without extended training in portion control: A follow-up to the Portion-Control Strategies Trial. *Appetite* 123: 334–342.

**Design Elements:** Assess Yourself icon: Aleksey Boldin/Alamy Stock Photo; Diversity Matters icon: Rawpixel Ltd/Getty Images; Wellness on Campus icon: Radius Images/Alamy Stock Photo; Take Charge icon: VisualCommunications/Getty Images; Critical Consumer icon: pagadesign/Getty Images.

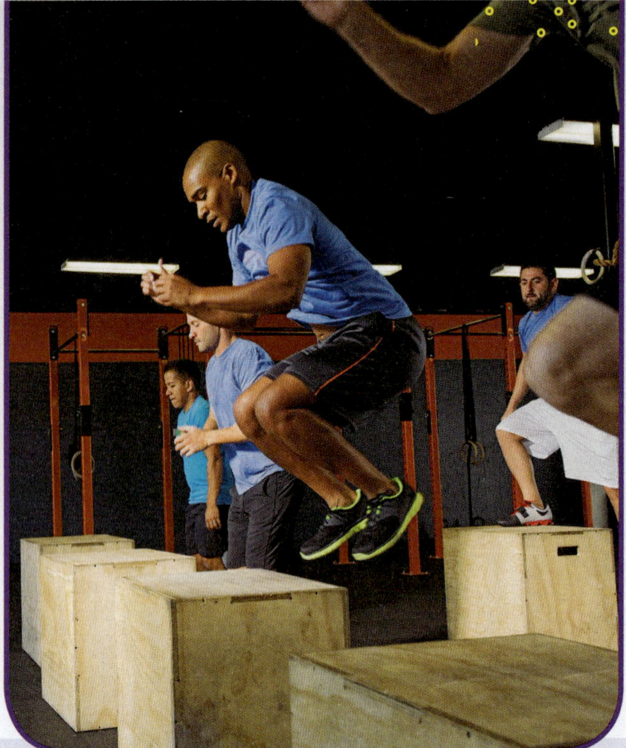
Erik Isakson/Getty Images

## CHAPTER OBJECTIVES

- Identify the major components of the cardiovascular system
- Describe the risk factors associated with cardiovascular disease
- Discuss the major forms of cardiovascular disease
- List the steps you can take to protect yourself against cardiovascular disease
- Explain the basic facts about cancer
- Discuss causes of cancer and how to avoid or minimize them
- Describe how cancer can be detected, diagnosed, and treated
- Describe common cancers as well as detection and treatment options for each

CHAPTER 13

# Cardiovascular Health and Cancer

**Cardiovascular disease (CVD)** refers to the development of diseases that affect the heart and blood vessels: cardiomyopathy (weakness of heart muscle), heart attack (blockage of a coronary artery), angina (chest pain from lack of blood flow to the heart muscle), and stroke (blockage or rupture of arteries that supply blood to the brain), as well as blood vessel diseases, arrhythmias (heart rhythm problems), and many other conditions affecting the heart's muscle, valves, or rhythms.

TERMS

**cardiovascular disease (CVD)** The collective term for various diseases of the heart and blood vessels.

**cardiovascular system (CVS)** The system that circulates blood through the body; consists of the heart and blood vessels.

As the country's leading cause of death, CVD claims about 2300 American lives every day. More than 92 million American adults have one or more types of CVD, and of these, over half are estimated to be 60 years of age or younger. Cancer is the second leading cause of death in the United States and is responsible for nearly one in four deaths, claiming about 600,000 lives annually. Although genes, age, and environmental factors play roles in the development of these diseases, CVD and cancer are also lifestyle diseases, linked to many lifestyle factors. The following sections provide information that can help you maintain a healthy heart for life and reduce your risks of developing cancer.

## THE CARDIOVASCULAR SYSTEM

The **cardiovascular system (CVS)** consists of the heart and blood vessels, which includes both arteries and veins. Together they transport blood throughout the body (Figure 13.1). When

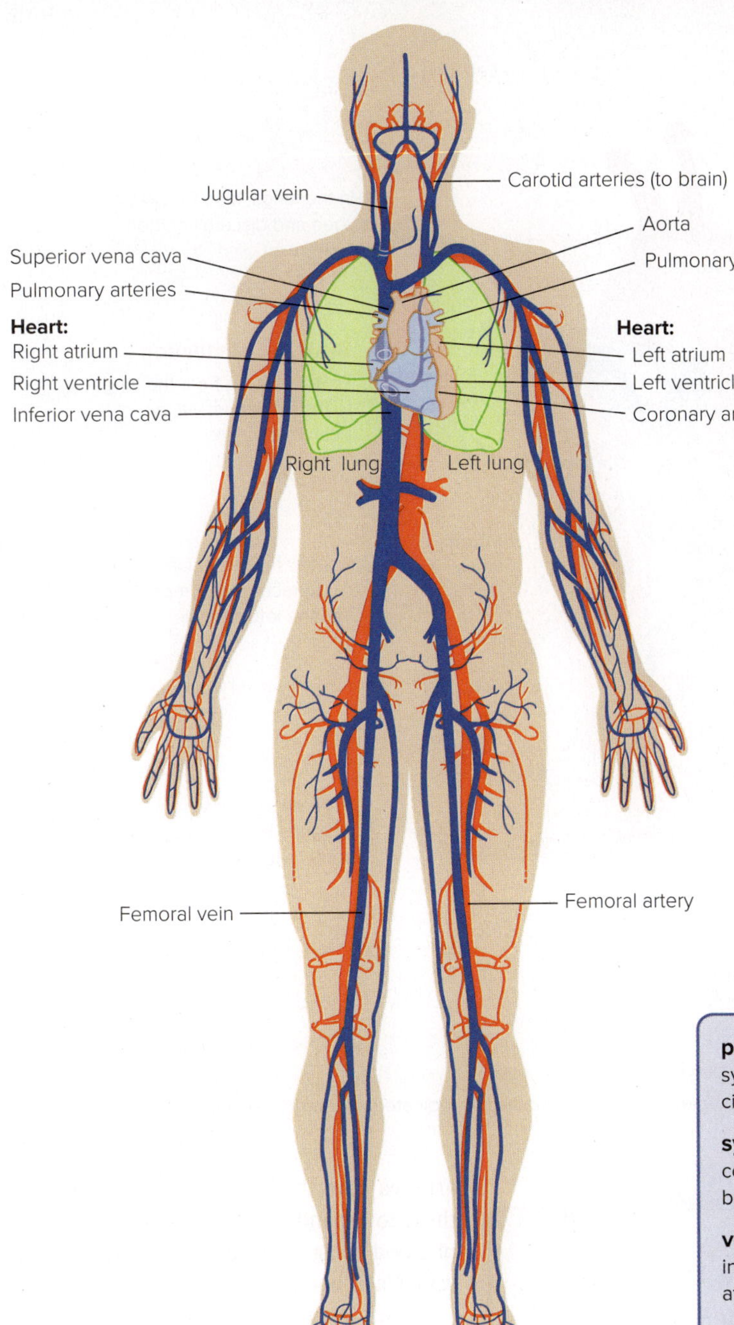


**FIGURE 13.1** **The cardiorespiratory system.**

the lungs are included, the system is known as the *cardiorespiratory* or *cardiopulmonary system*.

The heart is a four-chambered, fist-sized muscular organ located just beneath the sternum (breastbone). It pumps oxygen-poor blood to the lungs and delivers oxygen-rich blood to the rest of the body. Blood actually travels through two separate (but connected) circulatory systems. The right side of the heart pumps blood to the lungs in what is called **pulmonary circulation,** and the left side pumps blood through the rest of the body in the **systemic circulation.**

Oxygen-poor blood travels through the **superior vena cava** and **inferior vena cava** into the heart's right upper chamber, the **right atrium.** After the right atrium fills, blood flows into the heart's right lower chamber, the **right ventricle.** The right atrium and right ventricle are separated by the tricuspid valve. When the right ventricle is full, it contracts and pumps blood through the pulmonary arteries into the lungs. There, blood picks up oxygen and discards carbon dioxide. The newly oxygenated blood flows from the lungs through the pulmonary veins into the heart's **left atrium.** When the left atrium fills, it contracts and pumps blood into the **left ventricle.** When the left ventricle fills, it pumps blood through the aortic valve to the **aorta**–the body's largest artery–for distribution to the rest of the body. The path of blood flow through the heart and cardiorespiratory system is illustrated in Figure 13.2.

Each heartbeat consists of two basic parts: systole and diastole. During **systole,** the ventricles contract (ventricular systole) to pump blood out of the heart. During **diastole,** the heart relaxes and fills with blood.

**Blood pressure,** the force exerted by blood on the walls of the blood vessels, is created by the

**TERMS**

**pulmonary circulation** The part of the circulatory system controlled by the right side of the heart: the circulation of blood between the heart and the lungs.

**systemic circulation** The part of the circulatory system controlled by the left side of the heart: the circulation of blood between the heart and the rest of the body.

**vena cava** Either of two large veins (superior vena cava and inferior vena cava) through which blood is returned to the right atrium of the heart (plural, *venae cavae*).

**atrium** Either of the two upper chambers of the heart (left or right) in which blood collects before passing to the ventricles (plural, *atria).*

**ventricle** Either of the two lower chambers of the heart (left or right) that pump blood to the lungs and other parts of the body.

**aorta** The largest artery in the body; receives blood from the left ventricle and distributes it to the body.

**systole** The contraction phase of the heart.

**diastole** The relaxation phase of the heart.

**blood pressure** The force exerted by the blood on the walls of the blood vessels; created by the pumping of the heart and the resistance of the blood vessels.

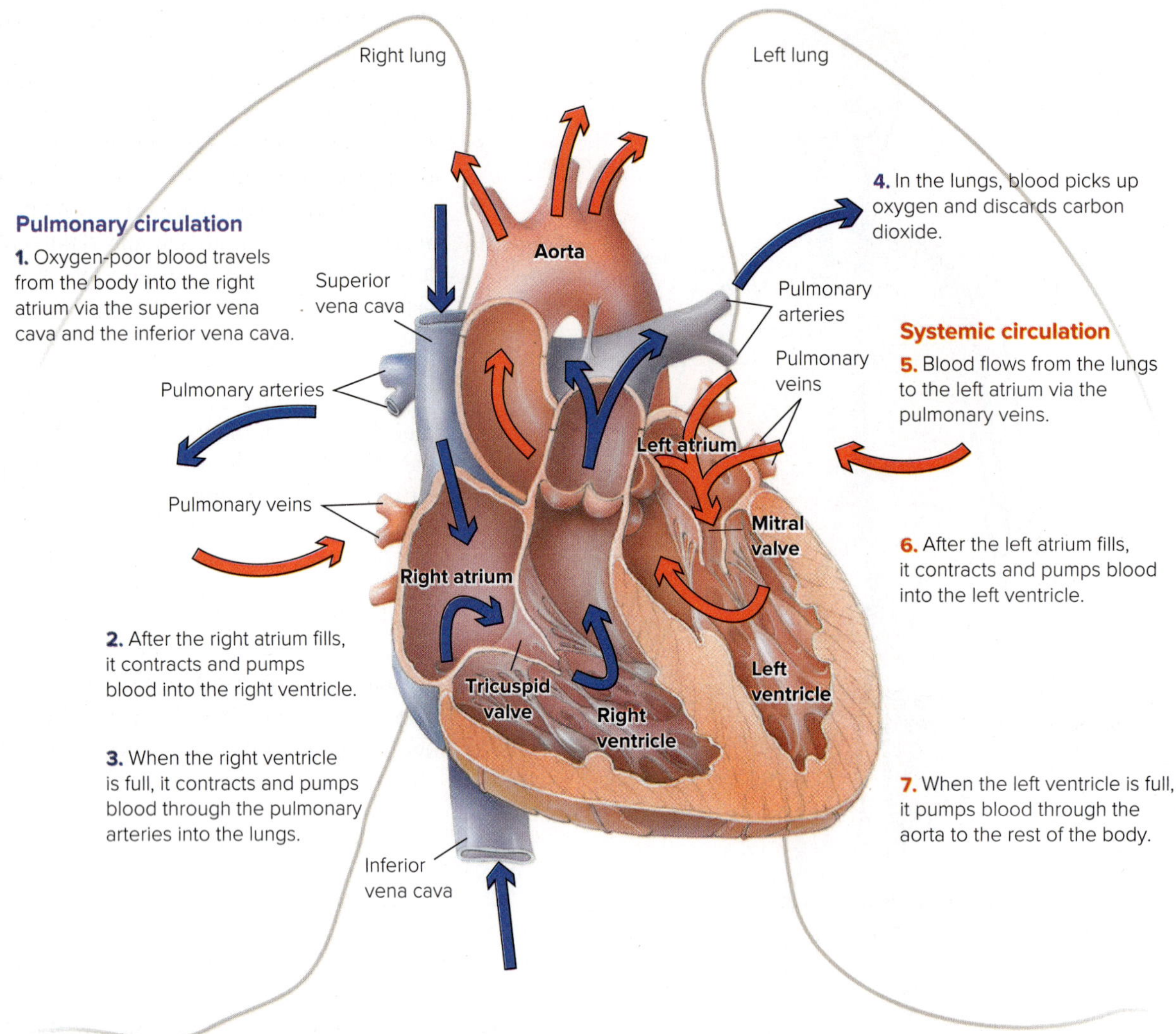


**FIGURE 13.2 Circulation in the heart.** Blue arrows indicate oxygen-poor blood; red arrows indicate oxygen-rich blood.

pumping action of the heart and the resistance of the blood vessels. This is an important concept because high blood pressure is treated by medicines that work on relaxing cardiac contractions as well as on reducing the resistance of the blood vessels. Blood pressure is reported as systolic pressure over diastolic pressure; for example, 120 over 80 mm Hg (or 120/80).

Blood vessels are classified by size and function. **Veins** carry blood to the heart, whereas **arteries** carry blood away from the heart. Veins have thin walls, but arteries have thick elastic walls that enable them to expand and relax with the pressure of blood being pumped through them during ventricular contraction.

After leaving the heart, the aorta branches into smaller and smaller vessels. The smallest arteries branch still further into **capillaries**—tiny vessels with walls only one cell thick. The capillaries deliver oxygen- and nutrient-rich blood to the tissues, and then pick up oxygen-poor, carbon-dioxide-laden blood. From the capillaries, this blood empties into small veins and then into progressively larger veins that return it to the heart to repeat the cycle.

Blood pumped through the chambers of the heart does not reach the cells of the heart, so the organ has its own network of arteries, veins, and capillaries. Two large vessels, the right and left **coronary arteries,** branch off the aorta and supply the heart itself with oxygenated blood (Figure 13.3). Blockage of blood flow within a coronary artery is the leading cause of heart attacks.

**QUICK STATS**

**In the U.S., 1 in every 5 deaths is due to heart disease.**

—CDC, 2022

**TERMS**

**vein** A vessel that carries blood to the heart.

**artery** A vessel that carries blood away from the heart.

**capillary** A small blood vessel that exchanges oxygen and nutrients between the blood and the tissues.

**coronary artery** A blood vessel branching from the aorta that provides blood to the heart muscle.

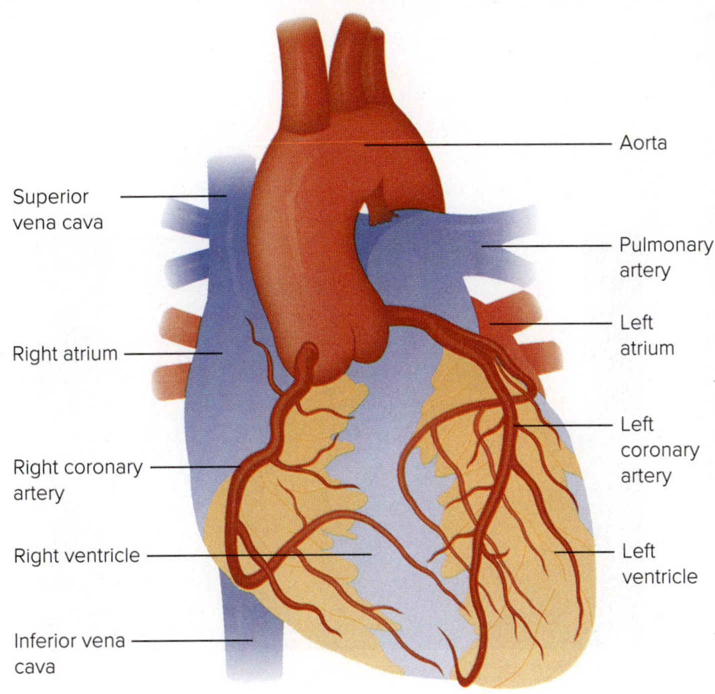


**FIGURE 13.3** **Blood supply to the heart.**

## MAJOR FORMS OF CARDIOVASCULAR DISEASE

Although deaths from cardiovascular disease have declined dramatically over the past 60 years, it remains the leading cause of death in the United States. According to the CDC, heart disease killed almost 697,000 Americans in 2020. Figure 13.4 shows the death rates among population groups due to heart disease in 2020, the most recent year for which data are available.

The main forms of CVD are atherosclerosis, coronary heart disease and heart attack, stroke, peripheral arterial disease, congestive heart failure, congenital heart disease, rheumatic heart disease, and heart valve disease. Many forms are interrelated and have elements in common; we treat them separately here for the sake of clarity. Hypertension, which is both a major risk factor and a form of CVD, is described later in the chapter.

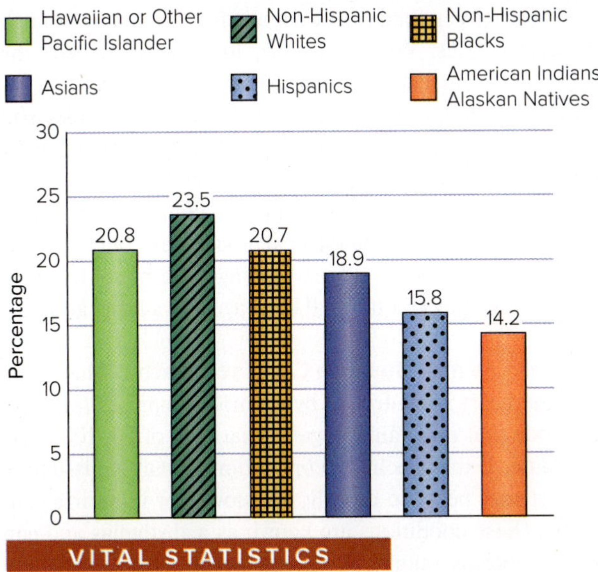


**FIGURE 13.4** **Percentage of U.S. deaths due to heart disease, by race/ethnicity.**

SOURCE: Centers for Disease Control and Prevention. 2022. About Multiple Cause of Death, 1999–2020. CDC WONDER Online Database website. Atlanta, GA: CDC.

### Atherosclerosis

A major precursor to heart attacks and other CVD is atherosclerosis, or thickening and hardening of the arteries. **Atherosclerosis** is a disease process in which arteries become narrowed by deposits of fat, cholesterol, and other substances (Figure 13.5). The process begins when the endothelial cells (cells that line the arteries) become damaged, often through a combination of factors such as smoking, high blood pressure, high insulin or glucose levels, and deposits of oxidized cholesterol particles. The body's response to this damage results in inflammation and changes in the artery lining that create a magnet for cholesterol particles, platelets, and other cells. These cells build up and cause a bulge in the wall of the artery. As these deposits, called **plaques,** accumulate in artery walls, the arteries lose their elasticity and their ability to expand and contract, restricting blood flow. Once narrowed by a plaque, an artery is vulnerable to blockage by blood clots. The risk of life-threatening clots, or heart attacks, increases if the fibrous cap covering a plaque ruptures.

If the heart, brain, or other organs are deprived of blood and the oxygen it carries, the effects of atherosclerosis can be deadly. Coronary arteries, which supply the heart with blood, are particularly susceptible to plaque buildup, a condition called **coronary heart disease (CHD)** or *coronary artery disease (CAD).* The blockage of a coronary artery causes a myocardial infarction, commonly described as a heart attack, and blockage of a cerebral artery (leading to the brain) causes a stroke. Blockage of an artery in a limb causes *peripheral arterial disease,* a condition that causes pain, numbness, and sometimes infection, and may require amputation of the affected limb.

The main risk factors for atherosclerosis are tobacco use, physical inactivity, high blood cholesterol levels, high blood pressure, diabetes, inflammatory conditions, and infections.

**TERMS**

**atherosclerosis** A form of cardiovascular disease in which the inner layers of artery walls are made thick and irregular by plaque deposits; arteries become narrow, and blood supply can be reduced.

**plaque** A deposit of fatty (and other) substances on the inner wall of an artery.

**coronary heart disease (CHD)** Heart disease caused by atherosclerosis in the arteries that supply blood to the heart muscle; also called *coronary artery disease (CAD).*

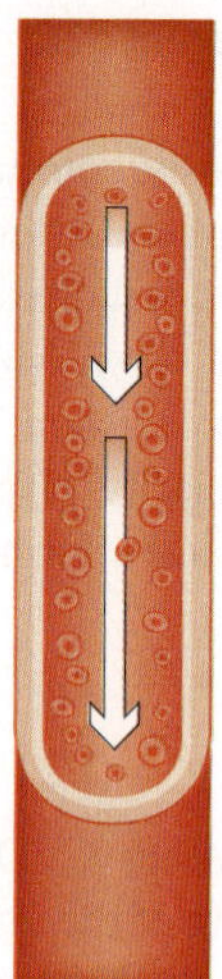

A healthy artery allows blood to flow freely.

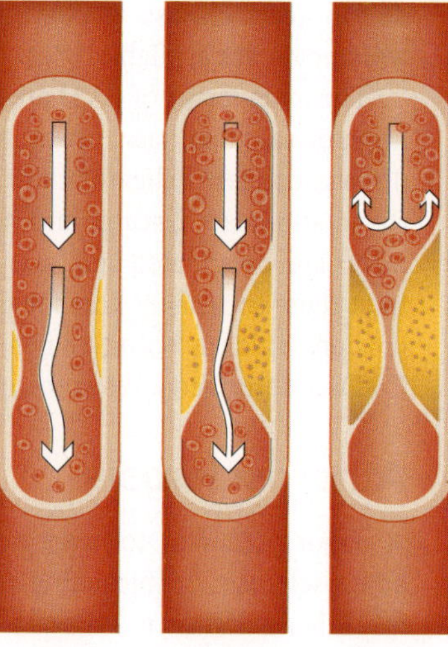

As plaque builds up in the arteries, the inside of the arteries begins to narrow, which lessens or blocks the flow of blood. Plaques can also rupture, causing a blood clot to form on the plaque and blocking the flow of blood.

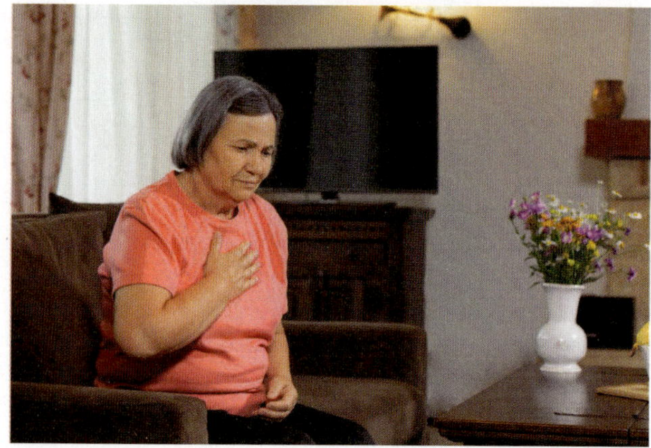

**FIGURE 13.5 Atherosclerosis: The process of cardiovascular disease.**

SOURCE: (left): Centers for Disease Control and Prevention. 2020. Heart Disease Facts. (https://www.cdc.gov/heartdisease/facts.htm) (right): Sanda Stanca/EyeEm/Getty Images

Atherosclerosis often begins in childhood: autopsy studies of young trauma victims have revealed atherosclerosis of the coronary arteries in adolescents. Healthy lifestyles can help delay its progression.

## Coronary Artery Disease and Heart Attack

The most common form of heart disease is CHD caused by atherosclerosis. When one of the coronary arteries becomes blocked, the result is a **heart attack,** or *myocardial infarction* (*MI*). During a heart attack, the heart muscle (the myocardium) is damaged and may die from lack of oxygenated blood. Although a heart attack may come without warning, it usually results from a chronic disease process.

Heart attack symptoms may include chest pain or pressure; arm, neck, or jaw pain; difficulty breathing; excessive sweating; nausea and vomiting; and loss of consciousness.

**TERMS**

**heart attack** Damage to, or death of, heart muscle, resulting from a failure of the coronary arteries to deliver enough blood to the heart; also known as *myocardial infarction (MI).*

**angina pectoris** Pain in the chest, and often in the left arm and shoulder, caused by the heart muscle not receiving enough oxygenated blood. The pain is usually brought on by exercise or stress.

**arrhythmia** A change in the heartbeat's normal, regular pattern.

**sudden cardiac death** A nontraumatic, unexpected death from sudden cardiac arrest, most often due to arrhythmia; in most instances, victims have underlying heart disease.

Most people having a heart attack suffer chest pain, but about one-third of heart attack victims do not. Women, older adults, and people with diabetes and certain forms of CVD are the most likely groups to experience heart attacks without chest pain.

### Angina

Arteries partially narrowed by disease may still be open enough to deliver sufficient amounts of oxygenated blood to the heart. However, during stress or exertion, the heart needs more oxygen than can be supplied by blood flow through narrowed arteries. When the need for oxygen exceeds the supply, chest pain, called **angina pectoris,** may occur.

Angina pain is usually felt as a tightness in the chest and heavy pressure behind the breastbone or in the shoulder, neck, arm, hand, or back. The pain is usually relieved by rest or medicine called nitroglycerin. Angina may be controlled in a number of ways (with drugs and medical procedures), but its course is unpredictable. Over a period ranging from hours to years, the narrowing may go on to full blockage and a heart attack.

### Arrhythmias and Sudden Cardiac Death

The pumping of the heart is controlled by electrical impulses from the sinus node that maintain a regular heartbeat of 60–100 beats per minute. If this electrical conduction system is disrupted, the heart may beat too quickly, too slowly, or in an irregular fashion. These conditions are known as **arrhythmias** and can cause symptoms ranging from imperceptible to severe and even fatal. Some new devices, such as wearable wristwatch heart-rate monitors, can allow for remote, real-time detection of cardiac arrhythmias.

**Sudden cardiac death,** also called *cardiac arrest,* is most often caused by an arrhythmia called *ventricular fibrillation,* a

## WELLNESS ON CAMPUS
# Are College Students at Risk for Heart Attacks?

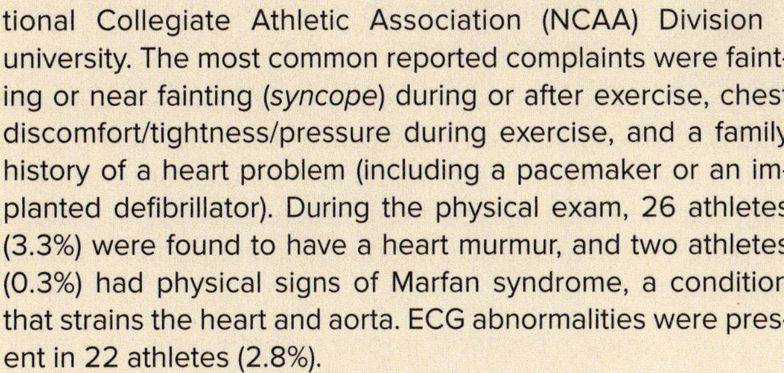

Do you know your blood pressure and cholesterol level? Are you prediabetic? If you don't know, you should find out. Although heart attack and strokes are rare events for college students, they do happen.

The college years are an important time to start looking at factors associated with cardiovascular disease. As adolescents, we think we are at low risk and engage in behaviors that worsen our risk factors. We may skip meals, avoid fruits and vegetables, sit on the couch or at a desk too much, smoke cigarettes, and drink alcohol. Young adults often lack knowledge about risk factors.

With busy schedules, college students often engage in behaviors that promote CVD risk. For some, studying and classes leave little time for physical activity. High-fat snack foods (cookies, cake, chips, and ice cream) often preempt nutrient-dense food (fruits, vegetables, and low-fat dairy foods). Dining halls have improved their nutritional outreach, posting signs about nutrition and offering healthy options, but many also offer all-you-can-eat buffets. College students also tend to gain weight. Men in college consume more fast food at lunch, which may explain why they gain more weight than women.

Men generally are at greater risk for CVD because they have lower HDL cholesterol and higher LDL cholesterol, blood pressure, fasting glucose, and BMI. Young adult males in college also engage in more of the behaviors that put them at risk.

## College Athletes

Sudden cardiac death is the number-one cause of death among college athletes during sports activities. To determine whether they are at risk for CVD, college athletes must undergo a screening examination before they participate in sports. The screening may include a questionnaire about the student's personal and family history, a physical exam, and sometimes an electrocardiogram (ECG or EKG) to detect cardiac abnormalities.

One study analyzed the data from the screening examinations of 790 athletes at a National Collegiate Athletic Association (NCAA) Division I university. The most common reported complaints were fainting or near fainting (*syncope*) during or after exercise, chest discomfort/tightness/pressure during exercise, and a family history of a heart problem (including a pacemaker or an implanted defibrillator). During the physical exam, 26 athletes (3.3%) were found to have a heart murmur, and two athletes (0.3%) had physical signs of Marfan syndrome, a condition that strains the heart and aorta. ECG abnormalities were present in 22 athletes (2.8%).

The study found that a physical examination and the history questionnaires would not have been informative enough without the ECGs. The questionnaires are vague and too broad to catch all students whose risk for sudden cardiac death is high. Although this school did have experience using ECGs, others do not have the physician expertise and institutional resources to properly interpret such tests. The study also found that of all college athletes, male basketball players carry the highest risk for sudden cardiac death.

A heart attack can occur at any age. Because so many young people are overweight or obese, the chances of cardiovascular diseases are greater than in the past.

SOURCES: Abshire, D. A., et al. 2016. Perceptions related to cardiovascular disease risk in Caucasian college males. *American Journal of Men's Health* 10(6): N136–N144; ACLS. 2020. *Cardiac Disease in the Young* (https://www.acls.net/cardiac-disease-in-the-young.htm); De Young, W. 2018. College students may not be as heart-healthy as they think. *The Conversation* (https://theconversation.com/college-students-may-not-be-as-heart-healthy-as-they-think-91730); Drezner, J. A., et al. 2015. Cardiovascular screening in college athletes. *Journal of the American College of Cardiology* 65(21): 2353–2355.

kind of heart rhythm that leads to ineffective blood flow. If ventricular fibrillation continues for more than a few minutes, it is generally fatal. Cardiac defibrillation, in which an electrical shock is delivered to the heart, can be effective in jolting the heart back into a normal rhythm. Training in the use of automated external defibrillators (AEDs) is available from organizations such as the American Red Cross and the American Heart Association. Sudden cardiac death most often occurs in people with CHD, and it occasionally occurs in young people such as college athletes during sports activities (see the box "Are College Students at Risk for Heart Attacks?").

**Helping a Heart Attack Victim** Most deaths from heart attacks occur within two hours of the first onset of symptoms. Unfortunately, many heart attack victims wait more than two hours before getting help. If you or someone you are with shows any of the signs of heart attack listed in the box "Warning Signs and Symptoms of Heart Attack, Stroke, or Cardiac Arrest," take immediate action. Call for help—even if the person denies something is wrong. Many experts also suggest that the heart attack victim *chew* and swallow one adult aspirin tablet (325 mg) as soon as possible after symptoms begin. Aspirin has an immediate anticlotting effect.

If the victim loses consciousness, a qualified person should immediately check for a pulse and, if no pulse is found, start administering emergency **cardiopulmonary resuscitation (CPR).** Another person should call 9-1-1 immediately. Damage to the heart muscle increases with time. If the person receives emergency care quickly enough, a clot-dissolving agent or emergency invasive procedure can be used to break up the clot in the coronary artery.

**TERMS**

**cardiopulmonary resuscitation (CPR)** A technique involving mouth-to-mouth breathing and/or chest compressions to keep oxygen flowing to the brain.

## TAKE CHARGE
## Warning Signs and Symptoms of Heart Attack, Stroke, or Cardiac Arrest

### Heart Attack Warning Signs and Symptoms

The most common symptoms of a heart attack are the following:

- *Chest pain or discomfort* is the most common symptom and is often experienced in the center or left side of the chest that usually lasts for more than a few minutes or goes away and comes back. It can feel like pressure, squeezing, fullness, or pain. It also can feel like heartburn or indigestion. It can be mild or severe.
- *Upper body discomfort* in one or both arms, the back, shoulders, neck, jaw, or upper part of the stomach (above the navel).
- *Shortness of breath* may be the only symptom, or it may occur before or along with chest pain or discomfort. It can occur when you are resting or doing mild physical activity.

But remember these additional facts:

- Heart attacks can start slowly and cause only mild pain or discomfort. Symptoms can be mild or more intense and sudden. Symptoms also may come and go over several hours.
- People who have high blood sugar (diabetes) may have no symptoms or very mild ones. Heart attacks without symptoms or with very mild symptoms are called silent heart attacks.
- Women are somewhat more likely than men to experience shortness of breath; nausea and vomiting; unusual tiredness (sometimes for days); and pain in the back, shoulders, and jaw.
- Other possible symptoms include breaking out in a cold sweat, light-headedness or sudden dizziness, or a change in the pattern of usual symptoms.

The signs and symptoms of a heart attack can develop suddenly or slowly—within hours, days, or weeks of a heart attack. If you think you or someone you know might be having heart attack symptoms or a heart attack, don't ignore it or feel embarrassed to call for help. **Call 9-1-1 right away.** Here's why:

- Acting fast can save a life. Every minute matters. Never delay calling 9-1-1 to do anything you think might help.
- An ambulance is the best and safest way to get to the hospital. Emergency medical services (EMS) personnel start lifesaving treatments right away. People who arrive at the hospital by ambulance often receive faster treatment.
- The 9-1-1 operator or EMS technician can give you advice. You might be told to chew (or crush) and swallow an aspirin, unless there is a medical reason for you not to take one.

### Stroke Warning Signs and Symptoms

The symptoms of stroke happen quickly:

- Sudden numbness or weakness of the face, arm, or leg (especially on one side of the body)
- Sudden confusion, trouble speaking, or understanding speech
- Sudden trouble seeing in one or both eyes
- Sudden trouble walking, dizziness, loss of balance or coordination
- Sudden severe headache with no known cause.

An acronym to help you remember the most common symptoms of a stroke is FAST (facial drooping, arm weakness, speech difficulty, and time to call 9-1-1). If you believe

**Detecting and Treating Heart Disease** Physicians have an expanding array of tools to evaluate the condition of the heart and its arteries. Currently the most common initial screening tool for CHD is the exercise stress test. During an exercise stress test, a patient runs or walks on a treadmill or pedals a stationary cycle while being monitored for abnormalities with an electrocardiogram (ECG). Changes in the heart's electrical activity while under stress can reveal heart problems and restricted blood flow. Exercise testing can also be performed in conjunction with imaging techniques such as nuclear medicine or echocardiography that provide pictures of the heart at or after stress, which can help pinpoint abnormal areas of the heart.

If symptoms or noninvasive tests suggest CHD, the next step is often a coronary **angiogram,** performed in a cardiac catheterization lab. In this test, a catheter (a small plastic tube) is threaded into an artery, usually in the wrist or groin, and advanced through the aorta to the coronary arteries. The catheter is then placed into the opening of the coronary artery and a special dye (contrast) is injected. The dye can be seen moving through the arteries via X-ray, and any narrowing or blockage can be identified. If a problem is found, it is commonly treated with a metal stent or **balloon angioplasty,** which is performed by specially trained cardiologists (Figure 13.6).

Other treatments, ranging from medication to major surgery, are also available. Along with a low-fat, Mediterranean-style diet, regular exercise, and smoking cessation, medical therapy can improve risk factors and biomarkers of health. A statin, or cholesterol-lowering medication, reduces lifetime

**TERMS**

**angiogram** A picture of the arterial system taken after injecting a dye that is opaque to X-rays.

**balloon angioplasty** A technique in which a catheter with a deflated balloon on the tip is inserted into an artery; the balloon is then inflated at the point of obstruction in the artery, pressing the plaque against the artery wall to improve blood supply.

someone is having a stroke, call 9-1-1 immediately. Ischemic strokes, the most common type, can be treated with a drug called t-PA, which dissolves blood clots. The drug must be administered within three hours, but to be evaluated and receive treatment in time, patients must get to the hospital within 60 minutes.

A transient ischemic attack (TIA) has the same signs and symptoms as a stroke. However, TIA symptoms usually last less than 1–2 hours (although they may last up to 24 hours). A TIA may occur only once in a person's lifetime or more often and can be a warning sign for future strokes. At first, it may not be possible to tell whether someone is having a TIA or stroke. All stroke-like symptoms require medical care.

### Sudden Cardiac Arrest Signs

In sudden cardiac arrest (SCA), the heart stops beating suddenly and unexpectedly, so blood stops flowing to the brain and other vital organs. The person suddenly becomes unresponsive and stops breathing, and if they do not receive treatment within minutes, death occurs. Usually, the first sign of SCA is loss of consciousness (fainting). At the same time, no heartbeat (or pulse) can be felt. Some people may have a racing heartbeat or feel dizzy or light-headed just before they faint. Within an hour before SCA, some people experience chest pain, shortness of breath, nausea, or vomiting.

If you are with someone who experiences these symptoms, begin CPR and call 9-1-1 immediately. Rapid treatment of SCA with a defibrillator can be lifesaving. A defibrillator is a device that sends an electric shock to the heart to restore its normal rhythm. Automated external defibrillators (AEDs) can be used by bystanders to save the lives of people who are having SCA. These portable devices often are found in public places, such as shopping malls, golf courses, businesses, airports, airplanes, convention centers, hotels, sports venues, and schools.

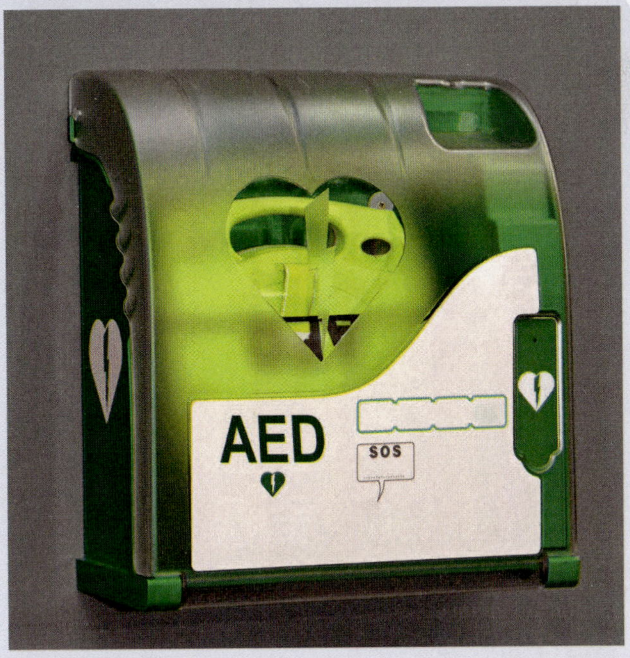

Baloncici/123RF

SOURCES: American Heart Association. 2020. *Heart Attack and Stroke Symptoms* (https://www.heart.org/en/about-us/heart-attack-and-stroke-symptoms); National Institute of Neurological Disorders and Stroke. 2013. *Know Stroke. Know the Signs. Act in Time* (http://stroke.nih.gov/materials/actintime.htm); National Heart, Lung, and Blood Institute. 2016. *What Is Sudden Cardiac Arrest?* (http://www.nhlbi.nih.gov/health-topics/sudden-cardiac-arrest).

risk of CHD by stopping or regressing plaque buildup in the heart arteries. Aspirin helps prevent platelets in the blood from sticking to arterial plaques and forming clots, and it also reduces inflammation.

Other prescription drugs can help control heart rate, dilate arteries, lower blood pressure, and reduce the strain on the heart—improving both the quality and length of life in heart patients. In **coronary bypass surgery,** surgeons remove a healthy blood vessel—usually a vein from the patient's leg—and graft it from the aorta to one or more coronary arteries to bypass a blockage.

## Stroke

For brain cells to function, they require a continuous supply of oxygen-rich blood. If brain cells are deprived of oxygenated blood for more than a few minutes, they will die. A **stroke,** also called a *cerebrovascular accident (CVA),* occurs when the blood supply to the brain is interrupted and brain tissue subsequently dies.

**Types of Strokes** There are two major types of strokes (Figure 13.7), described in the sections that follow.

**ISCHEMIC STROKE** An **ischemic stroke** is caused by a blockage in a blood vessel. There are two types of ischemic strokes: A

**TERMS**

**coronary bypass surgery** Surgery in which a blood vessel is grafted from the aorta to a point below an obstruction in a coronary artery, improving the blood supply to the heart.

**stroke** Impeded blood supply to some part of the brain, resulting in the destruction of brain cells; also called a *cerebrovascular accident (CVA).*

**ischemic stroke** Impeded blood supply to the brain caused by a clot obstructing a blood vessel.

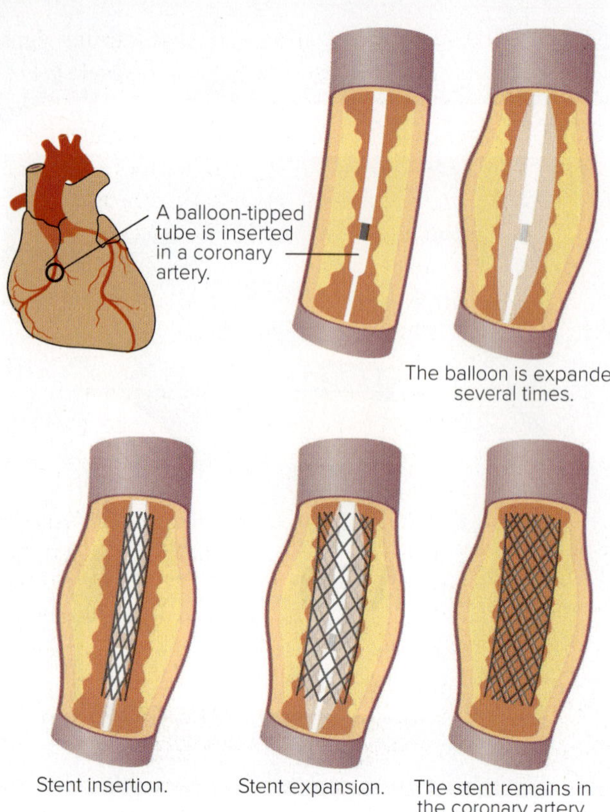


**FIGURE 13.6** **Balloon angioplasty and stenting.**

*thrombotic stroke* is caused by a **thrombus,** which is a blood clot that forms in a cerebral or carotid artery that has been previously narrowed or damaged by atherosclerosis. An *embolic stroke* is caused when an **embolus,** or a wandering blood clot, is carried through the bloodstream and becomes wedged in a cerebral artery. Ischemic strokes account for 87% of all strokes.

**HEMORRHAGIC STROKE** A **hemorrhagic stroke** occurs when a blood vessel in the brain bursts, spilling blood into the surrounding tissue. Cells normally nourished by the vessel are deprived of blood and cannot function. In addition, accumulated blood from the burst vessel may put pressure on surrounding brain tissue, causing damage and even death. There are two types of hemorrhagic strokes: In an *intracerebral hemorrhage,* a blood vessel ruptures within the brain. About 10% of strokes are caused by intracerebral hemorrhages. In a *subarachnoid hemorrhage,* a blood vessel on the brain's surface ruptures and bleeds into the space between the brain and the skull. About 3% of strokes are of this type.

**TERMS**

**thrombus** A blood clot that forms in a blood vessel that has already been damaged by plaque buildup; the clot may lead to stroke.

**embolus** A blood clot that breaks off from its place of origin in a blood vessel and travels through the bloodstream.

**hemorrhagic stroke** Impeded blood supply to the brain caused by the rupture of a blood vessel.

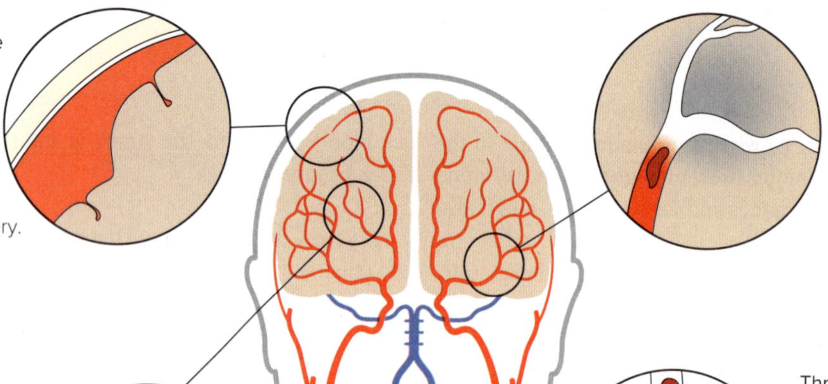
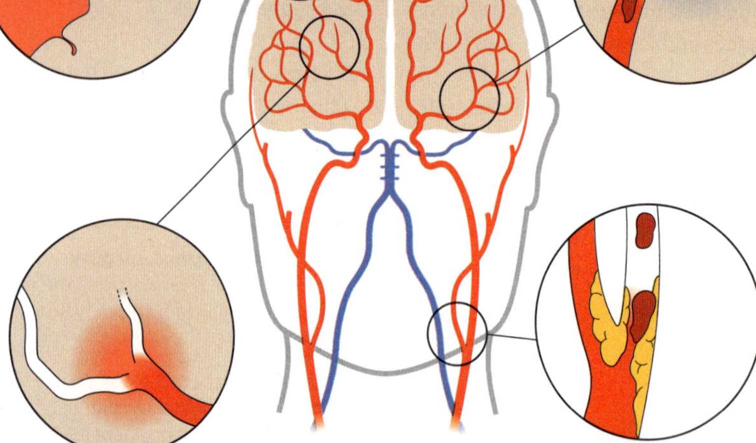


**FIGURE 13.7** **Types of stroke.**

SOURCE: "Harvard Health Letter", Harvard University, April 2000. Artwork by Harriet Greenfield, reprinted with permission.

Hemorrhages can be caused by head injuries or the bursting of a malformed blood vessel, or **aneurysm,** which is a blood-filled pocket that bulges out from a weak spot in the artery wall. Aneurysms in the brain may remain stable and never break. But when they do, the result is a hemorrhagic stroke. Aneurysms may be caused or worsened by hypertension.

**The Effects of a Stroke** The interruption of the blood supply to any area of the brain causes cell death in that region of the brain. Stroke survivors usually have some lasting disability. Which parts of the body are affected depends on the area of the brain that has been damaged. Brain cells control sensation and body movements, and so a stroke may cause paralysis, walking disability, speech impairment, memory loss, or changes in behavior. The severity of the stroke and how long the effects last depend on which brain cells have been injured, how widespread the damage is, how effectively the body can restore the blood supply, and how rapidly other areas of the brain can take over the functions of the damaged areas.

QUICK STATS

**About 795,000 Americans suffer strokes each year—1 every 40 seconds.**

—American Heart Association, 2022

**Detecting and Treating Stroke** Effective treatment requires the prompt recognition of symptoms and correct diagnosis of the type of stroke.

A quick way to recognize a stroke is to ask the person to do four simple things:

1. Ask the person to smile. If their smile droops on one side, or if they are unable to move or open one side of their mouth, they may be having a stroke.
2. Ask the person to hold their arms or legs out. If the person cannot move one arm/leg or hold one arm/leg still, it may be a sign of a stroke.
3. Ask the person to repeat a simple, short sentence, such as "Take me out to the ball game." If they have trouble speaking or cannot speak, a stroke is possible.
4. Ask the person whether they have any decreased sensation, numbness, or abnormal tingling in their legs, arms, or other body parts.

If someone has difficulty performing any of these tests, follow the steps described in the box "Warning Signs and Symptoms of Heart Attack, Stroke, or Cardiac Arrest."

Many people have strokes without knowing it. These "silent strokes" do not cause any noticeable symptoms while they are occurring. Although they may be mild, silent strokes leave their victims at a higher risk for subsequent and more serious strokes. They also contribute to loss of mental and cognitive skills.

Some stroke victims have a **transient ischemic attack (TIA),** or "ministroke," days, weeks, or months before they have a full-blown stroke. A TIA produces temporary stroke-like symptoms, such as weakness or numbness in an arm or a leg, speech difficulty, or dizziness. These symptoms are brief, often lasting just a few minutes, and do not cause permanent damage. TIAs should be taken as warning signs of a stroke, however, and anyone with a suspected TIA should get immediate medical attention.

A person with stroke symptoms should be rushed to the hospital. A **computed tomography (CT)** scan, which uses a computer to construct an image of the brain from X-rays, can assess brain damage and determine the type of stroke. If tests reveal that a stroke is caused by a blood clot—and if help is sought within a few hours of the onset of symptoms—the blockage can be treated with the same kind of clot-dissolving drugs that are used to treat coronary artery blockages. If the clot is dissolved quickly enough, brain damage is minimized and symptoms may disappear.

If detection and treatment of stroke come too late, rehabilitation and prevention of further events is the mainstay of treatment. Although dead brain tissue does not regenerate, nerve cells in the brain can make new pathways and over time regain some motor or speech functions.

Some people recover completely in a matter of days or weeks, but many stroke victims who survive must adapt to some disability.

## Peripheral Arterial Disease

**Peripheral arterial disease (PAD)** refers to atherosclerosis in the leg or arm arteries, which can eventually limit or completely obstruct blood flow. The same process that occurs in the heart arteries can occur in any artery of the body.

The risk of PAD is significantly increased in people with diabetes and people who use tobacco products.

Symptoms of PAD include claudication and a more difficult time fighting infections or healing ulcerations that can form in the leg or foot. *Claudication* is aching or fatigue in the affected leg with exertion, particularly walking, and often resolves with rest. Claudication occurs when leg muscles do not get adequate blood and oxygen supply. *Rest pain* occurs when the limb artery is unable to supply adequate blood and oxygen even when the body is not physically active. This occurs when the artery is significantly narrowed or completely blocked. If blood flow is not restored quickly, cells and tissues

TERMS

**aneurysm** A sac or outpouching formed by a distention or dilation of the artery wall.

**transient ischemic attack (TIA)** A small stroke; usually a temporary interruption of blood supply to the brain, causing numbness or difficulty with speech.

**computed tomography (CT)** The use of computerized X-ray images to create a cross-sectional depiction (scan) of tissue density.

**peripheral arterial disease (PAD)** Atherosclerosis in the arteries in the legs (or less commonly, the arms) that can impede blood flow and lead to pain, infection, and loss of the affected limb.

die; in severe cases, amputation may be needed. PAD is the leading cause of amputation in people over age 50. The likelihood of needing an amputation is increased in those who continue to use tobacco products, and PAD in people with diabetes tends to be extensive and severe.

## Congestive Heart Failure

With weakening of the heart muscle, the heart cannot maintain its regular pumping rate and force, and this can cause fluid buildup, an indication of **congestive heart failure** or **cardiomyopathy.** When extra fluid seeps through capillary walls, edema (swelling) results, usually in the legs and ankles, but sometimes in other parts of the body as well. Fluid can collect in the lungs and interfere with breathing, particularly when a person is lying down. This condition is called **pulmonary edema.**

Treatment includes reducing the workload on the heart, modifying fluid and salt intake, and using drugs that help the body eliminate excess fluid. Heart transplant can be a solution for some patients with severe heart failure, but the need greatly exceeds the number of donor hearts available. About 5.7 million Americans suffer from heart failure.

The risk of heart failure increases with age, and being overweight is a significant independent risk factor. Experts suggest that the incidence of heart failure will increase dramatically over the next few decades as our population ages and becomes increasingly obese.

## Other Forms of Heart Disease

Other, less common, forms of heart disease include congenital heart defects, rheumatic heart disease, and heart valve disorders.

### Congenital Heart Defects

About 1% of births each year in America, equivalent to 40,000 children, have a defect or malformation of the heart or major blood vessels. These conditions are collectively referred to as **congenital heart defects,** and they cause nearly 13,500 deaths a year in children under 1 year of age. Most common congenital defects can be accurately diagnosed and treated with medication or surgery. The most common congenital defects are holes in the wall that divides the chambers of the heart, which can cause mixing of oxygenated and deoxygenated blood and ineffective circulation. Another common defect is *coarctation of the aorta*—a narrowing, or constriction, of the aorta.

**Hypertrophic cardiomyopathy** occurs in approximately 1 out of every 500 people in the United States and is the most common cause of sudden death among athletes younger than age 35. This disease is characterized by an unusually thick, or hypertrophied, heart muscle, which can lead to ineffective blood flow to the body and abnormal heart rhythms. People with hypertrophic cardiomyopathy are at high risk for sudden death, mainly due to serious arrhythmias. Hypertrophic cardiomyopathy is most commonly diagnosed using echocardiography. Possible treatments include medications, surgery to reduce the thickened heart muscle, and even an implanted internal defibrillator for patients at high risk of sudden cardiac death.

### Rheumatic Heart Disease

**Rheumatic fever,** a consequence of certain types of untreated streptococcal throat infections, is a leading cause of heart failure worldwide, but is relatively uncommon in the United States. Rheumatic fever can permanently damage the heart muscle and heart valves, a condition called *rheumatic heart disease (RHD).* Symptoms of strep throat include the sudden onset of a sore throat, painful swallowing, fever, swollen glands, headache, nausea, and vomiting. If left untreated, up to 3% of strep infections progress into rheumatic fever. Rheumatic fever affects primarily children between the ages of 5 and 15 years.

### Heart Valve Disorders

Age, previous heart attacks, congenital defects, and certain types of infections can cause abnormalities in the valves between the chambers of the heart. Heart valve problems generally fall into two categories—the valve failing to open fully or failing to close completely. In either case, blood flow through the heart is impaired.

The most common heart valve disorder is **mitral valve prolapse (MVP),** which occurs in about 3% of the population. MVP is characterized by a billowing of the mitral valve, which separates the left ventricle and left atrium, during ventricular

### Ask Yourself

**QUESTIONS FOR CRITICAL THINKING AND REFLECTION**

Has anyone you know ever had a heart attack? If so, was the onset gradual or sudden? Were appropriate steps taken to help the person (for example, did anyone call 9-1-1, give CPR, or use an AED)? Do you feel comfortable dealing with a cardiac emergency? If not, what can you do to improve your readiness?

### TERMS

**congestive heart failure (cardiomyopathy)** A condition resulting from the heart's inability to pump enough blood to keep up with the body's metabolic needs; blood backs up in the veins leading to the heart, causing an accumulation of fluid in various parts of the body.

**pulmonary edema** The accumulation of fluid in the lungs.

**congenital heart defect** A defect or malformation of the heart or its major blood vessels, present at birth.

**hypertrophic cardiomyopathy** An inherited condition in which there is an enlargement of the heart muscle, especially the muscle between the two ventricles.

**rheumatic fever** A disease, mainly of children, characterized by fever, inflammation, and pain in the joints. It often damages the heart valves and muscle, a condition called rheumatic heart disease.

**mitral valve prolapse (MVP)** A condition in which the mitral valve billows out during ventricular contraction, allowing leakage of blood from the left ventricle into the left atrium.

contraction. In severe cases, blood leaks backward from the ventricle into the atrium and the heart has to work harder for the same amount of forward blood flow. Most people with MVP have no symptoms and need no treatment.

## RISK FACTORS FOR CARDIOVASCULAR DISEASE

Factors associated with an increased risk of developing cardiovascular disease are grouped into two main categories: major risk factors and contributing risk factors. Some lifestyle risk factors can therefore be changed; these are called modifiable risk factors. Others are beyond our control, while some require more research to fully understand. To prevent heart disease later in life, it is very important to establish healthy eating and exercise habits at a young age.

### Major Risk Factors That Can Be Changed

The American Heart Association (AHA) identifies certain factors that can increase the risk of developing CVD. Those that can be changed include tobacco use, high blood pressure, unhealthy blood cholesterol levels, physical inactivity, obesity, and diabetes. Diet is important, too. Most Americans, including young adults, have at least one major risk factor for CVD.

**Tobacco Use** Annually, nearly one in five deaths can be attributed to smoking. People who smoke a pack of cigarettes a day have twice the risk of heart attack faced by nonsmokers; smoking two or more packs a day triples the risk. When smokers have heart attacks, they are two to three times more likely than nonsmokers to die from them. Cigarette smoking also doubles the risk of stroke.

**High Blood Pressure** High blood pressure, or **hypertension,** is a risk factor for many forms of cardiovascular disease, including heart attacks and stroke.

Blood pressure, the force exerted by the blood on the vessel walls, is created by the pumping action of the heart and the resistance of the arteries. High blood pressure occurs when too much force is exerted against the walls of the arteries. Many factors affect blood pressure, such as exercise or excitement. Short periods of high blood pressure are normal, but chronic high blood pressure is a health risk.

Health care professionals measure blood pressure with a stethoscope and an instrument called a *sphygmomanometer.*

**Ask Yourself**

**QUESTIONS FOR CRITICAL THINKING AND REFLECTION**

How often do you think about the health of your heart? Do certain situations make you aware of your heart rate, or make you wonder how strong your heart is?

**Table 13.1 Blood Pressure Classification for Healthy Adults**

| CATEGORY[a] | SYSTOLIC (mm Hg) | | DIASTOLIC (mm Hg) |
|---|---|---|---|
| Normal[b] | below 120 | and | below 80 |
| Elevated | 120–129 | and | below 80 |
| Hypertension[c] | | | |
| Stage 1 | 130–139 | or | 80–89 |
| Stage 2 | at least 140 | or | at least 90 |

[a]When systolic and diastolic pressures fall into different categories, the higher category should be used to classify blood pressure status.

[b]The risk of death from heart attack and stroke begins to rise when blood pressure is above 115/75.

[c]Based on the average of two or more readings taken at different physician visits. In people older than 50, systolic blood pressure greater than 140 mm Hg is a much more significant CVD risk factor than diastolic blood pressure.

SOURCE: Whelton, P. et al. 2018. 2017 ACC/AHA/AAPA/ABC/ACPM/AGS/APhA/ASH/ASPC/NMA/PCNA Guideline for the prevention, detection, evaluation, and management of high blood pressure in adults: A report of the American College of Cardiology/American Heart Association Task Force on Clinical Practice Guidelines. *Journal of the American College of Cardiology* (71)6: e13–e115.

At home you can track your own blood pressure by using an electronic blood pressure monitor, and new technologies can measure blood pressure using wearable devices (see box "Digital Health Approach to Cardiovascular Disease"). A normal blood pressure reading for a healthy adult is below 120 mm Hg systolic and below 80 mm Hg diastolic (Table 13.1).

**HEALTH RISKS** High blood pressure is called a silent killer because it usually has no symptoms. A person may have high blood pressure for years without realizing it. But during that time, it slowly damages vital organs and increases the risk of heart attack, congestive heart failure, stroke, kidney failure, and blindness. The risk of death from heart attack or stroke begins to rise even within the "normal" range when blood pressure is above 120 over 80 mm Hg, with a significant focus by doctors on targeting lower blood pressures than goals used in the past. People with blood pressure in the range referred to as elevated are at increased risk of heart attack and stroke.

An appropriate blood pressure target for risk reduction may depend on a person's age and other risk factors for cardiovascular disease. Traditionally, the treatment target was to reduce blood pressure below the cutoff for hypertension (140 over 90 mm Hg). However, a panel of experts recently reviewed all current trials and published updated guidelines in late 2017. Available data show that intensive blood pressure control with

**TERMS**

**hypertension** Sustained abnormally high blood pressure.

## TAKE CHARGE
## Digital Health Approach to Cardiovascular Disease

### Online Information

Online health information is changing the relationship between physicians and patients. Online references, patient communities, review sites, and electronic social networks have empowered patients to better understand their health and their health care choices.

Some cardiovascular diseases flare up quickly or allow but a brief time to attempt treatment, so a digital health approach could be especially useful. How can technology help detect diseases and make medical treatment more precise and individualized? A recent collaboration between Apple and Stanford University evaluated a smartwatch-based sensor for irregular heart rate and screening of atrial fibrillation. Because wearing a watch is convenient, the study could enroll over 400,000 participants in 8 months. When the algorithm detected an irregular heart rate, patients were immediately notified to see a physician about possible atrial fibrillation. This otherwise clinically silent condition could now be acted on immediately—patients could initiate treatment and reduce their risk of stroke.

### Ambient Sensor Data

Managing chronic diseases also demands digital health interventions. We can keep tabs on our conditions through internet-connected scales, blood pressure cuffs, and other devices that are also available to health care professionals. They allow for more frequent checks to track progress and change. These devices also make measurements in our natural environments, instead of in a doctor's office. Currently, large health care systems such as the Veterans Health Administration and Kaiser Permanente Health Plan are implementing such devices for chronic disease management. Since the start of the Covid-19 pandemic, the Centers for Medicare and Medicaid Services (CMS) made a change to allow Medicare reimbursement for telehealth visits. This prompted a dramatic increase, from 13,000 to 1.7 million Medicare beneficiaries per week using telemedicine.

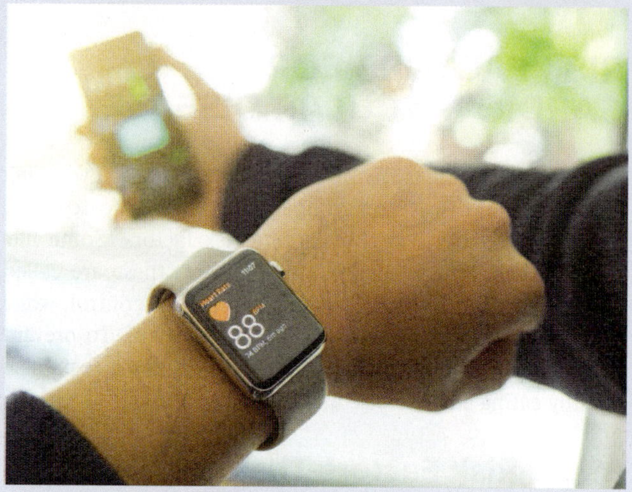


KANUT PHOTO/Shutterstock

### Patient-Generated Health Data

Devices communicate with health care providers and also help us generate our own health data. Various smartphone applications, smartwatches, and other wearables provide information ranging from activity levels, ambient noise measurements, and menstrual cycle tracking to heart rate, food consumption, continuous blood glucose monitoring, and blood pressure measurements. Given the strong relationships among cardiovascular disease, lifestyle, and chronic disease, our self-generated data can be essential in making medical decisions and tracking progress in lifestyle modifications. In a pre–Covid-19 pandemic national survey, 56% of individuals reported sharing their health tracking data with physicians.

SOURCE: Perez, M. V., et al. 2019. Large-scale assessment of a smartwatch to identify atrial fibrillation. *New England Journal of Medicine* 381: 1909–1917; Day, S., et al. 2019. Digital Health Consumer Adoption Report 2019. *Stanford Medicine Center for Digital Health and Rock Health Report.* Verma, S. 2020. Early impact of CMS expansion of Medicare telehealth during COVID-19. *Health Affairs* (https://www.healthaffairs.org/do/10.1377/hblog20200715.454789/full/).

new, lower targets (systolic pressure below 120 mm Hg) reduces the risk of heart attack, stroke, and death. Future research may help identify criteria to set more individualized blood pressure targets for each person.

**PREVALENCE** Hypertension is common. Under the newly updated blood pressure guidelines, about 46% of adults have hypertension (defined as systolic pressure of 120–129 mm Hg and diastolic pressure of less than 80 mm Hg). The incidence of high blood pressure increases with age, but it does occur among overweight children and young adults. Women can sometimes develop hypertension during pregnancy (after which the blood pressure will usually return to normal). High blood pressure is also more common in women taking oral contraceptives, especially in obese and older women and women who have used oral contraceptives for a long time.

> QUICK STATS
>
> **About half of U.S. adults have high blood pressure; only a quarter have it under control.**
>
> —Centers for Disease Control and Prevention, 2021

**TREATMENT** Currently, primary hypertension cannot be cured, but it can be controlled and managed. Because hypertension has no early warning signs, it is crucial to have your blood pressure tested at least once every two years (and more often if you have other CVD risk factors). Experts advise anyone with elevated blood pressure to monitor their blood pressure several times each week.

Lifestyle changes are recommended for everyone with hypertension. These changes include weight reduction, regular exercise, a healthy diet, and moderation of salt and alcohol use. The DASH diet (see Chapter 10) is recommended specifically for people with high blood pressure.

Nearly 80% of dietary salt in the typical American diet is found in processed food and drinks. It follows, then, that the easiest way to achieve population-wide reduction is for the food industry to lower the amount of salt added to food products. Reductions in supplemental salt in restaurant food have also been suggested; some cities now require warnings listed on dishes with high amounts of sodium. Self-prepared meals offer the greatest control over dietary salt intake. For people whose blood pressure is not adequately controlled with lifestyle changes, medication can be prescribed.

### High Cholesterol

*Cholesterol* is a fatty, waxlike substance that circulates through the bloodstream. It is an important component of cell membranes, sex hormones, vitamin D, the fluid that coats the lungs, and the protective sheaths around nerves. Adequate cholesterol is essential for the proper functioning of the body. Excess cholesterol, however, can clog arteries and increase the risk of CVD. There are two primary sources of cholesterol: the liver, which manufactures it, and dietary sources.

**GOOD VERSUS BAD CHOLESTEROL** Cholesterol is carried in the blood in protein-and-lipid packages called **lipoproteins.** Two types of lipoproteins influence an individual's risk of heart disease. **Low-density lipoproteins (LDLs)** (18–27 nm) shuttle cholesterol from the liver to the organs and tissues that require it. LDLs are known as "bad" cholesterol because, if the body has more than it can use, the excess cholesterol is deposited in the blood vessels. They can then be oxidized by free radicals, which speeds inflammation and damage to artery walls and increases the likelihood of a blockage. Recently discovered medications, called PCSK9 inhibitors, target the liver's handling of LDL cholesterol and greatly reduce blood LDL cholesterol levels, thus reducing the risk of heart attacks and strokes. **High-density lipoproteins (HDLs)** are "good" cholesterol. They shuttle unused cholesterol back to the liver for recycling. By removing cholesterol from blood vessels, HDLs help protect against atherosclerosis.

**BLOOD CHOLESTEROL GUIDELINES** An estimated 95 million American adults have total cholesterol levels of 200 mg/dl or higher (see Table 13.2). The recommended screening test measures total cholesterol, LDL cholesterol, HDL cholesterol, and triglycerides (another blood fat). It is recommended once every five years for all adults, beginning at age 20.

In general, high LDL, total cholesterol, and triglyceride levels, combined with low HDL levels, are associated with a higher risk for CVD. You can reduce this risk by lowering LDL, total cholesterol, and triglycerides. Raising HDL may be important because high HDL levels seem to offer protection from CVD even in cases where total cholesterol is high. This appears to be especially true for women.

The 2013 ACC and AHA guidelines on the treatment of high blood cholesterol recommend evaluation of a person's risk of developing atherosclerotic cardiovascular disease over the next 10 years (ASCVD risk), and treatment based on a risk score.

In 2018, the ACC/AHA updated the guidelines to incorporate an LDL goal of less than 70 mg/dl for patients at very high ASCVD risk. Patients with borderline ASCVD risk scores should have the extent of coronary artery calcium evaluated on CT scans. The guidelines also offer recommendations for people to modify their lifestyles either prior to developing or while already suffering from high cholesterol. These lifestyle guidelines include maintaining a healthy diet, engaging in regular aerobic exercise, avoiding tobacco products, and maintaining a healthy weight. These recommendations are vitally important

**Table 13.2 People Who Benefit from Treatment of High Cholesterol**

| |
|---|
| 1. People aged 75 and under with known cardiovascular disease, including previous heart attacks, chest pain due to partially clogged arteries, history of invasive treatment for clogged arteries, previous stroke, or previous clogged arteries in the limbs. |
| 2. People aged 21 and over with high LDL levels, 190 mg/dl or greater. |
| 3. People aged 40–75 with a history of diabetes, an LDL level 70–189 mg/dl, and no known history of cardiovascular disease. |
| 4. People aged 40–75 without diabetes or known cardiovascular disease but with a high risk of developing it over the next 10 years and an LDL level over 70 mg/dl.* |

*10-year cardiovascular risk is calculated using a tool available on the AHA website (https://professional.heart.org/professional/GuidelinesStatements/ASCVDRiskCalculator/UCM_457698_ASCVD-Risk-Calculator.jsp).

SOURCES: Stone, N.J., et al. 2013 ACC/AHA guideline on the treatment of blood cholesterol to reduce atherosclerotic cardiovascular risk in adults. *Journal of the American College of Cardiology* 63(25): 2889–2934.

**TERMS**

**lipoproteins** Protein and lipid substances in the blood that carry fats and cholesterol; classified according to size, density, and chemical composition.

**low-density lipoprotein (LDL)** A lipoprotein containing a moderate amount of protein and a large amount of cholesterol, which tends to become deposited on artery walls and increase the risk of heart disease; also known as "bad" cholesterol.

**high-density lipoprotein (HDL)** A lipoprotein containing relatively little cholesterol that helps transport cholesterol out of the arteries and thus protects against heart diseases; also known as "good" cholesterol.

in managing the risk of CVD and are often the first step in managing high cholesterol—before any medications are prescribed.

If lifestyle modifications have not adequately lowered cholesterol levels, statin therapy is recommended at different intensity doses. *High-intensity* therapy is defined as a statin dosage that reduces the LDL level by greater than or equal to 50%, whereas *moderate-intensity* therapy reduces LDL level by 30–50%. Statins may also decrease CVD risk even in those without high cholesterol levels. Of course, with any medication, side effects must be weighed against the potential benefits. The primary side effect seen with statins is muscle cramping, or muscle inflammation, which is usually mild and can be avoided by switching to a different kind of statin.

**BENEFITS OF CONTROLLING CHOLESTEROL** Some studies have shown that people can cut their heart attack risk by about 2% for every 1% that they reduce their total blood cholesterol levels. Current research indicates that treating elevated LDL and raising HDL levels not only reduces the likelihood that arteries will become clogged but also may reverse deposits on artery walls.

### Physical Inactivity

An estimated 40–60 million Americans are sedentary and at high risk for developing CVD. Exercise is a key component in the fight against heart disease. Exercise lowers CVD risk by helping to decrease blood pressure and resting heart rate, increase HDL levels, maintain desirable weight, improve the condition of blood vessels, and prevent or control diabetes. One study found that women who accumulated at least three hours of brisk walking each week cut their risk of heart attack and stroke by more than 50%.

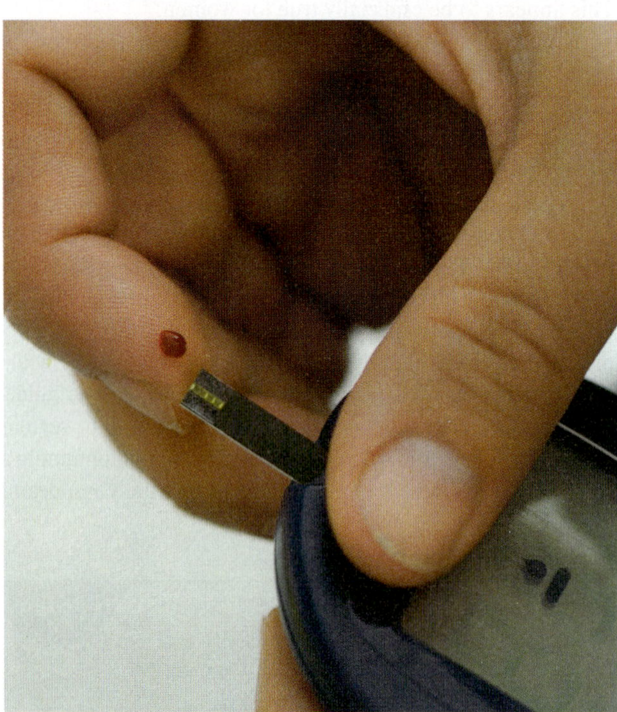

Blood glucose monitoring is important in managing diabetes and its associated risks. Michael Krasowitz/Photographer's Choice/Getty Images

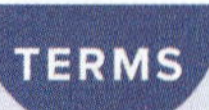

**TERMS**

**body mass index (BMI)** A calculated measure of human body shape; the ratio of mass (in kilograms) divided by height (in meters) squared: weight/height$^2$

### Obesity

As your weight increases, your risk of CVD increases. Death from CVD is two to three times more likely in obese people (**body mass index, or BMI** $\geq$ 30) than it is in lean people (BMI = 18.5–24.9), and for every 5-unit increase in BMI, a person's risk of death from coronary heart disease increases by 30%. The higher your BMI at age 18, the more likely you will eventually die from CVD.

### Insulin Resistance and Metabolic Syndrome

As people gain weight and become less active, their muscles, fat, and liver become less sensitive to the effect of insulin—a condition known as *insulin resistance*. As the body becomes increasingly insulin resistant, the pancreas must secrete more and more insulin (hyperinsulinemia) to keep glucose levels within a normal range. Eventually even high levels of insulin may become insufficient, and blood glucose levels start to rise (hyperglycemia), setting the stage for prediabetes and, if not addressed, eventually for type 2 diabetes.

Those who have insulin resistance tend to have several other related risk factors. This cluster of abnormalities is called *metabolic syndrome* or *insulin resistance syndrome* (Table 13.3). Metabolic syndrome significantly increases the risk of CVD—more so in women than in men. It is estimated that about 34% of the adult U.S. population has metabolic syndrome.

**Table 13.3** Characteristics of Metabolic Syndrome*

| FACTOR | CRITERIA |
|---|---|
| Large waistline (abdominal obesity) | 35 or more inches (88 cm) for women<br>40 or more inches (102 cm) for men |
| High triglyceride level | 150 mg/dl or higher<br>Or taking medication to treat high triglycerides |
| Low HDL level | Less than 50 mg/dl for women<br>Less than 40 mg/dl for men<br>Or taking medication to treat low HDL |
| High blood pressure | 130/85 mm Hg or higher (one or both numbers)<br>Or taking medication to treat high blood pressure |
| High fasting blood sugar | 100 mg/dl or higher<br>Or taking medication to treat high blood sugar |

*A person having three or more factors listed here is diagnosed with metabolic syndrome.

SOURCE: Adapted from National Heart, Lung, and Blood Institute 2015. *How Is Metabolic Syndrome Diagnosed?* (http://www.nhlbi.nih.gov/health/health-topics/topics/ms/diagnosis).

To reduce your risk of developing metabolic syndrome, choose a healthy diet and get plenty of aerobic exercise. Regular physical activity increases your body's sensitivity to insulin, improves cholesterol levels, and decreases blood pressure. Reducing calorie intake to prevent weight gain or losing weight if needed also reduces insulin resistance. The amount and type of carbohydrate intake is also important. Diets high in simple carbohydrates, such as white sugar and white flour (high-glycemic-index foods), can raise levels of glucose and triglycerides while lowering HDL, thus contributing to metabolic syndrome and CVD. This is particularly true for people who are already sedentary and overweight. For people prone to insulin resistance, eating more protein, vegetables, and fiber while limiting fat, added sugars, and starches may be beneficial.

**Diabetes** As described in Chapter 12, *diabetes mellitus* is a disorder characterized by elevated blood glucose levels due to an insufficient supply of insulin or inadequate response to insulin. Diabetes doubles the risk of CVD for men and triples the risk for women. The most common cause of death in adults with diabetes is CVD.

People with diabetes have higher rates of other CVD risk factors, including hypertension, obesity, and unhealthy blood lipid levels (typically, high triglyceride levels and low HDL levels). The elevated blood glucose and insulin levels that occur in diabetes can damage the endothelial cells that line the arteries, making them more vulnerable to atherosclerosis. Diabetics also often have platelet and blood coagulation abnormalities that increase the risk of heart attack and stroke. People with prediabetes (when the blood sugar levels are elevated but not high enough to diagnose diabetes) also face an increased risk of CVD.

In people with prediabetes, a healthy diet and exercise are the most effective tools in preventing diabetes. For people with diabetes, a healthy diet, exercise, and careful control of glucose levels are recommended to reduce the chances of developing complications. Even people whose diabetes is under control face a high risk of CVD, so control of other risk factors is critical.

QUICK STATS

**24% of men and 22% of women have metabolic syndrome.**

— National Library of Medicine, 2021

## Contributing Risk Factors That Can Be Changed

Other cardiovascular disease risk factors that can be changed include triglyceride levels, metabolic syndrome, inflammation, psychological and social factors, and alcohol and drug use.

**High Triglyceride Levels** Like cholesterol, **triglycerides** are blood fats that are obtained from food and manufactured by the body. High triglyceride levels are a reliable predictor of heart disease, especially if associated with other risk factors, such as low HDL levels, obesity, and diabetes. Factors contributing to elevated triglyceride levels include excess body fat, physical inactivity, cigarette smoking, type 2 diabetes, excessive alcohol intake, very high-carbohydrate diets, and certain diseases and medications.

For people with borderline high triglyceride levels, increased physical activity, reduced intake of added sugars, and weight reduction can help bring levels down into the healthy range. For people with high triglyceride levels, drug therapy with the addition of omega-3 fatty acids (found in fish) or fibrates may be recommended if initial strategies are ineffective.

**Inflammation** Inflammation plays a key role in the development of CVD. When an artery is injured by hypertension, smoking, cholesterol, or other factors, the body's response is to produce inflammation. A substance called *C-reactive protein (CRP)* is released into the bloodstream during the inflammatory response, and high levels of CRP indicate an elevated risk of heart attack and stroke. It has also been proposed that CRP by itself may harm the coronary arteries. Gum disease involves another type of inflammation that may moderately influence the progress of heart disease. Lifestyle changes and certain drugs can reduce CRP levels.

**Psychological and Social Factors** Many of the psychological and social factors that influence other areas of wellness are also important risk factors for CVD.

**STRESS** Excessive stress can strain the heart and blood vessels over time and contribute to CVD. When you experience stress, stress hormones activate the sympathetic nervous system. As described in Chapter 2, the sympathetic nervous system causes the fight, flight, or freeze response. This response increases heart rate and blood pressure so that more blood is distributed to the heart and other muscles in anticipation of physical activity. Blood glucose concentrations and cholesterol also increase to provide a source of energy, and the platelets become activated so that they will be more likely to clot in case of injury. If you are healthy, you can tolerate the cardiovascular responses that take place during stress. But if you already have CVD, stress can lead to adverse outcomes such as abnormal heart rhythms (arrhythmias) and heart attacks.

**CHRONIC HOSTILITY AND ANGER** Certain traits in a hard-driving personality—hostility, cynicism, and anger—are associated with increased risk of heart disease.

**DEPRESSION** Depression is common in people with coronary heart disease (CHD). People with depression may be more likely to smoke or be sedentary. They may not

TERMS

**triglyceride** A type of blood fat that can be a predictor of heart disease.

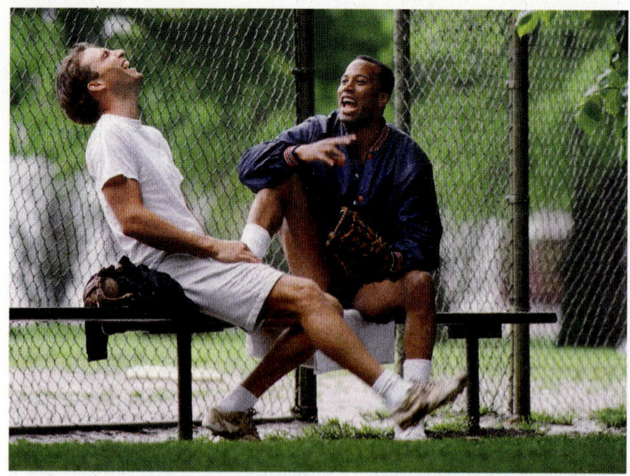

A strong social support network is a major antidote to stress and can help promote and support a healthy lifestyle that includes opportunities for exercise and relaxation. Corbis/Alamy Stock Photo

consistently take prescribed medications, and they may not cope well with having an illness or undergoing a medical procedure. Depression also causes physiological changes; for example, it elevates basal levels of stress hormones, which induce a variety of stress-related responses.

**ANXIETY** Evidence suggests that chronic anxiety and anxiety disorders (such as phobias and panic disorder) are associated with up to a threefold increased risk of CHD, heart attack, and sudden cardiac death. There is also some evidence that, similar to people with depression, people with anxiety are more likely to have a subsequent adverse cardiac event after having a heart attack.

**SOCIAL ISOLATION** Social isolation and low social support (living alone, or having few friends or family members) are associated with an increased incidence of CHD and poorer outcomes after the first diagnosis of CHD. Elderly men and women who report less emotional support from others before they have a heart attack are almost three times more likely to die in the first six months after the heart attack. A strong social support network is a major antidote to stress. Friends and family members can also promote and support a healthy lifestyle.

**LOW SOCIOECONOMIC STATUS** Low socioeconomic status and educational attainment are social factors associated with an increased risk of CVD. These complex associations are likely due to a variety of factors, including lifestyle, diet, and access to health care, among others.

**Alcohol and Drugs** Excessive drinking raises blood pressure and can increase the risk of stroke and heart failure. Stimulant drugs, particularly cocaine and methamphetamines—and associated stimulants, such as designer drugs including Ecstasy (MDMA)—can also cause serious cardiac problems, including heart attack, stroke, and sudden cardiac death. See Chapters 8 and 9 for more information about the use of alcohol and drugs.

## Major Risk Factors That Can't Be Changed

A number of major risk factors for cardiovascular disease cannot be changed. These include family history of CVD (genetics), aging, male gender, and ethnicity.

**Genetics** Multiple genes contribute to the development of CVD—and its associated risk factors, such as high cholesterol, hypertension, diabetes, and obesity. Having favorable genes decreases your risk of developing CVD; having an unfavorable set of genes increases your risk.

It is important to let your doctor know of any history of heart disease in your relatives.

**Age** About 70% of all heart attack victims are aged 65 and over, and about 80% who suffer fatal heart attacks are over 65. For people over 55, the incidence of stroke more than doubles in each successive decade. However, even people in their thirties and forties, especially men, can have heart attacks.

**Gender** Although CVD is the leading killer of both men and women in the United States, men face a greater risk of heart attack than women earlier in life. Until age 55, men also have a greater risk of hypertension. The incidence of stroke is also higher for males than females, until age 65. Estrogen production, which is highest during the childbearing years, may protect against CVD in premenopausal women. By age 75, however, this gender gap nearly disappears.

**Race and Ethnicity** Rates of heart disease vary among racial and ethnic groups in the United States, with African Americans having much higher rates of hypertension, heart disease, and stroke than other groups (see the box "Gender, Race/Ethnicity, and Cardiovascular Disease").

A complication to all this information is growing awareness of race bias throughout the history of scientific studies. Because these populations are heterogeneous, we cannot use racial and ethnic categories easily. Also problematic is attributing cardiovascular health issues to genetics when environmental factors may play a greater role in explaining disease.

## Possible Risk Factors Currently Being Studied

In recent years, other possible risk factors for cardiovascular disease have been identified. Homocysteine levels track with stress and inflammation. Homocysteine appears to damage the lining of blood vessels, resulting in inflammation and the development of fatty deposits in artery walls. These changes can lead to the formation of clots and blockages in arteries.

Several infectious agents have been identified as possible culprits in the development of CVD. *Chlamydia pneumoniae,* a common cause of flu-like respiratory infections, has been found in sections of clogged, damaged arteries but not in

# DIVERSITY MATTERS

## Gender, Race/Ethnicity, and Cardiovascular Disease

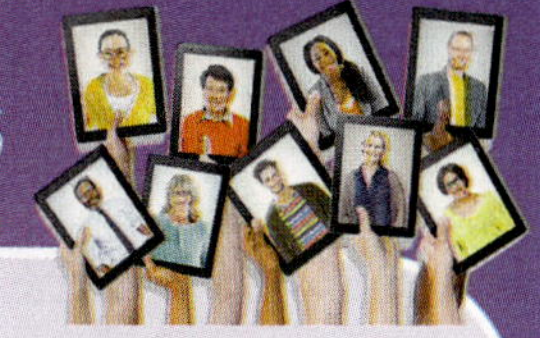

Cardiovascular disease is the leading cause of death for all Americans, but differences exist between men and women and among racial/ethnic groups in the incidence, diagnosis, and treatment of this deadly disease.

### CVD in Women

CVD has been thought of as a "man's disease," but it actually kills more women than men. Polls indicate that women vastly underestimate their risk of dying of a heart attack and overestimate their risk of dying of breast cancer. Approximately 1 in 4 women dies of CVD, whereas 1 in 38 dies of breast cancer. And although CVD typically does not develop in women younger than age 50, recent research suggests that the number of CVD deaths in women aged 35–45 may be increasing.

The hormone estrogen, produced naturally by a woman's ovaries until menopause, improves blood lipid concentrations and reduces other CVD risk factors. For several decades, many physicians encouraged menopausal women to take hormone therapy (HT), which includes estrogen, to relieve menopause symptoms and presumably to reduce their risk of CVD. However, some studies found that HT may actually *increase* a woman's risk for heart disease and other health problems, including breast cancer. However, these studies were mostly in women older than 60 years. Further analysis of old studies and newer studies revealed that the increased risk of CVD in women who started HT was age dependent; women in the early stages of menopause or ages 50–59 did not appear to have excess risk. These findings suggest that outcomes may depend on several factors, including the timing of hormone use. The U.S. Preventive Services Task Force and the American Heart Association recommend that HT not be used to protect against CVD.

When women have heart attacks, they are more likely than men to die within a year and are less likely than men to report the usual symptoms of a heart attack, such as chest pain. Additionally, women are likely to report fewer specific symptoms, which may obscure the diagnosis. These symptoms include fatigue; weakness; shortness of breath; nausea; vomiting; and pain in the abdomen, neck, jaw, and back. Women are also more likely to have pain at rest, during sleep, or with mental stress. A woman who experiences these symptoms should be persistent in seeking accurate diagnosis and appropriate treatment.

Careful diagnosis of cardiac symptoms is also key in avoiding unnecessary invasive procedures in cases of stress cardiomyopathy ("broken heart syndrome"), which occurs much more commonly in women than in men. The exact cause is unknown, but it is thought that hormones and neurotransmitters associated with a severe stress response stun the heart, producing heart-attack-like symptoms and decreased pumping function of the heart. Although the heart pumping function usually recovers, the patient's long-term mortality risk becomes similar to that of someone who has had an acute heart attack.

Women should be aware of their CVD risk factors and consult with a physician to assess their risk and determine the best way to prevent CVD.

### CVD in African Americans and Other Racial/Ethnic Groups

Although cardiovascular disease is the leading cause of death for all Americans, African Americans, Native Americans, and Mexican Americans are at higher risk for developing CVD than Euro-Americans and Asian Americans. Why would African Americans have lower CVD prevalence but higher death rates than other groups? One reason could be that these statistics come from self-reporting, and African Americans may report fewer doctor visits where they were told they had heart disease. The reasons for these disparities likely include both genetic and environmental factors.

The rate of hypertension among African Americans is among the highest in the world. African Americans tend to develop hypertension at an earlier age than non-Hispanic whites, and their average blood pressures are much higher. African Americans have a higher risk of stroke; have strokes at younger ages; and, if they survive, have more significant stroke-related disabilities. Some experts recommend that African Americans take antihypertensive drugs if their blood pressure reaches 130/80 rather than the typical 140/90 cutoff for hypertension—especially if they have diabetes or kidney disease.

A number of genetic and biological factors may contribute to CVD in African Americans. For instance, a higher sensitivity to dietary sodium may lead to elevated blood pressure. African Americans may also experience less dilation of blood vessels in response to stress, an attribute that also raises blood pressure for all racial/ethnic groups.

Another important CVD risk factor more common in Blacks than in whites is diabetes. However, Latinos are even more likely to develop it and insulin resistance, and at a younger age, than African Americans. There is variation within the Latino population, however; a higher prevalence of diabetes occurs among Mexican Americans and Puerto Ricans and a relatively lower prevalence among Cuban Americans.

It is important to note that environmental factors are increasingly being recognized as significant contributors to health care disparities. Racial and ethnic minorities are more likely than non-Hispanic whites to be poor, and low income is associated with reduced access to health care and healthy dietary options for CVD prevention. People who live in low-income neighborhoods experience longer delays between the onset of heart attack symptoms and reaching a hospital. Lower educational attainment is associated with low income, which often means less access to information about preventive health care, such as diet and stress management. Populations with low incomes tend to smoke more, consume more salt, and exercise less than those with higher incomes.

Discrimination may also play a role in CVD. Physicians and hospitals may treat the medical problems of diverse people racial minorities differently from those of whites. Discrimination, low income, and other forms of deprivation may also increase stress, which is linked with hypertension and CVD. Lack of insurance coverage and less-advanced medical technologies in hospitals that serve minority and low-income neighborhoods may also play a role.

All Americans, regardless of background, are advised to have their blood pressure checked regularly, exercise on a regular basis, eat a healthy diet, manage stress, and avoid tobacco products. Tailoring your lifestyle to any risk factors that may be especially relevant for you can also be helpful in some cases. Discuss your particular risk profile with your physician to help identify the lifestyle changes most appropriate for you.

## Ask Yourself

**QUESTIONS FOR CRITICAL THINKING AND REFLECTION**

What risk factors do you have for cardiovascular disease? Which ones are factors you control? If you have risk factors you cannot change (such as a family history of CVD), were you aware that you can make lifestyle adjustments to reduce your risk? Do you think you will make them?

sections of healthy arteries. Similarly, Covid-19 has been linked to severe cardiovascular complications, including increased rates of heart failure (3–33%), cardiogenic shock or low blood pressure due to decreased heart pumping function (9–17%), heart attacks (0.9–11%), arrhythmias (9–17%), and blood clots (23–27%) among hospitalized patients. Other factors currently under investigation include a specific type of LDL called lipoprotein(a) or Lp(a), LDL particle size, blood levels of iron, and blood levels of uric acid.

# PROTECTING YOURSELF AGAINST CARDIOVASCULAR DISEASE

You can take several important steps now to lower your risk of developing cardiovascular disease (Figure 13.8). CVD can begin very early in life. Reducing CVD risk factors when you are young can pay off with many extra years of life and health.

## Eat Heart-Healthy

For most Americans, eating a heart-healthy diet involves decreasing saturated and trans fat intake, eating a high-fiber diet, reducing sodium intake, avoiding excessive alcohol consumption, and eating foods rich in omega-3 fatty acids.

In addition to these familiar guidelines, a few specifics pertain to heart health: (1) Plant stanols and sterols, found in some types of trans-fat-free margarines and other products, reduce the absorption of cholesterol in the body and help lower LDL levels. (2) Folic acid, vitamin B-6, and vitamin B-12 lower homocysteine levels, and folic acid has also been found to reduce the risk of hypertension. (3) Diets rich in calcium may help prevent hypertension and possibly stroke by reducing insulin resistance and platelet aggregation. (4) There appears to be a close association between vitamin D deficiency and cardiovascular disease. However, studies have failed to show benefits to the replacement of low vitamin D levels with supplemental dietary vitamin D. (5) Replacing some animal proteins with soy protein (such as tofu) may help reduce the effects of saturated fat. (6) Healthy carbohydrates are important for people with insulin resistance, prediabetes, or diabetes. Finally, (7) reduced calorie intake also helps control body weight—an extremely important risk factor for CVD.

A diet plan that reflects many of the recommendations described here was released as part of a study called Dietary Approaches to Stop Hypertension, or DASH. The DASH study found that a diet low in fat and high in fruits, vegetables, and low-fat dairy products reduces blood pressure. It also follows the recommendations for lowering the risk of heart disease, cancer, and osteoporosis. See Chapter 10 for details about the DASH diet plan.

## Exercise Regularly

You can significantly reduce your risk of CVD with a moderate amount of physical activity. In addition to aerobic exercise for building and maintaining cardiovascular health,

**Do More**

- Eat a diet rich in fruits, vegetables, whole grains, and low-fat or fat-free dairy products. Eat five to nine servings of fruits and vegetables each day.
- Eat several servings of high-fiber foods each day.
- Eat two or more servings of fish per week; try a few servings of nuts and soy foods each week.
- Choose unsaturated fats rather than saturated and trans fats.
- Be physically active; do both aerobic exercise and strength training on a regular basis.
- Achieve and maintain a healthy weight.
- Develop effective strategies for handling stress and anger. Nurture old friendships and family ties, and make new friends; pay attention to your spiritual side.
- Obtain recommended screening tests and follow your physician's recommendations.

**Do Less**

- Don't use tobacco in any form: cigarettes, smokeless tobacco, cigars and pipes, bidis and clove cigarettes.
- Limit consumption of trans fats and saturated fats.
- Limit consumption of salt to no more than 2300 mg of sodium per day (1500 mg if you have or are at high risk for hypertension).
- Avoid exposure to environmental tobacco smoke.
- Avoid excessive alcohol consumption—no more than one drink per day for women and two drinks per day for men.
- Limit consumption of added sugars and refined carbohydrates.
- Avoid excess stress, anger, and hostility.

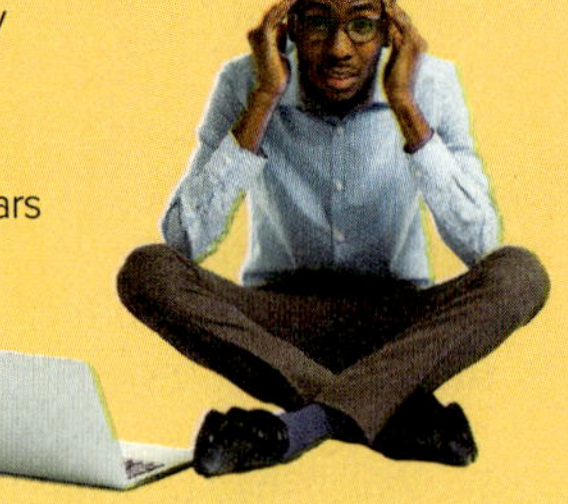

**FIGURE 13.8 Strategies for reducing your risk of cardiovascular disease.** Jessica Peterson/Rubberball/Getty Images; Vladyslav Starozhylov/Alamy Stock Photo

## BEHAVIOR CHANGE STRATEGY
### Reducing the Saturated and Trans Fats in Your Diet

The American Heart Association recommends that no more than 1% of the calories in your diet come from trans fats. Similarly, the *2015–2020 Dietary Guidelines* from the U.S. Department of Agriculture and U.S. Department of Health and Human Services recommend that Americans avoid trans fats from industrial sources completely and consume only small amounts from natural sources. Hydrogenated fats, products made with them, and deep-fried fast food can be high in trans fats. Although food manufacturers are phasing out trans fats, it's important to read labels to see how much a product contains. If a product contains less than 0.5% trans fat, the manufacturer is allowed to list trans fat content as 0%.

For saturated fats, the Dietary Guidelines for Americans recommend that intake be reduced to less than 10% of total calories. The American Heart Association recommends further reductions, down to less than 7% of total calories from saturated fat.

#### Monitor Your Current Diet

To see how your diet measures up, keep track of everything you eat for three days. Information about the calorie and fat content of foods is available on many food labels and online.

At the end of the monitoring period, record the calories and grams of trans and saturated fat for the foods you've eaten. Determine the percentage of daily calories as fat that you consumed for each day: Multiply grams of the type of fat by 9 (fat has 9 calories per gram) and then divide by total calories. For example, if you consumed 30 grams of saturated fats and 2100 calories on a particular day, then your saturated fat consumption as a percentage of total calories would be calculated as $30 \times 9 = 270$ calories of fat $\div$ 2100 total calories $= 0.13$, or 13%. If you have trouble obtaining all the data you need to do the calculations, you can still estimate whether your diet is high in saturated fat by seeing how many servings of foods high in unhealthy fats you typically consume on a daily basis. As described in Chapter 13, saturated fats are found in animal products, including meat and dairy products, as well as in tropical oils. Sources of healthy dietary fats that are most often recommended are liquid vegetable oils, fish, and nuts.

#### Make Healthy Changes

To reduce your intake of unhealthy fats, set a limit on the number of daily servings of foods high in saturated and trans fats that you have and continue to monitor your consumption. To plan healthy changes, take a close look at your food record. Do you choose many foods high in unhealthy fats? Do you limit your portion sizes to those recommended by MyPlate.gov? Try making healthy substitutions. Instead of a grilled ham and cheese sandwich, try a turkey sandwich with an oil-based dressing or sliced avocado. If you frequently eat in fast-food restaurants, find an appealing alternative—and recruit some friends to join you.

When you choose foods that are rich in saturated fat, *watch your portion sizes carefully.* Choose cuts of meat that have the least amount of visible fat, and trim off what you see. And balance your choices throughout the day. For example, if your lunch includes a cheeseburger and fries, choose a vegetarian pasta dish for dinner. Plan your diet around a variety of whole grains, vegetables, legumes, and fruits, which are nearly always low in unhealthy fats and high in nutrients; try nuts and fish for dietary sources of healthy fats. See Chapter 13 for more details about a heart-healthy diet and for a list of alternatives to some popular foods.

---

strength training helps reduce body fat and improves lipid levels and glucose metabolism.

The more exercise you get, the less likely you are to develop or die from CVD. Many studies, involving thousands of people, have shown that people who did regular aerobic exercise lowered their resting blood pressure by 2–4% on average. Lowered blood pressure itself reduces the risk of other kinds of cardiovascular disease.

> **Ask Yourself**
>
> **QUESTIONS FOR CRITICAL THINKING AND REFLECTION**
>
> Do you know what your blood pressure and cholesterol levels are? If not, is there a reason you don't know? Is something preventing you from getting this information about yourself? How can you motivate yourself to have these easy but important health checks?

## Avoid Tobacco Products

The number-one risk factor for CVD that you can control is smoking. Recent research has shown that vaping, or smoking electronic cigarettes, carries substantial risks for lung injury and cardiovascular disease. The dose of nicotine in e-cigarettes is often considerably more than a standard cigarette. See Chapter 9 for detailed information about the effects of smoking and strategies for quitting.

## Manage Your Blood Pressure, Cholesterol Levels, and Stress/Anger

If you have no CVD risk factors, have your blood pressure measured by a trained professional at least once every two years. Yearly tests are recommended if you have risk factors. If your blood pressure is high, follow your physician's advice on how to lower it.

All people aged 20 and over should have their cholesterol checked at least once every five years.

# BASIC FACTS ABOUT CANCER

**Cancer** is a group of diseases characterized by abnormal, uncontrolled multiplication of cells, which can ultimately cause death if left untreated.

## Tumors

Most cancers take the form of tumors, although not all tumors are cancerous. A **tumor** (or *neoplasm*) is a mass of tissue that serves no physiological purpose. It can be benign, like a wart, or malignant, like most lung cancers.

**Benign** (noncancerous) **tumors** are made up of cells similar to the surrounding normal cells and are enclosed in a membrane that prevents them from penetrating neighboring tissues. They are dangerous only if their physical presence interferes with body functions. A benign brain tumor, for example, can cause death if it blocks the blood supply to the brain.

The term **malignant tumor** is synonymous with cancer. A malignant tumor can invade surrounding structures, including blood vessels, the **lymphatic system,** and nerves. It can also spread to distant sites via blood and lymphatic circulation, producing invasive tumors almost anywhere in the body. A few cancers, such as leukemia (cancer of the blood), typically do not produce a mass but still have the fundamental property of rapid, uncontrolled cell proliferation.

Cancer begins when a change (or mutation) in a cell allows the cell to grow and divide when it should not. In adults, cells normally multiply at a rate just sufficient to replace dying cells. In contrast, a malignant cell divides into new cells without regard for normal control mechanisms and gradually produces a mass of abnormal cells, or a tumor. A pea-sized mass is made up of about a billion cells, so a single tumor cell must divide many times before the tumor grows to a noticeable size.

Eventually a tumor becomes large enough to cause symptoms or to be detected directly. In the breast, for example, a tumor may be felt as a lump or seen on an X-ray called a mammogram. In less accessible locations, like the lung, a tumor may be noticed only after it has grown considerably and may then be detected only by an indirect symptom, such as a persistent cough or unexplained bleeding. In the case of leukemia, changes in the blood are eventually noticed as increasing fatigue, infection, or abnormal bleeding. Once there is a suspicion of cancer, a patient will have a **biopsy** to confirm the diagnosis.

TERMS

**cancer** The abnormal, uncontrolled multiplication of cells.

**tumor** A mass of tissue that serves no physiological purpose; also called a *neoplasm*.

**benign tumor** A tumor that is not cancerous.

**malignant tumor** A tumor that is capable of spreading and thus is cancerous.

**lymphatic system** A system of vessels that returns proteins, lipids, and other substances from fluid in the tissues to the circulatory system.

**biopsy** The removal of a small piece of body tissue to allow for microscopic examination; a needle biopsy uses a needle to remove a small sample of tissue, but some biopsies require surgery.

**metastasis** The spread of cancer cells from one part of the body to another.

**staging** Classifying the extent of a cancer in a patient at the time of diagnosis.

**remission** A period during the course of cancer in which there are no symptoms or other evidence of disease.

**five-year survival rate** The percentage of patients diagnosed with a certain disease who will be alive five years after the date of diagnosis; used to estimate the prognosis of a particular disease.

## Metastasis

**Metastasis** is the spread of cancer cells from one part of the body to another. Metastasis occurs because cancer cells do not cling to each other as strongly as normal cells do and therefore may migrate from the site of the *primary tumor* (the cancer's original location). After cancer cells break away, they can pass through the lining of lymph or blood vessels to invade nearby tissue. This traveling and seeding process is called *metastasizing,* and the new tumors are called *secondary tumors* or *metastases.* The ability of cancer cells to metastasize makes early cancer detection critical. To cure cancer, every cancerous cell must be removed or destroyed. Once cancer cells enter either the lymphatic system or the bloodstream, it is extremely difficult to stop their spread to other organs of the body.

## The Stages of Cancer

The classifying process, called **staging,** is determined by the extent or spread of the cancer. To identify a cancer's stage, physicians assess the size or extent of the primary tumor, whether the cancer has invaded nearby lymph nodes, and whether metastases are present. By judging the extent of each criterion, physicians can determine the cancer's stage, establish how severe it is, and choose the most appropriate treatment.

## Remission

A significant number of cancer cases go into **remission,** which in some cases continues for years, or indefinitely. In remission, signs and symptoms of cancer disappear, and the disease is considered to be under control. Remission typically results from treatment; rarely do cancer patients enter remission spontaneously.

## The Incidence of Cancer

Each year more than 1.9 million people in the United States are diagnosed with cancer. Most will be cured or will live many years past their initial cancer diagnosis. In fact, the American Cancer Society (ACS) estimates that the **five-year survival rate**

| New cases | Deaths | Female |
|---|---|---|
| 10,880 (1%) | 7,570 (3%) | Brain and other nervous system |
| 42,600 (5%) | 2,570 (0.9%) | Melanoma of the skin |
| 31,940 (3%) | 1,160 (0.4%) | Thyroid |
| 118,830 (13%) | 61,360 (21%) | Lung and bronchus |
| 287,850 (31%) | 43,250 (15%) | Breast |
| 12,660 (1%) | 10,100 (4%) | Liver and intrahepatic bile duct |
| 29,240 (3%) | 23,860 (8%) | Pancreas |
| 28,710 (3%) | 4,960 (2%) | Kidney and renal pelvis |
| 70,340 (8%) | 24,180 (8%) | Colon and rectum |
| 19,880 (2%) | 12,810 (5%) | Ovary |
| 65,950 (7%) | 12,550 (4%) | Uterine corpus |
| 24,840 (3%) | 9,980 (4%) | Leukemia |
| 36,350 (4%) | 8,550 (3%) | Non-Hodgkin lymphoma |
| 934,870 | 287,270 | All sites* |

| Male | New cases | Deaths |
|---|---|---|
| Oral cavity and pharynx | 38,700 (4%) | 7,870 (2%) |
| Melanoma of the skin | 57,180 (6%) | 5,080 (2%) |
| Lung and bronchus | 117,910 (12%) | 68,820 (21%) |
| Esophagus | 16,510 (2%) | 13,250 (4%) |
| Liver and intrahepatic bile duct | 28,600 (3%) | 20,420 (6%) |
| Pancreas | 32,970 (3%) | 25,970 (8%) |
| Kidney and renal pelvis | 50,290 (5%) | 8,960 (3%) |
| Colon and rectum | 80,690 (8%) | 28,400 (9%) |
| Urinary bladder | 61,700 (6%) | 12,120 (4%) |
| Prostate | 268,490 (27%) | 34,500 (10%) |
| Leukemia | 35,810 (4%) | 14,020 (4%) |
| Non-Hodgkin lymphoma | 44,120 (5%) | 11,700 (4%) |
| All sites* | 983,160 | 322,090 |

VITAL STATISTICS

**FIGURE 13.9 Estimated number of new cancer cases and deaths by sex and by site, United States, 2022.** Estimated new cases are based on 2004–2018 incidence data reported by the North American Association of Central Cancer Registries (NAACCR). Estimated deaths are based on 2005–2019 US mortality data, National Center for Health Statistics. The numbers do not take into account the impacts of Covid-19.
*All sites, including others not listed here

SOURCE: "Cancer Facts and Figures, 2022." Atlanta, GA: American Cancer Society. 2022.

for all cancers diagnosed between 2011 and 2017 is 68% among white people and 63% among Black people. These statistics exclude more than 5 million cases of the curable types of skin cancer. Figure 13.9 shows the number of new cases of cancer each year and the number of deaths by sex and by cancer site.

Overall, men are more likely than women to die of cancer because men generally have a higher rate of tobacco and alcohol use, have greater occupational exposure to carcinogens, and take fewer preventive measures, like keeping regular contact with health care providers.

For 60 years, the number of cancer deaths increased steadily in the United States, largely due to a wave of lethal lung cancers among men caused by smoking. Heart-related damage from smoking reverses more quickly and more significantly than does cancer-related damage from smoking.

The overwhelming majority of skin cancers could be prevented by protecting the skin from excessive sun exposure, and the majority of lung cancers could be prevented by avoiding exposure to tobacco smoke. Thousands of cases of colon, breast, and uterine cancers could be prevented by improving diet and controlling body weight. Regular screenings and self-examinations have the potential to save an additional 100,000 lives per year.

# THE CAUSES OF CANCER

Although scientists do not know everything about what causes cancer, they have identified genetic, environmental, and lifestyle factors that increase the risk of developing cancer (see the box "Race/Ethnicity, Poverty, and Cancer").

## The Role of DNA

Heredity and genetics are important factors in a person's cancer risk. Certain genes may predispose some people to cancer, and specific genetic mutations have been associated with cancer.

Some mutations are inherited; others are caused by agents including radiation, certain viruses, and chemical substances. The most prominent example of an inherited genetic mutation associated with increased cancer risk involves the *BRCA* gene. Defects in these genes cause breast cancer and increase the risk of ovarian, pancreatic, and prostate cancers.

Genetic analysis of DNA from a blood sample can identify mutant copies of *BRCA1* and *BRCA2.* Women with a family history of breast cancer must still be monitored closely, even if they carry normal versions of *BRCA1* and *BRCA2.* The cancer-causing genetic defect in the family could be located on another gene.

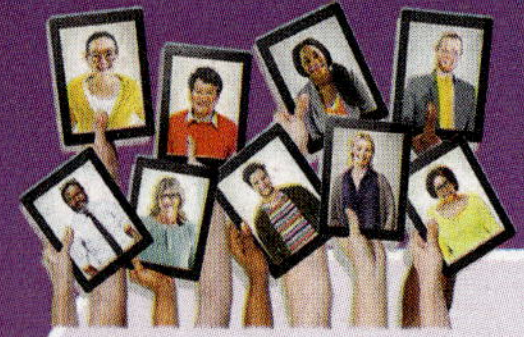

## DIVERSITY MATTERS
## Race/Ethnicity, Poverty, and Cancer

Rates of cancer have declined among all U.S. racial and ethnic groups in recent years, but significant disparities still exist:

- Among U.S. racial and ethnic groups, African American men have the highest incidence of and death rates from cancer.
- White women have a higher incidence of breast cancer, but African American women have the highest breast cancer death rate. African American women are more likely to have aggressive tumors, less likely to receive regular mammograms, and more likely to experience delays in follow-up.
- African American men have a higher rate of prostate cancer than any other U.S. group and more than twice the prostate cancer death rate of other groups. African American men are less likely than white men to undergo prostate-specific antigen (PSA) testing for prostate cancer.
- Latinas have the highest incidence of cervical cancer, but African American women have the highest cervical cancer death rate. Language barriers and problems accessing screening services are thought to particularly affect Latinas, who have relatively low rates of Pap testing.
- Asian Americans and Pacific Islander Americans have among the highest rates of liver and stomach cancers. Koreans, especially, suffer from stomach cancer; incidence and death rates are roughly twice as high as those among Japanese, who have the next-highest rates. Recent immigration helps explain these higher rates because these cancers are usually caused by infections that are more prevalent in Asian countries of origin.

The American Cancer Society's *Cancer Facts & Figures* features a special section on cancer among American Indian or Alaska Native (AIAN) people. Consisting of more than 750 tribes, the AIAN population is hard to generalize about. They are also the most misclassified group, and so the numbers describing their disease burdens are likely underestimated.

Still, statistical generalizations provide a starting point from which to glimpse the health care challenges of these communities and efforts made by them. Nationally, AIAN people are reported to have a higher incidence than Euro-Americans for lung, colorectal, and kidney cancers, as well as cancers of the stomach and cervix. Because their cancers are generally diagnosed at later stages, the survival rates are lower than for Euro-American people. Later-stage diagnoses reflect less access to high-quality health care. In addition to long-standing inequalities in treatment, AIAN people cope with higher burdens of major cancer risk factors such as smoking, obesity, and cancer-causing infections.

SOURCES: American Cancer Society. 2022. *Cancer Facts and Figures*. Atlanta, GA: American Cancer Society; Iqbal, J., et al. 2015. Differences in breast cancer stage at diagnosis and cancer-specific survival by race and ethnicity in the United States. *Journal of the American Medical Association* 313(2): 165–173.

## Tobacco and Alcohol Use

Smoking is responsible for about one-third of all cancer deaths, including 84% of lung cancer deaths for men and 81% of such deaths for women. In addition to lung and bronchial cancer, tobacco use is linked to cancers of the larynx, mouth, pharynx, esophagus, stomach, pancreas, liver, kidneys, bladder, and cervix, and directly causes acute myelogenous leukemia.

After tobacco use and excess body weight, alcohol ranks third as a preventable lifestyle risk factor for cancer. Even light drinkers (those who have no more than one drink a day) have an increased risk of some cancers.

## Dietary Factors

How important is diet in cancer prevention? The foods you eat contain many biologically active compounds, and your food choices may either increase your cancer risk by exposing you to potentially dangerous compounds or reduce your risk through consumption of potentially protective ones (Figure 13.10).

These dietary factors may affect cancer risk:

- ***Dietary fat and meat.*** Diets high in fat and meat may contribute to colon, stomach, and prostate cancers. Certain types of fats may be riskier than others. Omega-6 polyunsaturated fats are associated with a higher risk of some cancers; omega-3 fats are not.
- ***Foods cooked at high temperatures.*** High levels of the chemical acrylamide (a probable human carcinogen) are found in starch-based foods that have been fried or baked at high temperatures, especially french fries and certain types of snack chips and crackers.
- ***Fiber.*** Further study is needed to clarify the relationship between fiber intake and cancer risk, but experts still recommend a high-fiber diet for its overall positive effect on health.
- ***Fruits and vegetables.*** Researchers have identified nutrients in food components that may act against cancer. Some may prevent carcinogens from forming in the first place or block them from reaching or acting on target cells. Others boost enzymes that detoxify carcinogens and render them harmless. Some essential nutrients help reduce the harmful effects of carcinogens; for example, vitamin C, vitamin E, selenium, and the **carotenoids** (vitamin A precursors) may help block cancer by acting as antioxidants.

**TERMS**

**carotenoid** Any of a group of yellow-to-red plant pigments that can be converted to vitamin A by the liver; many act as antioxidants or have other anticancer effects. The carotenoids include beta-carotene, lutein, lycopene, and zeaxanthin.

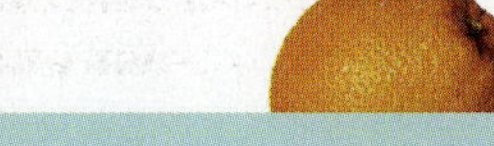

**Do More**

- Eat a varied, plant-based diet that is high in fiber-rich foods such as legumes and whole grains.
- Eat 7–13 servings of fruits and vegetables every day, favoring foods from the following categories:
  - Cruciferous vegetables
  - Citrus fruits
  - Berries
  - Dark green leafy vegetables
  - Dark yellow, orange, or red fruits and vegetables
- Be physically active.
- Maintain a healthy weight.
- Practice safer sex (to avoid HPV infection).
- Protect your skin from the sun with appropriate clothing and sunscreen.
- Perform regular self-exams (skin self-exam for all, testicular self-exam for men, breast self-awareness for women).
- Obtain recommended screening tests and discuss with your physician any family history of cancer.

**Do Less**

- Don't use tobacco in any form:
  - Cigarettes
  - Smokeless tobacco
  - Cigars and pipes
  - Bidis and clove cigarettes
- Avoid exposure to environmental tobacco smoke.
- Limit consumption of fatty meats and other sources of saturated fat.
- Avoid excessive alcohol consumption.
- Don't eat charred foods, and limit consumption of cured and smoked meats and meat and fish grilled in a direct flame.
- Avoid occupational exposure to carcinogens.
- Limit exposure to UV radiation from sunlight.
- Avoid tanning lamps or beds.

**FIGURE 13.10 Strategies for reducing your risk of cancer.** MRS.Siwaporn/Shutterstock; Stockbyte/Stockdisc/Getty Images; Stockbyte/Stockdisc/Getty Images; Robyn Mackenzie/123RF

Many other anticancer agents in the diet, known as **phytochemicals,** are substances in plants that help protect against chronic diseases. One of the first to be identified was sulforaphane, a potent anticarcinogen found in broccoli. Sulforaphane induces the cells of the liver and kidney to produce higher levels of protective enzymes, which then neutralize dietary carcinogens. Most fruits and vegetables contain beneficial phytochemicals, and researchers are just beginning to identify them.

## Inactivity and Obesity

The American Cancer Society recommends maintaining a healthy weight throughout life with a balanced diet and physical activity. About 5% of cancers in men and 11% of cancers in women can be attributed to excess body weight. A higher body mass index at age 25 increases one's risk of cancer later in life. Obesity in middle and later age has been shown to increase risk for many cancers. Evidence suggests that weight gain in early adulthood also puts us at risk—in women, particularly for endometrial and postmenopausal breast cancers, and in men, for colorectal cancer (Figure 13.11), but also generally for cancers of the gallbladder, liver, kidney, and esophagus.


May affect tumor growth regulators
Fat cells
Can raise levels of estrogen, insulin, and other hormones
Can trigger persistent inflammation
Excess hormones and inflammation tell cells to divide more rapidly than normal
Dividing cells can form tumors


**FIGURE 13.11 How excess body fat can lead to cancer.** Fat cells affect hormone levels, inflammation, and many cellular processes that may influence whether a cancer develops and how it progresses.

## Carcinogens in the Environment

Some carcinogens occur naturally in the environment, like viruses and the sun's UV rays. Others are manufactured or synthetic substances that show up occasionally in the general environment but more often in the work environments of specific industries. The ACS estimates that about 6% of cancer deaths stem from exposure to carcinogens in the environment—about 4% from occupational exposure and about 2% from exposure to naturally occurring or human-made pollutants in the larger environment.

**TERMS**

**phytochemical** A naturally occurring substance found in plant foods that may help prevent chronic diseases such as cancer and heart disease; *phyto* means "plant."

**Microbes** About 15–20% of the world's cancers are caused by microbes, including viruses, bacteria, and parasites, although the percentage is much lower in industrialized countries like the United States. Certain types of human papillomavirus are known to cause oropharyngeal cancer, cervical cancer, and other cancers, and the *Helicobacter pylori* bacterium has been linked to stomach cancer. The Epstein-Barr virus, best known for causing mononucleosis, is also suspected of contributing to Hodgkin lymphoma, cancer of the nasopharynx, and some stomach cancers. Human herpes virus 8 has been linked to Kaposi's sarcoma and certain types of lymphoma. Hepatitis viruses B and C cause as many as 80% of the world's liver cancers.

**Ingested Chemicals** Some compounds, like the nitrates and nitrites found in processed meat, are potentially dangerous. Although nitrates and nitrites are not themselves carcinogenic, they can combine with substances in the stomach and be converted to nitrosamines, which are highly potent carcinogens. Foods cured with nitrites, or by salt or smoke, have been linked to esophageal and stomach cancer, and they should be eaten sparingly.

**Environmental and Industrial Pollution** Pollutants in the air have long been suspected of contributing to the incidence of lung cancer. The best available data indicate that less than 2% of cancer deaths are caused by general environmental pollution, but estimates from the WHO are higher, suggesting that 19% of the world's cancers are caused by such substances in our air and water. Exposure to carcinogenic materials in the workplace is a more serious problem. Occupational exposure to specific carcinogens may account for about 4% of cancer deaths. In the United States, decreasing industry and government regulation mean that industrial sources of cancer risk may increase.

**Radiation** All sources of radiation are potentially carcinogenic, including medical X-rays, radioactive substances (radioisotopes), and UV rays from the sun. Successful efforts have been made to reduce the amount of radiation needed for mammograms, dental X-rays, and medical X-rays. Sunlight is an important source of radiation, and care should be taken to avoid excessive exposure.

QUICK STATS

**Worldwide, nearly 10 million people died of cancer in 2021.**

—World Health Organization, 2021

## DETECTING, DIAGNOSING, AND TREATING CANCER

Early cancer detection often depends on our willingness to be aware of changes in our own bodies and to make sure we keep up with recommended screening tests.

TERMS

**chemotherapy** The treatment of cancer with chemicals that selectively destroy cancerous cells.

### Ask Yourself

**QUESTIONS FOR CRITICAL THINKING AND REFLECTION**

What do you think your risks for cancer are? Do you have a family history of cancer, or have you been exposed to carcinogens? How about your diet and exercise habits? What can you do to reduce your risks?

### Detecting Cancer

Self-monitoring is the first line of defense. By being aware of the risk factors in your own life, your immediate family's cancer history, and your own history, you may bring a problem to the attention of a physician long before it would have been detected at a routine physical. In addition to self-monitoring, the ACS recommends routine cancer checkups, as well as specific screening tests for certain cancers (Table 13.4).

### Diagnosing Cancer

Methods for determining the exact location, type, and extent of a cancer continue to improve. A biopsy may confirm the type of tumor. Several diagnostic imaging techniques have replaced exploratory surgery for some patients: magnetic resonance imaging (MRI), CT scanning, and ultrasonography. MRI uses a huge electromagnet to detect hidden tumors by mapping, on a computer screen, the vibrations of different atoms in the body. CT scanning uses X-rays to examine the brain and other parts of the body. Ultrasounds use ultrasonic waves to produce images, often in breast and liver tumors.

### Treating Cancer

The ideal cancer therapy would kill or remove all cancerous cells while leaving normal tissue untouched. This is possible, when superficial tumors of the skin are surgically removed. Usually the tumor is less accessible, and some combination of surgery, radiation therapy, and chemotherapy must be applied instead. Some patients choose to combine conventional therapies with alternative treatments.

For most cancers, surgery is a definitive treatment. Surgically removing all the cancerous cells from the body can result in a long-lasting cure. This is particularly true for early cancers of the breast, prostate, lung, and colon. When the cancer is more advanced or involves nearby lymph nodes, patients may require chemotherapy or radiation therapy in addition to surgery.

**Chemotherapy,** or the use of medications to kill cancer cells, has been in use since the 1940s. Normal cells, which usually grow slowly, are not significantly destroyed by these drugs. However, some normal tissues such as intestinal, hair,

## Table 13.4 Early Detection of Cancer in Average-Risk Asymptomatic People

| SITE/TESTS AND PROCEDURES | DESCRIPTION | LINKS FOR MORE INFORMATION |
|---|---|---|
| **BREAST** | | |
| Mammography | Mammograms are the best way to find breast cancer early, when it is easier to treat. These imaging tests, which involve low-dose X-rays, are recommended every 1 to 2 years for women starting as early as age 40 and especially between 50 and 74, or as long as they are in good health. | CDC:<br>www.cdc.gov/cancer/breast/basic_info/screening.htm<br>NCI:<br>www.cancer.gov/types/breast/mammograms-fact-sheet<br>www.cancer.gov/types/breast/patient/breast-screening-pdq |
| Breast awareness | Routine examination of the breasts by health care providers or by women themselves starting in their 20s has not been shown to reduce deaths from breast cancer. However, any lump or other unusual change in the breast needs to be promptly reported to a doctor. | ACS:<br>www.cancer.org/treatment/understandingyourdiagnosis/examsandtestdescriptions/mammogramsandotherbreastimagingprocedures/index |
| **CERVIX** | | |
| Pap and HPV cytology tests | Pap tests can find abnormal cells in the cervix that may turn into cancer, and they can find cervical cancer early, when the chance of a cure is high. Testing every 3 to 5 years should begin at age 21 and end at age 65, if results have been normal. Women who have been vaccinated against HPV still need HPV tests. | CDC:<br>www.cdc.gov/cancer/cervical/basic_info/screening.htm<br>NCI:<br>www.cancer.gov/types/cervical/pap-hpv-testing-fact-sheet<br>www.cancer.gov/types/cervical/patient/cervical-screening-pdq |
| **COLON** | | |
| Colonoscopy and sigmoidoscopy | A sigmoidoscopy every 5 years or a colonoscopy at least every 10 years between the ages of 45 and 75 can reduce the likelihood of death from colorectal cancer and can detect abnormal polyps that can be removed before they turn into cancer. The virtual colonoscopy has not been shown to reduce deaths from colorectal cancer. | CDC:<br>https://www.cdc.gov/cancer/colorectal/pdf/QuickFacts-BRFSS-2016-CRC-Screening-508.pdf<br>ACS:<br>https://www.cancer.org/cancer/colon-rectal-cancer/detection-diagnosis-staging/acs-recommendations.html |
| High-sensitivity fecal occult blood test (FOBT) | This yearly multiple-stool, take-home test reduces death from colorectal cancer and is recommended for people between ages 50 and 75. If a positive result is found, the test is followed by a colonoscopy or sigmoidoscopy. | ACS:<br>www.cancer.org/healthy/findcancerearly/examandtestdescriptions/faq-colonoscopy-and-sigmoidoscopy |
| **LUNG** | | |
| Low-dose computed tomography (LDCT) | This imaging test has been shown to reduce lung cancer deaths among heavy smokers (30 pack-years*) between ages 55 and 74 who still smoke or have quit within the last 15 years. | CDC:<br>www.cdc.gov/cancer/lung/basic_info/screening.htm<br>NCI:<br>www.cancer.gov/types/lung/patient/lung-screening-pdq |
| **OVARY AND UTERUS** | | |
| CA-125 blood test, transvaginal ultrasound | There is no evidence that any screening test reduces deaths from ovarian cancer. However, these tests can help in diagnosing ovarian cancer. Women should report any unexpected bleeding or spotting to a doctor. | CDC:<br>www.cdc.gov/cancer/ovarian/basic_info/screening.htm<br>NCI:<br>www.cancer.gov/types/ovarian/patient/ovarian-screening-pdq |
| **PROSTATE** | | |
| Prostate-specific antigen (PSA) | Although this blood test, which is often accompanied by a digital rectal exam, can detect prostate cancer at an early stage, it is more likely to lead to overdiagnosis and overtreatment than to reduce deaths from prostate cancer. Starting at age 50, men should talk to a doctor about the pros and cons of this test. African American men and men whose father or brother had prostate cancer before age 65 should talk to a doctor about this test starting at age 45. | CDC:<br>www.cdc.gov/cancer/prostate/basic_info/screening.htm<br>NCI:<br>www.cancer.gov/types/prostate/psa-fact-sheet |

*A pack-year is calculated by multiplying the number of packs of cigarettes smoked per day by the number of years the person has smoked. For example, smoking 2 packs per day for 10 years is equal to 20 pack-years; smoking one-half pack per day for 10 years is equal to 5 pack-years.

SOURCES: Adapted from American Cancer Society. 2022. *Find Cancer Early* (https://www.cancer.org/healthy/find-cancer-early.html); Centers for Disease Control and Prevention (CDC). 2020. *Cancer Prevention and Control: Cancer Screening Tests* (http://www.cdc.gov/cancer/dcpc/prevention/screening.htm); National Cancer Institute (NCI); American Cancer Society 2021. *Cancer Facts and Figures 2021* (https://www.cancer.org/content/dam/cancer-org/research/cancer-facts-and-statistics/annual-cancer-facts-and-figures/2021/cancer-facts-and-figures-2021.pdf).

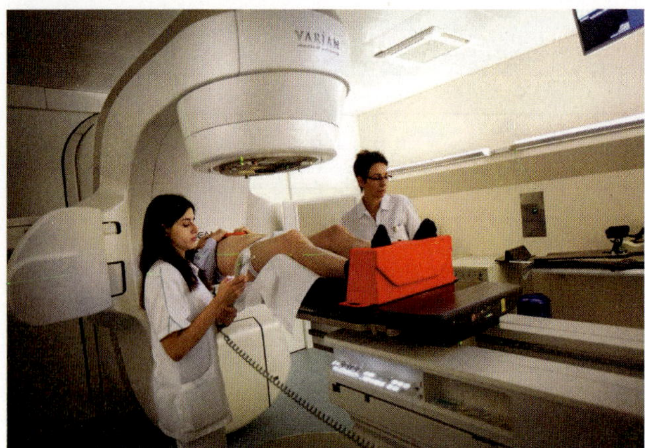

Radiation treatment for prostate cancer involves a machine that swings around the patient in a 360-degree fashion so that he gets beams of radiation from every direction. AMELIE-BENOIST/BSIP/Alamy Stock Photo

and blood-forming cells are always growing, and damage to these tissues produces the unpleasant side effects of chemotherapy, including nausea, vomiting, diarrhea, and hair loss.

Chemotherapy can be used in a variety of settings, depending on the type of cancer and the timing of drug administration. When the goal of treatment is cure (that is, completely eradicating all cancer cells), chemotherapy is often given either before or after surgery. Patients with cancers that are not thought to be curable (that is, not all cancer cells can be destroyed) can still benefit from chemotherapy. This is often referred to as *palliative chemotherapy.*

Radiation therapy uses a beam of X-rays or gamma rays directed at the tumor to kill tumor cells. With sophisticated techniques, the harmful rays are directed precisely at cancerous cells, in order to minimize damage to surrounding normal cells. Radiation therapy can be performed on an outpatient basis.

QUICK STATS

**16.9 million Americans with a history of cancer were alive in January 2019.**

—American Cancer Society, 2019

TERMS

**carcinoma** Cancer that originates in epithelial tissue (skin, glands, and lining of internal organs).

**sarcoma** Cancer arising from bone, cartilage, or striated muscle.

**lymphoma** A tumor originating from lymphatic tissue.

**leukemia** Cancer of the blood or the blood-forming cells.

**oncologist** A specialist in the diagnosis and treatment of cancer.

**hematologist** A specialist in the diagnosis and treatment of blood disorders, including cancers such as leukemia and lymphoma.

## COMMON TYPES OF CANCER

Cancers are classified according to the types of cells that give rise to them:

- **Carcinomas** arise from *epithelia*—tissues that cover external body surfaces, line internal tubes and cavities, and form the secreting portion of glands. This type of cancer is the most common. Major sites include the skin, breast, uterus, prostate, lungs, and gastrointestinal tract.
- **Sarcomas** arise from connective and fibrous tissues such as muscle, bone, cartilage, and the membranes covering muscles and fat.
- **Lymphomas** are cancers of the lymph nodes, part of the body's infection-fighting system.
- **Leukemias** are cancers of the blood-forming cells, which reside chiefly in the bone marrow.

Cancers vary greatly in how easily they can be detected and how well they respond to treatment. For example, certain types of skin cancer are easily detected, grow slowly, and are easy to remove; virtually all of these cancers are cured. Cancer of the pancreas, by contrast, is difficult to detect or treat, and few patients survive the disease. In general, it is difficult for an **oncologist** or **hematologist** to predict how a specific cancer will behave because each one arises from a unique set of changes in a single cell. In the sections that follow, we look more closely at the most common cancers and their causes, as well as how they are detected and treated.

### Lung Cancer

Lung cancer accounts for about 12% of all new cancer diagnoses and is the most common cause of cancer death in the United States: It is responsible for about 130,000 deaths each year. Since 1987, lung cancer has surpassed breast cancer as the leading cause of cancer death in women.

**Risk Factors** The chief risk factor for lung cancer is tobacco smoke, which currently accounts for 32% of all cancer deaths and 80% of lung cancer deaths. When smoking is combined with exposure to other carcinogens, such as asbestos particles or certain pollutants, the risk of cancer can be multiplied by a factor of 10 or more.

The smoker is not the only one at risk. Environmental tobacco smoke (ETS) is a human carcinogen.

**Detection and Treatment** Lung cancer is difficult to detect at an early stage and hard to cure even when detected early. Symptoms of lung cancer do not usually appear until the disease has advanced to the invasive stage. Signs and symptoms such as a persistent cough, chest pain, or recurring bronchitis may be the first indication of a tumor's presence. Spiral

## Ask Yourself

**QUESTIONS FOR CRITICAL THINKING AND REFLECTION**

Most people think of cancer as a death sentence, but is that necessarily true? Have you or has anyone you know had an experience with cancer? If so, what was the outcome? Have you ever considered whether you might be at increased risk for some types of cancer? Have you taken any steps to reduce your risk?

CT scans, a computer-assisted body imaging technique, can detect lung cancer in high-risk patients much earlier than chest X-rays. Besides CT scanning, a diagnosis can usually be made by chest X-ray or by studying the cells in sputum.

If caught early, localized cancers can be treated with surgery alone. The majority of patients are diagnosed with advanced disease, however, and radiation and chemotherapy are often used in addition to surgery. The five-year survival rate for all stages combined is only 22%. Phytotherapy, gene therapy, and immunotheraphy (vaccines) are being studied in hopes of improving these statistics.

## Colon and Rectal Cancer

Although effective screening methods exist, colon and rectal cancer is the fourth most common type of cancer, killing an estimated 53,000 Americans in 2022.

**Risk Factors** Age is a key risk factor for colorectal cancer; the vast majority of cases are diagnosed in people aged 45 and over. Heredity also plays a role. Many cancers arise from preexisting **polyps,** which are small growths on the wall of the colon that may gradually develop into malignancies. The tendency to form colon polyps appears to be determined by specific genes, so many colon cancers may be due to inherited gene mutations.

**QUICK STATS**

**86% of diagnosed cancers occur in people aged 50 and over.**

—American Cancer Society, 2021

Excessive alcohol use and smoking may increase the risk of colorectal cancer. Regular physical activity appears to reduce a person's risk, whereas obesity increases risk. A diet rich in fruits, vegetables, and whole grains is associated with lower risk. However, research findings on whether dietary fiber prevents colon cancer have been mixed. Studies have suggested a protective role for folic acid, magnesium, vitamin D, and calcium; in contrast, high intake of refined carbohydrates, simple sugars, and smoked meats and fish may increase risk.

Regular use of nonsteroidal anti-inflammatory drugs such as aspirin and ibuprofen may decrease the risk of colorectal cancer and other cancers of the digestive tract.

**Detection and Treatment** If identified early, precancerous polyps and early-stage cancers can be removed before they become malignant or spread. Because polyps may bleed, common warning signs of colorectal cancer are bleeding from the rectum and a change in bowel habits.

Regular screening tests are recommended beginning at age 45 (earlier for people with a family history of the disease or who are otherwise at high risk). A yearly stool blood test can detect small amounts of blood in the stool long before obvious bleeding would be noticed. More involved screening tests are recommended at 5- or 10-year intervals. These tests include a sigmoidoscopy or colonoscopy, during which a flexible fiber-optic device is inserted through the rectum and the colon is examined and polyps biopsied or removed. Screening is effective, and studies demonstrate that it can prevent up to 76–90% of colorectal cancers. Still, only about half of U.S. adults have undergone any of these tests.

Surgery is the primary treatment for colorectal cancer. Radiation and chemotherapy may be used before surgery to shrink a tumor or after surgery to destroy any remaining cancerous cells. The five-year survival rate ranges from 91 to 72% for colorectal cancers detected early and 65% overall.

## Breast Cancer

Breast cancer is the most common cancer in women. In men, breast cancer occurs rarely. In the United States, about one woman in eight will develop breast cancer during her lifetime. In 2022, 287,850 new breast cancer diagnoses were expected in the United States, and about 43,250 were expected to die from it. Worldwide, it is the second leading cause of cancer death in women.

Fewer than 2% of breast cancer cases occur in women under age 35, but incidence rates increase quickly with age. About 50% of cases are diagnosed in women aged 45–65.

**Risk Factors** Genetics plays a very important role in breast cancer. A woman who has two close relatives with breast cancer is about three times more likely to develop the disease than a woman without close relatives with it. Even though genetic factors are important, inherited mutations in breast cancer susceptibility genes account for only approximately 5–10% of all breast cancer cases.

Other risk factors include early onset of menstruation, late onset of menopause, having no children or having a first child after age 30, current use of hormone replacement therapy, obesity, and alcohol use. Estrogen exposure can increase the risk for breast and uterine cancer. Estrogen circulates in a woman's body in high concentrations between puberty and menopause. Fat cells also produce estrogen, and estrogen levels are higher in obese women. Alcohol can interfere with estrogen metabolism in the liver and increase estrogen levels in the blood. A dramatic drop in rates of breast cancer from 2001 to 2004 was attributed in part to reduced use of hormone replacement therapy by women

**TERMS**

**polyp** A small, usually harmless mass of tissue that projects from the inner surface of the colon or rectum.

over age 50. Millions of women stopped taking the hormones after research from the Women's Health Initiative linked hormone replacement therapy with an increased risk of breast cancer and heart disease.

Eating a low-fat, vegetable-rich diet, exercising regularly, limiting alcohol intake, and maintaining a healthy body weight can minimize the chance of developing breast cancer, even for women at risk from family history or other factors. Despite some popular myths, studies have shown that breast cancer incidence is not increased by underwire bras, antiperspirants, breast implants, or abortions.

**Early Detection** A cure is most likely if breast cancer is detected early, so regular screening is a good investment, even for younger women. The ACS recommends the following for the early detection of breast cancer:

- ***Mammography.*** A **mammogram** is a low-dose breast X-ray that can identify about 80–90% of breast cancers at an early stage, before physical symptoms develop. The ACS recommends that women at average risk for breast cancer begin annual mammograms at age 40; between age 45 and 54, women should have mammograms every year. Women over the age of 55 may choose to have mammograms every year or two. Some controversy surrounds the best age to start mammographic screening. Some groups have argued that the rates of false-positive mammograms are higher between ages 40 and 50; thus, the U.S. Preventive Services Task Force, for example, advises that women should wait until age 50 to begin routine screening.

- ***Breast awareness.*** The ACS no longer recommends breast self-exams (BSEs) or clinical breast exams, but many doctors still do, and a woman should be familiar with her breasts and alert her health care provider to any changes right away. The following are warning signs of breast cancer but can also be caused by other conditions: A new lump in the breast or underarm; thickening or swelling of part of the breast; irritation or dimpling of breast skin; redness or flaky skin in the nipple area of the breast; pulling in of the nipple or pain in the nipple area; nipple discharge other than breast milk, including blood; any change in the size or the shape of the breast; and pain in any area of the breast.

Additional screenings may be recommended for women at increased risk for breast cancer. Studies show that MRI may be better than mammography at detecting breast abnormalities in some women. The ACS recommends both an annual mammogram and an annual MRI for women who are at high risk for breast cancer, such as those who carry a *BRCA* mutation. **Ultrasonography** (use of sound waves to create images of soft tissue) is not a standard screening tool for breast cancer, but it is often used as a follow-up test if a mammogram reveals an abnormality in breast tissue.

**TERMS**

**mammogram** A low-dose X-ray of the breasts used to check for early signs of breast cancer.

**ultrasonography** An imaging method in which sound waves are bounced off body structures to create an image on a TV monitor; also called *ultrasound.*

**monoclonal antibody** An antibody designed to bind to a specific cancer-related target.

**Treatment** If a lump is detected, it may be scanned by ultrasonography and biopsied to see if it is cancerous. In most cases, the lump is found to be a cyst or other harmless growth, and no further treatment is needed. If the lump contains cancer cells, a variety of surgeries may be indicated, ranging from a lumpectomy (removal of the lump and surrounding tissue) to a mastectomy (removal of the breast).

Analyzing the tumor specimen with special stains can help predict the risk of breast cancer recurrence and help identify women who will benefit most from additional therapy; women can then make more informed treatment decisions. Treatment with **monoclonal antibodies,** such as trastuzumab, is an option for about 15–20% of patients diagnosed with breast cancer.

If the tumor is discovered before it has spread to the adjacent lymph nodes or outside the breast, the patient has a 99% chance of surviving more than five years. The relative survival rate for all stages is 90% at five years.

**Strategies for Prevention** A number of drugs have been proposed for the prevention of breast cancer, especially in high-risk patients. A family of drugs called *selective estrogen receptor modulators* (*SERMs*) acts like estrogen in some tissues of the body but blocks estrogen's effects in others. One SERM, tamoxifen, has long been used in breast cancer treatment because it blocks the action of estrogen in breast tissue. In 1998, the U.S. Food and Drug Administration (FDA) approved the use of tamoxifen to reduce the risk of breast cancer in healthy women who are at high risk for the disease. However, the drug has serious potential side effects, including increased risk of blood clots and uterine cancer. Another SERM, raloxifene, was approved in 2007 for the reduction of invasive breast cancer risk in postmenopausal women at high risk for breast cancer. Compared to tamoxifen, raloxifene has been shown to pose a slightly lower risk of blood clots and uterine cancer, but the risk is still higher than that of a placebo. Raloxifene has also been shown to improve bone mineral density.

## Prostate Cancer

The prostate gland is located at the base of the bladder in men and completely surrounds the urethra; if enlarged, it can block the flow of urine. Prostate cancer is the most common cancer in men and the second leading cause of cancer death in men. In the United States in 2022, over 268,400 new cases and more than 34,000 deaths were estimated.

**Risk Factors** Age is the strongest predictor of risk, with approximately 60% of cases of prostate cancer diagnosed in men over age 65. Inherited genetic predisposition may be responsible for 5–10% of cases, and men with a family history of the disease should be particularly vigilant about screening. African American men and Jamaican men of

African descent have the highest rates of prostate cancer of any groups in the world. Both genetic and lifestyle factors may be involved.

Diets that are high in calories, dairy products, and animal fats and also low in plant foods have been implicated as possible culprits, as have obesity, inactivity, and a history of sexually transmitted diseases. Type 2 diabetes and insulin resistance are also associated with prostate cancer. Soy foods, tomatoes, and cruciferous vegetables are being investigated for their possible protective effects.

**Detection** Warning signs of prostate cancer can include changes in urinary frequency, weak or interrupted urine flow, painful urination, and blood in the urine.

Techniques for early detection include a digital rectal examination and the **prostate-specific antigen (PSA) test.** The ACS recommends that men be provided information about the benefits and limitations of the tests and that both the exam and the PSA test be offered annually, beginning at age 50, for men who are at average risk of prostate cancer, do not have any major medical problems, and have a life expectancy of at least 10 years. Men at high risk, including African Americans and those with a family history of the disease, should consider beginning screening at age 45. Men with multiple family members who have been diagnosed with the disease should consider beginning screening at age 40.

**Treatment** Treatments vary based on the stage of the cancer and the patient's age. A small, slow-growing tumor in an older man may be treated with watchful waiting and no initial therapy because he is more likely to die from another cause before his cancer becomes life-threatening. More aggressive treatment would be indicated for younger men or those with more advanced cancers. Treatment may involve *radical prostatectomy* (surgical removal of the prostate). Although this has an excellent cure rate, it is major surgery and often results in **incontinence** or erectile dysfunction. Minimally invasive surgery, which utilizes a laparoscopic or robotic approach, can sometimes be performed with fewer complications and quicker recovery.

A less invasive alternative involves surgical implantation of radioactive seeds. Radiation from the seeds destroys the tumor and much of the normal prostate tissue but leaves surrounding tissue relatively untouched. Alternative or additional treatments include external radiation, hormonal therapy, cryotherapy, and chemotherapy. Several new treatments for advanced prostate cancer have recently been approved by the FDA, including a cancer vaccine, known as sipuleucel-T.

Survival rates for all stages of this cancer have improved steadily since 1940; the five-year survival rate is nearly 100%.

## Cancers of the Female Reproductive Tract

Several types of cancer can affect the female reproductive tract, and a few of these cancers are relatively common.

**Cervical Cancer** Cancer of the cervix can occur in women in their twenties and thirties. In the United States, approximately 14,000 women are diagnosed with cervical cancer each year, and the disease kills more than 4000 women annually.

Cervical cancer is largely a sexually transmitted infection or disease. Virtually all cases of cervical cancer stem from infection by the human papillomavirus (HPV), a group of about 100 related viruses that also cause common warts and genital warts. When certain types of HPV are introduced into the cervix, usually by an infected sex partner, the virus infects cervical cells, causing them to divide and grow. If unchecked, this growth can develop into cervical cancer. Cervical cancer is associated with multiple sex partners and is extremely rare in women who have not had heterosexual intercourse. Smoking, immunosuppression, and prolonged use of oral contraceptives also have been associated with increased risk.

Screening for the changes in cervical cells that precede cancer is done chiefly by means of the **Pap test.** During a pelvic exam, loose cells are scraped from the cervix and examined under a microscope to see whether they are normal. If cells are abnormal but not yet cancerous, the patient has a condition commonly referred to as *cervical dysplasia.* Sometimes such abnormal cells spontaneously return to normal, but in about one-third of cases the cellular changes progress toward malignancy. If this happens, the abnormal cells must be removed, either surgically or with a cryoscopic (ultra-cold) probe or localized laser treatment. When abnormal cells are in a precancerous state, the small patch of dangerous cells can be removed completely.

Without timely surgery, the malignant cells invade the cervical wall and spread to the uterus and adjacent lymph nodes. At this stage, chemotherapy and radiation may be used to kill the cancer cells, but chances for a complete cure are reduced. Even when a cure can be achieved, it often requires surgical removal of the uterus.

Because the Pap test is highly effective, all women between ages 25 and 65 should be tested. The recommended schedule for testing depends on risk factors, the type of Pap test performed, and whether the Pap test is combined with HPV testing. According to a 2018 study, following the introduction of the HPV vaccine in 2006, the rates of invasive cervical cancer dropped by 29% in younger women. Women who receive one of the vaccines should continue to receive routine Pap tests because the vaccines do not protect against all types of the virus.

**Uterine, or Endometrial, Cancer** Cancer of the lining of the uterus (the *endometrium*) most often occurs after the

TERMS

**prostate-specific antigen (PSA) test** A screening test for prostate cancer that measures blood levels of prostate-specific antigen (PSA).

**incontinence** The inability to control the flow of urine.

**Pap test** A scraping of cells from the cervix for examination under a microscope to detect cancer.

age of 55. Uterine cancer strikes approximately 66,000 American women annually and kills about 13,000 women each year. The risk factors are similar to those for breast cancer, including prolonged exposure to estrogen, early onset of menstruation, late menopause, never having been pregnant, and obesity. Type 2 diabetes is also associated with increased risk. The use of oral contraceptives or hormone therapies that contain estrogen plus progestin does not appear to increase risk.

Endometrial cancer often presents with abnormal vaginal bleeding in a postmenopausal woman. It is treated surgically, commonly by *hysterectomy,* or removal of the uterus. Radiation treatment, hormones, and chemotherapy may be used in addition to surgery. The 5-year relative survival rate for uterine cancer is 84% for white women and 63% for Black women, partly because white women are more likely to be diagnosed with early-stage disease; however, survival is substantially lower for Black women for every stage of diagnosis.

**Ovarian Cancer** Although ovarian cancer is rare compared with cervical or uterine cancer, it causes more deaths than the other two combined. In 2022, it was estimated that 20,000 new cases of ovarian cancer would be diagnosed in the United States and 13,000 women would die from it. There are often no warning signs of ovarian cancer. Early symptoms may include increased abdominal size and bloating, urinary urgency, and pelvic pain. It cannot be detected by Pap tests or any other simple screening method and is often diagnosed late in its development, when surgery and other therapies are unlikely to be successful.

The risk factors are similar to those for breast and endometrial cancers: increasing age (most ovarian cancer occurs after age 60), never having been pregnant, a family history of breast or ovarian cancer, obesity, and specific genetic mutations including *BRCA1* and *BRCA2.* A high number of ovulations appears to increase the chance that a cancer-causing genetic mutation will occur, so anything that lowers the number of lifetime ovulation cycles–pregnancy, breastfeeding, or use of oral contraceptives–reduces a woman's risk of ovarian cancer.

Women with symptoms or who are at high risk because of family history or because they harbor a mutant gene may be offered screening with a pelvic exam, ultrasound, and blood test. Ovarian cancer is treated by surgical removal of both ovaries, the fallopian tubes, and the uterus. Radiation and chemotherapy are sometimes used in addition to surgery. When the tumor is localized to the ovary, the five-year survival rate is more than 93%. However, it is diagnosed this early only 19% of the time. For all stages, the five-year survival rate is only 49%.

**TERMS**

**melanoma** A malignant tumor of the skin that arises from pigmented cells, usually a mole.

**ultraviolet (UV) radiation** Light rays of a specific wavelength emitted by the sun; most UV rays are blocked by the ozone layer in the upper atmosphere.

**basal cell carcinoma** Usually benign skin cancer of the base of the outermost layer of the skin.

**squamous cell carcinoma** Malignant cancer of the surface of the outermost layer of the skin.

## Skin Cancer

Skin cancer is the most common type of cancer, but it is often not included in cancer incidence and mortality statistics because many types of skin cancer are easily curable. Of the millions of cases of skin cancer diagnosed each year, about 1% are of the most serious type, **melanoma.**

**Risk Factors** Almost all cases of skin cancer can be traced to excessive exposure to **ultraviolet (UV) radiation** from the sun, including longer-wavelength ultraviolet A (UVA) and shorter-wavelength ultraviolet B (UVB) radiation. UVB radiation causes sunburns and can damage eyes and the immune system. UVA is less likely to cause an immediate sunburn, but it damages connective tissue and leads to premature aging of the skin, giving it a wrinkled, leathery appearance. (Tanning lamps and tanning salon beds emit mostly UVA radiation.) Both UVA and UVB radiation have been linked to the development of skin cancer, and the National Toxicology Program has declared both solar and artificial sources of UV radiation, including sunlamps and tanning beds, to be known human carcinogens.

Both severe, acute sun reactions (sunburns) and chronic low-level sun reactions (suntans) can lead to skin cancer. White people are about three times more likely than Hispanic people and 30 times more likely than Black or Asian/Pacific Islander people to develop a melanoma.

Severe sunburns in childhood have been linked to a significantly increased risk of skin cancer in later life, so children in particular should be protected. According to the Skin Cancer Foundation, the risk of skin cancer doubles in people who have had five or more sunburns in their lifetime. Because of damage to the ozone layer of the atmosphere (discussed in Chapter 15), there is a chance that we may all be exposed to increased UV radiation in the future. Other risk factors for skin cancer include having many moles (particularly large ones), spending time at high altitudes (fewer layers of atmosphere filter UV radiation), and a family history of the disease.

**Types of Skin Cancer** There are three main types of skin cancer, named for the types of skin cells from which they develop. **Basal cell carcinoma** and **squamous cell carcinoma** together account for about 95% of the skin cancers diagnosed each year. They are usually found in chronically sun-exposed areas, such as the face, neck, hands, and arms. They usually appear as pale, waxlike, pearly nodules or red, scaly, sharply outlined patches. These cancers are often painless, although they may bleed, crust, and form an open sore on the skin.

Melanoma is by far the most dangerous skin cancer because it spreads so rapidly. It can occur anywhere on the body, but the most common sites are the back, chest, abdomen, and lower legs. A melanoma usually appears at the site of a preexisting mole. The mole may begin to enlarge, become mottled or varied in color (colors can include blue, pink, and white), or develop an irregular surface or irregular borders. Tissue invaded by melanoma may also itch, burn, or bleed easily.

## CRITICAL CONSUMER
### Sunscreens and Sun-Protective Clothing

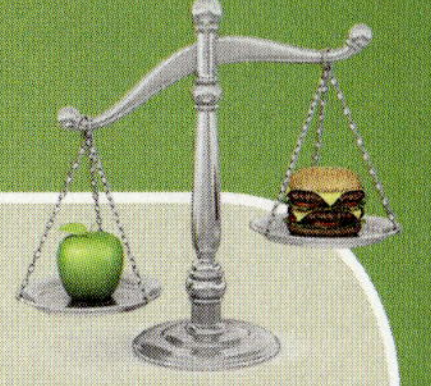

With consistent use of proper clothing, sunscreens, and common sense, you can lead an active outdoor life *and* protect your skin against most sun-induced damage.

#### Clothing

- Wear long-sleeved shirts and long pants. Dark-colored, tightly woven fabrics provide reasonable protection from the sun. Another good choice is clothing made from special sun-protective fabrics; these garments have an ultraviolet protection factor (UPF) rating, similar to the sun protection factor (SPF) rating for sunscreens.

- Wear a hat. A good choice is a broad-brimmed hat or a legionnaire-style cap that covers the ears and neck. Wear sunscreen on your face even if you are wearing a hat.

- Wear sunglasses. Exposure to UV rays can damage the eyes and cause cataracts.

#### Sunscreen

- Use a sunscreen and lip balm with an SPF of 15 or higher. An SPF rating refers to the amount of time you can stay out in the sun before you burn, compared with not using sunscreen. For example, a product with an SPF of 30 would allow you to remain in the sun without burning 30 times longer, on average, than if you didn't apply sunscreen. If you're fair-skinned, have a family history of skin cancer, are at high altitude, or will be outdoors for many hours, use a sunscreen with an even higher SPF. A higher SPF does not mean you can use less.

- Choose a broad-spectrum sunscreen that protects against both UVA and UVB radiation. The SPF rating of a sunscreen currently applies only to UVB, but a number of ingredients, especially titanium dioxide and zinc oxide, are effective at blocking most UVA radiation.

- Use a water-resistant sunscreen if you swim or sweat a great deal. Under FDA regulations, sunscreens cannot be labeled as "waterproof" or "sweatproof" because these claims overstate the products' actual effectiveness. Labels for "water resistant" must specify whether they provide the labeled SPF protection for 40 or 80 minutes of swimming or sweating. Also be sure to reapply sunscreen after activities, such as swimming, that could remove sunscreen.

- If you have acne, look for a sunscreen that is labeled "noncomedogenic," which means that it will not cause pimples.

- Shake sunscreen before applying. Apply it 30 minutes before exposure to allow it time to bond to the skin. Reapply sunscreen frequently and generously to all sun-exposed areas (many people overlook their temples, ears, and sides and backs of their necks). Most people use less than half as much as they need to attain the full SPF rating. One ounce of sunscreen is enough to cover an average-size adult in a swimsuit. Reapply sunscreen every two hours.

- If you're taking medications, ask your physician or pharmacist about possible reactions to sunlight or interactions with sunscreens. Medications for acne, allergies, and diabetes are just a few of the products that can trigger reactions. If you're using sunscreen and an insect repellent containing DEET, use extra sunscreen (DEET may decrease sunscreen effectiveness).

#### Time of Day and Location

- Avoid sun exposure between 10:00 a.m. and 2:00 p.m., when the sun's rays are most intense. Clouds allow as much as 80% of UV rays to reach your skin. Stay in the shade when you can.

- Consult the day's UV Index, which predicts UV levels on a 0–11+ scale, to get a sense of the amount of sun protection you'll need. Take special care on days with a rating of 5 or above. You can download a free UV index app from the U.S. Environmental Protection Agency or find index ratings from the National Weather Service.

- UV rays can penetrate at least 3 feet below the surface of water, so swimmers should wear water-resistant sunscreens. Snow, sand, water, concrete, and white-painted surfaces are also highly reflective of UV rays.

#### Tanning Salons

- Stay away from tanning salons! Despite advertising claims to the contrary, the lights used in tanning parlors are damaging to your skin. Tanning beds and lamps emit mostly UVA radiation, increasing your risk of premature skin aging (such as wrinkles) and skin cancer.

**Prevention** One major step you can take to protect yourself against all forms of skin cancer is to avoid lifelong overexposure to sunlight. Blistering, peeling sunburns from unprotected sun exposure are particularly dangerous, but suntans—whether from sunlight or from tanning lamps—also increase your risk of developing skin cancer later in life. People of every age, especially babies and children, need to be protected from the sun with **sunscreens** and protective clothing. For a closer look at sunlight and skin cancer, see the box "Sunscreens and Sun-Protective Clothing."

**Detection and Treatment** Make it a habit to examine your skin regularly. Most spots, freckles, moles, and blemishes on your body are normal; you were born with some of them, and others appear and disappear throughout your life. But if you notice an unusual growth, discoloration, sore that

> **TERMS**
>
> **sunscreen** A substance used to protect the skin from UV rays; usually applied as a lotion, cream, or spray.

## TAKE CHARGE
## Testicle Self-Examination

The best time to perform a testicular self-exam is after a warm shower or bath, when the scrotum is relaxed.

First, stand in front of a mirror and look for any swelling of the scrotum. Then examine each testicle with both hands. Place the index and middle fingers under the testicle and the thumbs on top. Roll the testicle gently between the fingers and thumbs. Don't worry if one testicle seems slightly larger than the other; that's common. Also, expect to feel the epididymis, which is the soft, sperm-carrying tube at the rear of the testicle.

Perform a self-exam each month. If you find a lump, swelling, or nodule, see a physician right away. The abnormality may not be cancer, but only a physician can make a diagnosis.

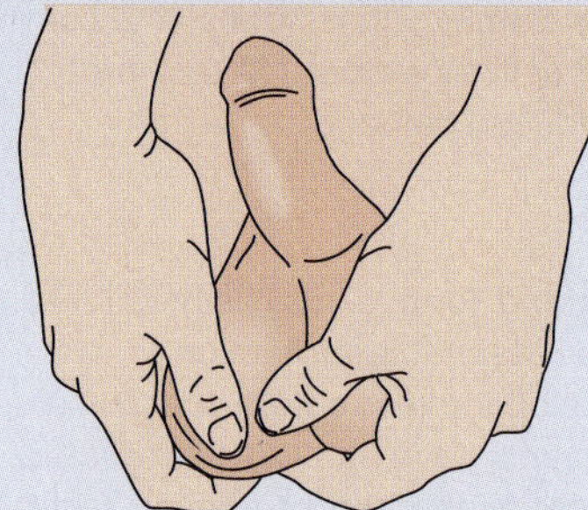

Other possible signs of testicular cancer include a change in the way a testicle feels, a sudden collection of fluid in the scrotum, a dull ache in the lower abdomen or groin, a feeling of heaviness in the scrotum, or pain in a testicle or the scrotum.

SOURCES: Mayo Clinic. 2021. *How to Do a Testicular Self Examination* (https://www.mayoclinic.org/tests-procedures/testicular-exam/about/pac-20385252); Mayo Clinic. 2021. *General Information about Testicular Cancer* (https://www.mayoclinic.org/diseases-conditions/testicular-cancer-care/symptoms-causes/syc-20352986).

does not heal, or mole that undergoes a sudden or progressive change, see your physician or dermatologist immediately.

Figure 13.12 illustrates the characteristics of a possible melanoma—asymmetry; border irregularity; color variations; a diameter greater than ¼ inch; and changes in the size, shape, or color of the mole. If someone in your family has had multiple skin cancers or melanomas, consult a dermatologist for a complete skin examination and discussion of your particular risk.

In the past decade, the FDA has approved several new therapies for metastatic melanoma. For example, ipilimumab is a monoclonal antibody that activates the body's anticancer immune response and was approved for patients with previously untreated metastatic melanoma. Since then, other immune therapies have also proven to be beneficial. For melanoma, the five-year survival rate is 99% if the tumor is localized, but in cases of distant-stage disease, it can be as low as 30%. Improvements in survival continue to happen with the use of the new immune-based treatments.

A—Asymmetry: Is one half unlike the other?

B—Border irregularity: Does it have an uneven, scalloped edge rather than a clearly defined border?

C—Color variation: Is the color uniform, or does it vary from one area to another, from tan to brown to black, or from white to red to blue?

¼ in.

D—Diameter larger than ¼ inch: At its widest point, is the growth as large as, or larger than, a pencil eraser?

Ordinary Mole

Changing in size, shape, and color

E—Evolving: A mole or skin lesion that looks different from the rest or has any change in size, shape, color, elevation, or another trait, or any new symptom such as bleeding, itching, or crusting.

**FIGURE 13.12 The ABCDE test for melanoma.** To see a variety of photos of melanoma and benign moles, visit the National Cancer Institute's Visuals Online site (http://visualsonline.cancer.gov).

## Testicular Cancer

Testicular cancer is relatively rare, accounting for only 1% of cancers in U.S. men (about 10,000 cases and 460 deaths per year), but it is the most common cancer in men ages 20–35. It is much more common among European Americans than among Latinos, Asian Americans, or African Americans. It is also relatively common among men whose fathers had testicular cancer. Men with undescended testicles are at increased risk for testicular cancer, and for this reason that condition should be corrected in early childhood.

Self-examination may help in the early detection of testicular cancer (see the box "Testicle Self-Examination"). Tumors

### Ask Yourself

**QUESTIONS FOR CRITICAL THINKING AND REFLECTION**

Has anyone you know had cancer? If so, what type of cancer was it? What were its symptoms? Based on the information presented so far in this chapter, did the person have any of the known risk factors for the disease?

## Ask Yourself

**QUESTIONS FOR CRITICAL THINKING AND REFLECTION**

For men, do you know how to perform self-examinations, such as testicular exams? For women, do you have breast self-awareness, which means familiarity with the appearance and feel of your breasts? Has your doctor ever given you instructions on self-exams? Given what you know about yourself and your family's medical history, do you think self-exams could be important for you?

are treated by surgical removal of the testicle and, if the tumor has spread, by chemotherapy; radiation treatment is used only rarely. The five-year survival rate for testicular cancer is 96% if *regional*, beyond the primary tumor and reaching nearby tissues, organs, or lymph nodes.

## TIPS FOR TODAY AND THE FUTURE

A growing body of research suggests that you can take an active role in preventing many cancers by adopting a wellness-focused lifestyle.

**RIGHT NOW YOU CAN:**

- Make an appointment to have your blood pressure and cholesterol levels checked.
- Plan to replace one high-fat and one high-sugar item in your diet with one that is high in fiber. For example, replace a doughnut with a bowl of whole-grain cereal.
- Buy multiple bottles of sunscreen and put them in places where you will most likely need them, such as your backpack, gym bag, or car.
- Check the cancer screening guidelines in this chapter and make sure you are up-to-date on your screenings.
- If you are a woman, develop breast self-awareness. If you are a man, do a testicular self-exam.

**IN THE FUTURE YOU CAN:**

- Track your eating habits for one week and then compare them to the DASH eating plan. Make adjustments to bring your diet closer to the DASH recommendations.
- Learn where to find information about daily UV radiation levels in your area, and learn how to interpret the information. Many local newspapers and television stations (and their websites) report current UV levels every day.
- Gradually add foods with abundant phytochemicals to your diet.

## SUMMARY

- The cardiovascular system circulates blood throughout the body. The heart pumps blood to the lungs via the pulmonary artery and to the body via the aorta.
- The six major risk factors for CVD that can be changed or controlled are tobacco use, high blood pressure, unhealthy cholesterol levels, inactivity, overweight or obesity, and diabetes.
- Hypertension occurs when blood pressure exceeds normal levels most of the time. It weakens the heart, scars and hardens arteries, and can damage the eyes and kidneys.
- High LDL and low HDL cholesterol levels contribute to clogged arteries and increase the risk of developing CVD.
- Physical inactivity, obesity, and diabetes are interrelated and are associated with high blood pressure and unhealthy cholesterol levels.
- Risk factors that can be changed include high triglyceride levels, metabolic syndrome, inflammation, and psychological and social factors.
- Risk factors that can't be changed include being over 65, being male, being African American, and having a family history.
- Atherosclerosis is a gradual hardening and narrowing of arteries that can lead to restricted blood flow and complete blockage.
- Heart attacks are usually the result of a long-term disease process. Warning signs of a heart attack include chest discomfort, shortness of breath, nausea, and sweating.
- A stroke occurs when the blood supply to the brain is cut off by a blood clot or hemorrhage. A transient ischemic attack (TIA) may be a warning sign of an impending stroke.
- Congestive heart failure occurs when the heart's pumping action becomes less efficient and fluid collects in the lungs or in other parts of the body.
- Dietary changes that can protect against CVD include decreasing your intake of fat and cholesterol, and increasing your intake of fiber by eating more fruits, vegetables, and whole grains.
- CVD risk can be reduced by exercising regularly, avoiding tobacco and environmental tobacco smoke, managing your blood pressure and cholesterol levels, and developing effective ways of handling stress and anger.
- Cancer is the abnormal, uncontrolled multiplication of cells; it can cause death if untreated.
- A malignant tumor can invade surrounding structures and spread to distant sites via the blood and lymphatic system, producing additional tumors.
- A malignant cell divides without regard for normal growth. As tumors grow, they produce signs or symptoms that are determined by their location in the body.
- Mutational damage to a cell's DNA can lead to rapid and uncontrolled growth of cells; mutagens include radiation, viral infection, and chemical substances in food and air.
- Cancer-promoting dietary factors include meat, especially red and processed meat; certain types of fats; and alcohol.
- Diets high in fruits and vegetables are linked to a lower risk of cancer.

# BEHAVIOR CHANGE STRATEGY
## Incorporating More Fruits and Vegetables into Your Diet

You know that fruits and vegetables are good for you, but did you know that they help fight cancer? They contain specific cancer-fighting compounds (phytochemicals) that help slow, stop, or even reverse the process of cancer. The National Cancer Institute (NCI) reports that people who eat five or more servings a day of fruits and vegetables have half the risk of cancer compared to those who eat fewer than two. According to the NCI, at least seven to nine servings per day is optimal.

Most Americans need to double the amount of fruits and vegetables they eat every day. Monitor your diet for one or two weeks to assess your current intake. Here are some tips to help you incorporate these foods into your diet.

### Breakfast

- Drink pure fruit juice every morning.
- Add raisins, berries, or sliced fruit to cereal, pancakes, or waffles. Top bagels with tomato slices.
- Try a fruit smoothie made from fresh or frozen fruit and orange juice or low-fat yogurt.

### Lunch

- Choose vegetable soup or salad with your meal.
- Replace potato chips or french fries with carrots, cucumbers, celery, bell pepper, or jicama.
- Add extra fruits or vegetables to salads—oranges, melons, tomatoes, dried cranberries.
- Add vegetables such as roasted peppers, cucumber slices, shredded carrots, avocado, or salsa to sandwiches.
- Drink tomato or vegetable juice instead of soda (watch for excess sodium and sugar).

### Dinner

- Choose a vegetarian main course, such as stir-fry or vegetable stew. Have at least two servings of vegetables with every dinner.
- Microwave vegetables and sprinkle them with a little olive oil and fresh garlic.
- Substitute vegetables for meat in casseroles, pasta, and chili.
- At the salad bar, pile your plate with steamed or raw vegetables and use low-fat or nonfat dressing.

### Snacks and On the Go

- Keep ready-to-eat fruits and vegetables on hand (apples, plums, pears, and carrots).
- Keep small packages of dried fruit in the car (try dried apples, apricots, peaches, pears, and raisins).
- Make ice cubes from pure fruit juice and drop them into regular or sparkling water.
- Freeze grapes for a cool summer treat.

### The All-Stars

Different fruits and vegetables contribute different vitamins, phytochemicals, and other nutrients, so be sure to get a variety. The following types of produce are particularly rich in nutrients and phytochemicals:

- Cruciferous vegetables (e.g., broccoli, cauliflower, cabbage, bok choy, brussels sprouts, kohlrabi, turnips)
- Citrus fruits (e.g., oranges, lemons, limes, grapefruit, tangerines)
- Berries (e.g., strawberries, raspberries, blueberries)
- Dark green leafy vegetables (e.g., spinach, chard, collards, beet greens, kale, mustard greens, romaine and other dark lettuces)
- Deep yellow, orange, and red fruits and vegetables (e.g., carrots, pumpkin, sweet potatoes, winter squash, red and yellow bell peppers, apricots, cantaloupe, mangoes, papayas)

- Other possible causes of cancer include inactivity and obesity, certain viruses and chemicals, and radiation.
- Self-monitoring and regular screening tests are essential to early cancer detection.
- Methods of cancer diagnosis include MRI scanning, CT scanning, and ultrasound.
- Treatment methods usually consist of some combination of surgery, chemotherapy, and radiation.
- Lung cancer kills more people than any other type of cancer. Tobacco smoke is the primary cause.
- Colon and rectal cancers are linked to age, heredity, obesity, and a diet rich in processed meat and low in fruits and vegetables. Most colon cancers arise from preexisting polyps.
- Breast cancer affects about one in eight women in the United States. Although there is a genetic component to breast cancer, diet and hormones are also risk factors.
- Prostate cancer is chiefly a disease of aging; diet and lifestyle probably are factors in its occurrence. Early detection is possible through rectal examinations and PSA blood tests.
- Cancers of the female reproductive tract include cervical, uterine, and ovarian cancers. The Pap test is an effective screening test for cervical cancer.
- Abnormal cellular changes in the skin, often a result of exposure to the sun, cause skin cancer, as does chronic exposure to certain chemicals. Skin cancers include basal cell carcinoma, squamous cell carcinoma, and melanoma.
- Testicular cancer can be detected early through self-examination.

## FOR MORE INFORMATION

*American Academy of Dermatology.* Provides information about skin cancer prevention.

http://www.aad.org

*American Cancer Society.* Provides a wide range of free materials on the prevention, diagnosis, and treatment of cancer.

http://www.cancer.org

*American Heart Association (AHA).* Provides information about hundreds of topics relating to cardiovascular disease.

http://www.heart.org

*American Institute for Cancer Research.* Provides information about lifestyle and cancer prevention, especially nutrition.

http://www.aicr.org

*Dietary Approaches to Stop Hypertension (DASH).* Provides information about the design, diets, and results of the DASH study, including tips on how to follow the DASH diet at home.

http://www.nhlbi.nih.gov/health-topics/dash-eating-plan

*EPA/Sunwise.* Provides information about the UV index and the effects of sun exposure, with links to sites with daily UV index ratings for cities in the United States and other countries.

https://www.epa.gov/sunsafety

*The Heart: The Engine of Life.* An online museum exhibit containing information about the structure and function of the heart, how to monitor your heart's health, and how to maintain a healthy heart.

https://www.fi.edu/heart-engine-of-life

*MedlinePlus: Blood, Heart, and Circulation Topics.* Provides links to reliable sources of information on cardiovascular health.

https://www.nlm.nih.gov/medlineplus/bloodheartandcirculation.html

*MedlinePlus Cancer Information.* Provides news and links to reliable information on a variety of cancers and cancer treatment.

http://www.nlm.nih.gov/medlineplus/cancers.html

*National Cancer Institute.* Provides information about treatment options, screening, and clinical trials.

http://www.cancer.gov

*National Comprehensive Cancer Network (NCCN).* Presents treatment guidelines for physicians and patients related to the treatment of various cancers; these guidelines were developed by a group of leading cancer centers.

http://www.nccn.org

*National Heart, Lung, and Blood Institute.* Provides information about and interactive applications for a variety of topics relating to cardiovascular health and disease, including cholesterol, smoking, obesity, hypertension, and the DASH diet.

http://www.nhlbi.nih.gov/

*National Heart, Lung, and Blood Institute–What Is Cholesterol?* Provides information about cholesterol, the diagnosis of elevated cholesterol, and treatments.

http://www.nhlbi.nih.gov/health-topics/high-blood-cholesterol

*National Stroke Association.* Provides information and referrals for stroke victims and their families as well as a stroke risk assessment.

http://www.stroke.org

*National Toxicology Program.* The federal program that creates regular reports listing the substances known or reasonably assumed to cause cancer in humans.

http://ntp.niehs.nih.gov

*Oncolink/The University of Pennsylvania Cancer Center Resources.* Contains information about different types of cancer and answers to frequently asked questions.

http://www.oncolink.org

See also the listings for Chapters 2, 3, 4, and 13–15.

## SELECTED BIBLIOGRAPHY


American Cancer Society. 2021. Pattern of DNA damage links colorectal cancer and diet high in red meat. *NCI Staff Blog* (https://www.cancer.gov/news-events/cancer-currents-blog/2021/red-meat-colorectal-cancer-genetic-signature).

American Cancer Society. 2022. *About Breast Cancer.* Atlanta, GA: American Cancer Society (https://www.cancer.org/cancer/breast-cancer.html).

American Cancer Society. 2022. *Cancer Facts and Figures 2022.* Atlanta, GA: American Cancer Society (https://www.cancer.org/content/dam/cancer-org/research/cancer-facts-and-statistics/annual-cancer-facts-and-figures/2022/2022-cancer-facts-and-figures.pdf).

American Cancer Society. 2022. *Key Statistics for Basal and Squamous Cell Skin Cancers.* Atlanta, GA: American Cancer Society (https://www.cancer.org/cancer/basal-and-squamous-cell-skin-cancer/about/key-statistics.html).

American Cancer Society. 2022. *Key Statistics for Melanoma Skin Cancer.* Atlanta, GA: American Cancer Society (https://www.cancer.org/cancer/melanoma-skin-cancer/about/key-statistics.html).

American Cancer Society. 2022. *Key Statistics for Testicular Cancer.* Atlanta, GA: American Cancer Society (https://www.cancer.org/cancer/testicular-cancer/about/key-statistics.html).

American Cancer Society. 2022. *Special Section: Ovarian Cancer.* Atlanta, GA: American Cancer Society (https://www.cancer.org/cancer/ovarian-cancer/about/key-statistics.html).

American Heart Association. 2020. *2020 Heart Disease and Stroke Statistical Update Fact Sheet At-a-Glance* (https://www.heart.org/-/media/files/about-us/statistics/2020-heart-disease-and-stroke-ucm_505473.pdf?la=en).

Arana, J. E., et al. 2018. Post-licensure safety monitoring of quadrivalent human papillomavirus vaccine in the Vaccine Adverse Event Reporting System (VAERS), 2009–2015. *Vaccine* 36(13): 1781–1788.

Auger, N., et al. 2020. Outcomes of Takotsubo syndrome at 15 years: A matched cohort study. *American Journal of Medicine* 133(5): 627–634.

Beil, L. 2017. Deflating cancer: New approaches to low oxygen may thwart tumors. *Science News* 191(4): 24–27.

Bouvard, V., et al. 2015. Carcinogenicity of consumption of red and processed meat. *Lancet Oncology* 16(16): 1599–1600.

Bucholz, E. M., et al. 2016. Life expectancy after myocardial infarction, according to hospital performance. *New England Journal of Medicine* 375(14): 1332–1342.

Cao, S., et al. 2015. The health effects of passive smoking: An overview of systematic reviews based on observational epidemiological evidence. *PLoS One* 10(10): e0139907.

Castellsaqué, X., et al. 2016. HPV involvement in head and neck cancers: Comprehensive assessment of biomarkers in 3680 patients. *Journal of the National Cancer Institute* 108(6): djv403.

Centers for Disease Control and Prevention. 2019. *Diabetes Home: Diabetes Quick Facts* (http://www.cdc.gov/diabetes/basics/quick-facts.html/).

Centers for Disease Control and Prevention. 2019. *Heart Disease Statistics and Maps* (http://www.cdc.gov/heartdisease/facts.htm).

Centers for Disease Control and Prevention. 2019. *National Diabetes Statistics Report: Estimates of Diabetes and Its Burden in the United States* (https://www.cdc.gov/diabetes/pdfs/data/statistics/national-diabetes-statistics-report.pdf).

Chung, M. K., et al. 2021. Covid-19 and cardiovascular disease: From bench to bedside. *Circulation Research* 128: 1214–1236.

Clarke, L. 2022. Tennis great Chris Evert shares ovarian cancer diagnosis 'as a way to help others.' *The Washington Post,* January 15 (https://www.washingtonpost.com/sports/2022/01/15/chris-evert-ovarian-cancer/).

Clark, R., et al. 2018. Plasma cytokines and risk of coronary heart disease in the PROCARDIS study. *Open Heart* 5(1): e000807.

Corrales, L., et al. 2020. Lung cancer in never smokers: The role of risk factors other than tobacco smoking. *Critical Reviews in Oncology/Hematology* 148: 102895 (https://pubmed.ncbi.nlm.nih.gov/32062313/).

Farvid, M. S., et al. 2016. Fruit and vegetable consumption in adolescence and early adulthood and risk of breast cancer: Population based cohort study. *British Medical Journal* 353: i2343.

Gilkes, D. M. 2016. Implications of hypoxia in breast cancer metastasis to bone. *International Journal of Molecular Sciences* 17(10): 1669. DOI:10.3390/ijms17101669.

Guan, W., et al. 2015. Race is a key variable in assigning lipoprotein(a) cutoff values for coronary heart disease risk assessment: The Multi-Ethnic Study of Atherosclerosis. *Arteriosclerosis, Thrombosis, and Vascular Biology* 35(4): 996–1001.

Guo, F., L. E. Cofie, and A. B. Berenson. 2018. Cervical cancer incidence in young U.S. females after Human Papillomavirus Vaccine introduction. *American Journal of Preventive Medicine* 55(2): 197–204.

Haberg, A. K., et al. 2016. Incidental findings and their clinical impact; the HUNT MRI study in a general population of 1006 participants between 50–66 years. *PLoS One* 11(3): e0151080.

Han, X., et al. 2015. Body mass index at early adulthood, subsequent weight change and cancer incidence and mortality. *International Journal of Cancer* 135(12): 2900–2909.

Heinl, R. E., et al. 2016. Comprehensive cardiovascular risk reduction and cardiac rehabilitation in diabetes and the metabolic syndrome. *Canadian Journal of Cardiology* 32(10S2): S349–S357.

Holyoake, T. L., and D. Vetrie. 2017. The chronic myeloid leukemia stem cell: Stemming the tide of persistence. *Blood* 129(12): 1595–1606.

Kaiser, J. 2016. Tests of blood-borne DNA pinpoint tissue damage: Assays spot cell death from diabetes, cancer, and more. *Science* 351(6279): 1253.

Li, X., et al. 2016. Effectiveness of prophylactic surgeries in *BRCA1* or *BRCA2* mutation carriers: A meta-analysis and systematic review. *Clinical Cancer Research* DOI: 10.1158/1078-0432.CCR-15-1465.

Lloyd-Jones, D. M., et al. 2016. 2016 ACC expert consensus decision pathway on the role of non-statin therapies for LDL-cholesterol lowering in the management of atherosclerotic cardiovascular disease risk: A report of the American College of Cardiology Task Force on Expert Consensus Documents. *Journal of the American College of Cardiology* 68(1): 92–125.

Lloyd-Jones, D. M., et al. 2017. 2017 focused update of the 2016 ACC expert consensus decision pathway on the role of non-statin therapies for LDL-cholesterol lowering in the management of atherosclerotic cardiovascular disease risk: A report of the American College of Cardiology Task Force on Expert Consensus Decision Pathways. *Journal of the American College of Cardiology* 70(14): 1785–1822.

Makhnoon, S., et al. 2022. Are beliefs about the importance of genetics for cancer prevention and early detection associated with high risk cancer genetic testing in the U.S. population? *Preventive Medicine Reports* 27(101781) (https://doi.org/10.1016/j.pmedr.2022.101781).

Maron, M. S., et al. 2016. Occurrence of clinically diagnosed hypertrophic cardiomyopathy in the United States. *American Journal of Cardiology* 117(10): 1651–1654.

Moore, S. C., et al. 2016. Leisure-time physical activity and risk of 26 types of cancer in 1.44 million adults. *JAMA Internal Medicine* 176(6): 816–825.

Mpekris, F., et al. 2017. Role of vascular normalization in benefit from metronomic chemotherapy. *Proceedings of the National Academy of Sciences of the United States of America* 114(8): 1994–1999.

Murphy, S. L., et al. 2015. Deaths: Final data for 2012. *National Vital Statistics Reports* 63(9).

Myers, E. R., et al. 2015. Benefits and harms of breast cancer screening: A systematic review. *Journal of the American Medical Association* 314(15): 1615–1634.

National Cancer Institute. 2017. Liquid biopsy: Using DNA in blood to detect, track, and treat cancer. *Cancer Currents Blog* (https://www.cancer.gov/news-events/cancer-currents-blog/2017/liquid-biopsy-detects-treats-cancer).

National Cancer Institute, National Institutes of Health. 2011. *Radon and Cancer* (http://www.cancer.gov/cancertopics/factsheet/Risk/radon).

National Center for Health Statistics. 2016. *Health, United States, 2015: With Special Feature on Racial and Ethnic Health Disparities.* Hyattsville, MD: National Center for Health Statistics.

National Heart, Lung, and Blood Institute. 2015. *How Is Metabolic Syndrome Diagnosed?* (http://www.nhlbi.nih.gov/health/health-topics/topics/ms/diagnosis).

National Human Genome Research Institute. 2021. *A Brief Guide to Genomics Fact Sheet* (https://www.genome.gov/about-genomics/fact-sheets).

National Toxicology Program. 2016. *Report on Carcinogens,* 15th ed. Research Triangle Park, NC: USDHHS Public Health Service (https://ntp.niehs.nih.gov/whatwestudy/assessments/cancer/roc/index.html).

Oswald, L. B., et al. 2022. Smoking is related to worse cancer-related symptom burden. *The Oncologist,* 27(2): e176–e184.

Pham, T., et al. 2016. The effect of serum 25-hydroxyvitamin D on elevated homocysteine concentrations in participants of a preventive health program. *PLos One* 11(8): e061368.

Razdan, S. N., et al. 2016. Quality of life among patients after bilateral prophylactic mastectomy: A systematic review of patient-reported outcomes. *Quality of Life Research* 25(6): 1409–1421.

Rothwell, P. M., et al. 2016. Effects of aspirin on risk and severity of early recurrent stroke after transient ischaemic attack and ischaemic stroke: time-course analysis of randomised trials. *Lancet* 388(10042): 365–375.

Saeed, A., D. L. Dixon, and E. Yang. 2020. Racial disparities in hypertension prevalence and management: A crisis control? *Journal of the American College of Cardiology Expert Analysis* (https://www.acc.org/latest-in-cardiology/articles/2020/04/06/08/53/racial-disparities-in-hypertension-prevalence-and-management).

Semsarian, C., et al. 2015. New perspectives on the prevalence of hypertrophic cardiomyopathy. *Journal of the American College of Cardiology* 65(12): 1249–1254.

Shi, S., et al. 2017. Depression and risk of sudden cardiac death and arrhythmias: a meta-analysis. *Psychosomatic Medicine* 79(2): 153–161.

Siegel, R. L., K. D. Miller, and A. Jemal. 2020. Cancer statistics, 2020. *CA: A Cancer Journal for Clinicians* 68(1) (https://acsjournals.onlinelibrary.wiley.com/doi/full/10.3322/caac.21590).

Sonnenburg, J. L., and F. Bäckhed. 2016. Diet–microbiota interactions as moderators of human metabolism. *Nature* 535: 56–64.

SPRINT Research Group. 2015. A randomized trial of intensive versus standard blood-pressure control. *New England Journal of Medicine* 373(22): 2103–2116.

Stone, N. J., et al. 2013. ACC/AHA guideline on the treatment of blood cholesterol to reduce atherosclerotic cardiovascular risk in adults: A report of the American College of Cardiology/American Heart Association Task Force on Practice Guidelines. *Journal of the American College of Cardiology.*

Torre, L. A., et al. 2016. Cancer statistics for Asian Americans, Native Hawaiians, and Pacific Islanders, 2016: Converging incidence in males and females. *CA: A Cancer Journal for Clinicians* 66(3): 182–202.

U.S. Department of Health and Human Services. 2014. *The Health Consequences of Smoking—50 Years of Progress: A Report of the Surgeon General.* Atlanta, GA: U.S. Department of Health and Human Services, Centers for Disease Control and Prevention, National Center for Chronic Disease Prevention and Health Promotion, Office on Smoking and Health.

U.S. Departments of Health and Human Services and Agriculture. 2015. *2015-2020 Dietary Guidelines for Americans* (http://health.gov/dietaryguidelines/2015/guidelines/).

Virani, S. S., et al. 2021. Heart disease and stroke statistics—2021 update. A report from the American Heart Association. *Circulation* 143: e254–e743.

Watkins, D. A., et al. 2017. Global, regional, and national burden of rheumatic heart disease, 1990–2015. *New England Journal of Medicine* 377: 713–722.

Whelton, P. K., et al. 2017. 2017 ACC/AHA/AAPA/ABC/ACPM/AGS/APhA/ASH/ASPC/NMA/PCNA guideline for the prevention, detection, evaluation, and management of high blood pressure in adults. A report of the American College of Cardiology/American Heart Association Task Force on Clinical Practice Guidelines. *Journal of the American College of Cardiology* S0735-1097(17): 41519-1.

Widmer, R. J., et al. 2015. The Mediterranean diet, its components, and cardiovascular disease. *American Journal of Medicine* 128(3): 229–238.

Willershausen, I., et al. 2013. Association between chronic periodontal and apical inflammation and acute myocardial infarction. *Odontology,* April 21.

Wolf, A. M. D., et al. 2018. Colorectal cancer screening for average-risk adults: 2018 guideline update from the American Cancer Society. *CA: A Cancer Journal for Clinicians.* DOI: 10.3322/caac.21457.

World Health Organization. 2022. *Fact Sheet: Cancer* (https://www.who.int/news-room/fact-sheets/detail/cancer.

Xie, X., et al. 2015. Effects of intensive blood pressure lowering on cardiovascular and renal outcomes: Updated systematic review and meta-analysis. *Lancet* S0140-6736(15): 00805-3.

Zhang, Z. M., et al. 2016. Race and sex differences in the incidence and prognostic significant of silent myocardial infarction in the Atherosclerosis Risk in Communities (ARIC) study. *Circulation* 133(22): 2141–2148.

**Design Elements:** Assess Yourself icon: Aleksey Boldin/Alamy Stock Photo; Diversity Matters icon: Rawpixel Ltd/Getty Images; Wellness on Campus icon: Radius Images/Alamy Stock Photo; Take Charge icon: VisualCommunications/Getty Images; Critical Consumer icon: pagadesign/Getty Images.

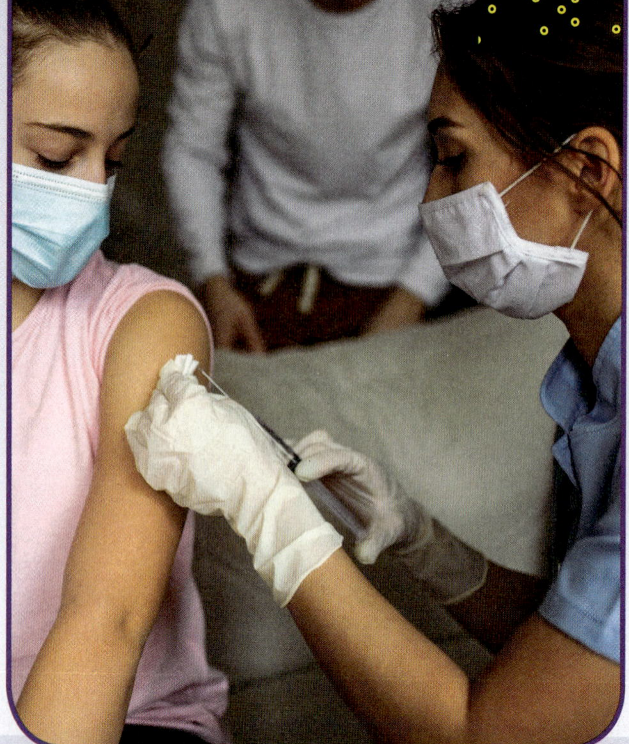
Sneksy/Getty Images

## CHAPTER OBJECTIVES

- Explain the body's physical and chemical defenses against infection
- Describe the step-by-step process by which infectious diseases are transmitted
- Identify the major types of pathogens, the diseases they cause, and possible treatments for them
- Discuss steps you can take to support your immune system

CHAPTER 14

# Immunity and Infection

Countless microscopic organisms live around, on, and in us. Although most microbes are beneficial, many of them can cause **infections.** But the constant vigilance of our immune system keeps them at bay and our bodies healthy. The immune system protects us not just from **pathogens** (disease-causing organisms) but also from cancers, some of which are linked to persistent infections and chronic inflammation. The reemergence of old scourges such as tuberculosis and the appearance of new viruses such as coronavirus disease 2019 (Covid-19) highlight the importance of understanding both the immune system and pathogens. This chapter introduces you to the mechanisms of immunity and infection; we also discuss strategies for keeping ourselves healthy.

TERMS

**infection** Invasion of the body by a microorganism.

**pathogen** An organism that causes disease.

## THE BODY'S DEFENSE SYSTEM

Our bodies have very effective ways of protecting themselves against invasion by foreign organisms. The immune system is the body's collective set of defenses that includes surface barriers as well as the specialized cells, tissues, and organs that carry out the immune response. The first line of defense is a formidable array of physical and chemical barriers. When these barriers are breached, cellular processes of the immune system come into play. Together these defenses provide an effective response to nearly all the invasions that our bodies experience.

### Physical and Chemical Barriers

The skin, the body's largest organ, prevents many microorganisms from entering the body. Although many bacterial and fungal organisms live on the surface of the skin, few can penetrate it except through a cut or break.

All body cavities and passages that are exposed to the external environment are lined with mucous membranes, which secrete mucus and contain cells designed to prevent unwanted organisms and particles from passing through or penetrating them. These areas include the mouth, nostrils, eyelids, bronchioles, vagina, and other organs of the respiratory, digestive, and urogenital tracts. Skin and mucous membranes are made of epithelial tissue, which consists of one or more layers of closely packed cells. They act as both physical and chemical barriers to potential invaders. The fluids that cover epithelial tissue, such as tears, saliva, and vaginal secretions, are rich in enzymes and other proteins that break down and destroy many microorganisms.

The respiratory tract is lined not only with mucous membranes but also with cells having hairlike protrusions called *cilia*. The cilia sweep foreign matter up and out of the respiratory tract. Particles that are not caught by this mechanism may be expelled from the system by a cough.

## The Immune System: Cells, Tissues, and Organs

Beyond surface barriers, the **immune system** operates through a remarkable information network involving billions of white blood cells that protect the body when a threat arises. We produce these white blood cells continuously throughout life.

The immune system is actually two interacting systems; both consist of cells that can recognize pathogenic microorganisms. The cells of the *innate immune system* are the first to respond to those pathogens. The T cells and B cells of the *adaptive immune system* have the remarkable ability both to accelerate and to improve the effectiveness of their responses. The complete elimination of a pathogen involves the coordinated activities of both systems.

**Cells of the Innate Immune System** The cells of the innate immune system recognize pathogens as "foreign" and kill them. They respond the same way no matter how many times a pathogen invades. The innate immune system includes *neutrophils,* white blood cells that ingest and destroy pathogens; *eosinophils,* white blood cells that fight parasitic infections; *macrophages,* scavenger cells that engulf and destroy bacteria and dying cells; *natural killer cells,* which directly destroy virus-infected cells and cells that have turned cancerous; and *dendritic cells,* which initiate the adaptive immune response.

**Cells of the Adaptive Immune System** The cells of the adaptive immune system are white blood cells called **lymphocytes.** The two main types of lymphocytes are T cells and B cells.

**Antigens and Antibodies** All your body cells display "self" markers that tell lymphocytes: *I belong to this body.* Invading microbes display markers that identify them as "nonself" or foreign. Nonself markers that trigger an immune response are called **antigens.** Each bacterial cell or virus has many antigens. **Antibodies** are specialized proteins that can recognize and neutralize specific invaders such as viruses and bacteria.

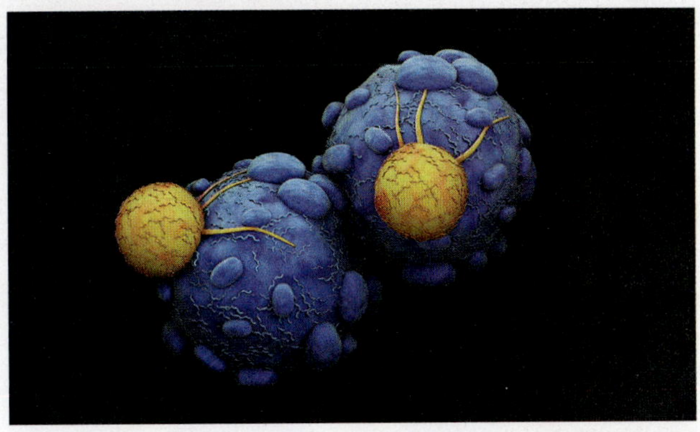

A dendritic cell is a white blood cell that engulfs foreign cells and displays their antigens in a way that makes these antigens recognizable by B and T cells. This process activates the B and T cells, signaling them to proliferate and respond to the specific invader. The dendritic cell shown in this scanning electron micrograph is magnified 2700 times. luismmolina/Getty Images

**T Cells and B Cells** Each T and B cell has receptors that allow it to recognize one specific antigen. The immune system produces T and B cells with many receptor types, each capable of recognizing a different antigen. Thus the immune system can recognize nearly all disease-causing microbes. When a B cell lymphocyte or T cell lymphocyte encounters the antigen for which it is specific, they attack the invading organisms. **B cells** become plasma cells that secrete antibodies. **T cells** differentiate into helper T cells, killer T cells, or suppressor T cells (also called regulatory T cells). B and T cells can mount a rapid and powerful response should they encounter the same invader months or even years in the future.

**The Inflammatory Response** When injured or infected, the body reacts by producing an inflammatory response. Macrophages engulf the invading microbe and produce substances that signal danger to other immune system cells. The resulting inflammatory response causes blood vessels to dilate and fluid to flow out of capillaries into the injured tissue. White blood cells are drawn to the area and attack the invaders, in many cases destroying them. At the

**TERMS**

**immune system** The body's collective system of defenses that includes surface barriers as well as the specialized cells, tissues, and organs that carry out the immune response.

**lymphocyte** A type of white blood cell that carries out important functions in the immune system.

**antigen** A substance that triggers the immune response.

**antibody** A specialized protein, produced by plasma cells, that can recognize specific antigens.

**B cell** A type of lymphocyte that produces antibodies.

**T cells** Cells responsible for cell-mediated adaptive immune reactions. Helper T cells activate macrophages and promote activation of B cells and killer T cells. Killer T cells kill cells infected with viruses, other intracellular pathogens, and tumor cells.

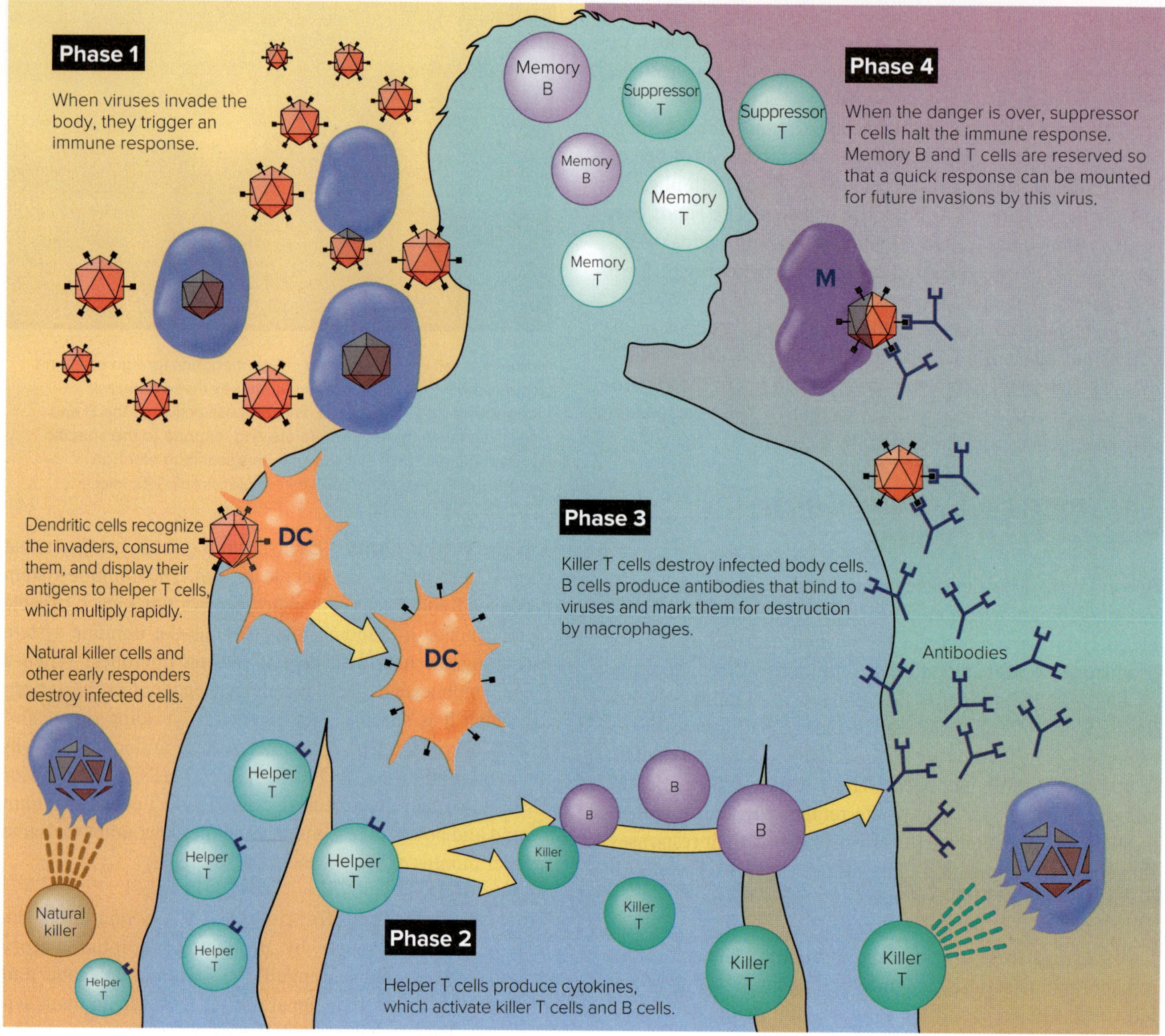


**FIGURE 14.1 The immune response.** Once invaded by a pathogen, the body mounts a complex series of reactions to destroy the invader. Pictured here are the phases of the immune response as the body works to destroy a virus.

site of infection there may be *pus*—a collection of dead white blood cells and debris resulting from the encounter.

**The Immune Response** The activities of the innate and adaptive immune systems are integrated to generate a coordinated and usually highly effective immune response. Figure 14.1 illustrates how this happens:

- ***Phase 1: Recognition.*** If a pathogen breaches the body's physical and chemical barriers (e.g., skin, cilia, and mucus), it initiates the first phase of the immune response by arousing dendritic cells at the site of pathogen entry. They engulf the pathogen and migrate to nearby lymphoid tissue. There the dendritic cells activate helper and killer T cells by presenting fragments of pathogen proteins to T cells. Antigen carried into lymphoid tissue also activates B cells, which can produce plasma cells to attack a specific type of invader.

- ***Phase 2: Proliferation.*** The activated helper and killer T cells multiply, amplifying the immune response to the pathogen. Helper T cells produce special growth stimulants called cytokines, signaling molecules that regulate immunity, inflammation, and production of blood cells and platelets; they further stimulate the activation and proliferation of killer T cells and B cells.

- ***Phase 3: Elimination.*** The activated T and B cells then become either memory cells or effector cells. The effector cells eliminate the pathogen. If the infecting pathogen is a virus or an intracellular bacterium, then killer T cells destroy body cells that are infected with that pathogen. Activated B cells become memory B cells or antibody-producing plasma cells. The antibodies bind to extracellular pathogens (those outside body cells) and mark them for destruction by macrophages and natural killer cells.

- *Phase 4: Slowdown.* Regulatory T cells inhibit lymphocyte proliferation and induce lymphocyte death, causing a slowdown of the immune response. This process restores memory T and B cells, which can initiate a rapid response if the same pathogen reappears.

**Immunity** Usually, after an infection, a person is immune to the same pathogen. This **immunity,** or insusceptibility, occurs because lymphocytes created during phase 2 of the immune response are reserved as memory T and B cells. They continue to circulate in the blood and lymphatic system for years. If the same antigen enters the body again, the memory T and B cells recognize and destroy it before it can cause illness. The ability of memory lymphocytes to remember previous infections and improve immune defenses if the same microbe is encountered in the future is called **adaptive immunity.**

**The Lymphatic System** The lymphatic system consists of a network of vessels that carry a clear fluid called lymph. It also includes organs and structures, such as the spleen and the lymph nodes, that function as part of the immune system. The lymphatic vessels pick up excess fluid from body tissues. This fluid may contain microbes and dead or damaged body cells. Macrophages, dendritic cells, and lymphocytes congregate in the lymph nodes. If immune cells in a lymph node recognize an antigen, the adaptive immune response is triggered. As the immune response progresses, a lymph node actively involved in fighting an infection may fill with cells and swell. Physicians use the location of swollen lymph nodes as a clue to an infection's location.

## Immunization

The ability of the immune system to remember previously encountered organisms and retain its ability to destroy or neutralize them is the basis for **immunization.** When a person is immunized, the immune system is primed with an antigen similar to the pathogenic organism. The body responds by producing antibodies, which prevent serious infection if the person is exposed to the disease organism itself. Thus, immunization (vaccination) activates the immune system and launches a natural immune response. The preparations used to alert the immune system are known as **vaccines.** Visit the Centers for Disease Control and Prevention (CDC) Vaccines & Immunizations website (www.cdc.gov/vaccines) for updates and the recommendations for children, travelers, pregnant women, and adults with special health risks. Some vaccines require multiple doses or periodic booster shots to maintain effectiveness, so it is important to keep up with the recommended vaccine schedule.

Immunization has become a source of public debate among people who question whether vaccinations do more harm than good. They worry about the efficacy and safety of certain types of vaccinations. Public health officials are concerned because decreases in vaccination rates can result in outbreaks of dangerous infectious diseases, especially since international travel makes it easy for pathogens to cross borders from countries with low vaccination rates, leading to large outbreaks.

**Types of Vaccines** Vaccines can be made in several ways. In some cases, microbes are cultured in the laboratory in a way that attenuates (weakens) them. These live, attenuated organisms are used in vaccines against diseases such as measles, mumps, and rubella (German measles). In other cases, when it is not possible to generate attenuated organisms, vaccines are made from pathogens that have been killed but that still retain their ability to stimulate the immune system to produce antibodies. Vaccines composed of killed viruses are used against influenza viruses, among others.

A recent advancement in vaccine technology is the **messenger RNA (mRNA) vaccine** used in several Covid-19 vaccines. The mRNA instructs the recipient's cells to produce harmless parts of a pathogen such as a virus. These in turn stimulate the immune system to produce antibodies.

**Vaccine Efficacy and Safety** In the past century, vaccines have helped to increase the average American life span by 30 years–and with an excellent safety record. Nevertheless, misinformation about vaccines has spread (particularly on the internet and in popular media), raising concerns about their efficacy and safety. The success of vaccines in preventing disease has been well established, but their role in human health is underappreciated.

Most childhood vaccines are effective enough to prevent disease in most people. For a small proportion of people, the vaccine does not provoke a strong enough immune response to avoid disease. Protection from infection is provided by those around them, as long as they live, work, and travel around people who have been vaccinated and are themselves protected. The same is true for people who cannot be vaccinated due to young age or underlying medical conditions (such as cancer treatment).

### Ask Yourself

**QUESTIONS FOR CRITICAL THINKING AND REFLECTION**

What are your views on government-required child vaccinations? What has shaped your views on this issue?

**TERMS**

**immunity** Resistance to infection.

**adaptive immunity** Immunity to infection acquired by the activation of antigen-specific lymphocytes in response to infection or immunization. Adaptive immunity results in immunological memory.

**immunization** The process of conferring immunity to a pathogen by administering a vaccine to a person.

**vaccines** A preparation of killed or weakened microorganisms, inactivated toxins, or components of microorganisms that is administered to stimulate an immune response; a vaccine protects against future infection by the pathogen.

**messenger RNA (mRNA) vaccine** A preparation of genetic material that after injection spurs the body to produce parts of a virus and in turn antibodies that protect against it.

## SPECIAL FEATURE
# Vaccine Hesitancy

Vaccine hesitancy—the reluctance or refusal to get vaccinated—is a problem not only in the United States; the World Health Organization declared it one of 10 major threats to global health.

### The Safety and Effectiveness of Vaccines

We have recently passed through the worst of the Covid-19 pandemic. Since the start of the Covid-19 vaccine rollout in December 2020, 264.5 million Americans have received at least one dose of vaccine; adverse effects related to Covid-19 vaccination have occurred at a rate of 0.006%. Covid-19 has taken the lives of over one million U.S. people.

People who are vaccinated are less likely to become infected with Covid-19. Data collected by the CDC found that, in October 2021, unvaccinated people were 10 times more likely to be infected and 20 times more likely to die from Covid-19 than were fully vaccinated people. The vaccinated are less likely to transmit the virus to others, which is especially important when they come into contact with those at high risks for severe illness, such as the elderly, people with underlying health conditions, the immunocompromised, and others ineligible for the vaccine.

In September 2022, 90.5% of adult Americans had received at least one dose of vaccine, and almost 52% had received at least one booster; in a survey of unvaccinated Americans in the beginning of 2022, around half said they would "definitely not" get the vaccine.

### Who Are the Unvaccinated?

Unvaccinated people may have difficulties finding time off or transportation to get vaccinated, or they may worry about vaccine safety and are waiting for more information. The unvaccinated are also less likely to trust institutions, such as government and health care systems. Uninsured people under age 50, political conservatives, and white evangelical Christians are the three least-vaccinated groups, with around 25% saying they will refuse vaccination. Roughly 40% of rural adult residents, African American adults, and Hispanic adults say the government has not done enough to help their communities during the Covid-19 pandemic—and vaccination has lagged among these groups.

Since the mid-2000s, numerous factors have resulted in rural hospital closures, creating "health care deserts," which limit the ability of health care systems to reach unvaccinated rural residents. For Black Americans, who have been disproportionately affected by higher rates of illness and death from Covid-19, distrust in the health care system is rooted both in history and present-day experiences with the health care system, including less health insurance and access to care, differences in quality of care, and stereotyping by providers.

### Misinformation and the Media

Polarized news sources, social media, and the speed of developments around the virus and the vaccines all help create a fertile environment for the spread of misinterpretation and deliberate disinformation. In one survey, 20% of Americans believed at least one of the following false vaccine claims: that the vaccine alters DNA, contains a tracking microchip, contains tissue of aborted fetuses, or causes infertility. Belief in such vaccine falsehoods was significantly associated with lower vaccination rates and greater vaccine resistance.

### What Will Increase Vaccination Rates?

In the 1950s, demand for the polio vaccine exceeded supply. State vaccine mandates for schools were met with little resistance. The rise of large social programs throughout the 1950s and 1960s, designed to lift people from poverty and expand access to education and health care, fostered the belief all members of society shared and benefited from a greater good. Today, vaccine refusal may be symptomatic of the erosion of this precious belief.

By the end of 2021, another public health success story: federal clinics have opened in diverse communities, and churches, barbershops, and beauty salons could also become sites of vaccination. Efforts targeting racial inequities are leading to Latino and African Americans vaccination rates rising.

**SOURCES:** Leonhardt, D. 2022. The Morning Newsletter, October 4 (https://messaging-custom-newsletters.nytimes.com/template/oakv2?campaign_id=9&emc=edit_nn_20221004&instance_id=73673&nl=the-morning&productCode=NN®i_id=79877247&segment_id=108899&te=1&uri=nyt%3A%2F%2Fnewsletter%2F5c7c35c2-3cb8-5d60-89bf-b05bad46a1ac&user_id=08d5f82afdf84c870d5eeb8f2f58f703). Centers for Disease Control and Prevention. 2022. *Covid-19: Reported Adverse Events* (https://www.cdc.gov/coronavirus/2019-ncov/vaccines/safety/adverse-events.html); Centers for Disease Control and Prevention. 2022. *COVID Data Tracker* (https://covid.cdc.gov/covid-data-tracker/#rates-by-vaccine-status); Kirzinger, A., et al. 2021. KFF COVID-19 Vaccine Monitor: November 2021. Kaiser Family Foundation (https://www.kff.org/coronavirus-covid-19/poll-finding/kff-covid-19-vaccine-monitor-november-2021/); Centers for Disease Control and Prevention. 2022. *Immunization* (https://www.cdc.gov/nchs/fastats/immunize.htm).

Keeping vaccination rates consistently high over time is necessary to maintain protection. Before the development of the measles vaccine in 1963, nearly everyone in the United States got measles, and hundreds died from measles every year. In the five years before the vaccine was introduced, about 400–500 deaths and 48,000 hospitalizations from measles occurred annually. Following widespread vaccination, the United States was declared measles-free in 2000, meaning measles is not constantly present. However, outbreaks have continued to occur, with infection brought into the United States by unvaccinated travelers (Americans or foreign visitors) who get measles while they are in other countries.

Vaccines are approved by the Advisory Committee on Immunization Practices—the advisors for the CDC—and the Committee on Infectious Diseases—the advisors for the American Academy of Pediatrics (AAP). Both the AAP and the CDC advisory committees have expert knowledge in virology, microbiology, statistics, epidemiology, and pathogenesis—knowledge necessary for reviewing and evaluating studies on vaccine efficacy and safety. (See the special feature on vaccine hesitancy.)

To further ensure their safety, vaccines are tested before being licensed in greater numbers of people for longer periods of time than are drugs. Each Covid-19 vaccine was tested in 30,000–40,000 people. Additionally, safety mechanisms such as the Vaccine Adverse Event Reporting System (VAERS) and the Vaccine Safety Datalink Project monitor adverse events reported after licensure. Side effects from immunization are usually mild, such as soreness at the injection site. It is estimated that an allergic reaction may occur in 1 in 1.5 million doses. Any risk from a vaccine must be balanced against the risk posed by the diseases it prevents.

QUICK STATS

**Since the HPV vaccine's introduction, HPV infections that cause most HPV cancers and genital warts among young adult women have dropped 81%.**

—CDC, 2022

For more on the safety, efficacy, and testing of vaccines, visit the CDC Vaccines & Immunizations website (www.cdc.gov/vaccines) and the website for the American Academy of Pediatrics (www.aap.org).

## Allergy: A Case of Mistaken Identity

**Allergies** affect an estimated 50 million Americans. In a person with an allergy, the immune system reacts to a harmless substance as if it were a harmful pathogen. Allergy symptoms—stuffy nose, sneezing, wheezing, skin rashes, and so on—usually are due to the immune response. An **allergen** is a molecule that elicits an exaggerated immune response. Common allergens include pollen, animal dander, dust mites and cockroaches, molds and mildew, foods, and insect stings.

QUICK STATS

**About 7% of U.S. children and 8% of U.S. adults currently have asthma.**

—Centers for Disease Control and Prevention, 2019

### The Allergic Response

Allergies are an adverse response to environmental antigens that are not pathogenic. The body's response is to release large amounts of **histamine,** a chemical associated with inflammation. In the nose, histamine may cause congestion and sneezing; in the eyes, itchiness and tearing; in the skin, redness, swelling, and itching; in the intestines, bloating and cramping; and in the lungs, coughing, wheezing, and shortness of breath. In some people, an allergen can trigger an **asthma** attack. Symptoms—wheezing, tightness in the chest, shortness of breath, and coughing—often occur immediately, within minutes of exposure, but inflammatory reactions may take hours or days to develop and then may persist for several days. The symptoms may be mild and occur only occasionally, or they may be severe and occur daily.

Asthma is caused by both chronic inflammation of the airways and spasm of the muscles surrounding the airways. The spasm causes constriction, and the inflammation causes the airway linings to swell and secrete extra mucus, which further obstructs the passages.

An asthma attack is initiated by an irritating stimulus in the bronchial tubes. The stimulus may be an inhaled allergen, such as pollen, dust mites, mold, animal dander, or cockroach droppings, or it can be a nonallergen stimulus, such as exercise, cold air, pollutants, tobacco smoke, infection, or stress. In women with asthma, hormonal changes that occur as menstruation starts may increase vulnerability to attacks. Both environmental and genetic factors contribute to the development of asthma.

**Anaphylaxis** is the most serious—although rare—acute allergic reaction to an antigen that the body has become hypersensitive to (e.g., a bee sting). Anaphylaxis results from a release of histamine throughout the body that can be life threatening. Symptoms may include swelling of the throat, extremely low blood pressure, fainting, heart arrhythmia, and seizures. Anaphylaxis is a medical emergency, and treatment requires immediate injection of epinephrine. People at risk for anaphylaxis should wear medical alert identification and keep self-administrable epinephrine readily available.

### Climate Change and Allergies

The predicted global changes in climate are likely to exacerbate allergies, including allergic rhinitis and asthma. Global warming is influencing plant and fungal reproduction and thus is influencing both spatial and temporal production of allergens. If warm weather periods lengthen, then the period of pollen release also will be prolonged and the amount of pollen released may increase. Thus, politicians and policymakers must become involved in reducing the impact of climate change on human health.

TERMS

**allergy** An immune response to normally innocuous foreign chemicals and proteins that is characterized by specific symptoms such as sneezing, rash, and swelling; also called *hypersensitivity*.

**allergen** A substance, such as pollen, that triggers an allergic reaction.

**histamine** A chemical released from cells in response to an allergen and responsible for dilation and increased permeability of blood vessels.

**asthma** A disease in which chronic inflammation and periodic constriction of the airways cause wheezing, shortness of breath, and coughing.

**anaphylaxis** A severe systemic hypersensitive reaction to an allergen characterized by difficulty breathing, low blood pressure, heart arrhythmia, seizure, and sometimes death.

**Dealing with Allergies** If you suspect you might have an allergy, visit your physician or an allergy specialist. You may be able to avoid or minimize exposure to allergens by changing your environment or behavior. For example, removing carpets from the bedroom and using special bedding can reduce dust mite contact. Also, medications are available for allergy sufferers. Many over-the-counter antihistamines are effective at controlling symptoms, and prescription corticosteroids delivered by aerosol markedly reduce allergy symptoms. A third approach is immunotherapy, in which a person is desensitized to a particular allergen through the administration of gradually increasing doses of the allergen over a period of months or years.

# THE SPREAD OF DISEASE

The immune system is operating at all times, maintaining its vigilance when you're well and fighting invaders when you're sick.

## Symptoms and Contagion

The symptoms you experience during an illness are related to the phase of infection and the actions of your immune system. During the first phase of infection, or **incubation period,** when viruses or bacteria are actively multiplying before the immune system has gathered momentum, you may not have any symptoms of the illness, but you may be contagious. During the second and third phases of the immune response, you may still be unaware of the infection, or you may "feel a cold coming on." Symptoms first appear during the *prodromal period,* which follows incubation. If you have acquired immunity, the infection may be eradicated during the incubation period or the prodromal period. In this case it does not develop into a full-blown illness.

Many symptoms of an illness are actually due to the body's immune response rather than to the actions or products of the invading organism. For example, fever is caused by macrophages and other cells' releasing certain cytokines during the immune response. These cytokines travel in the bloodstream to the brain and cause the body's thermostat to be reset to a higher level. The resulting elevated temperature helps the body fight against pathogens by enhancing immune responses.

You may be contagious before you experience any symptoms, and you are contagious as long as your body is releasing infectious microbes. For example, adults who have contracted the flu can infect other people beginning one day *before* symptoms develop and up to five to seven days *afterward.* Children may pass the flu virus for longer than seven days. Symptoms appear one to four days *after* infection.

Some people can be infected with the flu virus and yet perceive no symptoms. Mathematical models suggest that asymptomatic carriers contribute to the spread of a variety of diseases, such as influenza, Ebola, and others. The possibility that asymptomatic people can be infectious is an important reason that everyone should remain up to date on vaccines.

**TERMS**

**incubation period** The period when bacteria or viruses are actively multiplying inside the body's cells; usually a period without symptoms of illness.

**reservoir** A long-term host in which a pathogen typically lives.

**vector** An insect, rodent, or other organism that carries and transmits a pathogen from one host to another.

**systemic infection** An infection spread by the blood or lymphatic system to large portions of the body.

## The Chain of Infection

Infectious diseases are transmitted from one person to another through a series of steps. New infections can be prevented by interfering with any step in this process. The chain of infection has six major links:

1. ***Pathogen.*** The infectious disease cycle begins with a pathogen that enters the body.
2. ***Reservoir.*** The pathogen has a natural environment—called a **reservoir**—in which it typically lives. A person who is the reservoir for a pathogen may be ill or may be an asymptomatic carrier who, although having no symptoms, can spread infection.
3. ***Portal of exit.*** To transmit infection, the pathogen must leave the reservoir through some portal of exit. In the case of a human reservoir, portals of exit include saliva, the mucous membranes, blood, feces, and nose and throat discharges.
4. ***Means of transmission.*** Transmission can occur directly or indirectly. In *direct transmission,* the pathogen is passed from one person to another without an intermediary. Most common respiratory infections and many intestinal infections are passed directly. Other means of direct transmission include sexual contact and contact with blood. In *indirect transmission,* animals or insects such as rats, ticks, and mosquitoes serve as **vectors,** carrying the pathogen from one host to another. Pathogens can also be transmitted via contaminated soil, food, or water or from inanimate objects; they can also float in the air for long periods, suspended on tiny particles of dust or droplets that can travel long distances before they are inhaled.
5. ***Portal of entry.*** To infect a new host, a pathogen must have a portal of entry into the body. Pathogens can enter through direct contact with or penetration of the skin or mucous membranes, inhalation, or ingestion. Pathogens that enter the skin or mucous membranes can cause a local infection of the tissue, or they may penetrate into the bloodstream or lymphatic system, thereby causing a **systemic infection.** Agents that cause sexually transmitted infections usually enter the body through the mucous membranes lining the urethra (in males) or the cervix (in females).
6. ***The new host.*** Once in the new host, a variety of factors determine whether the pathogen will establish itself and

cause infection. People with a strong immune system or resistance to a particular pathogen are less likely to become ill than are people with poor immunity. If conditions are right, the pathogen will multiply and produce disease in the new host. In such a case, the new host may become a reservoir from which a new chain of infection can be started.

Interrupting the chain of infection at any point can prevent disease. Strategies for breaking the chain include both public health measures and individual action. For example, a pathogen's reservoir can be isolated or destroyed, as when a sick individual is placed under quarantine or when insects or animals carrying pathogens are killed. Public sanitation practices, such as sewage treatment and the chlorination of drinking water, can also kill pathogens. Transmission can be disrupted through strategies like hand washing and the use of face masks. Immunization and the treatment of infected hosts can stop the pathogen from multiplying, producing a serious disease, and being passed on to a new host.

## Epidemics and Pandemics

The rapid spread of a disease or health condition is called an **epidemic.** Although the word is usually used to refer to infectious diseases, it is also used for health conditions that are not caused by an infectious organism. For example, it is often said that obesity and diabetes have reached epidemic proportions in the United States.

An important underlying premise of the concept of "epidemic" is that the occurrence of the disease is greater than what is expected normally. Thus, the common cold, which occurs with great frequency, is never classified as an epidemic. Conversely, the term *epidemic* is used to refer to outbreaks of diseases that are not widespread. For example, when 10 infants died in California in 2010 from whooping cough, the incident was referred to as an epidemic.

A **pandemic** is an epidemic that has spread across a large area, such as an entire nation, a continent, or even the world. The term *pandemic* refers exclusively to infectious disease. Human history has been punctuated by numerous pandemics of various diseases, including bubonic plague, smallpox, and influenza. The probability of pandemics has increased over the past century because people have engaged in more global travel and integration, migrated to cities, changed land use, and exploited the natural environment more. These trends will probably continue and intensify. At the time of writing, late 2022, the number of worldwide deaths projected from Covid-19 is over 6.5 million.

Not all widespread infectious diseases are pandemics. An infectious disease is said to be **endemic** when it habitually exists in a certain region.

**Covid-19** Covid-19 is a respiratory illness caused by the coronavirus SARS-CoV-2, and it spreads from person to person. Coronaviruses are a large, diverse family of viruses common in people and in different species of animals, including camels, cattle, cats, dogs, ferrets, and bats. Some coronaviruses commonly cause mild upper-respiratory tract illnesses. But when they jump from animal to human hosts they can cause serious illness, partly because humans lack immunity to the new virus.

Covid-19 can lead to potentially serious illness, pneumonia sometimes requiring oxygen or mechanical ventilation. The receptor binding site of SARS-CoV-2 binds to the host cell receptor with a higher affinity than does that of SARS-CoV (which causes SARS illness), and that may explain its rapid spread. Covid-19 cases can range from mild to severe.

Covid-19 symptoms vary tremendously: fever, cough, fatigue, shortness of breath; and less routinely, headache, muscle aches and pains, sore throat, nausea, diarrhea, chills, loss of taste, loss of smell. About half of patients report neurological symptoms.

Several Covid-19 vaccines available in the United States have been extremely effective in preventing hospitalization and death from Covid-19. Due to the rise of highly contagious variants, Covid-19 cases reached a peak in January 2022, with over 800,000 new U.S. cases a day. The good news is that these new variants appear to be getting milder. As more individuals are exposed multiple times to Covid-19 as children, they will be protected as adults, as is the case with other common respiratory viruses.

**H1N1 Influenza** Before the Covid-19 outbreak, the last global pandemic was the 2009 outbreak of H1N1 influenza A virus. Initially called swine flu, this new strain of virus had never before been identified as a cause of human illness. Like Covid-19, H1N1 is an infectious respiratory illness. But it comes from any of several different types and strains of influenza viruses, rather than the single, novel virus that causes Covid-19. The influenza A virus mutates frequently during replication, and it can also exchange genes with other influenza A viruses, including strains that infect domestic and wild animals. The H1N1 strain resulted from a combination of genes from four viruses: two from swine flu viruses, one from an avian (bird) flu virus, and one from a human flu virus. The WHO continues to track trends globally, and the

### Ask Yourself

**QUESTIONS FOR CRITICAL THINKING AND REFLECTION**

Think about the last time you were sick with a cold, the flu, or an intestinal infection. Can you identify the reservoir from which the infection came? What vector, if any, transmitted the illness to you? Did you pass the infection to anyone else? If so, how?

**TERMS**

**epidemic** A rapidly spreading disease or health-related condition.

**pandemic** A widespread epidemic.

**endemic** Occurring regularly in a certain region.

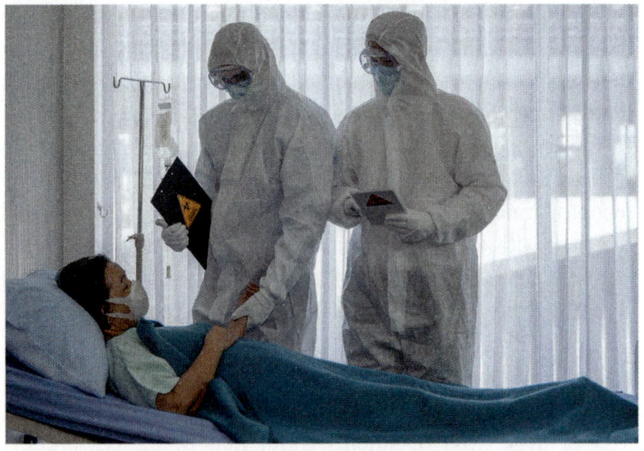

Treating someone with a highly infectious disease like the Covid-19 or Ebola virus involves a careful and meticulous process of putting on and taking off protective gear. The use of protective gear is one strategy for breaking the chain of infection. Mongkolchon Akesin/Shutterstock

CDC continues to recommend H1N1 vaccination for persons aged 6 months to 24 years and people aged 25–64 years who are at high risk.

## PATHOGENS, DISEASES, AND TREATMENTS

Most microorganisms do not cause disease at all. Some that potentially can cause disease are readily dealt with by the body's defenses discussed earlier in the chapter. However, some microorganisms cause infectious disease even in a healthy person. Worldwide, infectious diseases are responsible for more than 11 million deaths each year. The pathogens that cause infectious diseases include bacteria, viruses, fungi, protozoa, and parasitic worms (Figure 14.2). Infections can occur almost anywhere in or on the body. Examples of common infections are bronchitis, which is an infection of the airways (bronchi); meningitis, infection of the tissue surrounding the brain and spinal cord; and conjunctivitis (pinkeye), infection of the layer of cells surrounding the eyes.

### Bacteria

The most abundant living things on earth are **bacteria.** Bacteria are often classified by their shape: bacilli (rod-shaped), cocci (spherical), spirochete (spiral-shaped), or vibrios (comma-shaped).

**TERMS**

**bacterium** A microscopic single-celled organism with a cell wall (plural, *bacteria*). Bacteria may be helpful or harmful to humans.

**pneumonia** Inflammation of the lungs, typically caused by infection or exposure to chemical toxins or irritants.

**meningitis** Infection of the meninges (membranes covering the brain and spinal cord).

Bacteria play very important roles in human health. For example, our gut microbiota include at least a thousand different species of bacteria. Remarkably, the genetic material of all these bacteria adds up to more than 150 times as many genes as appear in our genome. These bacteria have several important functions, including assisting the digestion of certain foods and the production of vitamin K and some B vitamins, and controlling the growth of pathogenic bacteria by stimulating the mucosal immune system. In addition, there is evidence from studies of mice that gut microbiota influence the development of autoimmune disease. We also have bacteria in our skin and in our reproductive tracts. About 100 species of bacteria can cause disease in humans.

Pathogenic bacteria cause disease when they release toxins or grow in tissues that are normally sterile, such as the bladder. They can enter the body through a cut in the skin, an insect bite, contaminated food or drink, sexual activity, or any of several other means.

**Pneumonia** **Pneumonia** is an inflammation of the lungs. Although it can be caused by viruses or fungi, bacterial pneumonia is the most common and the most treatable. Pneumonia often follows another illness, such as a cold or the flu, but the symptoms are typically more severe–fever, chills, shortness of breath, increased mucus production, and cough. Pneumonia is one of the 10 leading causes of death for Americans; people most at risk for severe infection include those under age 2 or over age 75 and those with chronic health problems such as heart disease, asthma, or HIV. Worldwide, pneumonia is the leading cause of death for children under 5 years of age.

The most common cause of bacterial pneumonia is *Streptococcus pneumoniae*, or pneumococcus. A vaccine is available for pneumococcal pneumonia and is recommended for all adults age 65 and over and others at risk. Other bacteria that may cause pneumonia include *Haemophilus influenzae, Chlamydia pneumoniae,* and *Mycoplasma pneumoniae.* Mycoplasma is a very small bacterium; *M. pneumoniae* causes a mild form of pneumonia often called "walking pneumonia." Outbreaks of infection with mycoplasmas are relatively common among young adults, especially in crowded settings such as dormitories. Bacterial pneumonia can be treated with antibiotics.

**Meningitis** Inflammation of the *meninges,* the protective membranes covering the brain and spinal cord, is called **meningitis.** Inflammation is usually caused by infection of the fluid surrounding the brain. Most cases of meningitis are viral. Viral meningitis is usually mild and resolves without medical intervention. Bacterial meningitis, however, can be life threatening and requires immediate treatment with antibiotics. Symptoms of meningitis include fever, a severe headache, stiff neck, sensitivity to light, and confusion. Symptoms can appear quickly or over a few days. Immediate treatment is needed because death can occur within hours. *Neisseria meningitidis* (meningococcus) and *Streptococcus pneumoniae* (pneumococcus) are the leading causes of bacterial

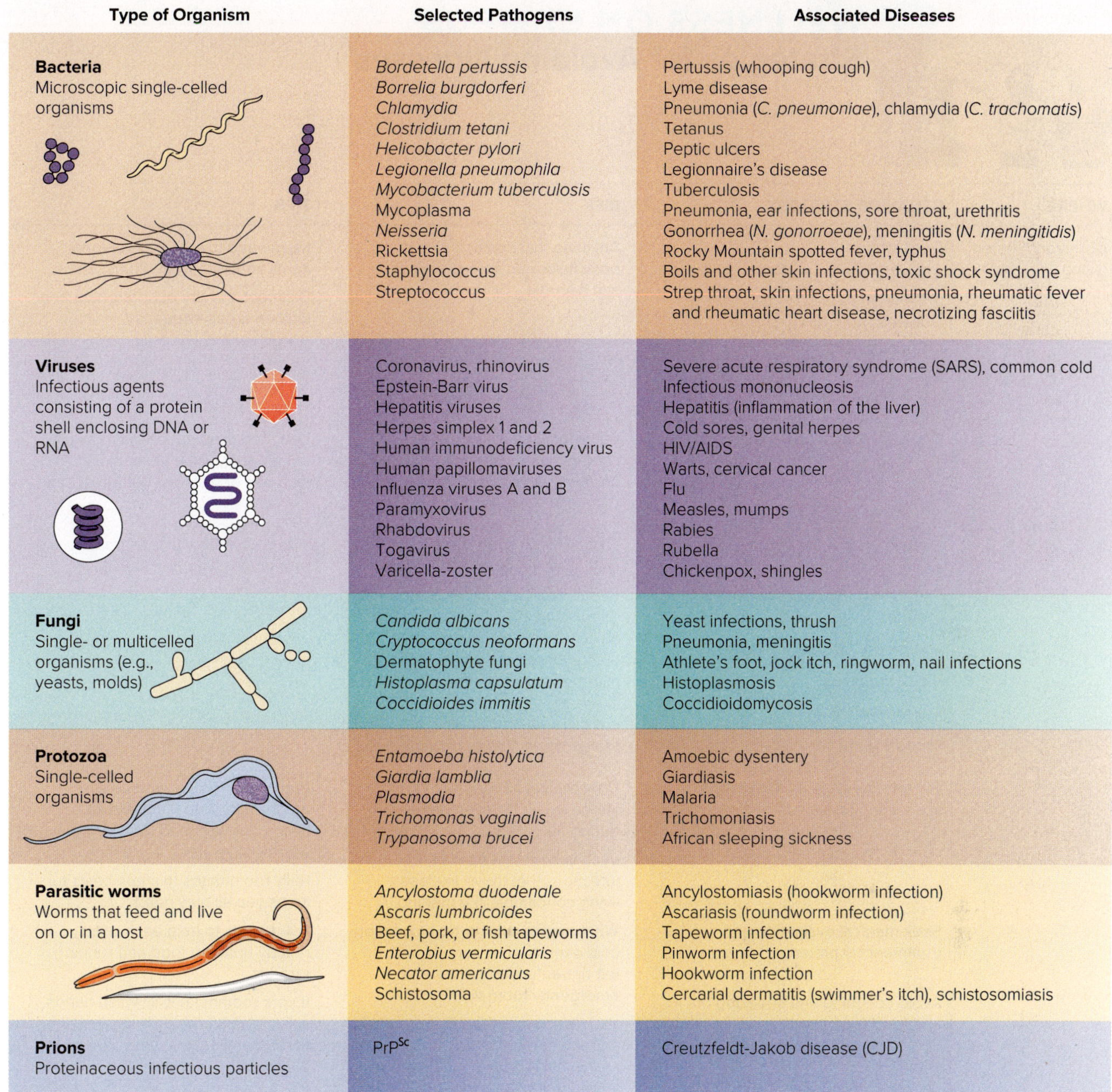

| Type of Organism | Selected Pathogens | Associated Diseases |
|---|---|---|
| **Bacteria**<br>Microscopic single-celled organisms | *Bordetella pertussis*<br>*Borrelia burgdorferi*<br>*Chlamydia*<br>*Clostridium tetani*<br>*Helicobacter pylori*<br>*Legionella pneumophila*<br>*Mycobacterium tuberculosis*<br>Mycoplasma<br>*Neisseria*<br>Rickettsia<br>Staphylococcus<br>Streptococcus | Pertussis (whooping cough)<br>Lyme disease<br>Pneumonia (*C. pneumoniae*), chlamydia (*C. trachomatis*)<br>Tetanus<br>Peptic ulcers<br>Legionnaire's disease<br>Tuberculosis<br>Pneumonia, ear infections, sore throat, urethritis<br>Gonorrhea (*N. gonorroeae*), meningitis (*N. meningitidis*)<br>Rocky Mountain spotted fever, typhus<br>Boils and other skin infections, toxic shock syndrome<br>Strep throat, skin infections, pneumonia, rheumatic fever and rheumatic heart disease, necrotizing fasciitis |
| **Viruses**<br>Infectious agents consisting of a protein shell enclosing DNA or RNA | Coronavirus, rhinovirus<br>Epstein-Barr virus<br>Hepatitis viruses<br>Herpes simplex 1 and 2<br>Human immunodeficiency virus<br>Human papillomaviruses<br>Influenza viruses A and B<br>Paramyxovirus<br>Rhabdovirus<br>Togavirus<br>Varicella-zoster | Severe acute respiratory syndrome (SARS), common cold<br>Infectious mononucleosis<br>Hepatitis (inflammation of the liver)<br>Cold sores, genital herpes<br>HIV/AIDS<br>Warts, cervical cancer<br>Flu<br>Measles, mumps<br>Rabies<br>Rubella<br>Chickenpox, shingles |
| **Fungi**<br>Single- or multicelled organisms (e.g., yeasts, molds) | *Candida albicans*<br>*Cryptococcus neoformans*<br>Dermatophyte fungi<br>*Histoplasma capsulatum*<br>*Coccidioides immitis* | Yeast infections, thrush<br>Pneumonia, meningitis<br>Athlete's foot, jock itch, ringworm, nail infections<br>Histoplasmosis<br>Coccidioidomycosis |
| **Protozoa**<br>Single-celled organisms | *Entamoeba histolytica*<br>*Giardia lamblia*<br>*Plasmodia*<br>*Trichomonas vaginalis*<br>*Trypanosoma brucei* | Amoebic dysentery<br>Giardiasis<br>Malaria<br>Trichomoniasis<br>African sleeping sickness |
| **Parasitic worms**<br>Worms that feed and live on or in a host | *Ancylostoma duodenale*<br>*Ascaris lumbricoides*<br>Beef, pork, or fish tapeworms<br>*Enterobius vermicularis*<br>*Necator americanus*<br>Schistosoma | Ancylostomiasis (hookworm infection)<br>Ascariasis (roundworm infection)<br>Tapeworm infection<br>Pinworm infection<br>Hookworm infection<br>Cercarial dermatitis (swimmer's itch), schistosomiasis |
| **Prions**<br>Proteinaceous infectious particles | $PrP^{Sc}$ | Creutzfeldt-Jakob disease (CJD) |

**FIGURE 14.2 Pathogens and associated infectious diseases.**

meningitis, particularly in adolescents and young adults (see the box "Strategies for Avoiding Illnesses").

The disease is fatal in 10–15% of cases, and 10–20% of people who recover have permanent disabilities, including brain damage, seizures, and hearing loss. Worldwide, meningitis kills about 170,000 people each year, particularly in the so-called meningitis belt in sub-Saharan Africa.

## Strep Throat and Other Streptococcal Infections

**Streptococcus** is the genus name of a group of bacteria that cause several diseases in humans. Streptococcal pharyngitis, or strep throat, is characterized by a red, sore throat with white patches on the tonsils, swollen lymph nodes, fever, and headache. Typically the streptococcus bacterium is spread from an infected individual through close contact via respiratory droplets. If left untreated, strep throat can develop into the more serious rheumatic fever. A particularly virulent type of streptococcus can invade the bloodstream, spread to other parts of the body, and produce dangerous systemic illness. If you have a streptococcal infection, you can minimize the risk

**TERMS**

**streptococcus** Any of a genus (*Streptococcus*) of spherical bacteria; streptococcal species can cause skin infections, strep throat, rheumatic fever, pneumonia, scarlet fever, and other diseases.

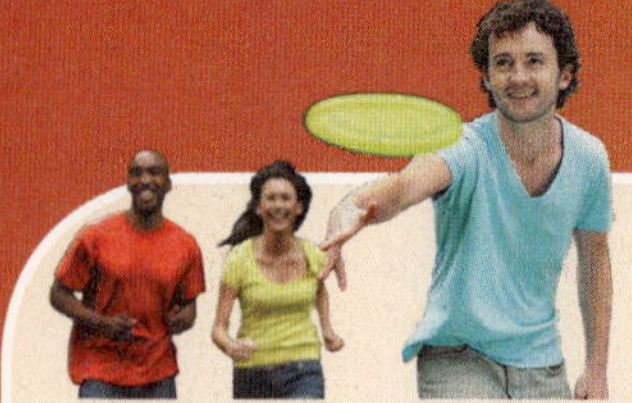

## WELLNESS ON CAMPUS
### Strategies for Avoiding Illnesses

| WHERE | BEHAVIOR STRATEGY | RISK | TIPS |
|---|---|---|---|
| Dormitory/Shared Living | Don't share:<br>• Deodorant<br>• Makeup<br>• Towels<br>• Sponges<br>• Razors<br>• Toothbrushes | Anything that contacts skin or body fluids can spread viruses and bacteria | Keep hand towels and personal items separate from others' items<br>Disinfect and dry out bathroom and kitchen areas frequently |
| | Don't do dishes in the bathroom | Bathroom surfaces are quickly contaminated with pathogens like norovirus and *Salmonella* | Use food preparation area sink. If unavailable, use a clean plastic dish pan or disinfect bathroom sink |
| | Routinely clean the dorm room: sweep, dust, vacuum, disinfect | Pathogens and allergens like mold can cause respiratory problems | Hire a cleaner with fees from roommates who don't clean |
| | The dirtiest areas of a dorm room include:<br>• Desk and dresser surfaces<br>• Door handles<br>• Light switches<br>• Bed sheets | Bed sheets and pillowcases collect dead skin cells, body oils and fluids, which can cause acne; allergens and dust mites can cause allergies, eczema, and asthma. Bed linens can also house *Staphylococcus* bacteria and viruses that cause the common cold and stomach flu | |
| | Get vaccines and flu shot before school and flu season begin | Unvaccinated college students increase risk for everyone else during flu season<br>Vaccines protect from other infections that thrive in close living conditions, like meningitis | Prepare for illness with OTC medications and a first-aid kit instead of having to hunt for them when you're sick<br>Rally roommates to share costs for items you all may need |
| | Seek medical evaluation and treatment for prolonged symptoms | What may appear to be a common cold can be more serious and, if left untreated, can require an emergency room visit | Ask friends to help each other rest by bringing food and running errands |
| | Avoid coughing and sneezing on, and touching others | You can contract the flu from someone 6 feet away | If your roommate is ill, wash hands, surfaces, handles, use separate towels, and stay on your side of the room |
| Gym or swimming pool | Wipe away sweat and disinfect exercise equipment at the gym | Sweat and spittle can spread pathogens like staphylococcus bacteria and influenza virus | Stock a dedicated gym bag with disinfectant wipes, clean towels, and flip-flops. Regularly clean the bag! |
| | Wear flip-flops or waterproof sandals in locker rooms, bathrooms, and communal showers; dry feet well afterward | Warmth and moisture help *tinea pedis* thrive and promote fungal infections like athlete's foot and nail fungus and HPV, which can cause viral infections like plantar warts | Forgot your flip-flops? Clean and thoroughly dry your feet after contact with floors. Avoid contact with floors if your feet have open cuts or wounds |
| Classroom | Don't go to class sick | You may infect other students, teachers, and staff | Know the attendance policies of your university and classes<br>Save absences for when you're actually sick<br>Know how to access health services and where the health center or clinic is |

| WHERE | BEHAVIOR STRATEGY | RISK | TIPS |
|---|---|---|---|
| Dining halls or other food environments | Don't share cups, water bottles, or eating utensils | Viruses spread easily through saliva | |
| | Don't eat old food or food that's been sitting out long | Resist that old slice of pizza. Food left out at temperatures between 40˚F and 140˚F (the temperature range known as the "danger zone") allow the rapid growth of bacteria like *Staphylococcus aureus*, *Salmonella enteritidis*, *E. coli*, and *Campylobacter* within two hours | Cool and store leftovers within two hours |
| | | Bacteria such as *Listeria monocytogenes* can grow on foods in the refrigerator | |
| | Don't eat food in classrooms, libraries, computer labs, or study areas | Surfaces in rooms not meant for eating are likely more contaminated than those in dining halls, which are washed and disinfected more regularly | Disinfect surfaces with wipes if you must eat in a communal non-eating room |
| On you | Frequently clean and disinfect your germiest objects:<br>• Cell phone<br>• Computer keyboard<br>• Bookbag, purse<br>• Headphones (earbuds) | These items tend to come with us everywhere we go, but don't get cleaned or disinfected nearly as often as they should. One in six cell phones tested positive for *E. coli* (from fecal matter); one in four had *Staphylococcus aureus* | Sanitize cell phones and earbuds daily with sanitation wipes; throw your bookbag in the washing machine; disinfect purses |
| | | Computer keyboards commonly house *E. coli* and *Staphylococcus aureus*; viruses may also be transmitted on keyboards. Crumbs found in keyboards encourage bacterial growth | |
| | | Bookbags and purses come in frequent contact with floors—even restroom floors; avoid laying them on beds, surfaces where you eat, or near your face and mouth | |
| | | Potential pathogens like *Staphylococcus* and others can greatly multiply on headset devices after one hour of use | |
| | Greetings: Offer an "elbow-bump" over a handshake or high-five, or just say hello | Handshakes transmit lots of germs, and students who regularly shake hands have been shown to get sick more often than those who don't. High-fives transmit half the germs of a handshake, and fist bumps 1/20th | Carry a small bottle of hand sanitizer in your bookbag supplies |
| | Masking: Wear a mask when required and as needed, in indoor settings and/or large groups | Covid-19 and other illnesses are transmitted by respiratory droplets. In many countries it was the norm to wear masks, even before the Covid-19 pandemic, to reduce the spread of illnesses | KN95, N95, KF94, and surgical masks are more effective than cloth masks, but cloth masks are better than nothing |

SOURCES: KidsHealth. 2022. Talking to Your Partner About Condoms (https://kidshealth.org/en/teens/talk-about-condoms.html); American Sexual Health Association. 2020. Talking to a Partner (http://www.ashasexualhealth.org/sexual-health/talking-about-sex/).

of spreading it by washing your hands well, especially before preparing foods, and by staying home until at least 24 hours after starting antibiotics.

### Toxic Shock Syndrome and Other Staphylococcal Infections

**Staphylococcus** (staph) bacteria are commonly found on the skin and in the nasal passages of healthy people. For example, *Staphylococcus aureus* occurs on 15–40% of people who show no signs of disease. Occasionally, however, staphylococci enter the body and cause an infection, ranging from minor skin infections such as boils to very serious conditions such as blood infections and pneumonia. The risk of a serious staph infection is higher in persons with certain medical conditions, including people suffering from malnutrition, alcoholism, intravenous drug use, diabetes, or kidney failure.

*Staphylococcus aureus* is responsible for many cases of toxic shock syndrome (TSS). The bacteria produce a toxin that causes a massive proliferation of T cells that can bind to it. The staphylococcus toxins are referred to as "super antigens" because the massive proliferation of T cells results in excessive production of pro-inflammatory cytokines. This "cytokine storm" causes tissue damage, widespread coagulation of blood in the blood vessels, and ultimately organ failure.

A serious antibiotic-resistant infection is caused by a staphylococcus bacterium known as methicillin-resistant *Staphylococcus aureus* (MRSA). Many cases of MRSA infection occur in hospitalized patients, and these infections tend to be severe. They include infections of surgical wounds, pneumonia, urinary tract infections, and blood infections. MRSA is also common in the community (outside hospital settings), where it usually infects the skin, causing painful lesions that resemble infected spider bites. The spread of MRSA infection is associated with places where people are in close contact with one another. Athletes are particularly at risk and should keep any cuts or abrasions covered. The best defense against MRSA is good hygiene and frequent hand washing.

### Tuberculosis

Caused by the bacterium *Mycobacterium tuberculosis,* **tuberculosis (TB)** is a chronic bacterial infection that usually affects the lungs, though it can affect other organs as well. TB is spread via the respiratory route. Symptoms include coughing, fatigue, night sweats, weight loss, and fever. Between 10 and 15 million Americans have been infected with *M. tuberculosis* and continue to carry it. The immune system usually prevents the disease from becoming active. In 2020, a total of 7174 new cases of TB were reported—an incidence of 2.2 cases per 100,000 population.

TB is a leading cause of death in people with HIV infection. Many strains of tuberculosis respond to antibiotics, but only over a course of treatment lasting 6–12 months. Failure to complete treatment can lead to relapse and the development of strains of antibiotic-resistant bacteria. Multidrug-resistant TB (MDR TB) is resistant to at least two of the best anti-TB drugs. Extensively drug-resistant TB (XDR TB) is resistant to those drugs as well as some second-line drugs. XDR TB is relatively rare, but patients with this form of TB have fewer and less effective treatment options.

**QUICK STATS**

**Each year, almost 3 million Americans become infected with antibiotic-resistant bacteria and fungi, and 35,000 die as a direct result of these infections.**

—Centers for Disease Control and Prevention, 2019

**TERMS**

**staphylococcus** Any of a genus (*Staphylococcus*) of spherical, clustered bacteria commonly found on the skin or in the nasal passages; staphylococcal species may enter the body and cause conditions such as boils, pneumonia, toxic shock syndrome, and severe skin infections.

**tuberculosis (TB)** A chronic bacterial infection that usually affects the lungs.

### Tick-Borne Infections

Some diseases are transmitted via insect vectors. Lyme disease is one such infection, and it accounts for more than 30,000 reported cases per year, although the actual number may be as high as 300,000. It is spread by the bite of a tick that is infected with the spiral-shaped bacterium *Borrelia burgdorferi.* Ticks acquire the bacterium by ingesting the blood of an infected animal. They can then transmit the microbe to their next host. Lyme disease has been reported in 48 states, but significant risk of infection is found in only about 100 counties in 10 states located in the northeastern and mid-Atlantic seaboard, the upper north-central region, and parts of northern California.

Symptoms of Lyme disease vary but typically occur in three stages. In the first stage, about 80% of victims develop a bull's-eye-shaped red rash expanding from the area of the bite, usually about two weeks after the bite occurs. The second stage occurs weeks to months later in 10–20% of untreated patients. Symptoms may involve the nervous and cardiovascular systems and can include impaired coordination, partial facial paralysis, and heart rhythm abnormalities. These symptoms usually disappear within a few weeks. Lyme disease can also cause fetal damage or death at any stage of pregnancy. Lyme disease is treatable at all stages, although arthritis symptoms arising in the third stage may not resolve completely. Lyme disease is preventable by avoiding contact with ticks, for example by wearing tick-repellent clothing or applying tick-repellent sprays, or by removing a tick before it has had the chance to transmit the infection.

Rocky Mountain spotted fever and typhus are caused by the *rickettsia* bacterium and are also transmitted via tick bites. Rocky Mountain spotted fever is characterized by sudden onset of fever, headache, and muscle pain, followed by development of a spotted rash. Ehrlichiosis, another tick-borne disease, typically causes less severe symptoms.

### Other Bacterial Infections

The following are a few of the many other infections caused by bacteria:

- ***Ulcers.*** Up to 90% of ulcers are caused by infection with the bacterium *Helicobacter pylori.* If tests show the presence of *H. pylori,* antibiotics often cure the infection and the ulcers.

- ***Tetanus.*** Also known as lockjaw, tetanus is caused by the bacterium *Clostridium tetani,* which thrives in deep puncture wounds and produces a deadly toxin. The toxin causes muscular stiffness and spasms, and infection is fatal in about 30% of cases. Due to widespread vaccination, tetanus is rare in the United States. Worldwide, however, approximately 31,000 newborns die each year through infection by unsterile cutting of the umbilical cord.

- ***Clostridium difficile.*** Another type of *Clostridium* bacteria, called *Clostridium difficile* (*C. diff*), has joined MRSA as a major emerging threat in American health care settings, particularly hospitals. It causes inflammation of the colon, resulting in diarrhea, fever, and nausea. Bacterial spores can live outside the body for long periods and can be found on objects like medical equipment, bathroom fixtures, and bed linens, as well as on people's hands. Most cases of *C. diff* infection respond to a new class of antibiotics that selectively kills *C. diff* without affecting the many bacterial species that populate the normal, healthy intestine.

- ***Pertussis.*** Also known as whooping cough, pertussis is a highly contagious respiratory illness caused by the bacterium *Bordetella pertussis.* Pertussis is characterized by bursts of rapid coughing, followed by a long attempt at inhalation that is often accompanied by a high-pitched whoop. Those at high risk include infants and children who are too young to be fully vaccinated and those who have not completed the primary vaccination series. A booster shot is recommended at 11–12 years or during adolescence and thereafter every 10 years. Adults account for about 24% of whooping cough cases.

- ***Urinary tract infections (UTIs).*** Infection of the bladder and urethra is most common among sexually active women, but UTIs can occur in anyone. The bacterium *Escherichia coli* (*E. coli*) is the most common infectious agent, responsible for about 80% of all UTIs.

- ***Travelers' diarrhea (TD).*** Symptoms include abdominal cramps, nausea, vomiting, and fever. If left untreated, bacterial TD lasts about 3–7 days. Treatments include fluid and electrolyte replenishment and antimotility drugs such as loperamide. Antibiotic treatment of bacterial TD is discouraged because of the possibility of triggering a different infection.

### Antibiotic Treatments

**Antibiotics** are drugs that either inhibit the growth of bacteria or kill them. Antibiotics both naturally occur and are manufactured synthetically. antibacterial antibiotics are categorized based on their mechanism of action. The majority of antibiotics inhibit the synthesis of the bacterial cell wall. The second largest group interferes with the production of bacterial proteins. A third class prevents the replication of the bacterial DNA.

Antibiotics have saved millions of lives. However, their overuse and misuse has led to the emergence of antibiotic-resistant bacteria. A bacterium can become resistant from a chance genetic mutation or through the transfer of genetic material from one bacterium to another. When exposed to antibiotics, resistant bacteria can grow and flourish while the antibiotic-sensitive bacteria die off. Antibiotic-resistant strains of many common bacteria, including strains of gonorrhea, salmonella, and tuberculosis, have developed. Antibiotic resistance is a major factor contributing to the rise in problematic infectious diseases. The CDC estimates that about 30% of antibiotic prescriptions in the United States are unnecessary.

Resistance is promoted when people fail to take the full course of an antibiotic or when they inappropriately take antibiotics for viral infections. Another possible source of resistance is the use of antibiotics in agriculture, which is estimated to account for 50–80% of the 25,000 tons of antibiotics used annually in the United States.

You can help prevent the development of antibiotic-resistant strains of bacteria by using antibiotics properly. Don't ask your doctor for an antibiotic every time you get sick. Antibiotics are helpful for bacterial infections but are ineffective against viruses. If you take an antibiotic for a viral infection, your illness will not improve. Use antibiotics as directed, and finish the full course of medication even if you begin to feel better. Doing so helps ensure that all targeted bacteria are killed off. Never take an antibiotic without a prescription. Finally, avoid "antibacterial" soap products. Aside from being ineffective, antibacterial soaps may also be harmful because they can potentially create antibiotic-resistant bacteria.

## Viruses

A **virus** is a microscopic organism consisting of genetic material covered by a protein coat. Viruses lack the enzymes essential to energy production and protein synthesis in normal animal cells, and they can replicate only inside the cells of another organism—acting as a parasite. Once a virus is inside the host cell, it sheds its protein covering and exploits the host's cellular machinery to produce more viruses like itself. Most contagious diseases are caused by viruses.

### The Common Cold

A cold may be caused by any of more than 200 viruses. Rhinoviruses and coronaviruses cause a large percentage of all colds among adults. Cold viruses

**TERMS**

**antibiotic** A synthetic or naturally occurring substance that kills or inhibits the growth of bacteria, fungi, or protozoa.

**virus** A very small infectious agent composed of nucleic acid (DNA or RNA) surrounded by a protein coat; lacks an independent metabolism and reproduces only within a host cell.

have been with us forever, but their DNA mutates frequently. Cold viruses are almost always transmitted by hand-to-hand contact. To lessen your risk of contracting a cold, wash your hands frequently.

If you catch a cold, over-the-counter (OTC) cold remedies may relieve your symptoms, but they do not eliminate the virus. Sometimes it is difficult to determine whether your symptoms are due to a virus (as in colds, flu, and some sinus infections), a bacterium (as in other sinus infections), or an allergy, but knowing the cause is important for appropriate treatment. For example, antibiotics will not affect a viral infection but will help treat a bacterial sinus infection.

**Influenza** Commonly called the flu, **influenza** is an infection of the respiratory tract caused by the influenza virus. (Many people use the term "stomach flu" to describe gastrointestinal illnesses, but these infections are actually caused by organisms other than influenza viruses.) Influenza is more serious than the common cold, usually including a fever and extreme fatigue. Most people who get the flu recover within one to two weeks, but some develop potentially life-threatening complications, such as pneumonia. The highest rates of infection occur in children. Influenza is highly contagious and is spread via respiratory droplets.

The most effective way to prevent the flu is through annual vaccination. Because flu viruses are constantly changing, the influenza vaccine composition is revised every year. Although the WHO recommends specific vaccine viruses (usually three or four) to be included in the flu vaccines, each country decides its own vaccine composition. In the United States, the FDA makes the final decision. The CDC recommends vaccination for all people aged 6 months and over.

**Measles, Mumps, and Rubella** Due to effective vaccines, three viral childhood illnesses that have decreased in the United States are measles, mumps, and rubella. Worldwide, more than 140,000 people die each year from measles. Measles is a highly contagious disease. Before the introduction of vaccines, more than 90% of Americans contracted measles by age 15. Rubella can be transmitted by a pregnant woman to her fetus, causing miscarriage, stillbirth, or severe birth defects, including deafness, eye and heart defects, and mental impairment. Mumps generally causes swelling of the parotid (salivary) glands, located just below and in front of the ears. This virus can also cause meningitis and, in males, inflammation of the testes.

**Chickenpox, Cold Sores, and Other Herpesvirus Infections** The **herpesviruses** are a large group of viruses. Once infected, the host is never free of the virus. The virus lies latent within certain cells and becomes active periodically, producing symptoms. Herpesviruses are particularly dangerous for people with a depressed immune system. The family of herpesviruses includes the varicella-zoster virus, which causes chickenpox and shingles; herpes simplex virus (HSV) types 1 and 2, which cause cold sores and the sexually transmitted infection herpes; and Epstein-Barr virus (EBV), which causes infectious mononucleosis.

Two herpesviruses that can cause severe infections in people with AIDS or who have a suppressed immune system are cytomegalovirus (CMV), which infects the lungs, brain, colon, and eyes, and human herpesvirus 8 (HHV-8), which has been linked to Kaposi's sarcoma, a cancer of the connective tissue.

**Viral Hepatitis** **Hepatitis** is inflammation of the liver. Hepatitis is usually caused by one of the three most common hepatitis viruses. Hepatitis A virus (HAV) causes the mildest form of the disease and is usually transmitted by food or water contaminated by sewage or an infected person. Hepatitis B virus (HBV) is usually transmitted sexually. Hepatitis C virus (HCV) can also be transmitted sexually, but it is much more commonly passed through direct contact with infected blood via injection drug use or—prior to the development of screening tests—blood transfusions. HBV and, to a lesser extent, HCV can also be passed from a pregnant woman to her child.

Symptoms of acute hepatitis infection can include fatigue, **jaundice,** abdominal pain, loss of appetite, nausea, and diarrhea. Most people recover from hepatitis A within a month or so. However, 5–10% of people infected with HBV and 70–85% of people infected with HCV become chronic carriers of the virus, capable of infecting others. Some chronic carriers remain asymptomatic, while others slowly develop chronic liver disease, cirrhosis, or liver cancer.

The extent of HCV infection has been recognized only recently. Most infected people are unaware of their condition. To ensure proper treatment and prevention, testing for HCV may be recommended for people who have injected drugs (even once); received a blood transfusion or a donated organ prior to July 1992; engaged in high-risk sexual behavior; or had body piercing, tattoos, or acupuncture involving unsterile equipment.

**Human Papillomavirus (HPV)** The more than 200 types of HPV cause a variety of warts (noncancerous skin tumors), including common warts on the hands, plantar warts on the soles of the feet, and genital warts around the genitalia. Depending on their location, warts may be removed using OTC preparations or professional methods such as laser surgery or cryosurgery. Because HPV infection is chronic, warts can reappear despite treatment. HPV causes the majority of cases of cervical cancer.

**TERMS**

**influenza** Infection of the respiratory tract by the influenza virus, which is highly infectious and prone to variation; the form changes rapidly; commonly known as the flu.

**herpesvirus** A large family of viruses responsible for cold sores, mononucleosis, chickenpox, shingles, and the sexually transmitted infection herpes; causes latent infections.

**hepatitis** Inflammation of the liver, which can be caused by infection, drugs, or toxins.

**jaundice** Increased bile pigment levels in the blood, characterized by yellowing of the skin and the whites of the eyes.

**Treating Viral Illnesses** Antiviral drugs typically work by interfering at some segment of the viral life cycle; for example, they may prevent a virus from entering body cells or from successfully reproducing within cells. Antivirals are currently available to fight infections caused by SARS-CoV-2, HIV, influenza, herpes simplex, varicella-zoster, HBV, and HCV.

## Fungi

A **fungus** is an organism that reproduces by spores. Only about 50 of the 148,000 species of fungi cause disease in humans. Some fungal diseases are extremely difficult to treat. First, our normal defenses must contend with fungal infections to skin, nails, and the respiratory tract. Second, external treatments are difficult because, unlike bacteria, fungi are similar enough in their cellular chemistry to humans that it is difficult to kill fungi without harming the infected human.

*Candida albicans* is a common fungus found naturally in the vagina of most women. When excessive growth occurs, the result is itching and discomfort, commonly known as a yeast infection.

Other common fungal conditions, including athlete's foot, jock itch, and ringworm, affect the skin. These three conditions are usually mild and easy to cure.

Fungi can also cause systemic diseases that are severe, life threatening, and extremely difficult to treat. Fungal infections can be especially deadly in people with impaired immune systems.

## Protozoa

**Protozoa** are single-celled organisms that can cause a range of diseases in humans. Millions of people in developing countries suffer from protozoal infections.

**Malaria,** caused by a parasitic protozoan of the genus *Plasmodium,* is a major killer worldwide. Half the world's population live in areas where malaria is a problem. In 2019, 229 million people had malaria, and 409,000 people died of it. Insecticide-treated bed nets reduce malarial infections, and they have reduced the deaths of children under age 5 by about 20%. Children under 5 account for 61% of all malaria deaths. Several antimalarial drugs can prevent or treat the disease, but drug resistance is an increasing problem.

**Giardiasis** is caused by *Giardia lamblia,* a protozoan responsible for most cases of protozoal travelers' diarrhea. Giardiasis is characterized by nausea, diarrhea, bloating, and abdominal cramps, and it is among the most common waterborne diseases in the United States. People may become infected with *Giardia* if they consume contaminated food or water or pick up the parasite from the contaminated surface of an object such as a bathroom fixture, diaper pail, or toy.

## Parasitic Worms

**Parasitic worms** are the largest organisms that can enter the body to cause infection. Intestinal parasites, such as the tapeworm and hookworm, cause a variety of relatively mild infections. Pinworm, the most common worm infection in the United States, primarily affects young children.

## Emerging Infectious Diseases

Emerging infectious diseases are infections that have increased in incidence or may increase in the near future. They include both known diseases that have experienced a resurgence, such as tuberculosis and cholera, and diseases that were previously unknown or confined to specific areas, such as the Zika, Ebola, and Covid-19.

**Selected Infections of Concern** Although the chances of the average American contracting an exotic infection are very low, emerging infections are a concern to public health officials and represent a challenge to all nations in the future.

**ZIKA DISEASE** Zika virus is transmitted by several species of *Aedes* mosquitoes. It can also spread through sex with an infected partner, and it can pass from a pregnant woman to her fetus.

In most people, Zika symptoms are very mild, lasting a week or less, and may include fever, rash, and joint pain. However, a small proportion of people infected with Zika develop a neurological condition called Guillain-Barré syndrome, usually characterized by muscle weakness. This condition typically resolves within a few weeks or several months. Zika can also cause birth defects including microcephaly (small head size), impaired growth, eye defects, hearing loss, and possibly other problems.

**EBOLA** Ebola virus disease (EVD) is caused by Ebola virus, which is transmitted to people from wild animals. Infected people can then transmit the virus to others through direct contact with blood or body fluids or objects that have been contaminated. EVD is a severe infection with an average fatality rate of about 50%. Ebola is rare, but outbreaks have occurred periodically since it was first identified in 1976. There is no vaccine; it is treated with supportive care (including providing intravenous fluids and electrolytes, maintaining

**TERMS**

**fungus** A single-celled or multicelled organism that reproduces by spores and feeds on organic matter; examples include molds, mushrooms, and yeasts. Fungal diseases include yeast infections, athlete's foot, and ringworm.

**protozoan** A microscopic single-celled organism that often produces recurrent, cyclical attacks of disease; plural, *protozoa.*

**malaria** A severe, recurrent, mosquito-borne infection caused by the parasitic protozoan *Plasmodium.*

**giardiasis** An intestinal disease caused by the parasitic protozoan *Giardia lamblia.*

**parasitic worm** A pathogen that causes intestinal and other infections; includes tapeworms, hookworms, pinworms, and flukes.

oxygen and blood pressure, and treating other infections if they occur). The spread of the infection is controlled by identifying and isolating the sick and their close contacts. The outbreak in West Africa that raged 2014–2016 was the largest in history, with 11,310 deaths. The WHO declared the end of the 10th Ebola outbreak in the Democratic Republic of Congo in June 2020.

**WEST NILE VIRUS** West Nile virus (WNV) is carried by birds and then passed to humans when mosquitoes bite first an infected bird and then a person. In the United States, West Nile virus has caused infections in humans in 47 states and the District of Columbia. Eighty percent of infected people do not develop a serious condition.

**PATHOGENIC *ESCHERICHIA COLI*** *E. coli* bacteria live in the intestines of humans and animals and are an essential component of gut immunity. However, some strains of *E. coli* cause diarrhea; six types cause disease. Since 2006, there have been 45 multistate outbreaks of *E. coli*-caused disease. These outbreaks have been caused by contaminated foods including lettuce, spinach, sprouts, hazelnuts, processed meats, frozen foods, poultry, flour/cake mix, and beef sold both in grocery store chains and in restaurants. However, people also can become infected in other ways, such as by swallowing contaminated swimming pool water and through contact with an infected animal–for example, by petting an animal and then not washing hands before eating. Pets and animals at exhibits such as petting zoos can be healthy but carry pathogens on their bodies that can be passed to humans.

### Factors Contributing to Emerging Infections

What's behind this rising tide of infectious diseases? Contributing factors are complex and interrelated. New or increasing drug resistance has been found in organisms that cause malaria, tuberculosis, gonorrhea, influenza, AIDS, and pneumococcal and staphylococcal infections. Some bacterial strains now appear to be resistant to all available antibiotics.

Another factor is poverty. More than 1 billion people live in extreme poverty, and half the world's population has no regular access to essential drugs. Population growth, urbanization, overcrowding, and migration (including the movement of refugees) also spread infectious diseases.

A poor public health infrastructure is often associated with poverty and social upheaval, but problems such as contaminated water supplies can occur even in industrial countries. Inadequate vaccination has led to the reemergence of diseases such as diphtheria, pertussis, measles, and mumps. Natural disasters such as hurricanes also disrupt the public health infrastructure, leaving survivors with contaminated water and food supplies and no shelter from disease-carrying insects.

International tourism and trade open the world to infectious agents. Covid-19 was reported to WHO on December 31, 2019, based on an unknown illness affecting workers at a seafood market in the city of Wuhan, China. It took over three months to reach the first 100,000 confirmed cases of the virus, and only 12 days to reach the next 100,000.

Mass production of food increases the likelihood that a chance contamination can lead to mass illness.

Other causes can be traced to human behaviors–for example, the widespread use of injectable drugs rapidly transmits HIV infection and hepatitis. Changes in sexual behavior over the past 40 years have led to a proliferation of old and new sexually transmitted infections. The use of day care facilities for children has led to increases in the incidence of several infections that cause diarrhea.

The lengthening of warm periods and a change to shorter or milder winters may enable pathogenic species and, for some pathogens, their insect vectors to expand their range into countries or states where they once had not existed or had been rare.

### Immune Disorders

Considering the complexity of the immune system, it is not surprising that the system sometimes fails to operate properly, resulting in disease.

When the immune system breaks down, "self" may be misread and attacked as "nonself," and the result is an autoimmune disease. In most autoimmune diseases, the immune system targets or destroys specific tissues. For example, in type 1 diabetes, the insulin-producing cells of the pancreas are destroyed. In multiple sclerosis, the protective coating around nerves is destroyed. In Hashimoto's thyroiditis, the thyroid gland is destroyed. In rheumatoid arthritis, the membranes lining the joints are destroyed.

Cancer cells are cells that mutate and multiply uncontrollably. The immune system detects cells that have recently become abnormal and destroys them just as it would a foreign cell. However, some types of cancer cells actually suppress immune responses.

## SUPPORTING YOUR IMMUNE SYSTEM

The immune system does an amazing job of protecting you from illness, but you can help ensure its optimal functioning by choosing healthy behaviors. Here are some general guidelines for supporting your immune system:

- Get enough sleep: People who sleep fewer than six hours per night have compromised immune function.
- Maintain regular eating patterns. Recent research suggests that eating–even anticipating eating–switches on immune cell activity to potentially incoming pathogens or "bad" bacteria. This activity may explain why disruptions to circadian rhythms and regular eating patterns could increase chronic inflammation in the gut.
- Wash your hands frequently. Use regular soap and wash thoroughly by scrubbing at least 20–30 seconds. When soap and water are not available, use hand sanitizer.
- Avoid contact with people who are contagious with an infectious disease.

## Ask Yourself

**QUESTIONS FOR CRITICAL THINKING AND REFLECTION**

Have you ever had any of the illnesses described in the preceding sections? How were you exposed to the disease? Could you have taken any precautions to avoid it?

- Make sure you drink water only from clean sources. Unpurified water from lakes and streams can carry pathogens, even if it appears pristine.
- Avoid contact with disease carriers such as rodents, mosquitoes, and ticks. Never touch or feed wild animals.
- Make sure you have received all your recommended vaccinations, and keep them up to date. Your physician can tell you exactly what immunizations you need and when you should have them.

# THE MAJOR STIs

**Sexually transmitted infections (STIs)** spread from person to person mainly through sexual activity. STIs are a particularly insidious group of illnesses because a person can be infected and be able to transmit the disease, yet not look or feel sick. The Centers for Disease Control and Prevention (CDC) estimates that the cost of STIs to the health care system in the United States is almost $16 billion per year.

**QUICK STATS**

**HIV/AIDS-related death is ranked as the ninth leading cause of death among Americans aged 25–34 years.**

—National Center for Health Statistics, 2021

The following seven STIs pose major health threats: HIV/AIDS, chlamydia, gonorrhea, human papillomavirus (HPV), herpes, hepatitis, and syphillis.

STIs are caused by a number of organisms, including bacteria, viruses, protozoa, and parasites. STIs can cause serious complications if left untreated and can result in long-term consequences, including chronic pain, infertility, stillbirths, genital cancers, and death. Additionally, women exposed to STIs while pregnant may place their fetus and newborn at risk for infection. The rates of many STIs in the United States have reached record highs—in some instances, much higher than those of other industrialized nations.

Those aged 15–24 account for half of STI cases in the United States. With the rise of dating apps, the increasing anonymity of sexual encounters, coupled with the stigma of STIs and our reluctance to talk about them, may also play a role in higher STI rates. Trends also show increased condom use with first sexual activity.

## HIV and AIDS

HIV causes AIDS. With recent advances in the treatment of **human immunodeficiency virus (HIV),** people infected with the virus are now living almost as long as people not infected with it. Adequate treatment is not accessible, however, for most people worldwide. Untreated HIV infection may advance to **acquired immunodeficiency syndrome (AIDS)** within 8–10 years of diagnosis. This stage of HIV infection is defined by a severely compromised immune system and the presence of opportunistic infections.

Many experts believe that the global HIV epidemic peaked in the late 1990s, at about 3.5 million new infections per year, compared with an estimated 1.5 million new infections in 2020. Disparities exist for incident infections and access to treatment in youth, women, and other key populations. Youth aged 15–24 represent 16% of the global population (see the box "HIV/AIDS around the World") and one-third of incident HIV infections.

In the United States in 2019, 1.2 million people were living with HIV. U.S. populations disproportionately burdened with HIV include those living in the southern United States, gay men and other men who have sex with men (as described by the CDC's classification), transgender women, African Americans, Latinos, and youth.

### What Is HIV Infection?

**HIV infection** is a chronic disease that progressively damages the body's immune system, making an otherwise healthy person less able to resist a variety of infections and disorders. Normally, when a virus or other pathogen enters the body, it is targeted and destroyed by the immune system. But HIV attacks the immune system itself, invading and taking over **CD4 T cells** (white blood cells that fight infection), macrophages, and other essential elements of the immune system. HIV enters a human cell and converts its own genetic material, RNA, into DNA. It then inserts this DNA into the chromosomes of the host cell. The viral DNA is not only instrumental in producing new copies of HIV, but it also seriously reduces immune functions.

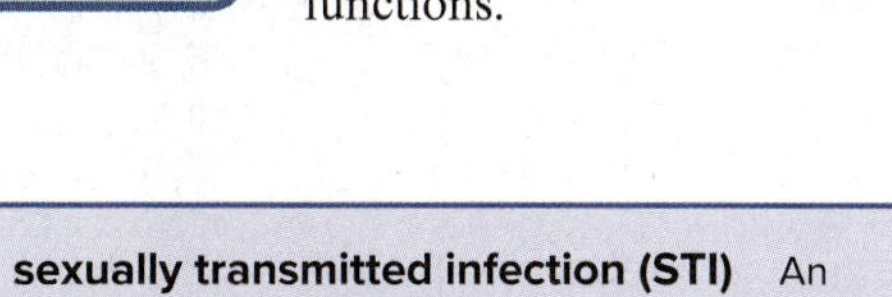

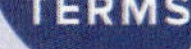

**TERMS**

**sexually transmitted infection (STI)** An infection that is transmitted mainly by sexual contact; some can also be transmitted by other means.

**human immunodeficiency virus (HIV)** The virus that causes HIV infection and AIDS.

**acquired immunodeficiency syndrome (AIDS)** An advanced stage of HIV infection.

**HIV infection** A chronic, progressive viral infection that damages the immune system.

**CD4 T cell** A type of white blood cell that helps coordinate the activity of the immune system; the primary target of HIV infection. A decrease in the number of these cells correlates with the severity of HIV-related illness.

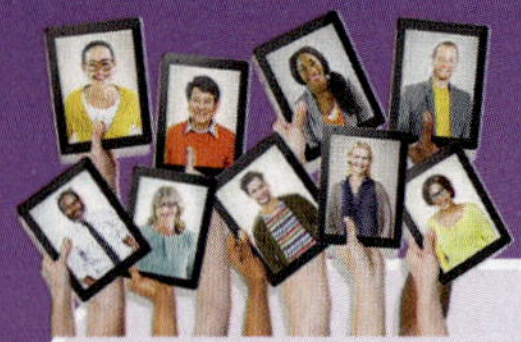

## DIVERSITY MATTERS
## HIV/AIDS around the World

We are nearly four decades removed from the first reports of cases of what we now know as AIDS. Those cases appeared in the gay community in California and New York, hemophiliacs, individuals who had received blood transfusions, injection drug users, women living with HIV, and their newborn infants. Between 55.9 and 110 million people have been infected, and tens of millions have died from HIV/AIDS–related causes since the start of the epidemic.

### Global Disparities in HIV/AIDS

The vast majority of cases have occurred in economically emerging countries, where heterosexual contact is the primary means of transmission. Sadly, HIV continues to disproportionately affect racial and ethnic minority populations and the poor. Approximately 5000 women ages 15–24 are infected with HIV weekly. The gender imbalance is even more pronounced in sub-Saharan Africa, the hardest-hit region, where six in seven new infections appear in adolescent girls ages 15–19, despite their comprising only 10% of the population. For adolescents, HIV falls among the top 10 causes of death overall and among the top five causes for younger adolescent girls aged 10–14. Factors at the root of this disparity include harmful gender norms and inequalities, violence, poverty, and lack of access to sexual and reproductive health services.

Other key populations at risk worldwide include gay men and other men who have sex with men, people who inject drugs, sex workers, transgender people, prisoners, clients of sex workers, and other sex partners of at-risk populations. These groups are often marginalized and stigmatized, reducing their access to services, which in turn increases rates of infection. In 2020, key populations and their partners accounted for 65% of new HIV cases globally—up to 93% and 39% in and outside sub-Saharan Africa, respectively. The risk of HIV infection was 25 times higher among gay men and other men who have sex with men, 26 times higher among sex workers, 34 times higher among transgender people, and 35 times higher among persons who inject drugs.

### HIV/AIDS Prevention and Treatment Gains and Challenges

Despite the ongoing tragedy of the epidemic, strides have been made in treatment and prevention measures. In 2020, around 84% of people living with HIV knew their status; among them, 87% were accessing HIV treatment and 90% were virally suppressed. Due to these scaled-up efforts, the rate of new infections and deaths has declined in some regions. AIDS-related deaths have decreased 64% since the peak in 2004. Treating HIV with effective drugs not only prolongs life and decreases suffering, but it also reduces the spread of the virus because individuals who have received treatment and maintain an undetectable viral load effectively have no risk of transmission to individuals without HIV.

Efforts to combat AIDS are complicated by political, economic, and cultural barriers. Education and prevention programs are often hampered by resistance from social and religious institutions and by the taboo on openly discussing sexual issues. Moreover, approximately 50% of adolescents cannot make decisions about their health. Condoms are not commonly used in many countries, and even when they are, women may not have agency to negotiate their use. Empowering women is a crucial priority in reducing the spread of HIV. In particular, reducing sexual violence against women, promoting financial independence, and increasing women's education and employment opportunities are essential.

Successful prevention approaches include STI treatment and education, public education campaigns about safer sex, and syringe exchange programs for injection drug users. Efforts are ongoing to improve access to barrier protective devices such as condoms. Male circumcision has been shown to reduce the risk of heterosexually acquired HIV infection in men by about 60%; voluntary adult male circumcision is recommended by the World Health Organization (WHO) as part of HIV prevention programs in regions with HIV epidemics among heterosexuals and with high HIV and low male circumcision prevalence. The partial protection provided by circumcision does not eliminate the need for condom use. The effectiveness of condoms for HIV prevention may be greater than 95%, but this depends on correct and consistent use.

Despite progress, according to the Joint United Nations Programme on HIV/AIDS (UNAIDS), without a scale-up in prevention and treatment efforts, the epidemic will continue to outrun the

Immediately following infection with HIV, billions of infectious particles are produced every day. For a time, the immune system keeps pace, also producing billions of new cells. Unlike the virus, however, the immune system cannot make new cells indefinitely; as long as the virus keeps replicating, it wins in the end. The destruction of the immune system is signaled by the loss of CD4 T cells. As the number of CD4 cells declines, an infected person may begin to experience mild to moderately severe symptoms. A person is diagnosed with AIDS when the number of CD4 cells in the blood drops below a certain level (200/μl). People with AIDS are vulnerable to several serious **opportunistic (secondary) infections**.

The first weeks after being infected with HIV are called the *acute infection* phase. Most, but not all, infected people develop

**TERMS**

**opportunistic (secondary) infection** An infection caused when organisms take the opportunity presented by a acute (initial) infection to multiply and cause a new, different infection.

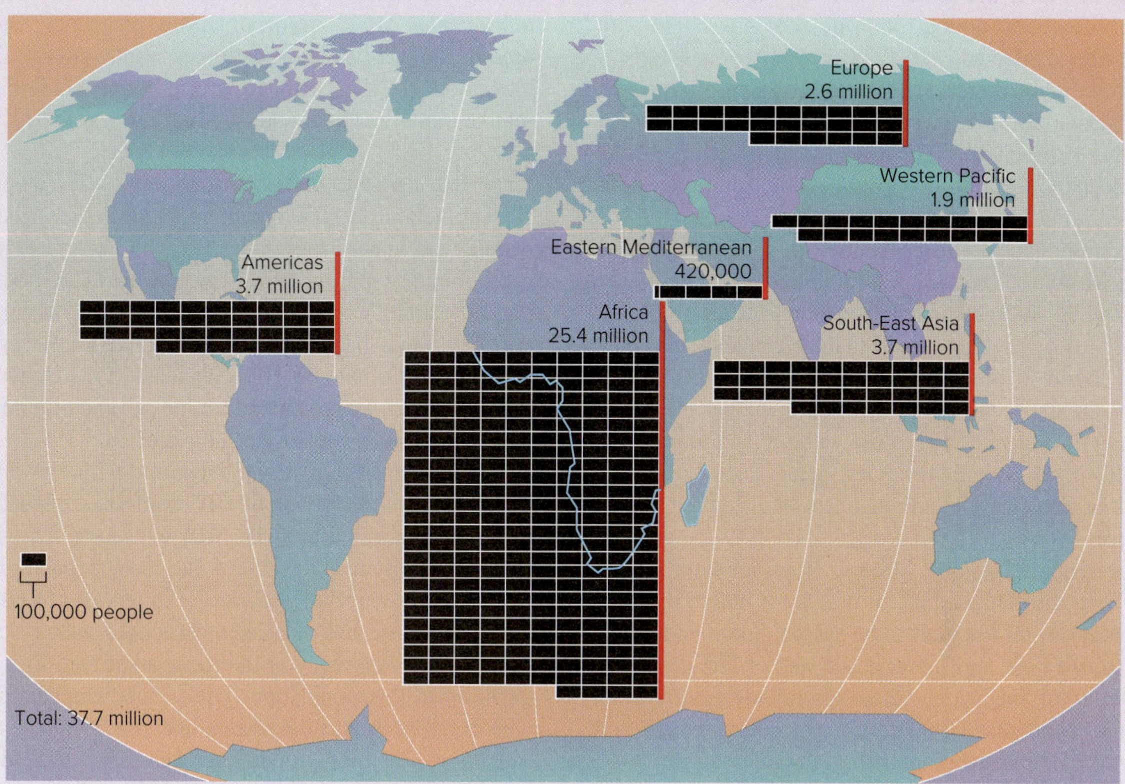


Approximate number of people living with HIV/AIDS in 2020.

response. There is a historic obligation to end the AIDS epidemic. UNAIDS launched a fast-track strategy in 2014 that aimed to greatly step up the response in low- and middle-income countries, with the goal of ending the epidemic by 2030. For 2030, UNAIDS set a 95-95-95 treatment target:

- 95% of people living with HIV know their status.
- 95% of people living with HIV who know their status are receiving treatment.
- 95% of people on treatment have suppressed viral loads. However, we still have miles to go.

The United States continues to be involved in the global strategy for closing treatment and prevention gaps. The President's Emergency Plan for AIDS Relief (PEPFAR), the Global Fund, and other organizations helped save more than 21 million lives by providing antiretroviral therapies to over 18 million people.

**SOURCES:** UNAIDS. World Health Organization. 2021. Number of people (all ages) living with HIV (https://apps.who.int/gho/data/view.main.22100WHO); USAID. 2015. *Condom Fact Sheet* (https://www.usaid.gov/sites/default/files/documents/1864/condomfactsheet.pdf); U.S. President's Emergency Plan for AIDS Relief. 2021. *Latest Global Program Results* (https://www.state.gov/wp-content/uploads/2021/12/PEPFAR-Latest-Global-Results_WAD-2021.pdf); UNAIDS. 2019. *Women and HIV: A Spotlight on Adolescent Girls and Young Women* (https://www.unaids.org/sites/default/files/media_asset/2019_women-and-hiv_en.pdf).

flulike symptoms about two to four weeks after being exposed to the virus. During this phase, people have large amounts of HIV in the bloodstream and genital fluids, making it easier to transmit the virus. Several months later, infected people develop antibodies to the virus, so commonly available tests will show a positive result. The next phase of HIV infection is the chronic **asymptomatic** (symptom-free) stage, also called the *latency* phase. This period can last from 2 to 20 years, averaging 11 years in untreated adults. During this time, the virus progressively infects and destroys the cells of the immune system. Even if they are symptom-free, people infected with HIV can transmit the disease to others if untreated.

**Transmitting the Virus** HIV lives only within cells and blood and blood products, semen, vaginal and cervical secretions, and breast milk, not outside the body. It is transmitted

**TERMS**

**asymptomatic** Showing no signs or symptoms of a disease.

by blood and blood products, semen, vaginal and cervical secretions, and breast milk. It cannot live in air, in water, or on objects or surfaces such as toilet seats, eating utensils, or telephones. A person is not at risk of HIV infection by being in the same classroom, dining room, or even household with someone who is infected.

The three main routes of HIV transmission are specific kinds of sexual contact, direct exposure to infected blood, and contact between an HIV-infected woman and her child during pregnancy, childbirth, breastfeeding, or premastication (prechewing food for a child).

HIV is more likely to be transmitted by anal or vaginal intercourse without a condom than by other sexual activities. During vaginal intercourse, male-to-female transmission is more likely to occur than female-to-male transmission. HIV has been found in preejaculatory fluid, which means that transmission can occur before ejaculation. Being the receptive partner during anal intercourse without a condom is the riskiest of all sexual activities. Oral-genital contact carries some risk of transmission, although less than anal or vaginal intercourse.

The presence of lesions, blisters, or inflammation from other STIs in the genital, anal, or oral areas makes it two to nine times easier for the virus to be passed. Spermicides may also cause irritation and increase the risk of HIV transmission. Studies of the widely used spermicide nonoxynol-9 (N-9) have found that frequent use may cause vaginal and rectal irritation, increasing the risk of transmission of HIV and other STIs.

The risk of HIV transmission during oral sex is generally considered to be low but may be increased if a person has oral sores or other damage to the gums or tissues in the mouth.

Studies in economically emerging nations with high rates of HIV infection have found that circumcised males have a lower risk of HIV infection than uncircumcised males.

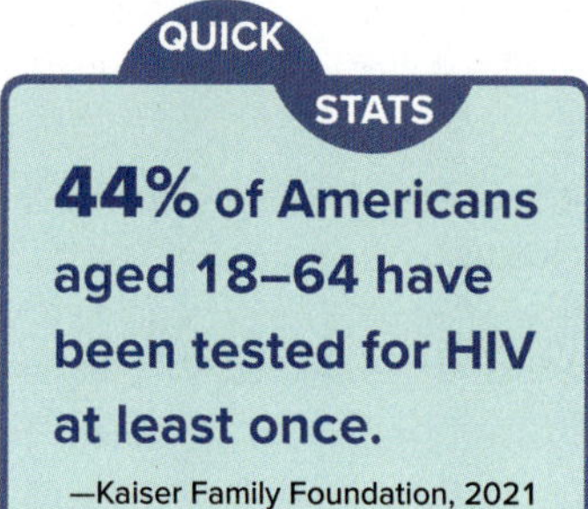


Direct contact with the blood of an infected person is another major route of HIV transmission. Needles and syringes used to inject drugs (including heroin, cocaine, anabolic steroids, and opioid medications) are usually contaminated with the user's blood.

In the past, before effective screening was available, some people were infected with HIV through blood transfusions and other medical procedures involving blood products. All blood in licensed U.S. blood banks and plasma centers is now screened thoroughly for blood-borne pathogens, including HIV. However, the blood supply is much less safe in the rest of the world. The WHO estimates that 0.001% of high- and 0.07% of low-income countries have transfusion transmissible HIV in their blood donor supply.

A small number of health care workers have acquired HIV on the job. Most of these cases involve needle sticks, in which a health care worker is accidentally stuck with a needle used on an infected patient. The likelihood of a patient's acquiring HIV infection from a health care worker is almost negligible; the risk of health care workers' acquiring HIV from infected patients is much greater.

The final major route of HIV transmission is mother-to-child transmission (MCT), also called *vertical* or *perinatal transmission.* MCT can occur during pregnancy, childbirth, breastfeeding, or premastication. Without intervention, the likelihood of HIV perinatal transmission is 15–45%; with intervention, the likelihood is reduced to less than 1%.

**Key Populations Affected by HIV** The populations most vulnerable to HIV infection include people aged 25–34, people who inject drugs, and men who have sex with other men. Young people aged 13–24 are the least likely to be aware they have an HIV infection, and the most likely to report that they have never been tested for HIV. In 2020, this age group made up 20% of all new HIV diagnoses in the United States. Young African American and Latino gay and other men who have sex with men were especially affected.

Among Americans newly diagnosed with HIV infection, the most common means of HIV exposure is sexual activity between men (Figure 14.3). Men who have sex with men (MSM) represent about 2% of the male population in the United States, but they account for most cases of HIV. Drug and alcohol use has also been associated with risky sexual behavior and is directly or indirectly associated with HIV acquisition in this population. Use of methamphetamine and club drugs, as well as the recreational use of erectile dysfunction drugs, has been associated with risky sexual behavior and HIV infection in MSM.

Data from the 2021 HIV Surveillance Report indicate that 7% of newly diagnosed HIV cases are attributable to injection drug use. People who inject drugs are particularly at risk from unsafe injection practices and high-risk sex, including condomless sex with casual partners and exchanging sex for money or drugs. These findings highlight the importance of educating people who

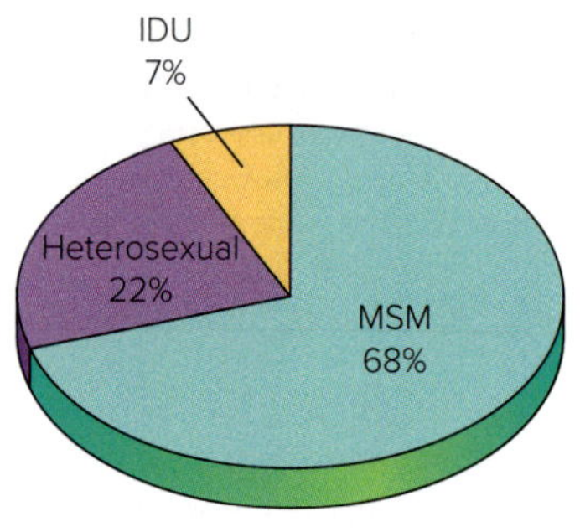


**FIGURE 14.3 Routes of HIV transmission among Americans newly diagnosed with HIV infection in 2020.**

SOURCE: Centers for Disease Control and Prevention. 2021. *HIV Surveillance Report,* vol. 33 (https://www.cdc.gov/hiv/library/reports/hiv-surveillance/vol-33/index.html.)

inject drugs about HIV acquisition. Topics should include safe injection practices, how to get substance use disorder counseling, and medication-assisted treatment.

In the United States, high rates of HIV infection occur in males, certain racial and ethnic groups, and poor people. In 2020, African Americans and Latinos represented 42% and 27% of new HIV cases even though they make up only 12% and 19% of the U.S. population, respectively. The majority of these infections occurred among men, particularly those reporting male-to-male sexual contact. These patterns of HIV infection reflect complex social, economic, and behavioral factors. Reducing the rates of HIV transmission and AIDS death in nondominant racial and ethnic groups, women, and high-risk groups requires addressing problems of poverty, discrimination, and substance use disorder. HIV prevention programs must be tailored to meet the special needs of high-risk underserved communities and must include testing, education, and equal access to health care.

**Symptoms** As described earlier, in the days or weeks following infection with HIV, most people develop symptoms, which can include fever, fatigue, rashes, headache, swollen lymph nodes, body aches, night sweats, sore throat, nausea, and ulcers in the mouth. Symptoms of primary infection can last from a few days to more than a month. Because these symptoms are similar to those of many common viral illnesses, the condition often goes undiagnosed.

Diagnosis of HIV at this very early stage of infection is extremely beneficial. People with early-stage HIV can engage in HIV care, receive highly active antiretroviral regimes to decrease viral load, and make lifestyle changes such as the correct and consistent use of condoms to decrease the likelihood of HIV transmission.

Other than the initial flulike symptoms, most people have few if any symptoms in the first months or years of HIV infection. As the immune system weakens, however, a variety of symptoms can develop—persistent swollen lymph nodes; lumps, rashes, sores, or other growths on or under the skin or on the mucous membranes; persistent yeast infections; unexplained weight loss; fever and drenching night sweats; dry cough and shortness of breath; persistent diarrhea; easy bruising and unexplained bleeding; profound fatigue; memory loss; difficulty with balance; tremors or seizures; changes in vision, hearing, taste, or smell; changes in mood and other psychological symptoms; and persistent or recurrent pain. Many of these symptoms can also occur with a variety of other illnesses.

People with HIV infection are highly susceptible to opportunistic infections, as noted earlier. The infection most often seen in the United States among people with HIV is ***Pneumocystis* pneumonia,** a fungal infection. **Kaposi's sarcoma,** a previously rare form of cancer, is common in persons with AIDS. Women with HIV infection may have frequent and difficult-to-treat vaginal yeast infections. Cases of tuberculosis (TB) are increasingly being reported in people with HIV.

**Diagnosis** Three general types of HIV diagnostic tests are currently available. **HIV antibody tests** are performed on blood or oral fluids to check whether the body is producing antibodies against the HIV virus. **Combination HIV antigen/antibody tests** look both for antibodies and for an HIV antigen known as p24 (part of the virus itself). **Nucleic acid tests (NATs)** test directly for HIV RNA in the blood; the test is expensive and not routinely used for initial screening.

If you get an HIV test within three months after a potential HIV exposure and the result is negative, get tested again in three months, or earlier if at greater risk for HIV. Testing for HIV is recommended for everyone (see the box "Know Your Status: Getting an HIV Test").

If a person is diagnosed with HIV, the next step is to determine the disease's severity. The infection itself can be monitored by tracking the viral load (the amount of virus in the body) with blood tests that measure HIV RNA (NAT tests).

A diagnosis of AIDS, the most severe form of HIV infection, is given if a person is living with HIV and either has developed an infection defined as an AIDS indicator or has a severely damaged immune system (as measured by CD4 T cell counts).

The CDC recommends that states provide opportunities for people to receive confidential HIV testing and counseling services. In the United States, every state has laws that require doctors, clinics, and laboratories to report all diagnosed cases of HIV and AIDS to public health authorities, who use this information to track and prevent the spread of the disease. Despite efforts to safeguard confidentiality and prohibit discrimination, mandatory reporting of HIV infection remains controversial. If people believe they are risking their jobs, friends, or social acceptability, they may be less likely to get tested or disclose partners to public health authorities. It is important that we reduce the stigma of HIV infection. You can find resources and a helpful infographic at https://www.cdc.gov/hiv/basics/hiv-stigma/index.html.

**Treatment** Although there is no known cure for HIV infection, medications can significantly alter the course of the disease and extend life. The drop in the number of U.S. AIDS deaths since 1996 is in large part due to the increasing use of highly effective antiretroviral drugs.

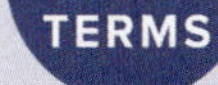


***Pneumocystis* pneumonia** A fungal infection common in people infected with HIV.

**Kaposi's sarcoma** A form of cancer characterized by purple or brownish lesions that are generally painless and occur anywhere on the skin; usually appears in persons infected with HIV.

**HIV antibody test** A blood test to determine whether a person has been infected with HIV; becomes positive within weeks or months of exposure.

**combination HIV antigen/antibody test** A blood test that detects the presence of HIV p24 antigen, an early marker for HIV infection, as well as HIV antibodies.

**HIV nucleic acid test (NAT)** A test used to detect the presence of HIV RNA and to determine the viral load (the amount of HIV in the blood).

## CRITICAL CONSUMER
# Know Your Status: Getting an HIV Test

### Who and How Often?

The CDC recommends that everyone between the ages of 13 and 64 be tested for HIV at least once as part of routine health care. The CDC hopes that routine HIV testing will increase the likelihood that people with HIV will be diagnosed earlier. People with certain risk factors should be tested more often. The CDC recommends testing at least once a year for anyone who answers yes to any of the following:

- Are you a man who has had sex with another man?
- Have you had sex—anal or vaginal—with a partner who is positive for HIV?
- Have you had more than one sex partner since your last HIV test?
- Have you injected drugs and shared needles or "works" (e.g., water or cotton) with others?
- Have you exchanged sex for drugs or money?
- Have you been diagnosed with or sought treatment for another STI?
- Have you been diagnosed with or received treatment for hepatitis or TB?
- Have you had sex with someone who could answer yes to any of the above questions or someone whose sexual history you don't know?

In addition, CDC guidelines state that sexually active gay and bisexual men may benefit from more frequent testing (e.g., every three to six months).

### Physician or Clinic Testing

Your physician, student health clinic, Planned Parenthood, or public health department can arrange your HIV test. Testing usually costs $50–$100, but public clinics often charge little or nothing. The standard test involves drawing a sample of blood that is sent to a lab, where it is checked using one or more of the available test types. For accuracy and early diagnosis, the CDC recommends laboratory tests done in the following sequence:

1. Combination test; if it is positive for antibodies and/or p24 antigen, this is followed by
2. Specialized antibody test, which confirms which type of HIV is present
3. If findings from the second test are indeterminate or contradictory, a NAT test is done to confirm if HIV RNA is present

It may take a week or more for the results of these tests to become available, and you'll be asked to call or come in personally to obtain your results, which should also include appropriate counseling.

Alternative tests are available at some clinics. Rapid oral tests use oral fluid, which is collected by swabbing the inside of the mouth. Rapid tests are available at some locations. These tests involve the use of blood or oral fluid and can provide results in as little as 20 minutes. If a rapid test is positive for HIV infection, a confirming test will be performed. Most rapid tests are antibody tests, which may be less likely than combination tests to detect HIV infection in the first few weeks following exposure. Similarly, blood tests may detect infection earlier than oral fluid tests, because the level of antibodies in oral fluid is lower than in blood.

Before you get an HIV test, be sure you understand what will be done with the results. Results from confidential tests may still become part of your medical record and are required to be reported to state and federal public health agencies. If you decide you want to be tested anonymously, ask your physician about an anonymous test, or use a home test.

### Home Testing

Home test kits vary in cost; however, you should be able to purchase a kit for $40–$70. Avoid test kits sold on the internet that are not approved by the U.S. Food and Drug Administration (FDA). As of this printing, the only "in home" HIV testing devices approved by the FDA were Home Access and OraQuick. Positive results with either test kit need to be confirmed with follow-up testing. To use the Home Access test, you prick a finger with a supplied lancet, blot a few drops of blood onto blotting paper, and mail it to the company's laboratory. In about a week (or within three business days for more expensive "express" tests), you call a toll-free number to find out your results. Anyone testing positive is routed to a trained counselor, who can provide emotional and medical support. The OraQuick HIV test, manufactured by Orasure, was approved by the FDA in July 2012. This home test is the first rapid HIV test approved for home use. Like the Orasure test available to clinics, the OraQuick home test uses a sample taken from the mouth and returns results in 20 minutes. The results of home test kits are completely anonymous. Anyone testing positive should call a medical doctor or the OraQuick Consumer Support Center for counseling and routes to care.

### Understanding the Results

A negative test result means that no evidence of infection was found—no antibodies or, if you had a combination test, p24 antigens. However, as noted earlier, it may take three weeks or even longer for the infection to be detectible. Therefore, an infected person may get a false-negative result. If you test negative but your risk of infection is high, ask about obtaining an NAT test, which allows for very early diagnosis. If you engage in any risky behaviors, get retested frequently.

A positive result means that you are infected. Seek medical care and counseling immediately. Rapid progress is being made in treating HIV, and treatments are potentially much more successful when started early. For more information about testing, visit the CDC National HIV, STD, and Hepatitis Testing website (www.hivtest.org).

SOURCES: Centers for Disease Control and Prevention. 2021. *Getting Tested* (https://www.cdc.gov/hiv/basics/hiv-testing/getting-tested.html). Centers for Disease Control and Prevention. 2020. *HIV Testing 101* (https://www.cdc.gov/hiv/pdf/library/factsheets/hiv-testing-101-info-sheet.pdf); HIV.gov. 2020. *HIV Testing Overview* (https://www.hiv.gov/hiv-basics/hiv-testing/learn-about-hiv-testing-overview); Centers for Disease Control and Prevention and Association of Public Health Laboratories. 2014. *Laboratory Testing for the Diagnosis of HIV Infection: Updated Recommendations* (http://dx.doi.org/10.15620/cdc.23447); U.S. Food and Drug Administration. 2018. *Testing for HIV* (http://www.fda.gov/BiologicsBloodVaccines/SafetyAvailability/HIVHomeTestKits/ucm126460.htm).

The main types of antiviral drugs used against HIV/AIDS are reverse transcriptase inhibitors, protease inhibitors, integrase inhibitors, and entry inhibitors. These drugs either block HIV from replicating itself or prevent it from infecting other cells. Research has shown that using combinations of antiviral drugs can sometimes reduce HIV in the blood to undetectable levels. A healthy person diagnosed with HIV who takes HIV medications as prescribed and has achieved HIV suppression, or undetectable levels of HIV in the blood, has effectively no risk of transmitting HIV to an uninfected partner. More than 30 drugs are now available to treat HIV, including several once-a-day tablets (containing a combination of HIV medications). Patients with low CD4 T cell counts can take a variety of antibiotics to help prevent opportunistic infections such as pneumonia and other bacterial and fungal infections.

HIV treatment is also challenging because taking the combination drugs is complicated, and the drugs have short-term side effects that may cause people to stop taking them. Drug resistance develops quickly if the medicines are taken incorrectly or inconsistently. The drugs can also have long-term side effects, including serious health problems in some individuals. The National Institutes of Health (NIH) has issued guidelines for HIV treatment that help patients and their doctors with decisions about the optimal retroviral treatment.

**Prevention** Research on the development of a safe, effective, and inexpensive vaccine to stop the spread of HIV worldwide has been ongoing.

Effective approaches to prevention include abstinence, correct and consistent condom use with all sexual acts, and needle exchange programs for persons who use intravenous drugs. There are now several FDA-approved drugs for preexposure prophylaxis (PrEP), including an injectable drug. These medications are taken by people who do not have HIV but are at high risk for it. In some cases, medications are also used to prevent infection in people who have been exposed to HIV, such as victims of sexual assault and health care workers with potential exposure to HIV-positive blood or other body fluids. This type of treatment, called PEP, should begin as soon as possible after exposure, but always within 72 hours.

**How Can You Protect Yourself?** Although AIDS cannot be cured, infection can be prevented. You can protect yourself by avoiding behaviors that may bring you into contact with HIV.

In a sexual relationship, the current and past behaviors of you and your partner determine the amount of risk involved. If you are uninfected and in a mutually monogamous relationship with another uninfected person, you are not at risk for HIV. For anyone not involved in a long-term, mutually monogamous relationship, abstinence from any sexual activity that involves the exchange of semen, pre-ejaculate, vaginal fluids, or rectal fluids is the only sure way to prevent HIV infection (Figure 14.4). Use of a condom reduces the risk of transmitting HIV during all forms of intercourse.

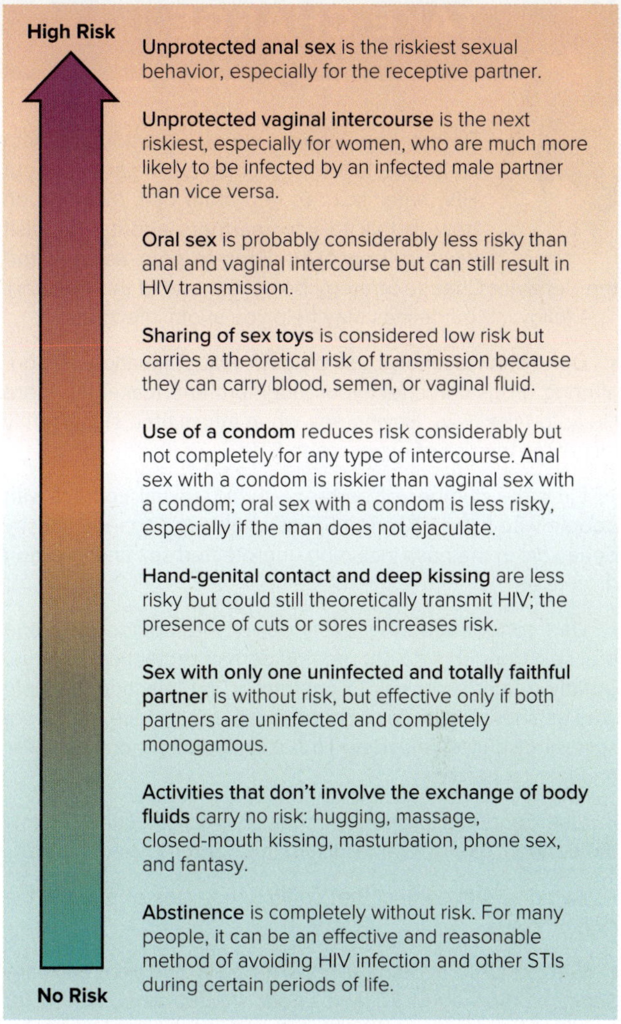

People who inject drugs should avoid sharing needles, syringes, filters, or anything that might have blood on it. Needles can be decontaminated with a solution of bleach and water, but this is not a foolproof procedure, and HIV can survive in a syringe for a month or longer. HIV can also survive boiling.

Once you know your status, education on risk reduction and individual responsibility can lead the way to ending this epidemic (see the box "Preventing STIs").

High Risk

**Unprotected anal sex** is the riskiest sexual behavior, especially for the receptive partner.

**Unprotected vaginal intercourse** is the next riskiest, especially for women, who are much more likely to be infected by an infected male partner than vice versa.

**Oral sex** is probably considerably less risky than anal and vaginal intercourse but can still result in HIV transmission.

**Sharing of sex toys** is considered low risk but carries a theoretical risk of transmission because they can carry blood, semen, or vaginal fluid.

**Use of a condom** reduces risk considerably but not completely for any type of intercourse. Anal sex with a condom is riskier than vaginal sex with a condom; oral sex with a condom is less risky, especially if the man does not ejaculate.

**Hand-genital contact and deep kissing** are less risky but could still theoretically transmit HIV; the presence of cuts or sores increases risk.

**Sex with only one uninfected and totally faithful partner** is without risk, but effective only if both partners are uninfected and completely monogamous.

**Activities that don't involve the exchange of body fluids** carry no risk: hugging, massage, closed-mouth kissing, masturbation, phone sex, and fantasy.

**Abstinence** is completely without risk. For many people, it can be an effective and reasonable method of avoiding HIV infection and other STIs during certain periods of life.

No Risk

**FIGURE 14.4 What's risky and what's not: The approximate relative risk of HIV transmission in various sexual activities.** (For additional information about the risk of acquiring HIV from certain types of exposures, visit https://www.cdc.gov/hiv/risk/index.html.)

## Chlamydia

*Chlamydia trachomatis* causes **chlamydia,** the most prevalent bacterial STI in the United States. Anyone can be susceptible to chlamydia, but, as with most STIs, women bear the greater burden because of possible complications and consequences of the disease. Rates of chlamydia in women were almost two times those in men in 2019. For women, the highest rates of infection occur among 15- to 24-year-olds. For men, the

TERMS

**chlamydia** An STI transmitted by the bacterium *Chlamydia trachomatis.*

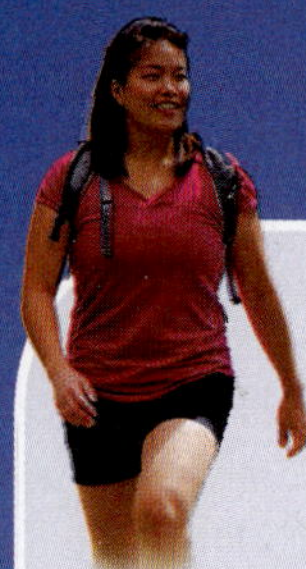

## TAKE CHARGE
## Preventing STIs

Before you begin a sexual relationship with someone, talk with your potential partner about HIV, safer sex, and condom use. (For tips on how to talk to your partners about STIs, visit www.gytnow.org/talking-to-your-partner/and the Behavior Change Strategy box at the end of this chapter). The following guidelines may help you avoid infection:

- Don't drink alcohol or use drugs in sexual situations. Mood-altering drugs can affect your judgment and make you more likely to take risks. Having sex when intoxicated significantly increases the risk of exposure to STIs.
- Limit the number of partners. Avoid sexual contact with people who have HIV or an STI or who have engaged in risky behaviors in the past, including unprotected sex and injection drug use.
- Use condoms during every act of intercourse including oral sex. Condoms do not provide perfect protection, but they greatly reduce your risk of contracting an infection. Multiple studies show that regular condom use can reduce the risk of several diseases, including HIV, chlamydia, gonorrhea, HPV, and genital herpes.
- Use condoms properly for maximum protection. Follow the condom use guidelines listed in Chapter 7.
- Avoid sexual contact that could cause cuts or tears in the skin or tissue.
- Get periodic screening tests for STIs and HIV. Sexually active women aged 25 and under should be screened for gonorrhea and chlamydia at least annually, and older women at risk for STIs should be offered screening. Gay men and other MSM should be tested for STIs at least annually or more frequently depending on risk behaviors. A Pap test is recommended at age 21 and every three to five years thereafter, depending a woman's age and on whether a Pap test is combined with HPV screening. More frequent screening may be recommended for women who have compromised immune systems or abnormal screening results.
- Get vaccinated. All sexually active people should be vaccinated against hepatitis B. All MSM should be vaccinated against hepatitis A. Young people aged 26 years and under should consider getting vaccinated against HPV; talk to your provider about HPV vaccination if you are age 26–45 and at risk for HPV. The vaccine protects against the strains that cause most (but not all) cases of cervical cancer and genital warts.
- Get prompt treatment for any STIs you contract. Make sure your partner gets tested and receives treatment, too. In some parts of the country, expedited partner therapy may allow your health care provider to give you a prescription or medications for your partner (consult your health care provider to see if this is available in your area). Don't have sex until both of you have completed your treatment.
- If you inject drugs of any kind, don't share needles, syringes, or anything that might have blood on it. If your community has a syringe exchange program, use it. Seek treatment.
- If you are at risk for HIV infection, don't donate blood, sperm, or body organs. Don't have unprotected sex or share needles or syringes. Consider talking to your provider to see if PrEP is right for you. Get tested for HIV soon, and get treatment. People with HIV who receive early treatment generally feel better and live longer than those who delay.

highest rates occur among 20- to 24-year-olds. African Americans have chlamydia infection rates about six times higher than those of Euro-Americans.

If left untreated, chlamydia can lead to pelvic inflammatory disease (PID). Chlamydia also greatly increases a woman's risk for infertility and ectopic (tubal) pregnancy. The CDC currently recommends annual chlamydia testing for all sexually active women aged 25 and under and for older women who are at increased risk.

Chlamydia can also lead to infertility in men. In sexually active men, chlamydia is the most common cause of epididymitis, which is inflammation of the sperm-carrying ducts. Up to half of all cases of urethritis in men are caused by chlamydia.

**TERMS**

**gonorrhea** A sexually transmitted bacterial infection caused by the bacterium *Neisseria gonorrhoeae* that usually affects mucous membranes.

Infants of infected mothers can acquire the infection through contact with the pathogen in the birth canal during delivery.

**Diagnosis and Treatment** Chlamydia can be diagnosed through laboratory tests on the parts of the body that were exposed to the bacteria. Once chlamydia has been diagnosed, the infected person and their partner(s) are given antibiotics—usually doxycycline for a week or azithromycin in a single dose, which can cure uncomplicated infection. Testing and treatment of partners is important. When it is unlikely that a partner will seek medical treatment, the CDC recommends that extra medication or an extra prescription be given to the patient to provide to their partner. This strategy, called *expedited partner therapy,* is legal and encouraged in some states under certain circumstances.

## Gonorrhea

**Gonorrhea** is caused by the bacterium *Neisseria gonorrhoeae,* which flourishes in mucous membranes and is transmitted through sexual contact with the penis, vagina, mouth, or anus of an infected partner. The microbe cannot thrive outside the human body and dies within moments of exposure to light and air.

Because the infection often causes no symptoms, many cases go undetected, and the number of new infections may be much higher. The incidence rates peak among 15- to 24-year-olds. Like chlamydia, gonorrhea can cause the syndromes urethritis, cervicitis, PID, epididymitis, and proctitis. An infant passing through the birth canal of an infected mother may contract *gonococcal conjunctivitis,* an eye infection that can cause blindness if not treated.

**QUICK STATS**

**U.S. rates of chlamydia and gonorrhea are highest among adolescents and young adults.**

—Centers for Disease Control and Prevention, 2021

In males, the incubation period for gonorrhea is generally two to seven days. The first symptoms are due to urethritis, which causes urinary discomfort and discharge from the penis. The lips of the urethral opening may become inflamed and swollen. In some cases, the lymph glands in the groin become enlarged and swollen. Up to half of infected males have very minor symptoms or none at all.

Most females with gonorrhea are asymptomatic. Those who have symptoms often experience pain with urination, increased vaginal discharge, pain or bleeding with intercourse, and lower abdominal pain.

Rectal gonorrhea infections in men and women may be associated with pus or blood in the feces or rectal pain and itching. Pharyngeal infections in men and women often do not cause symptoms; however, they may be associated with sore throat or pus on the tonsils.

**Diagnosis and Treatment** Gonorrhea is detectable by several tests, which are performed at the sites of sexual exposure. Depending on the test, samples of urine, urethral, vaginal, cervical, throat, or rectal fluids may be collected by the patient or provider. The current recommended treatment for gonorrhea is ceftriaxone, injected in a single dose. The dose accounts for concerning trends in antimicrobial resistance and the challenge of treating gonorrhea at anatomic sites such as the throat.

## Pelvic Inflammatory Disease

**Pelvic inflammatory disease (PID)** is a major complication in 10–40% of women who have been infected with either gonorrhea or chlamydia and have not received treatment. PID occurs when the initial infection travels upward beyond the cervix into the uterus, oviducts, ovaries, and pelvic cavity. PID may be serious enough to require hospitalization and sometimes surgery. Even if the disease is treated successfully, about 25% of affected women will have long-term problems, such as a continuing susceptibility to infection, ectopic pregnancy, infertility, and chronic pelvic pain.

PID is the leading cause of infertility in young women, often going undetected until the inability to become pregnant leads to further evaluation. Infertility occurs in 8% of women after one episode of PID, 20% after two episodes, and 40% after three episodes. The risk of ectopic pregnancy, a medical emergency that can be fatal if not treated quickly, increases significantly in women who have had PID.

Women under age 25 are much more likely to develop PID than are older women. Risk factors include having a new or multiple sex partners, having a sex partner who has other sex partners at the same time, inconsistent use of condoms, prior history of an STI, vaginal douching, and intrauterine device use in the first three weeks after insertion.

Symptoms of PID vary greatly. Some women may be asymptomatic; others may have abdominal pain, fever, chills, nausea, and vomiting. Early symptoms are essentially the same as those described for chlamydia and gonorrhea. Symptoms often begin or worsen during or soon after a woman's menstrual period. Many women have abnormal vaginal bleeding—either bleeding between periods or heavy and painful menstrual bleeding.

**Diagnosis and Treatment** Diagnosis of PID is made on the basis of symptoms, physical examination, ultrasound, and laboratory tests. **Laparoscopy** may be used to confirm the diagnosis and obtain material for cultures.

A combination of antibiotics are usually started immediately; in severe cases, the woman may be hospitalized and given intravenous antibiotics. It is especially important that all partners receive treatment. As many as 60% of the male contacts of women with PID are infected, up to half of whom are asymptomatic.

## Human Papillomavirus

**Human papillomavirus (HPV)** infection can cause several diseases, including common warts, **genital warts**, and genital cancers. HPV causes virtually all cervical cancers, as well as

**TERMS**

**pelvic inflammatory disease (PID)** An ascending infection that progresses from the vagina and cervix to the uterus, oviducts, and pelvic cavity.

**laparoscopy** A method of examining the internal organs by inserting a tube containing a small light through an abdominal incision.

**human papillomavirus (HPV)** The pathogen that causes human warts, including genital warts, as well as anal and genital cancers.

**genital warts** A sexually transmitted viral infection characterized by growths on the genitals; also called *genital HPV infection* or *condyloma.* Persistence of HPV infection predisposes the infected person to some forms of genital cancers.

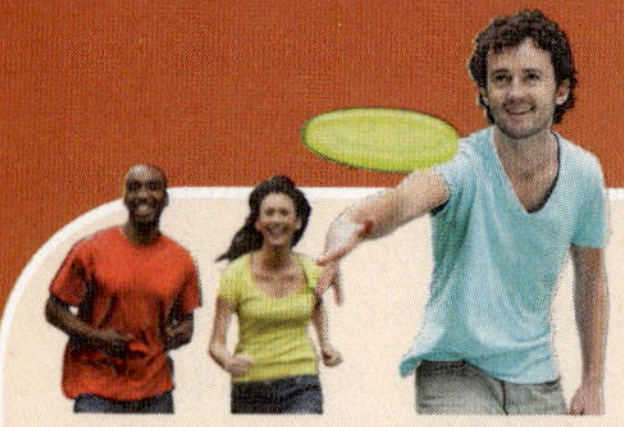

## WELLNESS ON CAMPUS
## College Students and STIs

### Why Do College Students Have High Rates of STIs?

- Risky sexual behavior is common. The National College Health Association found that fewer than half of college students used condoms consistently, and nearly a quarter of students reported more than one sex partner.
- College students underestimate their risk of STIs. Although students may have considerable knowledge about STIs, they often feel the risks do not apply to them—a dangerous assumption.
- Students may be infected but don't know it. Surveys by the National College Health Association found that despite reported access to sexual health services, less than a quarter of students reported ever being tested for HIV. Just over half of students completed the HPV vaccine series.

### What About Dating Apps?

- In this digital age, dating applications have expedited partner access with the click of a button or swipe.
- Some studies have shown an increase in risky sexual contacts and STIs with the use of dating apps for partner meetups. A number of factors are likely at play, including the ability to access new partner networks with varying levels of risk, which may increase the likelihood of STI exposure.
- Some apps allow users to disclose their STI, HIV, and PrEP use status upfront; however, this is not a reliable way to screen your partners.

### What Can Students Do to Protect Themselves against STIs?

- Take charge of your sexual health. The only person you can count on to stay safe is you!
- Limit your number of sex partners. Even people who are always in a monogamous relationship can end up with extensive potential exposure to STIs if, over the years, they have many relationships.
- Use barrier protection consistently, and don't assume it's safe to stop after you've been with a partner for several months. HIV infection, HPV infection, herpes, and chlamydia can be asymptomatic for months or years and can be transmitted at any time. If you haven't been using condoms with your current partner, start now.
- Stay healthy, and follow up with a provider regularly. If you are at risk for HIV, talk to your provider about PrEP. If there is a possibility that you have been exposed to HIV, talk to your doctor about post-exposure prophylaxis (PEP). Get tested for HIV and STIs regularly, and know your status.
- Enjoy sexuality on your own terms. Don't let the expectations of friends and partners cause you to ignore your own feelings. Let your own wellness be your first priority. If you choose to be sexually active, learn about safer sex practices.
- Get to know your partner, and talk to them before becoming intimate. Be honest about yourself, and encourage your partner to do the same. But practice safer sex no matter what.

SOURCES: American College Health Association. 2022. *American College Health Association-National College Health Assessment III: Reference Group Executive Summary Fall 2021*. Silver Spring, MD: American College Health Association. Beymer, M. R., R. E. Weiss, R. K. Bolan, et al. 2014. Sex on demand: Geosocial networking phone apps and risk of sexually transmitted infections among a cross-sectional sample of men who have sex with men in Los Angeles County. *Sexually Transmitted Infections* 90: 567–572; Cabecinha, M., C. H. Mercer, K. Gravningen, et al. 2017. Finding sexual partners online: Prevalence and associations with sexual behaviour, STI diagnoses and other sexual health outcomes in the British population. *Sexually Transmitted Infections* 93: 572–582.

anal, penile, vulvar, vaginal, and some forms of oropharyngeal cancers (the oropharynx includes the back of the mouth and the throat). Genital HPV is usually spread through sexual activity, including oral sex.

HPV is the most common STI in the United States. About 13 million Americans become infected with HPV each year. In all, more than 80% of sexually active people will have been infected with HPV by age 50. HPV is especially common in young people, with some of the highest infection rates among college students (see the box "College Students and STIs"). Many young women contract HPV infection within three months of becoming sexually active.

There are more than 200 different strains of HPV, and different strains cause different types of infection. More than 40 types are likely to cause genital infection. Types 6 and 11 cause 90% of visible genital warts. There are at least 14 other HPV strains, including 16 and 18, that are considered high-risk strains for cancer and are most often implicated in anogenital cancers (anal, cervical, penile, vaginal, and vulvar cancers). Three HPV vaccines are licensed in the United States. Each protects against HPV 16 and 18, the most common cancer-causing HPV types. In addition, the 4vHPV vaccine protects against HPV 6 and 11, two common wart-causing HPV types. The 9vHPV vaccine has the added benefit of protection from five different cancer-causing strains of the HPV virus. All three vaccines are licensed for use in females, and two (4vHPV and 9vHPV) are licensed for use in males. The CDC recommends vaccination for all girls and boys aged 11–12, although the vaccine can be given as early as age 9. The vaccine is most effective when given prior to exposure to genital HPV, as this virus is so common that many young people will be exposed to it shortly after becoming sexually active. For people not vaccinated as children, or those who are inadequately vaccinated, catch-up vaccination is recommended up to age 26 for women and 21 for men.

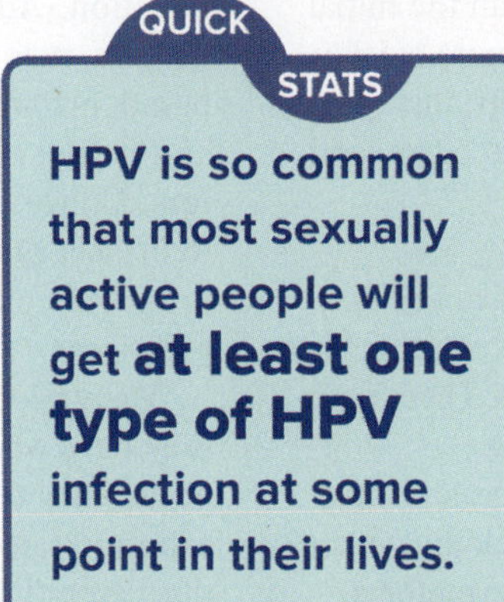


Most people infected with HPV have no visible warts or other symptoms and are not aware that they are infected and contagious to others. The good news is that the immune system usually clears the virus on its own, and infection disappears without any treatment. But in some cases, the infection persists and causes genital warts or cancers.

The types of HPV that cause cervical cancer do not produce any visible changes on the external genitals. The types that cause genital warts can produce anything from a small bump to a large, warty growth. Untreated warts can grow together to form a cauliflower-like mass. In males, they appear anywhere on the genitals, including the penis and urethra, appearing first at the opening and then spreading inside. The growths may cause irritation and bleeding, leading to painful urination and a urethral discharge. Warts may also appear around the anus or within the rectum. In women, warts may appear on the labia or vulva and may spread to the *perineum,* the area between the vagina and the rectum. They may also appear on the cervix.

**Diagnosis and Treatment** Genital warts are usually diagnosed based on the appearance of the lesions. HPV infection of the cervix is often detected on routine Pap tests. Special tests are now available to detect the presence of cancer-causing HPV infections and to distinguish among the more common strains of HPV, as a part of cervical cancer screening.

Treatment of genital warts focuses on reducing the number and size of warts, although most warts disappear eventually, even without treatment. The currently available treatments do not eradicate HPV infection. Warts may be removed by cryosurgery (freezing), electrocautery (burning), or laser surgery. Cervical abnormalities that are cancerous or precancerous are treated surgically or with other techniques such as electrical excision, freezing, and laser.

Anyone who has ever had HPV infection should inform all partners and use condoms, even though they do not provide total protection. Whether or not they have had the vaccine, women should have regular pelvic exams and Pap tests according to current guidelines.

QUICK STATS

**In the United States, about one out of every eight people aged 14–49 years has genital herpes.**

—Centers for Disease Control and Prevention, 2021

## Genital Herpes

Up to one in eight adults aged 14–49 in the United States has **genital herpes.** Worldwide, genital herpes is extremely common, and it is a major factor in HIV transmission.

There are two types of herpes simplex viruses, HSV 1 and HSV 2. HSV 1 is usually associated with oral herpes (infection of the mouth) and genital herpes can be caused by HSV 1 or HSV 2. Many people wrongly assume that they are unlikely to pick up an STI if they limit their sexual activity to oral sex, but this is not true, particularly in the case of genital herpes. These infections are commonly acquired through oral sex, particularly among young people (infection from kissing is uncommon, though still possible). However, changes in sexual behaviors, specifically oral-genital contact, have contributed to an increased incidence of anogenital HSV 1 infections in young adults. The type of virus may determine how frequently genital outbreaks occur. Compared to individuals with HSV 1 genital infections, those with HSV 2 infections tend to have more frequent outbreaks of genital lesions and shed more virus without having symptoms.

Because HSV is asymptomatic in most people, the infection is often acquired from a person who does not know that they are infected.

Newborns can occasionally be infected with HSV, usually during passage through the birth canal of an infected mother. Such transmission is more likely to occur when HSV 2 infection was acquired by the mother during the third trimester of pregnancy.

The morbidity and mortality associated with neonatal HSV infection highlights the importance of disclosing HSV status to your medical provider team during pregnancy. The risk of mother-to-child HSV transmission during pregnancy and delivery is low (less than 1%) in women with long-standing herpes infection. A pregnant person whose partner has herpes should practice safer sex and abstain from sex in the late stages of pregnancy. Precautions mothers can take to protect their babies from infection include medications to prevent or treat outbreaks and a cesarean section if active lesions are present at the time of delivery.

Up to 90% of people who are infected with HSV have no symptoms. Those who develop symptoms often first notice them on average between 2 and12 days of having sex with an infected partner. (However, it is not unusual for the first outbreak to occur months or even years after initial exposure.) The first episode of genital herpes frequently causes flulike symptoms in addition to genital lesions. The lesions tend to be painful or itchy and can occur anywhere on the genitals, inner thighs, or anal area. Depending on their location, they can cause considerable pain with urination. Lymph nodes in the groin may become swollen and tender.

TERMS

**genital herpes** A sexually transmitted infection caused by the herpes simplex virus.

Recurrent episodes are usually less severe than the initial one, with fewer and less painful sores that heal more quickly. Outbreaks can be triggered by a number of events, including stress, illness, fatigue, sun exposure, sexual intercourse, and menstruation.

**Diagnosis and Treatment** Genital herpes can be diagnosed on the basis of clinical findings, but laboratory testing is helpful if there is any question about the diagnosis. There is no vaccine to prevent herpes, but research is ongoing.

There is no cure for herpes, but it can be managed. Antiviral drugs such as acyclovir can be taken at the beginning of an outbreak to shorten the severity and duration of symptoms.

## Hepatitis A, B, and C

**Hepatitis** (inflammation of the liver) can cause serious and sometimes permanent damage to the liver, which can result in death in severe cases. One of the many types of hepatitis is caused by hepatitis B virus (HBV). Like HIV, HBV is found in blood and blood products, semen, saliva, urine, and vaginal secretions. Hepatitis B is much more contagious than HIV infection; it is easily transmitted through any sexual activity that involves the exchange of body fluids. HBV is not usually spread by hugging, coughing, food or water, sharing eating utensils or drinking glasses, or casual contact. The primary risk factors for HBV infection are sexual exposure and injection drug use (IDU); having multiple sex partners greatly increases risk. HBV can also be transmitted through sharing needles, razor blades, and toothbrushes contaminated with blood. With a goal of decreasing new HBV infections, preventing transmission, and reducing health disparities, vaccine recommendations were recently revisited. The Advisory Committee on Immunization Practices (ACIP) voted to recommend HBV vaccination for all adults under age 60, older adults with risk factors, and others desiring protection.

Other forms of viral hepatitis can also be sexually transmitted. Hepatitis A (HAV) is of particular concern for people who engage in anal sex; a vaccine is available and is recommended for all people at risk. There are no chronic infections associated with HAV.

Large population-based studies have demonstrated an association between hepatitis C virus (HCV) and individuals who engage in high-risk sexual encounters. Though fewer people in the United States acquire acute HCV infection annually, more chronic cases of HCV infection and subsequent deaths are noted than for cases of HBV. Most U.S. cases of HCV are associated with IDU. Other risks include receipt of infected blood products, needle-stick injuries in health care settings, and birth from a mother with HCV infection. Additionally, high-risk sexual exposure; sharing needles, razor blades, and toothbrushes contaminated with blood; high-risk health care procedures involving injections; and receipt of a tattoo in an unregulated facility are risk factors. Unlike HAV and HBV, there are no vaccines available to protect against HCV. If you inject drugs, talk to your doctor about counseling, treatment services, and safe injection practices.

Many people infected with HBV never develop symptoms; they have what are known as silent infections. If symptoms occur, they tend to appear an average of 90 days after HBV exposure (anywhere from 30–150 days). Mild cases of hepatitis cause flulike symptoms such as fever, body aches, chills, and loss of appetite. As the illness progresses, there may be nausea, vomiting, dark-colored urine, abdominal pain, and jaundice. Some people with hepatitis also develop a skin rash and joint pain or arthritis. Acute HBV infection can sometimes be severe, resulting in prolonged illness or even death.

Most adults who have acute HBV infection recover completely within a few weeks, but infections can persist for up to 6 months. About 5% of adults who are infected with HBV become chronic carriers of the virus, capable of infecting others for the rest of their lives. Some chronic carriers remain asymptomatic, whereas others develop chronic liver disease. Chronic hepatitis can cause cirrhosis, liver failure, and liver cancer.

**Diagnosis and Treatment** Hepatitis is diagnosed by blood tests used to analyze liver function, detect the infecting organism, and detect antibodies to the virus. Over the past few years, there has been a surge in safe and effective treatments to cure HCV; thus, testing and managing the care of infected individuals may help to curb this problem. There is no cure for HBV infection and no specific treatment for acute infections; antiviral drugs and immune system modulators may be used for chronic HBV infection.

Vaccination against HBV is recommended for all infants and children as well as previously unvaccinated adults.

## Syphilis

**Syphilis,** a disease that once caused death and disability for millions, can now be treated effectively with antibiotics. In 2020, there were more than 41,600 new cases of primary and secondary syphilis (early syphilis) reported in the United States, and almost 134,000 people received new diagnoses for any stage of syphilis. In 2020, 53% of primary and secondary syphilis cases were in MSM. The prevalence of HIV coinfection in MSM is also higher than in men who have sex with women or in women.

Syphilis is caused by a spirochete called *Treponema pallidum,* a thin, corkscrew-shaped bacterium. It requires warmth and moisture to survive and dies quickly outside the human body. The disease is usually acquired through sexual contact, although infected pregnant people can transmit it to their fetuses. The pathogen passes through any break or opening in the skin or mucous membranes and can be transmitted by vaginal or anal intercourse or oral contact with a syphilitic lesion.

**TERMS**

**hepatitis** Inflammation of the liver, which can be caused by infection, drugs, or toxins; some forms of infectious hepatitis can be transmitted sexually.

**syphilis** A sexually transmitted bacterial infection caused by the spirochete *Treponema pallidum.*

> ## Ask Yourself
>
> **QUESTIONS FOR CRITICAL THINKING AND REFLECTION**
>
> Have you ever had sex and regretted it later? If so, what were the circumstances and what influenced you to act the way you did? Were there any negative consequences? What preventive strategies can you use in the future to make sure it doesn't happen again?

Syphilis progresses through several stages, though not always in sequence. *Primary syphilis* is characterized by an ulcer called a **chancre** that appears within 10–90 days after exposure. The chancre is usually found at the site where the organism entered the body, such as the genital area, but it may also appear in other sites such as the mouth, breasts, or fingers. Chancres contain large numbers of bacteria and make the disease highly contagious when present; they are often painless and typically heal on their own within a few weeks. If the disease is not treated during the primary stage, about a third of infected individuals progress to chronic stages of infections.

*Secondary syphilis* is usually characterized by a skin rash that appears three to six weeks after the chancre. The rash may cover the entire body or only a few areas, but the palms of the hands and soles of the feet are usually involved. The rash is highly contagious but usually heals within several weeks or months.

If the disease remains untreated, the symptoms of secondary syphilis may recur over a period of several years; affected individuals may then lapse into an asymptomatic latent stage in which they experience no further consequences of infection. However, in about 15–30% of untreated syphilis cases, the individual develops *late,* or *tertiary, syphilis,* with symptoms that can appear 10–30 years after infection. Late syphilis can damage many organs of the body (brain, nerves, eyes, heart, blood vessels, liver, bones, and joints), possibly causing severe dementia, cardiovascular damage, blindness, and death.

*Neurosyphilis,* syphilis that invades the nervous system, can occur at any stage of the infection. Symptoms vary but may include headaches, vision or hearing loss, alterations in behavior, and disorders of movement. It is also possible that the patient has no overt symptoms at the time of diagnosis. *Ocular syphilis* is a clinical manifestation of neurosyphilis that can affect nearly any part of the eye structure. Symptoms may include decreased vision and the potential for permanent blindness. More than 200 cases of ocular syphilis were reported in 20 states in 2014–2015. Most of these cases were found in men who have sex with men who were infected with HIV, and few were found among heterosexual men and women without HIV.

Syphilis can traverse the placenta in pregnancy. If the mother does not receive treatment, the probable result is stillbirth, prematurity, or congenital deformity. In many cases, the infant is also born infected *(congenital syphilis)* and requires treatment.

**Diagnosis and Treatment** Syphilis is diagnosed with blood tests and by examination of infected tissues. Syphilis is a curable disease. Penicillin is the preferred antibiotic for treating syphilis at all stages, but damage from neurosyphilis and late syphilis can be permanent.

## Other Sexually Transmitted Infections

**Trichomoniasis** (often called *trich*) is the most prevalent nonviral STI in the United States; it is estimated to affect some 3.7 million individuals. The actual number of new infections is unknown; however, there were an estimated 6.9 million incident trichomoniasis infections in 2018 with 1.1 million (16%) among persons aged 15–24. The parasite that causes trichomoniasis, *Trichomonas vaginalis,* is highly transmissible during penile–vaginal sex. Nonsexual transmission is rare. Up to 85% of those infected may have no or minimal symptoms. Untreated infections might last for years. Women who become symptomatic with trichomoniasis develop a yellowish-green, diffuse, or foul-smelling vaginal discharge and severe itching and vulvar irritation. Men may develop inflammation of the urethra, epididymis, or prostate. *T. vaginalis* is not visible to the naked eye; however, a physician can check urine or urethral specimens and vaginal secretions for the presence of this organism. Treatment with oral metronidazole is the preferred regime for the management of trichomoniasis. Prompt treatment is important because studies suggest that trichomoniasis may increase the risk of HIV acquisition and transmission and, in pregnant people, premature delivery. If you or your partner has trichomoniasis, you should both receive treatment.

**Bacterial vaginosis (BV)** is the most common cause of abnormal vaginal discharge in women of reproductive age. BV occurs when healthful bacteria that normally inhabit the vagina become displaced by unhealthful species. BV is generally not considered an STI but may be associated with sexual activity—for example, change in partners, multiple partners, and women who have sex with women. Symptoms of BV include vaginal discharge with a fishy odor, and sometimes vaginal irritation. BV can place women at risk for other STIs, complications after some gynecological surgical procedures, and complications during pregnancy. BV is treated with topical and oral antibiotics.

**Pubic lice** (commonly known as *crabs*) and **scabies** are highly contagious parasitic infections. They are usually

> **TERMS**
>
> **chancre** The sore produced by syphilis in its earliest stage.
>
> **trichomoniasis** A protozoal infection caused by *Trichomonas vaginalis,* most commonly transmitted sexually.
>
> **bacterial vaginosis (BV)** A condition that may be linked to sexual activity; caused by an overgrowth of certain bacteria inhabiting the vagina.
>
> **pubic lice** Parasites that infest the hair of the pubic region; commonly called crabs.
>
> **scabies** A contagious skin disease caused by a type of burrowing parasitic mite.

treated with topical medicines, but oral medications are sometimes needed as well. Lice infestation can require repeated treatment.

## WHAT YOU CAN DO ABOUT SEXUALLY TRANSMITTED INFECTIONS

Take responsibility for your health and contribute to a reduction of STIs in three major areas: education, diagnosis and treatment, and prevention.

### Education

Educational campaigns about HIV/AIDS and other STIs have paid off in changing attitudes and sexual behaviors. Levels of awareness about HIV transmission among the general population are quite high, although some segments of the population are harder to reach and continue to engage in high-risk behaviors. Learning about STIs is still up to every person individually, as is applying that knowledge to personal situations.

### Diagnosis and Treatment

Early diagnosis and treatment of STIs can help you avoid complications and help prevent the spread of infection. The following actions are important:

- ***Be alert for symptoms.*** If you are sexually active, be alert for any sign or symptom of disease, such as a rash, a discharge, sores, or pain. Although only a physician can make a proper diagnosis of an STI, you can perform a genital self-examination between checkups to look for early warning signs of disease, such as bumps, sores, blisters, warts, or unusual discharge.

- ***Get vaccinated.*** Every young, sexually active person should be vaccinated against hepatitis B; vaccines are available for all age groups. The CDC also recommends that men who have sex with men, people who inject drugs, people living with HIV, and persons at risk for hepatitis A infection be vaccinated against hepatitis A, and males and females aged 9–26 be vaccinated against HPV.

- ***Get tested.*** Everyone aged 13–64 should be tested for HIV. If you are a sexually active woman aged 25 or younger, you should be receiving annual gonorrhea and chlamydia screening. High-risk men should receive annual or more frequent STI testing depending on risk, even if no symptoms are present. If you have a risky sexual encounter, see a physician as soon as possible.

- ***Inform your partners.*** Telling a partner that you have exposed them to an STI isn't easy. Despite the awkwardness and difficulty, it is crucial that your sex partner or partners be informed and urged to seek testing and/or treatment as quickly as possible.

#### TIPS FOR TODAY AND THE FUTURE

Your immune system is a remarkable germ-fighting network, but it needs your help to be vigilant about exposure, treatment, and prevention. STIs can have serious, long-term effects.

**RIGHT NOW YOU CAN:**

- Make sure that you have plenty of soap in your bathroom and kitchen. It should not be antibacterial soap.
- Start getting at least 15 more minutes of sleep each night.
- Make an appointment with your health care provider if you are worried about possible STI infection.
- Resolve to discuss condom use with your partner if you are sexually active and are not already using condoms.

**IN THE FUTURE YOU CAN:**

- Stock up on hand sanitizer and tissues. Put them in your backpack, car, locker, and other places where you might need to wash your hands when soap and water won't be available.
- Make an appointment with your physician to ensure your immunizations are up to date.
- Learn how to communicate effectively with a partner who resists safer sex practices or is reluctant to discuss their sexual history. Support groups and educational classes can help.

- ***Get treatment.*** Treatments for STIs are safe, and most are inexpensive. If you are receiving treatment, follow instructions carefully and complete all the medication as prescribed. Don't stop taking the medication just because you feel better or your symptoms have disappeared. If you have an STI, your partner needs to be tested and, if necessary, receive treatment. It is recommended that you return for follow-up testing to make sure that you have not been reinfected and that your infection is cured.

### Prevention

If you choose to be sexually active, think about prevention *before* you have a sexual encounter or find yourself in the heat of the moment. Find out what your partner thinks before you become sexually involved. By thinking and talking about responsible sexual behavior, you are caring for yourself, your potential partner, and your future children.

## SUMMARY

- The immune system includes both surface barriers and the cells that mount the immune response.
- Physical and chemical barriers to microorganisms include skin, mucous membranes, and the cilia lining the respiratory tract.

# BEHAVIOR CHANGE STRATEGY
## Talking about Condoms and Safer Sex

The time to talk about safer sex is before you begin a sexual relationship. But even if you've been having condomless sex with your partner, you can still start practicing safer sex now. The correct and consistent use of condoms can reduce the risk of acquiring many sexually transmitted infections.

There are many ways to bring up the subject of safer sex and condom use with your partner. Be honest about your concerns, and stress that protection against STIs means that you care about yourself and your partner. You may find that your partner shares your concerns and wants to use condoms. They may be happy and relieved that you have brought up the subject of safer sex.

However, if they resist the idea of using condoms, you may need to negotiate (see the dialogue suggestions). Stress that you both deserve to be protected and that sex will be more enjoyable when you aren't worrying about STIs. If you and your partner haven't used condoms before, buy some and familiarize yourselves with how to use them. Information on where to find condoms in your area and how to use a condom correctly can be found here: https://www.cdc.gov/condomeffectiveness/index.html. Once you feel more comfortable handling condoms, you'll be able to use them correctly and incorporate them into your sexual activity. Consider trying the female condom as well.

If your partner still won't agree to use condoms, think carefully about whether you want to have a sexual relationship with this person. Maybe they're not the right partner for you.

| IF YOUR PARTNER SAYS . . . | TRY SAYING . . . |
|---|---|
| "They're not romantic." | "Worrying about AIDS isn't romantic, and with condoms we won't have to worry." *or* "If we put one on together, a condom could be fun." |
| "I don't have any kind of disease! Don't you trust me?" | "Of course I trust you, but anyone can have an STI and not even know it. This is just a way to take care of both of us." |
| "I forgot to bring a condom. Let's just do it without a condom this time." | "It only takes one time to get pregnant or to get an STI. I just can't have sex unless I know I'm as safe as I can be." *or* "I never have sex without a condom. Let's go get some." *or* "I have some right here." |
| "I don't like sex as much with a rubber. It doesn't feel the same." | "This is the only way I feel comfortable having sex, but believe me, it'll still be good even with protection! And it lets us both just focus on each other instead of worrying about all that other stuff." *or* "They might feel different, but let's try." *or* "Sex won't feel good if we're worrying about diseases." *or* "How about trying the female condom?" |
| "But I love you." | "Being in love can't protect us from diseases." *or* "I love you, too. We still need to use condoms." |
| "But we've been having sex without condoms." | "I want to start using condoms now so we won't be at any more risk." *or* "We can still prevent infection or reinfection." |
| "I don't know how to use them." | "I can show you—want me to put it on for you?" |
| "No one else makes me use a condom!" | "This is for both of us . . . and I won't have sex without protection. Let me show you how good it can be—even with a condom." |
| "I'm [or you're] on the pill." | "But that doesn't protect us from STIs, so I still want to be safe, for both of us." |

SOURCES: KidsHealth. 2022. Talking to Your Partner About Condoms (https://kidshealth.org/en/teens/talk-about-condoms.html); American Sexual Health Association. 2020. Talking to a Partner (http://www.ashasexualhealth.org/sexual-health/talking-about-sex/).

- The immune response is carried out by white blood cells that are continuously produced in the bone marrow. Cells of the innate immune system include neutrophils, eosinophils, macrophages, dendritic cells, and natural killer cells. Cells of the adaptive immune system are lymphocytes–in particular, T cells and B cells.
- The immune response has four stages: recognition of the invading pathogen; replication of T cells and B cells; attack by killer T cells and macrophages; and suppression of the immune response.
- Immunization is based on the body's ability to remember previously encountered organisms.
- Allergic reactions occur when the immune system responds to harmless substances as if they were dangerous pathogens.
- The step-by-step process by which infections are transmitted from one person to another involves a pathogen, its reservoir, a portal of exit, a means of transmission, a portal of entry, and a new host. Infection can be prevented by breaking the chain at any point.
- Bacteria are single-celled organisms; some cause disease in humans. Significant bacterial infections include pneumonia, meningitis, strep throat, toxic shock syndrome, MRSA, tuberculosis, Lyme disease, and ulcers.

- Most antibiotics work by interrupting the production of new bacteria; they do not work against viruses. Bacteria can become resistant to antibiotics.

- Viruses cannot grow or reproduce themselves; viruses cause the common cold, influenza, measles, mumps, rubella, chickenpox, cold sores, mononucleosis, encephalitis, hepatitis, polio, and warts.

- Other infectious diseases are caused by certain types of fungi, protozoa, and parasitic worms.

- Autoimmune diseases occur when the body identifies its own cells as foreign.

- A healthy immune system can destroy mutant cells that may become cancerous.

- The immune system needs adequate nutrition and rest, moderate exercise, and protection from excessive stress. Vaccinations also help protect against disease.

- Human immunodeficiency virus (HIV) affects the immune system, making an otherwise healthy person less able to resist a variety of infections.

- HIV is carried in blood and blood products, semen, vaginal and cervical secretions, and breast milk. HIV is transmitted through the exchange of these fluids.

- There is currently no cure or vaccine for HIV. Drugs have been developed to slow the course of the disease and to prevent or treat certain secondary infections.

- HIV transmission can be prevented by making careful choices about sexual activity and not sharing drug needles.

- If you have been exposed to HIV, it is very important that you are seen by a provider. Post-exposure prophylaxis (PEP) medication is available to prevent HIV Infection after exposure, but timing is key.

- If you are at high risk for acquiring HIV, talk to your provider about PrEP for HIV prevention.

- Chlamydia causes epididymitis and urethritis in men; in women, it can lead to urethritis, cervicitis, pelvic inflammatory disease (PID), and infertility if untreated. Patients and their partners should be treated. In infants born to mothers with untreated chlamydia, it cause eye infections and pneumonia.

- Untreated gonorrhea can cause PID in women and epididymitis in men, leading to infertility. Patients and their partners should be treated. In infants born to mothers with untreated gonorrhea, infections of the eyes and other serious complications can occur.

- PID, usually a complication of untreated gonorrhea or chlamydia, is an ascending infection that progresses from the vagina and cervix to the uterus, oviducts, and pelvic cavity. It can lead to infertility, ectopic pregnancy, and chronic pelvic pain. Both the infected woman and her partners must receive treatment.

- Human papillomavirus (HPV) can cause genital warts and anogenital cancers. The virus can be transmitted by asymptomatic people. Even after treatment, a person may continue to carry the virus in healthy-looking tissue. The immune system often clears HPV on its own.

- Genital herpes is a common viral infection that can cause painful blisters on the genitals. The virus remains in the body for life and causes recurrent outbreaks.

- Hepatitis B (HBV) and C (HCV) are two of the many types of hepatitis virus that can cause inflammation of the liver. Both are transmitted through sexual and nonsexual contact. Following an initial infection, people can recover, but some become carriers and may develop serious complications.

- Vaccines are available to prevent HBV.

- Most U.S. HCV infections are found in persons who inject drugs. No vaccines are available to prevent HCV infection. Safe and effective medications are now available to cure hepatitis C.

- Syphilis is a highly contagious infection caused by the spirochete *T. pallidum*. It can be treated with antibiotics. The disease progresses through three stages. Untreated, it can lead to organ damage, deterioration of the central nervous system, and death. Patients and their partners should be treated.

- Trichomoniasis is a protozoal infection that is readily transmitted by penile-vaginal sex.

- Other diseases that can be transmitted sexually or are linked to sexual activity include bacterial vaginosis, pubic lice, and scabies. Any STI that causes sores or inflammation can increase the risk of HIV transmission.

## FOR MORE INFORMATION

*Alliance for the Prudent Use of Antibiotics.* Provides information about the proper use of antibiotics and tips for avoiding infections.

https://apua.org

*American Academy of Allergy, Asthma & Immunology.* Provides information and publications; pollen counts are available from the website.

http://www.aaaai.org

*American College of Allergy, Asthma & Immunology.* Provides information for patients and physicians; website includes an extensive glossary of terms related to allergies and asthma.

http://www.acaai.org

*American College Health Association (ACHA).* Offers free brochures on STIs, alcohol use, acquaintance rape, and other health issues.

http://www.acha.org/ACHA/Resources/Topics/Sexual_Health.aspx

*American Society for Microbiology.* Includes a library of images and an introduction to microbes.

http://www.asm.org

*Black AIDS Institute.* Provides public health information about a variety of topics including testing, treatment, vaccines, and health care access; focuses on the Black community.

http://www.blackaids.org

*CDC Female Condom Use.* Shows how to use a female condom.

https://www.cdc.gov/condomeffectiveness/Female-condom-use.html

*CDC Male Condom Use*. Shows the right way to use a male condom.

https://www.cdc.gov/condomeffectiveness/male-condom-use.html

*CDC National Center for Emerging and Zoonotic Infectious Diseases.* Provides extensive information on a wide variety of infectious diseases.

http://www.cdc.gov/ncezid/

*CDC National Prevention Information Network.* Provides extensive information and links for HIV/AIDS and other STIs.

http://www.cdcnpin.org

*CDC National STD and AIDS Hotlines.* Callers can obtain information, counseling, and referrals for testing and treatment. The hotlines offer information on more than 20 STIs and include Spanish and TTY services.

800-342-AIDS *or* 800-227-8922

800-344-SIDA (Spanish)

800-243-7889 (TTY, deaf access)

*CDC: Vaccines & Immunizations.* Provides information and answers to frequently asked questions about vaccines and immunizations.

http://www.cdc.gov/vaccines

*HIV Risk Reduction Tool.* CDC's online tool for estimating your risk for HIV with each sexual act.

https://hivrisk.cdc.gov/risk-estimator-tool/#-sb

*Joint United Nations Programme on HIV/AIDS (UNAIDS).* Provides information on the international HIV/AIDS situation.

http://www.unaids.org

*MedlinePlus: Sexually Transmitted Diseases.* Provides a clearinghouse of links and information on STIs and other sexual health topics; maintained by the CDC.

https://medlineplus.gov/sexuallytransmitteddiseases.html

*The NAMES Project Foundation, AIDS Memorial Quilt.* Includes the story behind the quilt, images of quilt panels, and information and links relating to HIV.

http://www.aidsquilt.org

*National Foundation for Infectious Diseases.* Provides information about a variety of diseases and disease issues.

http://www.nfid.org

*National HIV Curriculum.* Updates health care providers about HIV prevention, screening, diagnosis, and ongoing treatment and care.

https://www.hiv.uw.edu/

*National Institute of Allergy and Infectious Diseases.* Includes fact sheets about many topics relating to allergies and infectious diseases, including tuberculosis and sexually transmitted infections.

http://www.niaid.nih.gov

*National STD Curriculum.* Gives information about the epidemiology, pathogenesis, clinical manifestations, diagnosis, management, and prevention of STDs.

https://www.std.uw.edu/

*Planned Parenthood Federation of America.* Provides information about STIs, family planning, and contraception.

http://www.plannedparenthood.org

*World Health Organization: Infectious Diseases.* Provides fact sheets about many emerging and tropical diseases as well as information about current outbreaks.

http://www.who.int/topics/infectious_diseases/en

*World Health Organization (WHO): Sexually Transmitted Infections.* Provides information on international statistics and prevention efforts.

https://www.who.int/news-room/fact-sheets/detail/sexually-transmitted-infections-(stis)

## SELECTED BIBLIOGRAPHY


Abma, J. C., and G. M. Martinez. 2017. Sexual activity and contraceptive use among teenagers in the United States, 2011–2015. *National Health Statistics Reports;* no 104. Hyattsville, MD: National Center for Health Statistics (https://www.cdc.gov/nchs/data/nhsr/nhsr104.pdf).

AIDS.gov. 2021. *Pre-Exposure Prophylaxis (PrEP)* (https://hivinfo.nih.gov/understanding-hiv/fact-sheets/pre-exposure-prophylaxis-prep).

AIDS.gov. 2021. *The Basics of HIV Prevention* (https://hivinfo.nih.gov/understanding-hiv/fact-sheets/basics-hiv-prevention).

AIDS.gov. 2022. *Recommendations for the Use of Antiretroviral Drugs in Pregnant Women with HIV Infection and Interventions to Reduce Perinatal HIV Transmission in the United States* (https://clinicalinfo.hiv.gov/en/guidelines/perinatal/appendix-c-antiretroviral-counseling-guide-for-health-care-providers).

American Association of Blood Banks. 2022. *FAQs About Blood and Blood Donation* (https://www.aabb.org/for-donors-patients/faqs-about-blood-and-blood-donation).

American College Health Association. 2022. *American College Health Association National College Health Assessment III: Reference Group Executive Summary Fall 2021.* Hanover, MD: American College Health Association (https://www.acha.org/documents/ncha/NCHA-III_FALL_2021_REFERENCE_GROUP_EXECUTIVE_SUMMARY.pdf).

American College of Gynecology. 2021. *Cervical Cancer Screening* (https://www.acog.org/womens-health/infographics/cervical-cancer-screening).

American Sexual Health Association. 2022. *Diagnosing Herpes* (https://www.ashasexualhealth.org/herpes-testing/).

Boyle, P. 2021. mRNA technology promises to revolutionize future vaccines and treatments for cancer, infectious diseases. *Association of American Medical Colleges* (https://www.aamc.org/news-insights/mrna-technology-promises-revolutionize-future-vaccines-and-treatments-cancer-infectious-diseases).

Cabecinha, M., et al. 2017. Finding sexual partners online: Prevalence and associations with sexual behaviour, STI diagnoses and other sexual health outcomes in the British population. *Sexually Transmitted Infections* 93: 572–582.

Callaway, E. 2020. Coronavirus vaccines: Five key questions as trials begin. Some experts warn that accelerated testing will involve some risky trade-offs (https://www.nature.com/articles/d41586-020-00798-8).

Cantor, A. G., et al. 2016. Screening for syphilis: Updated evidence report and systematic review for the U.S. Preventive Services Task Force. *Journal of the American Medical Association* 315(21): 2328–2337.

Centers for Disease Control and Prevention. 2019. Clostridioides difficile *Infection* (https://www.cdc.gov/hai/organisms/cdiff/cdiff_infect.html).

Centers for Disease Control and Prevention. 2020. *HIV Testing* (https://www.cdc.gov/hiv/testing/index.html).

Centers for Disease Control and Prevention. 2020. *Populations at Greatest Risk* (https://www.cdc.gov/hiv/policies/hip/risk.html).

Centers for Disease Control and Prevention. 2021. *Antibiotic Prescribing and Use.* Atlanta, GA: U.S. Department of Health and Human Services (https://www.cdc.gov/antibiotic-use/common-illnesses.html).

Centers for Disease Control and Prevention. 2021. *Asthma* (https://www.cdc.gov/asthma/most_recent_national_asthma_data.htm).

Centers for Disease Control and Prevention. 2021. *E. coli (Escherichia coli)* (https://www.cdc.gov/ecoli/outbreaks.html).

Centers for Disease Control and Prevention. 2021. *Expedited Partner Therapy* (http://www.cdc.gov/std/ept/).

Centers for Disease Control and Prevention. 2021. HIV: Testing (https://www.cdc.gov/HIV/Basics/testing.html).

Centers for Disease Control and Prevention. 2021. *HIV in the United States: At a Glance* (https://www.cdc.gov/hiv/statistics/overview/ataglance.html).

Centers for Disease Control and Prevention. 2021. *HIV Surveillance Report, 2019*; vol. 32 (https://www.cdc.gov/hiv/library/reports/hiv-surveillance.html).

Centers for Disease Control and Prevention. 2021. Human Papillomavirus *(HPV)* (https://www.cdc.gov/hpv/parents/vaccine-for-hpv.html).

Centers for Disease Control and Prevention. 2021. *Pelvic Inflammatory Disease (PID): CDC Fact Sheet* (https://www.cdc.gov/std/pid/stdfact-pid-detailed.htm).

Centers for Disease Control and Prevention. 2021. *Sexually Transmitted Disease Surveillance 2019*. Atlanta: U.S. Department of Health and Human Services (https://www.cdc.gov/std/statistics/2019/default.htm).

Centers for Disease Control and Prevention. 2021. *Sexually Transmitted Infections Treatment Guidelines, 2021* (https://www.cdc.gov/std/treatment-guidelines/default.htm).

Centers for Disease Control and Prevention. 2021. *Surveillance for Viral Hepatitis-United States, 2019* (https://www.cdc.gov/hepatitis/statistics/2019surveillance/index.htm).

Centers for Disease Control and Prevention. 2021. *Tuberculosis (TB)* (https://www.cdc.gov/tb/statistics/tbcases.htm).

Centers for Disease Control and Prevention. 2022. *2021 Provisional Pertussis Surveillance Report* (https://www.cdc.gov/pertussis/downloads/pertuss-surv-report-2021_PROVISIONAL.pdf).

Centers for Disease Control and Prevention. 2022. *Genital Herpes - CDC Fact Sheet* (https://www.cdc.gov/std/herpes/stdfact-herpes.htm)

Centers for Disease Control and Prevention. 2022. *Genital HPV Infection Fact Sheet* (https://www.cdc.gov/std/hpv/stdfact-hpv.htm).

Centers for Disease Control and Prevention. 2022. *Hepatitis B Questions and Answers for Health Professionals* (https://www.cdc.gov/hepatitis/hbv/hbvfaq.htm#overview).

Centers for Disease Control and Prevention. 2022. *Influenza (Flu)* (https://www.cdc.gov/flu/index.htm).

Centers for Disease Control and Prevention. 2022. Lyme Disease (https://www.cdc.gov/lyme/datasurveillance/index.html?CDC_AA_refVal=https%3A%2F%2Fwww.cdc.gov%2Flyme%2Fstats%2Findex.html).

Centers for Disease Control and Prevention. 2022. Measles (Rubeola) (https://www.cdc.gov/measles/).

Centers for Disease Control and Prevention. 2022. *Pre-exposure Prophylaxis (PrEP)* (https://www.cdc.gov/hiv/clinicians/prevention/prep.html).

Centers for Disease Control and Prevention. 2022. *Recommended Adult Immunization Schedule* (https://www.cdc.gov/vaccines/schedules/downloads/adult/adult-combined-schedule.pdf).

Centers for Disease Control and Prevention. 2022. West Nile Virus (https://www.cdc.gov/westnile/).

Centers for Disease Control and Prevention. 2022. Zika Virus (https://www.cdc.gov/zika/index.html).

Coronavirus world map: Tracking the global outbreak. 2022. *The New York Times,* April 1 (https://www.nytimes.com/interactive/2021/world/covid-cases.html.)

Corum, J., and C. Zimmer. 2020. Bad news wrapped in protein: Inside the coronavirus genome. *The New York Times,* 3 April (https://www.nytimes.com/interactive/2020/04/03/science/coronavirus-genome-bad-news-wrapped-in-protein.html).

Dean, L. T., et al. 2018. The affordability of providing sexually transmitted disease services at a safety-net clinic. *American Journal of Preventive Medicine* 54(4): 552–558.

Do Prado, M. F., et al. 2012. Antimicrobial efficacy of alcohol-based gels with a 30-s application. *Letters in Applied Microbiology* 54(6): 564–567.

D'Amato, G., et al. 2015. Effects on asthma and respiratory allergy of climate change and air pollution. *Multidisciplinary Respiratory Medicine* 10: 39.

Fauci, A. S. 2019. Ending the HIV epidemic: A plan for the United States. *Journal of the American Medical Association* 321(9): 844–845.

Febo-Vazquez, I., C. E. Copen, and J. Daugherty. 2018. Main reasons for never testing for HIV among women and men aged 15–44 in the United States, 2011–2015. *National Health Statistics Reports;* no 107. Hyattsville, MD: National Center for Health Statistics.

Food and Drug Administration. 2019. FDA issues final rule on safety and effectiveness of consumer hand sanitizers. (https://www.fda.gov/news-events/press-announcements/fda-issues-final-rule-safety-and-effectiveness-consumer-hand-sanitizers).

Food and Drug Administration. 2020. *Women and HIV: Get the Facts on HIV Testing, Prevention, and Treatment* (https://www.fda.gov/consumers/free-publications-women/women-and-hiv-get-facts-hiv-testing-prevention-and-treatment).

Gargano, J., et al. 2022. Human papillomavirus. Chapter 5 in *Manual for the Surveillance of Vaccine-Preventable Diseases.* Centers for Disease Control and Prevention (https://www.cdc.gov/vaccines/pubs/surv-manual/chpt05-hpv.html).

Goulder, P. J., S. R. Lewin, and E. M. Leitman. 2016. Paediatric HIV infection: The potential for cure. *Nature Reviews Immunology* 16: 259–271.

Hay, P. E., et al. 2016. Which sexually active young female students are most at risk of pelvic inflammatory disease? A prospective study. *Sexually Transmitted Infections* 92(1): 63–66.

Henry J. Kaiser Family Foundation. 2021. *The Global HIV/AIDS Epidemic* (https://www.kff.org/global-health-policy/fact-sheet/the-global-hivaids-epidemic/).

Henry J. Kaiser Family Foundation. 2021. *The HIV/AIDS Epidemic in the United States* (https://www.kff.org/hivaids/fact-sheet/the-hivaids-epidemic-in-the-united-states-the-basics/).

Joint United Nations Programme on HIV/AIDS (UNAIDS). 2017. *UNAIDS Ending AIDS Progress towards the 90-90-90 targets* (http://www.unaids.org/sites/default/files/media_asset/Global_AIDS_update_2017_en.pdf)

Kamidani, S., and L. K. Pickering. 2019. Tetanus spores lie in wait for unvaccinated children. *American Academy of Pediatrics* (https://www.aappublications.org/news/2019/07/03/mmwr070319).

Kreisel, K., et al. 2017. Prevalence of pelvic inflammatory disease in sexually experienced women of reproductive age—United States, 2013-2014. *MMWR* 66(3): 80–83.

Kreisel, K. M., et al. 2021. Sexually transmitted infections among US women and men: Prevalence and incidence estimates, 2018. *Sexually Transmitted Diseases* 48(4): 208–214.

Markowitz, L. E., et al. 2016. Prevalence of HPV after introduction of the vaccination program in the United States. *Pediatrics* 137(3): e20151968.

Martinez, G. M., and J. C. Abma. 2020. Sexual activity and contraceptive use among teenagers aged 15–19 in the United States, 2015–2017. *NCHS Data Brief, 366.* Hyattsville, MD: National Center for Health Statistics (https://www.cdc.gov/nchs/products/databriefs/db366.htm).

McQuillan, G., et al., 2018. *Prevalence of Herpes Simplex Virus Type 1 and Type 2 in Persons Aged 14-49: United States, 2015-2016.* NCHS Data Brief no. 304 (https://www.cdc.gov/nchs/products/databriefs/db304.htm).

Medline Plus. 2022. Autoimmune diseases. *National Library of Medicine* (https://medlineplus.gov/autoimmunediseases.html).

Meites, E., et al. 2019. Human papillomavirus vaccination for adults: Updated recommendations of the Advisory Committee on Immunization Practices. *Morbidity and Mortality Weekly Report* 68: 698–702.

Moreira, E. D., Jr., et al. 2016. Safety profile of the 9-valent HPV vaccine: A combined analysis of 7 phase III clinical trials. *Pediatrics* 138(2): e20154387.

Murray, K. A., et al. 2015. Global biogeography of human infectious diseases. *Proceedings of the National Academy of Sciences* 112(41): 12746–12751.

National Institute of Allergy and Infectious Disease. 2020. *COVID-19, MERS & SARS* (https://www.niaid.nih.gov/diseases-conditions/covid-19).

National Institute of Neurological Disorders and Stroke. 2020. *Meningitis and Encephalitis Fact Sheet* (https://www.ninds.nih.gov/Disorders/Patient-Caregiver-Education/Fact-Sheets/Meningitis-and-Encephalitis-Fact-Sheet).

National Institutes of Health. n.d. *The HIV Life Cycle* (https://aidsinfo.nih.gov/understanding-hiv-aids/infographics/7/hiv-life-cycle).

National Institutes of Health: National Cancer Institute. 2021. *HPV and Cancer* (https://www.cancer.gov/about-cancer/causes-prevention/risk/infectious-agents/hpv-and-cancer#transmitted).

National Notifiable Disease Surveillance System. 2020. *Provisional 2019 Reports of Notifiable Diseases,* Week 52. Unpublished. Atlanta, GA: U.S. Department of Health and Human Services (https://www.cdc.gov/pertussis/downloads/pertuss-surv-report-2019-508.pdf).

Petrova, V. N., et al. 2019. Incomplete genetic reconstitution of B cell pools contributes to prolonged immunosuppression after measles. *Science Immunology* 4(4): eaay6125.

Poole, C. L., and D. W. Kimberlin. 2018. Antiviral approaches for the treatment of herpes simplex virus infections in newborn infants. *Annual Review of Virology* 5: 407–425.

Price, M. J., et al. 2016. Proportion of pelvic inflammatory disease cases caused by *Chlamydia trachomatis:* Consistent picture from different methods. *Journal of Infectious Diseases* 214(4): 617–624.

Rockefeller University Press. 2019. How sleep can fight infection. *ScienceDaily,* 12 February (www.sciencedaily.com/releases/2019/02/190212094839.htm).

Schwartz, N. G., et al. 2020. Tuberculosis—United States, 2019. *MMWR* 69(11): 286–289.

Seillet, C. et al. 2019. The neuropeptide VIP confers anticipatory mucosal immunity by regulating ILC3 activity. *Nature Immunology* 21(2): 168.

Spicknall, I. H., E. W. Flagg, and E. A. Torrone. 2021. Estimates of the prevalence and incidence of genital herpes, United States, 2018. *Sexually Transmitted Diseases* 48(4): 260–265.

Taniguchi, K., and M. Karin. 2018. NF-κB, inflammation, immunity and cancer: Coming of age. *Nature Reviews Immunology 18:* 309–324.

Taylor, D. J. 2016. Is insomnia a risk factor for decreased influenza vaccine response? *Behavioral Sleep Medicine* 14: 1–18.

Tobian, A., et al. 2019. Male circumcision for the prevention of HSV-2 and HPV infections and syphilis. *New England Journal of Medicine* 360: 1298–1309.

U.S. Department of Health & Human Services. 2021. *HIV Vaccines* (https://www.hiv.gov/hiv-basics/hiv-prevention/potential-future-options/hiv-vaccines).

U.S. Department of Health and Human Services. 2021. *HIV Overview: The HIV Life Cycle* (https://hivinfo.nih.gov/understanding-hiv/fact-sheets/hiv-life-cycle).

U.S. Food and Drug Administration. 2020. *Facts About In-Home HIV Testing* (https://www.fda.gov/consumers/consumer-updates/facts-about-home-hiv-testing).

U.S. Food and Drug Administration. 2020. *Patient Information—Gardasil 9* (http://www.fda.gov/downloads/BiologicsBloodVaccines/Vaccines/ApprovedProducts/UCM426460.pdf).

U.S. Preventive Services Task Force. 2016. Sero*logic Screening for Genital Herpes Infection US Preventive Services Task Force Recommendation Statement* (https://jamanetwork.com/journals/jama/fullarticle/2593575).

U.S. Preventive Services Task Force. 2020. *Hepatitis C Virus Infection in Adolescents and Adults: Screening* (https://www.uspreventiveservicestaskforce.org/uspstf/recommendation/hepatitis-c-screening).

UNAIDS. 2021. *Fact Sheet—World AIDS Day 2021* (https://www.unaids.org/en/resources/fact-sheet#:~:text=79.3%20million%20%5B55.9%20million%E2%80%93110,the%20start%20of%20the%20epidemic).

UNAIDS. 2022. *Global HIV & AIDS Statistics–Fact Sheet* (https://www.unaids.org/en/resources/fact-sheet). https://www.unaids.org/sites/default/files/media_asset/young-people-and-hiv_en.pdf

United Nations. 2022. *AIDS* (https://www.unaids.org/en).

Vásquez-Otero, O., et al. 2016. Dispelling the myth: Exploring associations between the HPV vaccine and inconsistent condom use among college students. *Preventive Medicine* 93: 147–150 (http://dx.doi.org/10.1016/j.ypmed.2016.10.007).

Wadman, M., et al. 2020. How does coronavirus kill? Clinicians trace a ferocious rampage through the *body, from brain to toes. Scien*ce, 17 April (https://www.sciencemag.org/news/2020/04/how-does-coronavirus-kill-clinicians-trace-ferocious-rampage-through-body-brain-toes).

World Health Organization. 2020. *Blood Safety and Availability* (https://www.who.int/news-room/fact-sheets/detail/blood-safety-and-availability)

World Health Organization. 2020. *Preventing HIV through Safe Voluntary Medical Male Circumcision for Adolescent Boys and Men in Generalized HIV Epidemics: Recommendations and Key Considerations* (https://www.who.int/publications/i/item/978-92-4-000854-0).

World Health Organization. 2020. The cost of inaction: COVID-19-related service disruptions could cause hundreds of thousands of extra deaths from HIV. (https://www.who.int/news-room/detail/11-05-2020-the-cost-of-inaction-covid-19-related-service-disruptions-could-cause-hundreds-of-thousands-of-extra-deaths-from-hiv).

World Health Organization. 2020. WHO Director-General's opening remarks at the media briefing on COVID-19, 11 March https://www.who.int/dg/speeches/detail/who-director-general-s-opening-remarks-at–media-briefing-on-covid-19—11-march-2020

World Health Organization. 2021. *Number of People (All Ages) Living with HIV Estimates by WHO Region* (https://apps.who.int/gho/data/view.main.22100WHO?lang=e).

World Health Organization. 2022. *Global HIV Programme: Mother-to-Child Transmission of HIV* (https://www.who.int/teams/global-hiv-hepatitis-and-stis-programmes/hiv/prevention/mother-to-child-transmission-of-hiv)

World Health Organization. 2022. *Global HIV Programme: Pre-*exposure Prophylaxis (PrEP) (https://www.who.int/teams/global-hiv-hepatitis-and-stis-programmes/hiv/prevention/pre-exposure-prophylaxis).

**Design Elements:** Assess Yourself icon: Aleksey Boldin/Alamy Stock Photo; Diversity Matters icon: Rawpixel Ltd/Getty Images; Wellness on Campus icon: Radius Images/Alamy Stock Photo; Take Charge icon: VisualCommunications/Getty Images; Critical Consumer icon: pagadesign/Getty Images.

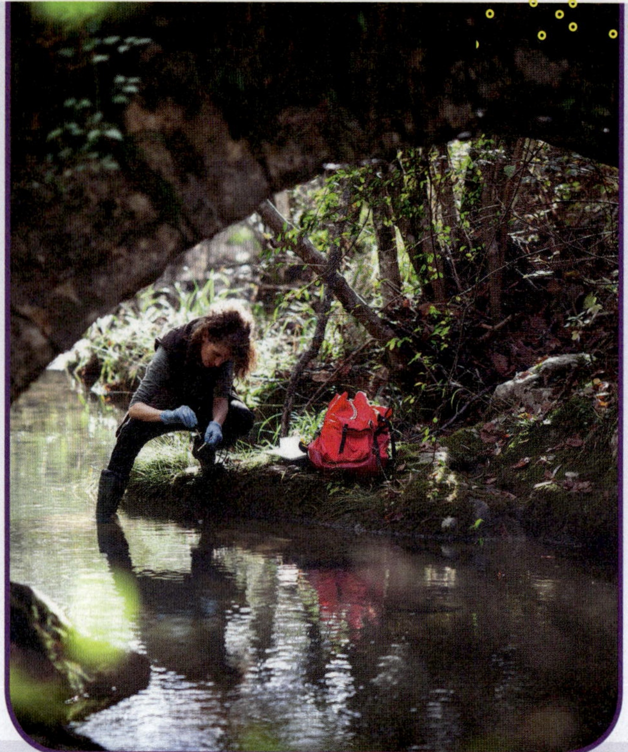
CasarsaGuru/Getty Images

## CHAPTER OBJECTIVES

- Explain the concept of environmental health and how it has developed
- Explain how population growth affects the earth's environment
- Explain the impact of energy use and production on the environment
- Describe the causes and effects of air and water pollution
- Describe the problem of solid waste disposal
- Identify environmental issues related to chemical pollution and hazardous waste
- Identify environmental issues related to radiation pollution
- Explain the concept of noise pollution and its impacts

CHAPTER 15

# Environmental Health

We are constantly reminded of our intimate relationship with everything that surrounds us—our **environment.** Although the planet provides us food, water, air, and everything else that sustains life, it also provides natural occurrences—earthquakes, tsunamis, hurricanes, drought, and changes in climate—that destroy life and disrupt society. Humans have always had to contend with the environment to survive. Today, we also have to find ways to protect the environment and our health from harmful byproducts of our way of life.

This chapter introduces the concept of environmental health and explains how the environment affects us. It also discusses the ways humans affect the planet and its resources—focusing in particular on energy use and production, air and water pollution, solid waste disposal, chemical and radiation pollution, and noise pollution.

> **TERMS**
>
> **environment** The natural and human-made surroundings in which we spend our lives.
>
> **environmental health** The collective interactions of humans with the environment and the short-term and long-term health consequences of those interactions.

## ENVIRONMENTAL HEALTH DEFINED

The field of **environmental health** grew out of efforts to control communicable diseases. These discoveries led to systematic garbage collection, sewage treatment, filtration and chlorination of drinking water, food inspection, and the establishment of public health enforcement agencies.

These efforts to control and prevent communicable diseases changed the health profile of the industrialized world. Americans rarely contract cholera, typhoid fever, plague, diphtheria, or other diseases that continue to kill large numbers of people in other parts of the world. The importance of vaccines can also be seen in the sharply dropping numbers of Covid-19

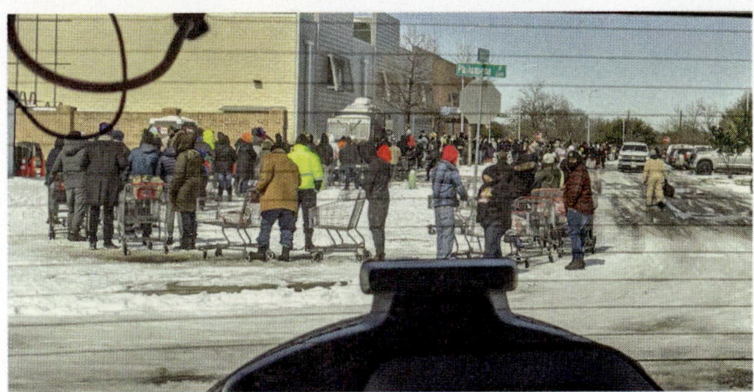

Natural events—such as the deep freeze in Texas 2021—can result in power outages for millions of people when they are all hooked up to the same big, centralized electricity generators. Bryan Klingner

cases in countries where Covid-19 vaccines are distributed and received in higher numbers. In 2021 the daily number of new Covid-19 cases in Britain dropped by 90% after its government began a strategy to vaccinate as many people as possible.

In the United States, a complex public health system is constantly at work behind the scenes attending to the details of these critical health concerns. Every time the system is disrupted, danger recurs. After any disaster that damages a community's public health system—whether a natural disaster such as a hurricane or a human-made disaster such as a terrorist attack—prompt restoration of basic health services becomes crucial to human survival. Every time we venture beyond the boundaries of our everyday world, whether traveling to a poorer country or camping in a wilderness area, we are reminded of the importance of these basics: clean water, sanitary waste disposal, safe food, and insect and rodent control.

QUICK
STATS
By 2050, the U.S. population will be nearly 400 million; its current population is 333 million.
—U.S. Census Bureau, 2022

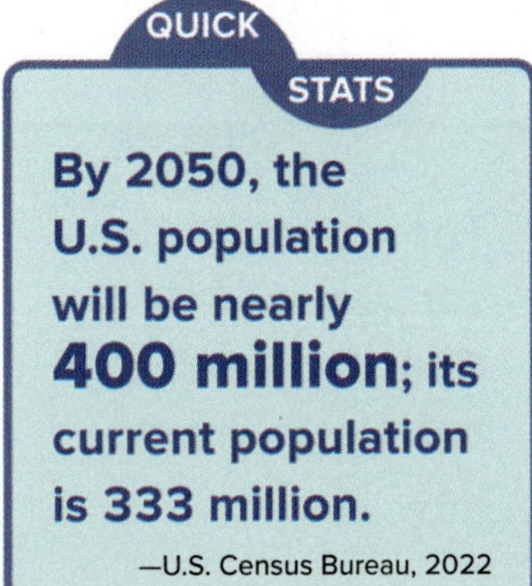

Environmental health encompasses all the interactions of humans with their environment and the health consequences of these interactions. Fundamental to this definition is a recognition that we hold the world in trust for future life on earth. Environmental pollutants contribute not only to infectious diseases and immediate symptoms, but to many chronic diseases as well. In addition, technological advances have increased our ability to affect and damage the environment. Further, rapid population growth (more than doubling in the past 50 years), which has resulted partly from past environmental improvements, means that ever more people are consuming and competing for resources, increasing human environmental impact.

Our responsibility is to pass on a world no worse, and preferably better, than the one we live in today. Although many environmental problems are complex and seem beyond the control of the individual, there are ways that every person can make a difference to the future of the planet.

**Ask Yourself**

**QUESTIONS FOR CRITICAL THINKING AND REFLECTION**

How often do you think about the environment's impact on your personal health? In what ways do your immediate surroundings (your home, neighborhood, school, workplace) affect your well-being? In what ways do you influence the health of your personal environment?

## POPULATION GROWTH AND CONTROL

Throughout most of history, humans have been a minor pressure on the planet. About 300 million people were alive in the year 1 CE (Common Era); by the time Europeans were settling in the Americas 1600 years later, the world population had increased gradually to a little over half a billion. But then it began rising exponentially—zooming to 1 billion by around 1800, more than doubling by 1930, and then doubling again in just 40 years (Figure 15.1).

The world's human population, currently around 7.8 billion, is increasing at a rate of about 80 million per year—approximately 150 people every minute. The average number of children per woman fell from 5 in 1950 to less than half that (2.4) in 2021. This decline in fertility has been happening in Western countries for decades and is now also happening in many of today's poor countries. In sub-Saharan Africa, Asia, and Latin America, women with more education are having fewer children; these regions nevertheless contribute the most to population size. Changes are also projected for the world's age distribution: For the first time in history, there are more older people than young children. By 2050, the number of people ages 80 and over will have tripled. Despite a slowing rate of growth, the population is still expanding. This expansion, particularly in the past 50 years, is believed to be responsible for most of the stress humans put on the environment.

No one knows how many people the world can support, but most scientists agree that there is a limit. An estimate from the Global Footprint Network is that we use as many ecological resources as if we lived on 1.6 earths. The primary factors that may eventually put a cap on human population are food, water, land, and energy.

Although it is apparent that population growth must be controlled, population trends are difficult to influence and manage. A variety of interconnecting factors fuel the current population explosion, including high birth rates, lack of family planning, and lower death rates.

To be successful, population management policies must change the condition of people's lives, especially through decreasing poverty, to remove the pressures to have large families. Research indicates that the combination of

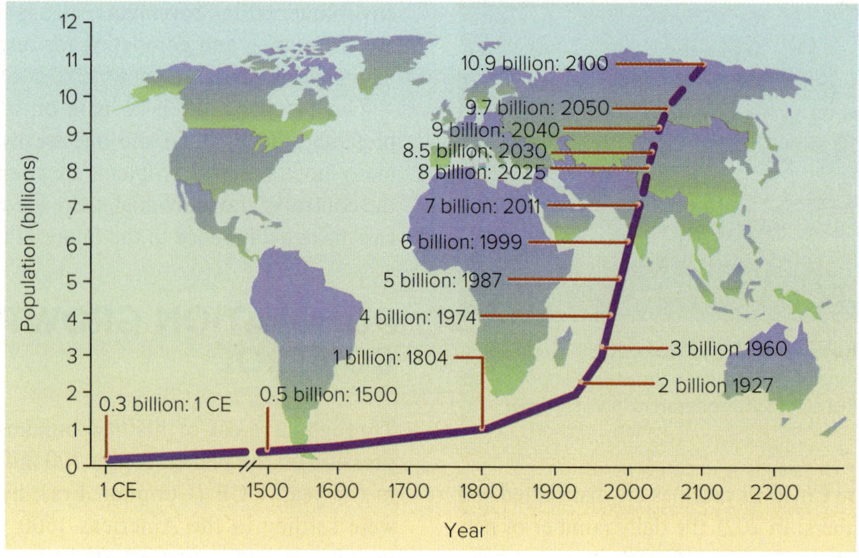


**FIGURE 15.1 World population growth.** The United Nations estimates that the world population will reach 8.5 billion in 2030, 9.7 billion in 2050, and 10.9 billion in 2100.

SOURCE: United Nations. 2019. *World Population Prospects: The 2019 Revision* (https://population.un.org/wpp/).

improved health, better education, and increased literacy and employment opportunities for women work together with family planning to decrease birth rates.

## ENVIRONMENTAL IMPACTS OF ENERGY USE AND PRODUCTION

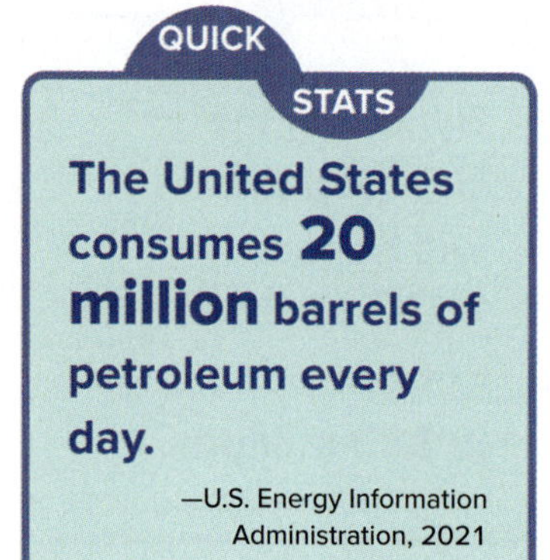


The United States and China are the biggest energy consumers (Figure 15.2). We use energy to create electricity, transport us, power our industries, and run our homes. About 80% of the energy we use comes from fossil fuels—oil, coal, and natural gas. The remainder comes from nuclear power and renewable energy sources such as hydroelectric, wind, and solar power.

Energy consumption is at the root of many environmental problems. Automobile exhaust and the burning of oil and coal by industry and by electric power plants are primary causes of the greenhouse effect, smog, and acid precipitation. Electric cars have a lower carbon footprint than gasoline cars, even accounting for the electricity used to charge them. The mining of coal and the extraction and transportation of oil and natural gas cause pollution on land and in water.

### Environmental Threats of Extreme Energy Sources

Despite improvements in energy efficiency, the combination of increasing global population and economic growth is expected to continue to drive up worldwide energy demand over time. At the same time, supplies of easily accessible oil will decline. In response, some energy companies have turned to what are often called "extreme energy sources." This term describes fossil fuels that are relatively difficult to access and extract from the environment. Technologies needed to access extreme energy sources include deepwater oil rigs, tar sands oil extraction, and drilling and hydraulic fracturing for natural gas extraction. Critics worry that these new technologies have been insufficiently studied and regulated and may pose significant new environmental risks.

Deepwater rigs extract oil that is buried deep under the ocean floor and can be difficult to manage. A tragic example was the Deepwater Horizon rig that exploded in April 2010 in the Gulf of Mexico. Oil gushed into the water at an estimated rate of 60,000 barrels a day. It took BP three months to plug the leak, after nearly 5 million barrels of oil had spilled. Chemical dispersants used to break up the oil had possible toxic effects and may have caused much of the oil to remain beneath the surface where it cannot be reached for cleanup. The long-term health effects to the remaining wildlife, and to humans, are not known.

Tar sands (or oil sands) are sand deposits that are saturated with a dense form of petroleum called bitumen. Making liquid fuel from the oil in tar sands is an energy-intensive process. The resulting product yields two to four times the amount of greenhouse gases per barrel compared to conventional oils. Canada has placed a priority on tar sands development, but critics note that these "dirty" deposits contain 240 gigatons of carbon, representing twice the amount of carbon dioxide emitted by all oil ever used. In

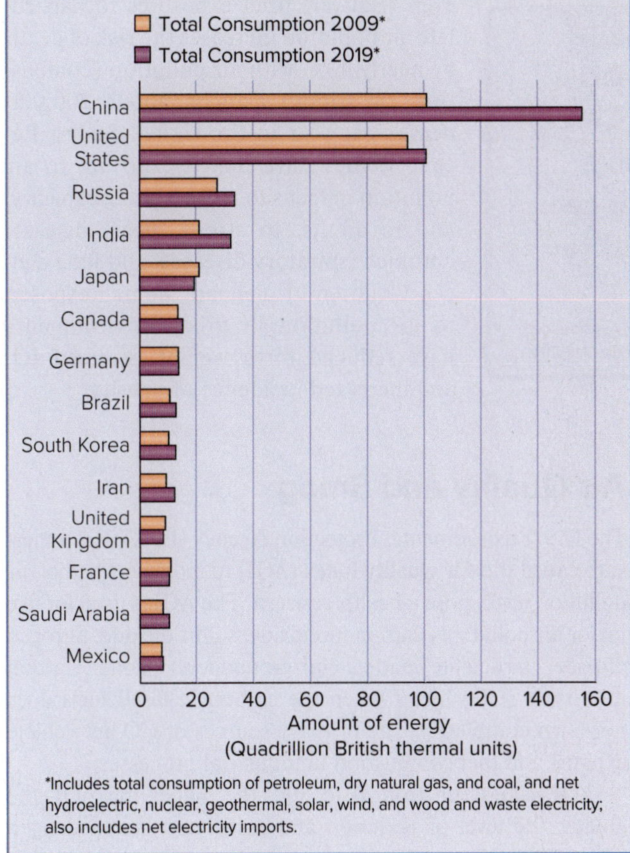


**FIGURE 15.2 Energy Consumption of Selected Countries.**

SOURCE: U.S. Energy Information Administration. 2021. *International Energy Statistics: Total Primary Energy Consumption (Quadrillion BTU): All Countries, 2019* (http://www.eia.gov/international/rankings/world?).

addition, Canada's tar sands oil will need to travel through thousands of miles of leak-prone pipelines across pristine wildlife habitats in both Canada and the United States, and when it reaches shipping terminals, huge increases in oil tanker ship traffic will endanger fragile marine habitats in both countries.

Hydraulic fracturing, or fracking, uses pressurized mixes of fluids to create cracks in rock formations deep underground, releasing natural gas. Health experts have raised concerns about the safety of the technique, especially since many of these wells are in residential areas, near homes and schools. Companies are not required to publicly disclose the specific chemicals used. In addition, the disposal of wastewater from the fracking process (which is done by injecting the fluid deep in the ground) has been linked to a dramatic increase in earthquakes in the central United States. Fracking pollutes the air, water, and soil and can cause noise and physical disturbances. This pollution is linked to preterm births, high-risk pregnancies, asthma, and other health problems. Despite this, there are few regulations in place to protect people from the effects of fracking. The storage of natural gas is also problematic. In 2015 a massive natural gas leak in Aliso Canyon, near Los Angeles, released over 100,000 tons of methane and ethane, causing major health problems to the local population and creating a carbon footprint even larger than the Deepwater Horizon spill.

## Renewable Energy

Sources of renewable energe are those naturally replenished and essentially inexhaustible, such as wind and sunlight. Together with technologies that improve energy efficiency, renewable energy sources contribute to sustainability–the capacity of natural or human systems to endure and maintain well-being over time. A common definition of *sustainable development* is development that meets society's present needs without compromising the ability of future generations to meet their needs.

*Wind power* uses wind to turn blades that run a turbine, which spins an electricity-producing generator. *Solar power* uses heat and light of the sun, for example, to generate steam that runs a turbine to produce electricity. *Geothermal power* taps heat in the earth's core; *biomass* is plant material that produces energy when burned; and *biofuels* are based on natural materials–alcohol or oil–that can be used as fuel.

World renewable energy production capacity increased by 56% from 2008 to 2010. By 2011, more than 118 countries had enacted some type of policy target or promotion policy related to renewable energy. Many of these targets called for 15–26% of energy or electricity to be provided by renewable sources by 2020. In 2020, despite the challenges of the Covid-19 pandemic, the annual renewable energy capacity additions increased 45% to almost 280 gigawatts, the highest increase since 1999.

## Alternative Fuels

The U.S. Department of Energy (DOE) is encouraging researchers and automobile manufacturers to produce vehicles that can run on alternative fuels such as ethanol.

Ethanol, a form of alcohol, is a renewable and largely domestic transportation fuel produced from fermenting plant sugars such as corn, sugarcane, and other starchy agricultural products. Ethanol use reduces the amount of imported oil required to produce gasoline, reduces overall greenhouse gas emissions from automobiles, and supports the U.S. agricultural industry.

Ethanol's critics show that corn-based ethanol requires more energy to produce than it yields when burned as fuel. Biodiesel, like ethanol, can be problematic depending on its material source. It is carbon neutral when the plants that are used to make it, such as soybeans and palm oil trees, absorb carbon dioxide as they grow and offset the carbon dioxide produced while making and using biodiesel. Most of the biodiesel used in the United States is made from soybean oil that is a by-product of processing soybeans for animal feed and numerous other food and nonfood products, and from waste animal fat and grease. However, in some parts of the world, natural vegetation and forests have been cleared and burned to grow soybeans and palm oil trees to make biodiesel, and these negative environmental and social effects can outweigh any benefit.

QUICK
STATS
137 million
Americans (43% of the nation) live where the air can be dangerous to breathe.
—American Lung Association's State of the Air, 2022

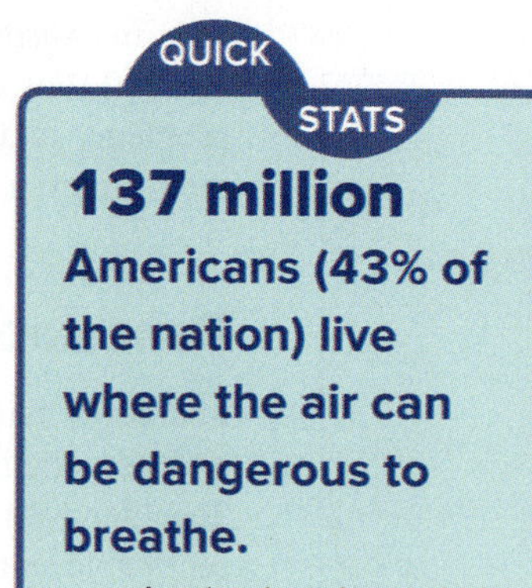

## Hybrid and Electric Vehicles

Hybrid electric vehicles (HEVs) use two or more distinct power sources to propel the vehicle, such as an onboard energy storage system (e.g., batteries), a traditional internal combustion engine, and an electric motor. Hybrid vehicles typically have greater fuel economy than conventional cars do, and they produce fewer polluting emissions. Hybrids also tend to run with less noise than conventional vehicles. Several hybrid models are currently available in the United States, and hybrids are gaining popularity with consumers and are being used more commonly in both corporate and government vehicle fleets. A second generation of all-electric vehicles (EVs) has recently been introduced to consumer markets, taking advantage of better battery storage performance and more "quick-charging" stations, and changing consumer perceptions of the convenience of EVs.

# AIR QUALITY AND POLLUTION

The World Health Organization (WHO) estimates that air pollution accounts for an estimated 4.2 million deaths per year. The air is polluted naturally by forest fires, pollen, dust storms, and other natural pollutants. Humans contribute to pollution with the by-products of our activities.

Air pollution is linked to a wide range of health problems, and the very young and older adults are among the most susceptible to its effects. For people with chronic ailments such as diabetes or heart failure, even relatively brief exposures to particulate air pollution increases the risk of death by nearly 40%, with air pollution (combustion emissions) causing about 200,000 deaths per year in the United States. Recent studies have linked exposure to air pollution in teens to reduced lung capacity, and in adults, to stroke, heart disease, chronic respiratory diseases, and lung cancer. Children of pregnant women exposed to air pollution in urban environments have reduced birth weight, reduced IQ, and increased incidence of obesity.

**TERMS**

**Air Quality Index (AQI)** A measure of local air quality and what it means for health.

**fossil fuels** Buried deposits of decayed animals and plants that are converted into carbon-rich fuels by exposure to heat and pressure over millions of years; oil, coal, and natural gas are fossil fuels.

**smog** Hazy atmospheric conditions resulting from increased concentrations of ground-level ozone and other pollutants.

**greenhouse effect** A warming of the earth due to a buildup of greenhouse gases in the atmosphere.

**greenhouse gas** A gas (such as carbon dioxide) or vapor that traps infrared radiation instead of allowing it to escape through the atmosphere, resulting in a warming of the earth (the *greenhouse effect*).

## Air Quality and Smog

The U.S. Environmental Protection Agency (EPA) uses a measure called the **Air Quality Index (AQI)** to indicate whether air pollution levels pose a health concern. The AQI is used for five major air pollutants carbon monoxide, sulfur dioxide, nitrogen dioxide, particulate matter, and ground-level ozone. Carbon monoxide (CO) forms when the carbon in **fossil fuels** does not burn completely. The primary sources of CO are vehicle exhaust and fuel combustion in industrial processes.

AQI values run from 0 to 500; the higher the AQI, the greater the level of pollution and associated health danger. When the AQI exceeds 100, air quality is considered unhealthful for groups sensitive to pollution, and for everyone as AQI values rise over 150.

The term **smog** was first used in the early 1900s in London to describe the combination of sulfurous smoke and fog. What we typically call *smog* today is a mixture of pollutants from car exhaust, power plants, and factory emissions. Heavy motor vehicle traffic, high temperatures, and sunny weather (UV radiation) can increase the production of ozone. Pollutants are also more likely to build up in areas with little wind or where a topographic feature such as a mountain range or valley prevents the wind from pushing out stagnant air.

## The Greenhouse Effect and Global Warming

Life on earth depends on a process known as the **greenhouse effect,** which contributes to a warm atmosphere. The temperature of the earth's atmosphere depends on the balance between the amount of energy the planet absorbs from the sun (mainly as high-energy UV radiation) and the amount of energy lost back into space (as lower-energy infrared radiation). Key components of temperature regulation are carbon dioxide, water vapor, methane, and other **greenhouse gases**—so named because, like the glass panes in a greenhouse, they let through visible light from the sun but trap some of the resulting infrared radiation and reradiate it back to the earth's surface. This process causes a buildup of heat

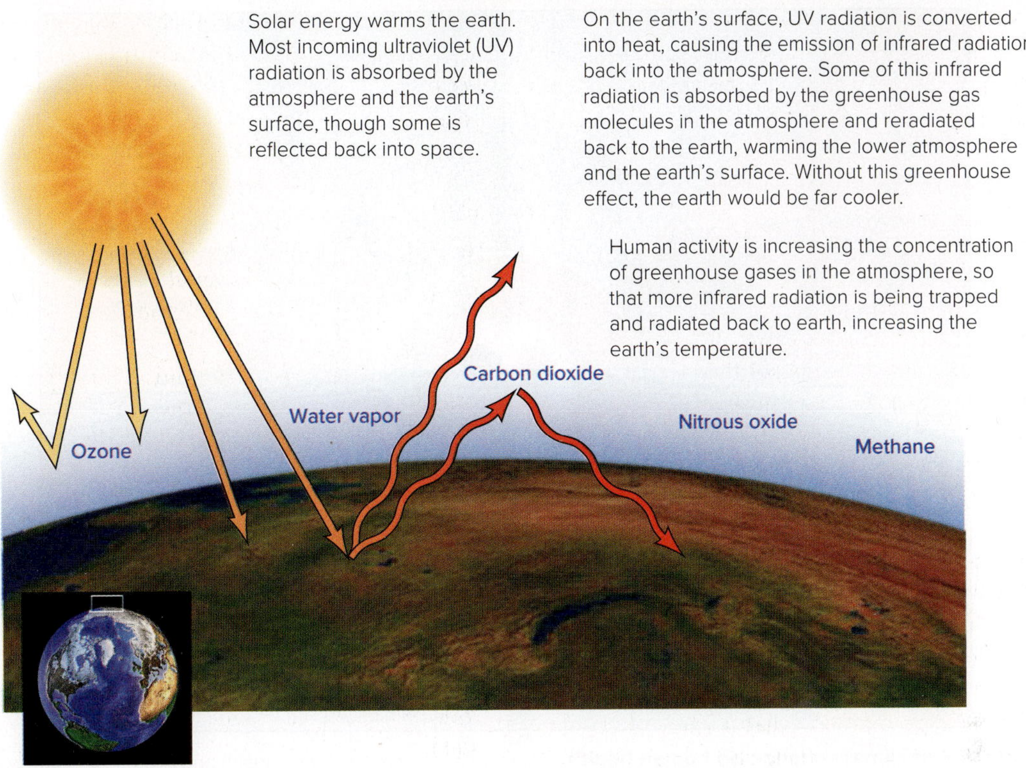


**FIGURE 15.3** **The greenhouse effect.** Key greenhouse gases that help trap heat energy in the lower atmosphere are carbon dioxide, methane, nitrous oxide, ozone, and water vapor. titoOnz/Alamy Stock Photo

(i.e., the greenhouse effect) that raises the temperature of the lower atmosphere (Figure 15.3).

There is scientific consensus that this natural process has been disrupted by human activity, causing **global warming** or *climate change*. The concentration of greenhouse gases is increasing because of human activity, especially the combustion of fossil fuels and emissions from agricultural production (Table 15.1).

An analysis of ice core samples shows that $CO_2$, methane, and nitrous oxide levels are now higher than at any time in at least the past 800,000 years. In that time period, $CO_2$ levels in the atmosphere ranged between 172 and 300 parts per million (ppm). But in recent decades we crossed over 400 ppm and to a record high of 421 ppm $CO_2$ in 2021. Experts believe $CO_2$ may account for about 60% of the greenhouse effect. The United States is responsible for one-third of the world's $CO_2$ emissions.

With rising temperatures, events such as droughts, floods, and wildfires have become much more common. More than ever previously recorded, the fires this past decade have burned more acres, spread more particulate matter and other debris, and destroyed forests, buildings, and human and animal life. Between 2017 and 2021, California burned in the largest and deadliest wildfires recorded—over 10 million acres. Fires have ravaged the United States West Coast, the Brazilian Amazon, and parts of Australia, the Arctic, Indonesia, Siberia, Portugal, and Argentina.

If global warming persists, experts say the impact may be devastating (Figure 15.4). Current and potential consequences include increased rainfall and flooding in some regions, and increased drought in others; increased mortality from heat stress, urban air pollution, and tropical diseases.

**Table 15.1** Sources of Greenhouse Gases

| GREENHOUSE GAS | SOURCES |
|---|---|
| Carbon dioxide | Fossil fuel and wood burning, factory emissions, car exhaust, deforestation |
| Chlorofluorocarbons (CFCs) | Refrigeration and air conditioning, aerosols, foam products, solvents |
| Methane | Cattle, wetlands, rice paddies, landfills, gas leaks, coal and gas industries |
| Nitrous oxide | Fertilizers, soil cultivation, deforestation, animal feedlots and wastes |
| Ozone and other trace gases | Photochemical reactions, car exhaust, power plant emissions, solvents |

**TERMS**

**global warming** An increase in the earth's atmospheric temperature when averaged across seasons and geographic regions; also called *climate change*.

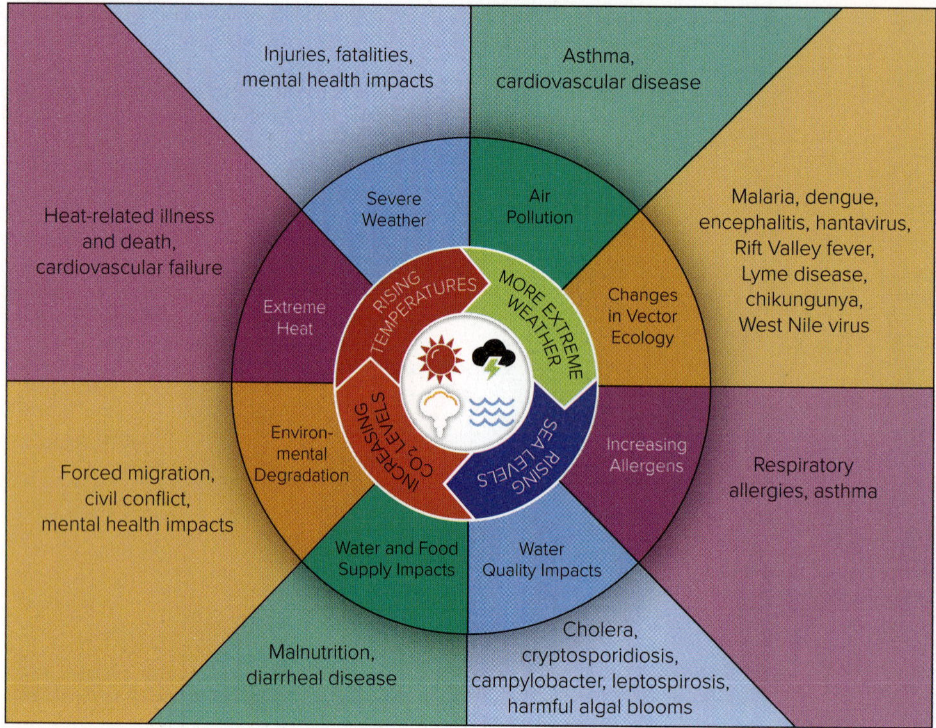


**FIGURE 15.4 Impact of climate change on human health.** Climate change can influence health and disease in many ways; the effects may vary based on location, age, socioeconomic status, and other factors.

SOURCE: Centers for Disease Control and Prevention. 2020. *Climate Effects on Health* (http://www.cdc.gov/climateandhealth/effects).

**Ask Yourself**

**QUESTIONS FOR CRITICAL THINKING AND REFLECTION**

How aware are you of the issues related to climate change, and where do you get your information? Do you think about how your lifestyle affects climate change on a day-to-day basis? Why do you think climate change is such a controversial and politically charged topic, especially in the U.S?

Deaths from extreme weather events such as hurricanes, tornadoes, droughts, and floods might also increase. A poleward shift of about 50–350 miles (150–550 km) will occur in the location of vegetation zones, affects crop yields, irrigation demands, and forest productivity. Alterations of ecosystems, result in possible species extinction. Arctic ice melts to some extent during the summer each year, but melting has increased by 20% since 1979.

At the 2015 United Nations Climate Change Conference in Paris, France, 195 countries made a landmark agreement to limit average global warming to 2°C above preindustrial temperatures, striving for a limit of 1.5°C. According to the Paris Agreement, each country is in charge of setting its own greenhouse emissions limits, so countries must pledge sufficient reductions in order for the Agreement to be effective. Progress has been made since 2015, but many countries are falling short of their reduction goals.

**TERMS**

**ozone layer** A layer of ozone molecules in the upper atmosphere that screens out UV rays from the sun.

**chlorofluorocarbons (CFCs)** Chemicals used as spray can propellants, refrigerants, and industrial solvents, which have been implicated in the destruction of the ozone layer.

## Thinning of the Ozone Layer

Another air pollution problem is the thinning of the atmosphere's **ozone layer,** a fragile, invisible layer about 10–30 miles above the earth's surface that shields the planet from the sun's hazardous UV rays. Since the mid-1980s, scientists have observed the seasonal appearance and growth of a hole in the ozone layer over Antarctica. Thinning over other areas has been noted more recently.

The ozone layer is being destroyed primarily by **chlorofluorocarbons (CFCs),** which are industrial chemicals used as coolants in refrigerators and air conditioners, as agents in some rigid foam products, as propellants in some aerosol sprays, and as solvents. When CFCs rise into the atmosphere, winds carry them toward the polar regions. During winter, circular winds form a vortex that keeps the air over Antarctica from mixing with air from elsewhere. CFCs react with airborne ice crys destroying ozone. When the polar vortex weakens in the summer, winds richer in ozone from the north replenish the lost Antarctic ozone.

About 30 years ago, an international agreement, the Montreal Protocol, engendered regulations on the production of ozone-depleting chemicals. Because of this, overall atmospheric ozone is no longer decreasing, and in 2019, the ozone hole was the smallest since 1982 (although variations in weather helped account for this). The Antarctic ozone layer has begun to show signs of healing, and although it will likely not return to its early-1980s state until about 2070 this is an example of science-based policy and international cooperation successfully tackling a global environmental issue.

Without the ozone layer to absorb the sun's UV radiation, life on earth would be impossible. The potential effects of increased long-term exposure to UV light for humans include skin cancer, cataracts and blindness, and reduced immune response.

## Indoor Air Quality (IAQ)

Although most people associate air pollution with the outdoors, homes and other buildings can harbor potentially dangerous pollutants. Some of these compounds trigger allergic responses, and others have been linked to cancer and developmental problems in children. Common indoor pollutants include the following: environmental tobacco smoke (ETS); carbon monoxide and other combustion by-products from woodstoves, fireplaces, kerosene heaters and lamps, and gas ranges; volatile organic compounds (VOCs), which are gases emitted from such household items as paints, lacquers, cleaning supplies, aerosols, building materials, furnishings, and office equipment; biological pollutants, such as bacteria, dust mites, mold, and animal dander, which can cause allergic reactions and other health problems; and indoor mold, a fungus that grows in damp places, such as on shower tiles and damp basement walls.

## Preventing Air Pollution

Here are a few ideas for how you can reduce air pollution:

- Cut back on driving or consider an EV or hybrid car. Ride your bike, walk, use public transportation, or carpool in a fuel-efficient vehicle.
- Keep your car tuned up and well maintained. Keep your tires inflated at recommended pressures, avoid quick starts, stay within the speed limit, limit air conditioning, and don't let your car idle unless absolutely necessary.
- Buy energy-efficient appliances and use them only when necessary. Run the washing machine, clothes dryer, and dishwasher only when you have full loads, do laundry in cold water. Clean refrigerator coils and clothes dryer lint screens frequently. Towel or air-dry your clothes and hair rather than using a dryer.
- Use energy-efficient lighting: halogen, light-emitting diode (LED), or compact fluorescent bulbs (not fluorescent tubes). For more information, see the box "High-Efficiency Lighting."
- Make sure your home is well-insulated with ozone-safe agents; use insulating shades and curtains to keep heat in during winter and out during summer.
- Plant and care for trees in your yard and neighborhood. Trees recycle carbon dioxide, and in so doing, trees work against global warming. They also provide shade and cool the air so that less air conditioning is needed.
- Before discarding a refrigerator, air conditioner, or humidifier, check with the waste hauler or your local government to ensure that ozone-depleting refrigerants will be removed prior to disposal.
- Keep your house adequately ventilated.
- Keep paints, cleaning agents, and other chemical products tightly sealed in their original containers.
- Don't smoke, and don't allow others to smoke in your home.
- Clean and inspect chimneys, furnaces, and other appliances regularly. Install carbon monoxide detectors.
- Always use an outside-venting hood when cooking.
- Use paints with low or no VOCs, and ventilate well when using high-VOC products.
- Keep areas mold free by fixing any leaks from the bathroom, roof, or basement.
- Use a HEPA air filter.

# WATER QUALITY AND POLLUTION

Few parts of the world have enough safe, clean drinking water, and yet few things are as important to human health.

## Water Contamination and Treatment

Many cities rely at least in part on wells that tap local groundwater, but often it is necessary to tap lakes and rivers to supplement wells. Because such surface water is more likely to be contaminated with both organic matter and pathogenic microorganisms, it is purified in water treatment plants before being piped into the community. At treatment facilities, the water is subjected to various physical and chemical processes, including screening, filtration, and disinfection (often with chlorine), before it is introduced into the water supply system. **Fluoridation,** a water treatment process that reduces tooth decay by 15–40%, has been used successfully in the United States for more than 60 years. However, there is controversy regarding its safety for human health, and many towns have banned its use in public water.

In most areas of the United States, water systems have adequate, dependable supplies; are able to control waterborne disease; and provide water with acceptable color, odor, and taste. However, problems occur. The Centers for Disease Control and Prevention (CDC) estimates that 1 million Americans become ill and 900–1000 die each year from microbial illnesses from drinking water.

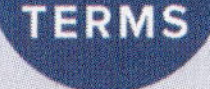


**fluoridation** The addition of fluoride to the water supply to reduce tooth decay.

## TAKE CHARGE
## High-Efficiency Lighting

Lighting accounts for about 15% of all residential electricity use. Switching to energy-efficient lighting is a good way to cut your home's energy use, lower your energy bills, and reduce your environmental footprint.

The Energy Independence and Security Act (EISA) of 2007 set national performance standards for lightbulbs for the first time, requiring that basic bulbs be at least about 25% more efficient; the standards were phased in by 2014. Traditional incandescent lightbulbs did not meet these new efficiency standards, so the use of other lighting choices has grown:

- ***Halogen incandescents.*** More energy-efficient incandescent bulbs that also last up to three times longer than traditional bulbs.
- ***Compact fluorescent lightbulbs (CFLs).*** Long-lasting fluorescents that work in many types of household fixtures. These bulbs contain a very small amount of mercury and require special handling if they are broken (visit www.epa.gov/cfl for specific cleanup and recycling instructions).
- ***Light-emitting diodes (LEDs).*** Rapidly expanding in household use, LEDs use only about 10% of the energy and last up to 50 times longer, compared to traditional bulbs.

Although the newer styles of lightbulbs can be more expensive than traditional incandescents, they save money because they require less energy to produce light. For example, a 17-watt (W) LED bulb produces as much light as a 75 W incandescent lightbulb. The new lightbulbs also last longer: CFLs last up to 10 times longer than conventional lightbulbs, and some LED bulbs last longer than 22 years. However, it is important to continue to actively conserve energy, even when using more energy-efficient technology. A "rebound effect" occurs when behavioral or other factors cause less gain in conservation than expected (for example, when people needlessly leave on lights because they know them to be more energy efficient).

To aid consumers in selecting bulbs, the Federal Trade Commission mandated Lighting Facts labels on all bulbs. Using these labels, you can compare types of bulbs and select the most appropriate one for your planned use. The brightness comparison is based on lumens rather than watts, because energy-efficient bulbs produce a brighter light with less energy—more lumens per watt than does a traditional incandescent bulb.

SOURCES: U.S. Energy Information Administration. 2020. *How Much Electricity Is Used for Lighting in the United States?* (http://www.eia.gov/tools/faqs/faq.cfm?id=99&t=3); Office of Energy Efficiency & Renewable Energy. 2014. *How Energy-Efficient Light Bulbs Compare with Traditional Incandescents* (http://energy.gov/energysaver/save-electricity-and-fuel/lighting-choices-save-you-money/how-energy-efficient-light)

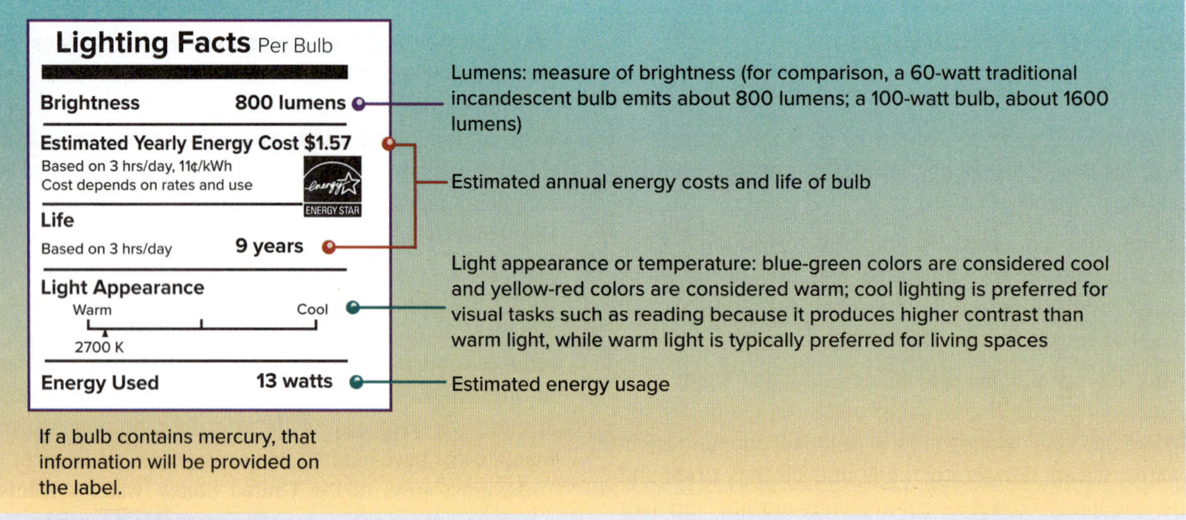


## Water Shortages

Water shortages are a growing concern in many regions of the world. Some parts of the United States, such as the desert West, are experiencing rapid population growth that outstrips the ability of local systems to provide adequate water to all. According to the World Health Organization, 2 billion people do not have safe drinking water, and 4.5 billion do not have access to safely managed sanitation. Less than 1% of the world's fresh water—about 0.007% of all the water on earth—is readily accessible for direct human use. Groundwater pumping and the diversion of water from lakes and rivers for irrigation are further reducing the amount of water available to local communities.

## Sewage

Most cities have sewage treatment systems that separate fecal matter from water in huge tanks and ponds and stabilize it so that it cannot transmit infectious diseases. After it is treated and biologically safe, the water is released back into the environment. The sludge that remains behind is often contaminated with **heavy metals** and is handled as hazardous waste.

Many cities have expanded sewage treatment measures to remove heavy metals and other hazardous chemicals. This action has resulted from many studies linking exposure to chemicals such as mercury, lead, and **polychlorinated biphenyls (PCBs)** with long-term health consequences, including cancer and damage to the central nervous system.

## Protecting the Water Supply

By reducing your own water use, you help preserve your community's valuable supply and lower your monthly water bill. By taking the following steps to keep the water supply clean, you reduce pollution overall and help protect the land, wildlife, and other people from illness.

- Take showers, not baths, to minimize your water consumption. Don't let water run when you're not actively using it while brushing your teeth, shaving, or hand-washing clothes or dishes.
- Install sink faucet aerators and water-efficient showerheads, which use two to five times less water with no noticeable decrease in performance.
- Replace old toilets and fix leaky faucets in your home.
- Don't pour toxic materials such as cleaning solvents, bleach, or motor oil down the drain. Store them until you can take them to a hazardous waste collection center.
- Don't pour old medicines down the drain or flush them down the toilet. Experts suggest that the best way to discard old medicines is to mix them with coffee grounds or cat litter, seal them in a container, and put them in the trash. Some pharmacies will take back unused or expired medications for disposal, and many communities have drop-off days for these drugs.

# SOLID WASTE POLLUTION

Humans living in the industrialized world generate huge amounts of waste, which must be handled appropriately if the environment is to be kept safe.

> **Ask Yourself**
>
> **QUESTIONS FOR CRITICAL THINKING AND REFLECTION**
>
> How would you describe the quality of the water where you live? Are there lakes or streams where you can safely swim or fish? What local information sources can you find about water quality in your area?

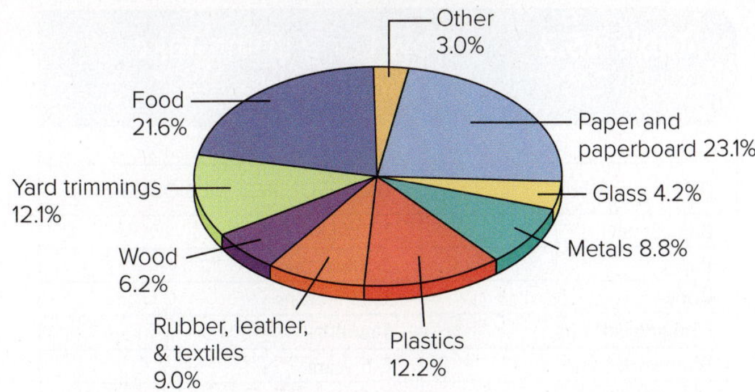


**FIGURE 15.5 Components of municipal solid waste, by weight, before recycling.**

SOURCE: U.S. Environmental Protection Agency. 2022. *Advancing Sustainable Materials Management: 2018 Fact Sheet* (Pub. No. 530-F-20-009). Washington, DC: EPA.

The bulk of the organic food garbage produced in American kitchens is now dumped into the sewage system by way of the mechanical garbage disposal. The garbage that remains is not hazardous from the standpoint of infectious disease because there is very little food waste in it, but it does represent an enormous disposal and contamination problem.

The biggest single component of household trash by weight is paper products, including junk mail, glossy mail-order catalogs, and computer printouts (Figure 15.5). Food, yard waste, and plastics are other significant components. About 1% of the solid waste is toxic; a new source of toxic waste is computer components. Burning, as opposed to burial, reduces the bulk of solid waste, but it can release hazardous material into the air. Manufacturing, mining, and other industries all produce large amounts of potentially dangerous materials that cannot simply be dumped.

## Disposing of Solid Waste

Since the 1960s, billions of tons of solid waste have been buried in **sanitary landfill** disposal sites. Sometimes protective liners are used around the site, and nearby monitoring wells are now required in most states. Layers of solid waste are regularly covered with thin layers of dirt until the site is filled. Some communities then plant grass and trees and convert the site into a park. Landfill is relatively stable; almost no decomposition occurs in the solidly packed waste.

Burying solid waste in landfills has several disadvantages. Burial is expensive and requires huge amounts of space. Waste can also contain chemicals such as pesticides, paints,

> **TERMS**
>
> **heavy metal** A metal with a high specific gravity, such as lead, copper, or tin.
>
> **polychlorinated biphenyl (PCB)** An industrial chemical used as an insulator in electrical transformers and linked to certain human cancers; banned worldwide since 1977 but persistent in the environment. Humans are exposed mainly through consumption of meat, fish, and dairy.
>
> **sanitary landfill** A disposal site where solid wastes are buried.

**Table 15.2** How Long Items Take to Biodegrade

| ITEM | TIME REQUIRED TO BIODEGRADE |
|---|---|
| Banana peel | 2–10 days |
| Paper | 2–5 months |
| Rope | 3–14 months |
| Orange peel | 6 months |
| Wool sock | 1–5 years |
| Cigarette butt | 1–12 years |
| Plastic-coated milk carton | 5 years |
| Aluminum can | 80–100 years |
| Plastic bottle | 450 years |
| Plastic six-pack holder ring | 450 years |
| Disposable diapers | 500 years |
| Plastic bag | 1000 years |
| Glass bottle | 1 million years |
| Styrofoam | Does not biodegrade |

and oils, which should not be released into the environment. Despite precautions, buried contaminants sometimes leak into the surrounding soil and groundwater.

*Biodegradation* is the process by which organic substances are broken down naturally by living organisms. These organic materials—including plant and animal matter, substances originating from living organisms, or artificial materials similar in nature to plants and animals—are put to use by microorganisms. The term **biodegradable** means that certain products can break down naturally, safely, and quickly into the raw materials of nature and then disappear back into the environment. If a product is **compostable,** it may break down through *biotic* processes—those involving living organisms—as well as *abiotic* processes, which involve nonliving factors such as climate and natural disasters. Table 15.2 shows the amount of time required for materials to biodegrade.

**Recycling** In **recycling,** many kinds of waste materials are collected and used as raw materials in the production of new products. Recycling is a good idea because it puts unwanted objects to good use, and it reduces the amount of solid waste sitting in landfills, some of which takes decades to decay naturally. However, the recycling industry took a hit in 2018 when China, the biggest importer of U.S. recycling, stopped accepting recyclable waste.

QUICK STATS

**The average American generates 4.9 pounds of trash per day; the recycling rate is about 32%.**

—U.S. Environmental Protection Agency, 2021

TERMS

**biodegradable** The ability of materials to break down via biotic processes—consumption by bacteria or fungi, or other biological processes.

**compostable** The ability of materials to break down via abiotic and biotic processes.

**recycling** The use of waste materials as raw materials in the production of new products.

If you have an electronic device to dispose of, look for an e-waste recycling program in your area. Many communities have recycling facilities that handle e-waste or host special e-waste collection events. Philip Laurell/Johner Images/Getty Images

**Discarded Technology: E-waste** A newer solid waste disposal problem involves the discarding of old computers, televisions, cell phones, and other electronic devices. Americans own roughly 24 electronic items per household and produce about 7 million tons of e-waste per year (42 pounds per person). Junked electronic devices are toxic because they contain varying amounts of lead, mercury, and other heavy metals. Many components of electronic devices are valuable, however, and can be recycled and reused. Local and state e-waste recycling programs are becoming more common, and private companies are getting into the e-waste recycling business. If you recycle your electronic devices, look for a "green" program or one that is certified by e-stewards, an organization that advocates for responsible e-waste recycling (www.e-stewards.org).

## Reducing Solid Waste

Researchers estimate that 80% of the nation's existing landfills will be filled within 20 years. By reducing your consumption, recycling more, reusing, and throwing away less, you can conserve landfill space. Here are some ideas to help you reduce solid waste:

- Limit your purchase and use of plastic products.
- Buy products with the least amount of packaging, or buy products in bulk. Buy products packaged in recyclable containers.
- Buy recycled or recyclable products. Avoid disposables; instead use long-lasting or reusable products such as refillable pens and rechargeable batteries.

## Ask Yourself

**QUESTIONS FOR CRITICAL THINKING AND REFLECTION**

What are your own waste-disposal habits? Do you recycle everything you can? Do you reuse items? Even if you are conscientious about the way you deal with waste, how could you improve your habits?

- Bring your own reusable mug, straw, and spoon to work or wherever you drink coffee or tea. Pack your lunch in reusable containers.
- To store food, use reusable plastic or glass containers and reusable wrap.
- If you receive something packaged with foam pellets, take them to a commercial mailing center that accepts them for recycling.
- Do not throw electronic items, batteries, or fluorescent lights into the trash. Take these to state-approved recycling centers.
- Start a compost pile for your organic garbage if you have a yard. If you live in an apartment, you can take your organic wastes to a community composting center, or use an indoor worm composting bin.

**QUICK STATS**

The Superfund National Priorities List includes **1333 sites** as of May 2022.

—U.S. Environmental Protection Agency, 2022

# CHEMICAL POLLUTION AND HAZARDOUS WASTE

New chemical substances are continually being introduced into the environment as pesticides, herbicides, solvents, and hundreds of other products. More people and wildlife are exposed to them than ever before.

## Asbestos

A mineral-based compound, asbestos was widely used for fire protection and insulation in buildings until the late 1960s. Microscopic asbestos fibers can be released into the air when this material is applied or when it later deteriorates or is damaged. These fibers can lodge in the lungs, causing **asbestosis,** lung cancer, and other serious lung diseases. Similar conditions expose workers to risk in the coal mining industry, from coal and silica dust (black lung disease), and in the textile industry, from cotton fibers (brown lung disease). The EPA has no general ban on asbestos.

## Lead

The CDC estimates that approximately half a million U.S. children aged 1–5 have blood lead levels above the cutoff at which the CDC recommends public health action. Many of these children live in poor, inner-city areas (see the box "Poverty, Gender, and Environmental Health"). No safe blood lead level has been identified for children. When lead is ingested or inhaled, it can permanently damage the central nervous system, cause mental impairment, hinder oxygen transport in the blood, and create kidney and digestive problems. Severe lead poisoning may cause coma or death. Lead exposure has been linked to attention-deficit/hyperactivity disorder (ADHD) in children. Lead can also build up in bones, where it may be released into the bloodstream during pregnancy or when bone mass is lost from osteoporosis.

Most environmental lead comes from lead-based paints. Lead paints were banned from residential use in 1978, but as many as 57 million American homes still contain them. In 2010, new guidelines were implemented requiring contractors to take special lead-containment measures when doing renovations, repairs, or painting. The use of lead in plumbing is now also banned, but some old pipes and faucets contain it; if these pipes and fixtures corrode, lead can leach into the water. The presence of lead pipes contributed to the drinking water crisis in Flint, Michigan. In 2014, the city changed water suppliers to one that produced higher levels of corrosive compounds but failed to add a required anticorrosive agent; lead from aging pipes leached into the drinking water. Researchers found that the incidence of elevated blood lead levels doubled in children in Flint after the water source change.

## Pesticides

**Pesticides** are chemicals that kill unwanted pests. Herbicides (plant killers) and insecticides (insect killers) are used extensively in agriculture, and they often have toxic effects in unwanted targets, such as beneficial insects and birds. Pesticide use has risks and benefits. For example, DDT was extremely effective in controlling mosquito-borne diseases in tropical countries and in increasing crop yields throughout the world, but it was found to harm wildlife. DDT also builds up in the food chain, increasing in concentration as larger animals eat smaller ones—a process known as **biomagnification** or *bioaccumulation.* DDT was banned in the United States in 1972.

Glyphosate (Roundup) is an herbicide that is widely used with genetically modified crops such as corn and soybeans

**TERMS**

**asbestosis** A lung condition caused by inhalation of microscopic asbestos fibers, which inflame the lung and can lead to lung cancer.

**pesticides** Chemicals used to kill agricultural and household pests, such as weeds, insects, and rodents.

**biomagnification** The accumulation of a substance in a food chain; also known as *bioaccumulation.*

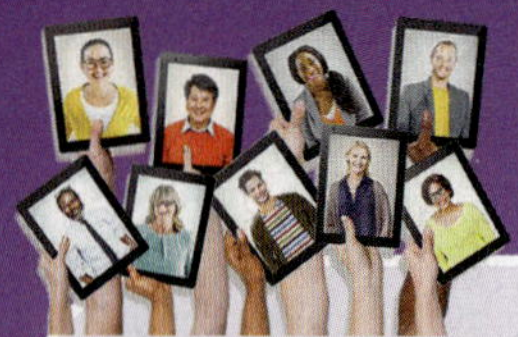

## DIVERSITY MATTERS
### Poverty, Gender, and Environmental Health

Residents of low-income and underrepresented communities are often exposed to more environmental toxins than residents of wealthier communities and they are more likely to suffer from health problems caused or aggravated by pollutants.

Low-income neighborhoods are often located near highways and industrial areas that have high levels of air and noise pollution; they are also common sites for hazardous waste production and disposal. Residents of substandard housing are more likely to come into contact with lead, asbestos, carbon monoxide, pesticides, and other hazardous pollutants associated with peeling paint, old plumbing, and poorly maintained insulation and heating equipment. In addition, low-income people are more likely to have jobs that expose them to asbestos, silica dust, and pesticides, and they are more likely to catch and consume fish contaminated with PCBs, mercury, and other toxins.

In the case of lead poisoning in children, the link among poverty, the environment, and health is abundantly clear. Because children may be at higher risk and more biologically vulnerable to lead exposure, elevated levels of lead show up in their test results. The CDC and the American Academy of Pediatrics recommend annual testing of blood lead levels for all children under age 6, with more frequent testing for children at special risk. In the Flint, Michigan, water crisis, the highest blood lead levels in children were found in the most socioeconomically disadvantaged neighborhoods. Causes include aging infrastructure, neglect by city officials, and the targeting of industry looking for cheap property. Additionally, poor residents suffer the consequences of lead exposure exponentially: even when diagnosed with high levels of poisoning and told how to improve the problem, families often cannot afford the medical treatments and the costs of repainting their houses.

Asthma is another health threat that appears to be linked with both environmental and socioeconomic factors. Although the number of Americans with asthma has been rising for 20 years, a recent study found a leveling and even decrease of incidence in children since 2013. Unfortunately, rates are still increasing in the poorest families. Researchers are not sure what causes asthma, but suspects include household pollutants, pesticides, air pollution, cigarette smoke, and allergens like cockroaches. These risk factors are likely to cluster in poor urban areas where inadequate health care may worsen the effects of asthma.

Gender also influences exposure to environmental hazards. In many societies, women are more often involved in day-to-day activities associated with the environment, including food preparation, agricultural work, and tasks around the home. These activities can expose women to indoor air pollution, water pollution, foodborne pathogens, agricultural chemicals, and waste contamination. Indoor pollutants, especially soot from burning wood, charcoal, and other solid fuels used for home heating and cooking, are a particular risk. Exposure to this particulate pollution increases the risk of respiratory diseases, lung cancer, and reproductive problems.

All humans are exposed to chemicals in air, food, and drinking water, and we all carry a load of chemicals in our bodies. Some of these chemicals accumulate in our bones, blood, or fatty tissues. Women are smaller than men, on average, and have a higher percentage of body fat, so chemicals that accumulate in fatty tissue may pose a relatively greater risk for women. By contrast, men may be more likely to work in industries that involve significant occupational exposures to disease-related toxins. For example, coal miners have an increased risk of lung cancer (black lung disease).

Although any chemical exposure can be a concern for health, women face the added risk of passing pollutants to a developing fetus during pregnancy or to an infant through breastfeeding. Even relatively low exposure to pollutants can result in a significant chemical body load in an infant or young child because of their small body size. And because infants and children are still developing, the effects of chemical exposure can be significant and devastating. It is not unusual for dangerous toxin exposures to be recognized first through noticeable effects on infants or children.

SOURCES: Muller, C., R. J. Sampson, and A. S. Winter. 2018. Environmental inequality: The social causes and consequences of lead exposure. *Annual Review of Sociology* 44 (https://doi.org/10.1146/annurev-soc-073117-041222); Akinbami, L. J., A. E. Simon, and L. M. Rosen. 2016. Changing trends in asthma prevalence among children. *Pediatrics* 137(1); Aelion, C. M., et al. 2013. Associations between soil lead concentrations and populations by race/ethnicity and income-to-poverty ratio in urban and rural areas. *Environmental Geochemistry and Health* 35(1): 1–12.

("Roundup-ready" crops). Glyphosate has been found in the majority of oat and wheat-based foods tested (i.e. cereal, pasta, breads, etc). In 2015, the World Health Organization listed glyphosate as a "probable human carcinogen." Organophosphate and organochlorine pesticides have been linked to mental problems in children, such as ADHD and low IQ. Pesticide exposure has also been linked to Alzheimer's and Parkinson's diseases, cancers, reproductive problems, depression, and respiratory problems.

## Mercury

A naturally occurring metal, mercury is a toxin that affects the brain and nervous system and may damage the kidneys and gastrointestinal tract, and increase blood pressure, heart rate, and heart attack risk. Mercury slows fetal and child development and causes irreversible deficits in brain function. Coal-fired power plants are the largest producers of mercury; other sources include mining

## CRITICAL CONSUMER
## Endocrine Disruption: A "New" Toxic Threat

In the 1970s and 1980s, scientists began to document strange occurrences in wildlife: disrupted reproduction, birth defects, tumors, and behavioral changes in birds, fish, and reptiles. The wildlife in and around the Great Lakes, an area with a history of industrial spills and contamination, was particularly affected. It was also becoming apparent that a drug given to pregnant women in the 1950s (a potent synthetic estrogen, DES) was causing infertility and rare reproductive cancers in their adult daughters.

In the mid-1990s, the influential book *Our Stolen Future* by Theo Colborn was published. Colborn suggested that toxic chemicals can cause effects other than acute toxicity (i.e., death), and that low amounts of these chemicals, over a long period of time, can cause disease. Even more concerning was the evidence that a fetus's exposure to chemicals during gestation can cause lasting changes and possible future disease in adulthood.

These chemicals, known also as **endocrine-disrupting chemicals (EDCs)** were altering the hormone systems of organisms. Most systems in the body rely on hormones, such as the immune, metabolic, and brain/nervous systems. A *hormone* is a chemical signal that is made in one area or organ of the body and travels to another to initiate effects. Estrogen, testosterone, and thyroid hormones are well-known examples.

Low levels of EDCs can disrupt these systems by mimicking or blocking natural hormones, causing abnormal effects. EDC exposure before and after birth may cause lifelong effects, including fertility problems, cancers, cardiovascular diseases, obesity, and mental disorders. These effects have been proven in laboratory animals and supported by observational (epidemiological) studies in humans.

Various manufactured chemicals, some in everyday products such as plastics, cosmetics, food packaging, flame retardants, pesticides, and others, are EDCs. These chemicals are known to contaminate household dust, drinking water, and food (especially meat and dairy products). Bisphenol A (BPA) is a chemical present in hard plastic (such as water bottles), the lining of canned foods, dental fillings, and cash register receipts. The chemical has been banned in children's products in California and the European Union, and many scientists believe it should be regulated more stringently in the United States.

Traditional methods of determining chemical toxicity usually test "gross" effects: death, deformities, and tumors. These methods typically do not test low (environmental) doses of chemicals; rather, they test at high doses and extrapolate down to find "safe" exposure levels. Often, EDCs have detrimental effects at low doses but not higher ones. Therefore, a new testing paradigm must be employed that addresses physiological effects at low doses. The modern environmental movement is new, and as our scientific knowledge of these chemicals evolves and improves, so must government testing and policies surrounding the issues of EDCs, for the continued protection of human health.

What can you do?

- Avoid personal and household products that contain EDCs (see https://www.ewg.org)
- Eat organic foods. Eat lower on the food chain.
- Avoid plastics, especially in contact with food and drinks. Do not microwave plastic containers.
- Dust, vacuum, and wipe down surfaces often.
- Avoid nonstick cookware and products.
- Avoid flame-retardant clothes and furniture.
- Avoid handling cash-register receipts. If you must, use gloves or wash your hands after handling receipts.
- Be especially cautious about exposing pregnant women, infants, and children to EDCs.
- Support legislation that will provide adequate testing and regulation of potential EDCs.

For more information visit https://www.niehs.nih.gov/health/topics/agents/endocrine/index.cfm

and smelting operations and the disposal of consumer products containing mercury.

## Other Chemical Pollutants

There are tens of thousands of chemical pollutants, and the extent of their toxic effects is just beginning to be understood (see the box "Endocrine Disruption: A 'New' Toxic Threat"). As mentioned earlier, hazardous wastes are commonly found in the home and should be handled and disposed of properly. They include automotive supplies (motor oil, antifreeze, transmission fluid), paint supplies (turpentine, paint thinner, mineral spirits), art and hobby supplies (oil-based paint, solvents, acids and alkalis, aerosol sprays), insecticides, batteries, computer and electronic components, and household cleaners containing sodium hydroxide (lye) or ammonia. These chemicals are dangerous when inhaled or ingested, when they contact the skin or the eyes, or when they are burned or dumped. Many cities provide guidelines about approved disposal methods and have hazardous waste collection days.

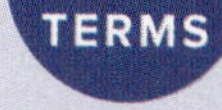


**endocrine-disrupting chemicals (EDCs)** Chemicals that disrupt the hormone systems of organisms.

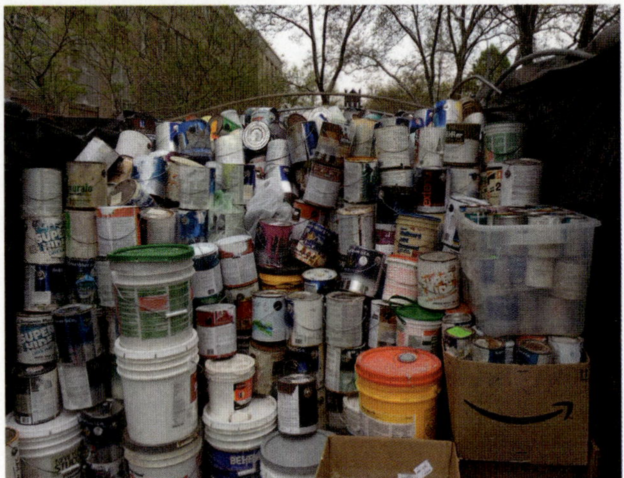

Many communities offer household hazardous waste drop-off programs for safe disposal of potentially harmful household chemicals. Zoran Milich/Moment Mobile/Getty Images

## Preventing Chemical Pollution

You can take steps to reduce the chemical pollution in your community. Just as important, by reducing and eliminating the number of chemicals in your home, you may save the life of a child or animal who might encounter one of those chemicals.

- When buying products, read the labels. Choose nontoxic, nonpetrochemical cleansers, disinfectants, polishes, and other personal and household products. Visit https://EWG.org.
- Eat and live organically. Avoid using chemical pesticides (weed, insect, and rodent killers) in the home and garden.
- Dispose of your household hazardous wastes properly. Contact your local environmental health office or health department for more information.
- Buy organic produce and produce that has been grown locally.
- If you must use pesticides or toxic household products, store them in a locked place where children and pets can't get to them. Don't measure chemicals with food preparation utensils, and wear gloves whenever handling them.
- If you have your house fumigated for pest control, be sure to hire a licensed exterminator. Keep everyone, including pets, out of the house while the crew works and, if possible, for a few days after.

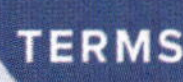

TERMS

**radiation** Energy transmitted in the form of rays, waves, or particles.

**radiation sickness** An illness caused by excess radiation exposure, marked by low white blood cell counts and nausea; possibly fatal.

**nuclear power** The use of controlled nuclear reactions to produce steam, which in turn drives turbines to produce electricity.

### Ask Yourself

**QUESTIONS FOR CRITICAL THINKING AND REFLECTION**

Are there any hazardous chemicals in your home, such as those found in cleaning products, solvents, paint, or batteries? Would you know what to do if one of these chemicals spilled? How would you clean it up?

# RADIATION POLLUTION

**Radiation** comes in several forms, such as UV rays, microwaves, or X-rays, and from several sources, such as the sun, electronics, uranium, and nuclear weapons. These forms of electromagnetic radiation differ in wavelength and energy, with shorter waves having the highest energy levels.

Of most concern to health are gamma rays, which are produced by radioactive sources such as nuclear weapons, nuclear energy plants, and radon gas. These high-energy waves are powerful enough to penetrate objects and break molecular bonds. Gamma radiation cannot be seen or felt, and its effects at high doses can include **radiation sickness** and death. At lower doses, chromosome damage, sterility, tissue damage, cataracts, and cancer can occur. Other types of radiation can also affect health. For example, exposure to UV radiation from the sun or from tanning salons can increase the risk of skin cancer. The effects of some sources of radiation, such as cell phones, remain controversial.

## Nuclear Weapons and Nuclear Energy

Nuclear weapons pose a health risk of the most serious kind to all species. Public health associations have stated that in the event of an intentional or unintentional discharge of these weapons, there could be millions of casualties. Reducing the stockpiles of nuclear weapons is a challenge and a goal for the 21st century.

Power-generating plants that use nuclear fuel also pose health problems. When **nuclear power** was first developed as an alternative to oil and coal, it was promoted as clean, efficient, inexpensive, and safe. In general, these claims have proven to be the case. Power systems in several parts of the world rely on nuclear power plants. However, despite safeguards and regulating agencies, accidents in nuclear power plants happen, many due to human error or following a natural disaster.

On March 11, 2011, a 9.0 magnitude earthquake 15 miles below Japan's Honshu Island, followed by a powerful tsunami, rocked Japan's northern Fukushima Prefecture and severely damaged the Fukushima Daiichi nuclear power plant complex. Seawater was used to cool the damaged reactors, resulting in the largest release of radiation into the Pacific Ocean in history.

An additional enormous problem is disposing of the radioactive wastes these plants generate. To date, no storage

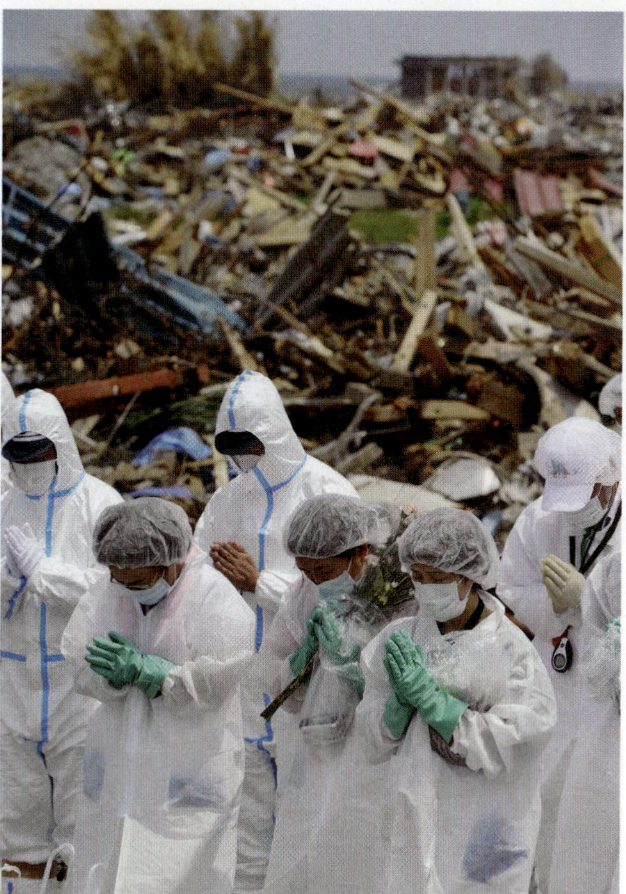

The 2011 Fukushima Daiichi nuclear disaster occurred when a tsunami, following a massive earthquake, flooded the low-lying rooms in which the plant's emergency generators were housed. The plant overheated, causing full meltdown in three of the six reactors.
Kyodo/AP Images

method has been devised that can provide infallible, infinitely durable shielding for nuclear waste. Despite these problems, nuclear power is gaining favor again as an alternative to fossil fuels.

**QUICK STATS**

**There are 93 nuclear reactors operating in the United States.**

—U.S. Energy Information Administration, 2022

## Medical Uses of Radiation

Another area of concern is the use of radiation in medicine.

No one should ever have a "routine" X-ray examination; each such exam should have a definite purpose, and its benefits and risks should be weighed carefully.

## Radiation in the Home and Workplace

There has been concern about electromagnetic radiation associated with common modern devices such as microwave ovens, computer monitors, and even high-voltage power lines. These forms of radiation do have effects on health, but research results are inconclusive.

### Ask Yourself

**QUESTIONS FOR CRITICAL THINKING AND REFLECTION**

Do you live in an area where radon is a problem? If so, has your home been checked for radon?

Another controversial issue today is the effect of radiation from cell phones on health. The California Department of Public Health recently issued a fact sheet on the possible risks of cell phone use and how to reduce radiation exposure. Cell phones use electromagnetic waves (radio frequency radiation) to send and receive signals. This radiation is not directional, meaning that it travels in all directions equally, including toward the user. Factors such as the type of digital signal coding in the network, the antenna and handset design, and the position of the phone relative to the head all determine how much radiation is absorbed by a user.

Another area of concern is **radon,** a naturally occurring radioactive gas found in certain soils, rocks, and building materials.

## Avoiding Radiation

The following steps can help you avoid unneeded exposure to radiation:

- Get only X-rays that you need, and keep a record of the date and location of every X-ray exam. Don't have a full-body CT (computed tomography) scan for routine screening; the radiation dose of one full-body CT scan is nearly 100 times that of a typical mammogram.
- Follow government recommendations for radon testing.
- Use sunscreen and clothing to protect yourself from the sun's UV radiation.

# NOISE POLLUTION

Prolonged exposure to sounds above 80–85 **decibels** (a measure of the intensity of a sound wave) can cause permanent hearing loss (Figure 15.6). Hearing damage can occur after eight hours of exposure to sounds

**TERMS**

**radon** A naturally occurring radioactive gas emitted from rocks and natural building materials that can become concentrated in insulated homes, causing lung cancer.

**decibel** A unit for expressing the relative intensity of sounds on a scale from 0 for the average least-perceptible sound to about 120 for the average pain threshold.

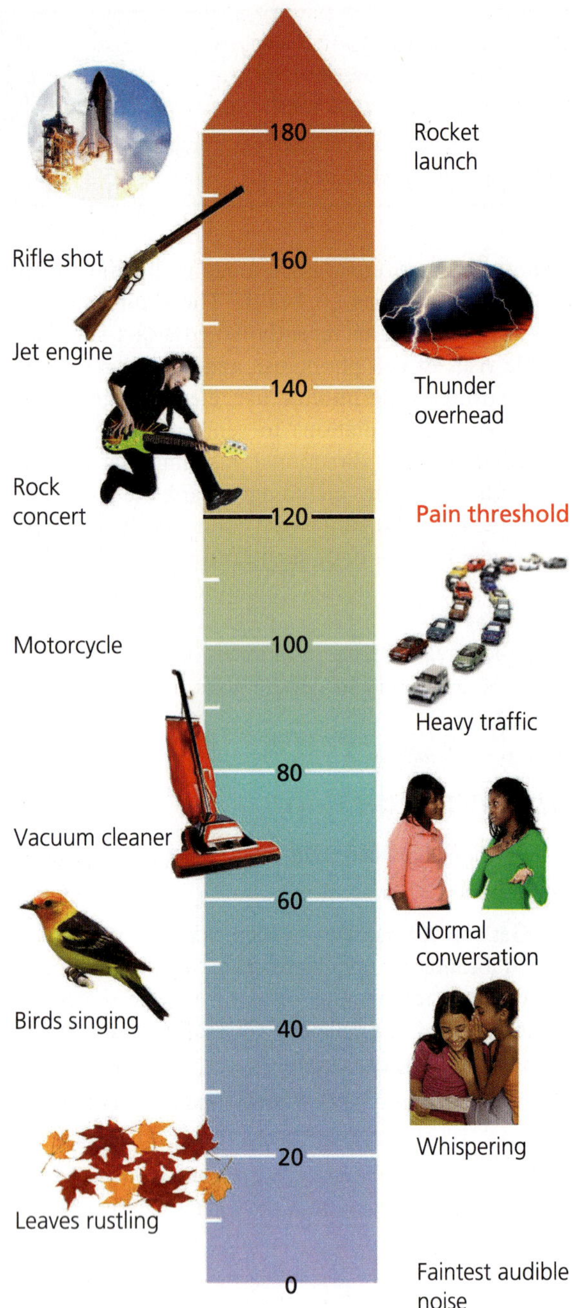


**FIGURE 15.6 The intensity of selected sounds.** Stocktrek/age fotostock; Stockbyte/Getty Images; Daxiao Productions/Shutterstock; Brand X Pictures/Getty Images; Pacific Northwest Photo/Shutterstock; Siede Preis/Photodisc/Getty Images; JupiterImages/Comstock Images/Getty Images; Stockbyte/Getty Images; Ken Karp/McGraw Hill; Jupiterimages/Stockbyte/Getty Images

louder than 80 decibels. Regular exposure for longer than one minute to more than 100 decibels can cause permanent hearing loss.

Noise pollution can cause chronic stress: it affects productivity and memory, increases stress hormone levels, and causes health effects such as cardiovascular problems and reduced immune function. Here are some ways to avoid exposing yourself to excessive noise:

- Wear ear protectors when working around noisy machinery.
- When listening to music on a headset set the volume below 60% of maximum. You should be able to hear people around you speaking in a normal tone of voice. Earmuff-style headphones may be easier on the ears than earbuds, which are inserted into the ear canal; headphones can be used up to one hour.
- For children, avoid toys that make loud noise.
- Avoid exposure to painfully loud sounds, and avoid repeated exposure to any sounds above 80 decibels.

## Ask Yourself

**QUESTIONS FOR CRITICAL THINKING AND REFLECTION**

How often do you listen to loud music? Do you ever use headphones? At what volume level do you like to listen? Do you think your listening habits pose a threat to your hearing? Would you let a child listen at the same volume level?

## TIPS FOR TODAY AND THE FUTURE

Environmental health involves protecting yourself from environmental dangers and protecting the environment from the dangers created by humans.

**RIGHT NOW YOU CAN:**

- Turn off the lights, televisions, and stereos in any unoccupied rooms.
- Turn off power strips when not in use.
- Turn down the heat a few degrees and put on a sweater, or turn off the air conditioner and change into cooler clothes.
- Reduce waste by reducing consumption of single-use items.
- Check your trash for recyclable items. Find out the recycling options in your area.

**IN THE FUTURE YOU CAN:**

- Replace burned-out lightbulbs with halogen, LED, or compact fluorescent lightbulbs.
- Have your car checked to make sure it runs as well as it can and puts out the lowest amount of polluting emissions possible.
- Go online and find one of the many calculators available that can help you estimate, and reduce, your environmental footprint.

## SUMMARY


- Environmental health encompasses all the interactions of humans with their environment and the health consequences of those interactions.
- The world's population is increasing rapidly, especially in developing countries. Factors that may eventually limit human population are food, availability of land and water, energy, and a minimum acceptable standard of living.
- Environmental damage from energy use and production can be limited through energy conservation and the development of nonpolluting, renewable sources of energy.
- Increased amounts of air pollutants are especially dangerous for children, older adults, and people with chronic health problems.
- Factors contributing to the development of smog include heavy motor vehicle traffic, hot weather, and stagnant air.
- Carbon dioxide and other natural gases act as a greenhouse around the earth, increasing the temperature of the atmosphere. Levels of these gases are rising through human activity; as a result, the world's climate is changing.
- The ozone layer that shields the earth's surface from the sun's UV rays has thinned and developed holes in certain regions.
- Indoor pollutants can trigger allergies and illness in the short term and chronic disease in the long term.
- Concerns with water quality focus on pathogenic organisms and hazardous chemicals from industry and households, as well as on water shortages.
- Sewage treatment prevents pathogens from contaminating drinking water; it often must also deal with heavy metals and hazardous chemicals.
- The amount of garbage is growing all the time; paper is the biggest component. Recycling can help reduce solid waste disposal problems, but reducing waste by reducing consumption is best.
- Potentially hazardous chemical pollutants include asbestos, lead, pesticides, mercury, and many household products. Proper handling and disposal are critical.
- Radiation can cause radiation sickness, chromosome damage, and cancer, among other health problems.
- Loud or persistent noise can lead to hearing loss, elevated blood pressure, and/or stress.


## FOR MORE INFORMATION

*California Department of Public Health: How to Reduce Exposure to Radiofrequency Energy from Cell Phones.* Fact sheet.

https://www.cdph.ca.gov/Programs/CCDPHP/DEODC/EHIB/CDPH%20Document%20Library/Cell-Phone-Guidance.pdf

*CDC National Center for Environmental Health.* Provides brochures and fact sheets about a variety of environmental issues.

http://www.cdc.gov/nceh/default.htm

*Clean Label Project.* Tests a variety of consumer foods and products for toxic chemicals.

https://cleanlabelproject.org

*DetoxMe.* Free smartphone app that helps reduce your exposure to potentially harmful chemicals where you live and work.

https://www.silentspring.org/detoxme/

*Earth Times.* An international online newspaper devoted to global environmental issues.

http://www.earthtimes.org

*Environmental Working Group.* Provides several consumer guides for reducing toxic chemical exposures.

https://ewg.org/consumer-guides

*Fuel Economy.* Provides information about the fuel economy of cars made since 1985 and tips on improving gas mileage.

http://www.fueleconomy.gov

*Global Footprint Network.* Calculates your personal ecological footprint based on your diet, transportation patterns, and living arrangements.

http://www.footprintcalculator.org/

*Green Vehicle Guide.* Provides information about EVs and other green vehicles.

https://www.epa.gov/greenvehicles

*Indoor Air Quality Information.* Provides information, publications, and contact info regarding IAQ.

https://www.epa.gov/indoor-air-quality-iaq.

*National Lead Information Center.* Provides information packets and specialist advice.

http://www.epa.gov/lead

*National Oceanic and Atmospheric Administration (NOAA): Climate.* Provides information about a variety of issues related to climate, including global warming, drought, and El Niño and La Niña.

http://www.noaa.gov/climate.html

*National Safety Council.* Provides information about lead, radon, indoor air quality, hazardous chemicals, and other environmental issues.

http://www.nsc.org/pages/home.aspx

*Pesticides in Produce: Consumer Reports Special Report.* Guidelines on how to minimize exposure to pesticides.

https://www.consumerreports.org/cro/health/natural-health/pesticides/index.htm

*The Post Carbon Institute: The Post Carbon Reader.* A collection of diverse and provocative articles on pressing environmental problems and what can be done about them.

http://www.postcarbon.org/pcr

*United Nations.* Several UN programs are devoted to environmental problems on a global scale; the websites provide information about current and projected trends and about international treaties developed to deal with environmental issues.

https://www.un.org/en/sections/issues-depth/population/

http://www.unep.org (Environment Programme)

*U.S. Department of Energy: Energy Efficiency and Renewable Energy (EERE).* Provides information about alternative fuels and tips for saving energy at home and in your car.

http://energy.gov/eere/office-energy-efficiency-renewable-energy

*U.S. Environmental Protection Agency (EPA).* Provides information about EPA activities and many consumer-oriented materials. The website includes special sites devoted to global warming, ozone loss, pesticides, and other areas of concern.

http://www.epa.gov

*Yale Environment 360.* An online magazine offering opinion, analysis, reporting, and debate on global environmental issues.

http://e360.yale.edu

There are many national and international organizations working on environmental health problems. A few of the largest and best known are listed here:

*Greenpeace*: 800-326-0959; http://www.greenpeace.org

*National Audubon Society*: 212-979-3000; http://www.audubon.org

*National Resources Defense Council*: 212-727-2700; http://www.nrdc.org

*National Wildlife Federation*: 800-822-9919; http://www.nwf.org

*Nature Conservancy*: 800-628-6860; http://www.nature.org

*Sierra Club*: 415-977-5500; http://www.sierraclub.org

*U.S. Green Building Council*: 800-795-1747; http://www.usgbc.org

*World Wildlife Fund–U.S.*: 800-960-0993; http://www.worldwildlife.org

## SELECTED BIBLIOGRAPHY


Aelion, C. M., et al. 2013. Associations between soil lead concentrations and populations by race/ethnicity and income-to-poverty ratio in urban and rural areas. *Environmental Geochemistry and Health* 35(1): 1-12.

Almukhtar, S., et al. 2019. The Great Flood of 2019: A complete picture of a slow-motion disaster. *The New York Times*, 11 September (https://www.nytimes.com/interactive/2019/09/11/us/midwest-flooding.html).

American Lung Association. 2022. *State of the Air, 2022* (http://www.lung.org/our-initiatives/healthy-air/sota/).

Centers for Disease Control and Prevention. 2017. Childhood blood lead levels in children aged <5 years—United States, 2009-2014. *Surveillance Summaries/MMRW* 66(3): 1-10.

Centers for Disease Control and Prevention. 2017. Surveillance for waterborne disease outbreaks associated with drinking water—United States, 2013-14. *MMWR* 66(44): 1216-1221.

Centers for Disease Control and Prevention. 2020. *Lead* (http://www.cdc.gov/nceh/lead).

Gore, A. C., et al. 2015. Executive summary to EDC-2: The endocrine society's second scientific statement on endocrine-disrupting chemicals. *Endocrine Reviews* 36(6): 593.

Gorski, I., et al. 2019. Environmental health concerns from unconventional natural gas development. *Oxford Research Encyclopedia of Global Public Health.*

Hatta-Attisha, M., et al. 2016. Elevated blood lead levels in children associated with the Flint drinking water crisis: A spatial analysis of risk and public health response. *American Journal of Public Health* 106(2): 283-290.

McDonald, B. C., et al. 2018. Volatile chemical products emerging as largest petrochemical source of urban organic emissions. *Science* 359(6377): 760-764.

National Oceanic and Atmospheric Administration. 2020. *Billion Dollar U.S. Weather Disasters, 1980-2016* (http://www.ncdc.noaa.gov/billions/).

Newell, K., et al. 2017. Cardiorespiratory health effects of particulate ambient air pollution exposure in low-income and middle-income countries: A systematic review and meta-analysis. *The Lancet: Planetary Health* 1(9): e368-e380 (https://www.thelancet.com/journals/lanplh/article/PIIS2542-5196(17)30166-3/fulltext?code=lancet-site).

REN21. 2018. *Renewables 2018 Global Status Report.* Paris: REN21 (http://www.ren21.net/status-of-renewables/global-status-report/).

Solomon, S., et al. 2016. Emergence of healing in the Antarctic ozone layer. *Science* 353(6296): 269-274.

United Nations Population Division, Department of Economic and Social Affairs. 2019. *World Population Prospects: Highlights.* New York: United Nations (https://www.un.org/development/desa/publications/world-population-prospects-2019-highlights.html).

U.S. Census Bureau. 2021. *Popclock* (https://www.census.gov/popclock/).

U.S. Energy Information Administration. 2020, August 10. *Gasoline and Diesel Fuel Update* (https://www.eia.gov/petroleum/gasdiesel/).

U.S. Energy Information Administration. 2020. *How Many Nuclear Power Plants Are in the United States, and Where Are They Located?* (https://www.eia.gov/tools/faqs/faq.cfm?id=207&t=3).

U.S. Energy Information Administration. 2020. *How Much Oil Is Consumed in the United States?* (https://www.eia.gov/tools/faqs/faq.cfm?id=33&t=6).

U.S. Energy Information Administration. 2021. *International Energy Rankings* (https://www.eia.gov/international/rankings/world).

U.S. Environmental Protection Agency. 2019. *Advancing Sustainable Materials Management: 2018 Fact Sheet* (https://www.epa.gov/sites/default/files/2021-01/documents/2018_ff_fact_sheet_dec_2020_fnl_508.pdf).

U.S. Environmental Protection Agency. 2020. *Superfund: National Priorities List* (https://www.epa.gov/superfund/).

U.S. Global Change Research Program. 2018. *Climate Change Impacts in the United States: The Fourth National Climate Assessment,* Washington, DC, USA (http://nca2018.globalchange.gov).

Walker, T. 2016. California methane gas leak "more damaging than Deepwater Horizon disaster." *Independent* (https://www.independent.co.uk/news/world/americas/california-methane-gas-leak-more-damaging-than-deepwater-horizon-disaster-a6794251.html).

World Health Organization. 2018. *A Global Overview of National Regulations and Standards for Drinking-Water Quality.* Geneva: WHO.


**Design Elements:** Assess Yourself icon: Aleksey Boldin/Alamy Stock Photo; Diversity Matters icon: Rawpixel Ltd/Getty Images; Wellness on Campus icon: Radius Images/Alamy Stock Photo; Take Charge icon: VisualCommunications/Getty Images; Critical Consumer icon: pagadesign/Getty Images.

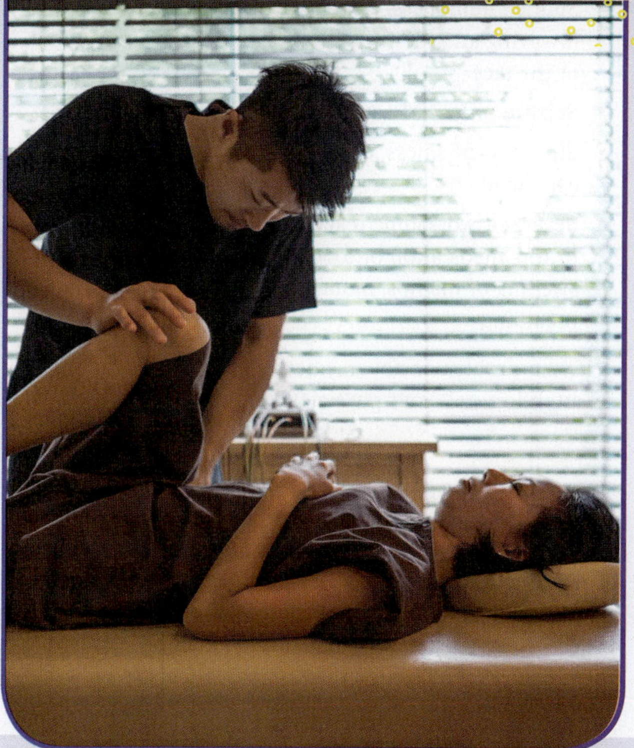
Andresr/Getty Images

## CHAPTER OBJECTIVES

- Understand options for self-care
- Understand options for professional care
- Describe the practices of conventional medicine
- Learn about integrative health practices
- Understand the costs of health care and how to pay for it

CHAPTER 16

# Conventional and Complementary Medicine

Today people are becoming more empowered and confident in their ability to solve personal health problems on their own. People who effectively manage their own health care gather information and learn skills from a variety of resources. They solicit opinions and advice in order to practice safe, effective self-care, and to make decisions about seeking professional medical care—whether conventional Western medicine or complementary and alternative medicine.

This chapter helps you develop skills needed to identify and manage medical problems and to make the health care system work effectively for you.

## SELF-CARE

Effectively managing medical problems involves developing several skills. First, you need to learn to closely examine your own body and assess your symptoms. You also must be able to decide when to seek professional advice and when you can safely deal with a problem on your own. You need to know how to safely and effectively self-treat common medical problems. Finally, you need to know how to develop a partnership with physicians and other health care providers and how to implement treatment plans.

### Self-Assessment

Symptoms are often the body's attempt to heal itself. For example, the pain and swelling that occur after an ankle injury immobilize and protect the injured joint so that healing can take place. A fever works to inhibit growth and reproduction of infectious agents. A cough can help clear the airways and protect the lungs. Understanding what a symptom means and what is happening in your body helps reduce anxiety about symptoms and enables you to practice safe self-care that supports your own healing mechanisms.

Carefully observing symptoms also helps you identify signals that indicate you need professional help. You should begin by noting when a symptom begins, how often and when it occurs, what makes it worse, what makes it better, and whether you have any associated symptoms or illnesses. You can also monitor your body's vital signs, such as temperature and heart rate. Medical self-tests for blood pressure, blood sugar, pregnancy detection, and urinary tract infections can also help you make more informed decisions about when to seek medical help and when to self-treat.

## Knowing When to See a Physician

Human responses to symptoms of injury and illness range from total denial to constant worry. In general, you should see a physician for symptoms that you would describe as follows:

- ***Severe.*** If a symptom is severe or intense, medical assistance is advised. Examples include significant pain, major injury and other emergencies.

- ***Unusual.*** If a symptom is peculiar and unfamiliar, it is wise to check it out with your physician. Examples include unexpected lumps, changes in a mole, problems with vision, difficulty swallowing, numbness, weakness, unexplained weight loss, or blood in the sputum (spit), urine, or stool.

- ***Persistent.*** If a symptom lasts longer than expected, seek medical advice. Examples in adults include fever for more than five days, a cough lasting longer than two weeks, a sore that doesn't heal within a month, and hoarseness lasting longer than three weeks.

- ***Recurrent.*** If a symptom returns again and again, medical evaluation is advised. Examples include recurring headaches, persistent abdominal pain, and backache.

Sometimes a single symptom is not a cause for concern, but when the symptom is accompanied by other symptoms, the combination suggests a more serious problem. For example, a fever accompanied by neck pain can suggest meningitis.

If you evaluate your symptoms and think you need professional help, you must decide how urgent the problem is. If it is a true emergency, you should go (or ask someone to take you) to the nearest hospital emergency department. Emergencies include the following:

- Major trauma or injury especially to the head, a suspected broken bone, deep wound, severe burn, eye injury, or animal bite
- Uncontrollable bleeding or internal bleeding, as indicated by blood in the sputum, vomit, or stool
- Intolerable and uncontrollable pain or severe chest pain
- Severe shortness of breath
- Persistent abdominal pain, especially if associated with nausea and vomiting
- Poisoning or drug overdose
- Sudden numbness, weakness, or loss of function involving an arm or leg, speech difficulty, or drooping of the face
- Seizure or loss of consciousness
- Stupor, drowsiness, or disorientation that cannot be explained
- Severe or worsening reaction to an insect bite or sting, or to a medication or food, especially if accompanied by swelling of the lips, mouth, or throat, or difficulty breathing

If your problem is not an emergency but still requires medical attention, call your physician's office.

## Self-Treatment

To help you make wise medical decisions, "A Self-Care Guide for Common Medical Problems" is provided in Appendix B. In most cases, your body can relieve your symptoms and heal the disorder, so patience and careful self-observation are often the best choices in self-treatment.

**Nondrug Options** Nondrug options are often easy, inexpensive, safe, and highly effective. For example, ice packs, massage, gentle yoga stretching, and neck exercises may at times be more helpful than drugs in relieving headaches and other pains. Getting adequate rest, increasing exercise, drinking more water, eating more or less of certain foods, using humidifiers, and changing ergonomics when sitting or working are some of the hundreds of nondrug options for preventing or relieving many common health problems. For a variety of disorders caused or aggravated by stress, the treatment of choice may be relaxation or other stress management strategies (see Chapter 2).

**Self-Medication** Self-treatment with nonprescription medications is an important part of health care. Nonprescription medications, also called **over-the-counter (OTC) medications**, are medicines that the U.S. Food and Drug Administration (FDA) has determined are safe when used according to label directions.

Hundreds of OTC products today use ingredients or dosage strengths that were available only by prescription a generation ago. With this increased consumer choice, however, consumers have an increased responsibility for using OTC drugs safely. Although many OTC products are effective, others are unnecessary or divert attention from better ways of coping. Many ingredients in OTC drugs—an estimated 70%—have not been proven to be effective, a fact the FDA recognizes. And any drug may have risks and side effects.

Follow these simple guidelines to self-medicate safely:

- Always read labels and follow directions carefully. The information on most OTC drug labels now appears in a standard format developed by the FDA (Figure 16.1). Ingredients, directions for safe use, and warnings are

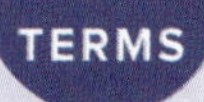


**over-the-counter (OTC) medication** A medication or product that can be purchased by a consumer without a prescription.

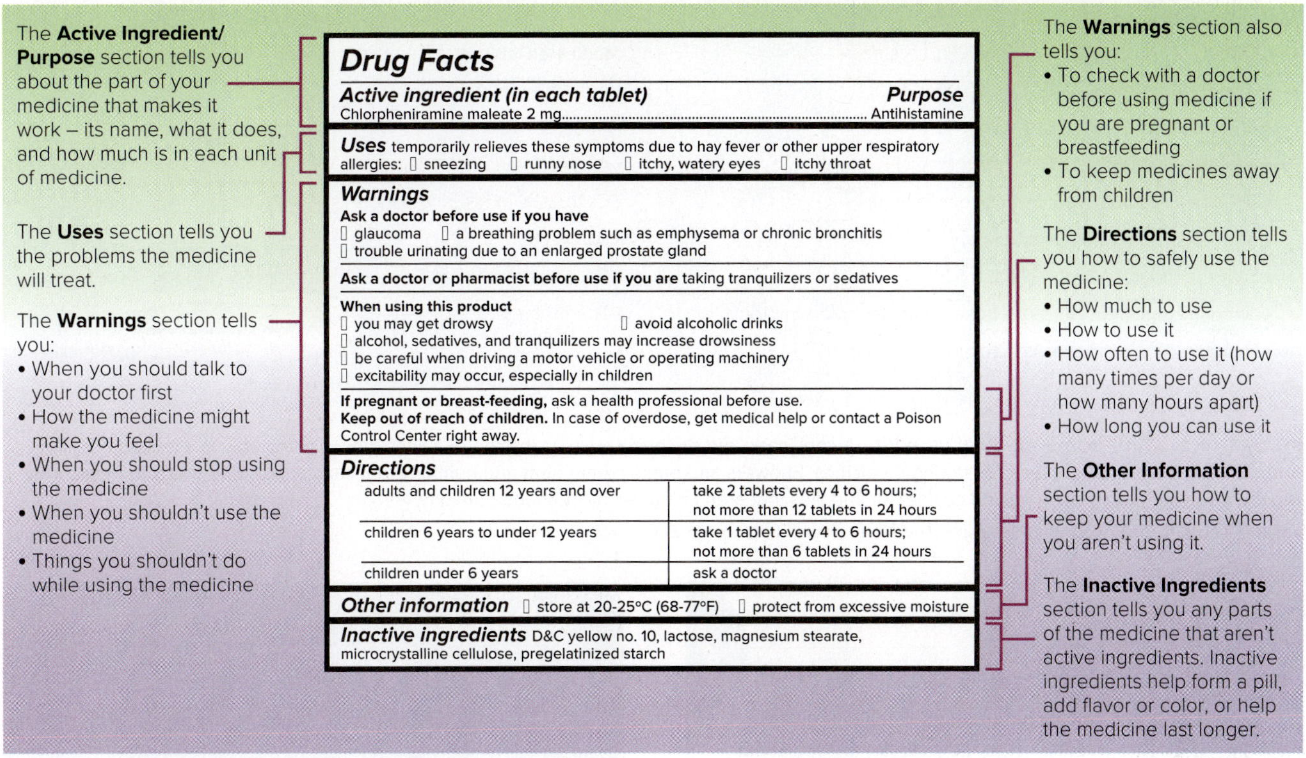

The **Active Ingredient/ Purpose** section tells you about the part of your medicine that makes it work – its name, what it does, and how much is in each unit of medicine.

The **Uses** section tells you the problems the medicine will treat.

The **Warnings** section tells you:

- When you should talk to your doctor first
- How the medicine might make you feel
- When you should stop using the medicine
- When you shouldn't use the medicine
- Things you shouldn't do while using the medicine

**Drug Facts**

***Active ingredient (in each tablet)*** — ***Purpose***

Chlorpheniramine maleate 2 mg.................... Antihistamine

***Uses*** temporarily relieves these symptoms due to hay fever or other upper respiratory allergies: ▯ sneezing ▯ runny nose ▯ itchy, watery eyes ▯ itchy throat

***Warnings***

**Ask a doctor before use if you have**
▯ glaucoma ▯ a breathing problem such as emphysema or chronic bronchitis
▯ trouble urinating due to an enlarged prostate gland

**Ask a doctor or pharmacist before use if you are** taking tranquilizers or sedatives

**When using this product**
▯ you may get drowsy ▯ avoid alcoholic drinks
▯ alcohol, sedatives, and tranquilizers may increase drowsiness
▯ be careful when driving a motor vehicle or operating machinery
▯ excitability may occur, especially in children

**If pregnant or breast-feeding,** ask a health professional before use.
**Keep out of reach of children.** In case of overdose, get medical help or contact a Poison Control Center right away.

***Directions***

| | |
|---|---|
| adults and children 12 years and over | take 2 tablets every 4 to 6 hours; not more than 12 tablets in 24 hours |
| children 6 years to under 12 years | take 1 tablet every 4 to 6 hours; not more than 6 tablets in 24 hours |
| children under 6 years | ask a doctor |

***Other information*** ▯ store at 20-25°C (68-77°F) ▯ protect from excessive moisture

***Inactive ingredients*** D&C yellow no. 10, lactose, magnesium stearate, microcrystalline cellulose, pregelatinized starch

The **Warnings** section also tells you:

- To check with a doctor before using medicine if you are pregnant or breastfeeding
- To keep medicines away from children

The **Directions** section tells you how to safely use the medicine:

- How much to use
- How to use it
- How often to use it (how many times per day or how many hours apart)
- How long you can use it

The **Other Information** section tells you how to keep your medicine when you aren't using it.

The **Inactive Ingredients** section tells you any parts of the medicine that aren't active ingredients. Inactive ingredients help form a pill, add flavor or color, or help the medicine last longer.

**FIGURE 16.1 Reading and understanding OTC drug labels.**

SOURCE: U.S. Food and Drug Administration. 2017. *The Over-the-Counter Medicine Label: Take a Look.*

clearly indicated. If you have any questions, ask a pharmacist or a qualified health care provider before using a product.

- Do not exceed the recommended dosage or length of treatment unless you discuss this with your health care provider.
- Use caution if you are taking other medications or supplements because OTC drugs and herbal supplements can interact with some prescription drugs. If you have questions about drug interactions, ask your health care provider or pharmacist *before* you take medicines in combination.
- Try to select medications with one active ingredient rather than a combination.
- When choosing medications, look for **generic drugs,** which contain the same active ingredient as brand-name products but generally at a much lower cost.
- Use a drug only if it is labeled clearly on its container, never when you can't read the label.
- If you are pregnant or nursing or have a chronic condition such as kidney or liver disease, consult your health care provider before self-medicating.
- The expiration date marked on many medications only estimates how long the medication is likely to be safe and effective. However, an extensive study by the FDA found that 90% of all prescription and OTC medications are potent well after their stated expiration dates. Exceptions include tetracycline and other antibiotics, nitroglycerine, and insulin. Expiration dates are very conservative. If a medicine is expired by more than a few months and you need to be certain that the medication is completely effective, you should purchase new medication. Because of environmental and safety concerns, never flush medicine down the toilet or sink, and do not discard medicine directly into the trash. You can dispose of old medicine by placing it in a sealed container with coffee grounds or cat litter, but the safest way to get rid of outdated medicines is to take them to a pharmacy or hospital. If you have any questions about a medicine's expiration date, ask a pharmacist.
- Store your medications in a cool, dry place away from direct light and out of the reach of children (Figure 16.2).
- Use special caution with aspirin. Because of an association with a rare but serious problem known as Reye's syndrome, aspirin should not be used by children or adolescents who may have the flu, chickenpox, or any other viral illness. Outdated aspirin that has an acidic odor should be discarded.

**TERMS**

**generic drug** A drug that is not registered or protected by a commercial trademark; a drug that does not have an exclusive brand name.

**Closet**

- Analgesic (relieves pain)
- Antacid (relieves upset stomach)
- Antihistamine (relieves allergy symptoms)
- Antibiotic ointment (reduces risk of infection)
- Antiseptic (helps stop infection)
- Fever reducer (adult and child)
- Decongestant (relieves stuffy nose and other cold symptoms)
- Hydrocortisone (relieves itching and inflammation)

**Medicine Cabinet**

- Adhesive bandages
- Adhesive tape
- Alcohol wipes
- Calibrated measuring spoon
- Disinfectant
- Gauze pads
- Thermometer
- Tweezers

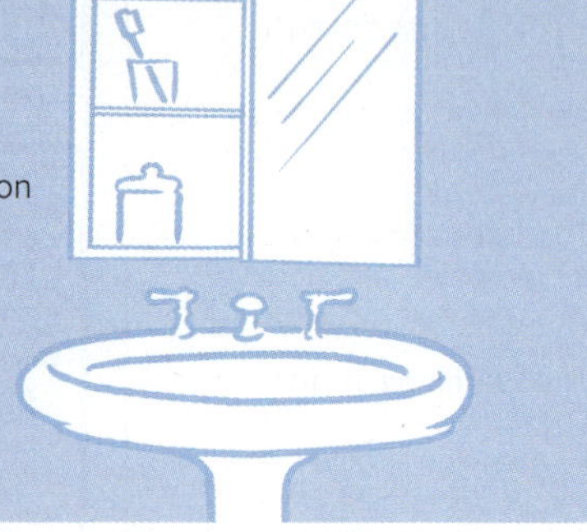

**FIGURE 16.2 Your home medical care kit.** A cool, dark, and dry place such as the top of a linen closet, preferably in a locked container and out of a child's reach, is best for storing medicines. Showers and baths create heat and humidity that can cause some drugs to deteriorate rapidly. Use your bathroom medicine cabinet for supplies that aren't affected by heat and humidity.

SOURCE: Lewis, C. 2000. Your medicine cabinet needs an annual checkup, too. *FDA Consumer*, March/April.

### Ask Yourself

**QUESTIONS FOR CRITICAL THINKING AND REFLECTION**

Do you often self-medicate for common medical problems, such as headaches or colds? If so, how careful are you about reading product labels and following directions? For example, would you know if you were taking two OTC medications that contained the same ingredient (such as acetaminophen or ibuprofen) at the same time?

## PROFESSIONAL CARE

When self-care is not appropriate or sufficient, seek professional medical care, whether by going to a hospital emergency department or by scheduling an appointment with your physician or another conventional health care provider. **Conventional medicine** is mainstream health care and medical practices taught in most U.S. medical schools and offered in most U.S. hospitals. In recent years, the majority of Americans have also sought health care from practitioners of **complementary and alternative medicine (CAM)**—defined as those therapies and practices that do not form part of conventional medicine. The most frequently used CAM therapies are nonvitamin, nonmineral dietary supplements, yoga, meditation, chiropractic, and massage therapy. (Table 16.1 shows that popularity among some of these therapies is increasing.) A Pew Research Center survey found that one-half of U.S. adults have tried CAM therapies—either instead of conventional medicine (20%) or in conjunction with it (29%). Younger adults are slightly more likely than people ages 65 and older to use it.

**Table 16.1 Complementary and Alternative Therapies Commonly Used by U.S. Adults**

| TYPE OF THERAPY | PERCENTAGE WHO USED THERAPY | |
|---|---|---|
| | 2012 | 2017 |
| Yoga | 9.5 | 14.3 |
| Meditation | 4.1 | 14.2 |
| Chiropractic | 9.1 | 10.3 |

SOURCE: Clark, T. C., et al. 2018. Use of yoga, meditation, and chiropractors among U.S. adults aged 18 and over. *NCHS Data Brief* 325. Hyattsville, MD: National Center for Health Statistics.

**TERMS**

**conventional medicine** A system of medicine emphasizing biological and physical scientific principles; diseases are thought to be caused by identifiable physical factors and characterized by a representative set of signs and symptoms; also called *biomedicine* or *standard Western medicine*.

**complementary and alternative medicine (CAM)** Health care practices and products that are not considered part of conventional, mainstream medical practice as taught in most U.S. medical schools and that are not available at most U.S. health care facilities; examples of CAM practices include acupuncture and herbal remedies.

**complementary medicine** Unconventional medical practices that are used together with conventional ones.

**alternative medicine** Unconventional medical practices that are used instead of conventional methods.

The term *CAM* includes both the terms **complementary** and **alternative medicine:** "Complementary" means an approach that combines nonmainstream and conventional medicine. "Alternative" refers to an approach that replaces conventional medicine. For example, when a conventional drug such as penicillin (an antibiotic) is used to fight an infection together with an unconventional remedy such as the herb echinacea (which enhances immunity to an infection), these treatments are considered complementary. However, if an unconventional remedy, such as a wrist band designed to apply pressure to an acupressure point, is used to prevent motion sickness instead of taking a conventional medication such as Dramamine (a drug used for motion sickness), the wrist bracelet is considered alternative.

## Ask Yourself

**QUESTIONS FOR CRITICAL THINKING AND REFLECTION**

What are your views about the use of CAM therapies? What events or information has shaped those views? Would you consider using complementary or alternative medicine?

*Integrative medicine* has become widely accepted in the United States. In integrative health conventional and complementary approaches are coordinated. The whole person is emphasized, rather than one isolated body part. A course of treatment will offer two or more interventions, such as medication along with yoga.

Consumers turn to integrative health or CAM for a variety of purposes related to health and well-being, such as boosting the immune system, lowering cholesterol levels, losing weight, quitting smoking, or enhancing memory. People with chronic conditions, including cancer, asthma, autoimmune diseases, and HIV infection, are particularly likely to try CAM therapies. Despite their popularity, many CAM practices remain controversial, and consumers need to be critically aware of safety issues. The National Center for Complementary and Integrative Health (NCCIH), formerly called the National Center for Complementary and Alternative Medicine, was established in 1992 to apply rigorous scientific methodology and standards for proving or disproving the safety and effectiveness of CAM.

# CONVENTIONAL MEDICINE

Referring to conventional medicine as "standard Western medicine" draws attention to the fact that it differs from various traditional medical systems that have developed in China, Japan, India, and other parts of the world. Calling it "biomedicine" reflects conventional medicine's foundation in the biological and physical sciences.

## Premises and Assumptions of Conventional Medicine

An important characteristic of Western medicine is the belief that disease is caused by identifiable and reproducible factors. Western medicine identifies the causes of disease as pathogens (such as bacteria and viruses), physical factors (such as trauma or toxins), genetic factors, or unhealthy lifestyles that result in changes at the cellular and molecular levels. In most cases, the focus of conventional medicine is primarily on the physical causes of illness rather than on mental or spiritual imbalance, which is more central to traditional medical systems, sometimes known as whole medical systems.

Another feature that distinguishes Western biomedicine from other medical systems is the concept that almost every disease is defined by a certain set of signs (*objective* physical manifestations) and symptoms (*subjective* effects perceived by a person), and that they are similar in most patients suffering from the disease.

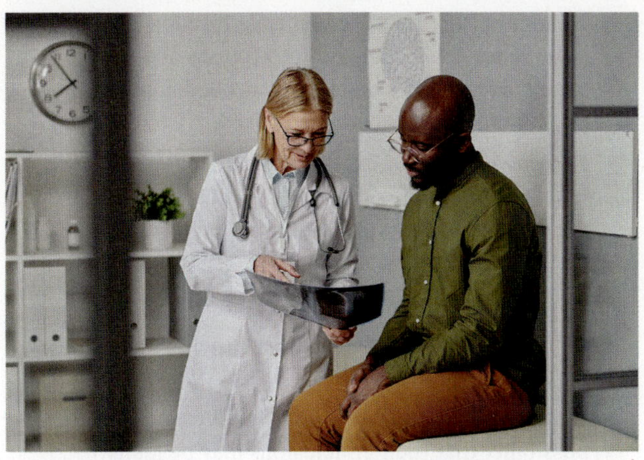

One feature that distinguishes Western biomedicine from other medical systems is the concept that almost every disease is defined by a certain set of signs and symptoms and that they are similar in most patients suffering from the disease. Pressmaster/Shutterstock

A disease can be caused by either internal or external factors. Internal factors include anatomic or physiologic abnormalities, and defective genetic, hormonal, and immune mechanisms. External causes include infections by bacteria and viruses, and some cases of traumatic injury. The public health measures of the 19th and 20th centuries–chlorination of drinking water, sewage disposal, food safety regulations, vaccination programs, education about hygiene, and so on–were an outgrowth of this orientation.

The implementation of public health measures is one way to control diseases; others include preventive lifestyle measures and the use of drugs and surgery. The discovery and development of sulfa drugs, antibiotics, and steroids in the 20th century, along with advances in chemistry that made it possible to identify the active ingredients in common plant-derived remedies, paved the way for the close identification of Western medicine with **pharmaceuticals** (medical drugs, both prescription and over-the-counter). Western medicine also relies heavily on surgery and advanced medical technology to discover the physical cause of an individual's disease and to correct, remove, or destroy it.

Western medicine is based on the scientific method for obtaining knowledge and explaining health-related phenomena. The resulting scientific explanations build on these kinds of evidence:

- ***Empirical.*** They are based on the evidence of the senses and on objective and systematic observation, carried out under carefully controlled conditions; they must be capable of verification by others through objective observation, which may include the use of technology (such as lab tests and physical measurement, such as blood pressure).
- ***Rational.*** They follow the rules of logic and are consistent with known facts.

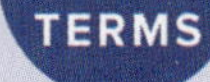

**pharmaceuticals** Medical drugs, both prescription and over-the-counter.

- ***Testable.*** Either they are verifiable through objective observation or they lead to predictions about what should occur under defined, controlled conditions (as in randomized controlled trials).
- ***Parsimonious.*** They explain phenomena using the fewest causes (for example, symptoms are attributed to the simplest explanation as supported by evidence).
- ***Generality.*** They explain phenomena among other patients who have similar signs and symptoms.
- ***Rigorously evaluated.*** They are continuously evaluated for agreement with the evidence and known principles.
- ***Tentative.*** Scientists are willing to entertain the possibility that their conclusions may be faulty if new and better evidence becomes available.

Western medicine uses the scientific method in health care practice by applying the research process, a highly refined and well-established approach to exploring the causes of disease and ensuring the safety and efficacy of treatments. Research ranges from case studies–descriptions of a single patient's illness and treatment–to **randomized controlled trials (RCTs)** conducted on large populations. RCTs are considered the highest level of evidence for treatment outcomes. Conclusions made based on an RCT may be enhanced by a relatively new standard of evidence, a **meta-analysis,** which mathematically combines data from two or more methodologically similar RCTs. If several RCTs show marginal or questionable conclusions, a meta-analysis determines which way "the scale will tip" by statistically combining the data from the studies.

The process of drug development is an example of rigorous scientific investigation. Drugs are developed and tested through an elaborate process that typically begins with preresearch in a laboratory and continues through trials with human participants, review and approval by the FDA, and monitoring of the drug's effects even after it is on the market. The production of Covid-19 vaccines in under a year is widely hailed as a monumental achievement; prior to that, the fastest vaccine development was the mumps vaccine, which took four years.

When results of research studies are published in medical journals, the community of scientists, physicians, researchers, and scholars has the opportunity to share the findings and enter a dialogue about the subject. Publication of research often prompts further research designed to replicate and confirm the findings, challenge the conclusions, or pursue related lines of thought or experimentation. How do we know if the health news we're reading or hearing is valid? Psychologists point to five criteria we use to decide whether information is true: compatibility with other known information; credibility of the source; whether others believe it; whether the information is internally consistent or logical; and whether there is supporting evidence. (See the box "Evaluating Health News.")

**TERMS**

**randomized controlled trial (RCT)** A scientific study in which subjects are randomly assigned to receive one of several clinical interventions. The intervention may be a control (e.g., a placebo, or "sugar pill"); another treatment that is being compared; or an existing, standard-of-care treatment.

**meta-analysis** A statistical recombination of data from two or more methodologically similar studies (usually RCTs) to form an overall conclusion; it has the benefit of including the outcomes of increased numbers of subjects who have varying responses.

## Pharmaceuticals and the Placebo Effect

In medical research, a placebo is often used when evaluating a new drug in a controlled trial (see Figure 16.3). A *placebo* is a biologically inactive substance that the subject cannot distinguish from the experimental drug. (For studies that don't involve drugs, such as surgery or acupuncture, a *sham* procedure may be used.) Either the experimental treatment or a placebo or sham procedure is administered randomly to subjects who are unaware which they are receiving (a "blinded" trial). By comparing the effects of the experimental treatment with the effects of the placebo or sham, researchers can evaluate whether the experimental treatment is more effective than the placebo.

Researchers have consistently found that 30–40% of all patients given a placebo show some improvement. A *placebo effect* occurs when a research subject improves after receiving a placebo; the placebo effect is the difference in outcome compared to no intervention at all (no placebo and no experimental treatment). The *treatment effect* is the difference in outcome between the placebo and the experimental treatment. If the subject does not respond better to the experimental treatment than to the placebo, then the improvement cannot be attributed to the specific actions or properties of the drug or procedure.

A placebo effect has been observed in treatment of a wide variety of conditions or symptoms, including coughing, seasickness, depression, migraines, and angina. In some cases, people given a placebo even report having the side effects associated with an actual drug.

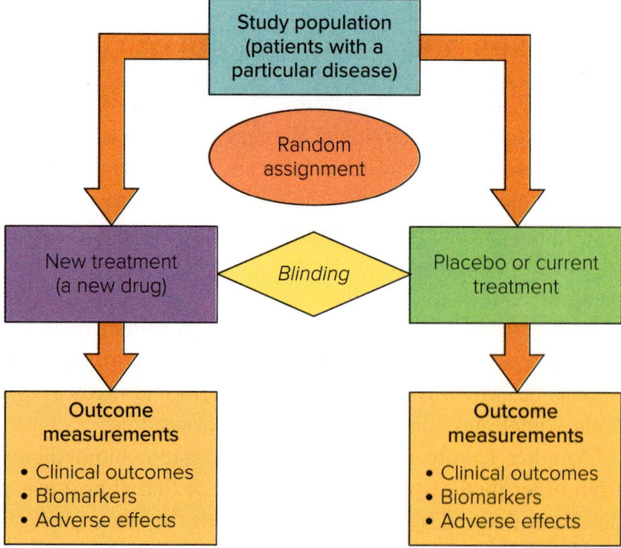


FIGURE 16.3 **How a randomized control trial works.**

## TAKE CHARGE
# Evaluating Health News

Health-related research published in scientific medical journals is often summarized for the public in the popular media, which may oversimplify, exaggerate, distort, or sensationalize the results. The following questions can help you evaluate the health information about conventional medicine and CAM that you will likely encounter in popular media:

1. *Is the report based on scientific studies?* Information or advice based on carefully designed research studies has more validity than opinions, anecdotes, or casual observations.
2. *What is the source of the information?* A study published in a respected peer-reviewed scientific journal has been examined by editors and researchers who are professionally prepared to evaluate the merits of a study and its results, and its application to actual patients. Most journals include information on the funding source and the authors' affiliations that may introduce a bias or conflict of interest. Studies sponsored by drug companies or other commercial groups are suspect. Sources sponsored by universities, government agencies, professional groups (such as MayoClinic.org and MedlinePlus.gov), and others that are rigorously peer-reviewed typically base their reports on scientific information and are considered more valid than commercial websites. Wikipedia is not considered a scientifically valid resource. When health information is critical, the consumer should review the original reference rather than rely solely on secondary interpretations.
3. *How many subjects were included in the study?* A study involving many subjects—hundreds or thousands of people—is more likely to yield reliable results than a study involving only a few subjects. Most quality studies include a "statistical power analysis" section that specifies how many subjects were necessary in order for the findings to be meaningful.
4. *Who were the subjects?* Research findings are more likely to apply to you if you share important characteristics with the study participants. For example, the results of a study on male smokers over age 60 may not be particularly meaningful for a 25-year-old female nonsmoker.
5. *What kind of study was it?* Randomized controlled trials (RCTs) and meta-analyses are considered the most valid. Epidemiological studies (which involve noncontrolled observations) may suggest useful information, but they cannot always establish cause-and-effect relationships. The following questions may help you to decide whether a study's results should be considered valid:
   - *Were the treatment group results compared to those of a control group or an already accepted therapy?*
   - *Were the subjects randomly assigned to the experimental groups?*
   - *Was the study blinded (to the subjects, the experimenters/evaluators, or both)?*
   - *Was it a multicenter study?* The results of several studies conducted in different places at different times can be mathematically combined as a meta-analysis. A well-conducted meta-analysis is considered one of the most valid types of studies.
6. *What do the statistics really say?* Are the results statistically significant? Statistical significance is usually reported as a p-value; when it is less than or equal to 0.05 or 5%, it is considered "statistically significant," meaning there is a 5% or lower probability that the findings were the result of chance. Does the study have the required number of subjects according to a statistical power analysis? Some studies report the effect size—the statistical difference in outcome between the treatment being tested and the control—instead of or in addition to a p-value. Most of the time the effect size is more revealing than the p-value.

   If study results are given in terms of relative risk—for example, a 50% reduction in the risk of developing a disorder—you should also consider the absolute risk of the condition. For example, if the absolute risk of developing a disorder is 2%, then a medication that reduced that risk by 50% (relative risk) would lower the risk to 1%: Out of 100 people *not taking* the medication, two on average would develop the disorder; out of 100 people *taking* the medication, one would develop the disorder.
7. *Is new health advice being offered?* If the media report new guidelines for health behavior or medical treatment, examine the source. Be suspicious of absolutes and overstated claims that use words such as "certainty," "always," and "never." Scientifically accurate reports use words such as "results show," "for many people," and "the evidence suggests." Reliable information sources should present the limitations of a study's results, describe how the results compare with those of other studies, and consider a great deal of evidence before offering health advice. Above all, use common sense, and check with your physician before making a major change in your health habits based on news reports.

For additional tips, visit NCCIH, *9 Questions to Help You Make Sense of Scientific Research* (https://nccih.nih.gov/health/know-science/make-sense-health-research), and NIH, *Understanding Risk: What Do Those Headlines Really Mean?* (https://permanent.access.gpo.gov/gpo64263/understanding_risk_0.pdf).

When a skilled and compassionate doctor or nurse can provide patients with confidence and hope, the positive aspects of the placebo effect can add to the benefits of treatment. Getting well, like getting sick, is a complex process. Anatomy, physiology, emotions, hope, beliefs, expectations, and prior experiences can contribute to the way the body reacts to medical treatments.

## The Providers of Conventional Medicine

Conventional medicine is practiced by a wide range of health care professionals in the United States. Several kinds of health care professionals are licensed to open their own practices, including medical doctors, osteopaths, dentists, podiatrists, psychologists, and optometrists.

- **Medical doctors** are practitioners who hold a doctor of medicine (MD) degree from an accredited medical school. They are commonly called "allopathic" physicians because of their historical practice philosophy: Treatment with opposites (the Greek prefix *allo-* means "difference," or "opposition"). For example, if the body is too warm, cool it down; if a patient is too stimulated, administer a tranquilizer. In the United States, becoming a practicing physician has several stages: premedical education in a college or university to earn a bachelor's degree; usually four years of medical school, which teaches basic medical skills and awards the doctor of medicine degree; and three to eight years of graduate medical study that includes an internship and a residency and possibly a specialty fellowship. The American Board of Medical Specialties currently recognizes and approves over 127 medical specialties and subspecialties.

TERMS

**medical doctor** A physician who holds the doctor of medicine (MD) degree from an accredited medical school; an *allopathic* physician.

**doctor of osteopathic medicine** A physician who holds the doctor of osteopathy (DO) degree from an accredited osteopathic medical school; osteopathy incorporates a whole-person approach and includes manipulating muscles and joints.

**dentist** A practitioner who holds a doctor of dental surgery (DDS) or doctor of medical dentistry (DMD) degree and whose practice includes the diagnosis, treatment, and prevention of diseases and injuries of the teeth, mouth, and jaws.

**psychologist** Health care provider who holds a PsyD or PhD degree; they treat mental health problems and usually do not prescribe medicine.

**optometrist** A practitioner who holds a doctor of optometry (OD) degree and is trained to examine the eyes, detect eye diseases, and prescribe corrective lenses.

**ophthalmologist** A practitioner who holds an MD or DO degree, has served a residency or fellowship specializing in diseases of the eye, and cares for all types of eye problems using drugs and surgery.

**nurse** A licensed health provider who is concerned with the diagnosis and treatment of human responses to actual or potential health problems and acts to promote, maintain, or restore health. Registered nurses (RNs) complete a bachelor of nursing degree. Licensed practical and vocational nurses complete a one- or two-year training program (LPN, LVN).

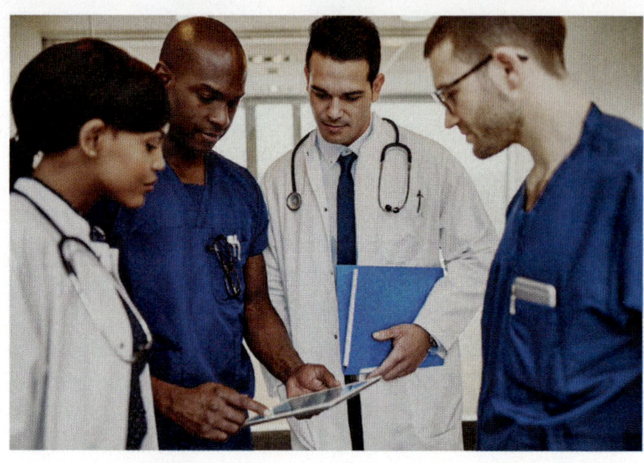

In Western medicine, treatment is usually provided by a team of health care professionals, often with different areas of specialization but with shared ideas and beliefs about the causes of illness.
langstrup/123RF

- **Doctors of osteopathic medicine** (DO) receive formal premedical education to earn a bachelor's degree; four years of osteopathic medical school leading to the DO degree; and residency and fellowship education similar to that of allopathic medical doctors over a comparable time frame. Like allopathic physicians, osteopathic physicians practice in all of the medical and surgical specialties and subspecialties, but osteopathic physicians may also practice and specialize in osteopathic manipulative treatment (manipulation of muscles and joints using stretching, pressure, and resistance).

- **Dentists** focus on the care of the teeth and mouth. They are graduates of four-year dental schools and hold the doctor of dental surgery (DDS) or doctor of medical dentistry (DMD) degree.

- **Psychologists** work with individuals, couples, families, or groups in many settings, such as private offices, hospitals, mental health organizations, schools, businesses, and nonprofit agencies. Many clinical and counseling psychologists hold a Doctor of Psychology (PsyD) or a Doctor of Philosophy (PhD) degree. Clinical psychologists, like psychiatrists, treat mental health problems but, unlike psychiatrists, are not medical doctors and usually do not prescribe medications.

- **Optometrists** are practitioners trained to examine the eyes, detect eye diseases, and treat certain vision problems, most often through the use of corrective lenses. They hold a doctor of optometry (OD) degree. All states permit optometrists to use certain drugs for diagnostic purposes, and most permit them to use drugs to treat minor eye problems. **Ophthalmologists** have an MD or DO degree and serve a residency or fellowship specializing in diseases of the eye. They care for all types of eye problems using drugs and surgery.

- **Nurses** or *registered nurses (RNs)* are practitioners concerned with the diagnosis and treatment of human responses to actual or potential health problems. They act to promote, maintain, or restore health. A nurse may receive advanced education to become a nurse practitioner (NP), a certified registered nurse anesthetist (CRNA), or a certified nurse midwife (CNM).

- **Physician assistants** (PAs) are nationally certified and state-licensed health care professionals who practice medicine as part of a team with physicians.

In addition to these practitioners, highly educated health care professionals include physical therapists, pharmacists, medical social workers, and registered dietitians.

QUICK STATS

**Employment of nurse practitioners is projected to increase by over 50% in the next decade.**

—U.S. Bureau of Labor Statistics, 2021

## Primary Care Physicians

The primary care disciplines include family practice, internal medicine, pediatrics, and gynecology. A primary care physician (PCP) is able to diagnose and treat the vast majority of common health problems and provide many preventive health services.

Recently, the United States ranked last in health equity, health care outcomes, and overall performance among 11 high-income countries. Most developed countries spend 12–17% of their health care budget on primary care; the U.S. spends 5.4%. Moreover, the unequal burdens faced by Black, Latino, and Indigenous people during the Covid-19 pandemic brought more attention to the huge racial gap in access to quality primary care. Patients from low-income, rural, and ethnically marginalized groups can have a hard time finding a local PCP and instead visit emergency rooms for care. To address some of these inequities, the National Academies of Sciences, Engineering, and Medicine put out a 2021 report advocating for an overhaul to our health care system: We should pay for primary care teams to care for people rather than doctors for delivering services; ensure that high-quality primary care is available to every person in every community; and train primary care teams where people live and work.

To select a PCP, begin by making a list of possible choices. If your insurance limits the health care providers you can see, check the plan's list first to see which doctors its network includes. If your health plan lets you choose a physician, ask for recommendations from family, friends, coworkers, local medical societies, and the physician referral service at a local clinic or hospital. You might also want to check online or call the offices of those on your list to find out the following: Is the physician covered by your health plan and accepting new patients? What are the office hours, and when is the physician or office staff available? What do patients do if they need urgent care or have an emergency? Which hospitals does the physician use? How many other physicians are available to cover when your PCP isn't available, and who are they? How long does it usually take to get a routine appointment? Does the office send reminders about preventive services and tests such as Pap tests? Does the physician (or a nurse or physician assistant) give advice online or over the phone for common problems and continued care of a diagnosed problem?

Schedule a visit with the physician you think you would most like to use. During that first visit, you'll get a sense of how well matched you are and how well he or she might meet your medical needs.

## Choosing a Specialist

You should be referred to a specialist when the services you need are outside the scope of your PCP's practice. The specialist may not be a physician but rather a physical therapist, audiologist, psychologist, or another type of practitioner. In most cases, your PCP will recommend the type of specialist you need based on your clinical findings; unless it's obvious, most of the time patients cannot accurately identify the appropriate medical discipline needed, since there are 145 medical specialties and subspecialties. In general, specialists are from the internal medicine subdisciplines, such as dermatology, gastroenterology, and neurology, or from the surgical subdisciplines, such as thoracic surgery, orthopedics, and neurosurgery. Some subdisciplines involve both internal medicine and surgery (gynecology, urology, and ophthalmology).

By the time of your visit, the specialist should have received a referral note from your PCP, your complete medical record, and access to all your recent lab tests and imaging studies as well as past tests that may be significant (e.g., MRIs of the spine years earlier). If your specialist refers you to another specialist, you should visit your PCP first, to keep him or her up to date on your symptoms and to discuss any questions you have about the next step in your specialized care.

## Getting the Most Out of Your Medical Care

The key to making the health care system work for you lies in good communication with your physician and other members of the health care team. Studies show that patients who interact more with physicians and ask more questions enjoy better health outcomes (see the box "Health Care Visits and Gender").

**The Physician–Patient Partnership** The physician–patient relationship is a *partnership* in which the physician acts more like a consultant and the patient participates more actively (see the box "Creating Your Own Health Record"). You should expect your physician to be attentive, caring, and able to listen and clearly explain health care matters to you. You also must do your part. You need to be assertive in a firm but nonaggressive manner. You need to express your feelings and concerns, ask questions, and, if necessary, be persistent. If your physician is unable to communicate clearly with you despite your best efforts, you probably need to change physicians.

TERMS

**physician assistant** A health provider who is nationally certified and licensed by his or her state to practice medicine as part of a team with physicians.

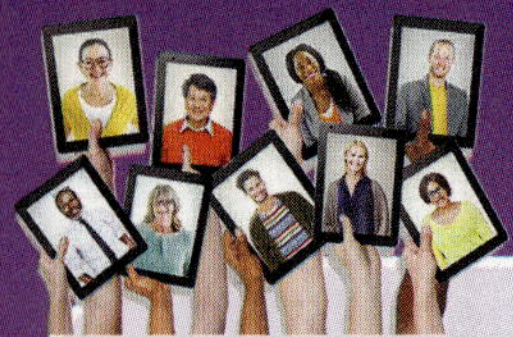

## DIVERSITY MATTERS
### Health Care Visits and Gender

Women are more likely than men to visit a health care provider. According to data from the National Center for Health Statistics covering all age groups, 20% of men report no health care visits in the past 12 months—nearly twice the 11% rate for women. A Kaiser Family Foundation survey of adults aged 18–64 found that 25% of men had not seen a provider within the past two years, compared to only 9% of women. Men also have lower rates of many preventive health services, including flu vaccinations and colon cancer screening, and are less likely than women to have a usual source of health care.

Women also seek a wider variety of health care alternatives. A recent book on women's yoga practices (Evans 2021) describes how Black women are disproportionately subjected to personal, cultural, and structural violence. They have had to get creative in finding paths to inner peace. The long history of self-care in strategies such as music, prayer, exercise, and particularly meditation and yoga can be seen in the memoirs of Black women such as Rosa Parks, and going back to days of enslavement.

Women generally use yoga, meditation, and chiropractors more than men. One explanation for this gender disparity may lie in the prenatal care and childbirth visits made by women of reproductive age. They may also need to make health care visits to obtain prescription contraceptives and have pelvic exams and Pap tests. Still, even when physician visits related to reproductive care are discounted, American men are less likely to report their symptoms and seek medical help.

Perhaps the way boys in the United States (and many other countries) are raised has something to do with their reluctance to seek preventive care (when no symptoms are present). One study of boys aged 15–19 in the United States reveals that they equated health with physical fitness. They saw no reason for preventive care and justified seeking any care only when a person was physically and severely ill. This belief system correlates with ideas of men as strong, tough, and able to ignore pain or symptoms of illness.

Ideally, everyone, regardless of gender or socioeconomic status, would get recommended health care screenings and immunizations. Without them, people may be unaware of asymptomatic conditions such as high cholesterol levels or high blood pressure. Preventive care throughout life is important for maximum wellness.

SOURCES: Clark, T. C., et al. 2018. Use of yoga, meditation, and chiropractors among U.S. adults aged 18 and over. *NCHS Data Brief* 325. Hyattsville, MD: National Center for Health Statistics (https://www.cdc.gov/nchs/data/databriefs/db325-h.pdf). Kaiser Family Foundation. 2015. *Gender Differences in Health Care, Status, and Use* (http://kff.org/womens-health-policy/fact-sheet/gender-differences-in-health-care-status-and-use-spotlight-on-mens-health); Evans, S. Y. 2021. *Black Women's Yoga History: Memoirs of Inner Peace*. New York: SUNY Press; Harvard Men's Health Watch. 2019. Mars vs. Venus: The gender gap in health. *Harvard Health Letter* (http://www.health.harvard.edu/newsletter_article/mars-vs-venus-the-gender-gap-in-health); Westwood, M., and J. Pinzon. 2008. Adolescent male health. *Paediatrics and Child Health* 13(1): 31–36.

**Your Physician Appointments** You may be offered the opportunity to see a physician assistant or nurse practitioner who works with your physician. This option may result in an earlier appointment where you may have more time to discuss your health concerns. Physicians are often pressed for time, so prepare for office visits by writing down your key concerns and questions, along with notes about your symptoms (when they started, how long they last, what makes them better or worse, what treatments you have already tried, and so on). Even well-informed, proactive patients often forget important information and questions during the dynamics of an office visit. If you're uncomfortable asking certain questions, practice discussing them ahead of time. Bring a list of all the medications you're taking—prescription, nonprescription, and herbal. Also bring any medical records or test results your physician may not already have.

Present your concerns at the beginning of the visit to set the agenda. Be specific and concise about your symptoms, and be open and honest about your concerns. Share your hunches with your physician—your guesses can provide vital clues. Ask questions if you don't understand something he or she says to you. Let your physician know if you are taking any drugs, are allergic to any medications, are breastfeeding, or may be pregnant. At the end of the visit, briefly repeat the physician's diagnosis, prognosis, the purpose of any tests, and instructions you have received to make sure you understand your next steps.

### Ask Yourself

**QUESTIONS FOR CRITICAL THINKING AND REFLECTION**

What sort of relationship do you have with your physician? Do you think he or she understands your needs and is familiar enough with your history? Are you satisfied with this relationship?

**The Diagnostic Process** The first step in the diagnostic process is the medical history, which includes primary reason for the visit, current symptoms, past medical history, and social history (job, family life, major stressors, living conditions, and health habits). Keeping up-to-date records of your medical history can help you provide your physician with key facts about your health.

The next step is usually the physical exam, which begins with a review of vital signs: blood pressure, heart rate (pulse), breathing rate, and temperature. Depending on your primary complaint, your physician may give you a complete physical or focus on specific areas, such as your ears, nose, and throat. Additionally, your physician may order medical tests. Physicians can order imaging studies (e.g., X-rays, MRIs, or CT

## WELLNESS ON CAMPUS
## Creating Your Own Health Record

What's your blood pressure? How about cholesterol level? What medicines are you taking? Many Americans believe that their medical records are compiled and maintained by some mysterious entity (probably called "them"), but this is not the case. The expanding use of computerized medical records may be useful within a particular clinic or health care system, but this does not mean that every person's individual medical history has been automatically collated into a single, easy-to-find source. Computerized health records maintained by one hospital or medical care system might not be accessible by another. We each need to be responsible for compiling our important medical records and keeping them safe and easily available to us or a caregiver in case we need the records for an emergency, or when traveling, moving, or looking for a new primary care provider. College is a good time to start doing this for yourself, and by sharing your health knowledge and assisting family members to do the same, you are playing a more active role in your family's health care.

Personal health records should be readily accessible in case of an emergency. Some personal computerized health record systems can be purchased online, or one can be devised individually. (You can find out about various personal health records on the U.S. government's HealthIT.gov website: http://www.healthit.gov/how-do-i/individuals.) Whether purchased or created individually, here's what your personal health record should contain:

- Your name, emergency contact, birth date, blood type, religious preference (if any), and the date this record was compiled or updated.
- All known allergies (including medications).
- A list of all chronic conditions and the dates of their diagnosis (e.g., diabetes, high blood pressure, asthma, emphysema).
- Any hereditary diseases.
- The names and dosages of all medications you take and reasons for taking them.
- The results of tests or procedures such as blood pressure, cholesterol, vision, and others.
- The dates and reasons for all past hospitalizations and operations. If the reasons were serious or may affect future treatments (e.g., major organ involvement; devices or materials implanted surgically), a hospital discharge summary should be included.
- The dates of physical exams and any major findings.
- Vaccination schedules.
- A print-out of all laboratory test results, and a written report of any imaging studies (e.g., X-rays, CT scans, MRIs), electrocardiograms (ECGs), and special tests such as audiograms and exercise stress tests. Check to verify that dates are included.

You have the right to all of your medical records—that is, to view them or request a copy or a summary of the information. To request copies, ask for an "authorization for the release of information form." Any fee should include only the cost of copying and postage (if you request mailing). If you see something in your medical record that you believe is incorrect or incomplete, you can request an amendment through your physician or a medical information professional, and you have the right for your amendment to be permanently included in your record.

SOURCES: MedlinePlus. *Personal Health Records* (www.nlm.nih.gov/medlineplus/personalhealthrecords.html); AHIMA Foundation. *myPHR* (http://www.ahimafoundation.org/).

scans), biopsies, blood and urine tests, or **endoscopies** to view, probe, or analyze almost any part of the body.

If your physician orders a test for you, be sure you know why you need it, what the risks and benefits are for you, how you should prepare for it (e.g., by fasting or discontinuing medications or herbal remedies), and what the test will involve. Also ask what the test results mean because no test is 100% accurate—**false positives** and **false negatives** can occur—and interpretation of some tests is subjective. You may want to obtain a second opinion, especially for serious conditions or major surgical procedures, or if you have significant unmet needs related to your medical care.

**Medical and Surgical Treatments** When starting any treatment, make sure you know the possible risks and side effects as well as the potential benefits.

Thousands of lives are saved each year by antibiotics, insulin, and other drugs, but we pay a price for having such powerful tools. A report from the National Academy of Medicine estimates that 1.5 million prescription-drug-related errors—called adverse drug events, or ADEs—occur each year in the United States. ADEs happen for several reasons:

- ***Medication errors.*** Physicians may overprescribe drugs, sometimes in response to pressure by patients. ADEs can occur if a physician prescribes the wrong drug or a dangerous combination of drugs. Such problems are especially prevalent among older adults, who typically take multiple medications.

**TERMS**

**endoscopy** A medical procedure in which a viewing instrument is inserted into a body cavity or opening.

**false positive** A test result that incorrectly detects a disorder or condition in a person who does not have the disorder or condition.

**false negative** A test result that fails to correctly detect a disease or condition.

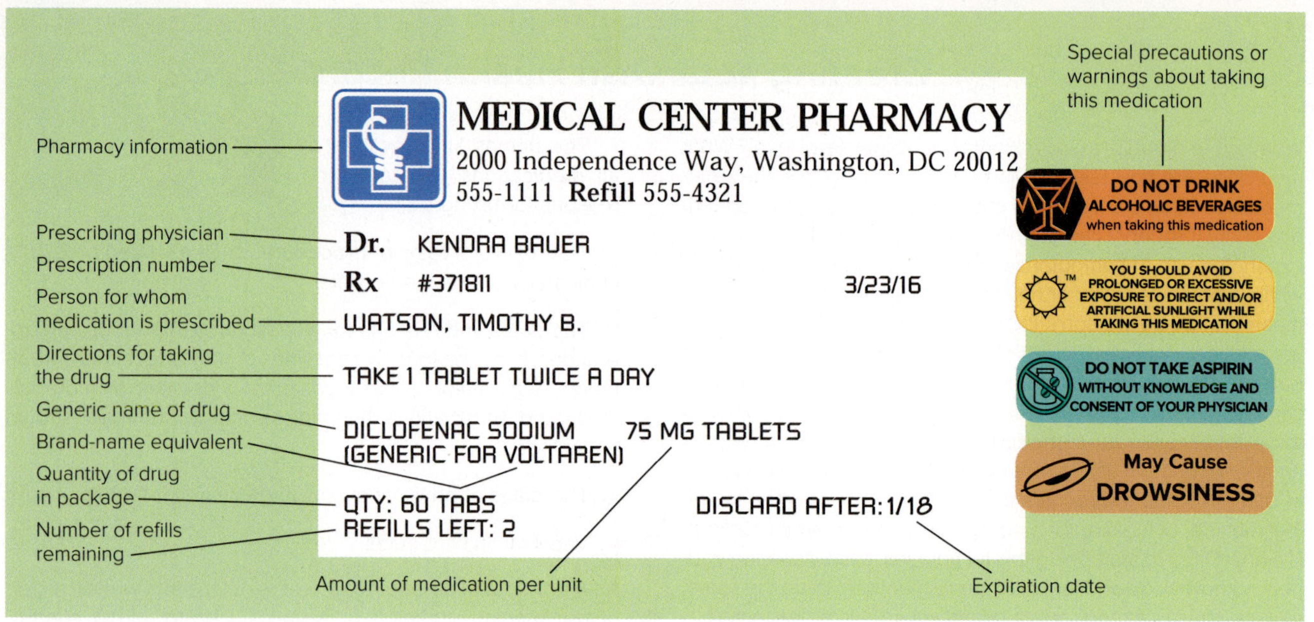


**FIGURE 16.4** **Reading and understanding prescription medication labels.**

The risk of ADEs increases greatly with the number of medicines you take. At the pharmacy, patients may receive the wrong drug or may not be given complete information about drug risks, side effects, and interactions. Problems can occur because of a physician's poor handwriting, misinterpretation of an abbreviated drug name, or similarities between the names and packaging of different drugs.

- ***Off-label drug use.*** Another potential problem is off-label use of drugs. Once a drug is approved by the FDA for one purpose, it can legally be prescribed (although not marketed) for purposes not listed on the label. Many off-label uses are safe and supported by some research, but both consumers and health care providers need to take special care with off-label use of medications. Physicians should explain their reason for prescribing an off-label drug.

- ***Online pharmacies.*** Although convenient, some online pharmacies may sell products or engage in practices that are illegal in the offline world, putting consumers at risk for receiving adulterated, expired, ineffective, or counterfeit drugs. The FDA recommends that consumers avoid sites that prescribe drugs for the first time without a physical exam, sell prescription drugs without a prescription, or sell medications not approved by the FDA. You should also avoid sites that do not provide access to a registered pharmacist to answer questions or that do not provide a U.S. address and phone number to contact if there's a problem. The National Association of Boards of Pharmacy sponsors a voluntary certification program for internet pharmacies. To be certified, a pharmacy must have a state license and allow regular inspections. Many experts recommend that consumers use online pharmacies only to obtain medicines prescribed by their usual health care providers.

- ***Costs.*** Spending on prescription drugs now the fastest-growing portion of U.S. health care spending. A recent RAND study found that prescription drugs in the United States cost, on average, over 2.5 times more than they do in 32 other nations. Many Americans have no or limited insurance coverage for prescription drug costs. Consumers may be able to lower their drug costs by using generic versions of medications, by joining a drug discount program, or by investigating mail-order or internet pharmacies.

Importing lower-cost drugs from Canada may be problematic. Canada imports U.S. drugs, and Health Canada—which provides regulation similar to the U.S. FDA—helps ensure the quality of Canadian-produced drugs, so safety should theoretically not be a concern for medicines from Canada. The past two presidential administrations and several states have actively pursued legislation to allow importation. However, no state proposal submitted to the Department of Health and Human Services to demonstrate safety and cost savings has been certified yet. U.S. regulators have found online sites advertising Canadian drugs but shipping fake or substandard versions of medications, and shipping costs can be high.

Patients share responsibility for their use of prescription drugs. Many people don't take their medications properly—skipping doses, taking incorrect doses, stopping too soon, or not taking the medication at all. An estimated 30–50% of the 4 billion prescriptions dispensed annually in the United States are not taken correctly and thus may not produce the desired results. Consumers can increase the safety and effectiveness of their treatment by carefully reading any prescription label (Figure 16.4) and fact sheets or brochures that come with the medication. Whenever you are given a prescription, ask the following questions: Are there nondrug alternatives? What is the name of the medication, and what is it supposed to do, within what period of time? Can I take a generic drug rather than a brand-name one? Is there written information about the medication?

If written information is provided, check it for the following: How and when do I take the medication, how much do I take, and for how long? What should I do if I miss a dose? What medications, foods, drinks, or activities should I avoid when taking this drug? What are the side effects, and what do I do if they occur?

Surgical procedures are performed more often in the United States than anywhere else in the world. Each year more than 70 million operations and related procedures are performed. About 20% are in response to an emergency such as a severe injury, and 80% are **elective surgeries,** meaning the patient can generally choose when and where to have the operation, if at all. Many elective surgeries can be done on an **outpatient** basis, so that the patient does not have to be admitted to a hospital for the procedure.

## INTEGRATIVE HEALTH

Increasingly, more conventional Western medical providers are receptive to integrative health, and they may approve or recommend safe and effective CAM in addition to conventional treatment. Whereas conventional Western medicine tends to focus on the body, on the physical causes of disease, and on ways to eradicate pathogens in order to restore health, CAM tends to focus on the mind, body, and spirit in seeking ways to prevent diseases and restore the whole person to balance so that he or she can regain health. This is referred to as **holistic health care**—considering the whole person as a mind-body-spirit entity when diagnosing, treating, or preventing any illness or disorder. The opposite of holistic is dualistic, which refers to treating the mind and body separately. Under dualism, it is believed that treating an individual's physical body is separate and different from treating an individual's mental state. Under holistic approaches, health is not achieved if the mental state is ignored, if the individual is spiritually isolated, or if the body has a disease; holistic health means that the needs of the body, mind, and spirit are balanced and in harmony.

Anecdotes and testimonials—about conventional or CAM treatments—are not adequate levels of evidence when it comes to your health. Nor are case reports alone sufficient to scientifically prove the effectiveness of a medical treatment. Caution is in order when choosing any mode of treatment that has not been scientifically evaluated for safety and effectiveness (see the box "Avoiding Health Fraud and Quackery"). Even though practitioners may not know precisely why or how a particular CAM procedure works—which is also often the case for conventional modalities—the standard of proof for safety and efficacy is the randomized controlled trial (RCT).

Here is a general introduction to the five categories of CAM (Figure 16.5) and a brief description of some of the more widely used therapies.

### Alternative Medical Systems

The nonconventional systems best known in the United States include traditional Chinese medicine and homeopathy. Traditional, or whole, medical systems have developed in many regions of the world, including in the Americas, the Middle East, India, Tibet, and Australia. These cultures formed complete systems of medical philosophy, theory, and practice. In many countries, these medical approaches continue to be used—frequently alongside conventional medicine and often by physicians trained in conventional medicine.

Alternative medical systems tend to have a number of concepts in common. For example, the concept of life force or energy exists in many cultures. In traditional Chinese medicine, the life force contained in all living organisms is called qi (sometimes spelled "chi"). Qi resembles the vis vitalis (Latin for "life force") of Greek, Roman, and European medical systems, and prana of ayurveda, a traditional medical system of India. Most traditional medical systems think of disease as a disturbance or imbalance not just of physical processes but also of forces or energies within the body, the mind, and thespirit. In traditional Chinese medicine, for example, the principle of balance is expressed as yin and yang, which are opposites that complement each other. Treatment aims at reestablishing equilibrium, balance, and harmony.

Because the whole patient, rather than an isolated body part or disease, is treated in most comprehensive alternative medical systems, it is rare that only a single treatment approach is used. Most commonly, multiple remedies and techniques are employed together and are adjusted according to the changes in the patient's health status.

**Traditional Chinese Medicine** In **traditional Chinese medicine (TCM)** the free and harmonious flow of qi defines health of the body, mind, and spirit. Illness occurs when qi is deficient or the flow of qi is blocked or disturbed. TCM is believed to restore the flow of blocked qi, treating illness by balancing energy, preventing disease, and supporting immunity.

Two major TCM treatment methods include **herbal remedies** and **acupuncture.** Chinese herbal remedies number about 5800 (compared with about 6800 prescription and

**TERMS**

**elective surgery** A nonemergency operation that the patient can choose to schedule.

**outpatient** A person receiving medical attention without being admitted to the hospital.

**holistic health care** Practice that takes into account the whole person—body, mind, and spirit—when assessing, treating, and preventing illnesses and maintaining health.

**traditional Chinese medicine (TCM)** The traditional medical system of China, which views illness as the result of a problem in the quality, quantity, balance, or flow of qi, the life force; therapies include acupuncture, herbal medicine, and massage.

**herbal remedy** A medicine prepared from plants.

**acupuncture** Insertion of thin needles through the skin at points along meridians—pathways through which qi is believed to flow.

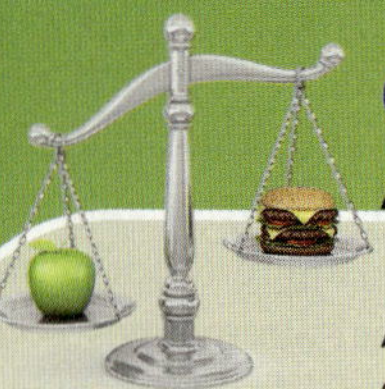

## CRITICAL CONSUMER
# Avoiding Health Fraud and Quackery

According to the Federal Trade Commission, consumers waste billions of dollars on unproven, fraudulently marketed, and sometimes useless health care products and treatments. In addition, individuals with serious medical problems may waste valuable time before seeking proper treatment. Worse yet, some of the products they're buying and using may cause serious harm. Health fraud often targets people with diseases that have no medical cure, and people who want shortcuts to improved health, weight loss, or enhanced personal appearance.

To help evaluate a product, you may talk to a physician or other licensed health professional who is impartial and knowledgeable about CAM modalities. Be wary of treatments offered by people who advise you to avoid seeking additional information or consulting others. Check with the Better Business Bureau or the local attorney general's office to see if other consumers have lodged complaints about a product or a product's marketer. You can also check with the appropriate health professional group such as the American Diabetes Association, American Cancer Society, or National Arthritis Foundation. Take special care with products and devices sold on television or online; the broad reach of the internet, combined with the ease of setting up and removing websites, makes online sellers particularly difficult to regulate.

If you think you have been a victim of health fraud or if you have an adverse reaction that you think is related to a particular supplement, you can report it to the appropriate agency:

- ***False advertising claims.*** Contact the FTC by phone (877-FTC-HELP), by mail (Consumer Response Center, Federal Trade Commission, Washington, DC 20580), or online (http://www.ftc.gov). You can also contact your state attorney general's office, your state department of health, or the local consumer protection agency (check a website or your local telephone directory).
- ***False labeling on a product.*** Contact the FDA district office consumer complaint coordinator for your geographic area. The FDA regulates safety, manufacturing, and product labeling.
- ***Adverse reaction to a supplement.*** If a health risk appears serious, call your physician immediately or go to an emergency clinic. You can also report your adverse reaction to FDA MedWatch by calling 800-FDA-1088 or by visiting the MedWatch website (http://www.fda.gov/Safety/MedWatch/).
- ***Unlawful internet sales.*** If you find a website that you think is misrepresenting or illegally selling drugs, medical devices, dietary supplements, or cosmetics, report it to the FDA. Problems can be reported to MedWatch or via the FDA website (http://www.fda.gov/ForConsumers/ProtectYourself).

| Domain | Characteristics | Examples |
|---|---|---|
| Alternative medical systems 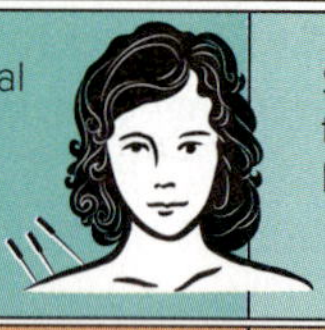 | Systems of health/healing theory and practice that have evolved independently and long before conventional biomedical approaches. | Traditional Chinese medicine, ayurvedic medicine, homeopathy, naturopathy. |
| Mind–body medicine | Practices that use thoughts, beliefs, and other mental activities to affect the health and functioning of the physical body (including the brain). | Meditation, hypnosis, prayer, guided imagery, art therapy, music therapy, emotive writing. 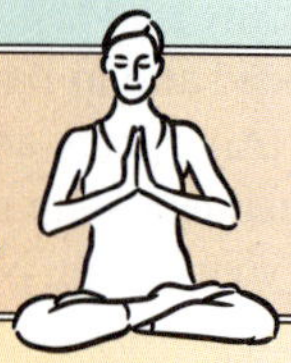 |
| Natural biologic products | Plant (herbals) and animal products used as medicinals and dietary supplements. 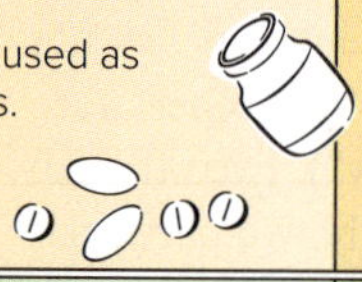 | Ginko biloba, shark cartilage, probiotics (live bacteria that may have beneficial health effects when ingested). |
| Manipulative and body-based practices | Methods for adjusting, moving, or touching the body to promote health and healing. | 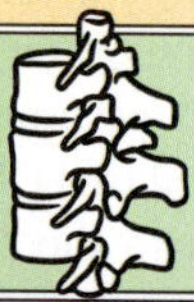 Chiropractic, osteopathic manual therapy, massage. |
| Other CAM practices 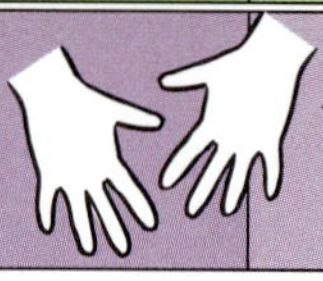 | Therapeutic methods involving energy modalities. | Magnet therapy, light therapy, Reiki, qigong, therapeutic touch. |

**FIGURE 16.5** The categories of CAM.

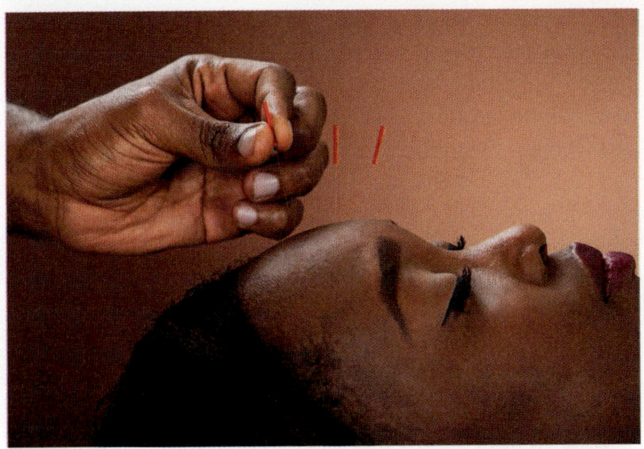

Acupuncture involves the insertion of needles at appropriate points in the skin to treat a variety of illnesses. andreypopov/123RF

many other OTC medications). Herbs, plant products, fungi (mushrooms), animal parts, and minerals may be used. These remedies, like everything else, have yin and yang properties or qi. When a disease is perceived to be due to a yin deficiency, remedies with more yin characteristics might be used for treatment. The use of a single medicinal substance is rare in Chinese herbal medicine; rather, several substances are combined in precise proportions, often to make a tea or soup.

An accumulating body of scientific evidence supports the medical use of acupuncture, expanding the acceptance of this CAM modality in the West and placing it on the border of conventional and nonconventional health care practice. In the Western view, acupuncture needles inserted through the skin at appropriate sites by highly trained professionals have an effect on nerves, muscles, and connective tissues that increases blood flow and stimulates the body's natural production of painkillers, hormones, and immune substances.

In TCM, acupuncture is viewed as correcting disturbances in the flow of qi. Qi is believed to flow through the body along several meridians, or pathways, and there are hundreds of acupuncture points located along these meridians.

The World Health Organization has compiled a list of more than 40 conditions for which acupuncture may be beneficial. A panel of experts at a National Institutes of Health (NIH) conference cited evidence that acupuncture was effective in relieving nausea and vomiting after chemotherapy and pain after surgery, including dental surgery. Newer studies show that acupuncture may help relieve the painful symptoms of fibromyalgia and reduce the joint pain and stiffness of osteoarthritis. There is insufficient evidence showing that acupuncture is effective for menstrual cramps, tennis elbow, carpal tunnel syndrome, asthma, and certain other conditions. Acupuncture is considered very safe, and over decades, few side effects have been reported. The FDA regulates acupuncture needles like other standard medical devices and requires that they be sterile.

**Homeopathy** As a CAM system of medical practice that has unconventional origins in Germany, **homeopathy** involves treating an individual with highly diluted substances intended to trigger the body's natural system of healing. The theory is that when given in very diluted, minute quantities, substances that produce symptoms of an illness in a healthy person will help bring about a cure in someone who is ill, and it will do this by stimulating the body's healing processes. A primary principle of homeopathy is "like cures like." Based on a patient's specific signs and symptoms, a homeopathic practitioner determines the most appropriate treatment; diluted remedies are typically administered in liquid form or applied to sweetened pellets. Although most homeopathic remedies are highly diluted, some products may be labeled as homeopathic but contain substantial amounts of active ingredients that can cause side effects or drug interactions.

Because treatments are highly individualized for each patient and difficult to explain using the conventional laws of chemistry, randomized controlled trials on homeopathy are difficult. Most clinical trials have concluded that at best there is only weak evidence of efficacy. Some states require homeopaths to be licensed and fulfill certain requirements before they are permitted to practice.

**Naturopathy** **Naturopathy** is based on the premise that the body has the ability to maintain and restore optimal health. Naturopathic doctors (NDs) use both CAM and conventional approaches holistically for prevention, diagnosis, and treatment and for helping their patients minimize risks and barriers to good health. The most frequently treated conditions include allergies, chronic pain, obesity, heart disease, fertility problems, and cancer. Naturopaths can perform minor surgery such as cyst removal and skin suturing. They are also trained to use prescription medications, although their education emphasizes natural modalities for healing.

## Mind–Body Medicine

Mind-body interventions make use of the integral connection between mind and body and the effect each can have on the other. They include many of the stress management techniques discussed in Chapter 2, including meditation, yoga, visualization, tai chi, and biofeedback. Psychotherapy, support groups, prayer, and music and art therapy are mind-body interventions. The placebo effect is one of the most widely known examples of mind-body interdependence. Many studies have shown evidence that mind-body interventions such as imagery, support groups, friendships, strong family relationships, meditation, prayer, and hypnotherapy can all have a positive impact on health.

**TERMS**

**homeopathy** An alternative system of practice that uses a holistic approach to diagnosis and treatment; involves administering minute doses of remedies that would, in larger quantities, produce symptoms similar to those of the illness.

**naturopathy** An alternative medical system based on supporting the body's ability to heal itself and maintain optimal health by removing barriers and creating an internal and external environment that promotes health and healing.

Clinical hypnosis is a focused state of awareness, perception, or consciousness that professionally trained practitioners use to treat a variety of physical and psychological conditions. **Hypnotherapy** is considered to be a CAM modality, although its use for certain conditions was accepted more than 40 years ago by the American Medical Association. Numerous evidence-based outcome studies have demonstrated its clinical usefulness, and brain-imaging technologies are helping to explain possible neurologic mechanisms.

Hypnotherapy involves the induction of a state of deep relaxation during which the patient is more likely to accept suggestions that can influence health and overcome conditions such as chronic pain, pain during surgery or childbirth, unhealthy habits, and anxiety and phobias. A number of NIH-sponsored reports found strong evidence for the effectiveness of hypnosis in reducing chronic pain stemming from a variety of medical conditions. Health professionals who are properly trained in hypnotherapy use this modality to augment their conventional treatments.

## Biologically Based Products

**Natural products,** also known as *biologically based therapies*, include substances derived from plant or animal sources. They consist primarily of herbal therapies or remedies, botanicals, and extracts from animal tissues (such as shark cartilage). A majority of the world's population relies on herbal remedies and other components of traditional, or indigenous, forms of medicine. Literature estimates that more than 95% of the U.S. public has used biologically based therapies at one point in their lifetime.

Well-designed clinical studies have been conducted on a number of natural products. A few commonly used herbals, their uses, and the evidence supporting their efficacy are presented in Table 16.2. Clinical trials with herbals such as St. John's wort, ginkgo biloba, and echinacea have shown only a few minor side effects. New studies are also evaluating the efficacy of varying dosages and their interactions with conventional drugs.

Although most drug–herb interactions are relatively minor compared to conventional drug–drug interactions, some can be potentially serious. For example, supplements containing kava kava have been linked to liver damage, and anyone who has liver problems, drinks large amounts of alcohol, or takes medications that can affect the liver is advised to consult a physician or pharmacist before using kava kava–containing supplements.

Another potential problem is the possibility of contaminants. In a sample of ayurvedic herbal medicine products, 20% were found to contain potentially harmful levels of lead, mercury, or arsenic. The content and potency of herbal preparations also varies.

Studies have shown that most people do not reveal their use of CAM therapies to their conventional health care providers, a problem that can have significant health consequences. Any herbs that are used in combination with conventional drugs should be evaluated for safety by a knowledgeable health care provider such as a pharmacist.

## Manipulative and Body-Based Practices

Touch and body manipulation are long-standing forms of health care. Manual healing techniques include the concept that misalignment or dysfunction in one part of the body can cause pain or dysfunction in that or another part.

**Chiropractic** The most commonly used CAM manual healing method is **chiropractic,** a method that focuses on the relationship between structure and function, primarily of the spine, joints, muscles, and the nervous system, to maintain or restore health. An important therapeutic procedure is the manipulation of joints, particularly those of the spinal column. However, chiropractors also use a variety of other techniques, including exercise, patient education and lifestyle modification, nutritional supplements, and orthotics (mechanical supports and braces).

Chiropractors, or doctors of chiropractic, are trained for a minimum of four years at accredited chiropractic colleges and can go on to postgraduate training in many countries. Although specifically listed by NCCIH as one of the manipulative and body-based practices of CAM, chiropractic is accepted by many health care and health insurance providers to a far greater extent than are many other types of CAM therapies. Based on research showing the efficacy of chiropractic management in acute lower-back pain, spinal manipulation has been included in the federal guidelines for the treatment of this condition, and electrodiagnostic tests show that chiropractic is effective in controlling back pain. Promising results have also been reported with the use of chiropractic techniques in neck pain and headaches.

A word of caution: Spinal manipulation must be performed only by a properly trained professional such as a chiropractor, osteopathic physician, or physical therapist who is specially trained and certified in orthopedic manual physical therapy (OMPT).

**TERMS**

**hypnotherapy** A mind–body technique that uses relaxation and imagery to help a patient imagine specific health outcomes and establish a belief that they can be achieved; commonly used for managing pain, phobias, and addictions.

**natural products** CAM therapies that include biologically based interventions and products; examples include herbal remedies, extracts from animal tissues, and dietary supplements.

**chiropractic** A CAM manipulative, body-based practice that focuses on disorders of the spine, and musculoskeletal and nervous systems, and the effects of these disorders on general health; the primary treatment is manipulation of the spine and other joints.

## Table 16.2 Commonly Used Herbals, Their Uses, Evidence for Their Effectiveness, and Contraindications

| BOTANICAL | USE | EVIDENCE | EXAMPLES OF ADVERSE EFFECTS AND INTERACTIONS |
|---|---|---|---|
| Cranberry (*Vaccinium macrocarpon*) | Prevention or treatment of urinary tract infections | Some evidence of a modest preventive effect in some women | None known |
| Dandelion (*Taraxacum officinale*) | As a "tonic" against liver or kidney ailments | No conclusive evidence | May cause diarrhea in some users; people with gallbladder or bile duct problems should not take dandelion |
| Echinacea (*Echinacea purpurea, E. angustifolia, E. pallida*) | Stimulation of immune functions; to prevent colds and flulike diseases; to lessen symptoms of colds and flu | Some trials showed that it prevents colds and flu and helps patients recover faster from colds | Might cause liver damage if taken over long periods of time (more than 8 weeks); because it is an immune stimulant, it is not advisable to take it with immune suppressants (e.g., corticosteroids) or during chemotherapy |
| Evening primrose oil (*Oenothera biennis L.*) | Reduction of inflammation | Long-term supplementation effective in reducing symptoms of rheumatoid arthritis | None known |
| Feverfew (*Tanacetum parthenium*) | Prevention of headaches and migraines | Most trials indicate that it is more effective than placebo | Should not be used by people allergic to other members of the aster family; has the potential to increase the effects of warfarin and other anticoagulants |
| Garlic (*Allium sativum*) | Reduction of cholesterol | Short-term studies have found a modest effect | May interact with some medications, including anticoagulants, cyclosporine, and oral contraceptives |
| Ginkgo (*Ginkgo biloba*) | Improvement of circulation and memory | Improves cerebral insufficiency and slows progression of senile dementia in some patients; improves blood flow | Could increase bleeding time; should not be taken with nonsteroidal anti-inflammatory drugs (NSAIDs) like aspirin or with anticoagulants; may cause gastrointestinal disturbance |
| Ginseng (*Panax ginseng*) | Improvement of physical performance, memory, immune function, and glycemic control in diabetes; treatment of herpes simplex 2 | No conclusive evidence exists for any of these uses | Interacts with warfarin and alcohol in mice and rats, so should probably not be used with these drugs; may cause liver damage |
| St. John's wort (*Hypericum perforatum*) | Treatment of depression | There is evidence that it is significantly more effective than placebo, is as effective as some standard antidepressants for mild to moderate depression, and causes fewer adverse effects | Known to interact with a variety of pharmaceuticals and should not be taken together with digoxin, theophylline, cyclosporine, indinavir, and serotonin reuptake inhibitors; reduces the effectiveness of oral contraceptives, antirejection drugs, and some medications used to treat infections, depression, asthmas, and seizure disorders. |
| Saw palmetto (*Serenoa repens*) | Improvement of benign prostatic hypertrophy | Studies show that saw palmetto may reduce mild prostate enlargement | Has no known interactions with drugs, but should probably not be taken with hormonal therapies |
| Valerian (*Valeriana officinalis*) | Treatment of insomnia | May help with some sleep disorders | Interacts with thiopental and pentobarbital and should not be used with these drugs |

**Exercise** Exercise for health maintenance, promotion, and disease prevention currently fits the definition of a CAM modality. However, this is changing due to an active campaign, Exercise Is Medicine (EIM), co-launched in 2007 by the American College of Sports Medicine and the American Medical Association. A study has found that 65% of Americans would be more interested in exercising to stay healthy if advised to do so by their physicians.

The EIM initiative encourages physicians to record a patient's exercise level as a routine vital sign during clinical visits, along with pulse, respiratory rate, temperature, and blood pressure. Those who are able will be advised to exercise for at least 30 minutes and to stretch and engage in light muscle training for an additional 10 minutes five days each week. The EIM website (www.exerciseismedicine.org) advises physicians, other health care providers, medical educators, and the public about the benefits of exercise. Through efforts such as this, exercise is likely to transition from a CAM modality to a conventional modality and to be taught in more U.S. medical schools and to be recommended and used as a treatment in U.S. health care institutions.

## Other CAM Practices

CAM practices also include traditional healing practices and energy therapies. Traditional healers may rely on touch as well as other senses, for example, sound—the chiming of a bell or the quality of a singing voice. These healers may incorporate counseling or psychological therapy in addition to prescribing herbal remedies.

**Energy therapies** are forms of treatment that use energy interactions between living organisms, energies produced by the organism itself, and those produced by outside sources such as electromagnetic energy. The recognition that the body produces electromagnetic fields has led to the development of many diagnostic procedures in Western medicine, including electroencephalography (EEG), electromyography (EMG), electrocardiography (ECG), and nuclear magnetic resonance imaging (NMRI). Energy therapies are based on the concept that energy surrounds and penetrates the body and can be influenced by movement, touch, pressure, or the placement of hands in or through the fields. Some evidence supports energy theory because the body's electromagnetic energy can be measured through ECG, EMG, and EEG technologies.

**Reiki** is an example of energy therapy; it is intended to correct disturbances in the flow of life energy (ki in the Japanese tradition) and enhance the body's healing powers through the use of specific hand positions on or near the patient's body. **Therapeutic touch** is derived from ancient techniques involving using the hands to detect and transmit energy (electromagnetic energy). It is based on the premise that healers can identify and correct energy imbalances by passing their hands over the patient's body.

**Magnetic therapies** include the application of therapeutic magnets to the body to manage pain, increase blood flow, and treat conditions such as arthritic pain. One animal study reported an increased rate of wound healing using magnets, but comprehensive literature reviews of studies on therapeutic magnets report little or no supporting evidence.

TERMS

**energy therapies** Forms of CAM treatment that use varying sources of energy originating either within the body or from outside sources to promote health and healing.

**Reiki** A CAM practice intended to correct disturbances in the flow of life energy and enhance the body's healing powers through the use of various hand positions on the patient.

**therapeutic touch** A CAM practice based on the premise that healers can identify and correct energy imbalances by passing their hands over the patient's body.

**magnetic therapies** A form of alternative medicine that uses magnets to treat pain and other health problems.

**tai chi** An ancient Chinese philosophy adapted as a CAM energy modality and practiced as exercise involving slow, continuous, meditative movements accompanied by deep breathing, and used for maintaining and restoring health.

## When Does CAM Become Conventional Medicine?

From one point of view, when ancient healers used the foxglove plant for medicinal purposes, it could be considered "alternative"—or even superstition. But when the plant's content, digitalis, was scientifically shown to be a useful pharmaceutical, it became a conventional medication for the treatment of heart disease. Because of modern research sponsored mostly by the NIH, a number of therapeutic alternatives have become mainstream medicine.

People of all backgrounds use CAM; use is greater among women than men and among those with higher levels of education and higher incomes. More than 42% of hospitals offer one or more CAM therapies, and 57 major U.S. universities have added integrative medical centers to their facilities. In addition, because of the widespread use of CAM among patients, U.S. medical schools include integrative medicine in their curricula, and the American Board of Physician Specialties recognizes it as a distinct medical discipline.

In 2017, yoga was the most practiced CAM in the United States—by 14% of adults, according to an NCCIH survey. Meditation also soared in popularity, tripling from 4% to 14% over five years. Other increasingly common CAM therapies in the United States include the following examples.

### Tai Chi and Fibromyalgia

A once mysterious and misunderstood disorder, fibromyalgia causes chronic pain throughout the body and general fatigue. It can be partially treated with drugs, but exercise is an important component of fibromyalgia therapy because it helps maintain or improve muscle strength and function. **Tai chi,** a CAM practice with origins in ancient China, uses slow, meditative movements

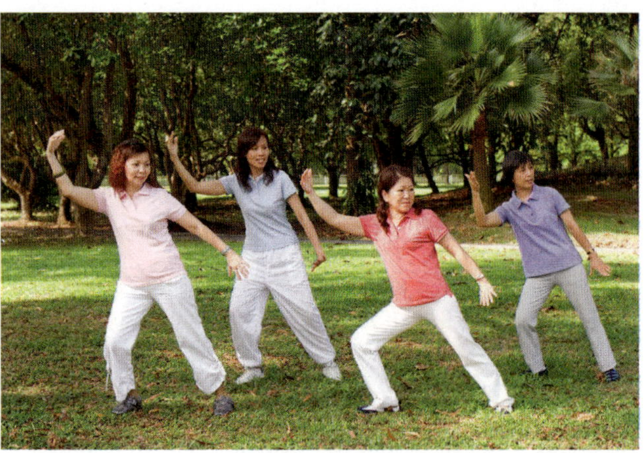

Tai chi combines gentle movements with mental focus, breathing, and relaxation. It has been shown to improve balance and stability and to help people with chronic conditions cope with pain. Phil Date/123RF

for maintaining and restoring health. Tai chi has long been known to offer many benefits, including gains in strength and flexibility, and it has also been shown to be helpful in pain management. A study published in the *New England Journal of Medicine* tracked the symptoms of two groups of fibromyalgia patients: one that learned a variety of tai chi movements and another that practiced stretching exercises and received wellness counseling. Over the course of the study, the patients who practiced tai chi reported significantly less pain than the other group, and the benefits lasted well beyond the study's end.

**CAM Therapies and Back Pain** CAM therapies are used more often for back pain than for any other condition. Over 80% of adults suffer from low-back pain at some point in their lives. A wide survey found that people tended to try chiropractic, massage, and acupuncture therapies for more severe cases and yoga, tai chi, and qigong for milder cases. Respondents said they elected to try CAM because conventional medical treatments weren't providing adequate pain relief. Nearly two-thirds said they experienced significantly reduced pain as a result of CAM therapy.

## Evaluating Complementary and Alternative Therapies

Compared to conventional medical therapies, CAM has less scientific information available about it and less regulation of associated products and providers. CAM therapies are more difficult to investigate than conventional therapies for several reasons. One problem is that most CAM therapies have a smaller effect size than conventional treatments, making experimental outcomes difficult to detect. Other difficulties include delayed effects (CAM therapies require longer studies and therefore more funding), variable effects (not all CAM therapies work equally well on everybody), and combination effects (several approaches used together may produce results not seen in a single approach–violating the traditional scientific tenet of parsimony). The bottom line is that it is important to take an active role when you are seeking medical information and advice in any modality, conventional or unconventional.

**Working with Your Physician** When a health issue might be serious, the NCCIH advises consumers not to seek complementary therapies without first consulting a conventional health care provider. Become informed and discuss conventional treatments that have been shown to be beneficial for your condition. If you are thinking of trying any complementary or alternative therapies, discuss these with your physician, pharmacist, or other conventional provider who is knowledgeable about your health status and is also informed about CAM or is willing to learn by consulting proper resources. If they are not informed about CAM, it may be helpful to share information from reliable, evidence-based sources with them. Areas to discuss with your physician or pharmacist include the safety of the treatment; evidence for its effectiveness; when the treatment should be administered; and cost.

If appropriate, schedule a follow-up visit with your physician to assess your condition and your progress after a certain amount of time using a complementary therapy. Keep a symptom diary to track your symptoms and gauge your progress. Symptoms such as pain and fatigue are difficult to recall with accuracy, so an ongoing symptom diary is an important tool. If your physician advises against CAM and can support the advice with good evidence, you should probably not use it. If you plan to pursue a therapy against your physician's advice, tell them. For supplements, particularly botanicals, pharmacists can also be an excellent source of information; inform them about any other unconventional or conventional medications you are taking.

**Questioning the CAM Practitioner** You can also get information from individual practitioners, educational programs, professional organizations, and state licensing boards. Ask about education, training, licensing, and certification. If appropriate, check with local or state regulatory agencies or the consumer affairs department to determine if any complaints have been lodged against the practitioner. Ask the practitioner why he or she thinks the therapy will be beneficial for your condition. Ask for a full description of the therapy and any potential side effects. In all cases, demand an evidence-based approach. Describe in detail any conventional treatments you are receiving or plan to receive. Ask how long the therapy should continue before it can be determined if it is beneficial. Ask about the expected cost of the treatment. Will your health insurance pay some or all of the costs?

If anything an unconventional practitioner says or recommends directly conflicts with advice from your physician, discuss it with your physician before making any major changes in your current treatment regimen or lifestyle.

> **Ask Yourself**
>
> **QUESTIONS FOR CRITICAL THINKING AND REFLECTION**
>
> Have you ever considered using a complementary or alternative treatment? If so, was it in addition to conventional treatment or instead of it? What kind of research did you do before having the treatment? What advice did your conventional health care provider give you about it?

# PAYING FOR HEALTH CARE

The U.S. health care system is one of the most advanced and comprehensive in the world, but it is also the most expensive (Figure 16.6). In 2020, Americans spent $4.1 trillion on health care, or more than $12,500 per person. Many factors contribute to the high cost of health care in the United States,

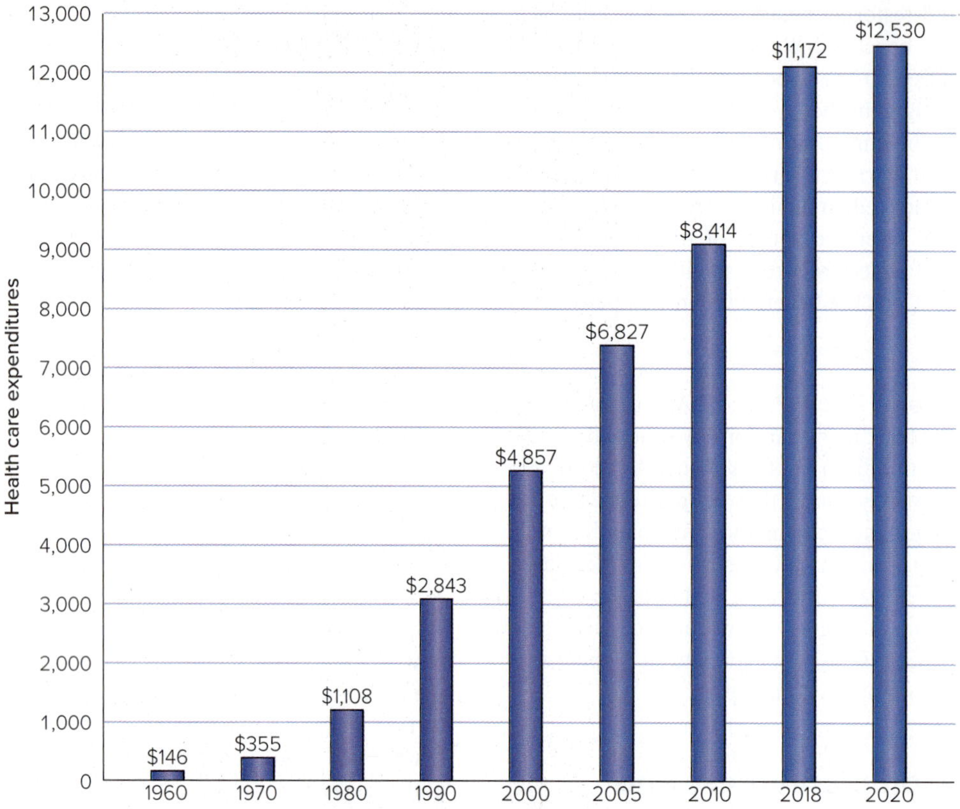


**FIGURE 16.6 Per-capita national health care expenditures, 1960–2018.**

SOURCE: Centers for Medicare & Medicaid Services. 2021. "National Health Expenditure Data: Historical." https://www.cms.gov/Research-Statistics-Data-and-Systems/Statistics-Trends-and-Reports/NationalHealthExpendData/NHE-Fact-Sheet.

including the cost of advanced equipment and new technology, expensive treatments for some illnesses, aging of the population, and the demand for profits by many commercial health enterprises. When we look at what rich countries spend on health per person and life expectancy in those countries, Americans spend far more money and live shorter lives (see Figure 20.7).

## The Affordable Care Act

The **Affordable Care Act (ACA)**, also called Obamacare, aims to tackle expanding health care costs, regulate the way insurance companies provide medical coverage, and encourage as many Americans as possible to get health coverage.

The ACA encourages healthy people to purchase insurance because more people paying into plans helps insurance companies keep **premiums** lower. An individual mandate had required that everyone buy a minimal insurance plan or pay a tax penalty. Although Congress repealed this mandate, a record-breaking 13.6 million new people enrolled in 2022. Contributing factors to this surge of enrollment were cost-lowering measures passed by Congress, increased advertising by the Biden administration, and disruptions to employer-provided insurance caused by the pandemic.

Two key provisions of the ACA are that it increases preventive services and it forbids insurance companies from discriminating on the basis of preexisting medical conditions. Preventive services include doctors' services, inpatient and outpatient hospital care, prescription drug coverage, pregnancy and childbirth, and mental health services. Before the ACA, a preexisting condition such as depression or diabetes–even pregnancy–could be the basis for insurance companies' rejecting a new patient. By some estimates, as many as 50 million Americans–the vast majority of them employed–had no health insurance.

Despite the ACA's successes and recent government subsidies, American Indians and Alaska Natives (AIAN), Native Hawaiians and Other Pacific Islanders (NHOPI), African Americans, and Hispanics are still more likely than Euro-Americans to be uninsured. In states that have not expanded Medicaid, uninsured rates have been higher for all people. More children under the age of 19 in poverty were uninsured in 2020 than in 2018.

TERMS

**Affordable Care Act** A U.S. law requiring most health insurance plans to include certain rights and protections (e.g., mental health and preventive services, no penalties for preexisting conditions, and the right to appeal health service charges). The law attempts to make health care more affordable for individuals and families.

**premium** The amount you pay each month for your insurance.

## How Health Insurance Works

Health insurance as required under the ACA protects you against costs incurred for medical expenses due to illness or injury. Depending on the policy, coverage may also include preventive services such as yearly exams; other physician services; medications; hospital stays; emergency department visits; physical, occupational, and speech therapy; vision care; dental coverage; and other expenses. Some insurance policies provide riders for specific CAM coverage for an additional charge. Policies differ based on the services covered, the amount of the **deductible** and **copayment,** and the limit of coverage. Of course, with many plans, the more services you add to the policy, the higher the premium. Coverage may be provided as an employment benefit or through a government-sponsored plan such as Medicaid (for certain disabled and low-income individuals) or Medicare (typically for individuals aged 65 and over and those with certain illnesses). See the box "Choosing a Health Insurance Plan."

Health insurance plans are either fee-for-service (indemnity) or managed care. With both types, the individual or his or her employer pays a basic premium, usually on a monthly basis; there are often other payments as well.

**Traditional Fee-for-Service (Indemnity) Plans** In a fee-for-service plan, or **indemnity plan,** you can go to any physician or hospital you choose. You or the provider sends the bill to your insurance company, which pays part of it. Usually you have to pay a deductible amount each year, and then the plan will pay a percentage–often 80%–of what it considers the "usual and customary" charge for covered services. You pay the remaining 20%, which is known as *coinsurance.*

**Managed Care Plans** **Managed care plans** have agreements with a network of specified physicians, hospitals, and health care providers to offer a range of services to plan members at reduced cost. In general, you have lower out-of-pocket costs and less paperwork with a managed care plan than with an indemnity plan, but you also have less freedom in choosing your health care providers. Most Americans with job-based insurance are covered by managed care plans. These include:

- **Health maintenance organizations (HMOs)** offer members a range of services for a set monthly fee. You choose a primary care physician who manages your care and refers you to specialists if you need them. If you go outside the HMO, you have to pay for the service yourself.
- **Preferred provider organizations (PPOs)** have arrangements with physicians and other providers who have agreed to accept lower fees.
- **Point-of-service (POS) plans** are options offered by many HMOs in which you can see a specialist or a physician outside the plan, but you will have to pay most or all of the cost unless your primary care physician referred you.

Many managed care plans try to reduce costs over the long term by paying for routine preventive care, such as regular checkups and screening tests and prenatal care; they may also encourage prevention by offering health education and lifestyle modification programs for members.

**Government Programs** Americans aged 65 and over and younger people with certain disabilities can be covered

### Ask Yourself

**QUESTIONS FOR CRITICAL THINKING AND REFLECTION**

What type of health insurance coverage do you have? If you are covered by your parents' or guardians' insurance, what are the plan's benefits? If you have coverage, do you know what types of medical services are fully or partially covered? What are your copayments and deductibles? If you were faced with a medical emergency, would you know how to contact and work with your insurer to make sure your costs were covered?

### TERMS

**deductible** The amount you pay for services before your insurance coverage begins. For example, if your deductible is $1000, the insurance company won't pay anything for services until your expenses total $1000. The insurance company may fully cover certain services before you've reached your deductible amount.

**copayment** The amount you pay for a particular health care service; your insurance provider pays the balance. For example, for a physical exam that costs $150, you might pay your doctor's office $25 at the time of service (your copayment), and the insurance company would pay $125. The copayment amount may vary according to the type of service you received.

**indemnity plan** A health insurance plan based on a fee for each service provided; the cost is shared between you and the insurance company, and you can go to any physician or hospital you choose.

**managed care plan** A health insurance plan that contracts with providers and health care facilities (the plan's "network") to provide care at reduced costs. There are three types of managed care plans: health management organizations (HMOs), preferred provider organizations (PPOs), and point of service (POS).

**health maintenance organization (HMO)** A type of prepaid health insurance plan that covers services within a network of physicians and other professionals who are contracted with the HMO.

**preferred provider organization (PPO)** A prepaid health insurance plan that contracts with physicians, other professionals, and hospitals to provide services for discounted fees. You can go to any provider including specialists without a PCP referral. Using nonparticipating providers results in higher costs to the patient.

**point-of-service (POS) plan** A type of plan where you pay less if you use physicians, other professionals, and hospitals that belong to the plan's network, but you are required to get a referral from a PCP before going to a specialist. A POS plan combines some of the essentials of both HMO and PPO plans.

## CRITICAL CONSUMER
### Choosing a Health Insurance Plan

Under the Affordable Care Act (ACA), a health insurance marketplace, also called a health exchange, facilitates the purchase of health insurance. But choosing a plan can be a complicated matter—confusing and intimidating. To organize your thinking about this decision, look for answers to the three questions discussed here.

#### 1. What Does the Plan Cover?

These are the 10 categories of health care services that health plans must cover to meet requirements of the ACA:

- Ambulatory patient services (care you get without being admitted to a hospital)
- Emergency services
- Hospitalization
- Maternity and newborn care
- Mental health and substance use disorder services including behavioral health treatment
- Prescription drugs
- Rehabilitative and habilitative services and devices (to help people with injuries, disabilities, or chronic conditions gain or recover mental and physical skills)
- Laboratory services
- Preventive services and chronic disease management
- Pediatric services, including oral and vision care

Insurance provided by large employers may differ slightly. You can ask for a summary of benefits and coverage to see what is covered.

#### 2. How Much Does the Plan Cost?

You pay for health insurance in two ways—through (1) your monthly premium and (2) the out-of-pocket expenses you pay when you receive care. Out-of-pocket expenses include deductibles, coinsurance, and copayments (see text for definitions). The higher the monthly premium you pay, the lower will be your out-of-pocket expenses.

For the ACA, the "metal categories"—bronze, silver, gold, and platinum—were created to help people choose a plan by simplifying the differences between costs and levels of coverage. As you consider your choices, note what the total cost of care includes: your premium plus out-of-pocket costs.

Generally, your monthly insurance payment is lowest in the bronze category, but deductibles are higher and you may have more out-of-pocket costs. Platinum plans typically have the highest premiums, but deductibles and out-of-pocket costs are low. If your income qualifies you for cost-sharing reductions, you can enroll in a silver plan where you get the best of both worlds: a lower premium and a lower deductible. Out-of-pocket costs will be lower as well.

| PLAN CATEGORY | THE INSURANCE COMPANY PAYS | YOU PAY |
|---|---|---|
| Bronze | 60% | 40% |
| Silver | 70% | 30% |
| Gold | 80% | 20% |
| Platinum | 90% | 10% |

The "metal categories" help you determine how you and your insurance plan share total costs.

SOURCE: https://www.healthcare.gov/choose-a-plan/plans-categories/.

#### 3. Which Doctors and Hospitals Are in Your Plan?

Every health insurance plan has a network of providers who agree to provide services to plan members for specific prices. As you've learned, plans vary in how restricted members are in relation to these networks. Some only allow members to receive services provided by doctors, specialists, or hospitals in the plan's network. Others are more flexible: They may charge less when plan members use doctors, hospitals, and other health care providers that belong to the plan's network; require members to get referrals to go outside the network; or allow members to use doctors, hospitals, and providers outside their network without a referral for an additional cost. It makes sense, then, to check the health plan and your doctor's office to make sure your desired providers are in the network of the plan you are considering.

You can get more information, browse plans, and apply for coverage at HealthCare.gov.

by **Medicare,** a federal health insurance program that helps pay for hospitalization, physician services, and prescription drugs. As a result of limits placed on payments, however, some physicians and managed care programs have stopped accepting Medicare patients. **Medicaid** is a joint federal-state health insurance program that covers some low-income people, especially children, pregnant women, and people with certain disabilities. The number of people and the number and cost of services covered by government programs has grown in recent years, challenging the ability of these programs to provide needed coverage.

**TERMS**

**Medicare** A federal health insurance program for people aged 65 and over and for younger people with certain disabilities.

**Medicaid** A federally subsidized state-run plan of health care for people with low income.

## TIPS FOR TODAY AND THE FUTURE

Most of the time, you can take care of yourself without consulting a health care provider. When you need professional care, you can still take responsibility for yourself by making informed decisions.

**RIGHT NOW YOU CAN:**

- Make sure that you have enough of your prescription medications on hand and that your prescriptions are up to date.
- If you take any supplements (dietary or herbal), ask your pharmacist if they can interact with any prescription drugs you are taking.
- Stock your home and car with basic first aid supplies.

**IN THE FUTURE YOU CAN:**

- Use professional and authoritative internet resources to thoroughly research complementary or alternative medical treatments you are using or considering to make sure they are considered safe and effective.
- Review your medical insurance needs by checking your coverage under your parents' or guardians' policy if you are under age 26 or by checking your state's online health insurance exchange, and contact your insurance agent if you have questions about your coverage.

## SUMMARY

- Informed self-care requires knowing how to evaluate symptoms. You should see a physician if symptoms are severe, unusual, persistent, or recurrent.
- Self-treatment doesn't necessarily require medication, but over-the-counter (OTC) drugs can be a helpful part of self-care.
- Conventional medicine is characterized by a focus on the physical causes of disease, the identification of signs and symptoms, the use of drugs and surgery for treatment, and the use of scientific thinking and research to understand diseases.
- Conventional practitioners include medical doctors, doctors of osteopathic medicine, podiatrists, optometrists, and dentists, as well as other highly trained professionals.
- The diagnostic process involves a medical history, a physical exam, and medical tests. Patients should ask questions about tests and treatments recommended by their providers.
- Safe use of prescription drugs requires knowledge of what the medication is supposed to do, how and when to take it, and the possible side effects.
- All surgical procedures carry risk; patients should ask many questions, including about alternatives.
- Complementary and alternative medicine (CAM) is defined as those therapies and practices that are not part of conventional health care and medical practice as taught in most U.S. medical schools and offered in most U.S. hospitals.
- *Integrative health* is a term used when both conventional and CAM methods are used to treat the whole person rather than, for example, just one organ system.
- CAM focuses on ways to restore the individual to optimal functioning using a body of knowledge based on the accumulated observations and experience of practitioners, often over decades or centuries, and, more recently, on the scientific evaluation of safety and efficacy.
- CAM practices can be classified into several broad categories: alternative medical systems, mind-body medicine, biologically based products, manipulative and body-based practices, and other CAM practices.
- Alternative medical systems such as traditional Chinese medicine and homeopathy are complete systems of medical philosophy, theory, and practice.
- Mind-body medicine includes meditation, biofeedback, group support, hypnosis, and prayer.
- Biologically based products include herbal remedies, vitamins, minerals, botanicals, animal tissue products, and dietary supplements.
- Manipulative and body-based practices include massage and other healing techniques; the most frequently used is chiropractic.
- Other CAM practices include traditional healing practices and energy therapies.
- Because there is currently less information available about CAM and less regulation of its providers and modalities, consumers should be proactive in researching and choosing treatments, using critical thinking skills, examining the available evidence-based information available, and exercising caution.
- The Affordable Care Act and other government reforms of the health care system (particularly the insurance industry) aim to make affordable health insurance coverage available to more Americans.
- Health insurance plans are usually described as either fee-for-service (indemnity) or managed care plans. Indemnity plans allow consumers more choice in medical providers, but managed care plans are less expensive.
- Government programs include Medicaid for people with low income and Medicare for those aged 65 and over or chronically disabled.

## FOR MORE INFORMATION

*Affordable Care Act.* Provides information on the Affordable Care Act and the Health Insurance Marketplace.

https://www.healthcare.gov

*Exercise Is Medicine.* Provides information on the initiative to promote physical activity, as well as a series of factsheets with guidelines on exercise for people with many different chronic conditions.

https://exerciseismedicine.org

## BEHAVIOR CHANGE STRATEGY
### Adhering to Your Physician's Instructions

Even though you sometimes have to entrust yourself to the care of medical professionals, you are still responsible for your own behavior. Following medical instructions and advice often requires the same kind of behavioral self-management that's involved in quitting smoking, losing weight, or changing eating patterns. For example, if you have an illness or injury, you may be instructed to take medication at certain times of the day, do special exercises or movements, or change your diet.

The medical profession recognizes the importance of patient adherence and encourages different strategies to support it, such as the following:

1. Use reminders placed at home, in the car, at work, on your computer screensaver, or elsewhere that improve follow-through in taking medication and keeping scheduled appointments. To help you remember to take medications:
   - Use one of the many quality apps available for your phone or computer. (Several of the best ones are listed and reviewed at http://www.singlecare.com/blog/best-medication-reminder-apps/)
   - Link taking the medication with some well-established routine, like brushing your teeth or eating breakfast.
   - Use a medication calendar, and check off each pill.
   - Use a medication organizer or pill dispenser.
   - Plan ahead; don't wait until you take the last pill to get a prescription refilled.
2. Use a journal or another form of self-monitoring to keep a detailed account of your health-related behaviors, such as taking pills on schedule, following dietary recommendations, following an exercise program, and so on.
3. Use a self-reward system so that desired behavior changes are encouraged, with a focus on short-term rewards.
4. Develop a clear image or explanation of how the medication or behavior change will improve your health, how you will look and feel, and your long-term well-being.

If these strategies don't help you stick with your treatment plan, you may need to consider other possible explanations for your lack of adherence. For example, are you confused about some aspect of the treatment? Do you find the schedule for taking your medications too complicated, or do the drugs have bothersome side effects that tempt you to avoid them? Do you feel that the recommended treatment is unnecessary or unlikely to help? Are you afraid of becoming dependent on a medication or that you'll be judged negatively if people know about your condition or treatment? A follow-up discussion with a health professional (your physician, physician assistant, nurse practitioner, dietitian, or physical therapist) and an examination of your attitudes and beliefs about your condition and treatment plan can also help improve your adherence.

*HealthIT.* Presents tips and tools related to health information technology.

https://www.healthit.gov

mobile*PDR*. App from the Prescribers' Digital Reference that offers information about drugs you may be prescribed.

https://www.pdr.net/

*National Center for Complementary and Integrative Health (NCCIH).* Provides background information and research results on many forms of CAM.

https://nccih.nih.gov

*U.S. Food and Drug Administration: For Consumers.* Provides materials about supplements, prescription and OTC drugs, and other FDA-regulated products.

http://www.fda.gov/consumers/

## SELECTED BIBLIOGRAPHY


Abrams, Z. 2021. Controlling the spread of misinformation. *Monitor on Psychology 52*(2): 44.

Academic Consortium for Integrative Medicine & Health. 2022. *Member Listing* (https://www.imconsortium.org/).

Agency for Healthcare Research and Quality. 2020. *The 10 Questions You Should Know* (https://www.ahrq.gov/questions/10questions.html).

American Academy of Family Physicians. 2022. *Patient Protection and Affordable Care Act (ACA)* (https://www.aafp.org/advocacy/advocacy-topics/health-care-coverage/aca.html).

American Association of Naturopathic Physicians. n.d. *About Naturopathic Medicine* (http://www.naturopathic.org/medicine).

American Board of Medical Specialties. 2022. *Guide to Medical Specialties* (https://www.abms.org/wp-content/uploads/2021/12/ABMS-Guide-to-Medical-Specialties-2022.pdf).

American Chiropractic Association. 2019. *Key Facts and Figures About the Chiropractic Profession* (www.acatoday.org/News-Publications/newsroom/key-facts/).

American Hospital Association. 2020. *Hospital Emergency Room Visits per 1,000 Population by Ownership Type* (http://kff.org/other/state-indicator/emergency-room-visits-by-ownership/).

Baer, H. A., et al. 2012. A dialogue between naturopathy and critical medical anthropology: What constitutes holistic health? Medical Anthropology Quarterly 26(2): 241–256.

Ball, P. 2020. The lightning-fast quest for COVID vaccines–and what it means for other diseases. *Nature: News Feature* (https://www.nature.com/articles/d41586-020-03626-1).

Buenz, E. J., R. Verpoorte, and B. A. Bauer. 2018. The ethnopharmacologic contribution to bioprospecting natural products. *Annual Review of Pharmacology and Toxicology* 58: 509–530.

Centers for Medicare & Medicaid Services. 2022. Marketplace 2022 open enrollment period report: Final national snapshot (https://www.cms.gov/newsroom/fact-sheets/marketplace-2022-open-enrollment-period-report-final-national-snapshot).

Clarke, T. C., et al. 2015. Trends in the use of complementary health approaches among adults: United States, 2002–2012. National Health Statistics Reports 79: 1–16.

Clark, T. C., et al. 2018. Use of yoga, meditation, and chiropractors among U.S. adults aged 18 and over. NCHS Data Brief, No. 325. Hyattsville, MD: National Center for Health Statistics. (https://www.cdc.gov/nchs/data/databriefs/db325-h.pdf).

Commonwealth Fund. 2015. The Problem of Underinsurance and How Rising Deductibles Will Make It Worse (http://www.commonwealthfund.org/publications/issue-briefs/2015/may/problem-of-underinsurance).

Cowen, V. S., and V. Cyr. 2015. Complementary and alternative medicine in US medical schools. Advances in Medical Education and Practice 6: 113–117.

Eissa, A., et al. 2022. Implementing high-quality primary care through a health equity lens. *Annals of Family Medicine* 20(2): 164–169.

Fleming, N. 2020. Coronavirus misinformation, and how scientists can help fight it. *Nature 583*: 155–156.

Fong, K. 2021. The U.S. health care system isn't built for primary care. *Harvard Business Review* (https://hbr.org/2021/09/the-u-s-health-care-system-isnt-built-for-primary-care).

Freed, M., T. Neuman, and J. Cubanski. 2021. 10 FAQs on prescription drug importation. *Kaiser Family Foundation* (https://www.kff.org/medicare/issue-brief/10-faqs-on-prescription-drug-importation/).

Ghildayal, N., et al. 2016. Complementary and alternative medicine use in the US adult low back pain population. *Global Advances in Health and Medicine* 5(1): 69–78.

Health Canada. 2022. *Drugs and Health Products* (https://www.canada.ca/en/services/health/drug-health-products.html).

Johns Hopkins Medicine 2022. *Types of Complementary and Alternative Medicine* (https://www.hopkinsmedicine.org/health/wellness-and-prevention/types-of-complementary-and-alternative-medicine).

Katz-Sanger, M. 2022. On more generous terms, Obamacare proves newly popular. *The New York Times* (https://www.nytimes.com/2021/12/22/upshot/on-more-generous-terms-obamacare-proves-newly-popular.html).

Keisler-Starkey, K., and Bunch, L. N. 2021. Health insurance coverage in the United States: 2020. (https://www.census.gov/library/publications/2021/demo/p60-274.html).

Kwok, J. Y. Y., et al. 2022. Stay mindfully active during the coronavirus pandemic: A feasibility study of mHealth-delivered mindfulness yoga program for people with Parkinson's disease. *BMC Complementary Medicine and Therapies* 22(37) (https://doi.org/10.1186/s12906-022-03519-y).

Lu, L., et al. 2022. Evidence on acupuncture therapies is underused in clinical practice and health policy. *British Medical Journal* 376: e067475.

Micozzi, M. S. 2018. *Fundamentals of Complementary and Alternative Medicine*, 6th ed. New York: Elsevier.

Mulcahy, A. W., et al. 2021. International prescription drug price comparisons. Santa Monica, CA: RAND Corporation (https://www.rand.org/pubs/research_reports/RR2956.html).

National Academies of Sciences Engineering and Medicine, Health and Medicine Division. 2021. *Implementing High-Quality Primary Care: Rebuilding the Foundation of Health Care*. National Academies Press

National Center for Complementary and Integrative Health. 2022. *Complementary, Alternative or Integrative Health: What's In a Name?* (https://www.nccih.nih.gov/health/complementary-alternative-or-integrative-health-whats-in-a-name).

National Center for Complementary and Integrative Health. 2020. *Placebo Effect* (https://nccih.nih.gov/health/placebo).

National Institutes of Health. 2021. *Dietary Supplements in the Time of COVID-19* (https://ods.od.nih.gov/factsheets/DietarySupplementsInTheTimeOfCOVID19-Consumer/).

National University of Natural Medicine. 2019. Licensing and scope of practice: How it affects your career as a naturopathic physician. (https://nunm.edu/2019/05/nd-licensing-and-scope/).

O'Malley, P. A. 2012. Preventing and reporting adverse drug events: Pharmacovigilance for the clinical nurse specialist. Clinical Nurse Specialist 26(3): 136–137.

Pew Research Center. 2017. Vast majority of Americans say benefits of childhood vaccines outweigh risks (https://www.pewresearch.org/internet/wp-content/uploads/sites/9/2017/02/PS_2017.02.02_Vaccines_FINAL.pdf).

Physicians' Desk Reference. 2017. *PDR for Nonprescription Drugs*, 71st ed. Montvale, NJ: Thomson Healthcare.

Society of Homeopaths. 2022. *What Is Homeopathy?* (https://homeopathy-soh.org/homeopathy-explained/what-is-homeopathy/).

Solis-Moreira, J. 2021. How did we develop a COVID-19 vaccine so quickly? *Medical News Today* (https://www.medicalnewstoday.com/articles/how-did-we-develop-a-covid-19-vaccine-so-quickly).

Tariq, R. A., et al. 2021. Medication errors and prevention. *National Center for Biotechnology Information* (https://www.ncbi.nlm.nih.gov/books/NBK519065/).

U.S. Bureau of Labor Statistics. 2021. Projections overview and highlights, 2020-30. *Monthly Labor Reivew* (https://www.bls.gov/opub/mlr/2021/article/projections-overview-and-highlights-2020-30.htm).

U.S. Food and Drug Administration. 2018. Understanding Unapproved Use of Approved Drugs "Off-Label" (https://www.fda.gov/patients/learn-about-expanded-access-and-other-treatment-options/understanding-unapproved-use-approved-drugs-label).

U.S. Food and Drug Administration. 2020. *Information for Consumers and Patients: Drugs* (https://www.fda.gov/drugs/resources-you-drugs/information-consumers-and-patients-drugs).

Wang, C., et al. 2010. A randomized trial of tai chi for fibromyalgia. New England Journal of Medicine 363(8): 743–754.

Wong, C. 2019. 5 Types of Complementary and Alternative Medicine *VeryWellHealth* (https://www.verywellhealth.com/types-of-complementary-and-alternative-medicine-88741).

World Health Organization. 2020. Managing the COVID-19 infodemic: Promoting healthy behaviours and mitigating the harm from misinformation and disinformation. *Statement* (https://www.who.int/news/item/23-09-2020-managing-the-covid-19-infodemic-promoting-healthy-behaviours-and-mitigating-the-harm-from-misinformation-and-disinformation).

**Design Elements:** Assess Yourself icon: Aleksey Boldin/Alamy Stock Photo; Diversity Matters icon: Rawpixel Ltd/Getty Images; Wellness on Campus icon: Radius Images/Alamy Stock Photo; Take Charge icon: VisualCommunications/Getty Images; Critical Consumer icon: pagadesign/Getty Images.

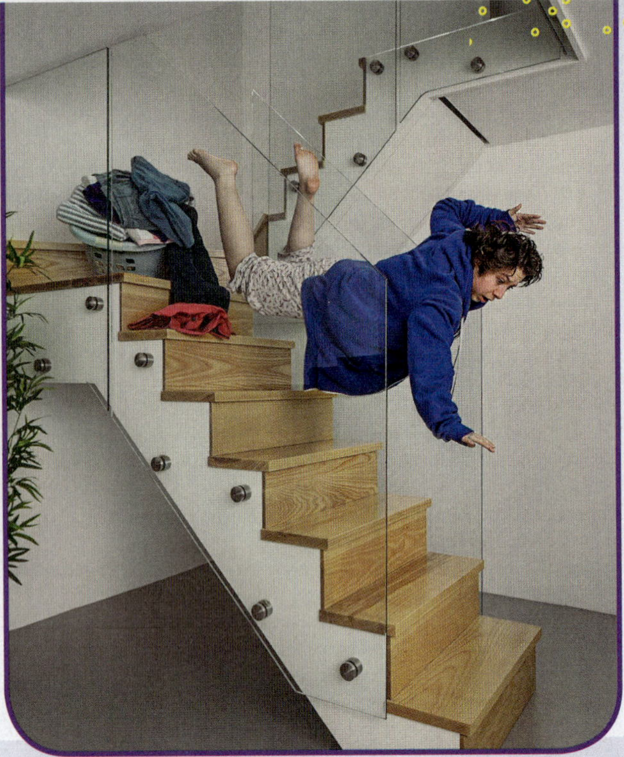
Justin Paget/Getty Images

## CHAPTER OBJECTIVES

- List the most common unintentional injuries and strategies for preventing them
- Discuss violence and intentional injuries, and how to protect yourself
- List strategies for helping others in an emergency

CHAPTER 17

# Personal Safety

Injuries, both intentional and unintentional, caused almost 201,000 deaths in 2020. This was the fourth leading cause of death for Americans in that year, up 16% from the previous year. The economic cost of injuries is high, with more than $4 trillion spent each year for medical care and rehabilitation of injured people. Injuries also cause emotional suffering for injured people and their families, friends, and colleagues.

Engineering strategies such as seat belts can help lower injury rates, as can the passage and enforcement of safety-related laws, such as those requiring tamper-proof containers for over-the-counter medications. Public education can also help prevent injuries.

If an injury occurs when no harm is intended, it is considered an **unintentional injury.** Motor vehicle crashes, falls, and fires often result in unintentional injuries. Public health officials prefer not to use the word *accidents* to describe unintentional injuries because it suggests events beyond human control. *Injuries* are predictable outcomes that can be controlled or prevented. In contrast, an **intentional injury** is one that is purposely inflicted.

Although Americans tend to express more concern about intentional injuries, unintentional injuries are far more common. Unintentional injuries are the leading cause of death for Americans ages 1 to 45 and usually rank third among the 10 leading causes of death; in 2020, however, Covid-19 ranked third. Because unintentional injuries are so common, they account for more **years of potential life lost** than any other cause of death. Let's look closely at the most common types of unintentional injuries.

TERMS

**unintentional injury** An injury that occurs when no harm was intended.

**intentional injury** An injury that is purposely inflicted by you or another person.

**years of potential life lost** The difference between an individual's life expectancy and their age at death.

## UNINTENTIONAL INJURIES

Unintentional injuries are the leading cause of death in the United States for people aged 1 to 45. Injury situations are categorized into four general classes based on where they occur: home injuries, motor vehicle injuries, leisure injuries, and work injuries. The greatest number of disabling injuries occur in the home; falls are the leading cause of nonfatal, unintentional injuries that are treated in hospital emergency departments. Wherever an injury occurs, however, your response can have a dramatic influence on the outcome.

### What Causes an Injury?

Most injuries are caused by a combination of human and environmental factors. Human factors are inner conditions or attitudes that lead to an unsafe state, whether physical, emotional, or psychological. A common human factor that leads to injuries is risk-taking behavior. People vary in the amount of risk they tend to take in life, but young men are especially prone to taking risks (see the box "Injuries among Young Men"). Some people take risks to win the admiration of their peers. Other people simply overestimate their physical abilities or enjoy attempting to defy the laws of nature. Alcohol and drug use is another common risk factor that leads to many injuries and deaths.

Psychological and emotional factors can also play a role in injuries. People sometimes act on the basis of inadequate or inaccurate beliefs about what is safe or unsafe. For example, a person who believes that seat belts trap people in cars when a crash occurs and decides not to wear a seat belt is acting on inaccurate information. However, many people who have accurate information still decide to engage in risky behavior. Young people often have unsafe attitudes, such as "I won't get hurt" or "It won't happen to me." Such attitudes can lead to risk taking and ultimately to injuries.

Environmental factors leading to injury are external conditions and circumstances. They may be natural (weather conditions, the undertow of the ocean at the beach), social (a drunk driver), work-related (defective equipment, a slippery surface), or home-related (faulty wiring). Making the environment safer is an important aspect of safety. Laws are often passed to try to make our environment safer. Examples include speed limits on highways, workplace safety requirements, and childhood immunizations.

**QUICK STATS**

**Since 1999, the age-adjusted drug-poisoning death rate has more than tripled, from 6.1 per 100,000 in 1999 to 21.6 per 100,000 in 2019.**

—National Center for Health Statistics, 2021

### Home Injuries

The most common fatal **home injuries** are the result of poisonings and falls (Table 17.1). The number of fatal injuries from firearms—in homicidal and suicidal shootings—has greatly increased.

**Poisoning** Overdose deaths began climbing before the Covid-19 pandemic, but the pandemic likely exacerbated the trend. In the latest data, the highest number of unintentional deaths due to drug poisoning occurred among people ages 35–44; people in the adjacent age groups (25–34 years and 45–54 years) followed closely behind. In 2021, about 13,500 deaths were attributed to prescription drug overdoses.

Prescriptions for opioid painkillers, such as codeine, hydrocodone, and morphine, are relatively easy to obtain. These drugs can quickly lead to addiction or overdose. Medications are safe only when used as prescribed. See Chapter 8 for more on opioids and the risk of addiction and overdose.

The most common type of gas poisoning is by carbon monoxide. Carbon monoxide gas is emitted by motor vehicle exhaust and heating equipment that runs on a fuel (e.g., gas, oil, kerosene, wood, charcoal). To prevent poisoning by gases, never operate or idle a vehicle in an enclosed space, like a garage, have your furnace inspected yearly, and use caution with any substance or device that produces potentially toxic fumes.

To be prepared for an unintentional poisoning, keep the national poison control hotline number (800-222-1222) in a convenient location or in your phone contacts. A call to the hotline will be routed to a local poison control center, which provides expert emergency advice 24 hours a day. If a poisoning occurs, act quickly. Remove the poison from contact with the victim's eyes, skin, or mouth, or move the victim away from contact with poisonous gases. Call the poison control center immediately. Do not follow the emergency instructions on product labels because they may be incorrect.

**Falls** Falls are the leading cause of death among people aged 65 and over. For people ages 44-64, falls are also a significant cause of unintentional death and injury. Most deaths from falls occur on stairs. Alcohol is a contributing factor in many falls. Strategies for preventing falls include the following:

- Install handrails and nonslip surfaces in the shower and bathtub.
- Keep floors, stairs, and outside areas clear of objects or conditions that could cause slipping or tripping, such as ice, snow, electrical cords, and toys.
- Put a light switch by the door of every room so that no one has to walk across a room to turn on a light. Use night lights in bedrooms (placed so as not to disrupt sleep), halls, stairs, and bathrooms.

**TERMS**

**home injuries** Unintentional injuries and deaths that occur in the home and on home premises to occupants, guests, domestic servants, and trespassers; falls, burns, poisonings, suffocations, unintentional shootings, drownings, and electrical shocks are examples.

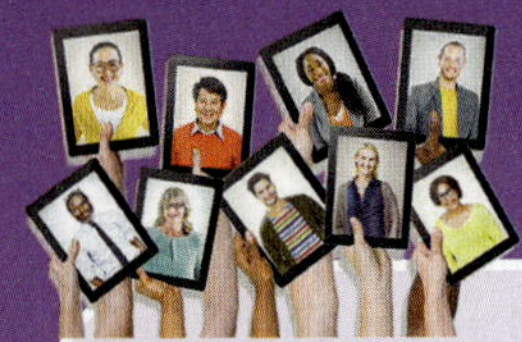

# DIVERSITY MATTERS

## Injuries among Young Men

Males significantly outnumber females in early deaths, whether unintentional or intentional. Women are more likely to *attempt* suicide, but men are more likely to actually kill themselves. Deaths due to drug poisoning have occurred in men more than twice as frequently as in women. Until recently, the number of men dying in crashes was more than twice the number of women, but the gap has narrowed since 2019. Since 1975, motorcyclist deaths have increased by more than 50% among all genders. Except among adults aged 70 and over, the nonfatal injury rate is substantially higher in males than in females—and it peaks among young adult males (see the figure). Gender stereotypes about men and injuries do not apply in every case. For example, in 2009 and 2010, female soldiers deployed to Afghanistan had more injuries and more severe ones than male soldiers. But speaking generally, why do men, especially young men, have such high rates of injury?

Nonfatal injury rate by age and sex.

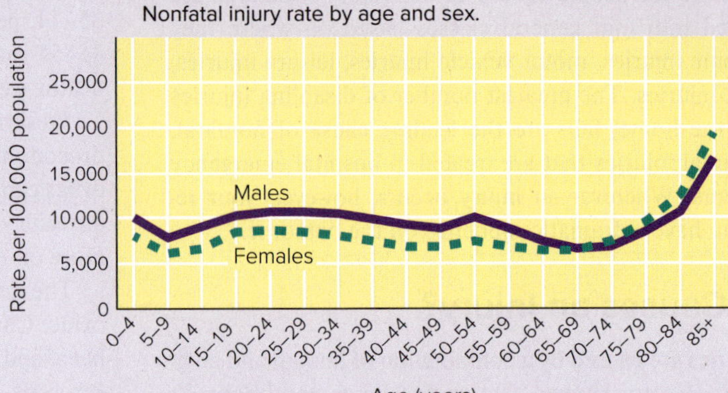


Some researchers suggest that the male hormone testosterone plays a role in risky and aggressive behavior. Differences in brain structure and brain activity may also influence how men and women respond to stressors and how quickly and to what degree they become verbally or physically aggressive in response to anger. Moreover, cultural ideologies that men should inhabit rigid social roles—for example, as the breadwinner, protector, or stoic warrior—can lead to emotional stress when men are faced with a reality that requires more flexibility. Ideologies that men are self-sufficient may conflict with notions about love and affection; thus, if a man cannot meet a partner's expectations for intimacy and a relationship fails, he may feel unable to ask for help and respond with a self-destructive reaction.

Men may also have greater exposure to injury. Compared with women, men drive more miles, have greater access to firearms, and are more likely to ride motorcycles, operate machinery, and have jobs associated with high rates of workplace injuries. They are also more likely to engage in sports and other recreational activities that are associated with high rates of injuries. Greater access to and use of firearms plays a role in higher rates of deaths among men from assault and suicide.

As gender dynamics change, the breadwinner role associated with men is now often shared with women. Both men and women work, and in some cases women are the sole breadwinners. Even as ideas about men as providers still prevail, fathers are expected to participate more fully in raising their children. In divorce cases, men are more likely to lose their home, children, and family, losses cited as factors in suicide.

SOURCES: Centers for Disease Control and Prevention. 2021. *Mortality 1999–2020 on CDC WONDER Online Database* (https://wonder.cdc.gov/controller/saved/D76/D266F024); Scourfield, J., and R. Evans. 2015. Why might men be more at risk of suicide after a relationship breakdown? Sociological insights. *American Journal of Men's Health* 9(5): 380–384; Stergiou-Kita, M., et al. 2016. Gender influences on return to work after mild traumatic brain injury. *Archives of Physical Medicine and Rehabilitation*. 97(2): S40–S45.

**Table 17.1** Leading Causes of Deaths from Unintentional Injury, 2020

| RANK | ALL AGE GROUPS TOTAL | 15–24 YEARS OLD | 25–34 YEARS OLD | 35–44 YEARS OLD |
|---|---|---|---|---|
| 1 | Poisoning* (97,034) | Poisoning (7,387) | Poisoning (22,636) | Poisoning (23,723) |
| 2 | Fall (43,292) | Motor vehicle traffic (6,741) | Drowning (702) | Motor vehicle traffic (6,031) |
| 3 | Motor vehicle traffic (40,698) | Drowning (652) | Motor vehicle traffic (7,929) | Fall (834) |
| 4 | Suffocation (19,810) | Fall (336) | Fall (596) | Drowning (635) |

SOURCE: Centers for Disease Control and Prevention, National Center for Health Statistics. 2022. *"Underlying Cause of Death 1999–2020." CDC WONDER Online Database* (http://wonder.cdc.gov/ucd-icd10.html).

* Mostly overdosing; also includes drug suicide, homicide, and other drug-induced causes

- When climbing a ladder, use both hands. Never stand higher than the third step from the top. When using a stepladder, make sure the spreader brace is in the locked position. With straight ladders, set the base out one foot for every four feet of height.
- Don't stand on chairs to reach things.
- If there are small children in the home, place gates at the top and bottom of stairs. Never leave a baby unattended on a bed or table.

**Fires** The National Fire Protection Association reported 356,500 home structure fires in 2020. Most fires begin in the kitchen, living room, or bedroom. Cooking is now the leading cause of home fire injuries; careless smoking is the leading cause of fire deaths, followed by problems with heating equipment and arson. A study of campus fire fatalities found that smoking materials left to smolder over time in a couch accounted for half of those fatalities in which smoking was involved.

To prevent fires, dispose of all cigarettes in ashtrays and never smoke in bed. Other strategies include proper maintenance of fireplaces, furnaces, heaters, chimneys, and electrical outlets, cords, and appliances. If you use a portable heater, keep it at least three feet away from curtains, bedding, and anything else that might catch fire. Never plug heaters into a surge protector or power strip, and never leave heaters on unattended.

Be prepared to handle fire-related situations. Plan at least two escape routes out of each room, and designate a location outside the home as a meeting place. For practice, stage a home fire drill; do this at night because that's when most deadly fires occur.

Install smoke detectors on every level of your home. Your risk of dying in a fire is almost twice as high if you do not use them. Clean the detectors and check the batteries once a month, and replace the batteries at least once a year. Be sure that all residents are familiar with the sound of the alarm; when it goes off, take it seriously. Get out as quickly as possible, and go to a designated meeting place. Don't stop for a keepsake or pet. If you think someone is still inside the burning building, tell the firefighters. Never go back inside a burning building.

If you're trapped in a room, feel the door. If it is hot or if smoke is coming in through the cracks, don't open it; use the alternative escape route. If you can't get out, go to the window and shout for help.

Smoke inhalation is the greatest cause of death and injury in fires. To avoid inhaling smoke, crawl along the floor away from the heat and smoke. Cover your mouth and nose, ideally with a wet cloth, and take short, shallow breaths.

If your clothes catch fire, don't run. Drop to the ground, cover your face, and roll back and forth to smother the flames. Remember: stop-drop-roll.

QUICK STATS

**About 76% of all injuries that require medical attention occur at home.**

—National Safety Council, 2022

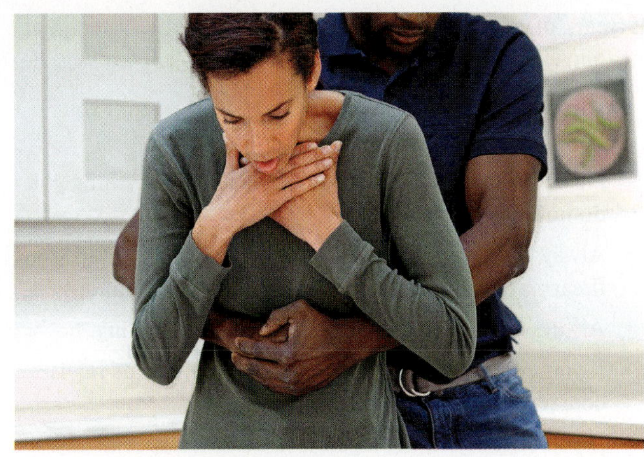

The Heimlich maneuver can save someone who is choking. Reach around the victim, making a fist and placing the thumb side of the fist just above the navel. Grasp your fist with the other hand and thrust upward and inward into the victim's abdomen. Continue with quick jerks until the object is expelled. Science Photo Library/Getty Images

**Suffocation and Choking** Suffocation and choking represented the fourth most common cause of death in the home. Elderly people and children are especially vulnerable. Children can suffocate if they put small items in their mouths, get tangled in their crib bedding, or get trapped in airtight appliances like old refrigerators. Keep small objects out of reach of children under age 3, and don't give them raw carrots, hot dogs, popcorn, gum, or hard candy. Examine toys carefully for small parts that could come loose. Don't give plastic bags or balloons to small children.

Adults can also become choking victims, especially if they fail to adequately chew food, or eat hurriedly or try to talk and eat at the same time. Many choking victims can be saved with the **Heimlich maneuver.** The American Red Cross recommends abdominal thrusts as the easiest and safest thing to do when an adult is choking. Back blows in conjunction with two-finger abdominal thrusts are an acceptable procedure for dislodging an object from the throat of an infant.

**Firearms** When researchers compared rates of firearm deaths in high-income countries, they found that although the rates in most countries had declined since 2003, those in the United States, already the highest, remained unchanged. Over one-third of all unintended U.S. firearm deaths and nonfatal injuries involve children and young adults under

TERMS

**Heimlich maneuver** A maneuver developed by Henry J. Heimlich, MD, to help force an obstruction from a person's windpipe or throat.

25 years of age. People who use firearms should remember the following:

- Always treat a gun as though it is loaded, even if you know it isn't.
- Never point a gun—loaded or unloaded—at anything you do not intend to shoot.
- Always unload a gun before storing it. Store unloaded firearms under lock and key, separate from ammunition.
- Always inspect firearms carefully before handling.
- If you ever plan to handle a gun, take a firearms safety course first.
- If you own a gun, use a gun lock designed specifically for that weapon.

Proper storage is critical. Do not assume that young children cannot fire a gun. Even children as young as 3 have enough finger strength to pull a trigger. One study estimated that 110 children aged 0–14 die each year as a result of unintentional firearm injuries. In the overwhelming majority of cases, victims and shooters are male, and the victim has either shot himself (one-third of cases) or been shot by another child.

VITAL STATISTICS

**Table 17.2** Lifetime Odds of Death Due to Selected Types of Injury

| INJURY TYPE | LIFETIME ODDS |
|---|---|
| Suicide | 1 in 88 |
| Opioid overdose | 1 in 92 |
| Motor vehicle crash | 1 in 107 |
| Fall | 1 in 106 |
| Homicide (assault by firearm) | 1 in 289 |
| Pedestrian incident | 1 in 543 |
| Motorcycle rider incident | 1 in 899 |
| Drowning | 1 in 1128 |
| Exposure to fire, flames, or smoke | 1 in 1547 |
| Choking on food | 1 in 2535 |
| Exposure to excessive natural heat | 1 in 8248 |
| Accidental gun discharge | 1 in 8571 |
| Electrocution, radiation, extreme temperatures, and pressure | 1 in 13,394 |
| Contact with sharp objects | 1 in 29,334 |
| Hornet/bee/wasp sting | 1 in 59,507 |
| Cataclysmic storm | 1 in 58,669 |
| Being bitten or attacked by a dog | 1 in 86,781 |
| Lightning strike | 1 in 138,849 |
| Airplane incident | Too few deaths in 2019 to calculate odds |

SOURCE: National Safety Council. 2022. *Lifetime Odds of Deaths for Selected Causes, U.S.* Itasca, IL: National Safety Council.

## Motor Vehicle Injuries

According to the National Highway Traffic Safety Administration (NHTSA), 4.5 million Americans were injured and 38,680 were killed in motor vehicle crashes in 2020. Despite fewer drivers on the road in 2020 due to the pandemic, fatalities were 7% higher than in 2019. The good news is that motor vehicle deaths in this country have decreased 25% in the past decade. Worldwide, motor vehicle crashes kill 1.35 million and injure up to 50 million people each year, placing motor vehicle injuries within the top 10 leading causes of death overall. Motor vehicle injuries also result in the majority of cases of paralysis due to spinal injuries, and they are the leading cause of severe brain injury in the United States. Table 17.2 illustrates how likely Americans are to die from motor vehicle crashes versus other types of injuries.

### Factors Contributing to Motor Vehicle Injuries

Common causes of motor vehicle injuries are speeding; aggressive driving; fatigue; inexperience; the use of cell phones, handheld devices, and other distractions; the use of alcohol and other drugs; and the incorrect use of seat belts and other safety devices. During the pandemic, fatal crashes increased even as miles traveled decreased.

QUICK STATS

**Motor vehicle deaths, injuries, and property damage cost Americans $463 billion in 2019.**

—National Safety Council, 2022

**DISTRACTED DRIVING** In 2019, motor vehicle crashes involving distracted drivers caused 3142 deaths and hundreds of thousands of injuries. Drivers in their twenties make up 25% of the distracted drivers in fatal crashes, according to the NHTSA. Distractions include visual-manual activity such as looking and using hands to type a text message (see the box "Cell Phones and Distracted Driving"), and cognitive tasks such as calculating numbers or formulating a sentence. Distractions can also intrude from outside the car—for example, billboards and roadside accidents—and from inside the car, as in the case of a conversation with a passenger, or eating, smoking, reaching for controls, preoccupation, and daydreaming.

**SPEEDING** After distracted and drunk driving, the next most common cause for car crashes is speeding and other errors in decision making (e.g., false assumption of others' actions, misjudgment of a gap or others' speed). As speed increases, momentum and the force of impact increase, and the time allowed for the driver to react (reaction time) decreases. Speed limits are posted to establish the safest maximum speed limit for a given area under ideal conditions; if visibility is limited or the road is wet, the safe maximum speed may be considerably lower.

**AGGRESSIVE DRIVING** Aggressive driving includes frequent, erratic, and abrupt lane changes; tailgating; running red lights or stop signs; passing on the shoulder; and blocking other cars trying to change lanes or pass.

## WELLNESS ON CAMPUS

# Cell Phones and Distracted Driving

A survey of nearly 5000 students from 12 colleges found that 91% reported phoning and/or texting while driving. This included 87% who text at traffic lights, 60% who text on city streets or in stop-and-go traffic, and 50% who send texts while driving on the freeway. Nearly half of the respondents said they were capable or very capable of safely talking on a cell phone while driving, but only 8.5% felt that other drivers were capable of doing so. These students overestimate their ability to multitask while driving.

The visual-manual distraction of locating, dialing, text messaging, browsing, and ending a call on handheld phones increases the risk of a crash by three times. Tasks that keep your hands and eyes from being engaged in driving the car have been shown to have a greater impact than cognitive distractions such as calculating numbers, formulating a sentence, listening to the radio, or talking with passengers. Many drivers assume that hands-free devices (like headsets, Bluetooth, and voice-control features on a phone or built into an automobile) are safer. However, research conducted by the National Safety Council has found that the cognitive distractions of using hands-free devices are just as unsafe.

Drivers using any phone—hands-free or handheld—have a tendency to look at objects without seeing them. Estimates indicate that drivers using cell phones fail to see up to 50% of the information in their driving environment. Distracted drivers experience what researchers call *inattention blindness*, similar to that of tunnel vision. Drivers look out the windshield, but they do not process everything that they need to know to effectively monitor their surroundings, seek and identify potential hazards, and respond to unexpected situations.

Drivers under age 25, who are the heaviest users of social media and cell phone technology, also generally have less skill in controlling vehicles and less efficiency in visual scanning, and they generally take more risks. Their lack of experience includes less ability to handle the effects of distraction, compared to the abilities of drivers aged 25 to 64.

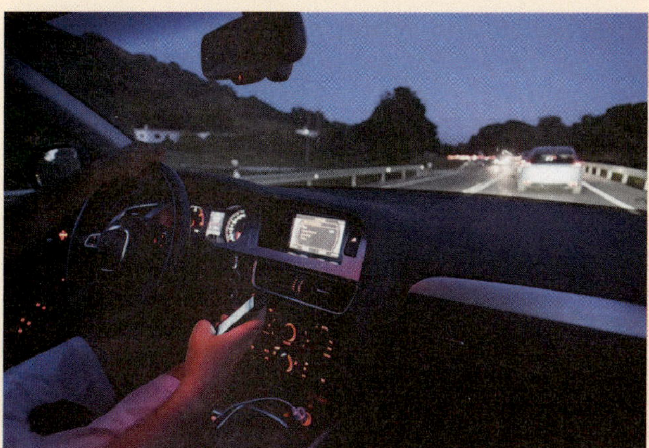

Ben Welsh/Design Pics/Getty Images

Phone applications designed to prevent distracted driving have had some success. However, they have not solved all the problems of breaking the driver's focus on the road. The technology still needs to find a balance between allowing specific contacts and phone functions to work and blocking those that have proven dangerous. Developers are still working to resolve these problems: (1) poor integration with other phone functions, (2) battery drainage, (3) integrating languages other than English, and (4) managing pop-up messages outside of texts, for example, Facebook Messenger and WhatsApp messages.

For people who live where cell phone use is legal while driving and who choose to use a phone regardless of the risk, the following strategies may increase safety:

- Minimize phone use while driving.
- Use a hands-free device so that you can keep both hands on the steering wheel.
- Be familiar with your phone and its functions, especially speed dial and redial.
- Store frequently called numbers on speed dial so that you can place calls without looking at the phone.
- If your phone has voice-activated dialing, use it.
- Let the person you are speaking with know you are driving, and be prepared to end the call at any time.
- Don't place or answer calls in heavy traffic or hazardous weather conditions.
- Don't take notes or look up phone numbers while driving.
- Time calls so that you can place them when you are at a stop.

Any kind of distraction—visual, manual, or cognitive—can contribute to an unsafe driving situation.

SOURCES: Hill, L., et al. 2015. Prevalence of and attitudes about distracted driving in college students. *Traffic Injury Prevention* 16(4): 362–367; National Highway Traffic Safety Administration. *Facts and Statistics: What Is Distracted Driving?* (https://www.nhtsa.gov/campaign/distracted-driving); National Safety Council. 2018. *Technologies Can Reduce Cell Phone Distracted Driving* (https://www.nsc.org/road-safety/safety-topics/distracted-driving/technology-solutions); Oviedo-Trespalacios, O., V. Truelove, and M. King. 2020. "It is frustrating to not have control even though I know it's not legal!": A mixed-methods investigation on applications to prevent mobile phone use while driving. *Accident Analysis & Prevention* 137 (https://doi.org/10.1016/j.aap.2019.105412).

**FATIGUE AND SLEEPINESS** Driving requires mental alertness and attentiveness. Studies have shown that sleepiness causes slower reaction times, reduced coordination and vigilance, and delayed information processing. Even mild sleep deprivation causes deterioration in driving ability comparable to that caused by a 0.05% blood alcohol concentration—a level considered hazardous while driving.

**ALCOHOL AND OTHER DRUGS** Alcohol is involved in about one-third of fatal crashes. Alcohol-impaired driving is illegal in all states and the District of Columbia. The legal limit for blood alcohol concentration (BAC) is 0.08%, but people can be impaired at much lower BACs. A driver with a BAC between 0.05% and 0.09% is nine times more likely to be involved in a crash than a person who has not been drinking. Because alcohol affects reason and judgment as well as the ability to make fast, accurate, and coordinated movements, a person who has been drinking will be less likely to recognize that they are impaired. Use of many over-the-counter and all psychoactive drugs is potentially dangerous if you plan to drive.

**SEAT BELTS, AIRBAGS, AND CHILD SAFETY SEATS** Although mandatory seat belt laws for adults are in effect in 49 states (excluding New Hampshire) and the District of Columbia, only 90% of motor vehicle occupants used seat belts in 2021, even though they are the single most effective way to reduce the risk of crash-related death. The good news is that seat belt usage was at its highest level ever. Of drivers not wearing seat belts who have been killed in automobile crashes, an estimated 60–70% would have survived if they had been wearing one. Some people think that if they are involved in a crash they are better off being thrown free of their vehicle. In fact, the chances of being killed are 25 times greater if you are thrown from a vehicle, whether it is due to injuries caused by hitting a tree or the pavement or by being hit by another vehicle. Seat belts not only prevent you from being thrown from the car at the time of the crash but also provide protection from second collisions: If a car is traveling at 65 miles per hour (mph) and hits another vehicle, the car stops first; then the occupants stop because they, too, are traveling at 65 mph. Second collisions occur when occupants hit something inside the car, such as the dashboard or windshield. Seat belts prevent these second collisions and spread the force of the first collision over the occupants' bodies.

Since 1998, all new cars and light trucks have been equipped with dual airbags—one for the driver and one for the front passenger. Many vehicles also offer side airbags, which further reduce the risk of injury. Advanced airbag systems include risk reduction technologies such as sensors to detect crash severity, seat position, passenger size, and whether a passenger is wearing a seat belt. Although airbags provide supplementary protection in the event of a collision, most are useful only in head-on collisions. They also deflate immediately after inflating and therefore do not provide protection in collisions involving multiple impacts. Airbags are not a replacement for seat belts; everyone in a vehicle should buckle up.

Airbags deploy forcefully and can injure a child or short adult who is improperly restrained or sitting too close to the dashboard, although second-generation airbags are somewhat safer for children than older devices. To ensure that airbags work safely, always follow these basic guidelines: Place infants in rear-facing infant seats in the back seat, transport children aged 12 and under in the back seat, always use seat belts and appropriate safety seats, and keep 10 inches between the airbag cover and the breastbone of the driver or passenger. If necessary, adjust the steering wheel or use seat cushions to ensure that an inflating airbag would hit you in the chest and not in the face.

Children who have outgrown child safety seats but are still too small for adult seat belts alone should be secured using booster seats that ensure that the seat belt is positioned low across the hips and thighs.

### Preventing Motor Vehicle Injuries

Defensive driving can also help you avoid a motor vehicle collision. Be aware of traffic conditions around you by checking your rearview and side mirrors frequently. Be aware of the driving behaviors of other drivers, especially those who may be following too closely, driving erratically, speeding, or frequently shifting lanes.

Never assume other drivers see you or that they anticipate an action you intend to make. Use your turn signals (even if you see no vehicles or pedestrians), make eye contact if possible, and allow enough road space and time for other drivers to prepare for and adjust to any action you take in traffic. Avoid driving in another driver's blind spot. Brake early, especially in poor weather conditions, allowing drivers behind you extra time for braking.

Take special care at intersections. Make sure you have time to complete your maneuver in the intersection. Always allow enough following distance. Use the three-second rule: When the vehicle ahead passes a reference point, count out three seconds. If you pass the reference point before you finish counting, drop back and allow more following distance. This rule works well at slower speeds when roads are dry and weather conditions are good. When traveling on highways or the interstate, use the four-second rule.

Slow down if weather or road conditions are poor.

### Motorcycles and Motor Scooters

About one in seven traffic fatalities involves someone riding a motorcycle. In recent years, riders aged 50 years and over have represented one-third of these fatalities. The data also reveal that, per mile traveled, motorcycle riders are 29 times more likely to die in a crash than occupants of a car or other motor vehicle. Injuries from motorcycle collisions are generally more severe than those involving automobiles because motorcycles provide little, if any, protection.

People riding motor scooters face additional challenges. Such vehicles usually have a maximum speed of 35–40 mph and have less power for maneuverability, especially in an emergency. Drivers should use caution and learn how to handle these vehicles in traffic.

Additional strategies for preventing motorcycle and motor scooter injuries include the following:

- For maximum visibility, wear light-colored clothing, drive with your headlights on, and correctly position yourself in traffic.

- Develop the necessary skills. (Skidding from improper braking is the most common cause of loss of control.)
- Wear a helmet marked with the DOT symbol, certifying that it conforms to federal safety standards established by the U.S. Department of Transportation.
- Protect your eyes with goggles, a face shield, or a windshield. Wear protective clothing.
- Drive defensively, particularly when changing lanes and at intersections, and never assume that other drivers can see you.

**Bicycles** Bicycle injuries result primarily from riders not knowing or understanding the rules of the road, failing to follow traffic laws, not having sufficient skill or experience to handle traffic conditions, or being intoxicated. Bicycles are considered vehicles; bicyclists must obey all traffic laws that apply to automobile drivers, including stopping at traffic lights and stop signs.

Research shows that wearing a helmet reduces the risk of head injury by 66–88%. Safe cycling strategies include the following:

- Wear safety equipment, including a helmet, eye protection, gloves, and proper footwear. To prevent clothes from tangling in the bike chain, secure the bottom of your pant legs with clips, and secure your shoelaces.
- Wear light-colored, reflective clothing. Equip your bike with reflectors, and use lights, especially at night or when riding in wooded or other dark areas.
- Ride with the flow of traffic, not against it, and follow all traffic laws. Use bike paths when they are available.
- Ride defensively; never assume that drivers can see you. Be especially careful when turning or crossing at corners and intersections. Watch for cars turning right.
- Stop at all traffic lights and stop signs. Know and use hand signals.

**Pedestrians** Since a low in 2009, motor vehicles deaths involving a pedestrian have increased 51% and now make up 17% of traffic fatalities. The highest rates of death and injury occur among children under age 15 and the elderly. Most incidents occur on open roads (not intersections), in urban areas, during dark lighting conditions. Pedestrian alcohol intoxication plays a significant role in up to half of all adult pedestrian fatalities, and researchers are also exploring the role of marijuana. Walking while distracted with a cell phone may also account for more injuries and deaths.

## Leisure Injuries

Most people enjoy some form of leisure activities, so it is not surprising that **leisure injuries** are a significant health-related problem in the United States. Specific safety strategies for activities associated with leisure injuries include the following:

- Don't swim alone, in unsupervised places, under the influence of alcohol, or for an unusual length of time. Use caution when swimming in unfamiliar surroundings or in water colder than 70°F. Check the depth of water before diving. Make sure that residential pools are fenced, and never allow children to swim unsupervised.
- Always use a **personal flotation device** (also known as a life jacket) when on a boat.
- For all sports and recreational activities, make sure facilities are safe, follow the rules, and practice good sportsmanship. Develop adequate skill in the activity, and use proper safety equipment, including, where appropriate, a helmet, eye protection, correct footwear, and knee, elbow, and wrist pads (see the box "Head Injuries in Contact Sports").
- If using equipment such as skateboards, snowboards, mountain bikes, or all-terrain vehicles, wear a helmet and other safety equipment, and avoid excessive speeds and unsafe stunts. Use playground equipment only for those activities for which it is designed.
- If you are active in excessively hot and humid weather, drink plenty of fluids, rest frequently in the shade, and slow down or stop if you feel uncomfortable. Danger signals of heat stress include excessive perspiration, dizziness, headache, muscle cramps, nausea, weakness, rapid pulse, and disorientation.
- Do not use alcohol or other drugs during recreational activities–such activities require coordination and sound judgment.

## Weather-Related Injuries

Although you can't control the weather, the best approach is to be prepared for inclement weather that may occur in your area. Even though conditions may seem harmless at times, they can become dangerous quickly.

- ***Heat.*** Extreme heat is the leading weather-related killer in the United States, according to the National Weather Service. Heat-related illness such as heat stroke and heat exhaustion can be fatal, especially for children, older adults, and people who are dehydrated. The CDC estimates that extreme heat kills more than 700 people in the United States each year. The best way to deal with excessive heat is to stay indoors as much as possible, with a fan or air conditioner on. Wear lightweight, light-colored clothing; drink plenty of water to stay hydrated; and avoid heavy meals.

**TERMS**

**leisure injuries** Unintentional injuries and deaths that occur in public places, or places used in a public way, not involving motor vehicles; include most sports and recreation deaths and injuries; examples are falls, drownings, burns, and heat and cold stress.

**personal flotation device** A device designed to save a person from drowning by buoying up the body while in the water.

## TAKE CHARGE
### Head Injuries in Contact Sports

Reports of bizarre behavior, suicides, and middle-aged dementia among former professional football players, boxers, and soccer players have focused worldwide media attention on sports concussions. Death from chronic traumatic encephalopathy (CTE), a disease caused by repetitive brain trauma, was the diagnosis for 87% of over 200 football players whose brains were donated for a 2017 study. (CTE can be diagnosed only by autopsy.) Of 111 brains donated by National Football League players, 110 were diagnosed with CTE.

CTE has been found in younger athletes as well. An amateur football player in his early twenties suffered a variety of symptoms before dying at age 25. He had received repeated concussions since starting to play football at age six and continuing through college. He was an above-average student, but because of his symptoms—first, ongoing headaches, insomnia, anxiety, and difficulty with memory and concentration; and later, apathy, feelings of worthlessness, and suicidal thoughts—he had to stop both playing football and attending college. The diagnosis at his autopsy was CTE.

Concussions, or mild traumatic brain injuries (MTBIs), can be diagnosed immediately or after some cognitive and neurological testing. An MTBI is a traumatic injury to the brain or spinal cord resulting from a direct blow to the head or indirect blows elsewhere that can cause violent brain movement in the skull. A concussion, for example, can result from a blow to the chest that makes the head snap forward. Symptoms include headache, nausea, vomiting, sleep disturbances, depression, and loss of concentration. Unconsciousness occurs in only 10% of concussions.

Forty million people worldwide suffer concussions every year. Concussions account for 5% of the nearly 225,000 sports injuries occurring in the United States each year. They are most common in football, hockey, skiing, wrestling, rugby, basketball, and soccer. In 2019, about 15% of all U.S. high school students reported one or more concussions related to sports or recreation. The incidence is higher in men than in women, but women are at greater risk when playing the same sport—for example, soccer. Concussions and their neurodegenerative fallouts also occur in soldiers and, generally, in people of all ages and careers if they have a fall or sustain an injury in a motor vehicle crash.

Although the National Football League continues to downplay the risk of injury in football, researchers and journalists have documented that repeated concussions in childhood sports can cause progressive damage to the brain.

Can we predict brain injuries before they become fatal? Researchers are working to predict injury risk—both of MTBI in the moment it happens and of CTE as it develops. For example, bioengineers at Stanford University outfitted athletes with mouth guards that monitored symptoms of MTBI and recorded more than 500 moments of impact during regular sporting events. This is especially significant because athletes often fail to recognize—let alone report—that they have suffered an injury. Because sustaining a second injury shortly after the first can result in much greater damage, an instantaneous indication of concussion should require medical professionals to pull a player to the sidelines.

What can individuals do to reduce their risk of concussion? Always wear a helmet when cycling, skiing, snowboarding, rock climbing, or skateboarding. Wearing seat belts and ensuring that car airbags are functioning properly can also help. Older adults can reduce their risk of concussions by keeping living spaces free of clutter, wearing stable footwear, and maintaining strength and balance through regular exercise.

Preventing concussions in contact sports is more challenging. The pre-participation physical examination can identify athletes with a history of concussion and assess their readiness to compete. Helmets in sports like football and hockey protect the skull from impact injuries (fractures and lacerations) but have little effect on the incidence or severity of concussions. Coaching fundamentals can teach athletes to avoid dangerous techniques such as spear blocking and tackling but do little to change the nature of high-impact collision sports. Professional officiating can cut down on dangerous play. Rule changes such as eliminating zone coverage in football or heading in soccer might reduce the concussion rate. Recognizing concussion injuries is important for preventing long-term disability. Finally, education can teach athletes about the symptoms and seriousness of concussions.

SOURCES: Centers for Disease Control and Prevention. 2021. *Traumatic Brain Injury and Concussion* (https://www.cdc.gov/traumaticbraininjury/index.html). Gregory, S. 2016. The NFL still won't tackle brain trauma at the Super Bowl. *Time,* February 6 (http://time.com/4210564/nfl-super-bowl-brain-trauma-cte/); Harmon, K. G., et al. 2013. American Medical Society for Sports Medicine Position Statement: Concussion in sport. *British Journal of Sports Medicine* 47(1): 15–26; Hernandez, F., et al. 2015. Six degree-of-freedom measurements of human mild traumatic brain injury. *Annals of Biomedical Engineering* 43(8): 1918–1934; McCarthy, M. 2016. Chronic traumatic encephalopathy is reported in 25 year old former American football player. *British Medical Journal* 352: 7027; Misra, A. 2014. Common sports injuries: Incidence and average charges. *ASPE Issue Brief,* March 17 (https://aspe.hhs.gov/pdf-report/common-sports-injuries-incidence-and-average-charges).

- ***Cold.*** Each year dozens of Americans die from exposure to cold temperatures. Conditions such as hypothermia (low body temperature) and frostbite (frozen skin or flesh) can be deadly. Most injuries and deaths in cold weather are due to a lack of preparedness or understanding of the dangers of low temperatures and wind chill. If you must go outdoors in very cold weather, dress in layers and cover your face, fingers, and ears to protect them from frostbite. Make sure your home and car are prepared with plenty of fuel, drinking water, warm clothes and blankets, batteries, and other emergency supplies.

• ***Wind.*** In extremely windy conditions, take cover in a sturdy shelter, preferably a permanent structure with a foundation. In a severe storm such as a tornado, move to the lowest portion of the building or to a small interior room away from windows. If you're outdoors when a severe storm or tornado strikes, lie flat in a low spot or ditch. Don't stay inside a car or hide under an open-sided structure such as a bridge; such structures can act as a funnel and intensify the wind.

• ***Lightning.*** About 400 Americans are struck by lightning every year, and about 10% of them die. Lightning can strike even when it's not raining, and it often strikes with no warning. If you hear thunder, you are close enough to the lightning's source to be struck. The National Weather Service recommends that you go indoors when conditions are right for lightning. You are safer in a house, as long as you avoid anything that conducts electricity, including corded telephones, electrical appliances, computers, plumbing, and metal doors and windows. If you are not near a building, the next best option is a car. If there is no shelter, stay low, such as in a ditch, and avoid bodies of water. Tents or pavilions should be avoided.

• ***Flooding.*** Stay away from rapidly rising or moving water; it can carry you away in an instant. Even fairly shallow water can sweep away a car if the current is fast enough. If you're near rapidly rising water, move to higher ground and call for help. Don't attempt to drive or walk through flooded streets, and don't traverse a bridge if it is being pounded by high, fast-moving water.

### Work Injuries

The Bureau of Labor Statistics estimates that in 2020 there were 4764 fatal injuries and over 2.7 million nonfatal workplace injuries and illnesses; of these, 1.2 million cases resulted in days away from work. Covid-19 was the leading cause of days away from work in 2020, with nurses and other medical staff experiencing the greatest increase in missed days. Overexertion and slips, trips, and falls were the next category of injuries, accounting for the most days away from work. Although people who do extensive manual labor and lifting on the job make up less than half the workforce, they account for more than 75% of all work-related injuries and illnesses.

Nonfatal injuries in the workplace declined in 2020, as did fatalities; at the same time, there was a 4000% increase of employer-reported respiratory illness cases, an effect of the pandemic. Transportation incidents accounted for the largest number of deaths, followed by slips and falls. Exposure to harmful substances, including unintentional overdose from nonmedical use of drugs, also led to more deaths in 2020. Other fatalities on the job involve crushing injuries, severe lacerations, burns, and electrocutions.

Back problems account for hundreds of thousands of work injuries each year, although it is estimated that twice as many workers experience some kind of minor back injury each year. According to the Bureau of Labor Statistics, back injuries account for almost one of five workplace injuries or illnesses.

> **Ask Yourself**
>
> **QUESTIONS FOR CRITICAL THINKING AND REFLECTION**
>
> Think of one injury you have suffered. What were you doing when you were injured? Could you have done anything to avoid or minimize it? How did the experience change your attitudes or behaviors?

Many back injuries that occur on the job could be prevented through the use of proper lifting techniques. Bend at the knees and hips, not at the waist. Remain in an upright position and crouch down if you need to lower yourself to grasp the object. Place feet securely about shoulder-width apart; grip the object firmly. Lift gradually, with straight arms. Avoid quick, jerky motions. Lift by standing up or pushing with your leg muscles. Keep the object close to your body. If you have to turn, change the position of your feet. Twisting is a common and dangerous cause of injury. Plan ahead so that your pathway is clear and turning can be minimized. Put the object down gently, reversing the steps for lifting.

Musculoskeletal injuries and disorders in the workplace include **repetitive strain injuries (RSIs).** RSIs are caused by repeated strain on a particular part of the body. Twisting, vibrations, awkward postures, and other stressors may contribute to RSIs. **Carpal tunnel syndrome** is one type of RSI that has increased in recent years due to increased use of computers, both at work and in the home (see the box "Repetitive Strain Injury" for more information).

## VIOLENCE AND INTENTIONAL INJURIES

According to the Federal Bureau of Investigation (FBI), more than 1.2 million violent crimes occurred in the United States in 2020, a 5.6% increase from 2019. Examples of violence are assault, sexual assault, domestic violence, suicide, child abuse, and homicide. Homicide increased 30% from 2019 to 2020, the largest single-year increase ever recorded in the country.

Research comparing the rates of violence in countries belonging to the Organisation for Economic Co-operation and Development (OECD) shows that the United States has much higher rates of violence than other countries (as do Mexico and Estonia), with 4–10 times the homicide death rates found in economically similar countries.

> **TERMS**
>
> **repetitive strain injury (RSI)** A musculoskeletal injury or disorder caused by repeated strain on the hand, arm, wrist, or other part of the body; also called *cumulative trauma disorder (CTD).*
>
> **carpal tunnel syndrome** Compression of the median nerve in the wrist, often caused by repetitive use of the hands, such as in computer use; characterized by numbness, tingling, and pain in the hands and fingers; can cause nerve damage.

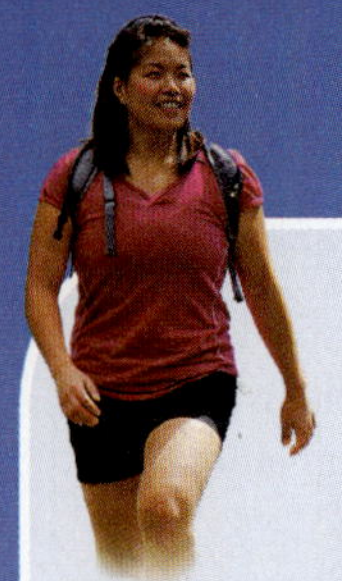

## TAKE CHARGE
### Repetitive Strain Injury

Repetitive strain injuries (RSIs) impact the musculoskeletal and nervous systems of the body and affect many people around the world. Other terms to describe this condition include *repetitive motion disorder (RMD), cumulative trauma disorder (CTD),* and *occupational overuse syndrome (OOS).*

An RSI can be caused by a combination of physical and psychosocial stressors, but the injury typically involves some kind of repetitive action or forceful exertion on the body over time. Pain in the extremities as well as the back and shoulders is commonly cited and tends to worsen with extended activity.

The task associated with an RSI may be something relatively simple and nonexertive like typing, writing, or clicking a computer mouse. One of the most common work-related injuries is *carpal tunnel syndrome (CTS),* which is characterized by pressure on the median nerve in the wrist that also affects tendons and ligaments in the forearm. Symptoms of CTS include numbness, tingling, burning, and/or aching in the hand, particularly in the thumb and the first three fingers. The pain may worsen at night and may shoot up from the hand as far as the shoulder. If it does not clear up on its own, immobilization of the joint at night can be helpful; other options may involve anti-inflammatory drugs or even surgery in extreme cases.

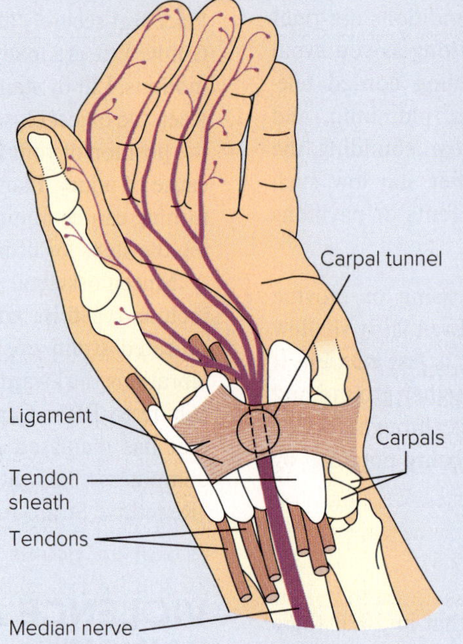


Examples of RSIs from physical activity by athletes include conditions commonly referred to as "golfer's elbow" or "tennis elbow," in which the joints are continually exposed to extreme stress in order to complete an action accurately with speed and force.

With new technologies being introduced every day, another type of RSI is now being recognized. Many people who use their thumbs to text suffer from a condition referred to as "texting thumb." Similarly, people who spend countless hours using handheld controls to play video games are experiencing "gamer's thumb."

In all cases, research indicates the primary risk factors are usually associated with poor posture, improper techniques for completing an activity, and overuse of a certain part of the body. The good news is that a person can make adjustments to reduce the risk of an RSI, either in what is being done or through modification of the environment. Warm up your wrists before you begin any repetitive motion activity, and take frequent breaks to stretch and flex your wrists and hands:

- Extend your arms out in front of you and stretch your wrists by pointing your fingers to the ceiling; hold for a count of five. Then straighten your wrists and relax your fingers for a count of five.
- With arms extended, make a tight fist with both hands and then bend your wrists so that your knuckles are pointed toward the floor; hold for a count of five. Then straighten your wrists and relax your fingers for a count of five.

Repeat these stretches several times, and finish by letting your arms hang loosely at your sides and shaking them gently for several seconds. It's also important to maintain a physically active lifestyle, take plenty of breaks to avoid hours of sedentary activity, stretch, apply proper ergonomic principles, and minimize other stress factors.

## Factors Contributing to Violence

Most intentional injuries and deaths are associated with an argument or a crime. However, there are many forms of violence, and no single factor can explain all of them.

**Social Factors** Rates of violence are not the same throughout society; they vary by geographic region, neighborhood, socioeconomic level, and many other factors. According to the FBI, murder rates were highest in the South in 2019, followed by the Midwest, West, and Northeast regions of the country. Neighborhoods that are disadvantaged in status, power, and economic resources typically experience the most violence. In 2018, 30% of violent crimes were committed by people under 25 years old.

People who feel they are a part of society (with strong family and social ties), who are economically integrated (having a reasonable chance at getting a decent job), and who grow up in areas with a feeling of community (with good schools, parks, and neighborhoods) are significantly less likely to engage in violence.

College campus environments can also contribute to violence. Because college campuses are transitory communities, some people may have less incentive to cooperate and coexist amicably.

**Violence in the Media** The mass media play a major role in exposing audiences of all ages to violence as an acceptable and effective means of solving problems. On average, children in the United States watch about four hours of television daily and may view as many as 10,000 violent acts on television and in movies each year.

Researchers have found that exposure to media violence at least temporarily increases aggressive feelings in children, making them more likely to engage in violent or fearful behavior; the direct, short-term effects on teens and adults are less clear. It makes sense for parents to be aware of the potential influence of the media on their children. A child may not clearly understand the distinctions between the fantasy world portrayed in the media and the complexities of the real world. Parents should monitor the TV shows, movies, video games, music, and other forms of media to which their children are exposed. Watching programs with children gives parents the opportunity to talk to them about violence and its consequences, to explain that violence is not the best way to resolve conflicts or solve problems, and to point out examples of positive behaviors such as kindness and cooperation.

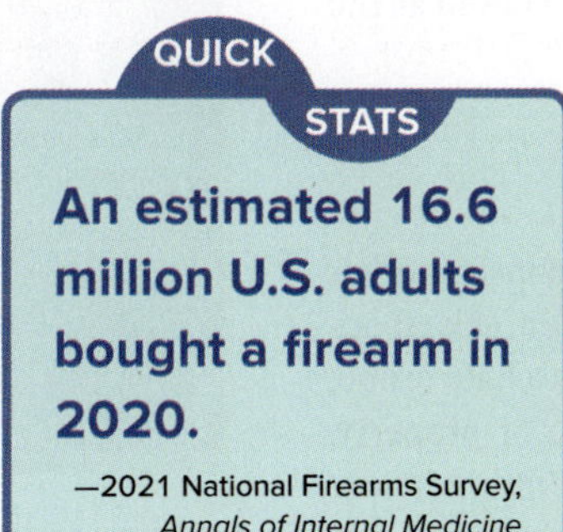


**Gender** In most cases, violence is committed by men. Males are nine times more likely than females to commit murder, and three times more likely than females to be murdered. Male college students are twice as likely as female students to be the victims of violence.

Women do commit acts of violence, including a small but substantial proportion of murders of spouses. This fact has been used to argue that women have the same capacity to commit violence as men, but most researchers note substantial differences. Men often kill their wives as the culmination of years of violence or after stalking them; they may kill their entire families and themselves at the same time. Women virtually never kill in such circumstances; rather, they kill their husbands after repeated victimization or while being beaten.

**Interpersonal Factors** Although most people fear attack from strangers, the majority of victims are acquainted with their attackers. More than half of murders of women and three-fourths of sexual assaults are committed by someone the woman knows. Crime victims and violent criminals tend to share many characteristics—that is, they are likely to be young, male, from a minority group, and poor. Being a victim of teasing, bullying, or social exclusion may lead to aggressive behavior or violence.

**Alcohol and Other Drugs** Substance misuse and dependence are consistently associated with interpersonal violence and suicide. Intoxication affects judgment and increases aggression in some people, causing a small argument to escalate into a serious physical confrontation. On college campuses, alcohol is involved in about 95% of all violent crimes.

**Firearms** Many criminologists argue that the high rate of homicide in the United States is directly related to the very widespread handgun ownership and the relative ease of obtaining firearms, considering that the United States is the only industrialized country so unregulated. Whereas most victims of assaults with other weapons don't die, the death rate from assault by handgun is extremely high. The use of a handgun can change a suicide attempt to a completed suicide and a violent assault to a murder.

## Assault

Assault is the use of physical force by a person or people to inflict injury or death on another. Homicide, aggravated assault, and robbery are examples of assault. Research indicates that the victims of assaultive injuries and their perpetrators tend to resemble one another in terms of ethnicity, educational background, psychological profile, and reliance on weapons.

## Homicide

According to the FBI, 21,500 Americans were murdered in 2020, a rate not seen since the 1990s. The spike in homicides in the past two years was largely concentrated in communities of low-income, marginalized ethnic groups. In 2020, African Americans were eight times as likely as Euro-Americans to be murder victims. Other demographics that describe people with the highest homicide victim rates are young people ages 20–29 and males. Males also account for 86% of all victims of firearm death and 87% of nonfatal firearm injuries. Firearm homicide rates are highest among teens and young adults 15–34 years of age, and among Americans of African, Indigenous, and Hispanic ancestry.

Most homicides are committed with a firearm, occur during an argument, and occur among people who know one another. Intrafamilial homicide, in which the perpetrator and the victim are related, accounts for about one of every eight homicides. Mass shootings receive a great deal of media coverage but represent a relatively small fraction of firearm-related deaths; 90% of homicides are single-victim incidents.

Deaths due to "legal interventions"—killings by police or other peace officers—are not technically classified as homicides. Newer methods that include such killings calculate that about 1000 people per year lose their lives in law enforcement-related incidents. In one study, Black men were 2.5 times more likely than white men to be killed by police; in another, Black people who were fatally shot were twice as likely as white people to be unarmed.

## Gang-Related Violence

Gangs are most frequently associated with large cities, but gang activity also extends to the suburbs and even to rural areas. It is estimated that about 1.4 million Americans belong to gangs. The average age for joining a gang is 14, so 40% of gang members are younger than 18 years of age.

Gangs are most common in areas where residents experience the most violent crime; have low income; and have high unemployment rates, population density, and crime rates. In these areas, young people may feel that legitimate success in life is out of reach and know that involvement in the drug market makes some gang members rich. Often gangs serve as a mechanism for companionship, self-esteem, support, and security. Indeed, gang membership may be viewed as the only possible means of survival in some areas.

## Hate Crimes

When criminal acts are motivated by bias against another person's race or ethnicity, national origin, religion, sexual orientation, or disability, the offense is classified as a hate crime. Hate crimes may be committed against people or property. Those committed against people may include intimidation, assault, and even rape or murder. Crimes against property most frequently involve graffiti, desecration of synagogues, cross burnings, and other acts of vandalism or property damage. FBI data indicate there were over 8000 hate crimes in 2020, but many go unfiled. In fact, according to the Department of Justice's Bureau of Justice Statistics, the actual number is closer to 250,000 hate crimes per year. In 2020, 65% of the reported hate crimes were based on race, ethnicity, or ancestry bias. Black Americans made up more than half of those victims. The murder of George Floyd followed by a social justice movement protesting violence and racism brought heightened media attention and may have contributed to increased targeting.

Similarly, as transgender rights are increasingly debated in the media, there has been greater visibility of–and hostility directed at–transgender people. A 2021 report found that transgender people are four times more likely than cisgender people to experience violent victimization, including rape. In 2021, one organization tracking murders of transgender people counted 50 killings, the highest since tracking began in 2013; the majority were Black and Latinx transgender women.

Another group recently targeted are Asian Americans. Over 2 million Asian Americans have experienced a hate crime, discrimination, or harassment since the coronavirus pandemic began. Asian American and Pacific Islander civil rights groups created a website, Stop AAPI Hate, for victims to safely report incidents in multiple languages and find resources.

Although hate crimes represent extreme, criminal responses committed out of fear, ignorance, or anger, they also fall on a continuum of prejudice that should be investigated. Prejudice is a learned behavior that represents systems of racism or bigotry larger than the individual. Hateful talk in the media, by politicians, or by others in our daily lives can escalate to racist sentiments and scapegoating in times of economic and social upheaval.

## School Violence

Approximately 423 homicide incidents between 1994 and 2016 occurred in relation to schools. Almost all involved a single victim, contrary to the perception that most school-related youth homicides occur in the context of a mass shooting. Gang-related activity (58%) and interpersonal disputes (44%) were the most common among known motives for single-victim, school-related homicides, reflecting broader community-wide causes of violence. As with other types of violence, both victims and offenders were predominantly young men. Homicide and suicide are the most serious but least common types of violence in schools; an estimated 764,600 nonfatal victimizations occurred at schools in 2019, including theft, vandalism, and assault.

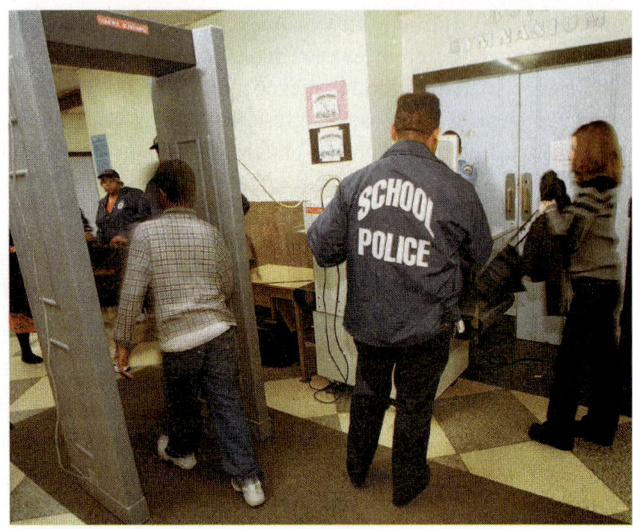

To increase safety, some high schools and middle schools (and even some elementary schools) have installed metal detectors. Dan Loh/Pool/AP Images

How risky is the school environment? rape, other sexual assaults, physical attacks or fights with a weapon, threats of attack with a weapon, and robbery with or without a weapon. Less than 3% of homicides of youths aged 5 to 19 occur at school. Total victimization rates for students aged 12 to 18 have declined both at school and away since 1992, and thefts and serious victimization declined both at and away from school.

Although schools are basically safe places, steps can be taken to identify at-risk youths and improve safety for all students. General characteristics of youths who have caused violent deaths in schools include the following: uncontrollable angry outbursts; violent and abusive language and behavior; isolation from peers; depression and irritability; access to and preoccupation with weapons; lack of support and supervision from adults.

## Workplace Violence

Data show that workplace violence has decreased by 35% in the past decade. OSHA reports that nearly 2 million American workers are victims of workplace violence each year, resulting in about 400 homicides. In about 60% of cases, workplace violence is committed by strangers; acquaintances account for nearly 40% of cases; and intimates account for 1%. Most perpetrators of workplace violence are white males over age 21. Women's leading cause of death in the workplace is homicide. Firearms are used in nearly 80% of workplace homicides, and the majority of these homicides occur during the commission of a robbery or other crime.

Workers at greater risk include those who exchange money with the public or work alone in small groups, such as delivery drivers; also health care professionals, public service workers, customer service agents, and law enforcement personnel have the most dangerous jobs.

## Terrorism

The FBI identifies terrorism as either international or domestic, and it can be motivated by right-wing, left-wing, and religious ideologies. Right-wing terrorist networks can be divided broadly into white supremacists, antigovernment extremists, and anti-woman incels (the "involuntary celibate" movement). Left-wing terrorists may oppose capitalism or perceived environmental abuses, or support social and political systems like anarchism, communism, or socialism. Religious terrorism uses violence in support of a religion, such as Islam, Judaism, or Christianity.

Since 1994, right-wing terrorism has been far more common in the United States than other forms, and it has grown significantly since 2014. Analyzing the 893 terrorist attacks and plots in the United States between 1994 and 2020, the Center for Strategic and International Studies found that far-right incidents accounted for 57% of them. Far-right terrorism was also more often responsible for greater fatalities per year than other forms. The deadliest homegrown right-wing terrorist attack in the United States—and the second deadliest in the country after 9/11—was the 1995 bombing of the Alfred P. Murrah Federal Building in Oklahoma City. More recent examples of far-right terrorism in the United States include the shooting of 10 people in a Buffalo, New York, grocery store by a white supremacist (2022); the racially motivated killing of 23 people in an El Paso, Texas, Walmart (2019); and the arrest of members of the antigovernment groups Proud Boys and Oath Keepers, who were charged with seditious conspiracy for their participation in the attack on the U.S. Capitol on January 6, 2021.

All forms of terrorism use technology to reach, radicalize, and recruit people who are receptive to extremist ideology through social media, messaging platforms, and online images, videos, and publications; at the same time, the anonymous nature of the internet greatly hinders law enforcement efforts. Be aware of your surroundings online and in public; don't overshare personal information; and if you see something suspicious, alert authorities.

## Family and Intimate-Partner Violence

Violence in families challenges some of our most basic assumptions. *Family violence* generally refers to a broad range of abusive acts committed by one family member toward another. Another category of abuse is **intimate-partner violence (IPV)**, formerly called domestic violence. IPV includes physical, sexual, or psychological harm imposed by a current or former spouse, or boyfriend, girlfriend, or other romantic or sexual partner. IPV is widespread. An estimated 36% of women and 33% of men experience IPV in their lifetimes. Around half of all women who identify as African American, American Indian/Alaska Native (AISN), and multiracial have experienced IPV in their lives.

Around 4 in 10 lesbian women, 6 in 10 bisexual women, 1 in 4 gay men, and 4 in 10 bisexual men have experienced IPV. A 2020 study found that transgender people were almost twice as likely to experience IPV as cisgender people. Child abuse consists of physical, sexual, or emotional abuse or neglect; an estimated one in four children experience some form of abuse or neglect in their lifetime.

**Physical Violence** Physical violence within intimate partnerships affects all genders and sexes, but women are disproportionately affected. Violence against intimate partners occurs at every level of society, although it is more common at lower socioeconomic levels. It occurs more frequently in relationships with a high degree of conflict—an inability to resolve arguments through negotiation and compromise.

The problem of physical violence in intimate relationships is apparent even among high school students. In a 2019 survey, 10% of college students reported physical violence in a partnered relationship since entering college: for men, the rate was 10%, for women 14%, and for students who identified as transgender, genderqueer, gender nonconforming, questioning, or something not listed on the survey (TGQN), 21.5%.

The need to control another person is at the root of much of abusive behavior. Early in a relationship, a person's tendency to be controlling may not be obvious. See the box "Recognizing the Potential for Abusiveness in a Partner (or Yourself)".

Studies have suggested a three-phase cycle of battering, consisting of a period of increasing tension, a violent explosion and loss of control, and a period of contrition and seeking forgiveness and promises that it will never happen again. The batterer is drawn back to this cycle over and over again but rarely achieves a change in behavior.

Abused people often stay in violent relationships for years. They may be economically dependent on their partners, feel trapped or fear retaliation if they leave, believe their children need a father, or suffer low self-esteem themselves. They may love or pity their partner, or they may believe they'll eventually be able to stop the violence. They often leave the relationship when they finally resolve their own ambiguous feelings.

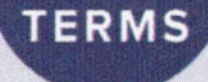


**intimate-partner violence (IPV)** Physical, sexual, or psychological harm by a current or former partner or spouse.

## TAKE CHARGE
## Recognizing the Potential for Abusiveness in a Partner (or Yourself)

There are no sure ways to tell whether someone will become abusive or violent toward an intimate partner, but you can look for warning signs. Remember that, although most abusive relationships involve male violence directed at a woman, anyone can be a victim or perpetrator of violence If you are concerned that a person you are involved with has the potential for violence, observe their behavior, and ask yourself these questions:

- What is this person's attitude toward women and LGBTQIA+ people? How does he treat his family members? How does he work with other students, colleagues, or bosses? How does he treat your friends?
- What is their attitude toward your autonomy? Do they respect the work you do and the way you do it? Or do they mock it, tell you how to do it better, or encourage you to give it up? Do they tell you they'll take care of you?
- How self-centered are they? Do they want to spend leisure time on your interests or theirs? Do they listen to you? Do they remember what you say?
- Are they possessive or jealous? Do they want to spend every minute with you? Do they cross-examine you about things you do when you're not together?
- What happens when things don't go the way they want them to? Do they blow up? Do they always have to get their way?
- Are they moody, mocking, critical, or bossy? Do you feel as if you're walking on eggshells when you're with them?
- Do you feel you have to avoid arguing with them?
- Do they drink too much or use drugs?
- Does he refuse to use condoms or take other precautions for safer sex?

Listen to your own uneasiness, and stay away from anyone who disrespects women, LGBT, and gender-nonconforming people, who wants or needs you intensely and exclusively, and who has a knack for getting their own way almost all the time.

If you are in a serious relationship with a controlling person, you may already have experienced abuse. (If you have put your partner in any of these situations, you are likely an abuser.) Consider the following questions:

- Does your partner constantly criticize you, blame you for things that are not your fault, or verbally degrade you?
- Do they humiliate you in front of others?
- Are they suspicious or jealous? Do they accuse you of being unfaithful or monitor your mail or phone calls?
- Do they track all your time? Do they discourage you from seeing friends and family?
- Do they prevent you from getting or keeping a job or attending school? Do they control your shared resources or restrict your access to money?
- Have they ever pushed, pulled, slapped, hit, kicked, bitten, or restrained you? Thrown an object at you? Used a weapon on you or pointed one at you?
- Have they ever destroyed or damaged your personal property or sentimental items, or threatened to do so?
- Have they ever forced you to have sex or to do something sexually you didn't want to do?
- Do they anger easily when drinking or taking drugs?
- Have they ever threatened to harm you or your children, friends, pets, or property?
- Have they ever threatened to blackmail you if you leave?

If you answered yes to one or more of these questions, you may be experiencing intimate-partner violence. (If you have seen any of these behaviors in yourself, seek immediate help to stop these behaviors.) If you believe you or your children are in imminent danger, look in your local telephone directory for a domestic violence shelter, or call 911. If you want information, referrals to a program in your area, or assistance, contact one of the organizations listed in the For More Information section at the end of the chapter.

**Stalking and Cyberstalking** **Stalking** is a crime under laws of all 50 states, the District of Columbia, the U.S. territories, and the federal government. In the United States, it is estimated that 10% of women and 2% of men are stalked each year by an intimate partner; about two-thirds of stalkers are men. Among bisexual women, almost a third have reported being stalked. About two of three female victims are stalked by current or former intimate partners; of these, a majority had been physically or sexually assaulted by that partner during the relationship. Weapons are used to threaten or harm victims in one out of five cases. Data indicate that the 18–24 age group experiences the highest rate of stalking and that stalking of trans, gay, and gender-nonconforming college students is greater than that experienced by the general population. A stalker's goal may be to control or scare the victim or to keep them in a relationship. Most stalking episodes last a year or less.

TERMS

**stalking** Repeatedly harassing or threatening a person through behaviors such as following a person, appearing at a person's residence or workplace, leaving written messages or objects, making harassing phone calls, or vandalizing property; frequently directed at a former intimate partner.

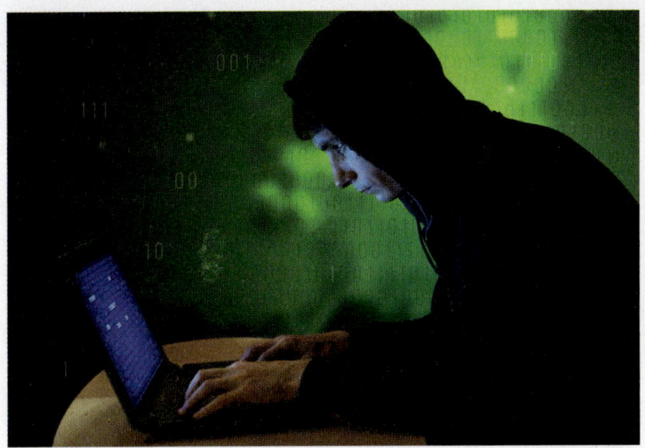

Set your social media profiles to "private." Artem Oleshko/Shutterstock

The use of the internet, email, chat rooms, Facebook, Instagram, and other electronic means to stalk another person is known as **cyberstalking.**

Cyberstalkers may send harassing or threatening messages to the victim, or they may encourage others to harass the victim—for example, by impersonating the victim and posting inflammatory messages and personal information on bulletin boards or in chat rooms. Guidelines for staying safe online include the following:

- Avoid using your real name on the internet. Select an age- and gender-neutral identity.
- Avoid filling out profiles for accounts with information that could be used to identify you.
- Do not share personal information in public spaces anywhere online or give it to strangers.
- Learn how to filter unwanted email messages.
- Always use unique passwords that contain many characters—preferably an alphanumeric combination to make it more difficult for someone to hack into your account.
- If you use a social networking site, set your profile to "private" if that is an option.
- If you experience harassment online, do not respond to the harasser. Log off or go to a different site. If harassment continues, contact the harasser's internet service provider (ISP). Save all communications for evidence, and contact your ISP and your local police department.

QUICK STATS

**Native Americans are twice as likely to experience a rape or sexual assault when compared to all races.**

—Rape, Abuse, & Incest National Network (RAINN), 2022

**Violence against Children** Violence is also directed against children. In 2018, one in seven children were abused or neglected in the United States. About 3.5 million children received preventive services from Child Protective Services. Nearly five children die every day as a result of abuse and neglect.

Parents who abuse children tend to have low self-esteem, to believe in physical punishment, to have a poor marital relationship, and to have been abused themselves (although many people who were abused as children do not grow up to abuse their own children). Poverty, unemployment, and social isolation are characteristics of families in which children are abused. External stressors related to socioeconomic and environmental factors are most closely associated with neglect, whereas stressors related to interpersonal issues are more closely associated with physical abuse. Single parents are at especially high risk for abusing their children. Very often one child, whom the parents consider different in some way, is singled out for violent treatment.

**Elder Abuse** Each year over 4 million older adults are abused, exploited, or mistreated by someone who is supposed to be giving them care and protection; only 1 in 24 incidents is reported. Most abusers are family members who are serving as caregivers. Elder abuse can take different forms: physical, sexual, or emotional abuse; financial exploitation; neglect; or abandonment. Abuse may become an outlet for frustration. Many observers believe that the solution to elder abuse is support for both the elder and caregiver in the form of greater social and financial assistance, such as adult day care centers and education and public care programs.

## Sexual Violence

The use of force and coercion in sexual interactions is one of the most serious problems in human relationships. The most extreme manifestation of sexual coercion—forcing a person to submit to another's sexual desires—is rape, but sexual coercion occurs in many subtler forms, including sexual harassment (see the box "The #MeToo Movement and Sexual Harassment").

**Sexual Assault: Rape** **Sexual assault** is any unwanted sexual contact, including fondling and molestation. Rape is one type of sexual assault. Removing the term *forcible* from the offense name, the FBI redefined **rape** in 2013 as "penetration, no matter how slight, of the vagina or anus with any body part or object, or oral penetration by a sex organ of another person, without consent of the victim." When the victim is younger than the legally defined age of consent, the act constitutes **statutory rape,** whether or not coercion is involved. Coerced sexual activity in which the victim knows or is dating

TERMS

**cyberstalking** The use of email, chat rooms, bulletin boards, or other electronic communication devices to stalk another person.

**sexual assault** Any unwanted sexual contact.

**rape** Unwanted penetration—oral, anal, or vaginal.

**statutory rape** Sexual interaction with someone under the legal age of consent.

## TAKE CHARGE
### The #MeToo Movement and Sexual Harassment

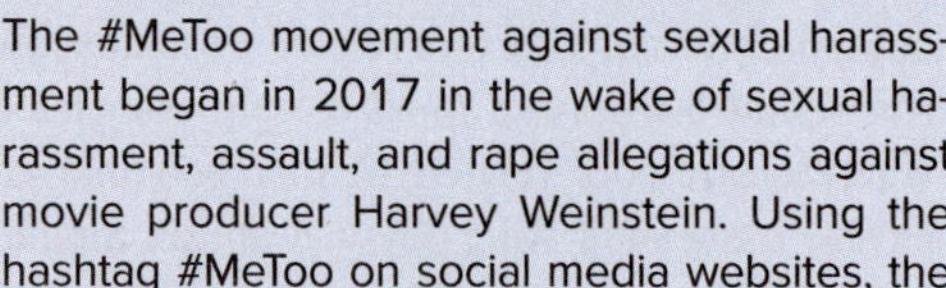

The #MeToo movement against sexual harassment began in 2017 in the wake of sexual harassment, assault, and rape allegations against movie producer Harvey Weinstein. Using the hashtag #MeToo on social media websites, the campaign encourages people to share stories of sexual abuse and misconduct perpetrated against them in order to demonstrate the magnitude of the problem. Beginning with Hollywood celebrities, the movement's popularity has spread to the media, music, and technology industries, scientific fields, academia, politics, and some religious institutions, resulting in the firing of numerous accused men in positions of power.

Although sexual harassment is forbidden by law, many cases go unreported. In a survey of 17,000 federal employees, 42% of women and 15% of men reported having been sexually harassed. If you are unsure what harassment is and whether you might be doing it, here are a few tips: Offer genuine compliments, but not about a person's body. Make conversation and jokes, but not those of a sexual nature. Greet others in a friendly way, not by whistling and leering. Be a kind, caring friend, coworker, or person; don't pat, rub, or touch someone without permission. Pursue friendships and romantic relationships, but not after the first one or two requests are turned down.

If you have been the victim of sexual harassment, you can take action to stop it. Be assertive with anyone who uses language or actions you find inappropriate. If possible, confront your harasser and tell him or her that the situation is unacceptable to you and you want the harassment to stop. Be clear. "Do not *ever* make sexual remarks to me" is an unequivocal statement. If assertive communication doesn't work, assemble a file or log documenting the harassment, noting the details of each incident and information about any witnesses who may be able to support your claims. You may discover others who have been harassed by the same person, which will strengthen your case. Then file a grievance with the harasser's supervisor or employer, such as someone in the dean's office if you are a student, or someone in the human resources office if you are an employee.

If your attempts to deal with the harassment internally are not successful, you can file an official complaint with your city or state Human Rights Commission or Fair Employment Practices Agency, or with the federal Equal Employment Opportunity Commission. You may also wish to pursue legal action under the Civil Rights Act or under local laws prohibiting employment discrimination. Often the threat of a lawsuit or other legal action is enough to stop the harasser.

the rapist is often referred to as **date rape,** or *acquaintance rape.* Most victims know their assailants, but fewer than 40% of all sexual crimes are reported. Because rape so often goes unreported, it is difficult to estimate how common it is and what demographic trends exist. Until the late 1980s, the popular understanding of rape was an event that occurs in a back alley with a stranger. Even people who had been raped in more common circumstances such as in a home or by someone they knew, and found their experience to be one of the worst of their lives, did not call it rape.

Although most people who experience sexual violence are women, some studies indicate that approximately a quarter of males (23.6%) experience some form of sexual violence over the course of their lifetime. This includes rape, being forced to penetrate an individual, sexual coercion, and unwanted sexual contact. Research on male rape victims has often focused on specific subpopulations such as incarcerated men, gay and bisexual men, and child sexual abuse cases. Few male victims report incidents, and when they do, it is after a significantly longer time than it takes females; it also takes males longer to seek medical and mental health treatment, and there are generally fewer resources set up for them.

Anyone can be a rape victim. Over 200,000 cases of rape are reported each year. One in five women have reported being raped, and 1 in 14 men have been made to penetrate someone else. Nearly half of bisexual women and one in eight lesbian women have experienced rape. Around 16% of women and 10% of men experienced sexual coercion by someone using pressure tactics, influence, or authority. More than a third of women and a fifth of men experienced unwanted sexual contact, like groping, in their lifetime. One-third of lesbian women and almost 60% of bisexual women reported unwanted sexual contact, as did a third of gay men and 20% of bisexual men.

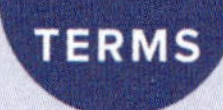


**date rape** Sexual assault by someone the victim knows or is dating; also called *acquaintance rape.*

People, in most cases men, who commit rape may be any age and come from any socioeconomic group. Some rapists are exploiters in the sense that they rape on the spur of the moment and mainly want immediate gratification. Some attempt to compensate for feelings of sexual inadequacy and an inability to obtain satisfaction otherwise. Others are more hostile and sadistic and are primarily interested in hurting and humiliating a particular person, in most cases a woman. Often the rapist is more interested in dominance, control, and power than in sexual satisfaction.

About 19% of rapes are committed by strangers, but acquaintances, current or former intimate partners, and nonspouse relatives make up the majority of perpetrators.

Most cases of date rape are never reported to the police, partly because of the subtlety of the crime. Usually no weapons are involved, and direct verbal threats may not have been made. Rather than being terrorized, the victim usually is attracted to the assailant at first. Victims of date rape tend to shoulder much of the responsibility for the incident, questioning their own judgment and behavior rather than blaming the aggressor.

**FACTORS CONTRIBUTING TO DATE RAPE** Although the general status of women in society has improved, the belief that nice women don't say yes to sex (even when they want to) and that real men don't take no for an answer is still prevalent among some groups.

Men and women also differ in their perception of romantic encounters and signals. In one study, researchers found that men interpreted women's actions on dates, such as smiling or talking in a low voice, as indicating an interest in having sex, whereas the women interpreted the same actions as being friendly.

Men who rape their dates tend to share certain attributes, including hostility toward women, a belief that dominance alone is a valid motive for sex, and an acceptance of sexual violence.

**DATE-RAPE DRUGS** Studies have shown that drugs are a factor in more than 60% of sexual assaults. The most common form of drug-facilitated sexual assault (DFSA) is alcohol; about 5% of DFSA victims are given date-rape drugs. Also called predator drugs, they include flunitrazepam (Rohypnol), gamma hydroxybutyrate (GHB), and ketamine ("Special K"). Rohypnol is not legal in the United States, but ketamine and GHB can be obtained legally because they are used for legitimate medical purposes.

These drugs have a variety of effects, including sedation; if slipped surreptitiously into a drink, they can incapacitate a person within about 20 minutes and make them more vulnerable to assault. Rohypnol, GHB, and other drugs also often cause anterograde amnesia, meaning victims have little memory of what happened while they were under the influence of the drug.

The Drug-Induced Rape Prevention and Punishment Act of 1996 adds up to 20 years to the prison sentence of any rapist who uses a drug to incapacitate a victim. Strategies such as the following can help ensure that your drink is not tampered with at a bar or party:

- Check with campus or local police to find out if drug-facilitated sexual assault has occurred in your area.
- Drink moderately and responsibly. Avoid group drinking and drinking games.
- Be wary of opened beverages—alcoholic or nonalcoholic—offered by strangers. When at an unfamiliar bar, watch the bartender pour your drink.
- Let your date be the first to drink from the punch bowl at a bar, club, or rave.
- If an opened beverage tastes, looks, or smells strange, do not drink it. If you leave your drink unattended, such as when you dance or use the restroom, get a fresh drink when you return to your table. Also, finish your food before leaving it unattended at the table.
- If you go to a party, club, or bar, go with friends. Arrange to arrive and leave together. Have a prearranged plan for checking on each other visually and verbally. If you feel giddy or lightheaded, get assistance.

Everyone can take actions that will reduce the incidence of acquaintance rape.

**DEALING WITH A SEXUAL ASSAULT** Experts disagree about whether a woman who is faced with a rapist should fight back or give in quietly to avoid being injured or to gain time in the hope of escaping. Each situation is unique, and a woman should respond in whatever way she thinks best. If you are threatened by a rapist and decide to fight back, here is what Women Organized Against Rape (WOAR) recommends:

- Trust your gut feeling. If you feel you are in danger, don't hesitate to run and scream. It is better to feel foolish than to be raped.
- Yell—and keep yelling. It will clear your head and start your adrenaline going; it may scare your attacker and also bring help. Don't forget that a rapist is also afraid of pain and afraid of getting caught.
- If an attacker grabs you from behind, use your elbows for striking their neck, sides, or stomach.
- Try kicking. Your legs are the strongest part of your body, and your kick is longer than their reach. Kick with the foot that is farther back and with the toe of your shoe. Aim low to avoid losing your balance.
- An attacker's most vulnerable spot is their knee; it's low, difficult to protect, and easily knocked out of place. Don't try to kick a rapist in the crotch; men will have better protective reflexes there.
- Once you start fighting, keep it up. Your objective is to get away as soon as you can.
- Remember that ordinary rules of behavior don't apply. It's OK to vomit, act crazy, or claim to have a sexually transmitted infection.

If you are raped, tell the first friendly person you meet what happened. Call the police, tell them you were raped, and give your location. Try to remember as many facts as you can about your attacker; write down a description as soon as possible. Don't wash or change your clothes, or you may destroy important evidence. The police will take you to a hospital for a complete exam; show the physician any injuries. Tell the police simply, but exactly, what happened. Be honest, and stick to the true account. If you decide that you don't want to report the rape to the police, be sure to see a physician as soon as possible. You need to be checked for pregnancy and sexually transmitted infections.

**THE EFFECTS OF RAPE** Rape victims suffer both physical and psychological injury. For most, physical wounds heal within a few weeks. Psychological pain may endure and be substantial. Even the most physically and mentally strong are likely to experience shock, anxiety, depression, shame, and a host of psychosomatic symptoms after being victimized. These psychological reactions following rape constitute rape trauma syndrome, which is characterized by fear, nightmares, fatigue, crying spells, and digestive upset. (Rape trauma syndrome is a form of posttraumatic stress disorder; see Chapter 3.) Self-blame is very likely; society has contributed to this tendency by perpetuating the myths that people can always defend themselves and that no one can be raped if they don't "want" to be. Fortunately these false beliefs are dissolving in the face of evidence to the contrary.

Many organizations offer counseling and support to rape victims. Look in the telephone directory under Rape or Rape Crisis Center for a hotline number to call. Your campus may have counseling services or a support group.

**Child Sexual Abuse** Child sexual abuse is any sexual contact between an adult and a child who is below the legal age of consent. Adults and older adolescents are able to coerce children into sexual activity because of their authority and power over them. Threats, force, or the promise of friendship or material rewards may be used to manipulate a child. Sexual contacts are typically brief and consist of genital manipulation; genital intercourse is much less common.

Sexual abusers are usually male, heterosexual, and known to the victim. The abuser may be a relative, a friend, a neighbor, or another trusted adult acquaintance. Child abusers are often pedophiles, people who are sexually attracted to children. They may have poor interpersonal and sexual relationships with other adults and feel socially inadequate and inferior. One highly traumatic form of sexual abuse is **incest:** sexual activity between people too closely related to legally marry.

Child sexual abuse is often unreported. Surveys suggest that as many as 27% of women and 16% of men were sexually abused as children. An estimated 150,000–200,000 new cases of child sexual abuse occur each year. It can leave lasting scars; victims are more likely to suffer as adults from low self-esteem, depression, anxiety, eating disorders, self-destructive tendencies, sexual problems, and difficulties in intimate relationships.

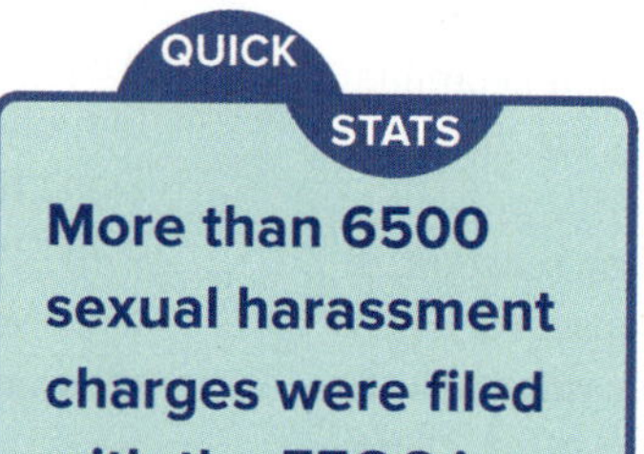

**QUICK STATS**

**More than 6500 sexual harassment charges were filed with the EEOC in 2020.**

—U.S. Equal Employment Opportunity Commission

If you were a victim of sexual abuse as a child and feel it may be interfering with your functioning today, you may want to address the problem. A variety of approaches can help, such as joining a support group of people who have had similar experiences, confiding in a partner or friend, or seeking professional help.

**Sexual Harassment** Unwelcome sexual advances, requests for sexual favors, and other verbal, visual, or physical conduct of a sexual nature constitute **sexual harassment** if such conduct explicitly or implicitly affects academic or employment decisions or evaluations; interferes with an individual's academic or work performance; or creates an intimidating, hostile, or offensive academic, work, or student living environment.

Extreme cases of sexual harassment occur when a manager, a professor, or another person in authority uses their ability to control or influence jobs or grades to coerce people into having sex or to punish them if they refuse. A hostile environment can be created by conduct such as sexual gestures, display of sexually suggestive objects or pictures, derogatory comments and jokes, sexual remarks about clothing or appearance, obscene letters, and unnecessary touching or pinching.

## What You Can Do about Violence

Violence in our society is a serious threat to our collective health and well-being. This is especially true on college campuses, which in a sense are communities in themselves but sometimes lack the authority or guidance to tackle the issue of violence directly (see the box "Gun Violence"). Schools are now providing training for conflict resolution and are educating people about the diverse nature of our society, thereby encouraging tolerance and understanding.

Reducing gun-related injuries may require changes in the availability, possession, and lethality of the 10–14 million firearms sold legally in the United States each year with the appropriate supporting documentation. As part of the Brady gun control law, computerized instant background checks are performed for about 60% of gun sales (those by federally licensed dealers) to prevent purchases by convicted felons, people with a history of mental instability, and certain other groups; however, broad loopholes

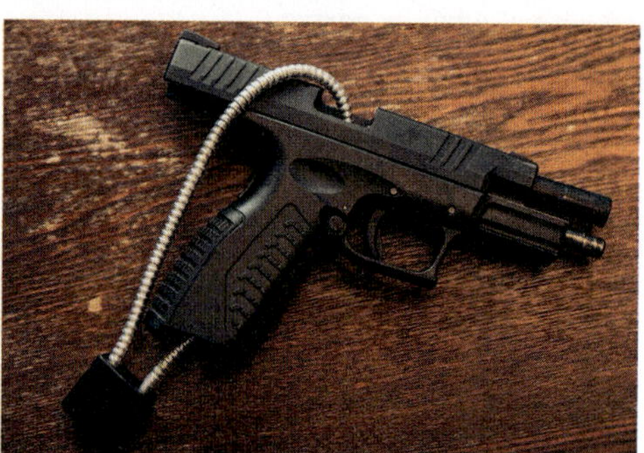

Using a gun lock can prevent firearm accidents. Tippman98x/Shutterstock

**TERMS**

**incest** Sexual activity between close relatives, such as siblings or parents and their children.

**sexual harassment** Unwelcome sexual advances, requests for sexual favors, and other conduct of a sexual nature that affects academic or employment decisions or evaluations; interferes with an individual's academic or work performance; or creates an intimidating, hostile, or offensive academic, work, or student living environment.

**Ask Yourself**

**QUESTIONS FOR CRITICAL THINKING AND REFLECTION**

Are you or is anyone you know a survivor of a violent act? If so, what were the circumstances surrounding the event? What was the outcome? How did the event affect your life or the life of the person you know?

## Gun Violence

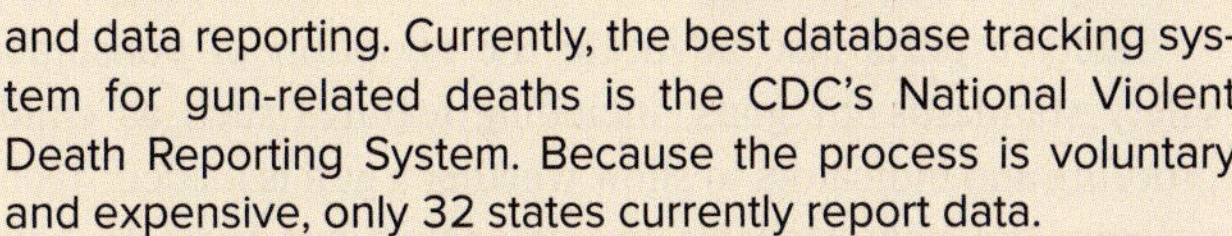

When Americans face health threats like a virus or disease, our health care providers take immediate action to control the epidemic. Should we take a similar approach to gun violence?

Statistics on gun violence are grim. In 2020, the CDC recorded the highest number of deaths from gun-related injuries: 45,222 people. It disproportionately affects young people, particularly males, and socially disadvantaged groups. Gun violence is a uniquely American problem. Making up only 5% of the world population, Americans nevertheless own 42% of privately held guns. In the United States there are more guns than people.

Should gun violence be viewed as any other contagion that can spread and endanger life? Special interest groups like the National Rifle Association have lobbied hard to prevent a public health approach. In response to attempts by the CDC to study gun violence in the mid-1990s, a Republican-Congress, pushed by gun lobbyists, passed the Dickey Amendment, which prohibits government-sponsored health institutions from using funds to "advocate or promote gun control." In 2016, over 140 medical institutions signed a letter to Congress urging it to lift restrictions on funding for gun violence research. That finally came to pass in 2018; the next year lawmakers approved funding for research. In 2021, Rochelle Walensky became the first CDC director in over 20 years to make a strong public statement about gun violence, calling it a "serious public health threat," possibly signaling that research will finally be prioritized.

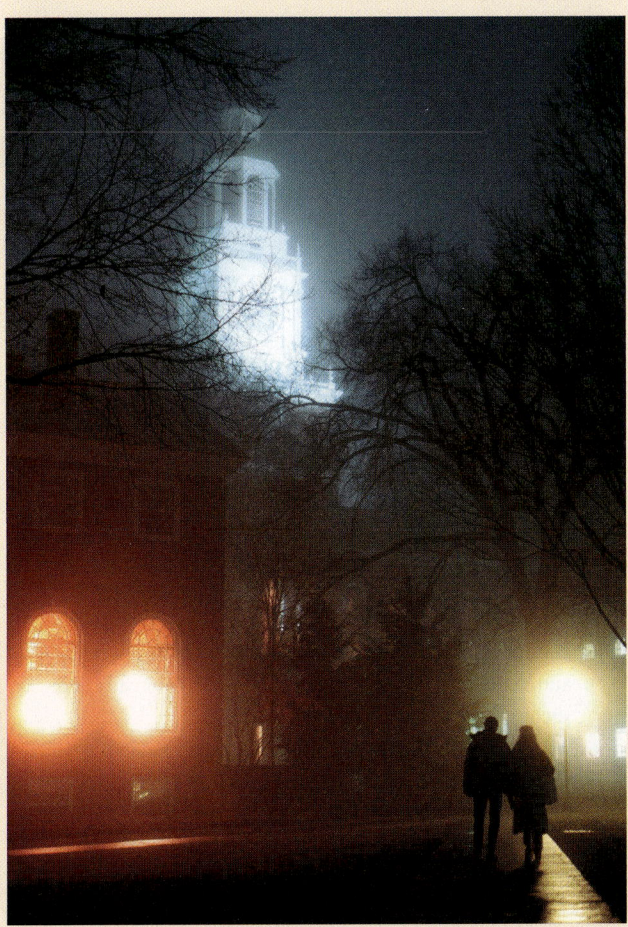

George Robinson/Alamy Stock Photo

The American Public Health Association (APHA) suggests we need better surveillance and data reporting. Currently, the best database tracking system for gun-related deaths is the CDC's National Violent Death Reporting System. Because the process is voluntary and expensive, only 32 states currently report data.

One consistent theme that emerges from the limited research in this country and from research abroad is that more firearms and more permissive laws are associated with more gun-related deaths, whereas fewer guns and more restrictive laws are associated with fewer gun fatalities. In states such as New York, New Jersey, and Rhode Island, where gun ownership was 5–10% in 2013, there were roughly 5 gun deaths per 100,000 residents. By contrast, states such as Idaho, Arkansas, and West Virginia had a gun ownership rate of 55–60% and a gun death rate of around 15 per 100,000 residents.

The AHPA calls for "commonsense" gun laws:

- Universal background checks for all, including purchasers online or at gun shows
- The reinstatement of the federal ban on high-powered assault rifles, which expired in 2004
- Expanded access to mental health services. It's important to note, however, that people with mental illnesses are more likely to be victims of gun violence, not perpetrators
- Expanded resources for school and community prevention strategies
- Greater investment in gun safety technologies

Since the 2012 shootings at Sandy Hook Elementary School in Connecticut, when 6 adults and 20 young children were killed by a 20-year-old gunman, a movement of young activists started to take shape. The #neveragain movement has blossomed as mass shootings continue to take out high school and college students, and politicians continue to listen to gun lobbyists. A poll by Harvard University's Institute of Politics shows that two-thirds of American voters under age 30 support stricter gun-control laws. They are marching, protesting, speaking up, and may be shifting the debate.

**SOURCES:** Alter, C. 2018. 'We just had a gun to our heads.' The Florida shooting survivors are transforming America's gun debate. *Time*, February 21 (http://time.com/5169436/florida-shooting-kids-gun-control-debate/); American Public Health Association. 2018. *Preventing Gun Violence* (https://www.apha.org/-/media/files/pdf/factsheets/160317_gunviolencefs.ashx?la=en&hash=AB71DE1BEDEBB2A797F8EC378E672791904FCF87); Gun Violence Archive. 2018. Past Summary Ledgers (http://www.gunviolencearchive.org/past-tolls); Lopez, G. 2018. America's gun problem, explained. *Vox* (https://www.vox.com/2015/10/3/9444417/gun-violence-united-states-america); Editors. 2021. Gun violence is an epidemic. Better data can help. *Bloomberg Opinion* (https://www.bloomberg.com/opinion/articles/2021-09-28/the-cdc-director-is-right-gun-violence-is-a-threat-to-public-health-ku413do3); National Public Radio. 2022. Treating gun violence as a "serious public health threat." *Consider This* From NPR (https://www.npr.org/2022/01/13/1072842699/treating-gun-violence-as-a-serious-public-health-threat); Zhang, S. 2018. Why can't the U.S. treat gun violence as a public-health problem? *The Atlantic* (https://www.theatlantic.com/health/archive/2018/02/gun-violence-public-health/553430/).

exist for purchasing guns from private sellers, at gun shows, or online, without background checks. In some states, waiting periods are required in addition to the background checks. Some groups advocate a complete and universal federal ban on the sale of all firearms, but most want "commonsense" reform, like universal background checks and bans on military-style assault weapons.

Safety experts also advocate the adoption of consumer safety standards for guns, including features such as childproofing and indicators to show whether a gun is loaded. Technologies are now available to personalize handguns to help prevent unauthorized use. Owner identification through magnetic encoding, touch memory, radio frequency, or fingerprint reading can prevent others from using a personalized handgun. Education about proper storage is also important. Surveys indicate that more than 34% of homes with children contain guns. Data also show that in only 39% of those homes are firearms stored properly: locked, unloaded, and separate from ammunition. Unfortunately, over 7000 children are admitted to U.S. hospitals with gunshot wounds each year. To be effective, any approach to firearm injury prevention must have the support of law enforcement and the community as a whole.

## PROVIDING EMERGENCY CARE

A course in **first aid** can help you respond appropriately when someone is injured. One important benefit of first aid training is learning what *not* to do in certain situations. For example, a person with a suspected neck or back injury should not be moved unless there are other life-threatening conditions. A trained person can assess emergency situations accurately before acting.

Emergency rescue techniques can save the lives of people who are choking, who have stopped breathing, or whose hearts have stopped beating. As described earlier, the Heimlich maneuver is used when a victim is choking. Pulmonary resuscitation (also known as rescue breathing, artificial respiration, or mouth-to-mouth resuscitation) is used when a person is not breathing. Cardiopulmonary resuscitation (CPR) is used when a pulse cannot be found. In 2010, the American Heart Association made significant changes in its CPR guidelines for laypersons. Previous guidelines were to clear the airway, check for breathing, and begin chest compressions (ABC). The current guidelines are to begin chest compressions, clear the airway, and check for breathing (CAB). Starting with compressions gets the blood circulating, which is critical to keeping the person alive until help arrives. Compressions should be delivered fast, about 100 times a minute. The American Heart Association also authorizes use of a hands-only CPR technique on a teen or adult who suddenly collapses due to cardiac arrest; learn more and watch training videos at the association's website (heart.org/handsonlycpr). Courses in first aid and CPR are offered by the American Heart Association and the American Red Cross.

A new feature of some of these courses is training in the use of automated external defibrillators (AEDs), which monitor the heart's rhythm and, if appropriate, deliver an electrical shock to restart the heart. Because of the importance of early use of defibrillators in saving heart attack victims, these devices are being installed in public places, including casinos, airports, and many office buildings.

As a person providing assistance, you are the first link in the **emergency medical services (EMS) system**, a system designed to network community resources for providing emergency care.

**TERMS**

**first aid** Emergency care given to an ill or injured person until medical care can be obtained.

**emergency medical services (EMS) system** A system designed to network community resources for providing emergency care.

### Ask Yourself

**QUESTIONS FOR CRITICAL THINKING AND REFLECTION**

What kinds of emergency training have you had? What kinds of skills do you have that would enable you to help someone who was hurt, was trapped, or needed some other kind of assistance?

### TIPS FOR TODAY AND THE FUTURE

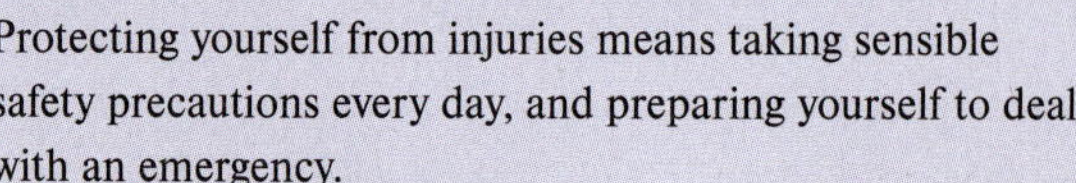

Protecting yourself from injuries means taking sensible safety precautions every day, and preparing yourself to deal with an emergency.

**RIGHT NOW YOU CAN:**

- Check your home for any object or situation that could cause an injury, such as a tripping hazard, top-heavy shelves, and so on.
- Test the batteries in your home's smoke detectors, and change them if necessary. Test the detectors to make sure they work properly.
- If you ride a bike, check your helmet to ensure that it fits properly and will protect you in a crash. If you have any doubts, throw it away and buy a new one.

**IN THE FUTURE YOU CAN:**

- Get trained in CPR, rescue breathing, and the use of an automated external defibrillator. If you have already had such training, take a refresher course.
- Be watchful for hazardous situations at your school or workplace. If you notice anything suspicious, report it to an appropriate person right away.
- Prepare for a poisoning emergency by putting the number of your local poison control hotline in a conspicuous place.

## SUMMARY

- Injuries are caused by a dynamic interaction of human and environmental factors.
- The home can contain many poisonous substances, including medications, cleaning agents, plants, and fumes from cars and appliances.
- Most fall-related injuries occur on stairs or steps. Alcohol, chairs, and ladders are also involved in a significant number of falls.
- Careless smoking and problems with cooking or heating equipment are common causes of home fires. Being prepared for fire emergencies means planning escape routes and installing smoke detectors.
- Performing the Heimlich maneuver can prevent someone from choking to death.
- The proper storage and handling of firearms can help prevent injuries; assume that any gun is loaded.
- Key factors in motor vehicle injuries include aggressive driving, speeding, a failure to wear seat belts, alcohol and drug intoxication, fatigue, and distraction.
- Motorcycle, motor scooter, and bicycle injuries can be prevented by developing appropriate skills, driving or riding defensively, and wearing proper safety equipment, especially a helmet.
- Many injuries during leisure activities result from the misuse of equipment, lack of experience, use of alcohol, and a failure to wear proper safety equipment.
- Most work-related injuries involve extensive manual labor; back problems and repetitive strain injuries are most common.
- Factors contributing to violence include poverty, the absence of strong social ties, the influence of the mass media, cultural attitudes about gender roles, problems in interpersonal relationships, alcohol and drug use, and the availability of firearms.
- Types of violence include assault, homicide, gang-related violence, hate crimes, school violence, workplace violence, terrorism, family and intimate-partner violence, and sexual violence.
- Physical abuse occurs at every socioeconomic level. The core issue is the abuser's need to control other people.
- Most rape victims are women, and most know their attackers.
- Child sexual abuse often results in serious trauma; usually the abuser is a trusted adult.
- Sexual harassment is unwelcome sexual advances or other conduct of a sexual nature that affects academic or employment performance or evaluations or that creates an intimidating, hostile, or offensive academic, work, or student living environment.
- Strategies for reducing violence include conflict resolution training, social skills development, and education programs that foster tolerance and understanding among diverse groups.
- Steps in giving emergency care include making sure the scene is safe for you and the injured person, conducting a quick examination of the victim, calling for help, and providing emergency first aid.

## FOR MORE INFORMATION

*American Association of Poison Control Centers.* Provides free, confidential, and expert advice related to poisoning.

800-222-1222

http://www.aapcc.org

*American Automobile Association Foundation for Traffic Safety.* Provides consumer information about all aspects of traffic safety; the website has online quizzes and extensive links.

http://www.aaafoundation.org/home

*American Bar Association: Domestic Violence.* Provides information about statistics, research, and laws relating to domestic violence.

https://www.americanbar.org/groups/domestic_violence/

*Consumer Product Safety Commission.* Provides information and advice about safety issues relating to consumer products.

http://www.cpsc.gov

*Governor's Highway Safety Association.* Provides up-to-date information about cell phone and texting laws, as well as general information and publications related to traffic safety.

http://www.ghsa.org/html/stateinfo/laws/cellphone_laws.html

*Insurance Institute for Highway Safety.* Provides information about crashes on the nation's highways, as well as reports on topics such as speeding and crashworthiness of vehicles.

http://www.iihs.org

*Learning for Justice.* Offers suggestions for fighting hate and promoting tolerance; sponsored by the Southern Poverty Law Center.

https://www.learningforjustice.org/

*National Center for Health Statistics (Centers for Disease Control and Prevention).* Monitors the health of the United States and provides up-to-date information and statistical data to the public and professionals.

http://www.cdc.gov/nchs

*National Center for Injury Prevention and Control.* Provides consumer-oriented information about unintentional injuries and violence.

http://www.cdc.gov/injury

*National Center for Victims of Crime.* An advocacy group for crime victims; provides statistics, news, safety strategies, tips on finding local assistance, and links to related sites.

http://www.victimsofcrime.org

*National Children's Alliance.* Helps local communities respond to allegations of child abuse.

http://nationalchildrensalliance.org

*National Fire Protection Agency.* Gives information about fire, electrical, and related hazards.

www.nfpa.org

*National Highway Traffic Safety Administration.* Supplies materials about reducing deaths, injuries, and economic losses from motor vehicle crashes.

http://www.nhtsa.gov

*National Safety Council.* Provides information and statistics about preventing unintentional injuries.

http://www.nsc.org

*National Violence Hotlines.* Provide information, referral services, and crisis intervention.

800-799-SAFE (7233) (domestic violence), http://www.thehotline.org

800-422-4453 (child abuse), http://www.childhelp.org

800-656-HOPE (4673) (sexual assault), http://www.rainn.org

*Occupational Safety and Health Administration.* Provides information about topics related to health and safety issues in the workplace.

http://www.osha.gov

*Prevent Child Abuse America.* Provides statistics, information, and publications relating to child abuse, including parenting tips.

http://www.preventchildabuse.org

*Rape, Abuse, and Incest National Network (RAINN).* Provides guidelines for preventing and dealing with sexual assault and abuse.

http://www.rainn.org

*World Health Organization: Violence and Injury Prevention and Disability.* Provides statistics and information about the consequences of intentional and unintentional injuries worldwide.

http://www.who.int/violence_injury_prevention

The following sites provide statistics and background information about violence and crime in the United States:

*Bureau of Justice Statistics:* http://www.bjs.gov

*Federal Bureau of Investigation:* http://www.fbi.gov

*National Criminal Justice Reference Service:* http://www.ncjrs.gov

## SELECTED BIBLIOGRAPHY


AAA Foundation for Traffic Safety. 2020. *Cannabis Use Among Drivers in Fatal Crashes in Washington State Before and After Legalization* (https://aaafoundation.org/cannabis-use-among-drivers-in-fatal-crashes-in-washington-state-before-and-after-legalization/).

Administration for Children & Families. 2020. Child abuse, neglect data released. *29th edition of the Child Maltreatment Report.* Washington, DC: U.S. Department of Health & Human Services (https://www.acf.hhs.gov/media/press/2020/2020/child-abuse-neglect-data-released).

Ahrens, M. and Evarts B. 2021. *Fire Loss in the United States During 2020.* National Fire Protection Association (https://www.nfpa.org/~/media/fd0144a044c84fc5baf90c05c04890b7.ashx).

Aizenman, N. 2017. Gun violence: How the U.S. compares with other countries. *National Public Radio,* October 6 (https://www.npr.org/sections/goatsandsoda/2017/10/06/555861898/gun-violence-how-the-u-s-compares-to-other-countries).

Bicycle Helmet Safety Institute. 2022. *Bicycle Helmet Laws* (https://www.helmets.org/mandator.htm).

Burch, A. D. S., and L. V. Ploeg. 2022. Buffalo shooting highlights rise of hate crimes against Black Americans. *The New York Times,* May 16 (https://www.nytimes.com/2022/05/16/us/hate-crimes-black-african-americans.html).

Bureau of Labor Statistics. 2021. Employer-related workplace injuries and illnesses—2020. *News Release.* Washington, DC: U.S. Department of Labor (https://www.bls.gov/news.release/pdf/osh.pdf).

Cantor, D., et al. 2020. *Report on the AAU Campus Climate Survey on Sexual Assault and Misconduct.* Association of American Universities. (https://www.aau.edu/sites/default/files/AAU-Files/Key-Issues/Campus-Safety/Revised%20Aggregate%20report%20%20and%20appendices%201-7_(01-16-2020_FINAL).pdf).

Centers for Disease Control and Prevention. 2019. *10 Leading Causes of Deaths by Age Group United States—2019* (https://wisqars.cdc.gov/cgi-bin/broker.exe).

Centers for Disease Control and Prevention. 2019. *Nonfatal Injury Reports, 2000–2019.* Atlanta, GA: Centers for Disease Control and Prevention (https://wisqars.cdc.gov/nonfatal-reports).

Centers for Disease Control and Prevention. 2020. *Global Road Safety* (https://www.cdc.gov/injury/features/global-road-safety/index.html).

Centers for Disease Control and Prevention. 2020. *Impaired Driving: Get the Facts. Injury Prevention and Control: Motor Vehicle Safety.* Atlanta, GA: Centers for Disease Control and Prevention (https://www.cdc.gov/motorvehiclesafety/impaired_driving/impaired-drv_factsheet.html).

Centers for Disease Control and Prevention. 2021. *Drug Overdose Deaths in the United States, 1999–2020.* NCHS Data Brief, no 428. Hyattsville, MD: National Center for Health Statistics (https://www.cdc.gov/nchs/products/databriefs/db428.htm)

Centers for Disease Control and Prevention. 2021. *Mortality in the United States, 2020.* NCHS Data Brief, no 427. Hyattsville, MD: National Center for Health Statistics (https://www.cdc.gov/nchs/products/databriefs/db427.htm#section_4).

Centers for Disease Control and Prevention. 2021. *Preventing Child Abuse and Neglect* (https://www.cdc.gov/violenceprevention/childabuseandneglect/fastfact.html).

Centers for Disease Control and Prevention. 2021. *Preventing Elder Abuse* (https://www.cdc.gov/violenceprevention/elderabuse/fastfact.html).

Centers for Disease Control and Prevention. 2021. *Violence Prevention* (https://www.cdc.gov/violenceprevention/firearms/fastfact.html).

Centers for Disease Control and Prevention. 2022. *Leading Causes of Death* (https://www.cdc.gov/nchs/fastats/leading-causes-of-death.htm).

Centers for Disease Control and Prevention. 2022. U.S. overdose deaths in 2021 increased half as much as in 2020 - but are still up 15%. Press release (https://www.cdc.gov/nchs/pressroom/nchs_press_releases/2022/202205.htm).

Federal Bureau of Investigation. 2020. *Crime in the United States, 2019.* U.S. Department of Justice (https://ucr.fbi.gov/crime-in-the-u.s/2019/crime-in-the-u.s.-2019/topic-pages/murder).

Federal Bureau of Investigation. 2021. *FBI Releases 2020 Crime Statistics.* Washington, DC: U.S. Department of Justice (https://www.fbi.gov/news/pressrel/press-releases/fbi-releases-2020-crime-statistics).

Federal Bureau of Investigation National Press Office. 2021. FBI releases updated 2020 hate crime statistics. Press release (https://www.fbi.gov/news/pressrel/press-releases/fbi-releases-updated-2020-hate-crime-statistics).

Fornaris, J. 2021. *Gangs in America* (https://storymaps.arcgis.com/stories/000d265de2a74cada1a21ff555b6dd3e).

Frederique, N. 2020. What do data reveal about violence in schools? National Institute of Justice (https://nij.ojp.gov/topics/articles/what-do-data-reveal-about-violence-schools).

Goodnough, A. 2021. Overdose deaths have surged during the pandemic, CDC data shows. *New York Times* (https://www.nytimes.com/2021/04/14/health/overdose-deaths-fentanyl-opiods-coronaviurs-pandemic.html).

Governors Highway Safety Association. 2021. *Child Passenger Safety Laws* (http://www.ghsa.org/html/stateinfo/laws/childsafety_laws.html).

Human Rights Campaign. 2022. *Fatal Violence Against the Transgender and Gender Non-Conforming Community in 2022* (https://www.hrc.org/resources/fatal-violence-against-the-transgender-and-gender-non-conforming-community-in-2022).

Institute of Education Sciences. 2021. *Report on Indicators of School Crime and Safety: 2020* (https://nces.ed.gov/pubs2021/2021092.pdf).

Institute of Education Sciences. 2022. *Incidence of Victimization at School and Away From School* (https://nces.ed.gov/programs/coe/indicator/a02?tid=4).

Johnson, K. 2021. FBI: Record surge in 2020 murders. USA Today (https://www.usatoday.com/story/news/politics/2021/09/27/fbi-reports-2020-murder-surge-biggest-single-year-jump/5886792001/).

Kaiser Family Foundation 2019. Intimate Partner Violence (IPV) Screening and Counseling Services in Clinical Settings (https://www.kff.org/report-section/intimate-partner-violence-ipv-screening-and-counseling-services-in-clinical-settings-issue-brief/#endnote_link_441373-1).

Kochanek, K.D., et al. 2017. Deaths: Final data for 2017. *National Vital Statistics Reports* 68(9) (https://www.cdc.gov/nchs/data/nvsr/nvsr68/nvsr68_09-508.pdf)

Lee, J., and K. Ramakrishnan. 2021. Anti-Asian hate affects upwards of 2 million adults (http://aapidata.com/blog/anti-asian-hate-2-million/).

Lucas, R. 2021. FBI data shows an unprecedented spike in murders nationwide in 2020. *National Public Radio* (https://www.npr.org/2021/09/27/1040904770/fbi-data-murder-increase-2020).

May, T. 2018. For Chinese pedestrians glued to their phones, a middle path emerges. The New York Times, June 8 (https://www.nytimes.com/2018/06/08/world/asia/china-pedestrians-smartphones-path.html).

Miller, M., Zhang, W., Azrael, D. 2021. Firearm Purchasing during the Covid-19 pandemic: Results from the 2021 National Firearms Survey. Annals of Internal Medicine (https://www.acpjournals.org/doi/full/10.7326/M21-3423).

Morgan, R. and Truman, J. 2020. Criminal Victimization, 2019. U.S. Department of Justice (https://www.bjs.gov/content/pub/pdf/cv19.pdf).

National Center for Education Statistics. 2020. Indicators of school crime and safety. Institute of Education Sciences (https://nces.ed.gov/programs/crimeindicators/ind_01.asp).

National Health Care Provider Solutions. 2015. AHA 2015 Guidelines Are Published: CPR Key Points (https://nhcps.com/aha-2015-cpr-guidelines-published-key-points/).

National Highway Traffic Safety Administration. n.d. *Distracted Driving* (https://www.nhtsa.gov/risky-driving/distracted-driving).

National Safety Council. 2022. *All Injuries: Overview* (https://injuryfacts.nsc.org/all-injuries/overview/).

National Safety Council. 2022. *Costs: Societal Costs* (https://injuryfacts.nsc.org/all-injuries/costs/societal-costs/).

National Safety Council. 2022. *Road Users: Pedestrians* (https://injuryfacts.nsc.org/motor-vehicle/road-users/pedestrians/).

Occupational Safety and Health Administration. 2002. *Fact Sheet: Workplace Violence* (https://www.osha.gov/sites/default/files/publications/factsheet-workplace-violence.pdf).

Office of Behavioral Safety Research. 2021. Update to special reports on traffic safety during the COVID-19 public health emergency: Fourth quarter data (Report No. DOT HS 813 135). National Highway Traffic Safety Administration (https://rosap.ntl.bts.gov/view/dot/56125).

Peeples, L. 2020. What the data says about police brutality and racial bias—and which reforms might work. *Nature* (https://www.nature.com/articles/d41586-020-01846-z)

Peitzmeier, S. M., et al. 2020, September 1. Intimate partner violence in transgender populations: Systematic review and meta-analysis of prevalence and correlates. *American Journal of Public Health* 110(9): e1–e14 (https://ajph.aphapublications.org/doi/10.2105/AJPH.2020.305774).

Pickrell, T. M., and E.-H. Choi. 2015. Seat Belt Use in 2014—Overall Results (Report No. DOT HS 812 113). Washington, DC: National Highway Traffic Safety Administration.

Rape, Abuse & Incest National Network (RAINN). 2022. *Campus Sexual Violence: Statistics* (https://www.rainn.org/statistics/campus-sexual-violence).

Rape, Abuse & Incest National Network (RAINN). 2022. *Perpetrators of Sexual Violence: Statistics* (https://www.rainn.org/statistics/perpetrators-sexual-violence).

Rape, Abuse & Incest National Network (RAINN). 2022. *Victims of Sexual Violence: Statistics* (https://www.rainn.org/statistics/victims-sexual-violence).

Reyns, B., B. Henson, and B. Fisher. 2012. Stalking in the twilight zone: Extent of cyberstalking victimization and offending among college students. Deviant Behavior 33(1): 1–25.

Ritchie, H. 2018. Is it fair to compare terrorism and disaster with other causes of death? Our World in Data blog (https://ourworldindata.org/is-it-fair-to-compare-terrorism-and-disaster-with-other-causes-of-death).

Schmidt, M. 2018. How to not sexually harass someone: A simple guide to decency (https://inland360.com/more-news/2018/10/how-to-not-sexually-harass-someone-a-simple-guide-to-decency/).

Schramm P. J., et al. 2021. Heat-related emergency department visits during the Northwestern heat wave—United States, June 2021. Morbidity and Mortality Weekly Report 70: 1020–1021.

Southern Poverty Law Center. 2021. Hate Crimes, Explained (https://www.splcenter.org/hate-crimes-explained).

Swogger, M. T., et al. 2012. Self-reported childhood physical abuse and perpetration of intimate partner violence: The moderating role of psychopathic traits. Criminal Justice and Behavior 39(7): 910–922.

This American Life. 2022. My lying eyes. Episode 770 (https://www.thisamericanlife.org/770/my-lying-eyes).

U.S. Bureau of Labor Statistics. 2021. *Employer-Reported Workplace Injuries and Illnesses, 2020*. U.S. Department of Labor (https://www.bls.gov/news.release/pdf/osh.pdf).

U.S. Bureau of Labor Statistics. 2021. *National Census Fatal Occupational Injuries, 2020*. U.S. Department of Labor (https://www.bls.gov/news.release/pdf/cfoi.pdf).

Walfield, S. M. 2021. Men cannot be raped: Correlates of male rape myth acceptance. *Journal of Interpersonal Violence* 36(13–14): 6391–6417.

Webster, D., Crifasi, C. K., and J. S. Vernick. 2014. Effects of the repeal of Missouri's handgun purchaser licensing law on homicides. Journal of Urban Health 91(2): 293–302.

Williams Institute. 2021. Press release: Transgender people over four times more likely than cisgender people to be victims of violent crime. University of California Los Angeles (https://williamsinstitute.law.ucla.edu/press/ncvs-trans-press-release/).

World Health Organization. 2021. *Road Traffic Injuries* (Fact Sheet No. 358) (http://www.who.int/mediacentre/factsheets/fs358/en/).

Xu, J. Q., et al. 2021. Deaths: Final data for 2019. *National Vital Statistics Reports;* 70(08). Hyattsville, MD: National Center for Health Statistics. DOI: https://dx.doi.org/10.15620/cdc:106058

**Design Elements:** Assess Yourself icon: Aleksey Boldin/Alamy Stock Photo; Diversity Matters icon: Rawpixel Ltd/Getty Images; Wellness on Campus icon: Radius Images/Alamy Stock Photo; Take Charge icon: VisualCommunications/Getty Images; Critical Consumer icon: pagadesign/Getty Images.

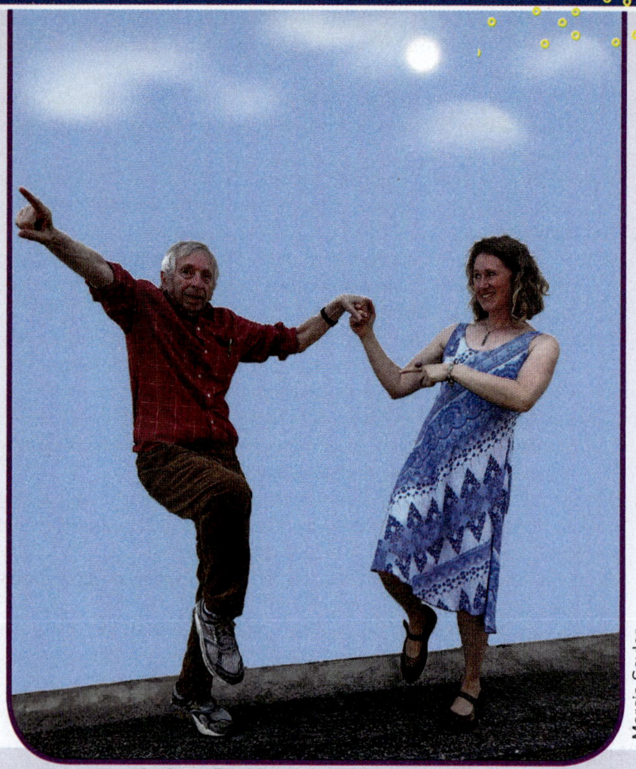
Marcia Seyler

Authors Paul Insel, aged 82, and Claire Insel, aged 42.

## CHAPTER OBJECTIVES

- List strategies for healthy aging
- Identify challenges that may accompany aging and explain how people can best confront them
- Explain the factors influencing life expectancy
- Understand the issues facing older adults in the United States

CHAPTER 18

# The Challenge of Aging

***Nor, indeed, are we to give our attention solely to the body; much greater care is due to the mind and soul; for they, too, like lamps, grow dim with time, unless we keep them supplied with oil.***

—On Old Age, Cicero (106–43 BCE)

In 2021, the number of Americans aged 100 or older was about 97,000, compared with only about 4000 centenarians in 1950. And it's not only the extremely old who are increasing in number. The percentage of Americans aged 65 and up has quadrupled since the beginning of the 20th century, from about 4% of the total population in 1900 to about 16% in 2020. In the United States, as in much of the world, people are living longer while birth rates are declining, resulting in a gradual but profound aging of our population.

**Aging** refers to the changes that occur in an organism over time. Aging is an inevitable process that begins at birth and ends when we die. Despite the inevitability of aging, there are many factors, some of which are in our control, that can modify the rate at which we age and the quality of our lives during our older years. There is no definitive age at which we become "old," but age 65 is commonly used in research and population statistics as the lower limit of old age. Throughout this text, the terms "older" and "elderly" refer to people aged 65 years and up.

## PERSPECTIVES ON AGING

In general, *biological aging* is associated with a reduction in the body's potential to repair and regenerate tissue. **Gerontology** is the scientific study of the physical changes that occur with aging. Despite an explosion of aging-related research, we have

> **TERMS**
>
> **aging** A normal process of getting older, which includes physical, mental, and social changes.
>
> **gerontology** The scientific study of the physical changes that occur with aging.

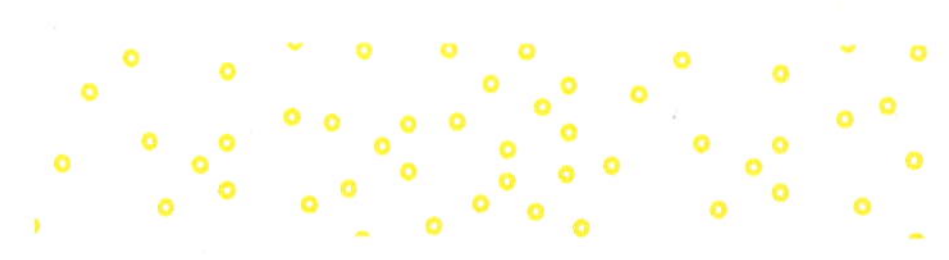

a long way to go before we fully understand the biological processes of aging. Current theories of aging fall into two main groups: programmed and damage related.

*Programmed aging* hypothesizes that our bodies age because of a hardwired pattern of shifts in gene expression that have been programmed through evolution. Advocates of this theory say that just as the growth of an embryo or a child occurs in a predetermined orderly manner, our genetic expression continues to change in a programmed manner throughout life, which ultimately results in the physical changes of aging and death.

*Damage-related aging* theories postulate that environmental exposures such as disease, toxins, and natural radiation cause genetic and cellular damage that eventually exceeds the capacity of our bodies' repair systems.

*Psychological aging* refers to the cognitive, emotional, and behavioral changes that naturally occur in humans over time. These include a gradual decline in cognitive processing speed, memory, and other mental functions, which occurs in most healthy older people. The normal cognitive changes associated with aging are relatively mild compared with the severe cognitive and behavioral deficits that occur in neurodegenerative diseases such as Alzheimer's disease.

Finally, *social aging* refers to the shifts in our relationships and societal roles as we age. These changes are often the result of major life events such as retirement, changes in income, deaths of family members and friends, or moving to a new location.

Old age can be a wonderful part of life's journey. Many people live out their later years in loving and stable relationships and are in good psychological and physical health until they reach very old age. Others experience great challenges during the aging process. These can include severe decline in physical abilities, lack of social support, financial adversity, loneliness, and loss of self-esteem. The "age-old" question has been, what can we do to slow the physical aging process and lengthen our healthy, happy life span? Research shows that if we optimize wellness starting from our early years, we have a much greater chance of thriving during old age. Our perception of old age also makes a difference. Studies reveal that people who view aging in a more positive light are much more likely to thrive than those who have a generally negative attitude toward aging.

Many diseases, such as cancer, cardiovascular disease, arthritis, diabetes, and progressive neurological disorders such as dementia, become increasingly common with advancing age. But none of these diseases is inevitable, and your odds of acquiring these diseases is less if you follow lifelong healthy habits. Not smoking, eating well, exercising regularly throughout life, maintaining strong social bonds, and avoiding chronic stress all reduce the risk of acquiring these and many other diseases.

Of course, even with the healthiest behavior and environment, biological aging inevitably occurs. It results from genetic and biochemical processes we don't yet fully understand, but which include accumulated DNA damage, genetically programmed aging, inflammation, changes and impairment in metabolism, and likely many other processes. These biological changes increase the risk for many diseases. Together, gradual aging and impairment from disease cause physiological changes throughout the body. Because of redundancy in most organ systems, the body's ability to function is not affected until damage is fairly extensive. Further research may help pinpoint the causes of aging and develop therapies to repair and even prevent damage to aging bodies.

**QUICK STATS**

**Today, 9% of people worldwide (727 million) are aged 65 and over. By 2050, experts estimate that will increase to 16%.**

—United Nations, World Population Aging, 2020

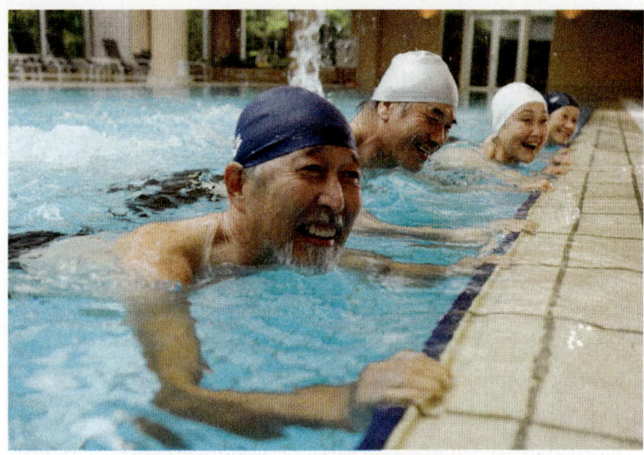

Regular exercise is a key to successful, healthy aging. Indeed/Taxi Japan/Getty Images

## Life-Enhancing Measures

Through good habits you can prevent, delay, lessen, or even reverse some of the negative changes associated with aging. Simple, daily practices can make a great difference to your level of energy and vitality now and throughout life. The following suggestions are mentioned throughout this text, but because they are profoundly related to health in later life, we highlight them here.

**Don't Smoke** The average pack-a-day smoker can expect to live about 13 to 14 fewer years than a nonsmoker. Furthermore, smokers suffer more illnesses and recover from illnesses more slowly than nonsmokers (see Chapter 9). About 8% of U.S. adults age 65 and up are current smokers. It is never too late to quit smoking, and although all the damage from a lifetime of smoking can't be undone, quitting has important and immediate health benefits.

**Challenge Your Mind** Your level of education and mental activity throughout life seems to reduce your risk for developing dementia in old age. Reading, writing, doing puzzles, learning a language, and studying music are good ways to stimulate the brain. The more complex the activity, the more protective it may be. However, the causal relationship between such activities and cognitive diseases is not fully understood. For example, some effects of mental exercise may be related to a buildup of cognitive reserve, your brain's ability to find alternative routes to get the job done. This may delay the onset of symptoms caused by a dementing disease, without actually changing the disease's underlying biological course.

**Develop Physical Fitness** Exercise significantly enhances psychological, cognitive, and physical health. A review of more than 70 scientific studies cited in the 2018 *Physical Activity Guidelines Advisory Committee Report* found that physically active people have a significantly lower risk of dying prematurely compared with inactive people. Poor fitness and low physical activity levels were found to be better predictors of premature death than smoking, diabetes, or obesity. The committee found that about 150 minutes (2.5 hours) of physical activity per week is sufficient to decrease the risk of death.

The positive effects of exercise include lower blood pressure and healthier cholesterol levels; better protection against heart attacks and an increased chance of survival if one occurs; sustained or increased lung capacity; weight control and increased muscle mass; maintenance of strength, flexibility, and balance; improved sleep; longer life expectancy; protection against osteoporosis and type 2 diabetes; increased effectiveness of the immune system; and maintenance of mental agility and flexibility, response time, memory, and hand–eye coordination.

The stimulus that exercise provides also seems to protect against the loss of **fluid intelligence,** which is the ability to find solutions to new problems. Fluid intelligence depends on rapidity of responsiveness, memory, and alertness. Individuals who exercise regularly are also less susceptible to depression and dementia.

Regular physical activity also fends off age-related *sarcopenia,* which is the loss of muscle mass (see Chapter 11). Gradual loss of skeletal muscle mass occurs in nearly all people over age 30, with a loss of about 12% of muscle mass by age 65 and a 30% loss by age 80. Recent studies have shown that physical activity, especially when it includes strength training, can reduce and even reverse the rate of loss of skeletal muscle mass that typically occurs with aging, which in turn decreases the risk for cardiovascular and many other chronic diseases.

**TERMS**

**fluid intelligence** The capacity to analyze new problems, reason, and identify patterns and relationships, independent of past knowledge.

**QUICK STATS**

**Among people ages 65 and older in 1965 only 5% had completed a bachelor's degree or more. By 2018, this share had risen to 33%.**

Administration for Community Living, 2021

## Ask Yourself

**QUESTIONS FOR CRITICAL THINKING AND REFLECTION**

Where would you wish to spend your "golden years"? Do you look forward to this stage of your life, or are you anxious about it? What influences have shaped your feelings about aging?

Regular physical activity is essential for healthy aging, as well as for vitality throughout life. A National Institute on Aging program offers four key types of exercises with the goals of improving endurance, strength, balance, and flexibility. Older adults with chronic conditions should seek guidance from their health care provider to find out what physical activities are effective, enjoyable, and safe given their particular strengths and challenges. For more about the beneficial effects of exercise for older adults, see the box "Can Exercise Delay the Effects of Aging?"

**Eat Wisely** Good health at any age is enhanced by eating a varied, nutrient-dense diet (see Chapter 10). For many adults, that means eating more fruits, vegetables, and whole grains while eating fewer foods high in saturated and trans fats and added sugars. Special guidelines for older adults include the following:

- Get enough vitamin B-12 (eggs, dairy products, meat) and extra vitamin D from fortified foods or supplements.
- Limit sodium intake to 1500 mg per day (3/4 teaspoon salt), and get enough potassium (4700 mg per day) from foods such as yams, winter squash, potatoes, avocados, white beans, and bananas. Older adults are particularly sensitive to the blood pressure–raising effects of excessive sodium intake.
- Eat foods rich in dietary fiber and drink plenty of water to help prevent constipation.
- Pay special attention to food safety. Older adults are often more susceptible to foodborne illness.
- Eat foods that are nutrient dense, including fruits and vegetables, and foods that contain healthy fats such as avocados, olive oil, and salmon.

**Maintain a Healthy Weight** A little less than one-third of older people are obese, which increases their risk for many chronic diseases, including cardiovascular disease, diabetes, and many cancers (see Chapter 13). On the other hand, being underweight has also been linked to increased risk of death in the elderly. Mortality rates in those over 65 years were lowest in people whose weight fell in the normal to slightly overweight range.

## TAKE CHARGE
## Can Exercise Delay the Effects of Aging?

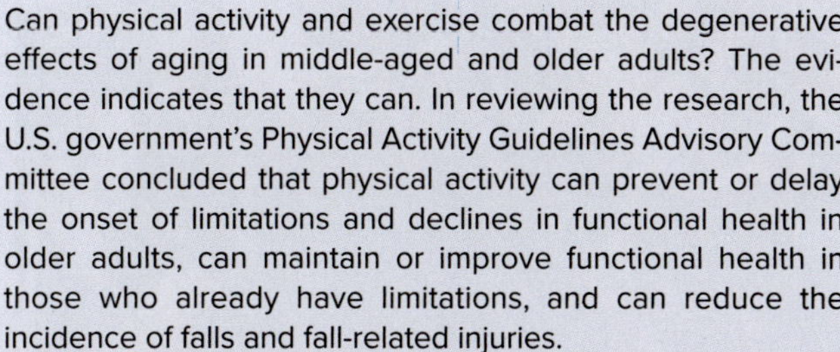

Can physical activity and exercise combat the degenerative effects of aging in middle-aged and older adults? The evidence indicates that they can. In reviewing the research, the U.S. government's Physical Activity Guidelines Advisory Committee concluded that physical activity can prevent or delay the onset of limitations and declines in functional health in older adults, can maintain or improve functional health in those who already have limitations, and can reduce the incidence of falls and fall-related injuries.

One mechanism by which physical activity prevents decline in functional health is through maintenance or improvement of the physiological capacities of the body, such as aerobic power, muscular strength, and balance. Declines in these physiological capacities occur with biological aging and are often compounded by disease-related disability. But evidence shows that older adults who participate in regular aerobic exercise are 30% less likely than inactive individuals to develop functional limitations (such as a limited ability to walk or climb stairs) or role limitations (such as a limited ability to be the family grocery shopper). Although studies found that both physical activity and aerobic fitness were associated with reduced risk of functional limitations, aerobic fitness was associated with a greater reduction of risk. Evidence also suggests that regular physical activity is safe and beneficial for older adults who already have functional limitations.

Numerous studies have shown that regular exercise—particularly strength training, balance training, and flexibility exercises—can improve muscular strength, muscular endurance, and stability and provide some protection against falls. Aerobic activity, especially walking, also helps reduce the risk of falls, and some evidence indicates that tai chi exercise programs are beneficial as well. Regular exercise not only reduces the incidence of falls but also greatly enhances mobility, allowing older people to live more independently and with greater confidence. Research also shows that regular physical activity can reduce anxiety and depression in older adults. Exercise stimulates blood flow to the brain and may help the brain to function more efficiently and improve memory. There is some evidence that exercise may stave off mental decline and the occurrence of age-related dementia.

Current physical activity recommendations for older adults from the American Heart Association and the American College of Sports Medicine include moderate- to vigorous-intensity aerobic activity, strength training, and flexibility exercises, as well as balance exercises for older adults at risk for falls. Unfortunately, only about 12% of people aged 65 and over get the recommended amounts of physical activity, and many get no exercise at all beyond the activities of daily living. Older adults are the least active group of Americans. Although it is important to exercise throughout life, the evidence indicates that older adults who become more active even late in life can experience improvements in physical fitness and functional health.

SOURCES: Physical Activity Guidelines Advisory Committee. 2018 *Physical Activity Guidelines Advisory Committee Report, 2018*. Washington, DC: U.S. Department of Health and Human Services; National Institute on Aging. 2021. *Exercise & Physical Activity: Getting Fit for Life* (https://www.nia.nih.gov/health/exercise-and-physical-activity-getting-fit-life).

**Control Drinking and Overdependence on Medications** Alcohol abuse ranks with depression as a common hidden mental health problem, affecting about 10% of older adults. Elders are especially vulnerable to the toxic effects of alcohol, in part because the ability to metabolize alcohol decreases with age. The same amount of alcohol will produce a higher blood alcohol level and more impairment in an elder compared with a young person. Alcohol overuse is often not identified in the elderly because the effects of alcohol or drug dependence can mimic disease, such as Alzheimer's disease.

Many people, including health professionals, don't realize that alcohol abuse is a common problem in the elderly. But in fact, widowers over age 75 have the highest rate of alcoholism of any group in the United States.

Opioid and benzodiazepine overuse is becoming increasingly common in the elderly. Misuse of these medications is especially dangerous for older people because they are more likely to have reduced kidney or liver function, so they are less able to break down medication and more likely to overdose.

Signs of potential alcohol or drug misuse include unexplained falls or frequent injuries, forgetfulness, depression, and malnutrition.

**Schedule Preventive Care** When detected early, many diseases, including hypertension, diabetes, glaucoma, and many types of cancer, can be successfully controlled by medication and lifestyle changes. Vaccinations in all life stages are life-saving: people age 65 and older make up about 90% of all deaths due to influenza, but flu vaccination greatly reduces death due to flu in people of all ages. For the elderly, vaccinations against Covid, influenza, pneumococcus pneumonia, and other serious diseases greatly enhance the quality and quantity of life. Recommended screenings and immunizations can protect against preventable chronic and infectious diseases (see Chapters 13–14).

**Recognize and Reduce Stress** Stress-induced physiological changes increase wear and tear on the body, and worsen cognitive decline in the elderly. Like people of all ages, elders benefit from reducing stress, getting enough sleep, not overworking, and avoiding substance misuse. The relaxation techniques described in Chapter 2 can help people of any age deal with stress.

**Nurture Social Connections** Research shows that social connectedness is strongly associated with a longer, healthier, and happier life. Indeed, studies have shown that loneliness and social isolation are major risk factors for mortality, ranking similarly to other well-known risk factors such as smoking and physical inactivity. Strong relationships with friends and family are life enhancing in a multitude of ways.

## DEALING WITH THE CHANGES OF AGING

Just as you can act to limit or delay some of the physical changes of aging, you can also prepare psychologically, socially, and financially for changes that may occur later in life.

### Changing Roles and Relationships

Retirement marks a major life change for many. Many people "retire" from their full-time job, but then continue to work part time. Others may retire, then start a new career. People who have well-developed leisure pursuits and meaningful relationships adjust better to retirement than those with few interests outside work. Although retirement may be a desirable milestone for most people, it may also be viewed as a threat to prestige, purpose, and self-respect.

Retirement and the end of child rearing also bring about changes in the relationship between marriage partners. The amount of time a couple spends together will likely increase, and activities will change. Couples may need a period of adjustment in which they get to know each other as individuals again. Discussing what types of activities each partner enjoys can help couples set up a mutually satisfying routine of shared and independent activities. But not all elderly people live as couples. Death of a spouse, divorce, and separation are all common reasons that older people become single. Older couples are much more likely to divorce or separate today than in the past. The loss of a spouse, whether through separation, divorce, or death, is one of the most serious stressors anyone can face. In particular, during the first three months after the death of a spouse, the risk of death for the surviving spouse increases by more than 60%. Loving social support from family, friends, and community support groups is critical for helping elders cope with major losses.

**Increased Leisure Time** Although retirement and freedom from child care responsibilities may confer the advantages of leisure time and freedom from work-related stress, many people who have spent most of their lives focused primarily on their careers may not know how to enjoy their free time. If you have developed diverse interests throughout life, retirement can be a joyful and fulfilling period of your life. It can provide opportunities for you to expand your horizons, try new activities, take classes, and meet new people. Volunteering in your community can enhance self-esteem through opportunities to contribute to society.

**The Economics of Retirement** Retirement may mean a severely restricted budget or possibly even financial disaster if you have failed to put aside adequate savings. Financial planning for retirement should begin early in life. People in their twenties and thirties should estimate how much money they need to support themselves comfortably, calculate their projected income, and begin a savings program. The earlier people begin such a program, the more money they will have at retirement.

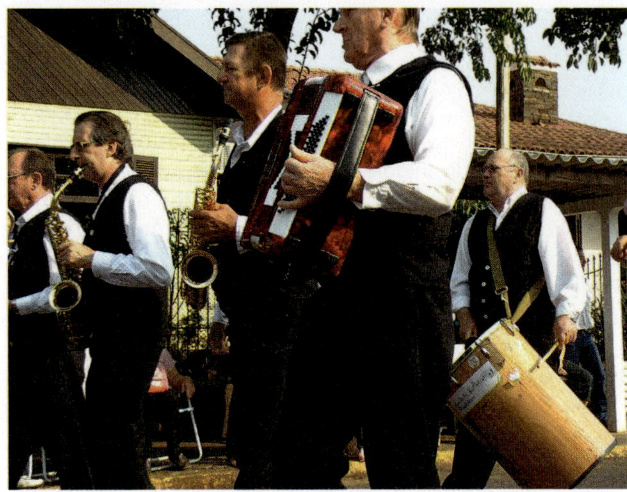

The retirement years can be the best part of your life socially, with increased opportunities to meet and interact with new and different people through social clubs. Claire Insel

Financial planning for retirement is especially critical for women. American women are much less likely than men to be covered by pension plans, 401(k) plans, and other retirement programs, reflecting the fact that women tend to have lower-paying jobs, work part time, or not have paid employment at all because of caregiving for children or elderly family members. Although the gap is narrowing, women currently outlive men by about five to six years, and they are more likely to develop chronic conditions that impair their daily activities later in life. The net result of these factors is that nearly twice as many women age 80 and over live in poverty compared with men of similar age.

### Adapting to Physical Changes

A person can do many things to minimize the effects of the physical changes associated with aging. However, some changes in physical functioning are inevitable, and successful aging involves anticipating and accommodating these changes. Adapting rather than giving up favorite activities may be the best strategy for dealing with physical limitations. Older people with limited strength may have to develop priorities for how to best use their energy. Paying close attention to the need for rest and sleep is crucial for enjoying life at all ages, but especially for elders. Coping with chronic health issues is, unfortunately, part of life for most elderly people. According to the National Council on Aging, approximately 80% of older adults have at least one chronic disease, and nearly as many have at least two. The most frequently occurring conditions in older people include arthritis, heart disease, cancer, diabetes, and hypertension.

**Hearing Loss** Loss of hearing occurs in virtually everyone as they age—a condition known as *presbycusis*, which can range from mild to severe. Hearing loss is the result of gradual deterioration of the tiny hair cells in the cochlea (a hollow bone in the inner ear) and is often compounded by factors such as exposure to loud noise, certain medications that can damage hearing, trauma, smoking, and diseases such as hypertension and diabetes. Hearing loss should be assessed and treated by a health care professional. Hearing aids are often effective in improving quality of life, and they may even help to decrease the risk for developing dementia. Some people resist wearing hearing aids because of cost or fear of social stigma, but the benefits of using hearing aids—or personal amplification devices (which are much less expensive and available without a prescription)—can make the adjustment to these devices well worth the effort.

QUICK STATS

**Over half of all people with glaucoma are unaware that they have the disease.**

World Glaucoma Association, 2022

**Vision Changes** Vision usually declines with age, often making it difficult to perform far-away activities like driving and up-close activities like reading. By the time we reach our forties, nearly all of us will have developed *presbyopia*—a gradual decline in the ability to focus on close objects. This decline occurs because the lens of the eye becomes stiffer as we age, making it difficult or impossible to focus on nearby objects. Other vision changes that typically occur with aging include having trouble distinguishing certain colors and taking longer to adjust to changes in light intensity. Vision loss in the elderly is also caused by common eye diseases, such as **glaucoma**, **age-related macular degeneration (AMD), cataracts**, and **diabetic retinopathy,** all of which can be detected with regular screening and treated with medication, laser treatments, or surgery.

Glaucoma is caused by increased fluid pressure within the eye. The optic nerve can be permanently damaged by this increased pressure, resulting in a loss of side vision and, if untreated, blindness. Medication, and laser and conventional surgery are other options. Of the more than 3 million Americans with glaucoma, only half know that they have it; those who have not been diagnosed lose the opportunity to control it and preserve their sight. People over age 60 and anyone with a family history of glaucoma are at a higher risk.

AMD is a slow disintegration of the *macula*—the tissue at the center of the retina where fine, straight-ahead detail is distinguished. AMD usually occurs after age 50 and is the leading cause of vision loss in Americans age 60 and up. Risk factors for AMD are age, family history, smoking, white race, excessive unprotected sun exposure, and poor diet. Some cases of AMD can be treated with injections or laser surgery.

*Cataracts* are a clouding of the lenses of the eyes. Risk factors for cataracts include older age, smoking, diseases such as diabetes and hypertension, eye injury or surgery, and excessive sunlight exposure. Surgery is usually very effective. *Diabetic eye disease* occurs in most people who have had diabetes for over two decades. Early diabetic retinopathy, which is treatable, often has no symptoms. It is crucial that people with diabetes have frequent eye examinations so that retinopathy and other eye diseases can be identified and treated before they result in permanent vision loss and blindness.

**Arthritis** About half of older people report having doctor-diagnosed **arthritis,** and many more elders have undiagnosed arthritis. Osteoarthritis is the most common.

It most often affects the hands and the weight-bearing joints of the body—the knees, ankles, hips, and spine. Risk factors for osteoarthritis include aging, previous trauma, chronic overuse of the joints, being overweight, and genetic factors.

The prevention and treatment of osteoarthritis are similar. These strategies include exercise (which can protect the joint by lubricating it and strengthening the muscles that surround it), weight management (which lightens the load on weight-bearing joints), and avoidance of heavy or repetitive use of the joint.

**Osteoporosis** As described in Chapter 10, **osteoporosis** is a condition in which bones become dangerously thin and fragile, making them very easy to break. Older women are at higher risk for osteoporosis than men, due in part to bone loss associated with postmenopausal decrease in estrogen. Osteoporosis normally does not cause pain, or any other symptoms, until a fracture occurs. Fractures of the hip and vertebrae are the most common and serious consequences of osteoporosis. The collapse of one or more vertebrae can cause loss of height, stooped posture, severe back pain, and breathing problems.

More than 50 million people in the United States either already have osteoporosis or are at high risk due to low bone mass that is not yet severe enough to meet criteria for osteoporosis. Women are at greater risk for osteoporosis than men because adult women typically have less overall bone mass than men. Bone loss accelerates in women during the first 5

TERMS

**glaucoma** An increase in pressure in the eye due to fluid buildup that can result in loss of side vision and, if left untreated, blindness.

**age-related macular degeneration (AMD)** A deterioration of the macula (the central area of the retina) leading to loss of vision in the center of the visual field, making it hard to read, drive, or recognize faces.

**cataracts** Opacity of the lens of the eye that impairs vision and can cause blindness.

**diabetic retinopathy** Damage to the blood vessels of the light-sensitive tissue at the back of the eye (retina) in people who have diabetes.

**arthritis** Inflammation and swelling of a joint or joints, usually causing pain and stiffness.

**osteoporosis** The loss of bone density, causing bones to become weak, porous, and more prone to fractures, usually at the hip, spine, or wrist.

to 10 years after the onset of menopause because of the drop in estrogen, a hormone that, among many other things, helps to maintain bone mass. That, combined with the fact that women tend to live longer than men, makes osteoporosis much more common in women, although men who live into their eighties and nineties often develop osteoporosis.

Risk factors for osteoporosis include female gender, older age, and race (Black and Latina women have lower rates of osteoporosis than white and Asian women). Other risk factors include tobacco use, excessive use of alcohol (more than two drinks per day), poor diet (especially long-term low calcium intake), lack of vitamin D, thyroid disease, a family history of osteoporosis or hip fracture, early menopause (before age 45), abnormal or irregular menstruation, a history of anorexia, and a thin, small frame. Thyroid medication, corticosteroid drugs (which are often used to treat conditions such as arthritis or asthma), and certain antiseizure drugs are among the many medications that can increase the risk of osteoporosis.

Preventing osteoporosis requires building as much bone as possible during your young years and then maintaining it as you age. Girls aged 9–18 are in their critical bone-building years, and they should eat foods rich in calcium and vitamin D and get adequate exercise. Weight-bearing activities must be performed regularly throughout life to have lasting effects. Strength training improves bone density, muscle mass, strength, and balance, protecting against both bone loss and falls, a major cause of fractures. Even the very elderly benefit from low-intensity strength training and weight-bearing exercises. These activities can improve bone density and can also improve balance, reducing the risk for falls. Bone mineral density scans use X-rays to gauge an individual's risk of fracture and help determine if any medical treatment is needed. Screening tests are recommended for women over 65, men over 70, and anyone over 50 who has had a fracture with minimal trauma or other risk factors. Below-normal bone density that is not severe enough to meet criteria for full-blown osteoporosis may be classified as *osteopenia,* which is usually treated with exercise, nutrition, and sometimes medication. Osteoporosis is treated with lifestyle modifications and medications.

**Increased Risk for Falls** Weakness, poor vision, impaired balance, cognitive deficits, and environmental hazards all contribute to the risk for falls in the elderly. Older people fall more often than younger adults, and the consequences of their falls tend to be much more severe. About one-fourth of all people age 65 and older have a significant fall each year. Even relatively minor falls can result in devastating, sometimes lethal, injuries in the elderly.

**QUICK STATS**

**Unpaid caregivers provide an estimated 15.3 billion hours of care to people with dementia, valued at nearly $257 billion.**

—Alzheimer's Association, 2021

**Changes in Sexual Functioning** The ability to enjoy sex can continue well into old age. Education about normal changes due to aging and how to manage them can help to reassure older people that enjoyable sexual activity is still possible. For example, the use of a lubricant is a simple but very effective solution for the typical vaginal dryness that occurs after menopause and contributes to difficulties with intercourse. Erectile dysfunction becomes more common as men age but is often treatable with a combination of counseling and medications. Sexually transmitted infections are on the rise in all age groups, including people over 50. Practicing safe sex, including using condoms, remains important at all ages.

## Psychological and Cognitive Changes

Beyond brain changes associated with normal aging, older people are also at increased risk for many types of degenerative neurological diseases.

**Cognitive Impairment** **Dementia** refers to a set of symptoms associated with cognitive decline, such as problems with memory, language, attention, problem solving, and decision making. Diseases that lead to progressive cognitive impairment include, among others, Alzheimer's disease (AD), vascular dementia, cerebrovascular disease, Lewy-body dementia (LBD), and frontotemporal lobe dementia. Symptoms of these diseases can include changes in memory, thinking, language, visuospatial function, judgment, and behavior. Early disease stages can sometimes be difficult to differentiate from normal aging, but eventually problems become more apparent, and the person may lose the ability to function independently. Some patients with relatively mild symptoms may fulfill criteria for a diagnosis of *mild cognitive impairment,* which is defined as objective cognitive impairment that can be detected with psychological testing, but the person is still able to function in most activities of daily life. For example, a patient may not recall as many details of a story as others, but she can still live alone, cook for herself, and enjoy a satisfying social life.

**Alzheimer's disease (AD)** is the most common disease leading to dementia and is the

**TERMS**

**dementia** A loss of cognitive functioning that can interfere with daily life and cause a loss of the ability to function independently.

**Alzheimer's disease (AD)** A disease characterized by the accumulation of beta-amyloid and tau in the brain, causing a progressive loss of memory and other brain functions, leading to dementia.

**Ask Yourself**

**QUESTIONS FOR CRITICAL THINKING AND REFLECTION**

Scientists have identified genes that strongly increase the risk for Alzheimer's disease. Would you want to know whether you carried these genes?

cause for an estimated 60–80% of all cases of dementia. AD is a progressive brain disorder that is characterized by a gradual accumulation of the proteins beta-amyloid and tau in the brain. These proteins, in combination with inflammation and other incompletely understood processes, eventually destroy brain cells, leading to impairment of memory, cognition, and other brain functions. AD probably begins 20 years or more before symptoms are first noticed. Once symptoms occur, the disease gradually progresses until the person loses the ability to walk, speak, or even swallow. AD is irreversible and eventually fatal. The diagnosis of early AD can be challenging, and doctors may use biomarkers in cerebrospinal fluid or neuroimaging to confirm that AD is the cause of the symptoms. Research is ongoing to develop a simple and accurate blood test to diagnose AD, but no such test is currently available.

Besides age, one of the strongest risk factors for late onset AD is the gene variant *APOE* ε4. Other major risk factors include type 2 diabetes, high blood pressure, high total cholesterol, obesity, and a history of head trauma. Many other genetic and environmental factors may also contribute to the risk for AD. Factors that seem to decrease the risk for AD include higher educational attainment and lifestyle factors such as regular physical activity, not smoking, healthy diet, avoiding excess alcohol use, and maintaining a healthy weight. Notice that these are the same lifestyle factors that seem to reduce the risk for heart disease, some cancers, stroke, and other serious diseases associated with aging.

**Vascular dementia,** or **vascular cognitive impairment,** is a broad term describing cognitive changes that occur due to cerebrovascular disease, which can impair blood flow to the brain, resulting in damage or death of brain tissue. Vascular dementia accounts for about 10% of all dementia, although many experts believe that vascular issues often coexist with and contribute to the brain damage seen in other types of dementia such as AD. The symptoms of vascular dementia vary widely, depending on the type of vascular insult and its location in the brain. Sometimes symptoms start or worsen after a major stroke, and in other cases symptoms develop gradually due to progressive occlusion of small vessels deep in the brain. High blood pressure, cigarette smoking, diabetes, and hyperlipidemia are some risk factors that may be treated to reduce the risk of vascular cognitive impairment.

**Lewy-body dementia** (LBD) is a progressive brain disorder in which Lewy bodies (abnormal protein deposits) build up in areas of the brain, causing changes in behavior, cognition, and movement. It is similar to AD in many ways but is more likely than AD to cause fluctuations in cognitive ability, attention, or alertness. People with LBD are also much more likely to have visual hallucinations than people with AD. Additionally, LBD is associated with Parkinson-like changes in walking and movement, sleep disorders, and autonomic problems, such as loss of blood pressure control and disturbed bladder and bowel function. Treatment of symptoms may provide some benefit for patients with LBD, but the disease is not curable.

*Mixed dementia* is the condition describing what most older people with significant cognitive impairment often have—several brain pathologies simultaneously, which may all contribute to the impairment. The most common scenario is a combination of AD and vascular brain changes.

**Depression** Depression is not a normal part of aging, and it is important to diagnose and treat. Distinguishing between depression and dementia can be difficult in the elderly because the two conditions share many of the same symptoms, such as cognitive impairment, social withdrawal, changes in sleep habits, difficulty concentrating, and loss of interest in previously enjoyable activities. Common triggers for depression in the elderly include unresolved grief, chronic health conditions, unrelieved pain, and changes in social and financial situation.

Many people are surprised to learn that suicide is relatively common among the elderly; in particular, white men aged 75 and over commit suicide more often than any other demographic group.

**Grief** Aging is usually associated with multiple significant losses: deaths of friends and family members, loss of physical strength and changes in appearance, loss of health, and often material losses. Grief is an emotional response to loss. Grief is a natural part of human experience but can be extremely painful and sometimes debilitating and slow to resolve. People of all ages often find help through in-person or online support groups with others who have experienced similar losses.

**QUICK STATS**

**Life expectancy for the highest versus the lowest-income Californians increased to 16 extra years in 2021, compared with 12 years in 2019.**

—Schwandt et al., 2022

## LIFE IN AN AGING SOCIETY

**Life expectancy** is a statistical average of the ages at death of a group of people over a certain period. In 2020, the overall life expectancy for the total U.S. population was 77.3 years. Those who survive to age 65 can expect to live to be even older. A man reaching age 65 today can expect to live, on average, until age 82. A woman turning age 65 today can expect to live, on average, until age 85. (See the box "Why Do Women Live Longer?")

**TERMS**

**vascular dementia** Cognitive changes that occur due to cerebrovascular disease, when brain cells die due to inadequate blood flow.

**cognitive impairment** Reduced mental functioning that may include memory, concentration, and judgment.

**Lewy-Body dementia** A progressive brain disorder in which Lewy bodies (abnormal protein deposits) build up in areas of the brain, causing changes in behavior, cognition, and movement.

**life expectancy** The average length of time a person is expected to live.

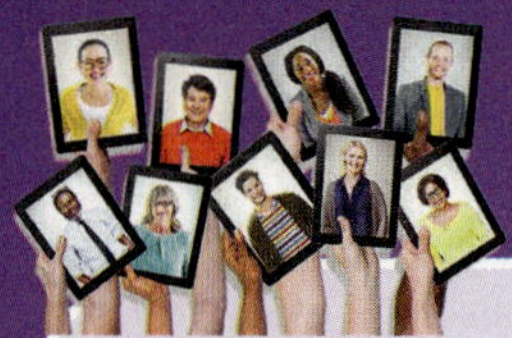

## DIVERSITY MATTERS
### Why Do Women Live Longer?

Women live longer than men in nearly every country around the world, even in places where maternal mortality rates are high. In the United States women on average can expect to live about five years longer than men (see the table in this box). As a consequence, the majority of people age 65 and older are women, with over 27 million older women versus about 22 million older men in the United States. Worldwide, women comprise more than 85% of the population that is more than 100 years old. From before birth through old age, human males have higher mortality rates than females. The female advantage in longevity is also seen in many other mammalian species, including great apes and most monkeys.

The reason for the gender gap in life expectancy is not entirely understood but is likely influenced by many biological, social, and lifestyle factors. The fact that females have two X chromosomes while males have only one, as well as differences in mitochondrial inheritance, may provide a genetic advantage that protects females from many diseases. In addition, the female hormone estrogen is also believed to be protective against many health conditions, especially cardiovascular disease. Conversely, the male hormone testosterone may have some negative effects on longevity. Interestingly, males who were castrated before puberty (who have very low levels of testosterone) seem to live much longer on average than men with normal testosterone levels. Hormonal levels may also help explain why men tend to have more visceral fat (fat surrounding the vital organs, such as the heart, that increases the risk for cardiac disease) than women do. Some experts believe that testosterone may also have a negative effect on the immune system.

In general, males are more likely to behave in ways that put them at higher risk for early death. Men are more likely to take more life-threatening risks than women, so they have higher rates of death due to trauma. Suicide rates are considerably higher in males than in females. Men are more likely to smoke and drink excessively than are women. Some experts hypothesize that women cope better with stress than men do.

The news for women is not all good, however, because not all their extra years are likely to be healthy years. They are more likely than men to suffer from chronic, but generally non-lethal, conditions like arthritis and osteoporosis. Women's longer life spans, combined with the fact that men tend to marry younger women and that widowed men remarry more often than widowed women do, mean there are many more single older women than men. Older men are more likely to live in family settings, whereas older women are more likely to live alone. For many reasons, older women are much more likely than older men to be poor.

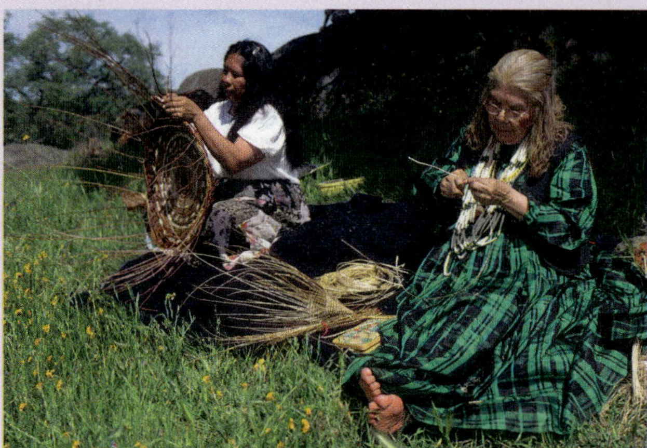

These Kashia Pomo women weave baskets together, which helps them stay active and maintain social and community ties, enhancing wellness as they age. inga spence/Alamy Stock Photo

U.S. Life Expectancy

| Year of Birth | Men | Women |
|---|---|---|
| ***U.S. LIFE EXPECTANCY AT BIRTH*** | | |
| 1900 | 46.3 | 48.3 |
| 1950 | 65.6 | 71.1 |
| 2000 | 74.1 | 79.3 |
| 2010 | 76.2 | 81.1 |
| 2019 | 76.3 | 81.4 |
| 2020 | 74.2 | 79.9 |
| ***ADDED EXPECTED YEARS FROM AGE 65*** | | |
| 1900 | 11.5 | 12.2 |
| 1950 | 12.8 | 15.0 |
| 2000 | 16.0 | 19.0 |
| 2010 | 17.7 | 20.3 |
| 2019 | 18.2 | 20.8 |
| 2020 | 17.0 | 19.8 |

SOURCES: National Center for Health Statistics. 2016. Health, United States, 2015. Hyattsville, MD: National Center for Health Statistics; World Health Organization. 2019. World Population Aging 2019. Geneva: World Health Organization; World Health Organization 2019. Female life expectancy. Centers for Disease Control. 2021. Mortality in the United States, 2020. *NCHS Data Brief 427* (https://www.cdc.gov/nchs/products/databriefs/db427.htm).

As life expectancy increases and the birth rate drops, a larger proportion of people will be elderly. Society will need to adapt to a population that is increasingly skewed toward older people. This will necessitate changes in every aspect of our culture, including economics, governmental policies, and changes in our general attitudes toward older adults.

## The Aging Minority

People age 65 and over are a large minority in the U.S. population. The number of U.S. elders exceeded 54 million and comprised about 16% of the total U.S. population in 2019.

The homeownership rate is about 80% for those aged 65–84, which is much higher than the homeownership rate for those under age 35 (about 38%). Older people's living expenses are often lower after retirement, which can help compensate for the decreased income that usually occurs. Unfortunately, the financial status of a substantial proportion of elders in the United States is precarious. Most older Americans rely on fixed sources of income, such as **Social Security** and pensions, that are eroded by inflation and are often not enough to live on comfortably.

QUICK STATS

**Approximately 42 million Americans have provided care to an adult aged 50 or over—without pay—in the prior 12 months.**

—AARP, 2020

Health care is the largest expense for older adults. On average, they visit a physician 10–12 times a year, are hospitalized more frequently, and require twice as many prescription drugs as the general population. Many elderly people with low incomes must choose between paying for medications and buying food. Health care costs are the most common reason for bankruptcy among Americans of all ages, including the elderly.

## Family and Community Resources for Older Adults

With help from friends, family members, and community services, people in their later years can often remain active and independent. Over half of noninstitutionalized older Americans live with a spouse some live with a family member other than a spouse, and about 27% live alone. Only about 3% of people age 65 and over live in institutional settings, but among those over age 85, about 8% live in a nursing home.

QUICK STATS

**For about half of seniors, Social Security provides at least 50% of their income; for about 1 in 4 seniors, it provides at least 90%.**

—Center on Budget and Policy Priorities, 2020

Most often, the bulk of the caregiving is provided by the elderly person's spouse, grown daughter, or daughter-in-law. Caregiving can be rewarding, but it is also hard work. When the experience is stressful and long term, family members may become emotionally and physically exhausted. Caregivers are often juggling work, school, child care, and other home responsibilities in addition to caring for their elderly loved one. Caregivers often need to cut back on work or school activities, or even quit altogether, when caregiving demands increase. There are a few forward-thinking corporations and schools that respond to the needs of their employees/students who are family caregivers by providing services such as flexible schedules, leaves, and even on-site adult care.

TERMS

**Social Security** A government program that provides financial assistance to retirees, disabled persons, and families of retired, disabled, or deceased workers, financed through taxes on businesses and workers.

## Government Aid and Policies

The federal government helps older Americans through several programs, such as food assistance, housing subsidies, Social Security, Medicare, and Medicaid. Funding for Social Security comes primarily from American workers who pay into the system, and it depends on a sufficient number of current workers to support the number of retired people who are receiving benefits. As longevity increases and birth rates decline in the United States, fewer workers will be supporting growing numbers of elderly beneficiaries.

Currently, there are about four working-age adults for every senior citizen in the United States, but this ratio will fall to about 2.6 to 1 by 2050, according to the Social Security Administration. For comparison, there were eight working-age adults for every senior citizen in 1945. Adjustments to the retirement age are being made to ease the strain on the Social Security system.

Medicare is a federal health insurance program for older adults and disabled persons. It provides basic health care coverage for acute episodes of illness that require skilled professional care. It pays for some preventive services, including an initial physical exam, vaccinations, and screenings for cardiovascular disease, certain cancers, and many other conditions. It does not pay for many office visits, dental care, or dentures. The vast majority of nursing home care, especially long-term care, is not covered by Medicare. About 1.3 million older people currently live in nursing homes, but Medicare pays less than 2% of nursing home costs, and private insurers pay less than 1%, creating a tremendous financial burden for nursing home residents and their families.

When their financial resources are exhausted, people may apply for Medicaid. Medicaid provides medical insurance to low-income people of any age.

### Ask Yourself

**QUESTIONS FOR CRITICAL THINKING AND REFLECTION**

What do you want your life to be like when you are older? Do you hope to retire, or keep working indefinitely? Where would you like to live? How much time do you spend thinking about these questions? What have you planned for your later years?

## WHAT IS DEATH?

Whether it is victims of a terrorist attack, an earthquake or a car crash, or a woman in her nineties dying peacefully with her family close by, images of death are all around us. Nevertheless, we rarely think about the inevitability of death in our own lives. Most of us live as if we are immortal. Accepting and dealing with death presents unique challenges to our sense of self, our relationships with others, and our understanding of the meaning of life itself.

Although pain and distress may accompany the dying process, facing death also presents an opportunity for growth as well as affirmation of the preciousness of our daily lives. Dealing with the death of a loved one can tear families apart, but it can also bring them together. The way we choose to confront death can greatly influence how we live.

Questions about the meaning of death and what happens when we die are central to the great religions and philosophies of the world. Some promise a better life after death. Others teach that everyone is evolving toward perfection or divinity, a goal reached after successive rounds of life, death and rebirth. Still others suggest that it is not possible to know what—if anything—happens after death and that any judgment about life's worth and meaning must be made on the basis of satisfactions or rewards we create for ourselves and those around us in our lifetimes.

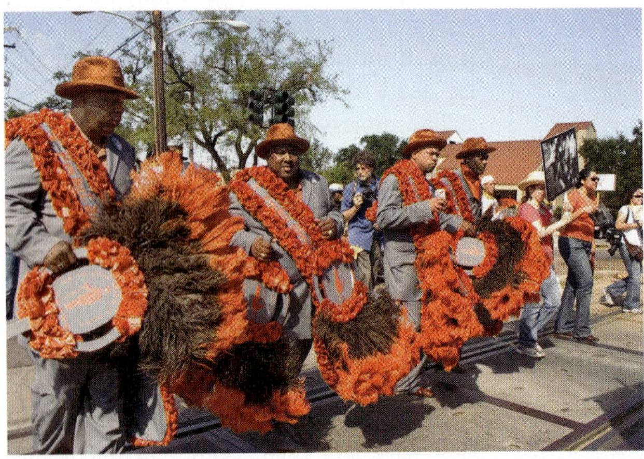

Ninette Maumus/Alamy Stock Photo

**TERMS**

**senescence** The biological process of aging.

**clinical death** The medical term applied to the point at which there is no longer blood flow in the body (the heart has stopped beating) and breathing has ceased.

**life support systems** Medical technologies, such as a ventilator, that allow vital body functions to be sustained artificially.

**brain death** A complete and irreversible cessation of brain activity indicated by various diagnostic criteria; this medical determination may be necessary when intensive hospital-based life support systems have been used to artificially sustain organ systems in the body.

Even for the most secular individuals, spiritual beliefs and traditions can shape attitudes and behaviors surrounding death. Spirituality and religion offer solace to the extent that they may provide some meaning in dying. Mourning rituals and ceremonies associated with various religions ease the pangs of grief for many people. Dying and death are more than biological events; they have social and spiritual dimensions.

**Senescence,** the biological process of aging, is complex, rooted in genetics, and universal in all mammals, including humans. Organisms age on both a cellular and a whole-organism level, ultimately resulting in death. Although scientific understanding of senescence is progressing, and average life spans are increasing, death remains an inevitable event for humans and nearly all other living beings.

### Defining Death

Traditionally death has been defined as cessation of the flow of vital body fluids. This cessation occurs when the heart stops beating and breathing ceases, referred to as **clinical death.** These traditional signs are adequate for determining death in most cases. However, over the past several decades, the use of cardiopulmonary resuscitation (CPR) and other medical techniques have brought many "dead" people (by the traditional definition) back to life. The use of ventilators, artificial heart pumps, and other **life support systems** allow many body functions to be sustained artificially. In such cases, making a determination of death can be difficult and often controversial. The concept of **brain death** was developed to determine whether a person is alive or dead when traditional signs are inadequate because of supportive medical technology. The way death is defined has significant legal, ethical, and social consequences, including potential effects on criminal prosecution, inheritance, treatment of the corpse, and even mourning.

The Uniform Determination of Death Act, developed in 1981, provides criteria for determining brain death, which is defined as the complete and irreversible loss of function of the entire brain, including the brain stem. The concept of brain death is particularly crucial for organ donation and transplantation. Medical technologies such as ventilators are used so that organs will remain viable over the hours or days that are needed to arrange for transplantation. Some organs—hearts, most obviously—must be harvested from a human being who is declared legally dead. Timing is critical in removing a heart from someone who has been declared dead and transplanting it into a person whose life can thereby be saved.

Safeguards are necessary to ensure that the determination of death occurs without regard to any plans for subsequent transplantation of the deceased's organs. Several thorough examinations need to be performed over a period of time in order to determine that both higher brain and brain-stem functions (which regulate heartbeat and breathing) have ceased irreversibly. The American Academy of Neurology has called for uniform legal standards for brain death in all states, as well as standard policies and practices regarding determination of brain death for all medical facilities throughout the United States.

As medical and technological advances occur, it has become increasingly clear that biological death consists of a series of events that occur over a period of time. In contrast to clinical death (irreversible cessation of heartbeat and breathing) or brain death, **cellular death** refers to a gradual process that occurs when heartbeat, respiration, and brain activity have stopped. Many cells throughout the body continue to survive for seconds, minutes, or hours after clinical and brain death, but gradually die as they utilize remaining oxygen and glucose. Cellular death encompasses the breakdown of metabolic processes and results in complete nonfunctionality at the cellular level. In a biological sense, therefore, death can be defined as the cessation of life due to irreversible changes in cell metabolism.

## Learning about Death

Our understanding of death changes as we grow and mature, as do our attitudes toward it. Very young children view death as an interruption and an absence, but their lack of a mature time perspective means that they do not understand death as final and irreversible. A child's understanding of death evolves greatly from about age 6 to age 9. During this period, most children begin to understand that death is final, universal, and inevitable. A person who consciously recognizes these facts is said to possess a **mature understanding of death.**

However, even individuals who possess a mature understanding of death commonly also hold nonempirical ideas about it. Such nonempirical ideas—that is, ideas not subject to scientific proof—deal mainly with the notion that human beings survive in some form beyond the death of the physical body. Does the self or soul continue to exist after the death of the physical body? If so, what is the nature of this afterlife? Developing personally satisfying answers to such questions, which involve what Speece and Brent term **noncorporeal continuity,** is also part of the process of acquiring a mature understanding of death.

In the United States, with its relative affluence and orderliness, death is not a part of the day-to-day existence of most young people. There are exceptions, however, especially among those who have grown up during the Covid-19 era, or in environments with high rates of violence or in places where deaths due to drug overdose are particularly frequent. However, even when death strikes those around us, many of us continue to feel a sense of invulnerability—that is, "It won't happen to me." By the time we reach old age, reminders of aging and death are frequent, especially as we experience the loss of many of our peers. The very old have often lost nearly everyone of significance in their lives. Coping with the death of loved ones and the loneliness that often follows, and preparing for our own impending death are central developmental tasks for the very elderly.

## Denying versus Acknowledging Death

The ability to find meaning and comfort in the face of mortality depends not only on having an understanding of the facts of death but also on our attitudes toward it. Many people avoid any thought or mention of death. The sick and old are often isolated in hospitals and nursing homes. Relatively few Americans have been present at the death of a loved one. Where the reality of death is concerned, "out of sight, out of mind" is often the rule of the day.

Although many commentators characterize the predominant attitude toward death in the United States as "death denying," others are reluctant to generalize so broadly. People often maintain conflicting or ambivalent attitudes toward death. Those who view death as a relief or release from insufferable pain may have at least a sense that death is sometimes welcomed, but few people wholly avoid or wholly welcome death. In the past several decades, attitudes toward death in our culture have begun to change slowly. The hospice movement (discussed later in this chapter) has provided support and guidance for many families who choose to be present during the dying process of their loved ones, often in their own homes.

Some cultures not only acknowledge the reality of death, but embrace it, even at times in a joyous way. For example, traditional Mexican culture honors the dead by remembering them often, especially during the annual holiday *Día de los*

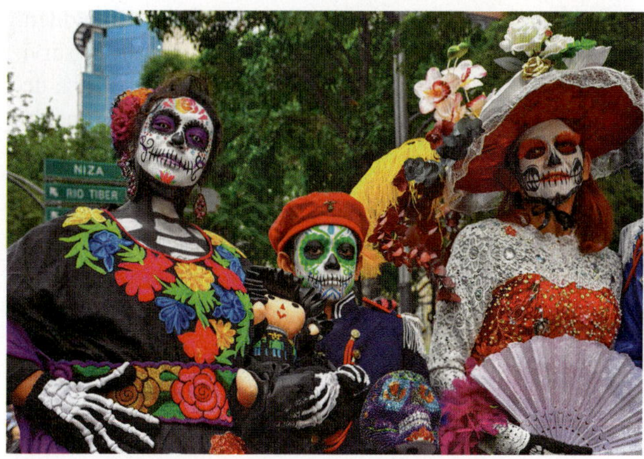


In Mexico, individuals publicly celebrate departed loved ones on the annual holiday *Día de los Muertos* (Day of the Dead). Eve Orea/ Shutterstock

**TERMS**

**cellular death** The breakdown of metabolic processes at the level of the body's cells.

**mature understanding of death** The recognition that death is universal and irreversible, that it involves the cessation of all physiological functioning, and that there are biological reasons for its occurrence.

**noncorporeal continuity** The notion that human beings survive in some form after the death of the physical body.

## Ask Yourself

**QUESTIONS FOR CRITICAL THINKING AND REFLECTION**

What situations or events make you think seriously about your own mortality? Is this something you consider now and then, or do you avoid thinking about death? What has influenced your willingness or reluctance to think about death?

*Muertos* (Day of the Dead), in which families include their departed loved ones in their celebrations. This holiday is festive, tinged with some sadness, but mostly full of love, fun, and good humor. Similar celebrations that honor the dead in a festive manner are common in many cultures throughout the world. In the United States, Halloween—originally celebrated in church liturgy to remember their faithful dead—is now just a "spooky" holiday; witches, ghosts, and scary entities of all types abound, but our own departed loved ones are not invited to the party. Although specific religions have their own ways of honoring the dead, the general American culture lacks outlets for remembering departed loved ones and honoring their place in our hearts.

# PLANNING FOR DEATH

Acknowledging the inevitability of death allows us to plan for it. Adequate planning can help ensure that a sudden, unexpected death is not made even more difficult for survivors. Even when death is not sudden, individuals with a debilitating illness may become unable to make decisions for themselves. Many decisions can be anticipated, considered, and discussed with close relatives and friends long before death occurs.

**TERMS**

**will** A legal instrument expressing a person's intentions and wishes for the disposition of their property after death.

**estate** The money, property, and other possessions belonging to a person.

**testator** The person who makes a will.

**intestate** Not having made a legal will.

**advance directive** Any legally recognized statement made by a competent person about their choices for medical treatment should he or she become unable to make such decisions or communicate them in the future.

**living will** A type of advance directive that allows individuals to provide instructions about the kind of medical care they wish to receive, or not receive, if they become unable to participate in treatment decisions.

**health care proxy** A type of advance directive that allows an individual to appoint another person as an agent in making health care decisions in the event he or she becomes unable to participate in treatment decisions; also known as a *durable power of attorney for health care.*

## Making a Will

Surveys indicate that less than half of adult Americans have a will. A **will** is a legal instrument expressing a person's intentions and wishes for the disposition of their property after death. It is a declaration of how your **estate**—that is, money, property, and other possessions—will be distributed after your death. During the life of the **testator** (the person making the will), a will can be changed, replaced, or revoked. When the testator dies, it becomes a legal instrument governing the distribution of the estate.

When a person dies **intestate**—that is, without having left a valid will—property is distributed according to rules set up by the state. You don't necessarily need an attorney to make a will. If your needs are simple, online wills or legal forms sold in stores can be adequate if you follow instructions carefully.

You can also help your family members by writing down information that would be crucial to them should you die or become incapacitated. This document should include information such as bank accounts, credit cards, insurance policies, the location of documents and keys, the names of professional advisers, passwords for online accounts, the names of people who should be notified of your death, and so on.

An **advance directive** is a legal document that states your preferences about medical treatment. Having an advance directive is worthwhile for adults of any age, not just for the elderly. Two forms of advance directives are legally important. First is the **living will,** which enables individuals to provide instructions about the kind of medical care they wish to receive or prohibit if they become incapacitated or otherwise unable to participate in treatment decisions. Most living wills also include your preferences regarding organ donation.

The second important form of an advance directive is the **health care proxy,** which is also known as a *durable power of attorney for health care.* This document allows you to appoint another person to make decisions about medical treatment if you become unable to do so. This decision maker may be a family member, a close friend, or an attorney with whom you have discussed your treatment preferences. The proxy is expected to act in accordance with your wishes as stated in an advance directive or as otherwise made known. If no proxy is chosen, most states assign the task to the patient's spouse, parents, or closest relative.

## Giving the Gift of Life

Each day about 17 people on transplant waiting lists die because not enough organs are available. As of August 2021, about 107,000 Americans were waiting for organ transplants.

There are several long-standing myths and fears about organ donation. A common unfounded fear is that if you are seriously injured or ill, physicians won't work as hard to save your life if they know you are a donor. Not true! Saving your life is always the first priority. Another common myth is that organ donation disfigures the body and makes an open-casket funeral impossible. In fact, donated organs are removed surgically, which does not change the appearance of the body for the funeral service. In addition, some people are concerned that their religion may prohibit organ donation. When in doubt, you can discuss this with your clergy. But nearly all organized religions approve of organ and tissue donation, and most consider it an act of great kindness and charity.

If you decide to become an organ donor, there are multiple ways to register. You can complete a **Uniform Donor Card** either physically or online (go to organdonor.gov). Alternatively, in many states you can indicate your wish on your driver's license. You can also register online through the nonprofit website Donate Life America (donatelife.net), which manages a national registry for organ donors. Regardless of how you register, you are free to revoke your decision to be a donor at any time. Surveys show that most Americans would donate a family member's organs if they knew that was what their loved one wanted.

QUICK STATS

**One deceased donor can save up to 8 lives through organ donation and can save or improve the quality of 75 more people's lives through tissue donation.**

—American Transplant Foundation, 2022

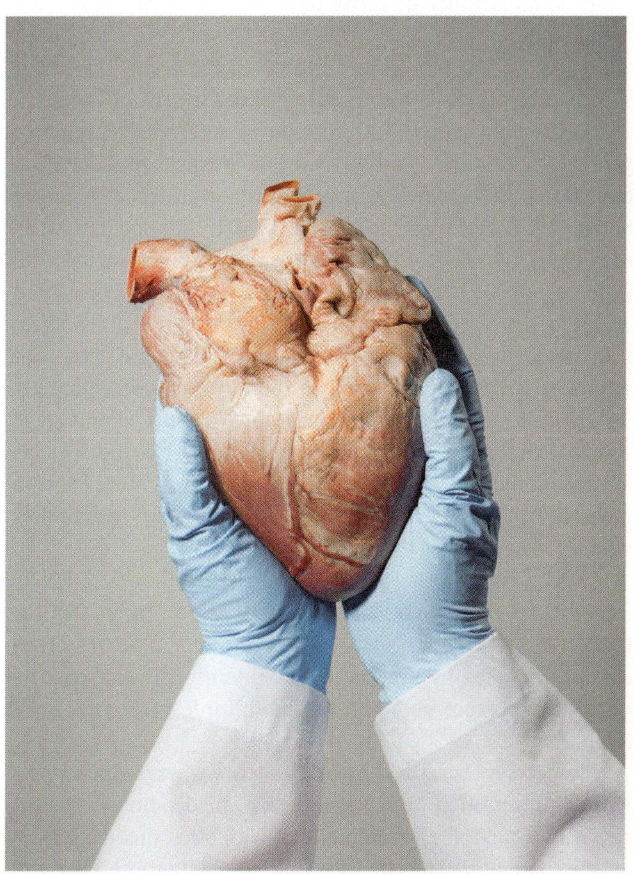

PM Images/Getty Images

## Considering Options for End-of-Life Care

Most of us will need caregiving for weeks, months, or even years as we near the end of our lives. The help needed can involve any combination of home care, residential facility care (such as assisted-living facilities), hospital stays, nursing home care, and hospice care. By becoming aware of the options, we and our families are empowered to make more informed and appropriate choices.

**Home Care** The majority of people express a preference for at-home care during the end of life. An obvious advantage of home care is the fact that the person is in a familiar setting, ideally in the company of family and friends. Family members are not always able to provide the level of care that is needed. When possible, however, home care is generally the most satisfying option as a person's life is reaching its end. In 2017, for the first time since the early part of the 1900s, more people who died a natural death were at home than in a hospital. Terminally ill people who wish to die at home, in their residential care facility, or in a more peaceful hospital environment are often aided by **hospice** programs, which are widely available throughout the United States and are providing a growing number of terminally ill patients much-needed assistance.

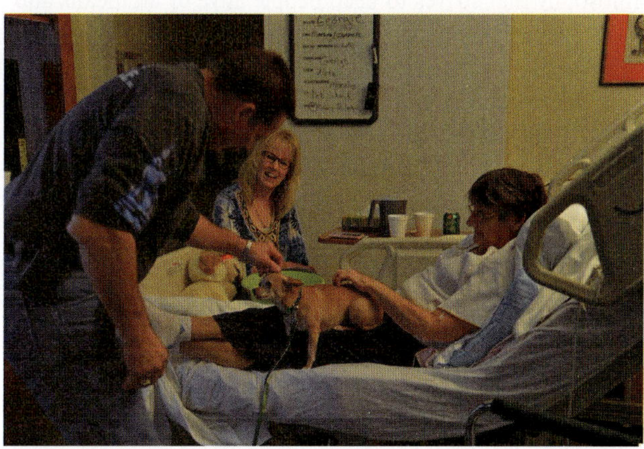

Hospice care focuses on relieving pain and other distressing symptoms in dying people and on providing support for family members. Jahi Chikwendiu/The Washington Post/Getty Images

TERMS

**Uniform Donor Card** A consent form authorizing the use of the signer's body parts for transplantation or medical research upon their death.

**hospice** A system of palliative care specifically for patients who are likely to die within six months, often at home, to optimize the quality of life for dying patients and their families.

Hospice is a system of **palliative care,** a collaborative, team-based approach to treatment that aims to prevent and relieve suffering in patients with serious or life-threatening illness. The overarching goal of palliative care is to improve the quality of life for the patient and their family during this period in their lives.

About two-thirds of hospice patients receive care in the place they call "home," which is most frequently their private residence, but also can be a nursing home or a residential care facility. It is also offered in hospitals and freestanding hospice facilities. Hospice care is available to people of all ages who are judged to be in their last six months of life. In addition to helping patients achieve a good and peaceful death, an important goal of hospice care is to help patients and families discover how much can be shared at the end of life through personal and spiritual connections.

**QUICK STATS**

**In 2020, 370 people received prescriptions under Oregon's Death with Dignity Act; 245 of those patients actually took the drugs and died as a result.**

—Oregon Public Health Division, 2021

## Difficult Decisions at the End of Life

When death is approaching, medical interventions may increase suffering without improving the quality, or even quantity, of life. The decision to stop doing tests and treatments is often a difficult one for patients and their families, especially if their loved one is not receiving hospice care. Out of a desire to do "everything possible," families may unintentionally subject their loved one to unnecessary suffering. A medical philosophy that strives to keep people alive by all means and at any cost is increasingly being questioned.

Ethical questions about a person's right to die became prominent with the landmark case of Karen Ann Quinlan in 1975. At age 22 she was admitted in a comatose state to an intensive care unit, where her breathing was sustained by a mechanical ventilator. When she remained in a **persistent vegetative state,** her parents asked that the respirator be disconnected, but the medical staff responsible for Karen's care denied their request. The request to withdraw treatment reached the New Jersey Supreme Court, which ruled that artificial respiration could be discontinued.

Since then, courts have ruled on removing other types of life-sustaining treatment, in certain circumstances. Notable was the 1998 case of Terri Schiavo, a married 26-year-old woman, who sustained a cardiac arrest that caused extensive brain damage. As a result, she entered a persistent vegetative state; she could breathe on her own but required a feeding tube for nutrition. She lacked awareness, showed no sign of voluntary movement, and her condition was irreversible. Contending that she would not want to continue living on life support, Terri's husband requested that her feeding tube be removed. Terri's parents contested the request, and a series of legal and political actions ensued, eventually involving the U.S. president and Congress. Finally, after Schiavo had spent 15 years in a persistent vegetative state, the U.S. Supreme Court intervened, allowing physicians to remove the feeding tube. Schiavo died two weeks later. Autopsy showed profound, irreversible brain damage. Cases like this highlight the importance of expressing your wishes about life-sustaining treatment, in an advance directive or other document, before the need arises.

**Withholding or Withdrawing Treatment** The right of a competent patient to refuse unwanted treatment is now generally established in both law and medical practice. The consensus is that there is no medical or ethical distinction between withholding (not starting) a treatment and withdrawing (stopping) a treatment once it has been started. The right to refuse treatment remains constitutionally protected even when a patient is unable to communicate. In this situation, decisions are made by the patient's designated power of attorney for health care, or closest family member, who must do their best to determine what the patient would have wanted under the current circumstances. Having a clear advance directive, written when the patient was competent to make health care decisions, is extremely helpful for families who are faced with these difficult decisions.

**Physician-Assisted Death and Voluntary Active Euthanasia** *Physician-assisted death* and *voluntary active euthanasia* refer to practices that intentionally hasten the death of a person; both require the full informed consent of the patient.

**Physician-assisted death (PAD)** occurs when a doctor provides a prescription for a lethal dose of medication (usually a sedative, sometimes in combination with other medications)—at the patient's request—with the understanding that the patient plans to use the medication to end their life. The

**TERMS**

**palliative care** A collaborative, team-based approach to treatment that aims to prevent and relieve suffering in patients with serious or life-threatening illness.

**palliative care** A collaborative, team-based approach to treatment that aims to prevent and relieve suffering in patients with serious or life-threatening illness.

**persistent vegetative state** A condition of extensive and irreversible brain damage with absence of higher brain function for an extended period. The person may have sleep-wake cycles, and occasional eyelid opening and movement, but lacks awareness or any cognitive function.

**physician-assisted death (PAD)** The practice of a physician intentionally providing, at the patient's request, a lethal overdose of drugs or other means for a patient to hasten death with the understanding that the patient plans to use them to end their life. The patient administers the drugs to himself or herself.

patient chooses if and when he or she wishes to take the fatal dose, usually in a home setting without the physician present. As of 2020, physician-assisted death is legal in California, Colorado, the District of Columbia, Hawaii, Maine, New Jersey, New Mexico, Oregon, Vermont, and Washington.

Oregon was the first state to legalize PAD following a citizens' initiative called the Death with Dignity Act. Even though PAD has been legally available in Oregon since 1994, the practice remains rare; in 2020 there were 40,226 total deaths in the state of Oregon, and only 245 (0.6%) were physician-assisted deaths. The majority of patients who have chosen to use PAD to end their lives have been in the late phases of terminal cancer.

In 1997 and again in 2006, the U.S. Supreme Court affirmed that individual states have the right to craft policy concerning PAD. The Supreme Court has also ruled on a related topic: the doctrine of **double effect** in the medical management of pain. The doctrine says that a harmful effect of treatment, even if it results in death, is permissible if the harm is not intended and occurs as a side effect of a beneficial action. The significance of this ruling as it relates to end-of-life care is that if the doctor's intent is to relieve a patient's severe pain, it is permissible to give the dose of medication needed to relieve the pain even if that dose, as a side effect, could cause respiratory depression, which could possibly hasten the patient's death. The doctrine of double effect allows physicians throughout the United States to do what is necessary to relieve a patient's pain, even if there is a chance that the medication may hasten death.

**Active euthanasia** is different from PAD, and it is illegal in the United States. Active euthanasia is defined as the intentional act of killing someone who would otherwise suffer from an incurable and painful disease. *Voluntary euthanasia* (also known as voluntary active euthanasia, or VAE) is the intentional termination of life at the patient's request by someone other than the patient, usually a doctor or nurse. This means that a mentally competent patient requests direct assistance to die and receives active assistance from a qualified medical practitioner. The difference between PAD and VAE is that PAD requires that patients ingest the medication themselves, whereas with VAE, the health professional can administer the medication to the patient.

Voluntary active euthanasia is legal under very strict guidelines in Belgium, Luxembourg, Canada, New Zealand, Spain, the Netherlands, and Colombia, but is currently unlawful in the United States and the rest of the world. In the United States, taking active steps to end someone's life is a crime—even if the motive is mercy.

When a person is near death and still having severe suffering despite optimal treatment, sometimes **palliative sedation** will be used. Palliative sedation involves giving a sedative medication that keeps the patient in an unconscious or semiconscious state until pain is brought under control or the patient dies as a result of their underlying disease. Palliative sedation is not meant to hasten death; rather it is used as a last resort when physician, patient, and family agree that this is the best way to relieve otherwise intractable suffering.

## Planning a Funeral or Memorial Service

Funerals, memorial services, and celebrations of life are rites of passage that commemorate a person's life and acknowledge their passing from the community. Funerals and memorials allow survivors to support one another as they cope with their loss and express their grief. The presence of death rites in nearly every human culture suggests that these ceremonies serve deep-seated human needs.

**Disposition of the Body** People generally have a preference about the final disposition of their own body. For most Americans, the choice is either burial or cremation, and often depends on cultural and religious norms. *Burial* involves a grave dug into the earth (often with a cement liner) or entombment in a mausoleum (a building that houses dead bodies or remains). If a body is to be buried and the family wishes that the body be viewed during a wake or in an open-casket funeral, **embalming** is generally done.

Green, or natural, burial is an increasingly common option in some parts of the United States. The intent is to allow the body to recycle naturally and to protect the surrounding environment. Bodies are placed in the ground wrapped in cloth or rapidly degrading wooden or cardboard coffins, with no cement vault. *Cremation* involves subjecting a body to intense heat, thereby reducing its organic components to a mineralized skeleton. The remaining bone fragments are then

### Ask Yourself

**QUESTIONS FOR CRITICAL THINKING AND REFLECTION**

Have you ever been involved in a funeral? What role did you play? Did you feel that the service reflected the values and beliefs of the deceased person? Did the service provide healing and comfort to family and friends? Did the experience cause you to think about your own funeral and what it should be like?

**TERMS**

**double effect** A situation in which a harmful effect occurs as an unintended side effect of a beneficial action, such as when medication intended to control a patient's pain has the unintended result of causing the patient's death.

**active euthanasia** A deliberate act intended to end another person's life; voluntary active euthanasia involves the practice of a physician's administering—at the request of a patient—medication or some other intervention that causes death.

**palliative sedation** The practice of using a sedative medication to keep a patient in an unconscious or semiconscious state until pain is brought under control or the patient dies as a result of the underlying disease.

**embalming** The process of removing blood and other fluids and replacing them with chemicals to disinfect and temporarily retard deterioration of a corpse; some of the chemicals used, such as formaldehyde, are toxic and carcinogenic.

## CRITICAL CONSUMER

### A Consumer Guide to Funerals

A traditional funeral with a casket costs about $8000, and many funerals cost $10,000 or more. When no preplanning has been done, as often occurs, family members have to make decisions under time pressure and in the grip of strong feelings. As a result, they may make poor decisions and spend more than they need to. To avoid these problems, millions of consumers are now making funeral arrangements in advance, comparing prices and services so that they can make well-informed purchasing decisions. Many people see funeral planning as an extension of will and estate planning.

Alternatives to traditional funerals exist. Cremation is now used in over 55% of deaths in the United States, with the rate of cremation increasing rapidly in recent years. According to the National Funeral Directors Association, by 2040 the U.S. cremation rate is projected to be over 78%, although cremation does have negative environmental effects, such as $CO_2$ emissions and release of toxic substances into the air. Cremation is a much less expensive alternative to a traditional burial. A direct cremation (no service or visitation at the funeral home) can cost as little as $600 in some cities and has a lower environmental impact than traditional burial. Cremated remains can be buried, placed in a columbarium niche, put into an urn kept by the family, interred in an urn garden, or scattered at sea or on land. Scattering ashes is regulated by a variety of federal, state, and local laws, so check these first. Whole-body donation (usually to a medical school) is another option chosen by many people for altruistic reasons, as well as for the fact that there is usually no cost.

Another alternative to an expensive traditional funeral is a more personalized, "do-it-yourself" family-centered funeral, with minimal costs because most of the tasks needed to care for the deceased person are provided by family and friends.

To ensure that you make the best possible decisions when planning a funeral, consider these options:

- Plan ahead. Think about what type of funeral you want and ask your loved ones about their preferences.
- Shop around. If you are going to use a funeral home, look for a few that belong to the National Funeral Directors Association (NFDA), and compare prices.
- Ask for a price list. The Funeral Rule requires funeral directors to give you an itemized price list when you ask either in person or over the telephone. Many funeral homes offer package funerals that cost less than individual items, but you may not need or want everything included in the package.
- Decide on the goods and services you want. Basic services include planning the funeral and coordinating arrangements with the cemetery or crematory. The casket is usually the single most expensive item; an average casket costs slightly more than $2000, but some caskets sell for as much as $10,000. You do not have to buy the casket from the funeral home you use. Many "big box" stores now sell caskets at much lower cost than funeral homes. Special body bags or very simple wood or cardboard caskets are also used and generally cost well under $1000.
- Resist pressure to buy goods and services you don't really want or need. Funeral directors are required to inform you that you need buy only those goods and services you want. If you feel you are being pressured, go elsewhere.
- In choosing a cemetery, consider its location, religious affiliation, the types of monuments allowed, and cost. Visit ahead of time to make sure it's suitable. Consider green burial if this option would have pleased your loved one. Use of a cemetery is optional for cremation.
- Once decisions have been made, put them in writing, give copies to family members, and keep a copy accessible. Review these decisions every few years and revise them if necessary.

SOURCE: National Funeral Directors Association. 2021. *Statistics* (https://www.nfda.org/news/statistics)

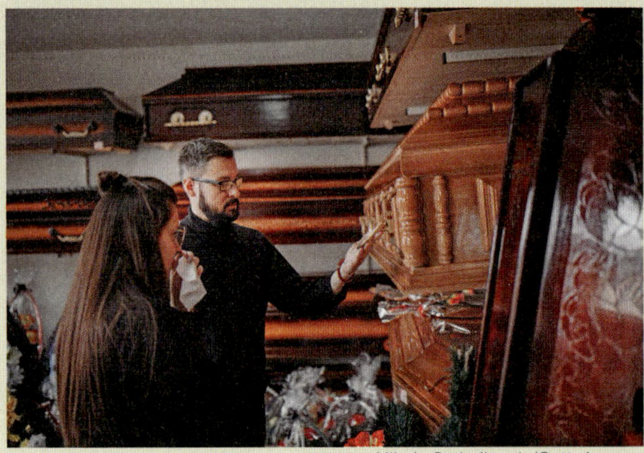

Nikola Stojadinovic/Getty Images

usually put through a cremulator, which reduces them to a granular state, often referred to as ashes (which actually resemble coarse sand). Only a decade ago, burial was more common than cremation in the United States, but now cremation is the more popular choice. Cremation is acceptable to many Christian sects and is the norm for most Hindus, Sikhs, Jains, and many Buddhists. In contrast, cremation is forbidden for Muslims, many Jewish sects, and the Eastern Orthodox Church (for more on cremation, see the box "A Consumer Guide to Funerals").

**Arranging a Service** A funeral or memorial service can be a healing experience that allows loved ones to share memories and support one another. The service is often led by clergy, but many nontraditional services are led by a family member or close friend. The more the service fits the personality of the deceased person and meets the practical and emotional needs of the family, the better.

People who have a terminal illness sometimes find comfort and satisfaction in helping to plan for their own memorial services. A memorial service can be the joint creation of the dying person and family members who wish to be part of the project. Making at least some plans ahead of time can help ease the burden on survivors, who will undoubtedly face a great number of tasks and decisions when the death occurs.

## COPING WITH IMMINENT DEATH

There is no one right way to live with or die of a life-threatening illness. Every disease has its own set of problems and challenges, and each person copes in their own way. Much of the suffering experienced by people with a life-threatening illness comes from overwhelming feelings of loss on all levels.

### The Tasks of Coping

In her groundbreaking 1969 book *On Death and Dying,* Elisabeth Kübler-Ross, a Swiss American psychiatrist and one of the first medical experts to focus on the topic of end of life, suggested that the response to an awareness of imminent death involves five psychological stages: denial, anger, bargaining, depression, and acceptance.

Today the notion of stages has been deemphasized in favor of highlighting the tasks that require attention in order to cope well with a life-threatening illness. Psychologist and author Charles Corr, for example, distinguishes four primary dimensions in coping with dying:

1. ***Physical.*** Satisfying bodily needs and minimizing physical distress
2. ***Psychological.*** Maximizing a sense of security, self-worth, autonomy, and richness in living
3. ***Social.*** Sustaining significant relationships and addressing the social implications of dying
4. ***Spiritual.*** Identifying, developing, or reaffirming sources of meaning and fostering hope

Some people with life-threatening illness respond with a fighting spirit that views the illness not only as a threat but also as a challenge. These people strive to inform themselves about their illness and take an active part in treatment decisions, as much as they are able. They attempt to continue to set and accomplish goals, maintain relationships, and sustain a sense of personal vitality, competence, and power despite life-threatening illness. Other people with terminal disease, particularly in the later stages, tend to withdraw, and they sometimes find their peace in quietly letting go of striving. For many dying people, the world around them becomes smaller and more intimate. They may find it most helpful to ease into a peaceful place, in the presence of calm and loving people who respect their need for quiet companionship.

> **Ask Yourself**
>
> **QUESTIONS FOR CRITICAL THINKING AND REFLECTION**
>
> What is your notion of a "good death"? In what setting does it take place, and who is there? In the last days of your life, what do you think you would want to say, and to whom? If you were terminally ill, what would be the most supportive things others could do for you?

### Supporting a Person in the Last Phase of Life

People often feel uncomfortable in the presence of a person who is in the final stage of life. How should we act? What can we say? Perhaps the most important and comforting thing we can do for a dying person is to simply be present. Sitting quietly and listening carefully, we can take our cues from the person who is dying. If the person is capable of speaking, and wishes to talk, attentive listening is an act of great kindness. If the person doesn't wish to talk, or is not able to, physical touch such as holding hands or putting a hand on the person's shoulder can be the most effective way to express your love and concern.

As death is drawing near, simple steps—such as repositioning the patient, covering him or her with a light blanket, dimming the room's lighting, playing soft favorite music, or holding hands—can provide great relief and reassurance in the last moments of apparent unresponsiveness before death finally comes.

## COPING WITH LOSS

Even if you have not experienced the death of someone close, you have likely experienced many losses related to life changes. The loss of a job, the ending of a relationship, transitions from one school or neighborhood to another—these are the kinds of losses that occur in all our lives. Such losses are sometimes called little deaths, and in varying degrees they all involve grief.

### Experiencing Grief

**Grief** is the reaction to loss. It encompasses thoughts and feelings as well as physical and behavioral responses. Mental distress may involve disbelief, confusion, anxiety, disorganization, and depression. The emotions that can be present in normal grief include not only sorrow and sadness, but also relief, anger, guilt, and self-pity, among others. Bereaved people experience a range of feelings, including conflicting ones. Observing the faces of families at the funeral of a beloved relative often reveals smiles and moments of laughter in addition to solemn expressions and tears. Recognizing that grief can involve many feelings—not just sadness—makes us more able to cope with it.

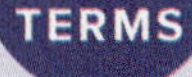


**grief** A person's reaction to loss as manifested physically, emotionally, mentally, and behaviorally.

## TAKE CHARGE
### Coping with Grief

- Recognize and acknowledge your loss.
- React to grief in the way that feels most natural to you. There is no "right" way to grieve.
- Take time for nature's process of healing. The odds are good that you will be functioning well again before long. Be patient with yourself.
- Know that powerful, overwhelming feelings will change with time. Grief is often experienced as a long series of ups and downs, with the intensity of feelings decreasing gradually over time.
- Beware of the lure of drugs and alcohol to reduce the pain of your grief, especially if you have had a substance use disorder in the past. Using alcohol or drugs to numb yourself will ultimately backfire and make your healing more difficult.
- Honor your loved one in a way that is meaningful to you. Consider creating a small memorial with a photo and flowers, start a scholarship in your loved one's name, plant a memorial tree, or write a song or poem in their honor.
- Consider joining a bereavement support group (in person or online) to connect with others who have had recent losses.
- Surround yourself with life: go out in nature, enjoy the healing companionship of a pet, connect with friends and family.
- If you are having difficulty functioning at school, work, or home after a few weeks, consider counseling or a support group.
- People who have had a recent loss are at higher risk for suicide. If you are having thoughts of suicide, or feeling hopeless, seek help right away.
- Care for yourself by finding time to eat, sleep, and move your body.
- Don't be afraid to let laughter and joy remain in your life. Experiencing positive feelings during mourning does not indicate a lack of respect or love for the deceased.

Common behaviors associated with grief include crying and talking repetitively about the deceased and the circumstances of the death. Bereaved people may be restless, as if not knowing what to do with themselves. Outward signs of grief may involve frequent sighing, crying, inappropriate laughter, insomnia, loss of appetite, and marked fatigue. Grief may also evoke a reexamination of religious or spiritual beliefs as a person struggles to make meaning of the loss. Guilt is a common emotion after the death of a loved one. People frequently blame themselves in some way for the death, or for not doing enough for the deceased, or for feeling a sense of relief that their loved one is gone. All such manifestations of grief can be present as part of our total response to **bereavement**—that is, the event of loss.

**Mourning** is closely related to grief and is often used as a synonym for it. However, mourning refers not so much to the *reaction* to loss but to the *process* by which a bereaved person adjusts to loss and incorporates it into their life. How this process is managed is determined, at least partly, by cultural and gender norms for the expression of grief.

**The Course of Grief** Grieving, like dying, is highly individual. In the first hours or days following a death, a bereaved person is likely to experience shock and numbness, as well as a sense of disbelief, especially if the death was unexpected. The cause or mode of death—natural, accidental, homicide, or suicide—influences how grief is experienced. Even when a death is anticipated, grief is not necessarily diminished when the loss becomes real.

The death of a loved one is frequently a severe physical as well as emotional stressor. For example, in the first day after the death of a loved one, the rate of heart attack in the survivor increases by as much as 21 times. The risk of death decreases gradually over time but still remains well above normal for several months after a loved one dies. After a death, grieving people often have difficulty sleeping, may neglect to eat nourishing food, and may forget to take their usual medications. These factors add to the health risks associated with recent loss. Recent loss also has a cognitive impact on many grievers. People often report that they feel confused and have difficulty concentrating following a significant loss.

After the initial shock begins to fade, the course of grief is characterized by anxiety, apathy, and pining for the deceased. The pangs of grief are felt as the bereaved person deeply experiences the pain of separation. Mourners often experience despair as they replay the events surrounding the loss, perhaps fantasizing that somehow everything could be undone.

As time goes on, the acute pain and emotional turmoil of grief begin to subside. Physical and mental balance are gradually reestablished. The bereaved person becomes increasingly reintegrated into their social world. Sadness doesn't go away completely, but it recedes into the background much of the time. Although reminders of the loss stimulate waves of active grieving from time to time, the main focus is the present, not the past. Adjusting to loss may sometimes feel like a betrayal of the deceased loved one, but it is healthy to engage again in ongoing life and the future (see the box "Coping with Grief").

**TERMS**

**bereavement** The period of sorrow that follows the death of a loved one.

**mourning** The process whereby a person actively copes with grief in adjusting to a loss and integrating it into their life.

Social support for the bereaved is as critical during the later course of grief as it is during the first days after a loss. In offering support, we can reassure the grieving person that grief is normal, permissible, and appropriate. The anniversary of the loved one's death, birthdays, and major holidays following a significant loss can reignite the intensity of grieving, and the support of others is especially important and appreciated during those times. Connecting with friends and family to acknowledge the loss and reaffirm your ongoing relationship can be extremely comforting throughout the grieving experience.

Bereaved people may find it helpful to share their stories and concerns through organized support groups. Hospices provide bereavement support groups and counseling free of charge, usually for 13 months after the death. Many online and in-person support groups are organized around specific types of bereavement, such as loss of a child or a parent, or the loss of a loved one to suicide.

There is no hard and fast "normal" amount of time that grief should last, but when the duration and intensity far exceed what is usually expected, it is often referred to as complicated grief. Rates of complicated grief in Western countries tend to be highest when a child is lost, or when the death was violent and unexpected (see the box "Surviving the Sudden or Violent Death of a Loved One"). A history of mood disorder such as depression, as well as previous or ongoing substance use disorder, increases the risk for prolonged grief. Psychotherapy, with or without medication, can be critical for someone who is suffering from prolonged and debilitating grief.

## Supporting a Grieving Person

When a person finds out that a loved one has died, the initial reaction may be profound shock and overwhelming distress. Such a person may initially respond best to the physical comfort of hugging and holding. Later, simply listening may be the most effective way to help someone who is grieving. Talking about the loss is an important way that many survivors cope with the changed reality, and they may need to tell their story over and over. The key to being a good listener is to avoid speaking too much, and to refrain from making judgments about whether the thoughts and feelings expressed by a survivor are right or wrong, good or bad. The emotions, thoughts, and behaviors evoked by loss may not be the ones we expect, but they can nonetheless be valid and appropriate within a survivor's experience of loss.

> **Ask Yourself**
>
> **QUESTIONS FOR CRITICAL THINKING AND REFLECTION**
>
> Have you ever been in a close relationship with a bereaved person? What kind of support did he or she seem to appreciate most? Why do you think that was the case? How did the experience affect you?

If a grieving friend or relative talks about suicide or seems in danger of causing harm to himself or herself or others, seek professional help right away. Most people are resilient and cope well with loss, but the recent loss of a loved one is a major risk factor for suicide and self-harm. Be alert to signs that a grieving person is in serious danger.

## When a Young Adult Loses a Friend

Among young people aged 18–24 in the United States, the leading causes of death tend to be sudden and unexpected: unintentional injuries, overdose, homicide, and suicide. Losing a close friend to an unexpected death can be particularly traumatic. As a friend, you may feel unsupported and left out of the family's grieving. Also, you may blame yourself in some way for your friend's death or feel you should have somehow prevented the tragedy. If you lose a friend, be sure to look for support from friends, family, clergy, or health professionals, especially if the intense sadness or guilt feelings last for more than a few days or weeks. Friends can often help each other by working together to create their own way of celebrating the life of their lost friend.

## Helping Children Cope with Loss

Children tend to cope with loss in a healthier fashion when they are included as part of their family's experience of grief and mourning. Although adults may be uncomfortable about sharing potentially disturbing or painful news with children, a child's natural curiosity usually negates the option of completely withholding information. Mounting evidence shows that it is best to include children from the beginning—as soon as a terminal prognosis is made, for example—to help them understand what is happening. Children should spend time with the dying person, if possible, to learn, share, offer, and receive comfort.

In talking about death with children, the most important guideline is to be honest. Offer an explanation at the child's level of understanding. Find out what the child wants to know. Keep the explanation simple, stick to basics, and verify what the child has understood from your explanation.

# COMING TO TERMS WITH DEATH

We may wish we could keep death out of view and protect ourselves and others from the pain associated with it. But this wish cannot be fulfilled. With the death of a beloved friend or relative, we are confronted with emotions and thoughts that relate not only to the immediate loss but also to our own mortality. Our exposure to death can offer opportunities for extraordinary growth in the midst of loss. Encounters with dying and death, painful as they may be, can help us more fully appreciate the infinite preciousness of life and love.

## TAKE CHARGE
# Surviving the Sudden or Violent Death of a Loved One

Coping with the death of a loved one is among the greatest challenges a person faces in a lifetime. When the death is due to sudden or violent causes, such as injury, homicide, suicide, or unintentional drug overdose, the challenges of grieving are multiplied many fold. Experts estimate that one out of three of us will experience the traumatic loss of a close friend or relative to sudden violent death. Motor vehicle crashes, by their nature sudden and unpredictable, are one of the most common causes of traumatic death in young people. Hardly anyone makes it through high school without losing at least one classmate in an automotive crash. A fatal car crash leaves behind many victims besides those who died. Friends and relatives are devastated by the loss of a beloved young person. Any occupants of the vehicle who survive the crash typically suffer from injuries and psychological trauma, in addition to their grief for the ones who died. Posttraumatic stress is a common outcome for survivors. If the driver was intoxicated, or otherwise at fault for the crash, survivors must also cope with that difficult knowledge. Feelings of anger and guilt are often mixed in with the sadness and loss.

Although homicide is far less common in the United States than motor vehicle crashes, young people who grow up in high-crime neighborhoods all too often experience the loss of relatives, friends, or acquaintances due to killings. When a loved one is murdered, grievers may agonize over the circumstances of the crime and imagine the horrible suffering their loved one might have endured. Survivors may be haunted by memories of the person's mangled body or may obsess over missing details of the crime. Survivors may also fear for their own safety. The police and legal system may add to the trauma through insensitivity at best, and offensive behavior toward survivors at worst.

People who survive a loved one's suicide or unintentional drug overdose also experience great suffering as a result of the stigma attached to these types of death. They often feel terrible guilt, wondering if they were in part responsible for their loved one's distress, or whether they could have done something to prevent the death. Perhaps the most difficult aspect of coping with sudden or violent death, and suicide in particular, is the societal stigma frequently directed at the survivors. The spouse or parent of someone who has committed suicide is often suspected of having been a source of the victim's unhappiness, or at least guilty for not sensing the trouble and doing something about it.

Thus, beyond the challenges of coping with a "natural" death, those who lose a loved one to a sudden or violent death face many additional sources of anguish. The sense of the world as a benevolent, safe, and predictable place is often lost when loved ones die in traumatic circumstances. Survivors often face questions of blame, legal issues, financial distress, and lack of social support. A grieving survivor may be called upon to relive the trauma and its horrifying memories over and over again during encounters with police and in legal proceedings. Moreover, friends and community members often avoid survivors, or respond with morbid curiosity or judgmental comments, rather than providing the loving support that is so desperately needed. Or they may back away from someone whose loss is too frightening to contemplate. The instinct to blame the deceased and the survivors for some aspect of a violent death is also common and often represents our attempt to reassure ourselves that if only we are vigilant, and do the right thing, this kind of tragedy won't happen to us or our loved ones.

Some experts refer to the grief experience related to violent loss as "traumatic grief," a term used by Marilyn Armour, a prominent researcher in the field. Traumatic grief involves symptoms of separation-related distress, resulting from the loss of a loved one, as well as symptoms of traumatic distress related to the horrible ordeal the mourner has experienced. Posttraumatic stress often complicates a survivor's ability to recover, and severe, prolonged grief may result. Finding meaning in a sudden and violent death is often much more challenging than in a death from old age or a lengthy illness. When someone dies of natural causes, the survivors are often comforted by the belief that at least their loved one is no longer suffering or that the person "died peacefully." In the case of violent death, there are no similar thoughts to soften the blow.

Despite the great challenges, most people who lose someone to a violent death do eventually recapture a sense of normalcy. Helping survivors starts with all of us reaching out with nonjudgmental love and kindness. For all survivors, the support of friends and community is crucial for regaining a sense of peace. A number of excellent organizations support survivors of loved ones whose deaths were through accidents, overdose, suicide, homicide, and other types of violence (see For More Information at the end of this chapter). Most of these organizations provide information about joining online and in-person support groups, as well as finding professional help for those who are having difficulty coping with traumatic loss.

## TIPS FOR TODAY AND THE FUTURE

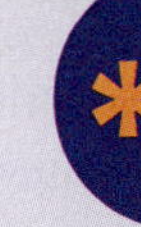

**RIGHT NOW YOU CAN:**

- Review your financial situation, and start thinking about a plan for the future.
- Think about any unhealthy habits you have, and resolve to change them.
- Speak to older people about what aging has meant to them, and see what lessons you can learn from them.
- Consider volunteering at an adult day care center or nursing home—share what you enjoy, such as music, reading, or arts and crafts.
- Think about life's impermanence and appreciate the now.
- Don't miss out on opportunities to let your friends and loved ones know that you care for them. Let your awareness of death guide you into leading a loving and purposeful life.
- Consider organ donation as a lasting gift of life to others. If you want to be an organ donor, make the appropriate arrangements now, as described in this chapter.

**IN THE FUTURE YOU CAN:**

- Keep moving! Adapt your physical activity to your current needs and interests. Keep making movement a fun habit.
- Continue an open dialogue with your loved ones about what brings meaning to your lives.
- Volunteering can be a source of satisfaction throughout life. Keep helping others in ways that you enjoy and are meaningful to you.
- Talk to your parents or grandparents about their wishes for the end of life. Let them know you care for them and want to be involved. Suggest that you look together at an advance directive form.
- Make a difference for a grieving friend or relative. Show that you care by your loving presence and your willingness to listen quietly.

## SUMMARY

- People who take charge of their health during their youth have greater control over the physical and mental aspects of aging.
- Biological aging takes place over a lifetime, but some other changes associated with aging are more abrupt.
- A lifetime of interests and hobbies helps maintain creativity and intelligence.
- Exercise and a healthful diet throughout life enhance physical and psychological health.
- Alcohol and drug misuse is a common but often hidden problem among older adults.
- Tobacco use shortens life and may cause severe health impairment for many years, even after quitting smoking.
- Keeping up with immunizations and participating in recommended health screening can help us live a longer, healthier life.
- Stress translates to wear and tear on the body; getting enough sleep, nurturing social connections, and practicing relaxation can be effective in reducing stress and increasing vitality and happiness.
- Retirement can be one of the most fulfilling and enjoyable times of life. Adjusting to new roles, participating in a variety of activities, having enough money to live comfortably, and having a sense of purpose in life are all important factors in successful retirement.
- Occasional slight confusion and forgetfulness are a part of normal aging, but more severe symptoms could be signs of a neurodegenerative disease, such as Alzheimer's disease, and should prompt a medical evaluation.
- People over age 65 form a large and growing minority in the United States and throughout the world.
- Family and community resources can help older adults stay active and independent.
- Government aid to older adults includes food assistance, housing subsidies, Social Security, Medicare, and Medicaid.
- The existence of death makes rational sense in terms of species survival and evolution; grappling with the philosophical and spiritual aspects of our own death is a major part of life's journey.
- Dying and death are more than biological events; they have social and spiritual dimensions.
- The traditional criteria for clinical death are the cessation of breathing and heartbeat. Brain death is an irreversible cessation of brain activity indicated by various diagnostic criteria.
- A mature understanding of death can include ideas about the survival of the human personality or soul after death. Problems arise when avoidance or denial of death fosters the notion that it happens only to others.
- A will is a legal instrument that governs the distribution of a person's estate after death.
- Advance directives, such as living wills, are used to express your wishes about the use of life-sustaining treatment and how you would wish to be treated if you could not speak for yourself.
- Palliative care is a team-based approach to improving the quality of life for seriously ill patients by controlling pain and relieving physical and psychological suffering.
- Choices about end-of-life care include making decisions about attempting to prolong life through artificial means or allowing natural death to occur if you have a terminal condition with no reasonable chance of recovery.
- The right of a competent patient to refuse unwanted treatment, or to terminate an undesired treatment, is now generally established in both law and medical practice.
- Physician-assisted death occurs when a physician prescribes medication at a patient's request, with the understanding that the patient plans to take the medicine to end their life. PAD is legal,

with strict regulations, in some states in the United States. Voluntary active euthanasia refers to the intentional ending of a patient's life, at their request, by someone other than the patient, such as a doctor or nurse.

- Living donors can donate a single kidney or parts of other organs. Living donations account for nearly 20% of organ transplantation.

- Bereaved people usually benefit from participating in a funeral or other type of memorial service to commemorate a loved one's life and death.

- For Americans, the decision about what to do with the body after death usually involves choosing between burial or cremation.

- Coping with dying involves physical, psychological, social, and spiritual dimensions.

- The gift of listening and loving touch can be especially important to someone who is dying.

- Grief encompasses thoughts and feelings as well as physical and behavioral responses. Complicated grief occurs when someone is debilitated by severe grief over a lengthy period of time.

## FOR MORE INFORMATION

*AARP.* Provides information about all aspects of aging, including health promotion, health care, and retirement planning.

http://www.aarp.org

*Administration on Aging.* Provides fact sheets, statistical information, and internet links to other resources on aging.

http://www.acl.gov

*Aging with Dignity: Five Wishes.* Source for an advance directive that includes designation of a health care proxy (durable power of attorney), and the kind of medical treatment you want or want to avoid.

http://fivewishes.org

*Alliance for Aging Research.* A nonprofit organization that supports medical and psychological research on aging.

http://www.agingresearch.org

*Alzheimer's Association.* Offers tips for caregivers and patients and information on the causes and treatment of Alzheimer's disease.

http://www.alz.org

*American Foundation for Suicide Prevention.* The "Find Support" section of this website has information for people whose lives have been touched by suicide, including support groups, individual help, and crisis care for those who are considering suicide, have attempted suicide, have lost someone to suicide, or have a loved one who has attempted suicide.

https://afsp.org/find-support/

*Arthritis Foundation.* Provides information about arthritis, including free brochures, referrals to local services, and research updates.

http://www.arthritis.org

*Bone Health and Osteoporosis Foundation.* Provides information about the causes, prevention, detection, and treatment of osteoporosis.

http://www.nof.org

*Caring Connections (a program of the National Hospice and Palliative Care Organization).* Extensive information about end-of-life -caregiving, hospice, and palliative care.

http://www.caringinfo.org

*Donate Life America.* Extensive information about organ donation and transplantation. This website allows you to add your information to be on the national registry of organ donors.

http://www.donatelife.net

*Family Caregiver Alliance.* Provides extensive educational material for caregivers, including written material in many languages, videos, and classes; provides support such as respite care; advocates for caregivers through public policy.

http://www.caregiver.org

*GRASP: Grief Recovery After a Substance Passing.* Website for friends and family of people who have died as a result of substance use. Local and online support groups are available.

http://grasphelp.org

*Healthy Aging: U.S. Department of Health and Human Services.* Lists numerous significant resources for all aspects of aging healthfully: brain and mental health, nutrition, exercise training, networking, how to locate benefits and find care, retirement planning, and many other aspects.

http://www.hhs.gov/aging/healthy-aging/index.html#

*Hospice Foundation of America.* Provides extensive information about hospice care, end-of-life care, grief, and grief support groups.

http://www.hospicefoundation.org

*Medicare.* Provides signup information; listings to compare doctors, providers, hospitals, plans, and suppliers available through the program; and details on costs and coverage.

http://www.medicare.gov

*National Council on Aging.* Provides helpful information about retirement planning, health promotion, and lifelong learning.

http://www.ncoa.org

*National Hospice and Palliative Care Organization (NHPCO).* Provides information about hospice care and advance directives, including an online national directory of hospices listed by state and city.

http://www.nhpco.org

*National Institute on Aging.* Provides fact sheets and brochures about aging-related topics.

http://www.nia.nih.gov

https://www.nia.nih.gov/health/exercise-physical-activity

*The Compassionate Friends.* Provides grief support after the death of a child, including local chapters and online support groups.

http://www.compassionatefriends.org

*The Dougy Center.* Offers education about childhood bereavement and support groups for bereaved children, teens, young adults, and parents.

http://www.dougy.org

The following organizations provide information about organ donation and donor cards:

*Donate Life America:* http://www.donatelife.net

*Health Resources and Services Administration:*

http://www.organdonor.gov

*United Network for Organ Sharing:* http://www.unos.org

# SELECTED BIBLIOGRAPHY


2021 Alzheimer's disease facts and figures. 2021. *Alzheimer's Dementia* (March) 17(3): 327–406. (https://pubmed.ncbi.nlm.nih.gov/33756057/).

AARP Public Policy Institute and National Alliance for Caregiving. 2020. *Caregiving in the United States 2020* (http://www.aarp.org/ppi/info-2020/caregiving-in-the-united-states.html).

Administration for Community Living. 2021. *2020 Profile of Older Americans* (https://acl.gov/sites/default/files/Aging%20and%20Disability%20in%20America/2020ProfileOlderAmericans.Final_.pdf).

Agronin, M. 2019. Sexual dysfunction in older adults. *Up To Date* (https://www.uptodate.com/contents/sexual-dysfunction-in-older-adults).

Alcohol Addiction Center. 2022. *Six Facts About Elderly Alcohol Abuse* (https://alcoholaddictioncenter.org/elder-alcohol-abuse/).

Alzheimer's Association. 2021. *Global Dementia Cases Forecasted to Triple by 2050* (https://www.alz.org/aaic/releases_2021/global-prevalence.asp)

American Transplant Foundation. 2019. *Facts and Myths* (http://www.americantransplantfoundation.org/about-transplant/facts-and-myths/).

America's Health Ratings. 2021. *Obesity in United States Summary* (https://www.americashealthrankings.org/explore/annual/measure/Obesity/state/ALL).

America's Health Ratings. 2021. *Poverty in United States Summary 2020* (https://www.americashealthrankings.org/explore/senior/measure/poverty_sr/state/ALL).

Armstrong, S. 2019. *Borrowed Time: The Science of How and Why We Age.* London: Bloomsbury Sigma.

Axelrod, J. et al. 2019. Isolated and struggling, many seniors are turning to suicide. *National Public Radio* (https://www.npr.org/2019/07/27/745017374/isolated-and-struggling-many-seniors-are-turning-to-suicide).

Binette, J. 2021. *Where We Live, Where We Age: Trends in Home and Community Preferences. A National Survey of Adults Age 18-Plus.* Washington, DC: AARP Research, November (https://www.aarp.org/research/topics/community/info-2021/2021-home-community-preferences.html).

Bleiberg, L. 2019. Congress approves over-the-counter hearing aids. AARP (https://www.aarp.org/health/conditions-treatments/info-2019/otc-hearing-aids.html).

Buchholz, K. 2021. *There Are Now More than Half a Million People Aged 100 or Older Around the World.* World Economic Forum (https://www.weforum.org/agenda/2021/02/living-to-one-hundred-life-expectancy/)

Burkle, C. M., et al. 2014. Why brain death is considered death and why there should be no confusion. *Neurology,* September 12 (epub).

Centers for Disease Control and Prevention. 2018. 10 *Leading Causes of Death by Age Group, U.S.-2018* (https://www.cdc.gov/injury/wisqars/LeadingCauses.html).

Centers for Disease Control and Prevention. 2020. *Alzheimer's Disease and Healthy Aging* (https://www.cdc.gov/aging/publications/features/dementia-not-normal-aging.html).

Centers for Disease Control and Prevention. 2021. *Arthritis* (https://www.cdc.gov/arthritis/data_statistics/arthritis-related-stats.htm).

Centers for Disease Control and Prevention. 2021. *COVID-19 Mortality Overview* (https://www.cdc.gov/nchs/covid19/mortality-overview.htm)

Centers for Disease Control and Prevention. 2021. *Current Cigarette Smoking Among Adults in the United States* (https://www.cdc.gov/tobacco/data_statistics/fact_sheets/adult_data/cig_smoking/index.htm)

Centers for Disease Control and Prevention. 2021. *Disability and Health Related Conditions* (https://www.cdc.gov/ncbddd/disabilityandhealth/relatedconditions.html).

Centers for Disease Control and Prevention. 2021. *Mortality in the United States, 2020* (https://www.cdc.gov/nchs/products/databriefs/db427.htm).

Centers for Medicare and Medicaid Services. 2021. *COVID-19 Nursing Home Data* (https://data.cms.gov/covid-19/covid-19-nursing-home-data).

Centers for Medicare and Medicaid Services. 2021. *National Health Expenditure Data 2020* (https://www.cms.gov/Research-Statistics-Data-and-Systems/Statistics-Trends-and-Reports/NationalHealthExpendData/NationalHealthAccountsHistorical).

Chin-Mei, L., and C. Lee. 2019. Association of hearing loss with dementia. *JAMA Network Open* (https://jamanetwork.com/journals/jamanetworkopen/fullarticle/2740068).

Cicero. 1923. *On Old Age. On Friendship. On Divination.* Translated by W. A. Falconer. Loeb Classical Library 154. Cambridge, MA: Harvard University Press.

Death with Dignity National Center. 2022. *Death with Dignity in Your State* (https://deathwithdignity.org/in-your-state/).

EthnoMed. 2018. Cultural relevance in end of life care. (https://ethnomed.org/clinical/end-of-life/cultural-relevance-in-end-of-life-care).

Family Caregiver Alliance. 2019. *Caregiver Statistics: Demographics* (https://www.caregiver.org/caregiver-statistics-demographics).

Fulmer, T., and D. Volmert. 2018. Reframing aging: Growing "old at heart." *Stanford Social Innovation Review* (https://ssir.org/articles/entry/reframing_aging_growing_old_at_heart#).

Gallup Poll. 2016. *Majority in U.S. Do Not Have a Will* (http://news.gallup.com/poll/191651/majority-not.aspx).

Glazier, A. 2018. Organ donation and the principles of gift law. *Clinical Journal of American Society of Nephrology* 13(8): 1283–1284.

Gollub, J., et al. 2019. Association of subclinical hearing loss with cognitive performance. *JAMA Otolaryngology Head Neck Surgery* (https://jamanetwork.com/journals/jamaotolaryngology/fullarticle/2755646?guestAccessKey=9854eff1-fb55-4f64-88a0-4fc1466f9475&utm_content=weekly_highlights&utm_term=112319&utm_source=silverchair&utm_campaign=jama_network&cmp=1&utm_medium=email).

Greer, D. M., et al. 2016. Variability of brain death policies in the United States. *JAMA Neurology* 73(2): 213–218.

Haberman, C. 2014. From private ordeal to national fight: The case of Terri Schiavo. *New York Times,* 20 April (https://www.nytimes.com/2014/04/21/us/from-private-ordeal-to-national-fight-the-case-of-terri-schiavo.html).

Harvard Men's Health Watch. 2019. *Don't Buy Into Brain Health Supplements.* Harvard Health Publishing (https://www.health.harvard.edu/mind-and-mood/dont-buy-into-brain-health-supplements).

Hellmuth, J., G. D. Rabinovici, and B. L. Miller. 2019. The rise of pseudomedicine for dementia and brain health. *Journal of the American Medical Association* 321(6): 543–544.

Horovitz, B. 2020. 5 million student caregivers need more resources and flexibility from school. *AARP* (https://www.aarp.org/caregiving/life-balance/info-2020/student-caregivers-need-support.html).

Kaiser Family Foundation. 2019. *An Overview of Medicare* (https://www.kff.org/medicare/issue-brief/an-overview-of-medicare/).

Kolata, G. 2019. More Americans are dying at home than in hospitals. *New York Times,* 11 December (https://www.nytimes.com/2019/12/11/health/death-hospitals-home.html).

Kristensen, P., Weisaeth, L., Heir, T. 2012. Bereavement and mental health after sudden and violent losses: A review. *Psychiatry* 75(1): 76–97.

Lewiecki, E. 2021. Osteoporotic fracture risk assessment. *Up to Date* (https://www.uptodate.com/contents/osteoporotic-fracture-risk-assessment?sectionName=Fracture%20risk%20assessment%20tool&search=osteoporosis%20screening%20guidelines&topicRef=2046&anchor=H4&source=see_link#H4).

Lewy Body Dementia Association. 2022. *What Is LBD?* (https://www.lbda.org/what-is-lbd/).

Ma, Y. et al. 2021. 24-hour urinary sodium and potassium excretion and cardiovascular risk. *New England Journal of Medicine* (https://www.nejm.org/doi/full/10.1056/NEJMoa2109794).

Mayo Clinic. 2018. *Living Wills and Advance Directives for Medical Decisions* (http://www.mayoclinic.org/healthy-lifestyle/consumer-health/in-depth/living-wills/art-20046303?pg51).

National Cancer Institute. 2020. *Grief, Bereavement, and Coping with Loss* (https://www.cancer.gov/about-cancer/advanced-cancer/caregivers/planning/bereavement-hp-pdq/#section/_149).

National Council on Aging. 2021. *Get the Facts on Elder Abuse* (https://www.ncoa.org/article/get-the-facts-on-elder-abuse).

National Council on Aging. 2021. *Get the Facts on Falls Prevention* (https://www.ncoa.org/article/get-the-facts-on-falls-prevention).

National Council on Aging. 2021. *Get the Facts on Healthy Aging* (https://www.ncoa.org/article/get-the-facts-on-healthy-aging).

National Council on Aging. 2021. *Top 10 Financial Scams Targeting Seniors* (https://www.ncoa.org/article/top-10-financial-scams-targeting-seniors0).

National Eye Institute. 2021. *Age-Related Macular Degeneration* (https://www.nei.nih.gov/learn-about-eye-health/eye-conditions-and-diseases/age-related-macular-degeneration).

National Eye Institute. 2021. *Diabetic Retinopathy* (https://www.nei.nih.gov/learn-about-eye-health/eye-conditions-and-diseases/diabetic-retinopathy).

National Funeral Directors Association. 2020. *Statistics* (https://www.nfda.org/news/statistics).

National Hospice and Palliative Care Organization. 2020. *History of Hospice Care* (https://www.nhpco.org/hospice-care-overview/history-of-hospice/).

National Institute on Aging. 2019. *Long Term Care: Residential Facilities, Assisted Living, and Nursing Homes* (https://www.nia.nih.gov/health/residential-facilities-assisted-living-and-nursing-homes).

National Institute on Aging. 2021. *Exercise & Physical Activity:* Getting Fit for Life (https://www.nia.nih.gov/health/exercise-and-physical-activity-getting-fit-life).

National Poll on Healthy Aging. 2019. *Thinking About Brain Health.* University of Michigan. (https://www.healthyagingpoll.org/report/thinking-about-brain-health).

NIH Osteoporosis and Related Bone Diseases National Resource Center. 2019. *Osteoporosis Overview* (https://www.bones.nih.gov/health-info/bone/osteoporosis/overview).

Oregon Death with Dignity Act. 2021. *Oregon Death with Dignity Act: 2020 Data Summary* (https://www.oregon.gov/oha/PH/PROVIDERPARTNERRESOURCES/EVALUATIONRESEARCH/DEATHWITHDIGNITYACT/Documents/year23.pdf).

Parkes, C., P. Laungani, and W. Young (Eds.). 2015. *Death and Bereavement across Cultures,* 2nd ed. New York: Routledge.

Partnership to Fight Chronic Disease. 2019. *What Is the Impact of Chronic Disease on America?* (http://www.fightchronicdisease.org/sites/default/files/pfcd_blocks/PFCD_US.FactSheet_FINAL1%20(2).pdf).

Press, D. 2021. Treatment of Alzheimer disease. *Up to Date* (https://www.uptodate.com/contents/treatment-of-alzheimer-disease?sectionName=ADUCANUMAB&search=alzheimer%27s%20diagnosis&topicRef=5071&anchor=H2549013834&source=see_link#H2549013834).

Rauch, J. 2019. *The Happiness Curve: Why Life Gets Better After 50.* London: Picador Publishing/Macmillan Publishers.

Rico-Uribe, L. et al. 2018. Association of loneliness with all-cause mortality: A meta-analysis. *PLoS One* (https://www.ncbi.nlm.nih.gov/pmc/articles/PMC5754055/).

Russell, J. A., et al. 2019. Brain death, the determination of brain death, and member guidance for brain death accommodation requests: AAN position statement. *Neurology* 92: 1–5.

Sacks, O. 2015. *Gratitude.* Canada: Knopf.

Schwandt, H., et al. 2022. Changes in the relationship between income and life expectancy before and during the COVID-19 pandemic, California, 2015–2021. *JAMA* 328(4): 360–366.

Slade, K., et al. 2020. The effects of age-related hearing loss on the brain and cognitive function. *Trends in Neurosciences* (https://www.cell.com/trends/neurosciences/fulltext/S0166-2236(20)30169-7).

Social Security Administration. 2021. *Fast Facts & Figures About Social Security, 2021* (https://www.ssa.gov/policy/docs/chartbooks/fast_facts/index.html).

Tufts Now. 2022. *Muscle Loss in Older Adults and What to Do About It* (https://now.tufts.edu/articles/muscle-loss-older-adults-and-what-do-about-it).

Tyrovolas, S, et al. 2019. Skeletal muscle mass in relation to 10 year cardiovascular disease incidence among middle aged and older adults: The ATTICA study. *Journal of Epidemiology and Community Health.* Published online 11 November (https://jech.bmj.com/content/early/2019/10/16/jech-2019-212268.full).

United Nations Department of Economic and Social Affairs. 2020. *World Population Ageing 2020 Highlights* (https://www.un.org/development/desa/pd/sites/www.un.org.development.desa.pd/files/files/documents/2020/Sep/un_pop_2020_pf_ageing_10_key_messages.pdf).

United States Census Bureau. 2021. *Income and Poverty in the United States: 2020* (https://www.census.gov/library/publications/2021/demo/p60-273.html).

United States Census Bureau. 2021. *Quarterly Residential Vacancies and Homeownership, Third Quarter 2021* (https://www.census.gov/housing/hvs/files/currenthvspress.pdf).

U.S. Department of Health and Human Services. 2018. *Physical Activity Guidelines for Americans,* 2nd ed. (https://health.gov/paguidelines/second-edition/pdf/Physical_Activity_Guidelines_2nd_edition.pdf).

U.S. Department of Health and Human Services. 2020. *Organ Donation Statistics* (https://www.organdonor.gov/statistics-stories/statistics.html).

Wilson, R., et al. 2021. Cognitive activity and onset age of incident Alzheimer disease dementia. *Neurology* (https://pubmed.ncbi.nlm.nih.gov/34261788/).

Zhu, X., et al. 2021. Inflammation, epigenetics, and metabolism converge to cell senescence and ageing: The regulation and intervention. *Nature* (https://www.nature.com/articles/s41392-021-00646-9#Abs1).

**Design Elements:** Assess Yourself icon: Aleksey Boldin/Alamy Stock Photo; Diversity Matters icon: Rawpixel Ltd/Getty Images; Wellness on Campus icon: Radius Images/Alamy Stock Photo; Take Charge icon: VisualCommunications/Getty Images; Critical Consumer icon: pagadesign/Getty Images.

# INDEX

Note: Page references followed by b indicate boxes; f for figures; t for tables. Boldface numbers indicate pages on which key terms are defined.

## A


ABCDE test, 338f
Abiotic processes, 390
Abortion, 160
  defined, **162**
  first-trimester
    aspiration, 163
    medical *vs.* aspiration abortion, 163
  induced, **162**
  personal considerations, 162
  politization of, 165
  postabortion considerations, 164
  public opinion, 165f
  second-trimester, 164
  spontaneous, 138, **162**
  United States
    in 2017, 161f
    fetal/maternal indicators, 162
    personal and social indicators, 162
    since 19th century, 161
Absorption of alcohol, 193
Abstinence, **158**
Academic resilience, 27
Academic stress, 31
Acamprosate, 205
Acceptable Macronutrient Distribution Ranges, 226
Acceptance, 43, 88
Accidents. *See also* Injuries
  due to sleepiness, 74–75
  in home, 425–28
  motor vehicle, 428–31
  workplace, 433
Acculturation, 51b
Acetaldehyde, 194b
Acetaldehyde dehydrogenase, 194b
Acetate, 194b
Acquaintance rape, 440
Acquired immunodeficiency syndrome, **361**. *See also* HIV/AIDS
Active euthanasia, **463**
Active labor, **140**
Acupuncture, 404, **411**
Acute stress, **29**. *See also* Stress
Acute stress disorder, **53**
Adaptive immune system, 345
Adaptive immunity, **347**
Added sugars, 228–29
Addiction
  behavioral
    compulsive buying/shopping, 173
    compulsive exercising, 172
    gambling disorder, 172
    gaming, 172
    internet, 173
    sex and pornography addiction, 172–73
    work addiction, 172
  defined, **170**
  development of, 172
  diagnosing, 171
  drug effects, 171
  impaired control, 171
  nicotine, 206–8
  nonmedical drug, use among Americans, 170t
  psychoactive drugs, 174t
  psychological/physical dependence, 171
  risky use, 171
  social problems, 171
Addictive behaviors, **170**
Additives, 209–10
  in food, 250
Addyi (flibanserin), 123
Adenosine, **71**
Adequate Intake (AI), 235
Adipose tissue, 284, **286**
Adolescent sexuality, 125
Adrenal glands, **114**
Adult sexuality, 125
Advance directive, **460**
Advertising, alcohol, 204b
Aerobic exercise
  aging and, 451b
  body composition, 286
  high-intensity interval training, 267b
Affirmations, 37
Affordable Care Act (ACA), 7–8
  choosing plans, 418
  defined, **418**
  major provisions, 418
Africa, HIV/AIDS in, 362b
African Americans. *See also* Black people
  cancer risk, 328b
  cardiovascular disease risk, 323b
  Covid-19, 10b
  diabetes, 291
  health disparities, 9
  vaccines, 348b
Age
  cancer risk, 328b
  cardiovascular disease risk and, 322
  and distracted driving, 428
  fatal injuries and, 426t
  sleep and, 72
Age-related macular degeneration (AMD), **453**
Aggression, 197. *See also* Violence
Aggressive driving, 428
Agility, 263
Aging
  associated changes, 452–55
  attitude toward, 449
  challenges during, 450
  defined, **448**
  dietary challenges, 243
  life-enhancing measures and, 449–52
  life expectancy and, 455–57
  perspectives on, 448–52
  policies and attitudes toward, 457
  sexuality, 116–17
Aging male syndrome, 117
Agoraphobia, **53**
Airbags, 430
Air pollution, 12, 384–87
  prevention of, 387
Air quality, 384–87
Air Quality Index, **384**
Al-Anon, 204
Alarm stage (GAS), 28, 28f
Alaska Natives
  diabetes, 291
  health disparities, 9
Alateen, 204
Alcohol consumption
  aggression and, 197
  among college students, 370b
  body and, 192–95
  cancer risk and, 328
  cardiovascular disease risk and, 322
  drinking and driving, 197–99
  driving and, 430
  emergency, 196b
  excessive use of, 201–6
  hangover, 196
  health benefits of, 201
  higher concentrations of, 196
  immediate effects, 195–97
  injuries and violence, 197
  long-term effects of, 199–200, 199f
  low concentrations of, 196
  other drugs, 197
  pedestrian injuries and, 431
  pregnancy and, 200–1
  premenstrual symptoms, 116
  prenatal care, 135–37
  problems, 206
  sex and ethnic differences, 205–6, 205t
  sexual decision making and, 197
  sexual response, 122
  for stress management, 38–39
  violence and, 435
Alcohol, defined, **192**
Alcoholic beverages, 192–93
Alcoholic energy drinks, 198b
Alcoholics Anonymous (AA), 186, 204
Alcohol misuse, **201**
  immediate and long-term effects of, 199f
Alcohol poisoning, 196
Alcohol-related neurodevelopmental disorder, **200**
Alcohol use disorder, **201**
  causes of, 203–4
  health effects, 202
  mild to severe, 201–2
  patterns and prevalence, 202
  and sleep, 78b
  social and psychological effects, 202
  treatment, 204–5
Allergens, **349**
Allergies
  climate change and, 349
  dealing with, 349–50
  defined, **349**
  response, 349
Allostatic load
  defined, **29**
  stress response and, 29
Alternative fuels, 383–84

Alternative medicine, **402**
Alzheimer's disease (AD), 8, **454-**55
Ambien (zolpidem), 179
Amenorrhea, **293**
American Academy of Pediatrics (AAP), 348, 392b
American Cancer Society (ACS), 326
American College of Sports Medicine, 270b
American Heart Association (AHA), 227-28
  on CVD risk factors, 317
American Indians. *See* Native Americans
American Psychiatric Association, 55
American Public Health Association, 443b, 468b
Amino acids, **225**
Ammonia in tobacco products, 210
Amniocentesis, **134**
Amniotic sac, **133**
Amphetamines, 39, 180
Anabolic steroids, **273**
Anal intercourse, 121
Anaphylaxis, 251, **349**
Androgens, **110**
Androgyny, **123**
Android pattern, 290
Andropause, 117
Anemia, **233**
Anesthetics, defined, **179**
Aneurysms, **315**
Anger, 321
  cardiovascular disease risk and, 325
  dealing with, 49-50
  explosive, 49
  managing, 49-50
  in other people, 50
Angina pectoris, **211, 310**
Angiograms, **312**
Annual percentage rate, 4b
Anorexia nervosa, **294**
  characteristics of, 294
  health risks of, 294
Antabuse, 194b
Anterograde amnesia, 179
Antibiotics, **357**
Antibodies, **345**
Antidepressants, 55, 58
Antigens, **345**
Antimanic drugs, 55
Antioxidants, **230**
Antipsychotic medications, 55
Antiretrovirals, 363b
Antivirals, 359
Anxiety
  cardiovascular disease risk and, 322
  defined, **52**
  exercise effects, 262
  panic disorder and, 52-53
  sleep disrupters, 77
  social media use and, 49
  in social situations, 63b
Anxiety disorders
  generalized anxiety disorder, 53
  obsessive-compulsive disorder, 53
  panic disorder, 52-53
  posttraumatic stress disorder, 53
  prevalence of, 52t
  social anxiety disorder, 52
  specific phobia, 52
  treatment of, 53
Anxious/avoidant attachment, 87
AOD use, 174b
Aorta, **307**
Aortic aneurysm, tobacco's effects, 211
Apgar score, **141**
*APOE* ε4, 455
Appreciation, 103
Apps, 300b
Arrhythmias, **310-**11
Arteries, coronary, **308**
Arthritis, **453**
Artificial (intrauterine) insemination, **130**
Asbestosis, **391**
Asian Americans
  alcohol misuse rates, 206
  diabetes, 291
  health disparities, 9
Aspiration abortion (D&C), **163**
Aspirin, 311, 401
Assault, 435. *See also* Sexual assault
Assault rifle bans, 443b, 468b
Assertiveness, **49**
Assisted reproductive technology (ART), **129**
Asthma, **349,** 392b
Asymptomatic phase, HIV, **363**
Atherosclerosis, 29, 310f
  causes of, 309
  defined, **309**
  tobacco use and, **210**
Athletes' dietary needs, 229, 243
Athletic performance, sleep habits and, 73
Attachment
  anxious/avoidant, 87
  defined, **87**
Attention-deficit/hyperactivity disorder (ADHD), **53-**54
Attentive listening, 93
Attunement, 92
Atypical sexual development, 117-18
Auditory hallucinations, 56
Authenticity, 43
Authoritarian parents, 102
Authoritative parents, 102
Auto accidents, 74-75
Automated external defibrillators, 313b
Automobile exhaust, 382
Autonomic nervous system, **24**
  functions of, 24
  parasympathetic division, 24
  physical reactions to stressors, 24
  return to homeostasis, 25
  sympathetic division, 24
Autonomy, **43**
Avoidant restrictive food intake disorder (ARFID), 296

## B

Background checks, 443b, 468b
Backlit digital book, 70b
Back pain, 417
Bacteria. *See also* Infectious diseases; Sexually transmitted infections
  infections, 357
  meningitis, 352-53
  pneumonia, 352
  streptococcal infections, 353-56
  tuberculosis, 356
Bacterial vaginosis, **373**
Bacterium, **352**
Balance, 264
Balloon angioplasty, **312,** 314f
Barbiturates, **178**
Barefoot shoes, 275b
Barrier methods, **146**
Basal cell carcinoma, **336**
Bath salts, 183
B cells, **345**
Bedtime goal, 79b
Beer, 193
Behavioral addiction
  compulsive buying/shopping, 173
  compulsive exercising, 172
  gambling disorder, 172
  gaming, 172
  internet, 173
  sex and pornography addiction, 172-73
  work addiction, 172
Behavioral model, 58-59
Behavior change. *See also* Wellness
  boosting self-efficacy, 14
  defined, **13**
  enhancing readiness to, 14-16
  motivation for, 13-14
  overcoming barriers to, 14
  personalized plan, creation of, 17-19, 17f
  relapse, dealing with, 16-17
  safer sex, 375b
  smoking cessation, 217
  social anxiety, 63b
  target behavior in, **13**
Benadryl, 197
Benign tumors, **326**
Benzedrine, 180
Benzodiazepines, **178**
Bereavement, **466**
Beverages, healthy eating patterns, 236
Biculturalism, 51b
Bicycles, 431
Billings method, 158
Binary, **108**
Binge drinking
  among college students, 203b
  defined, **197**
  overall costs, 202
Binge eating, weight management, **286**
Binge-eating disorder, **295**
Bioaccumulation, 391
Biodegradable, **390**
Biodegradation, 390t
Biodiesel, 383
Bioelectrical impedance analysis (BIA), 289
Biofeedback, 38
Biofuels, as renewable energy source, 383
Biological aging, 448
Biologically based therapies, 414
Biological model, 58
Biological sex, **109**
Biomagnification, **391**
Biomass, as renewable energy source, 383
Biomedicine. *See also* Conventional medicine
Biopsies, **326**
Biopsychosocial model, 59
Biotic processes, 390
Biotin, 231t
Bipolar disorder
  bipolar I disorder, 55
  bipolar II disorder, 55
  defined, **55**
Bipolar I disorder, 55
Bipolar II disorder, 55
Birth control. *See also* Contraception
  defined, **145**
  pills, 152
Bisphenol A, 393b
Black Americans
  alcohol misuse rates, 205-6
  vaccines, 348b
Black people, 10b. *See also* African American
Blastocyst, **132**
Blended family, 103
Blood alcohol concentration
  body weight and, 194, 195f
  defined, **194**
  dose-response relationship, 199f
  impact on driving, 430
  intoxication, 195f
  percentage of body fat, 194
  sex, 194

Blood pressure
cardiovascular disease risk and, 317, 325
classification, 317t
defined, **307**
health risks, 317–18
hypertension, 318
treatment, 318–19
Blood tests, 135
Body awareness techniques, 38
tai chi, 38
yoga, 38
Body-based practices, 414–16
manipulative, 414–16
Body composition. *See also* Weight management
adipose tissue, 286
bioelectrical impedance analysis (BIA), 289
defined, **263**
essential fat, 286
exercise, 260, 263
healthy, 290f
percent body fat, 287
scanning procedures, 289
skinfold measurement, 289
visceral fat, 287
Body dysmorphic disorder (BDD), 293
Body fat
distribution, 290
effects on BAC, 194
excessively low, 292–93
intake goals, 226t
wellness and, 290–93
Body image, **293**
problems, 293
Body mass index (BMI), **320**
biased, 288b
calculation, 288–89
classification and disease risk, 287t
defined, **288**
Body weight. *See* Weight management
Bones, female athlete triad effects, **293**
*Bordetella pertussis,* 357
*Borrelia burgdorferi,* 356
BPA, 393b
Brain, injuries, 432b
Brain damage, 200
Brain death, **458**
Braxton Hicks contractions, **132**
*BRCA1,* 327
*BRCA2,* 327
Breast awareness, 334
Breast cancer
detection and treatment, 331t
early detection, 334
prevention, 334
risk factors, 333–34
treatment, 334
Breastfeeding, 142
dietary challenges, 243
Breasts, 112
Breast self-exams, 334
Breathing, 37b
Broad-spectrum sunscreens, 337b
Brown fat, 134
Bulimia nervosa, **294**
characteristics of, 295
health risks of, 295
Burial, 463
Burnout, 31

## C

CA-125 blood test, 331t
Caffeinated alcoholic beverages, 198b
Caffeine
energy "shots,", 181
and homeostatic sleep drive, 71
prenatal care, 136
psychoactive drug, 181
as sleep disrupter, 77, 77t
Calcium, 232t, 233b
Calendar methods, 158
Calories, 225
in alcoholic beverages, 193
in food labels, 245b, 246
on menus and vending machines, 246
Cancer, 306
causes of, 327–30
defined, **326**
detection, diagnosis, and treatment, 330–32
exercise effects on risk, 261
female reproductive tract, 335–36
impact of alcohol misuse, 200
incidence of, 326–27
stages of, 326
types of, 332–39
*Candida albicans,* 259
Cannabis, products, 181–82
Capacity for intimacy, 43
Capillaries, **308**
Carbohydrates
complex, 228
defined, **228**
intake goals, 226t
recommended intake, 229
simple, 228
Carbon dioxide, 383
Carbon monoxide
air quality, 384
in cigarette smoke, 214
in hookah smoke, 214
in indoor air, 387
poisoning by, 425
Carcinogens, **209,** 329–30
Carcinomas, **332**
Cardiac arrest, 310. *See also* Heart attacks
symptoms of, 312b
warning signs, 312b
Cardiac arrhythmias, 74
Cardiac myopathy, **200**
Cardiopulmonary resuscitation (CPR), **311,** 444, 458
Cardiorespiratory endurance, **262–**63
Cardiorespiratory endurance exercise
frequency, 269
intensity, 269–70
progression, 271
time (duration), 271
type, 271
volume of activity, 271
warm-up and cool-down, 271
Cardiorespiratory endurance training, **262**
Cardiorespiratory functioning, exercise and, 259, 260f
Cardiorespiratory system, 307
Cardiovascular disease
defined, **306**
diabetes, 291
digital health approach to, 300b, 318b
exercise effects, 261
major forms of, 309–17
preventing, 324–25
risk factors for, 317–24
sleep and, 74
stress and, 29–30
tobacco use and, 210–11
Cardiovascular system
alcohol's effects, 200
anatomy, 306–8, 307f
defined, **306**
Caregiving, for older adults, 457
Carotenoids, **328, 329**
Carpal tunnel syndrome, **433,** 434b
Caskets, 464b
Cataplexy, 82
Cataracts, **453**
Caya, 156
CD4 T cells, **361**
Cell-free DNA, **134**
Cell health, 259–60
Cell phones, 395, 429b
Cellular death, **459**
Cemeteries, 464b
Center for Collegiate Mental Health, 57b
Centers for Disease Control and Prevention (CDC), 7
diabetes, 74
fetal alcohol syndrome (FAS), 200
sexually transmitted infections, 361
vaccines, 347
violent death reporting system, 443b, 468b
weight loss, 299
Central nervous system (CNS), **178**
depressants
club drugs, 179
effects, 179
types, 178–79
from use to misuse, 179
stimulants
amphetamines, 180
caffeine, 181
cocaine, 179–80
stimulant ADHD medications, 181
Cerebral cortex, **210**
Cerebrovascular accident. *See* Stroke
Cervical cap, **157**
Cervix, cancer of, 331t
Cesarean section, **141**
Chadwick's sign, 131
Chain of infection, 350–51
Chancres, **373**
Chantix, 217–18
Chemical barriers, 344–45
Chemical pollution
asbestos, 391
lead, 391
mercury, 392–93
pesticides, 391–92
prevention, 394
Chemotherapy, **330,** 332
Chest pain, 312b
Chickenpox, 358
Childbirth
choices in, 139
delivery, 139–41
labor, 139–41
postpartum period, 141–43
Children
anxious/avoidant attachment, 87
cope with loss, 467
drug use, 184
lead exposure, 392b
separation and divorce, 101
sexual abuse, 442
sexual behaviors, 125
tobacco's effects, 215
violence, 439
weight management, 283
Child safety seats, 430
Chiropractic, **414**
Chlamydia
defined, **367**
diagnosis and treatment, 368
*Chlamydia pneumoniae,* 322, 352
*Chlamydia trachomatis,* 367
Chlorofluorocarbons, 385t, **386**

Choking accidents, 427
Cholesterol, **227,** 261
  blood, 319–20
  cardiovascular disease risk and, 325
  controlling, 320
  good *vs.* bad, 319
  treatment of, 319t
Chorionic villi, 133
Chorionic villus sampling (CVS), **134**
Chronic bronchitis, **212**
Chronic diseases, defined, **6**
Chronic obstructive pulmonary disease, 212
Chronic stress
  and allostatic load, 29
  defined, **29**
Chronic traumatic encephalopathy, 432b
Cigarettes. *See also* Tobacco use
  lung cancer and, 211–12
  "reduced harm,", 210
  for stress management, 38
Cigarette smoke, 192
Cigarette tar, **209**
Cigars, 213–14
Circadian clock, 69f
Circadian rhythm, 79b
  changes in, 72
  defined, **68**
  disruptions, 70–71
  light, 68–69, 69f
  variation, 68
Circumcision, 362b
Cirrhosis, **200**
Cisgender, **109**
Climate change, 385
  allergies and, 349
  human health, 386f
Clinical death, **458**
Clitoris, **111**
*Clostridium difficile,* 357
*Clostridium tetani,* 357
Clothing, 275b
  for sun protection, 337b
Club drugs, 179
Cluster headaches, 30
Cocaine
  effects of, 179–80
  nasal mucosa/injected intravenously, 180
  uses during pregnancy, 180
Cocarcinogens, **209**
Codeine, 197
Cognitive appraisal, of potential stressor, 26
Cognitive-behavioral therapies (CBTs), 59
Cognitive distortion, **46,** 47b
Cognitive impairment, 454–**55**
Cognitive model, 59
Cognitive therapy, for psychological disorders, 59
Cohabitation, 99f
Coitus, **111**
*Coitus interruptus,* 158
Colborn, Theo, 393b
Cold-related injuries, 432
Cold sores, 358
Collectivist culture, 51b
College students
  alcohol use, 203b
  benefits to, 8
  cell phone use while driving, 429b
  contraception use, 159b
  dietary challenges, 243
  drug use/misuse, 174b
  pregnancy, 159b
  and risk for heart attacks, 311b
  sleep and, 72
  stalking, 438
  STI risk among, 370b
  wellness for, 11b
Colon cancer
  detection and treatment, 333
  risk factors, 333
Colonoscopies, 331t
Colorectal cancer, detection and treatment, 331t
Colostrum, **142**
Combination HIV antigen/antibody test, **365**
Combined hormonal pill, 152
Commitment, in family, 103
Common cold, 357–58
Communicating, about sexuality, 127b
Communication
  digital, 92–93
  effective, guidelines for, 94b
  in families, 103
  and gender role, 87
  honest, 49–50, 127
  in intimate relationships, 92–95
  nonverbal, 92
  open, 127
  skills, 93
  for stress management, 34
Compact fluorescent lightbulbs, 388b
Companionship, 88
Competitiveness, 91
Complementary and alternative medicine (CAM), **402**
  U.S. adults, 402t
Complementary medicine, **402**
Complete proteins, 225–26
Complex carbohydrates, 228
Compostable, **390**
Compulsions, **53**
Compulsive buying/shopping, 173
Compulsive exercising, 172
Computed tomography (CT), 289, **315**
Conception, **145**
  fertilization, 128–29
  process of, 128
  twins, 129
Concussions, 432b
Condoms
  college students' use, 159b, 370b
  discussing with partners, 375b
  female, 155
  with HIV/AIDS risk, 362b–363b
  male, 154–55
Conflict, in intimate relationships, 93–95
Conflict resolution, strategies for, 93–95
Congenital adrenal hyperplasia (CAH), 117
Congenital heart defects, **316**
Congenital malformation, **136**
Congestive heart failure, **316**
Consciousness, altered states of, **182**
Contact sports injuries, 432b
Contagion, 350
Contemplation, 15–16
Continuous positive airway pressure (CPAP) machine, 82
Contraception
  after pregnancy, 159–60
  among college students, 159b
  barrier methods, **146**
  behavioral methods of
    abstinence, 158
    fertility awareness, 158
    withdrawal, 158
  defined, **145**
  female condom, 155
  injectables, 153–54
  intrauterine device methods, **146**
  male condom, 154f
  types of, 146–47
  unintended pregnancies, 146f
Contraception, permanent
  female sterilization, 149–50
  male sterilization, 149
  vasectomy, 149
Contraceptive
  choosing, 147
  defined, **145**
Contraceptive effectiveness, 146f
Contraceptive failure rate, **147**
Contraceptive implants
  advantages, 151
  disadvantages, 151
  effectiveness, 151
  placement of, 151f
Contraceptive methods
  barriers to use, 148b
  convenience/comfort level, 148
  ease and cost, 148
  health risks, 148
  potential noncontraceptive benefits, 147
  relationship, 148
  religious/philosophical beliefs, 149
  STI risk, 148
Contraceptive sponge, **157**
Control, stress and, 36
Conventional medicine
  alternative therapies, 417
  back pain, 417
  CAM therapies, 417
  characteristics, 403
  defined, **402**
  evaluating complementary, 417
  eye care
    physician assistants (PAs), 407
    registered nurses (RNs), 406
  fibromyalgia, 416–17
  pharmaceuticals and placebo effect, 404
  premises and assumptions, 403–4
  premises and assumptions of, 403–4
  providers of, 406
    dentists, 406
    doctors of osteopathic medicine (DO), 406
    medical doctors, 406
    nurses, 406–7
    optometrists, 406
    physician assistants (PAs), 407
    psychologists, 406
  tai chi, 416–17
Cooking fires, 427
Coordination, 264
Copayment, **419**
Coping strategies, 33b
  alcohol and drugs, 38–39
  dietary patterns, 298
  with divorce, 101
  for loss of loved one, 465
  with terminal illness, 465
  tobacco use, 38
  unhealthy eating habits, 39
Copper T-380A, 150f
Core training exercises, 272
Coronary arteries, **308**
Coronary artery disease, 309–13
Coronary artery disease (CAD), 261
Coronary bypass surgery, **313**
Coronary heart disease, **210, 309**
Coronavirus (Covid-19) pandemic, 8
  dating, 96b
  symptoms, 351
  vaccines, 348b, 351
Corpora cavernosa, 113
Corpus spongiosum, 113
Cortisol, **24**
Cosmetic concerns of smoking, 212–13
Cottage cheese, 241
Coughing, sleep disruption due to, 77
Counterproductive strategy, 63b




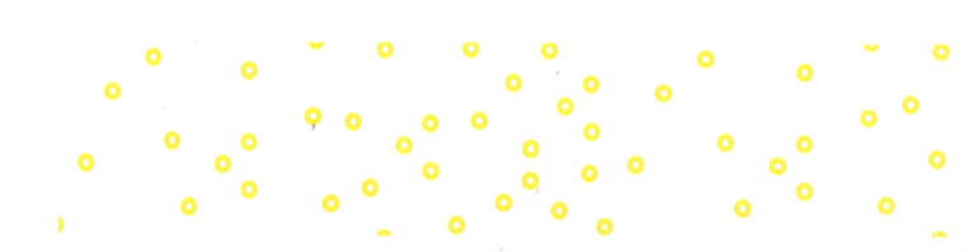

Covid-19, health inequality and, 10b. *See also* Coronavirus
Cowper's glands, **113**
Cranberry, 415t
C-reactive protein (CRP), 321
Creativity, 43
Credit cards, 4b
Cremation, 463
Cruciferous vegetables, **234**
Cultural wellness, 2, 2f
Culture, 109
  and psychological health, 51b
Cunnilingus, **120**
Cyberstalking, 438-**39**
Cytomegalovirus (CMV), 358

## D

Daily hassles, 31
Daily Values, **235,** 245b
Dairy products, 241
Damage-related aging, 449
DASH Eating Plan, 242, 258f
Date rape
  defined, **440**
  drugs, 441
  factors, 441
Dating, 95
Daytime sleepiness, 78
DDT, 391
Death and dying
  coping with, 465
  defined, 458-59
  mourning, 466
  planning for, 460-64
  understanding of, 459
Death in the United States, causes of, 6t, 7t
Deaths
  alcohol-related, 200
  climate change impacts, 386
  from injury, 426t
Decibel, **395**
Deductible, **419**
Deep sleep, 67
Deepwater Horizon spill, 383
Defense mechanisms, 47-**48,** 48t
Defibrillation, 313b
Delirium tremens, **202**
Delusions, 56
Dementia, **454**
  sleep problems and, 73
Dendritic cells, 345
Dentist, **406**
Denying death, 459-60
Department of Energy (U.S.), 383
Dependence, **171**. *See also* Addiction
Depersonalization, **181**
Depo-Provera injection, 153-54
Depressants, sedative-hypnotic, **178**
Depression
  aging and, 455
  cardiovascular disease risk and, 321-22
  defined, **54**
  exercise effects, 262
  sleep and, 72-73
  social media use and, 49
  symptoms, 54
DES, 393b
Dexedrine, 180
Diabetes
  risk factors, 291
  sleep apnea and, 74
  types of, 291
  warning signs, 291
Diabetes mellitus, 292f
  cardiovascular disease risk and, 321
  causes, 228
  defined, **291**
  race/ethnicity and, 323b
Diabetic retinopathy, **453**
*Día de los Muertos,* 459-60
*Diagnostic and Statistical Manual of Mental Disorders,* 5th edition, 295
Diagnostic process, 408-9
Dialectical behavior therapy (DBT), 60
Diaphragm, **156,** 156f
Diary writing, 36
Diastole, **307**
Dickey Amendment, 443b, 468b
Dietary Approaches to Stop Hypertension, 324
Dietary fiber, **229**
*Dietary Guidelines for Americans,* **235,** 235-39
Dietary patterns. *See also* Weight management
  cancer risk and, 328b
  challenges for, 243
  eating habits, 296-98
  emotions and coping strategies, 298
  exercise, 298
  food choices, quality of, 297-98
  physical activity, 298
  portion sizes, 297
  total calories, 296-97
Dietary Reference Intakes, **234,** 235
Dietary Supplement Health and Education Act (1994), 248b
Dietary supplements
  labels, 248b
  nutrition and, 246-47
Differentiation, 132
Digestion, **224**
Digestive system, 200, 225f
Digital communication, 92-93
Digital devices, 70b
Digital sleep trackers, 70b
Digital social networks, 32
Dilation and evacuation (D&E), **164**
Direct transmission, 350
Disability, sexuality in, 125
Discarded technology, 390
Discrimination, 323b
Distracted driving, 428
Distress, **28**
Disulfiram, 194b, 204
Diverse populations. *See* Ethnicity/race; Health disparities
Divorce, 101
DNA, 327
Doctor of osteopathic medicine, **406**
Dose-response function, 198
Double effect, **463**
Driving, alcohol use and, 197-99
Drug addiction, treatment
  family and friends cope, 187
  groups/peer counseling, 186
  harm reduction strategies, 186-87
  medication-assisted treatment, 185-86
  treatment centers, 186
Drug problem, 186b
Drugs, **169**. *See also* Medications
Drug therapy, for psychological disorders, 58
Drug use/misuse
  allure of drugs, 173
  avoiding
    alcohol, 136
    caffeine, 136
    drugs, 136
    infections, 136
    tobacco, 136
  cardiovascular disease risk and, 322
  college students, uses, 174b
  effects of
    brain chemistry, changes, 175-76
    physical factors, 176
    psychological factors, 176
    social factors, 176
  factors associated
    adolescents, 174
    dysfunctional family, 174
    male, 173-74
    poor, 174
    thrill-seeker, 174
    trouble at school, 174
    troubled childhood, 174
  inhalants, 183
  legal consequences, 175
  new psychoactive substances, 183-84
  prescription drug misuse, 183
  prevention
    drugs, 184
    families, 184
    legalizing drugs, 184
    misuse, 187-88
    society, 184
    treating drug addiction, 184-87
  race/ethnicity, 185b
  risks
    drug-related emergency department, 175t
    infection/injection drug use, 175
    intoxication, 175
    legal consequences, 175
    side effects, 175
    unexpected side effects, 175
    unknown drug constituents, 175
  for stress management, 38-39
  violence and, 435
*DSM-5,* 171
Dual-energy X-ray absorptiometry (DEXA), 289
Dual-photon absorptiometry, 289
Durable power of attorney for health care, 460
Dysmenorrhea, **115**
Dyspareunia, 122

## E

Eating disorders
  anorexia nervosa
    characteristics of, 294
    health risks of, 294
  binge-eating disorder, 295
  bulimia nervosa, 294-95
    characteristics of, 295
    health risks of, 295
  defined, **293**
  treatment, 296
Eating habits, 296-98. *See also* Dietary patterns
  unhealthy, 39
Eating patterns, **235**
Ebola virus disease (EVD), 359-60
Echinacea, 415t
E-cigarettes, 214
Economics of retirement, 452
ECT. *See* Electroconvulsive therapy (ECT)
Ectopic pregnancy, **137**-38
Education level, 3
  health disparities, 9
Education programs, STIs, 362b, 374
EEG. *See* Electroencephalogram (EEG)
Ehrlichiosis, 356
Ejaculation, **154**
Elder abuse, 439
Elective surgeries, **411**
Electric cars, 382
Electric vehicles, 384
Electrocardiogram, **268**
Electroconvulsive therapy (ECT), **55**

Electroencephalogram (EEG), **66,** 67f, 196
Electromagnetic waves, 395
Elimination, in immune response, 346
Embalming, **463**
Embolus, **314**
Embryo, **133**
Emergency contraception (EC), **159**-60
Emergency medical services (EMS) system, **444**
Emotional intelligence
  defined, **44**
  development of, 89-90
Emotional wellness, 2, 2f. *See also* Psychological health
  exercise effects, 262
Emotions, 298
  defined, **43**
Empathy, 86
Emphysema, **212**
Empirical knowledge, 403
Endemic, **351**
Endocrine-disrupting chemicals, 393b
Endocrine system, **24**
  and physical reactions to stressors, 24
End-of-life care, 461-62
Endometriosis, 129
Endometrium, **114**
Endoscopy, **409**
Endurance training, 263
Energy
  defined, **225**
  healthy calorie intake, 239
  nuclear, 394-95
Energy balance, **284**
Energy consumption, 382, 383f
Energy sources, 382-83
Energy therapies, **416**
Engaged life, 43-44
Environment
  carcinogens in, 329-30
  defined, **380**
  influence of, on health, 12
Environmental health
  air quality and pollution, 384-87
  chemical pollution and hazardous waste, 391-94
  energy use and, 382-84
  noise pollution, 395-96
  overview, **380**-81
  population growth and, 381-82
  radiation and, 394-95
  solid waste pollution, 389-91
  water quality and pollution, 387-89
Environmental pollution, 330
Environmental Protection Agency, 384
Environmental tobacco smoke (ETS), **214**-15, 387
Environmental wellness, 2f, 3
Eosinophils, 345
Epidemics, **351**
Epididymis, **110, 113,** 338b
Epidural injection, 141
Epinephrine, **24**
Episiotomy, **141**
Equipment for exercise, 274-76
Erectile disorder, **121**
Erikson, Erik, 44
Erogenous zones, **118**
Erotic fantasy, **120**
*Escherichia coli,* 360
Essential fat, **286**
Essential nutrients, **224**
Estate, **460**
Estradiol, 110
Estrogen, **110**
  breast cancer risk and, 328b
  cardiovascular disease risk and, 323b
  life expectancy and, 456b
Ethanol, 383
Ethnicity/race
  cancer risk and, 328b
  cardiovascular disease risk and, 322
  and Covid-19, 10b
  drinking patterns and, 205-6
  hate crimes, 436
  and health disparities, 8-9
  heart disease, 309f
  and psychological health, 51b
Ethyl alcohol, 192
Euphoria, **176**
Eustress, **28**
Evening primrose oil, 415t
E-waste, 390
Excretion of alcohol, 193-94
Exercise
  aging and, 451b
  as alternative medical approach, 415-16
  basic physical training principles, 268-69
  body composition, 260
  cardiorespiratory functioning, 259
  cardiovascular disease risk and, 324-25
  defined, **264**
  dietary patterns, 298
  disease prevention and management, 260-62
  eating and drinking for, 276
  erectile function, 122
  flexibility, 273-74
  health and fitness benefits of, 268f
  health benefits, 259-62
  immune function, 262
  injuries, 262
  for insomnia, 81
  low-back pain, 262
  medical clearance, 267-68
  metabolism and cell health, 259-60
  for muscular strength and endurance, 271-73
  physical fitness and, **262**
  premenstrual symptoms, 116
  prenatal care, 136
  resting metabolic rate, 284
  selecting activities, 269
  for stress management, 34
  wellness for life, 262
Exhaustion stage of GAS, 28, 28f
Expectations, 36
Experience, stressor and, 27
Exposure, **59**
External locus of control, 14

# F

Facebook, 92
Fallopian tube, 112
  ectopic pregnancy in, 137
Falls, 425-27, 451b
  risk for, 454
False negative, **409**
False positive, **409**
Families
  parenting styles, 101-2
  single-parent, 102-3
  stepfamilies/blended, 103
  successful, 103-4
  support of older adults, 457
  violence, 437-39
FAST acronym, 312b
Fat. *See also* Body fat
  cells, 284
  healthy eating patterns, 236
  recommended intake, 227-28
  sources of, 226-27
  types, 226-27
Fat-free mass, **263**
Fatigue, driving and, 430
Fat-soluble vitamin, 231t
Fatty acids, 227t
Fatty liver, 200
Fecal occult blood test, 331t
Federal programs for older adults, 457
Federal Trade Commission (FTC), 300
Feedback, in communication, 93
Fellatio, **120**
Female athlete triad, **293**
Female infertility, 129
Female orgasmic disorder (FOD), 121-22
Fermentation, 193
Fertility. *See also* Contraception
  defined, **147**
Fertility awareness-based method, 158
Fertilization
  defined, **128**
  egg, **128**
Fertilized egg, **128**
Fetal abnormalities, diagnosing
  invasive diagnostic tests, 134
  noninvasive screening tests, 134
  ultrasonography, 134
Fetal alcohol spectrum disorder (FASD), 201
Fetal alcohol syndrome (FAS), **136,** 200
Fetal development
  abnormalities, diagnosing, 134
  first trimester, 132-33
  second trimester, 133-34
  third trimester, 134
Feverfew, 415t
Fiber
  cancer risk and, 328
  dietary, **229**
  recommended intake, 230
  sources of, 230
  types of, 229-30
Fibromyalgia, 416-17
Fight, flight, or freeze reaction, **24**-26, 25f
Financial stress, 31
Financial wellness, 2f, 3, 4b
  retirement planning, 452
Firearms, 58
  deaths from, 427-28
  risk reduction, 443b
  violence and, 435
Fires, 427
First aid, **444**
Fish consumption, 250
Fitness. *See* Physical fitness
  managing, 276-80
Five-year survival rate, **326**
Flashbacks, **182**
Flavorings in tobacco products, 210
Flesh-eating strep, 356
Flexibility, **263**
Flint, Michigan, water contamination, 392b
Flooding, 433
Fluid intelligence, **450**
Flunitrazepam (Rohypnol), 179
Fluoridation, **387**
Fluoride, 232t, 233b
Flushing syndrome, 194b
Folate, 231t
Follicle, **114**
Food allergies, 250-**51**
Food and Drug Administration (U.S.), 248b, 366b
Food and Nutrition Board, 230
Food biotechnology, 250
Foodborne illness, 247
Food fats, 227
Food intolerances, 250-**51**
Food labels, 245-46, 245b
Food marketing and public policy, 286
Food package nutrient claims, 246t
Food perceptions and behaviors, 286

Foods. *See also* Dietary patterns
additives in, 250
antioxidants, 234
cancer risk and, 328
functional, 250
phytochemicals, 234
positive change, 238b
protein content of, 226t
Food safety, 135
Football players, 432b
Footwear, 275b
Forcing, 125
Fortified wine, 193
Fossil fuel, **384**
Foster friendships, 34
Fracking, 383
Fraternal (dizygotic) twins, **129**
Free radicals, **234**
Fruits
cancer risk and, 328-29
increasing consumption, 240
Fukushima Daiichi nuclear accident, 394
Functional fiber, **230**
Functional foods, 250
Functional health, 451b
Funeral Rule, 464b
Funerals, 463-64
Fungi, **359**

## G

GAD. *See* Generalized anxiety disorder (GAD)
Gambling disorder, 172
Gamer's thumb, 434b
Gaming addiction, 172
Gamma hydroxybutyrate (GHB), **179**
Gamma radiation, 394
Gang-related violence, 435-36
Garlic, 415t
GAS. *See* General adaptation syndrome (GAS)
Gasoline, 383
Gender
cardiovascular disease risk and, 322
defined, 8
health care visits and, 408b
in health hazards, 213
HIV/AIDS risk and, 362b
life expectancy and, 456b
sex, 109
sexual response and, 120
sleep and, 72
toxin exposure and, 392b
violence and, 435
Gender-affirming treatment, 124
*Gender and Our Brains* (Gina Rippon), 109
Gender dysphoria, 123
Genderfluid, **124**
Gender identity, 97-98
and health disparities, 9-11
Gender ideology, **109**
Gender nonconforming, 109, **123**
Gender role, 27, **87**
and communication, 87
defined, **27**
sexuality and, **109**
General adaptation syndrome (GAS)
alarm stage, 28, 28f
defined, **28**
resistance stage, 28, 28f
response to stressors, 28
stage of exhaustion, 28, 28f
Generality knowledge, 404
Generalized anxiety disorder (GAD), **53**
Generic drugs, **401**
Genes, **12, 129**
Genetically modified organisms, **250**
Genetic factors, 283-84
Genetics
cardiovascular disease risk and, 322
tobacco use, 208-9
Genital herpes, **371**-72
Genital warts, **369**
Genome, **12**
Genuineness, 86
Geographic location, and health-related disparities, 9
Geothermal, as renewable energy source, 383
Germ cells, **110**
Gerontology, **448**
Gestational carrier, 130
Gestational diabetes, 291
Gestational diabetes mellitus (GDM), **138**
GHB, **179**
Ghrelin, 285
*Giardia lamblia,* 359
Giardiasis, **359**
Gingivitis, 213
Ginkgo, 415t
Ginkgo biloba, 415t
Ginseng, 415t
Glaucoma, **453**
Global Footprint Network, 381
Global warming, 349, **385**
Glucose, **228**
Glycogen, **228**
Glyphosate, 391-92
Golfer's elbow, 434b
Gonads, **110**
Gonorrhea, **369**
Government aid, 457
Government policies, 457
Government programs for older adults, 457
Grains, 229b, 241
Green burial, 464b
Greenhouse effect, **384-**86, 385f
Greenhouse gases, **384-**86
Grief, 455
coping with, 466b
course of, 466-67
defined, **465**
Groundwater, 388
Group B streptococcus (GBS), 136
G-spot, 112
Guilt, and grief, 455
Gun violence, 443b. *See also* Firearms
Gut microbiota, 285
Gynecomastia, 116
Gynoid pattern, 290

## H

*Haemophilus influenzae,* 352
Hall, Jeffrey, 68
Hallucinogens
defined, **182, 202**
LSD (lysergic acid diethylamide), 182
MDMA (methylenedioxymethamphetamine), 182
PCP (phencyclidine), 182
Halogen incandescents, 388b
Hands-free device, 429b
Hangovers, 196
Harassment, sexual, 440b
Hardiness, 26
Hard liquor, 193
Harm reduction strategies, 186-87
Hate crimes, 436
Hatha yoga, 38
Headaches
cluster, 30
migraine, 30
stress and, 30
tension, 30
Head injuries, 432b
Health
defined, **1**
habits and, 12, 13
mental (*see* Psychological health)
and sleep, 72-75
stress and, 27-30
Health and Retirement Study, 264
Health at Every Size (HAES), 293
Health behaviors, personal, 12
Health care, access to, 12
Health care expenses, of older adults, 457
Health care proxy, **460**
Health claims, 248b, 405b
Health disparities
defined, **8**
disability, 9
geographic location, 9
income and education, 9
race and ethnicity, 8-9
sex and gender, 8
sexual orientation and gender identity, 9-11
Health fraud, avoiding, 412b
Health information, 405b
evaluation of, 15b
Health insurance, 419-20
Affordable Care Act (ACA), 7-8
Affordable Care Act provision, 420b
choosing plans, 420b
Medicare and Medicaid, 419
for obesity treatment, 5b
overview, 419-20
physician appointments, 419
students and, 8
Health issues for diverse populations, 8-11
Health maintenance organization (HMO), **419**
Health news, evaluating, 405b, 412b
Health problems, stress and
cardiovascular disease, 29-30
headaches, 30
immune function, altered, 30
psychological disorders, 30
Health promotion, 7-11
agencies for, 7
defined, **7**
health insurance options, 7-8
health issues for diverse populations, 8-11
national Healthy People initiative, 8
Health records, 409b
Health-related fitness, **262**
Health span, 6
defined, **6**
Healthy eating patterns
dietary guidelines, 236
supporting, 239
*Healthy People 2020,* 8
*Healthy People 2030,* 8
Healthy People initiative, 8
Healthy U.S.-style food patterns, 255f
Hearing loss, 453
Heart. *See also* Cardiovascular disease
anatomy, 307f
blood supply to, 309f
circulation in, 308f
healthy, 324
Heart attacks
college students at risk for, 311b
defined, **310**
responding to, 312b
symptoms, 310, 312b
warning signs, 312b
in women, 312b
Heart disease, 291. *See also* Cardiovascular disease
Heart rate, target for exercise, 270b

Heart valve disorders, 316-17
Heat-related injuries, 431
Heavy drinking, 197. *See also* Alcohol consumption; Binge drinking
Heavy metal, **389**
Hegar's sign, 131
Heimlich maneuver, **427**
*Helicobacter pylori*, 330, 357
Helmet use, 432b
Help. *See also* Social support
  friendship, 88
Hematologists, **332**
Hemorrhagic stroke, **314**-15
Hepatitis, **358, 372**
Hepatitis A virus (HAV), 358, 372
Hepatitis B virus (HBV), 358, 372
Hepatitis C virus (HCV), 358, 372
Herbal remedy, **411**
Herbicides, 391
Heroin, infection and injection drug, 175
Herpes simplex virus (HSV), 358
Herpesviruses, **358**
Heterosexual/straight, **97**
High, **170**
High-density lipoproteins (HDLs), 261, **319**
High-efficiency lighting, 388b
High-intensity interval training, 267b
High-intensity therapy, 320
Hispanic Americans
  alcohol misuse rates, 206
  diabetes risk, 291, 323b
Histamine, **349**
HIV/AIDS
  diagnosis, 365
  diagnosis and treatment, 362b
  global risks, 362b
  prevention, 362b, 367
  symptoms, 365
  transmission, 363-64, 364f
  treatment, 365-67
  vulnerable groups, 364-65
HIV antibody tests, **365,** 366b
HIV infection, **361**
HIV nucleic acid test (NAT), **365**
H1N1 influenza A virus, 351-52
Hodgkin lymphoma, 330
Holistic health care, **411**
Home Access HIV test, 366b
Home Access test kit, 366b
Home care, 461-62
Home fires, 427
Home HIV test kits, 366b
Home injuries
  choking, 427
  defined, **425**
  falls, 425-27
  firearms, 427-28
  fires, 427
  poisoning, 425
  suffocation, 427
Homeopathy, **413**
Homeostasis, defined, **25**
Homeostatic sleep drive, **71**
Home pregnancy tests, 131b
Home test kits, HIV, 366b
Homicides, 435
Homocysteine, 322
Homologous, **109**
Honesty, in intimate relationship, 89
Hookahs, **214**
Hooking up, 95, 96b
Hormone replacement therapy, 323b
Hormones, **24**
  chemical effects on, 393b
  reproductive life cycle, 110
  weight management, 285
Hormone therapy (HT), 117
Hospice, **461**
Hostility, 321
HPV cytology tests, 331t
Human chorionic gonadotropin (hCG), **131,** 131b
Human immunodeficiency virus (HIV), **361**. *See also* HIV/AIDS
Human papillomavirus (HPV), **369**-71
  overview, 358
Hybrid electric vehicles, 384
Hyde, Janet, 115
Hydraulic fracturing, 383
Hydrogenation, **227**
Hymen, **111**
Hyperactivity, 54
Hypertension, 309
  cardiovascular disease risk, 317
  defined, **317**
  race/ethnicity and, 323b
  sleep apnea and, 74
Hypertrophic cardiomyopathy, **316**
Hypnotherapy, **414**
Hypomanic episodes, 55
Hypothalamus, **114**
Hysterectomy, 336

## I

Ibuprofen, in dysmenorrhea, 115
Identical (monozygotic) twins, **129**
Illness, sexuality in, 125
Immune function, 262
Immune response
  elimination, 346
  proliferation, 346
  recognition, 346
  slowdown, 347
Immune system
  adaptive, 345
  defined, **345**
  innate, 345
  supporting, 360-61
Immunity, defined, **347**
Immunization
  defined, **347**
  principles of, 347-49
Impulsivity, 54
Inactivity. *See* Physical activity
Inattention blindness, 429b
Inattentive driving, 429b
Incest, **442**
Income, health disparities, 9
Incomplete proteins, 225-26
Incontinence, **335**
Incubation periods, **350**
Indemnity plan, **419**
Indirect transmission, 350
Indoor air quality, 387
Induced abortion, **162**
Induction abortion, **164**
Industrial pollution, 330
Infant mortality, **139**
Infants, tobacco's effects, 215
Infections, 136, **344**
Infectious diseases
  defined, **6**
  factors contributing, 360
  new concerns, 359-60
  pathogens and associated, 353f
Inferior vena cava, **307**
Infertility
  defined, **129**
  female, 129
  male, 129
  treating, 129-30
Inflammation, 321
  stress and, 29
Inflammatory response, 345-46
Influenza, **358**
Injectable naltrexone, 205
Injuries
  alcohol-related, 197, 430
  due to violence, 433-44
  home, 425-28
  leisure, 431
  motor vehicle, 428-31
  prevention of, 262
  sexual assault, 441
  unintentional (*see* Unintentional injuries)
  weather-related, 431-33
  workplace, 433
Innate immune system, 345
Insecticides, 391
Insoluble fiber, **230**
Insomnia, 74
  chronic, 79-81
  defined, **79**
  medications and, 78b
  symptoms, 79
  treatment of, 80-81
Instructors, exercise, 274-76
Insulin resistance, 261, 320-21
Integration, 46
Integrative health. *See also* Complementary and alternative medicine
  alternative medical systems, 411-13
  homeopathy, 413
  naturopathy, 413
  traditional chinese medicine, 411-13
Integrative medicine, 402
Intellectual wellness, 2, 2f
Intelligence, emotional, **44**
Intentional injury, defined, **424**
Intermittent explosive disorder (IED), 49
Internal locus of control, 14
Internet addiction, 173
Interpersonal stress, 31
Interpersonal wellness, 2, 2f
Intersex, **110**
Interval training, 267b
Intestate, **460**
Intimate-partner violence, **437**-39
Intimate relationships
  breakup in, 91
  challenges in, 89-91
  choosing partner, 95
  cohabitation, 99f
  communication in, 87
  conflict in, 93-95
  dating and, 95
  family life, 101-3
  friendships, 87-88
  love, sex, and, 88-89
  marriage, 98b
  nonsexual, 87-88
  peer relationships, 87-88
  sexual orientation and gender identity in, 97-98
  singlehood and, 98-99
  unhealthy, 91
  violence in, 91
Intoxication, **169,** 175. *See also* Alcohol consumption
  blood alcohol concentration, 195f
Intracerebral hemorrhage, 314
Intrauterine device (IUD)
  advantages, 150
  contraceptive implant, placement, 151f
  Copper T-380A, 150f
  disadvantages, 150-51
  effectiveness, 151
  methods, **146**

Intrauterine insemination, 130
Invasive diagnostic tests, 134
In vitro fertilization (IVF), **130**
Iodine, 232t
Iron, 232t
Ischemic stroke, **313–**14, 313b
Isometric (static) exercise, **272**
Isopropyl alcohol, 193
Isotonic (dynamic) exercise, **272**
Ivory Wave, 183

## J

Jadelle, 151
Jaundice, **358**
Jealousy, in relationship, 91
Job-related stressors, 31
Joint United Nations Programme on HIV/AIDS, 362b
Journal articles, 405b

## K

Kaposi's sarcoma, 330, **365**
k-complexes, 67
Kegel exercises, 136
Kilocalories, **225**
Klinefelter syndrome, 117
Kyleena, 151

## L

Labeling
  dietary supplements, 245b, 248b
  food products, 245b
  fraudulent, 412b
  over-the-counter drugs, 401
Labia majora, 111
Labia minora, 111
Labor
  cesarean delivery, 141
  defined, **139**
  first stage, 140
  induction, 138
  pain relief during delivery, 141
  second stage, 140
  third stage, 141
Lactation, **141**
Lacto-ovo-vegetarians, 242
Lacto-vegetarians, 242
Laparoscopy, **149, 369**
Latinos
  Covid-19, 10b
  health disparities, 9
Latinx, 10b
Lead poisoning, 391
Learning while sleeping, 80b
LED bulbs, 387
Left atrium, **307**
Left ventricle, **307**
Leisure injuries, **431**
Leisure time after retirement, 452
Leptin, 285
Lesbian, gay, bisexual, and transgender (LGBT), 124. *See also* Gender identity; Sexual orientation
  and health disparities, 9
Lesbian, gay, bisexual, transgender, questioning, intersex, and asexual (LGBTQIA+), 51
Leukemia, **332**
Leukoplakia, 213
Levonorgestrel, 160
Lewy-body dementia (LBD), 454, **455**
Life changes
  as source of stress, 31
  traumatic, 31
Life-enhancing measures, aging and
  control drinking, 451
  eat wisely, 450
  healthy weight, 450
  medications, overdependence on, 451
  mind, 449–50
  nurture social connections, 451–52
  physical fitness, 450
  preventive care, 451
  recognize and reduce stress, 451
  smoke, 449
Life expectancy, 3f
  aging and, **455**
  defined, **3**
  gender differences, 456b
  long and short, 3–7
  obesity and, 5b
Lifestyle choices
  defined, **6**
  healthy eating, 238b
  length and quality of life, 6t, 7t
Life support systems, **458**
Light beer, 193
Light-emitting diodes, 388b
Lightening, **132**
Lighting, 388b
Lighting Facts labels, 388b
Lightning injuries, 433
Liletta, 151
Linehan, Marsha, 60
Lipids, 226
Lipoproteins, **319**
Listening, in communication, 93
*Listeria monocytogenes,* 135
Lithium, 55
Liver, alcohol metabolism, 194b
Living together, 99–100
Living will, **460**
Locus of control, **14**
Loneliness, dealing with, 49
Long-acting reversible contraception (LARC), **150**
  contraceptive implants, 151
  intrauterine devices (IUDs), 150–51
Longevity, 261f
Love relationships, 88–89, 89f
  pleasure and pain of, 89
  transformation, 89
Low-back pain, 262
Low birth weight (LBW), **139**
Low-density lipoprotein (LDL) cholesterol, **227,** 261, **319**
Low-dose computed tomography, 331t
Loyalty, 88
Lubricants, water-based, 154
Lumens, 388b
Lunesta (eszopiclone), 179
Lung cancer
  black lung disease, 392b
  detection and treatment, 332–33
  early detection, 331t
  in nonsmokers, 214–15
  risk factors, 332
  tobacco use and, 211–12
Luteal phase, 115
Lyme disease, 356
Lymphatic system, **326,** 347
Lymphocytes, 29, **345**
Lymphomas, **332**

## M

Macronutrients, **224**
Macrophages, 345, 347
Magnesium, 232t
Magnetic resonance imaging (MRI), 289
Magnetic therapies, **416**
Mainstream smoke, **214**
Malaria, **359**
Male condom, **154–55,** 154f
Male infertility, 129
Malignant tumors, **326**
Malt liquor, 193
Mammography, 331t, 334
Managed care plan, **419**
Mania, **55**
Manipulative CAM techniques, 414–16
Marfan syndrome, 311b
Marijuana
  long-term effects, 182
  short-term effects and uses, 181–82
  use of, 39
  withdrawal from, 39
Marriage
  benefits of, 100
  cohabitation and, 99f
  equality, 98b
  issues and trends in, 100–1
  predictors of, 101
  retirement's effects, 452
  separation and divorce, 101
Maslow's hierarchy of needs, 42, 43f
Mass media
  tobacco use in, 209
  violence and death in, 434–35
Masturbation, **120**
Mature understanding of death, **459**
Maximal oxygen consumption, **269**
Meaningful life, 44
Measles, 347
Meat consumption
  cancer risk and, 328
  portion sizes, 240b
Medicaid, 8, 457
Medical abortion, **163**
Medical and surgical treatments, 409–11
Medical care
  conventional medicine, 403–11
  diagnostic process, 408–9
  integrative health care approaches, 411–17
  medical and surgical treatments, 409–11
  paying for, 417–20
  physician appointments, 408
  physician-patient partnership, 407
  professional care options, 402–3
  self-care, 399–401
Medical clearance for exercise, 267–68
Medical doctors, **406**
Medical records, 409b
Medicare, 457
Medications
  aging and, 451
  errors, 409–10
  for HIV/AIDS, 362b
  interactions with sunscreen, 337b
  radiation, 395
Medication therapy, 186
Meditation, 77
Mediterranean diet, 236, 257f
Medwatch program, 248b
Melanoma, **336**
Melatonin, **69,** 78b
Men. *See also* Gender
  alcohol misuse rates, 205
  clothing, 275b

Men (*continued*)
diabetes, 74
fatal injuries among, 426b
health care visits, 408b
puberty in, 116
risk for heart attacks, 311b
sex organs, 112–13
Menarche, **114**
Meningitis, **352,** 352–53
Menopause, **116**
weight management, 285
Menses, **114**
Menstrual cycle, **114**
follicular phase, 114
luteal phase, 115
menses, 114
ovulation, 114–15
Menstrual symptoms, 115
Mental health. *See* Psychological health
Mental health professional, choosing and evaluating, 61b
Menthol cigarettes, 210
Mercury, 392–93
Messages
angry, 93
nonverbal, 92
Messenger RNA (mRNA) vaccine, **347**
Meta-analysis, **404**
Metabolic rate, 260
Metabolic syndrome, 291, 320–21, 320t
Metabolism
of alcohol, 193–94, 194b
exercise effects, 259–60
weight management, 284–85
Metastasis, **326**
Methamphetamine, 180
Methane, 385t
Methanol, 193
Methedrine, 180
Methicillin-resistant *Staphylococcus aureus* (MRSA), 356
Methylenedioxypyrovalerone (MDPV), 184
#MeToo movement, 440b
METs, **270**
Mexican American, 51b
Microbes, 330
Micronutrients, **224**
Microsleep, **75**
Migraine headaches, 30
Mild cognitive impairment, 454
Mild traumatic brain injuries, 432b
Milex diaphragm, 156
Mind-body medicine, 413–14
Mindful breathing, 37b
Mindfulness, 60
aging and, 449–50
defined, **36**
for stress management, 36–38
Mindfulness-based stress reduction (MBSR), 37b
Mindfulness meditation, 37b
Minerals, **232**
Minimalist footwear, 275b
Ministroke, 315
Mirena, 151
Miscarriages, 162
Missed menstrual period, 131
Mitral valve prolapse, **316**
Mixed dementia, 455
Moderate-intensity therapy, 320
Momentary lapse, 75
Monoclonal antibody, **334**
Monounsaturated fatty acids, 227t
Mons pubis, 111
Montreal Protocol, 386
Mood disorders
bipolar disorder, 55
defined, **54**
depression, 54–55
Mood, sleep and, 72–73
Mood stabilizers, 55
Morbidity rate, **5**
Mortality, 200
Mortality rate, **5**
Mother-to-child transmission (MCT), 364
Motivation, for behavior change, 13–14
Motor behavior, disorganized, 56
Motor scooters, 430–31
Motor vehicle injuries
aggressive driving, 428
airbags, 430
alcohol and other drugs, 430
child safety seats, 430
distracted driving, 428
fatigue and sleepiness, 430
prevention, 430
seat belts, 430
speeding, 428
Mourning, **466**
Mucus method, 158
Mullerian ducts, 110
Multicenter studies, 405b
Multi-factor model
behavior, 286
culture, 296
fat cells, 284
food marketing and public policy, 286
genetic factors, 283–84
gut microbiota, 285
hormones, 285
metabolism, 284–85
sleep, 285
Mumps, 347
Murdock, Karla, 70b
Muscle dysmorphia, 293
Muscle relaxation, 37–38
Muscular endurance, **263**
Muscular strength, **263**. *See also* Strength training
Musculoskeletal pain, sleep and, 73
Mutuality, 88
*Mycobacterium tuberculosis,* 356
*Mycoplasma pneumoniae,* 352
Myocardial infarction, **211**
Myocardial infarction (MI), 310
Myocardium, 211
Myometrium, 112
MyPlate, **235,** 239f
dairy, 241
energy intake and portion sizes, 239–40
fruits, 240
grains, 241
oils, 241
physical activity, 241–42
protein foods, 241
solid fats and added sugars, 241
vegetables, 240–41

## N

Naltrexone, 204
Narcolepsy
defined, **82**
treatment, 82
Narcotics, 197
Narcotics Anonymous (NA), 186
National Center for Complementary and Integrative Health (NCCIH), 403
National Fire Protection Association, 427
National Football League, 432b
National Funeral Directors Association, 464b
National Highway Traffic Safety Administration (NHTSA), 428
National Highway Transportation Safety Administration, 197
National Institute on Drug Abuse (NIDA), 209
National Institutes of Health (NIH), 7, 54, 283
National Nutritional Foods Association, 248b
National Rifle Association, 443b
National Suicide Prevention Lifeline, 58
National Violent Death Reporting System, 443b
National Weather Service, 433
Native Americans
alcohol misuse rates, 205
diabetes, 291
health disparities, 9
Native Hawaiian, health disparities, 9
Natural killer cells, 345
Natural products, **414**
Naturopathic doctors (NDs), 413
Naturopathy, **413**
Necrotizing fasciitis, 356
Negative self-talk, 46, 47b
Negative thinking, 46
*Neisseria meningitidis,* 352
Nerve cell communication, 50f
Nervous system, **24**
and physical reactions to stressors, 24
Nervous tension, 23
Neuropeptides, 29
Neurostimulation, 58
Neurosyphilis, 373
Neurotransmitters, 38, **175**
Neutrophils, 345
#neveragain movement, 443b
Nexplanon, 151
Niacin, 231t
Nicotine
addiction, 206–8
defined, **206**
replacement products, 218–20
for stress management, 38
Nitrous oxide, 385t
Nocturnal emissions, **116**
Noise pollution, 395–96
Nonbinary, **123**
Noncomedogenic sunscreens, 337b
Noncorporeal continuity, **459**
Noninvasive screening tests, 134
Nonoxynol-9, 364
Non-rapid eye movement (NREM) sleep, **67**
Nonsteroidal anti-inflammatory drugs (NSAIDs), 115
Nonverbal communication, 92
Noradrenaline. *See* Norepinephrine
Norepinephrine, 24
Nuclear energy, 394–95
Nuclear power, **394**
Nuclear weapons, 394–95
Nurse, **406**
Nurture social connections, 451–52
Nutrient density, **225**
Nutrition
carbohydrates, 228–29
DASH Eating Plan, 242, 258f
defined, **224**
density, **225**
dietary challenges for, 243
Dietary Guidelines for Americans, 235–39
Dietary Reference Intakes (DRIs), 235
fat, 226–28
fiber, 229–30
minerals, 232–33
MyPlate, 239–42

personal guidelines, 244–51
plant-based diet, 242–43
proteins, 225–26
for stress management, 35
vitamins, 230
water, 233–34
Nutrition Facts panels, 245b

## O

Obamacare. *See* Affordable Care Act (ACA)
Obesity, 311b
cancer risk, 329
cardiovascular disease risk and, 320
and life expectancy, 5b
prevalence of, 284f
risk factor for, 291
sleep deprivation and, 74
weight management, 283
Obsessions, **53**
Obsessive-compulsive disorder (OCD), **53**
Occupational wellness, 2f, 3
Off-label drug use, 410
Oils (edible), 241
Omega-6/omega-3 fatty acids, 227t
Oncologist, **332**
*On Death and Dying* (Kübler-Ross), 465
One drink, **193**
Online dating, 95–97
Online help and apps, for psychological health issues, 60–61
Online information, 300b, 318b
evaluating, 405b
Online pharmacies, 410
Openness, in intimate relationship, 89
Ophthalmologist, **406**
Opioid overdose, 186b
Opioids, 39, **176**
overdose deaths, 178
sleepiness by, 78b
Opportunistic infections, **362**
Optimal health, 11
Optimism, **48**
Optometrist, **406**
Oral contraceptives (OCs), 115
defined, **152**
Oral-genital stimulation, 120–21
OraQuick HIV test, 366b
OraQuick test kit, 366b
Orasure test, 366b
Organic, **247**
Orgasm, 116, **120**
Orgasmic disorder, **121**
Orthorexia, 296
Osteoporosis, 116
defined, **233**
exercise effects on risk, 261
risk with aging, **453**–54
Other specified feeding or eating disorders (OSFED), **295**–96
*Our Stolen Future* (Colborn), 393b
Outpatient, **411**
Ovarian cancer, 331t, 336
Ovaries, 110, **112**
Overeaters Anonymous (OA), 300
Over-the-counter (OTC) medications, 300, **400,** 401f
Over-the-counter sleep aids, 78b
Overweight, 311b
defined, **287**
overcoming approaches, 299–302
*Overwhelmed* (Brigid Schulte), 27
Ovulation, 114–**15**
Ozone, 385t
Ozone layer, **386**
thinning of, 386–87

## P

Pacific Islander Americans, health disparities, 9
Pain management, sleep disrupters, 77
Paints, lead in, 391
Palliative care, **462**
Palliative chemotherapy, 332
Palliative sedation, **463**
Pandemics, **351**–52
Panic attacks, **53**
Panic disorder, **52**–53
Pantothenic acid, 231t
Pap tests, 331t, **335**
ParaGard, 150
Parasitic worms, **359**
Parasympathetic division, **24**
Parental leave, 102
Parenting, 101
styles, 101–2
Parents
authoritarian, 102
authoritative, 102
demandingness, 102
permissive, 102
responsiveness, 102
single, 102–3
uninvolved, 102
Paris Agreement, 386
Parsimonious knowledge, 404
Partners, discussing STIs with, 375b
Past experiences, stressors, 27
Pathogens
bacteria, 352–57
chain of infection, 350–51
defined, **247, 344**
fungi, 359
parasitic worms, 359
protozoa, 359
viruses, 357–59
PayPal, 4b
PCP (phencyclidine), 182
Pedestrian injuries, 431
Peer counseling, 186
for psychological health, 60
Peer pressure, 203b
Peer-reviewed journal articles, 405b
Pelvic inflammatory disease (PID), 129, **369**
Pelvis
external view of, 112f
internal view of, 111f
Penicillin, 373
Penis, 111, **112**
anatomy, 112f
external view of, 112f
sexual response cycle, 119f
Percent body fat, **287**
Perinatal transmission, 364
Perineum, **111**
Peripheral arterial disease, 309, **315**–16
Permissive parents, 102
Persistent symptom, 400
Persistent vegetative state, **462**
Personal contract, 18–19
Personal flotation device, **431**
Personal health records, 409b
Personality
defined, **26**
hardy, 26
and response to stress, 26–27
Personalized plan, creation of, 17–19, 17f
Pertussis, 357
Pessimism, **48**
Pesticides, **391**–92
Pharmaceuticals, **403**–4
Pharmacological therapy, for mental health issues, 58
Pheromones, 118
Phobia, specific, **52**
Phosphorus, 232t
Physical activity
aging and, 451b
defined, **264**
dietary patterns, 298
health and fitness benefits of, 268f
with healthy eating, 241–42
injuries during, 432b
during pregnancy, 137b
pyramid, 266f
time for, 265b
*Physical Activity Guidelines Advisory Committee Report,* 450
Physical barriers, 344–45
Physical changes, 452–54
Physical fitness, 78–79
aging and, 450
body composition, 263
cardiorespiratory endurance, 262–63
defined, **262**
flexibility, 263
muscular strength and endurance, 263
skill-related components of, 263–64
Physical separation, 101
Physical training principles
individual differences, 269
progressive overload, 268–69
rest and recuperation, 269
reversibility, 269
specificity, 268
Physical violence, 437
Physical wellness, 2, 2f
Physician appointments, 408
Physician assistants (PAs), **407**
Physician-assisted death (PAD), **462**–63
Physician-patient partnership, 407
Phytochemicals, **234, 329**
Pinworm, 359
Pipes, 213–14
lead in, 391
Pituitary gland, **114**
Placebo effect, **176,** 404
Placenta, **133**
Placental abruption, **138**
Placenta previa, **138**
Plant-based diet
plan, 242–43
types, 242
Plaques, **210, 309**
*Plasmodium,* 359
Pleasant life, 43
Plumbing, lead in, 391
Pluripotency, 132
*Pneumocystis* pneumonia, **365**
Pneumonia, 352, **352**
Point-of-service (POS) plan, **419**
Poisoning, 425
Poisoning, alcohol, 196
Poisons in tobacco, 209
Polychlorinated biphenyl (PCB), **389**
Polyps, **333**
Polyunsaturated fatty acids, 227t
Population control, 381–82
Population growth, 381–82, 382f
Pornography addiction, 172–79
Portals of exit and entry, 350

Portion sizes, 239-40, 240b
Positive attitude, 36
Positive psychology, 42-44, **43**
Postpartum depression, **142**
Postpartum period, childbirth, **141**
attachment, 142-43
breastfeeding, 142
postpartum depression, 142
Posttraumatic stress disorder (PTSD), 33, **53**
Potassium, 232t
Potassium citrate, 210
Poverty
health disparities, 9
HIV/AIDS risk and, 362b
toxin exposure and, 392b
Power, 263
Precontemplation, 15
Prediabetes, 291
Preeclampsia, **138**
Preferred provider organization (PPO), **419**
Pregnancy
alcohol consumption and, 200-1
changes during, 131-32
cocaine, 180
college students, 159b
complications/loss
ectopic pregnancy, 137-38
gestational diabetes, 138
infant mortality, 139
labor induction, 139
low birth weight, 139
placental abruption, 138
placenta previa, 138
preeclampsia, 138
preterm birth, 138
preterm labor, 138
spontaneous abortion, 138
stillbirth, 138
sudden infant death syndrome, 139
contraception after, 159-60
dietary challenges, 243
emotional responses to, 132
later stages of, 132
physical activity during, 137b
physiological changes, 130f
smoking cessation, 215
weight management, 285
woman's body, changes
breast tenderness, 131
emotional upset, 131
fatigue, 131
increased urination, 131
light bleeding, 131
missed menstrual period, 131
nausea, 131
sleepiness, 131
weight gain, 132t
Premature, **139**
Premature commitment, 90
Premature ejaculation, **121**
Premenstrual dysphoric disorder (PMDD), **115**
Premenstrual symptoms
alcohol/tobacco uses, 116
exercise, 116
limit salt intake, 116
nutritious diet, 116
Prozac/Zoloft, 116
relax/sleep, 116
Premenstrual syndrome (PMS), **115**
Premiums, insurance, **418**
Prenatal care, importance of
birth, preparing for, 137
blood tests, 135
environmental hazards, avoiding
alcohol, 136
caffeine, 136
drugs, 136
infections, 136
tobacco, 136
exercise, 136
physical activity, 137b
prenatal activity, 136
prenatal nutrition, 135
preparing, for birth, 136
regular checkups, 135
Prepuce, **111**
Prescription drugs, 301
Preterm birth, 138
Preterm labor, 138
Preventive care, 451
Primary care physician, choosing, 407
Primary syphilis, 373
Problem-solving ability, 36
Processed foods, refined grains in, 228, 229b
Professional care, 402-3
Professional help, for psychological disorders, 61-62
Progesterone, **110**
Progestin-only pills, 152
Programmed aging, 449
Progressive overload, **268-69**
Proliferation, in immune response, 346
Proof value, **193**
Prostaglandins, 115
Prostate cancer, 331t
detection, 335
risk factors, 334-35
treatments, 335
Prostate gland, **113**
Prostate-specific antigen test, 331t
Prostate-specific antigen (PSA) test, 331t, **335**
Proteins
complete and incomplete, 225-26
defined, **225**
food items, 226t
healthy choices, 241
intake goals, 226t
recommended intake, 226
role in nutrition, 225-26
Protozoa, **359**
Provigil, 82
Prozac, 116
Psychoactive drugs, 172t
defined, **169, 206**
Psychoactive drugs, groups of
central nervous system depressants
club drugs, 179
effects, 179
types, 178-79
from use to misuse, 179
central nervous system stimulants
amphetamines, 180
caffeine, 181
cocaine, 179-80
stimulant ADHD medications, 181
opioids, 176-78
Psychodynamic model, 59
Psychological aging, 449
Psychological defenses, 47-48. *See also* Defense mechanisms
Psychological disorders
anxiety disorders, 52-53
attention-deficit/hyperactivity disorder, 53-54
mood disorders, 54-55
prevalence of, 52t
schizophrenia, 55-56
stress and, 30
therapeutic models, 58-60
Psychological health
defense mechanisms, 47-48
defined, **42**
disorders (*see* Psychological disorders)
ethnicity, culture, and, 51b
Psychological wellness, exercise effects, 262
Psychologists, **406**
Psychoneuroimmunology (PNI), **29**
Psychosis, **180**
Psychotherapy, 413
for psychological disorders, 58-59
for stress-related problems, 39
Psyllium, 230
PTSD. *See* Posttraumatic stress disorder (PTSD)
Puberty, **114**
in females, 114
in males, 116
weight management, 285
Pubic lice, **373**
Public health, 3f
Pulmonary circulation, **307**
Pulmonary edema, **316**
Pulmonary heart disease, tobacco's effects, 211
Purge, **294**

## Q

Quackery, 412b
Quadruple marker screen (QMS), **134**
Qualified health claims, 248b
Quality of life, 3f
Queer, **97**
Questionnaires, patient history, 311b
Questionnaires, sleep, 76b
Quitting
benefits of, 216-17, 217t
options for
behavior change, 217
smoking cessation products, 217-20

## R

Race
Covid-19, 10b
and health disparities, 8-9
Racial categories in medicine, 10b
Radiation, 330
avoiding, 395
defined, **394**
home and workplace, 395
medical uses of, 395
Radiation pollution, 394-95
Radiation sickness, **394**
Radiation therapy, 332
Radical prostatectomy, 335
Radon, **395**
Randomized controlled trials, **404,** 404f
Rape, **125, 439**-42
effects of, 441-42
Rape, Abuse, and Incest National Network (RAINN), 126
Rapid eye movement (REM) sleep, **67**
Rapid HIV tests, 366b
Rational knowledge, 403
Realism, 43
Realistic self-talk, 46-47, 47b
Real social networks, 31-32
Reciprocity, 88
Recognition, in immune response, 346
Recommended Dietary Allowance, 235
Rectal cancer
detection and treatment, 333
risk factors, 333
Recuperation, 269
Recurrent symptom, 400
Recycling, **390**
"Reduced harm" cigarettes, 210
Refined grains, 228
Reflux, and sleep disruption, 76-77

Registered nurses (RNs), 406
Reiki, **416**
Reinforcement, **58**
Relative risk, 405b
Relaxation techniques, 38
Remission, **326**
Renewable energy sources, 383
Repetitive strain injury (RSI), **433,** 434b
Repetitive transcranial magnetic stimulation (rTMS), 55
Research, 405b
Reservoirs, 350, **350**
Resilience, defined, **27**
Resistance exercise, **272**
Resistance stage of GAS, 28, 28f
Respect, in friendship, 88
Response, **58**
Responsible sexual behavior
  agreed-on sexual activities, 127
  contraception use, 127
  open, honest communication, 127
  safe sex, 127
  sexual privacy, 127
  sober sex, 127–28
Rest, 269
Restaurants, 246
Resting metabolic rate (RMR), **284**
Restless leg syndrome (RLS)
  defined, **81**
  symptoms, 81
  treatment, 81
Retirement, 452
Reversibility, **269**
Reye's syndrome, 401
Rheumatic fever, **316**
Rheumatic heart disease, 316
Rh factor, **135**
Rh-immune globulin, 135
Rhinoviruses, 357
Rhythm method, 158
Riboflavin, 231t
Right atrium, **307**
Right ventricle, **307**
Risk factor, defined, **1**
Risk-taking behavior, 426b
Rocky Mountain spotted fever, 356
*Roe v. Wade,* 161, 165
Rogers, Carl, 86
Rohypnol, **179**
Role models, 14
Rosbash, Michael, 68
Rubella, 347


## S


Safe food handling, 249b
Safer sex, 375b
Safety
  emergency care and, 444
  home injuries, 425–28
  motor vehicle crashes, 428–31
  in sports and leisure activities, 431
  workplace, 433
Same-sex couples, 97
Same-sex marriage, 98b
Same-sex relationships, HIV/AIDS risk and, 362b
Sandy Hook Elementary School shootings, 443b
Sanitary landfill, **389**
Sarcomas, **332**
Sarcopenia, 450
SARS-CoV-2, 351
Saturated fatty acids, 227t
Saw palmetto, 415t
Scabies, **373**
Scanning technologies, 289
Schizophrenia
  in adolescence, 55
  defined, **55**
  delusions in, 56
  general characteristics of, 56
  hallucinations in, 56
  treatment, 56
School violence, 436
Scientific journals, 405b
Scrotum
  defined, **113**
  external view of, 112f
Seasonal affective disorder (SAD), **55**
Seat belts, 430
Secondary reinforcers, **208**
Secondary syphilis, 373
Sedation, **178**
Sedentary lifestyle, cancer risk, 329
Sedentary time, 265
Selective estrogen receptor modulators (SERMs), 334
Selenium, 232t
Self-acceptance, 2
Self-actualization, **43**
Self-assessment, need for medical care, 399–400
Self-care
  physician, needs, 400
  self-assessment, 399–400
  self-treatment, 400
    home medical care kit, 402f
    nondrug options, 400
    self-medication, 400–1
Self-concept
  defined, **43**
  development of, 45–46, 86–87
  integrated, 46
  negative, 46
  positive, 46
  stability, 46
Self-confidence, 2
  exercise effects, 262
Self-cutting, 57b
Self-disclosure, 93
Self-efficacy
  boosting of, strategies for, 14
  defined, **14**
  exercise effects, 262
Self-esteem, 2
  defined, **43**
  exercise effects, 262
  healthy level of, 45–47
  meeting challenges to, 46–47
Self-examination for testicular cancer, 338b
Self-harm, deliberate, 57b
Self-help, 60
Self-image, 43. *See also* Self-concept
Self-injury, 57b
Self-medication, 402f
Self-stimulation, 120
Self-talk, 14
  defined, **46**
  negative, 46, 47b
  realistic, 46–47, 47b
Self-treatment, 400
  home medical care kit, 402f
  nondrug options, 400
  self-medication, 400–1
Seligman, Martin, 43
Selye, Hans, 28
Semen, **113**
Seminal vesicle, **113**
Senescence, **458**
Sense of humor, 37
Separation distress, 101
Servings, standard drinks *versus,* 193
Set-point theory, 284
Severe symptom, 400
Sewage, 389
Sex. *See also* Gender
  blood alcohol concentration, 194
  cardiovascular disease risk and, 323b
  defined, 8
  drinking patterns and, 205–6
  health care visits, 408b
Sex addiction, 172–73
Sex chromosomes, **110**
  disorders of, 117
Sex reassignment, 124
Sexual anatomy
  from binary to spectrum, 109–10
  female sex organs, 110–12
  male sex organs, 112–13
Sexual arousal
  physical stimulation, 118
  psychological stimulation, 118
Sexual assault, **439**
  dealing with, 441
Sexual behaviors
  among college students, 370b
  anal intercourse, 121
  children, 125
  coitus, 121
  oral-genital stimulation, 120–21
  responsible, 127–28
  self-stimulation, 120
Sexual coercion, **125**–26
Sexual disorders
  causes of, 122
  common, 121–22
  defined, **121**
  health issues, 123
  treatment, 122–23
Sexual dysfunction, 121
Sexual harassment, 440b, **442**
Sexual intercourse, **111**
Sexuality
  aging and, 116–17, 454
  biological variations, 109
  communicating, 127b
  cultural norms, 109
  defined, **108**
  gender roles and, 123–24
  human, 114–18
  sexual orientation and, 123–24
  stimulation and response, 118
Sexually transmitted diseases (STDs). *See* Sexually transmitted infection (STI)
Sexually transmitted infections (STIs)
  bacterial vaginosis, 373
  chlamydia, 367–68
  defined, **145, 361**
  genital herpes, 371–72
  gonorrhea, 369
  hepatitis A, 369
  hepatitis B, 369
  hepatitis C, 369
  HIV/AIDS, 361–67
  human papillomavirus, 369–71
  pelvic inflammatory disease, 369
  pubic lice, 373–74
  syphilis, 372–73
  trichomoniasis, 373
Sexual orientation
  defined, **97, 109**
  and health disparities, 9–11
  origins of, 124
  in relationships, 97–98
Sexual relationship, engaging preparations, 126b
Sexual response cycle
  excitement phase, 118
  orgasmic phase, 120
  plateau phase, 118–20

Sexual response cycle (*continued*)
  resolution phase, 120
  stages of, 119f
Sexual stimulation
  physical stimulation, 118
  psychological stimulation, 118
Sexual violence, 439–42
Sham procedure, 404
Short-acting reversible contraception, 151
  cervical cap, 157
  contraceptive skin patch
    advantages, 153
    disadvantages, 153
    effectiveness, 153
  contraceptive sponge
    advantages, 157
    disadvantages, 157
    effectiveness, 157
  diaphragm with spermicide
    advantages, 156
    disadvantages, 156
    effectiveness, 157
  female condoms
    advantages, 155
    disadvantages, 155
    effectiveness, 155
  injectable contraceptives, 153
    advantages, 154
    disadvantages, 154
    effectiveness, 154
  male condoms
    advantages, 155
    disadvantages, 155
    effectiveness, 155
  oral contraceptives (OCs)
    advantages, 152
    combination pill, 152
    disadvantages, 152
    effectiveness, 152
    progestin-only pills, 152
  vaginal contraceptive ring
    advantages, 153
    disadvantages, 153
    effectiveness, 153
  vaginal spermicides
    advantages, 157
    disadvantages, 157–58
    effectiveness, 158
Shyness, 63b
Sidestream smoke, **210**
Sigmoidoscopies, 331t
Silver insurance plans, 420b
Simple carbohydrates, 228
Singlehood, 95–100
Single-parent family, 102–3
Sino-implant, 151
Skene's gland, **112**
Skill-related fitness, **263**
Skin cancer
  detection and treatment, 337–38
  prevention, 337
  risk factors, 336
  types of, 336
Skin cancers, 337b
Skinfold measurement, 289
Skyla, 151
SKYN, 155
Skype, 92
Sleep
  during adolescence, 72
  age on, effect of, 72
  apps, 70b
  architecture, 66
  brain activity during, 66
  case scenarios, 83b
  changes across life span, 71–72
  cycles, 67–68
  delayed sleep phase, 79b
  digital devices and, 70b
  disorders, 79–82
  exercise effects, 262
  gender and, 72
  and health, 72–75
  healthy sleep program, 75–79
  and learning, connection of, 80b
  natural sleep drives, 68–71
  NREM sleep, 67
  REM sleep, 67
  requirement for, 71
  routine, 80–81
  short sleepers, 71
  stages, 66–68
  for stress management, 38
  trackers, 70b
  weight management, 285
Sleep apnea, **72**
  in overweight people, 82
  treatments for, 82
Sleep diary, 75, 75f
Sleep disrupters
  anxiety, 77
  bedroom, 77
  caffeine, 77, 77t
  checklist, 76
  defined, **76**
  nasal congestion and cough, 77
  pain, 77
  reflux, 76–77
  stress, 77
  urination, 77
Sleep medications, 78b
Sleep spindles, 67
Slowdown, in immune response, 347
Slow-wave sleep, 67, **67**
"SMART" criteria, 17–18
Smartwatches, 300b, 318b
Smog, **384**
Smokeless tobacco, 213
Smoking cessation, 207f
  e-cigarettes unsupported for, 214
  immediate effects of, 210
  long-term effects of, 210–13
  media, 209
  pregnancy, 215
  products, 217–20
Social aging, 449
Social anxiety disorder, **52,** 63b
Social isolation, 322
Socialization, **87**
Social media, 203b, 440b
  balance in use of, 49
  and communication, 92–93
  psychological problems and, 49
Social networks, 92–93
  digital, 32
  real, 31–32
Social phobia. *See* Social anxiety disorder
Social Security, **457**
Social support, for stress management, 34
Socioeconomic status
  cardiovascular disease risk and, 322
  HIV/AIDS risk and, 362b
  of older adults, 457
  toxin exposure and, 392b
Sodium, 232t
  limiting intake, 450
Solar, as renewable energy source, 383
Solid waste pollution, 389–91
  components of, 389f
  disposing of, 389
    biodegradation, 390
    discarded technology, 390
    recycling, 390
  reducing, 390–91
Soluble fiber, **229**
Sonata (zaleplon), 179
Sound intensity, 396f
Soybean oil, 383
Specialist, choosing, 407
Specialist physicians, 407
Specificity principle, **268**
Specific phobia, **52**
Speed, 263
Speeding, 428
Sperm, **110**
Spermicide, **154**
SPF rating, 337b
Sphygmomanometer, 317
Spirituality, 465
Spiritual wellness, 2–3, 2f, 35–36, 103
Spontaneous abortion, 138, **162**
Sports injuries, 432b
Spying, in relationships, 93
Squamous cell carcinoma, **336**
Stability of self-concept, 46
Stage I sleep, 67
Stage II sleep, 67
Stage III sleep, 67
Stages of change model, 14–16, 16f
  action, 16
  contemplation, 15–16
  maintenance, 16
  precontemplation, 15
  preparation, 16
  termination, 16
Staging, **326**
Stalking, **438**–39
Standard drink, 193
*Staphylococcus aureus,* 356
Staphylococcus bacteria, 356
Statistical significance, 405b
Statutory rape, **439**
Stents, 314f
Stepfamilies, 103
Sterilization, **149**
Sternberg, Robert, 88
Stillbirth, 138
Stimulants, 39
  ADHD medications, 181
  defined, **179**
Stimulus, **58**
St. John's wort, 415t
Strength training
  choosing equipment, 272
  core training, 272
  frequency, 272–73
  intensity and time, 273
  for older adults, 457
  progression, 273
  sex differences in, 272
  supplements, 273
  types of, 271–72
  volume, 273
Strep throat, 353–56
Streptococcus, **353**
*Streptococcus pneumoniae,* 352
Stress
  acute, **29**
  aging and, 451
  cardiovascular disease risk and, 321, 325
  chronic, **29**
  college-related, 31
  coronavirus outbreak and, 31
  counterproductive coping strategies, 38–39
  daily hassles and, 31
  defined, **24**
  discrimination and, 32b




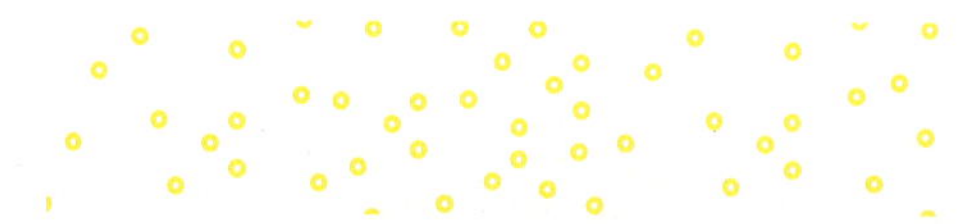

due to life changes, 31
exercise effects, 262
and health, 27-30
immigrants and, 32b
and immunity, 29
job-related, 31
long-term, 24
management, 34-39
racial/ethnic minorities and, 32b
short-term, 24
sleep disrupters, 77
sources of, 30-33
symptom of, 28f
Stressed power motivation, 26
Stressors, **23**
cognitive responses, 26
college, 31
job-related, 31
physical responses to, 24-25
psychological responses, 26-27
social, 31-32
transcultural, 51b
Stress response, defined, **23**
Stroke
defined, **313**
detecting and treating, 312b, 315
effects of, 315
exercise effects, 261
hypertension and, 323b
race/ethnicity and, 323b
symptoms of, 312b
tobacco's effects, 211
types of, 313-15, 314f
warning signs, 312b
Structure-function claims, 248b
Subarachnoid hemorrhage, 314
Subcutaneous fat, **286**
Substance abuse, 171
Substance Abuse and Mental Health Services Administration (SAMHSA)., 197
Substance misuse, **171**
diagnosing, 171
*DSM-5,* 171
Substance use disorders
defined, **171**
development of, 172
Sudden cardiac death, **310**-11
Sudden infant death syndrome (SIDS), **139**
Suffocation, 427
Sugars
added to foods, 228-29
reducing in diet, 236
in tobacco products, 210
Suicide
among older adults, 457
bipolar disorders and, 55
with firearms, 426b
gender differences, 426b
grief as risk factor, 455
help from mental health professional, 61b
myths about, 57t
protective factors, 58
risk factors, 57
warning signs, 56
Sunscreens, **337,** 337b
Superior vena cava, **307**
Support groups
for dealing with stress, 39
grief, 455
for psychological health, 60
Supportiveness, in relationship, 91
Supportive people, 14
Suprachiasmatic nucleus (SCN), **68**
Surgery, 301, 404
for cancer, 328b
colorectal cancer, 333
Sustainable development, 383
Sympathetic division, **24**
Symptothermal technique, 158
Synapse, 175
Syncope, 311b
Synesthesia, **182**
Syphilis, **372-**73
Syringe exchange programs, 362b
Systemic circulation, **307**
Systemic infections, **350**
Systole, **307**


## T


Tai chi, 38
defined, **416**
Take Off Pounds Sensibly (TOPS), 300
Tanning beds, 337b
Target behavior, **13**
Target heart rate zone, **269**
T cells, **345**
Temperature methods, 158
Tennis elbow, 434b
Tension headaches, 30
Tentative knowledge, 404
Teratogen, **136**
Terrorism, 437
Testable knowledge, 404
Testator, **460**
Testes, 110, **113**
Testicular cancer, 112, 338-39, 338b
Testosterone
defined, **110**
role in behavior, 426b
Tetanus, 357
Texting, 429b
Texting, and sleep problems, 70b
Texting thumb, 434b
Therapeutic touch, **416**
Thiamin, 231t
Thirdhand smoke, 215
Thrombotic stroke, 314
Thrombus, **314**
Tick-borne infections, 356
Time balancing, 91
Time management skills, strategies for improving of, 35
Time pressures, 31
Tobacco, defined, **206**
Tobacco use
accidental fires and, 427
aging and, 449
cancer risk and, 328
cardiovascular disease risk and, 317, 325
effects on sleep, 78b
FDA regulation of, 216
genetic factors, 208-9
nicotine addiction, 206-8
overview of health hazards, 209-14
premenstrual symptoms, 116
prenatal care, 136
quitting, 216-19
rationalizing dangers, 209
social and psychological factors, 208
for stress management, 38
Tolerable Upper Intake Level (UL), 235
Tolerance, **170**
for alcohol, 202
for nicotine, **208**
Total body electrical conductivity (TOBEC), 289
Total fiber, **230**
*Toward a Psychology of Being* (Abraham Maslow), 42, 43f
Toxic shock syndrome (TSS), 356
*Toxoplasma gondii,* 135
t-PA, 313b
Traditional Chinese medicine (TCM), **411**-13
Tranquilizer, **178**
Tranquilizers, 39
Trans fatty acids, **227,** 227t
Transgender, 8, **123**-24
Transient ischemic attack, 313b, **315**
Transmission of infection, 350
Traumatic stressors, 33
Travelers' diarrhea, 357
Treatment effect, 404
*Treponema pallidum,* 372
Triangular theory of love, 89f
Trichomoniasis, **373**
Triglycerides, 226, **321**
Trimester
defined, **130**
first, 132-33
second, 133-34
third, 134
Tropical oils, 227
Trust, in friendship, 88
Tubal sterilization, **149**
Tuberculosis, 356
Tumors, **326**
Tuning, 92
Turner syndrome, 117
Twins
fraternal (dizygotic), 129
identical (monozygotic), 129
Type 2 diabetes, 261


## U


Ulcers, 357
Ulipristal (Ella), 160
Ultrasonography, **134, 334**
Ultraviolet radiation, **336**
in greenhouse effect, 384
ozone layer, 386
Umbilical cord, **133**
UNAIDS, 362b
Unconditional positive regard, 86
Unequal commitment, 90
Unified sense of self, 45
Uniform Determination of Death Act, 458
Uniform Donor Card, **461**
Unintended pregnancy, 146f, **162**
Unintentional injuries
defined, **424**
home injuries, 425-28
intentional injuries *vs.,* 433-44
from leisure activities, 431
motor vehicle, 428-31
workplace, 433
Uninvolved parents, 102
Unrealistic expectations, 90-91
Unsaturated fatty acids, 227t
Unstressed affiliation motivation, 27
Unusual symptom, 400
UPF rating, 337b
Urethra, **111**
Urinary tract infections, 357
U.S. Department of Agriculture (USDA), 228
U.S. Food and Drug Administration, 58
USP Dietary Supplement Verification Program, 248b
Uterus, **112**
cancer of, 331t
UV index, 337b

## V

Vaccine Adverse Event Reporting System (VAERS), 349
Vaccines
  Covid-19, 351
  defined, **347**
  effectiveness, 348b
  efficacy, 347–49
  hesitancy, 348b
  messenger RNA (mRNA), **347**
  misinformation, 348b
  rates, 348b
  safety, 348b
  types of, 347
Vaccine Safety Datalink Project, 349
Vagina, 111
Vaginal contraceptive film (VCF), 157
Vaginal spermicides, 157–58
Vaginismus, 122
Valerian, 415t
Valium, 39, 197
Values
  defined, **45**
  development of, 45
Vaping, 207f
Vascular dementia, **455**
Vas deferens, **113**
Vasectomy, **149**
Vasocongestion, **118**
Vector, **350**
Vegetable proteins, 226
Vegetables
  cancer risk and, 328–29
  cruciferous, **234**
  fiber in, 230
  healthy intake, 240–41
  proteins in, 226
Vegetarians, **242**
  food patterns, 256f
Veins, **308**
Vending machines, 246
Venmo, 4b
Ventricular fibrillation, 310
Vertical transmission, 364
Vestibular bulbs, 111
Viable, **162**
Viagra, 122
Violence
  alcohol-related, 197
  factors contributing to, 434–35
  gang-related, 435–36
  school, 436
  sexual, 439–42
  workplace, 436–37
Viral hepatitis, 358
Viruses, **357**–59
Visceral fat, **287**
Vision changes, 453
Visualization, 14
Vitamin A, 231t
Vitamin B-6, 231t
Vitamin B-12, 231t
  aging and, 450
Vitamin C, 231t
Vitamin D, 135, 233b
  functions, 231t
Vitamin E, 231t
Vitamin K, 231t, 233b
Vitamins
  deficiencies, 230
  defined, **230**
  excesses, 230–32
  functions of, 230
Volatile organic compounds (VOCs), 387
Voluntary active euthanasia, 462–63
Volunteering, 34
Vulva, **110**
  external view of, 111f

## W

Waist-to-hip ratio (WHR), 290
Walking meditation, 37b
Walking pneumonia, 352
Warm-ups, 271
Water contamination, 387
Water intake, 233–34
Water pollution, 387–89
Water quality, 387–89
Water-resistant sunscreens, 337b
Water shortages, 388
Water-soluble vitamin, 231t
Water supply, 389
Water treatment, 387
Wearables, 300b
Weather-related injuries, 431–33
Websites
  chemical pollution, 394
  evaluating, 405b
  e-waste recycling, 390
  health information, 405b
  HIV testing, 366b
  toxic products, 393b
Weight gain, pregnancy, 132t
Weight loss approaches, 299
  plans and products, 299–300
  prescription weight loss drugs, 301
  programs, 300–1
Weight management
  aging and, 450
  approaches, 299–302
  apps and wearables for, 300b
  body fat and wellness, 291–93
  body image and eating disorders, 293–96
  body weight and composition principles, 286–90
  fat cells, 284
  food marketing, 286
  food perceptions and behaviors, 286
  genetic factors, 283–84
  gut microbiota, 285
  healthy lifestyle, adoption, 296–98
  hormones, 285
  metabolism, 284–85
  public policy, 286
  sleep, 285
  sleep deprivation and, 74
Weinstein, Harvey, 440b
Wellbutrin, 218
Wellness
  access to health care and, 12
  body fat and, 291–93
  cultural, 2, 2f
  defined, **1**
  dimensions of, 1–3, 2f
  emotional, 2, 2f
  environmental, 2f, 3
  factors, 11–12
  financial, 2f, 3, 4b
  intellectual, 2, 2f
  interpersonal, 2, 2f
  occupational, 2f, 3
  physical, 2, 2f
  spiritual, 2–3, 2f, 35–36
  students and, 11b
West Nile virus, 360
White Rush, 183
Whole-body donation, 464b
Whole grain, **228,** 229b
Wills, **460**
Wind, as renewable energy source, 383
Wind-related injuries, 433
Wines, 193
Withdrawal, contraceptive method, **158**
Withdrawal symptoms, drugs, **171**
  tobacco use, **208**
Wolffian ducts, 110
Women. *See also* Gender
  alcohol misuse rates, 205
  amphetamines, 180
  antidepressants, 55
  cardiovascular disease risk and, 323b
  climacteric, 116–17
  clothing, 275b
  depression, 54
  health care visits, 408b
  life expectancy, 456b
  orgasmic dysfunction, 122
  puberty in, 114
  sex organs, 110–12
  sexual arousal disorder, 121
  sexual response cycle, 119f
  sleep and, 72
Women Organized Against Rape (WOAR), 441
Work addiction, 172
Workaholics, 172
Work injuries, 433
Workplace
  radiation in, 395
  violence, 436–37
World Health Organization (WHO), 200, 362b, 384
Writing about stressful events, 36

## X

Xanax, 39
X-rays, 330

## Y

Years of potential life lost, **424**
Yoga, 38
Young adults, 27
Young, Michael, 68

## Z

Z-drugs, 179
Zeitgebers, **68**
Zika virus, 359
Zinc, 232t
Zoloft, 116
Zoom, 183
Zyban, 218
Zygote, 128



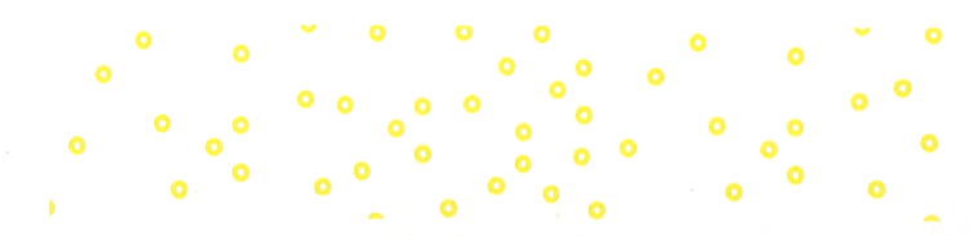